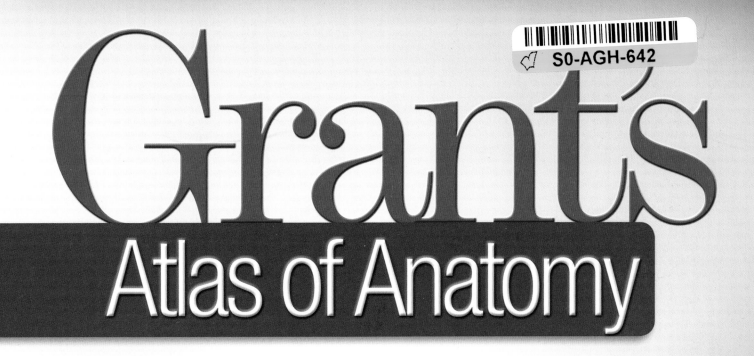

Grant's Atlas of Anatomy

THIRTEENTH EDITION

S0-AGH-642

Grant's
Atlas of Anatomy

THIRTEENTH EDITION

Anne M.R. Agur, B.Sc. (OT), M.Sc., Ph.D

Professor, Division of Anatomy, Department of Surgery, Faculty of Medicine
Department of Physical Therapy, Department of Occupational Therapy
Division of Biomedical Communications, Institute of Medical Science
Graduate Department of Rehabilitation Science, Graduate Department of Dentistry
University of Toronto
Toronto, Ontario, Canada

Arthur F. Dalley II, Ph.D.

Professor, Department of Cell & Developmental Biology
Adjunct Professor, Department of Orthopaedics and Rehabilitation
Vanderbilt University School of Medicine
Adjunct Professor of Anatomy
Belmont University School of Physical Therapy
Nashville, Tennessee

 Wolters Kluwer | Lippincott Williams & Wilkins
Health

Philadelphia • Baltimore • New York • London
Buenos Aires • Hong Kong • Sydney • Tokyo

Acquisitions Editor: Crystal Taylor
Product Manager: Julie Montalbano
Marketing Manager: Joy Fisher Williams
Designer: Holly McLaughlin
Compositor: SPi Global

Thirteenth Edition

By J.C.B. Grant:

First Edition, 1943   Second Edition, 1947   Third Edition, 1951
Fourth Edition, 1956   Fifth Edition, 1962   Sixth Edition, 1972

By J.E. Anderson:

Seventh Edition, 1978 Eighth Edition, 1983

By A.M.R. Agur:

Ninth Edition, 1991   Tenth Edition, 1999
Eleventh Edition, 2005

By A.M.R. Agur and A.F. Dalley:

Twelfth Edition, 2009

351 West Camden Street   Two Commerce Square
Baltimore, MD 21201   2001 Market Street
                                Philadelphia, PA 19103

Printed in China

Library of Congress Cataloging-in-Publication Data
Agur, A. M. R.
    Grant's atlas of anatomy / Anne Agur. — 13th ed.
        p. ; cm.
    Atlas of anatomy
    Includes bibliographical references and index.
    ISBN 978-1-60831-756-1
  I. Grant, J. C. Boileau (John Charles Boileau), 1886-1973. II. Title. III. Title: Atlas of anatomy.
    [DNLM: 1. Anatomy, Regional—Atlases. QS 17]
    611.0022'2—dc23

                                                                    2011040823

CCS0912

9 8 7 6 5 4 3 2

by Dr. Carlton G. Smith, M.D., Ph.D. (1905–2003)

Professor Emeritus, Division of Anatomy, Department of Surgery
Faculty of Medicine, University of Toronto, Toronto, Ontario, Canada

Dr. J.C. Boileau Grant in his office, McMurrich Building, University of Toronto, 1946. Through his textbooks, Dr. Grant made an indelible impression on the teaching of anatomy throughout the world. *(Courtesy of Dr. C. G. Smith.)*

The life of Dr. J.C. Boileau Grant has been likened to the course of the seventh cranial nerve as it passes out of the skull: complicated, but purposeful.[1] He was born in the parish of Lasswade in Edinburgh, Scotland, on February 6, 1886. Dr. Grant studied medicine at the University of Edinburgh from 1903 to 1908. Here, his skill as a dissector in the laboratory of the renowned anatomist, Dr. Daniel John Cunningham (1850–1909), earned him a number of awards.

Following graduation, Dr. Grant was appointed the resident house officer at the Infirmary in Whitehaven, Cumberland. From 1909 to 1911, Dr. Grant demonstrated anatomy in the University of Edinburgh, followed by two years at the University of Durham, at Newcastle-on-Tyne in England, in the laboratory of Professor Robert Howden, editor of *Gray's Anatomy*.

With the outbreak of World War I in 1914, Dr. Grant joined the Royal Army Medical Corps and served with distinction. He was mentioned in dispatches in September 1916, received the Military Cross in September 1917 for "conspicuous gallantry and devotion to duty during attack," and received a bar to the Military Cross in August 1918.[1]

In October 1919, released from the Royal Army, he accepted the position of Professor of Anatomy at the University of Manitoba in Winnipeg, Canada.

With the frontline medical practitioner in mind, he endeavored to "bring up a generation of surgeons who knew exactly what they were doing once an operation had begun."[1] Devoted to research and learning, Dr. Grant took interest in other projects, such as performing anthropometric studies of Indian tribes in northern Manitoba during the 1920s. In Winnipeg, Dr. Grant met Catriona Christie, whom he married in 1922.

Dr. Grant was known for his reliance on logic, analysis, and deduction as opposed to rote memory. While at the University of Manitoba, Dr. Grant began writing *A Method of Anatomy, Descriptive and Deductive,* which was published in 1937.[2]

In 1930, Dr. Grant accepted the position of Chair of Anatomy at the University of Toronto. He stressed the value of a "clean" dissection, with the structures well defined. This required the delicate touch of a sharp scalpel, and students soon learned that a dull tool was anathema. Instructive dissections were made available in the Anatomy Museum, a means of student review on which Dr. Grant placed a high priority. Illustrations of these actual dissections are included in *Grant's Atlas of Anatomy*.

The first edition of the *Atlas*, published in 1943, was the first anatomical atlas to be published in North America.[3] *Grant's Dissector* preceded the *Atlas* in 1940.[4]

Dr. Grant remained at the University of Toronto until his retirement in 1956. At that time, he became Curator of the Anatomy Museum in the University. He also served as Visiting Professor of Anatomy at the University of California at Los Angeles, where he taught for 10 years.

Dr. Grant died in 1973 of cancer. Through his teaching method, still presented in the Grant's textbooks, Dr. Grant's life interest—human anatomy—lives on. In their eulogy, colleagues and friends Ross MacKenzie and J. S. Thompson said, "Dr. Grant's knowledge of anatomical fact was encyclopedic, and he enjoyed nothing better than sharing his knowledge with others, whether they were junior students or senior staff. While somewhat strict as a teacher, his quiet wit and boundless humanity never failed to impress. He was, in the very finest sense, a scholar and a gentleman."[1]

This edition of *Grant's Atlas* has, like its predecessors, required intense research, market input, and creativity. It is not enough to rely on a solid reputation; with each new edition, we have adapted and changed many aspects of the *Atlas* while maintaining the commitment to pedagogical excellence and anatomical realism that has enriched its long history. Medical and health sciences education, and the role of anatomy instruction and application within it, continually evolve to reflect new teaching approaches and educational models. The health care system itself is changing, and the skills and knowledge that future health care practitioners must master are changing along with it. Finally, technologic advances in publishing, particularly in online resources and electronic media, have transformed the way students access content and the methods by which educators teach content. All of these developments have shaped the vision and directed the execution of this thirteenth edition of *Grant's Atlas*, as evidenced by the following key features.

Classic "Grant's" images updated for today's students. A unique feature of *Grant's Atlas* is that, rather than providing an idealized view of human anatomy, the classic illustrations represent actual dissections that the student can directly compare with specimens in the lab. Because the original models used for these illustrations were real cadavers, the accuracy of these illustrations is unparalleled, offering students the best introduction to anatomy possible. Over the years and in this edition, we have made many changes to the illustrations to match the shifting expectations of students, adding more vibrant colors and updating the style. All figures were carefully analyzed to ensure that label placement remained effective and that the illustration's relevance was still clear.

Schematic illustrations. Full-color schematic illustrations and orientation figures supplement the dissection figures to clarify anatomical concepts, show the relationships of structures, and give an overview of the body region being studied. The illustrations conform to Dr. Grant's admonition to "keep it simple": extraneous labels were deleted, and some labels were added to identify key structures and make the illustrations as useful as possible to students.

Legends with easy-to-find clinical applications. Admittedly, artwork is the focus of any atlas; however, the *Grant's* legends have long been considered a unique and valuable feature of the *Atlas*. The observations and comments that accompany the illustrations draw attention to salient points and significant structures that might otherwise escape notice. Their purpose is to interpret the illustrations without providing exhaustive description. Readability, clarity, and practicality were emphasized in the editing of this edition. Clinical comments, which deliver practical "pearls" that link anatomic features with their significance in health care practice, appear in blue text within the figure legends. New clinical comments have been added in this edition, providing even more relevance for students searching for medical application of anatomical concepts.

Enhanced diagnostic imaging and surface anatomy. Because medical imaging has taken on increased importance in the diagnosis and treatment of injuries and illnesses, diagnostic images are used liberally throughout the chapters, and a special imaging section appears at the end of each chapter. Over 100 clinically relevant magnetic resonance images (MRIs), computed tomography (CT) scans, ultrasound scans, and corresponding orientation drawings are included in this edition. Labeled surface anatomy photographs with ethnic diversity continue to be an important feature in this new edition.

Updated and improved tables. Tables help students organize complex information in an easy-to-use format ideal for review and study. In addition to muscles, tables featuring nerves, arteries, and other relevant structures are included. The table format in this edition received a substantial update; a consistent color code is used to clearly demarcate columns. Tables are strategically placed on the same page as the illustrations that demonstrate the structures listed in the tables.

Logical organization and layout. The organization and layout of the *Atlas* have always been determined with ease-of-use as the goal. Although the basic organization by body region was maintained in this edition, the order of plates within every chapter was scrutinized to ensure that it is logical and pedagogically effective. Sections within each chapter further organize the region into discrete subregions; these subregions appear as headings on the pages. Readers need only glance at these headings to orient themselves to the region and subregion that the figures on the page belong to. A chapter table of contents comprises the first page of each chapter.

Helpful learning and teaching tools. The thirteenth edition of *Grant's Atlas* offers a wide range of online resources for both the student and the instructor on Lippincott Williams & Wilkins' thePoint site: http://thePoint.lww.com/GrantsAtlas13e. Students have access to an online e-book, an interactive atlas containing all of the atlas images, an interactive question bank, and selected video clips from the best-selling *Acland's Video Atlas of Human Anatomy* collection. For instructors, online ancillaries include an interactive atlas with slide-show and image-export functions as well as an image bank.

We hope that you enjoy using this thirteenth edition of *Grant's Atlas* and that it becomes a trusted partner in your educational experience. We believe that this new edition safeguards the *Atlas's* historical strengths while enhancing its usefulness to today's students.

Anne M.R. Agur
Arthur F. Dalley II

ACKNOWLEDGMENTS

Starting with the first edition of this *Atlas* published in 1943, many people have given generously of their talents and expertise and we acknowledge their participation with heartfelt gratitude. Most of the original carbon-dust halftones on which this book is based were created by Dorothy Foster Chubb, a pupil of Max Brödel and one of Canada's first professionally trained medical illustrators. She was later joined by Nancy Joy, who is Professor Emeritus in the Division of Biomedical Communications, University of Toronto. Mrs. Chubb was mainly responsible for the artwork of the first two editions and the sixth edition; Miss Joy, for those in between. In subsequent editions, additional line and halftone illustrations by Elizabeth Blackstock, Elia Hopper Ross, and Marguerite Drummond were added. In recent editions, the artwork of Valerie Oxorn and the surface anatomy photography of Anne Rayner of Vanderbilt University Medical Center's Medical Art Group have augmented the modern look and feel of the atlas.

Much credit is also due to Charles E. Storton for his role in the preparation of the majority of the original dissections and preliminary photographic work. We also wish to acknowledge the work of Dr. James Anderson, a pupil of Dr. Grant, under whose stewardship the seventh and eighth editions were published.

The following individuals also provided invaluable contributions to previous editions of the atlas and are gratefully acknowledged: C.A. Armstrong, P.G. Ashmore, D. Baker, D.A. Barr, J.V. Basmajian, S. Bensley, D. Bilbey, J. Bottos, W. Boyd, J. Callagan, H.A. Cates, S.A. Crooks, M. Dickie, C. Duckwall, R. Duckwall, J.W.A. Duckworth, F.B. Fallis, J.B. Francis, J.S. Fraser, P. George, R.K. George, M.G. Gray, B.L. Guyatt, C.W. Hill, W.J. Horsey, B.S. Jaden, M.J. Lee, G.F. Lewis, I.B. MacDonald, D.L. MacIntosh, R.G. MacKenzie, S. Mader, K.O. McCuaig, D. Mazierski, W.R. Mitchell, K. Nancekivell, A.J.A. Noronha, S. O'Sullivan, W. Pallie, W.M. Paul, D. Rini, C. Sandone, C.H. Sawyer, A.I. Scott, J.S. Simpkins, J.S. Simpson, C.G. Smith, I.M. Thompson, J.S. Thompson, N.A. Watters, R.W. Wilson, B. Vallecoccia, and K. Yu.

THIRTEENTH EDITION

We are indebted to our colleagues and former professors for their encouragement—especially Dr. Keith L. Moore for his expert advice and Drs. Daniel O. Graney, Lawrence Ross, Ryan Splittgerber, Lily Cabellon, and Douglas J. Gould for their invaluable input.

We extend our gratitude to our medical illustrator Valerie Oxorn, whose artistic skills and anatomical insights made substantial contributions to this edition. We would also like to acknowledge Jennifer Clements, Art Director at Lippincott Williams & Wilkins, who managed the art program for this edition.

Special thanks go to everyone at **Lippincott Williams & Wilkins**—especially Crystal Taylor, Acquisitions Editor, and Julie Montalbano, Product Manager. All of your efforts and expertise are much appreciated.

We would like to thank the hundreds of instructors and students who have over the years communicated via the publisher and directly with the editor their suggestions for how this *Atlas* might be improved. Finally, we would like to acknowledge the reviewers who reviewed previous editions of the *Atlas* as well as the following reviewers who reviewed the twelfth edition and provided expert advice on the development of this edition in particular:

FACULTY REVIEWERS

Belinda Beck, Griffith University, Queesnsland, Australia
Juliette Cooper, University of Manitoba, Winnipeg, Manitoba, Canada
Donald Fletcher, East Carolina State University, Greenville, North Carolina
Georgina Fyfe, Curtin University, Perth, Australia
Doug Gould, The Ohio State University, Columbus, Ohio
Rod Green, Latrobe University, Victoria, Australia
Jan Smit, Queen's University Belfast, United Kingdom
Mark Stringer, University of Otago, New Zealand
Marjan Vandersteen, Universiteit Hasselt, Diepenbeek, Belgium
Bruce Wainman, McMaster University, Hamilton, Ontario, Canada
Robert Whitaker, University of Cambridge, United Kingdom

STUDENT REVIEWERS

Merrian Brooks
Tameka Byrd
Daniel Choi
Terry Dean
Stephen Goldberg
Peter Hakim
Andrew Jensen
Daniel Kou
Malini Kumar
Janelle Lum
Leah Phillabaum

We hope that readers and reviewers will find many of their suggestions incorporated into the twelfth edition and will continue to provide their valuable input.

Anne M.R. Agur
Arthur F. Dalley II

CONTENTS

CONTENTS

6 Upper Limb 481

7 Head 611

8 Neck 751

9 Cranial Nerves 817

LIST OF TABLES

CHAPTER 1

1.26 Courtesy of Dr. E.L. Lansdown, University of Toronto, Canada

1.36A Courtesy of Dr. D.E. Sanders, University of Toronto, Canada

1.36C Courtesy of Dr. E.L. Lansdown, University of Toronto, Canada

1.36 Courtesy of I. Verschuur, Joint Department of Medical Imaging, UHN/Mount Sinai Hospital, Toronto, Canada

1.43B,E Courtesy of I. Verschuur, Joint Department of Medical Imaging, UHN/Mount Sinai Hospital, Toronto, Canada

1.43C and 1.52 Moore KL, Dalley AF, Clinically Oriented Anatomy, 5th ed, 2006:170 (Fig. 155). A is based on Torrent-Guasp F, Buckberg GD, Clemente C et al. The Structure and Function of the Helical Heart and Its Buttress Wrapping. I. The normal macroscopic structure of the heart. Sem. Thor. Cardiovasc Surgery. 13 (4): 301–319, 2001.

1.46D Dean D, Herbener TE. Cross-Sectional Human Anatomy, 2000:25 (Plate 2.9).

1.49C Courtesy of I. Verschuur, Joint Department of Medical Imaging, UHN/Mount Sinai Hospital, Toronto, Canada

1.50B,D Courtesy of I. Morrow, University of Manitoba, Canada

1.51B Courtesy of Dr. J. Heslin, Toronto, Canada

1.52C Feigenbaum H, Armstrong WF, Ryan T. Feigenbaum's Echocardiography. 5th ed, 2005:116.

1.57 Courtesy of I. Verschuur, Joint Department of Medical Imaging, UHN/Mount Sinai Hospital, Toronto, Canada

1.64B Courtesy of Dr. E.L. Lansdown, University of Toronto, Canada

1.79A-F MRIs courtesy of Dr. M.A. Haider, University of Toronto, Canada

1.80A-C MRIs courtesy of Dr. M.A. Haider, University of Toronto, Canada

1.81AB MRIs courtesy of Dr. M.A. Haider, University of Toronto, Canada

CHAPTER 2

2.7B Lockhart, RD, Hamilton, GF., Fyfe FW. Anatomy of the Human Body, Philadelphia, Lippincott, 1959.

2.9 Clay JH, Pounds DM. Basic Clinical Massage Therapy: Integrating Anatomy and Treatment. 2nd ed, 2008:275. (Fig. 7.2)

2.26B MRI courtesy of Dr. M.A. Haider, University of Toronto, Canada

2.32C Dudek RW, Louis TM, *High-Yield Gross Anatomy,* 4th edition, 2010:106. (Fig. 11.2)

2.34A Dudek RW, Louis TM, *High-Yield Gross Anatomy,* 4th edition, 2010:103. (Fig. 11.1)

2.34B Courtesy of Dr. J. Heslin, Toronto, Canada

2.34C,D Courtesy of Dr. E.L. Lansdown, University of Toronto, Canada

2.36 Courtesy of Dr. J. Heslin, Toronto, Canada

2.42A Courtesy of Dr. C.S. Ho, University of Toronto, Canada

2.42B Courtesy of Dr. E.L. Lansdown, University of Toronto, Canada

2.45A Courtesy of Dr. E.L. Lansdown, University of Toronto, Canada

2.45B Courtesy of Dr. J. Heslin, Toronto, Canada

2.47 Courtesy of Dr. K. Sniderman, University of Toronto, Canada

2.53B Courtesy of A. M. Arenson, University of Toronto, Canada

2.59D Courtesy of Dr. G.B. Haber, University of Toronto, Canada

2.61AB Courtesy of Dr. J. Heslin, Toronto, Canada

2.63AB Courtesy of Dr. G.B. Haber, University of Toronto, Canada

2.66B Radiograph courtesy of G.B.Haber, University of Toronto, Canada; photo courtesy of Mission Hospital Regional Center, Mission Viejo, California

2.73B Courtesy of M. Asch, University of Toronto, Canada

2.72B Courtesy of E.L. Lansdown, University of Toronto, Canada

2.68B (right) Courtesy of M. Asch, University of Toronto, Canada

2.91A-C Courtesy of Dr. M.A. Haider, University of Toronto, Canada

2.91D The Visible Human Project; National Library of Medicine; Visible Man Image number 1625.

2.91E,G Dean D, Herbener TE. Cross Sectional Human Anatomy, 2000:45,53 (Plates 3.9, 3.13)

2.92A-D Courtesy of Dr. M.A. Haider, University of Toronto, Canada

2.93A-D Courtesy of Dr. M.A. Haider, University of Toronto, Canada

CHAPTER 3

3.7 Snell, R. Clinical Anatomy by Regions, 9th edition, 2011. (Figs. 7.39 and 7.41)

3.13C Dudek RW, Louis TM, *High-Yield Gross Anatomy,* 4th edition, 2010:189. (Fig. 18.4)

3.24 (left) from Dauber W, Pocket Atlas of Human Anatomy Rev 5e, NY, Thieme 2007, p. 195

3.26C,D Bickley LS, Bates' Guide to Physical Examination and History Taking, 10th edition, p. 563.

3.33B,C Bickley LS, Bates' Guide to Physical Examination and History Taking, 10th edition, p. 540, 541

3.33D Courtesy of RE Bristow, Johns Hopkins School of Medicine, Baltimore, MD

3.68A-D Courtesy of Dr. M.A. Haider, University of Toronto, Canada

3.68E Courtesy of The Visible Human Project; National Library of Medicine; Visible Man Image number 1940

3.69 Uflacker R. Atlas of Vascular Anatomy: An Angiographic Approach, 1997:611.

3.70A-C Courtesy of Dr. M.A. Haider, University of Toronto, Canada

3.71 MRIs courtesy of Dr. M.A. Haider, University of Toronto, Canada

3.72A-G MRIs courtesy of Dr. M.A. Haider, University of Toronto, Canada; sectioned specimens from The Visible Human Project; National Library of Medicine; Visible Woman Image numbers 1870 and 1895

3.73AB Courtesy of Dr. M.A. Haider, University of Toronto, Canada.

3.74A-D Ultrasounds courtesy of A.M. Arenson, University of Toronto, Canada

3.75D Reprinted with permission from Stuart GCE, Reid DF. Diagnostic studies. In Copeland LJ (ed.): Textbook of Gynecology. Philadelphia, WB Saunders, 1993.

CHAPTER 4

4.1B Courtesy of D. Salonen, University of Toronto, Canada

4.7B,D,F and 4.8E Courtesy of Drs. E. Becker and P. Bobechko, University of Toronto, Canada

4.8C,D Courtesy of E. Becker, University of Toronto, Canada

4.11A,B Courtesy of J. Heslin, Unitersity of Toronto, Canada

4.11C,D Courtesy of D. Armstrong, University of Toronto, Canada

4.12C Courtesy of D. Salonen, University of Toronto, Canada

4.15B and 4.16B Courtesy of E. Becker, University of Toronto, Canada

4.40C Clay JH, Pounds DM. Basic Clinical Massage Therapy: Integrating Anatomy and Treatment. 2003:92 (Fig. 3.40)

4.49B Courtesy of D. Salonen, University of Toronto, Canada

4.56AB Courtesy of The Visible Human Project; National Library of Medicine; Visible Man 1168.

4.56C Courtesy of D. Armstrong, University of Toronto, Canada

4.57A,B Courtesy of The Visible Human Project; National Library of Medicine; Visible Man 1715.

4.58A,B Courtesy of The Visible Human Project; National Library of Medicine; Visible Man 1805.

4.59A-D Courtesy of D. Salonen, University of Toronto, Canada

CHAPTER 5

5.3B,D Courtesy of P. Babyn, University of Toronto, Canada

5.8A-D A and B are based on Foerster, O.: The Dermatomes in Man. Brain 56(1):1-39, 1933.C and D are based on Keefan JJ, Garrett FD. The segmental distribution of the cutaneous nerves in the limbs of man. Anat Rec 1948;102:409

5.12B Rassner: Dermatologie. Lehrbuch und Atlas © Urban & Schwarzenberg Verlag München. (Appeared in Moore KL, Dalley AF. Clincally Oriented Anatomy. 4th Ed., 1999:527.)

5.14B Courtesy of Dr. E.L. Lansdown, University of Toronto, Canada

5.22A-D Modified from Clay JH, Pounds DM. Basic Clinical Massage Therapy: Integrating Anatomy and Treatment. 2002:301 (Plate 9.2).

5.22E,H Modified from Clay JH, Pounds DM. Basic Clinical Massage Therapy: Integrating Anatomy and Treatment. 2002:280,312 (Figs. 8.10, 9.10)

5.34A Courtesy of E. Becker, University of Toronto, Canada

5.39C Daffner RH. Clinical Radiology: The Essentials. Baltimore: Williams & Wilkins, 1993:491 (Fig. 11.99)

5.40B Courtesy of Dr. D. Salonen, University of Toronto, Canada

5.51 (inset) Courtesy of Dr. Robert Peroutka, Cockeysville, MD

5.56A,B Courtesy of Dr. P. Bobechko, University of Toronto, Canada

5.56C Courtesy of Dr. D. Salonen, University of Toronto, Canada

5.57B,C Courtesy of Dr. D. Salonen, University of Toronto, Canada

5.58 Courtesy of Dr. P. Bobechko, University of Toronto, Canada

5.59B,C Courtesy of Dr. D. Salonen, University of Toronto, Canada

5.65C,D Clay JH, Pounds DM. Basic Clinical Massage Therapy: Integrating Anatomy and Treatment. 2002:352,354 (Figs. 10.16 & 10.18)

5.73A Courtesy of Dr. D. K. Sniderman, University of Toronto, Canada

5.81B and 5.86A Courtesy of Dr. E. Becker, University of Toronto, Canada

5.86B Courtesy of Dr. P. Bobechko, University of Toronto, Canada

5.87B Courtesy of E. Becker, University of Toronto, Canada

5.89B Courtesy of Dr. W. Kucharczyk, University of Toronto, Canada

5.90B Courtesy of Dr. W. Kucharczyk, University of Toronto, Canada

5.98C Courtesy of Dr. P. Bobechko, University of Toronto, Canada

5.100C Courtesy of The Visible Human Project; National Library of Medicine; Visible Man 2105.

5.100D-F MRIs courtesy of Dr. D. Salonen, University of Toronto, Canada

5.102C Courtesy of The Visible Human Project; National Library of Medicine; Visible Man 2551.

5.102D-F MRIs courtesy of Dr. D. Salonen, University of Toronto, Canada

Table 5.3 (unnumbered figures) Dudek RW, Louis TM, *High-Yield Gross Anatomy,* 4ᵗʰ edition, 2010:228. (Table 21-1)

CHAPTER 6

6.7A,B Based on Foerster, O.: The Dermatomes in Man. Brain 56(1):1-39,1933. (Appeared in Moore KL, Dalley AF. Clinically Oriented Anatomy. 4th ed, 1999:682,683.)

6.7C,D Based on Keegan JJ, Garrett FD. The segmental distribution of the cutaneous nerves in the limbs of man. Anat Rec 1948;102:409

6.10 Tank W, Gest TR: KWW Atlas of Anatomy. Baltimore: Lippincott Williams & Wilkins, 2008. Pl. 2-53, p. 82.

6.21L Courtesy of D. Armstrong, University of Toronto, Canada

6.24C Courtesy of D. Armstrong, University of Toronto, Canada

6.29B Rowland LP, Merritt's Textbook of Neurology, 9th ed. Baltimore, Williams & Wilkins, 1995

6.31ABD Clay JH, Pounds DM. Basic Clinical Massage Therapy: Integrating Anatomy and Treatment. 2002:113,136,132 (Plates 4.4, 4.31, 4.24)

6.33B,D Clay JH, Pounds DM. Basic Clinical Massage Therapy: Integrating Anatomy and Treatment. 2002:144,138 (Figs. 4.44, 4.33)

6.48A Courtesy of E. Becker, University of Toronto, Canada

6.48C,E Courtesy of D. Salonen, University of Toronto, Canada

6.48D Courtesy of R. Leekam, University of Toronto and West End Diagnostic Imaging, Canada

6.53C Courtesy of E. Becker, University of Toronto, Canada

6.54 Radiographs courtesy of J. Heslin, Toronto, Canada;

6.55B Courtesy of D. Salonen, University of Toronto, Canada

6.56B Courtesy of E. Becker, University of Toronto, Canada

6.63A, 6.64A, 6.65A, 6.66A Clay JH, Pounds DM. Basic Clinical Massage Therapy: Integrating Anatomy and Treatment. 2002:170 (Plate 5.3)

6.72A-D Clay JH, Pounds DM. Basic Clinical Massage Therapy: Integrating Anatomy and Treatment. 2002:174 (Plate 5.55)

6.83 Clay JH, Pounds DM. Basic Clinical Massage Therapy: Integrating Anatomy and Treatment. 2002:127 (Plate 5.5)

6.89F Courtesy of E. Becker, University of Toronto, Canada

6.92A,B Courtesy of E. Becker, University of Toronto, Canada

6.93B Courtesy of D. Armstrong, University of Toronto, Canada

6.99 A-C Courtesy of D. Salonen, University of Toronto, Canada

6.100C-E Courtesy of D. Salonen, University of Toronto, Canada

6.101A-C Courtesy of D. Salonen, University of Toronto, Canada

6.102 B Courtesy of R. Leekam, University of Toronto and West End Diagnostic Imaging, Canada

6.35A,B Clay JH, Pounds DM. Basic Clinical Massage Therapy: Integrating Anatomy and Treatment. 2002:170,171,173,179 (Plates 5.3, 5.4, 5.6, and Fig. 5.1)

CHAPTER 7

7.1B,E,F Courtesy of Dr. D. Armstrong, University of Toronto, Canada

7.7A,B Courtesy of Dr. E. Becker, University of Toronto, Canada

7.29A-C Courtesy of Dr. D. Armstrong, University of Toronto, Canada

7.35A,B Courtesy of I. Verschuur, Joint Department of Medical Imaging, UHN/Mount Sinai Hospital, Toronto, Canada

7.38D Courtesy of Dr. W. Kucharczyk, University of Toronto, Canada

7.39B Melloni,R. Melloni's Illustrated Review of Human Anatomy by Structures-Arteries, Bones, Muscles, Nerves, Veins, 1988, p. 198

7.42A-D Modified from Girard, Louis, Anatomy of the Huma Eye. II. The Extra-ocular Muscles. Teaching Films, Inc. Houston, TX

7.45C Melloni,R. Melloni's Illustrated Review of Human Anatomy by Structures-Arteries, Bones, Muscles, Nerves, Veins, 1988, p. 189.

7.46A Courtesy of J.R. Buncic, University of Toronto, Canada

7.56 CTs and MRIs from Langland OE, Langlais RP, Preece JW. Principles of Dental Imaging, 2002:278 (Figs. 11.32A, B; 11.33A, B).

7.65A Langland OE, Langlais RP, Preece JW. Principles of Dental Imaging, 2002:334 (Fig. 14.1).

7.65B Courtesy of M.J. Phatoah, University of Toronto, Canada.

7.66E Courtesy of Dr. B. Libgott, Division of Anatomy/Department of Surgery, University of Toronto, Ontario, Canada

7.67B,C Woelfel JB, Scheid RC. Dental Anatomy: Its Relevance to Dentistry. 6th ed, 2002:86,46 (Figs. 3.5 & 3.6).

7.76B Courtesy of D. Armstrong, University of Toronto, Canada

7.76C Courtesy of E. Becker, University of Toronto, Canada

7.77C Courtesy of E. Becker, University of Toronto, Canada

7.78B Modified from Paff, GH Anatomy of the Head & Neck. Philadelphia: WB Sanders Co., 1973. figs 238–240, p. 142–143.

7.84D Courtesy of Welch Allyn, Inc. Skaneateles Falls, NY. (Appeared in Moore KL, Dalley AF. Clinically Oriented Anatomy. 4th ed, 1999:966 (Fig. 8.2)

7.94B-D Courtesy of W. Kucharczyk, University of Toronto, Canada

7.95B Courtesy of Dr. W. Kucharczyk, University of Toronto, Canada

7.96A-C All photos courtesy of The Visible Human Project; National Library of Medicine; Visible Man 1107 and 1168.

7.99–7.102, 7.104, 7.105B,C and 7.106 Colorized from photographs provided courtesy of Dr. C.G. Smith, which appears in Smith CG. Serial Dissections of the Human Brain. Baltimore: Urban & Schwarzenber, Inc. and Toronto: Gage Publishing Ltd., 1981 (© Carlton G. Smith)

7.103A-F MRIs courtesy of Dr. D. Armstrong, University of Toronto, Canada

7.107A-E MRIs courtesy of Dr. D. Armstrong, University of Toronto, Canada

7.108A-F MRIs courtesy of Dr. D. Armstrong, University of Toronto, Canada

7.109A-C MRIs courtesy of Dr. D. Armstrong, University of Toronto, Canada

7.53 Illustrations from Clay JH, Pounds DM. Basic Clinical Massage Therapy: Integrating Anatomy and Treatment. 2002:76,74,79 (Figs.3.17, 3.15, 3.19).

7.64 (bottom left illustration) Clay JH, Pounds DM. Basic Clinical Massage Therapy: Integrating Anatomy and Treatment, 2002:80 (Fig. 3.22).

CHAPTER 8

8.5B Courtesy of J. Heslin, University of Toronto, Canada

8.7 Modified from Clay JH, Pounds DM. Basic Clinical Massage Therapy: Integrating Anatomy and Treatment. 2003:90,91 (Figs. 3.36, 3.48)

8.12A Modified from Clay JH, Pounds DM. Basic Clinical Massage Therapy: Integrating Anatomy and Treatment. 2003:88 (Fig. 3.34)

8.15B Courtesy of Dr. D. Armstrong, University of Toronto, Canada

8.24B Modified from Clay JH, Pounds DM. Basic Clinical Massage Therapy: Integrating Anatomy and Treatment. 2003:92 (Fig. 3.40)

8.25A Clay JH, Pounds DM. Basic Clinical Massage Therapy: Integrating Anatomy and Treatment. 2003:101,128 (Figs. 3.53, 4.17)

8.25B Clay JH, Pounds DM. Basic Clinical Massage Therapy: Integrating Anatomy and Treatment. 2ⁿᵈ ed, 2008:103. (Fig. 3.40)

8.25C Clay JH, Pounds DM. Basic Clinical Massage Therapy: Integrating Anatomy and Treatment. 2ⁿᵈ ed, 2008:140. (Fig. 4.17)

8.25D Clay JH, Pounds DM. Basic Clinical Massage Therapy: Integrating Anatomy and Treatment. 2ⁿᵈ ed, 2008:67. (Fig. 3.6)

8.28 Clay JH, Pounds DM. Basic Clinical Massage Therapy: Integrating Anatomy and Treatment. 2003:96,100,104 (Figs. 3.48, 3.52, 3.56)

8.34A Abrahams P. The Atlas of the Human Body. San Diego, CA: Thunder Bay Press, 2002, p. 86.

8.34B From Liebgott B. The Anatomical Basis of Dentistry. Philadelphia, PA: Mosby, 1982.

8.41A Rohen JW, Yokochi C, Lutjen-DrecollE, Romrell LJ. Color Atlas of Anatomy: A Photographic Study of the Human Body. 5th ed, 2002.

8.41C Courtesy of Dr. D. Salonen, University of Toronto, Canada.

8.44A-C Courtesy of Dr. D. Salonen, University of Toronto, Canada;

8.46B Courtesy of Dr. E. Becker, University of Toronto, Canada

8.47 Siemens Medical Solutions USA, Inc.

CHAPTER 9

9.23A-F Courtesy of Dr. W. Kucharczyk, University of Toronto, Canada

9.24A-C Photos courtesy of Dr. W. Kucharczyk, University of Toronto, Canada

Thorax

Clavicular head of pectoralis major

Suprasternal (jugular) notch

Deltoid

Clavicle

Anterior axillary fold

Sternum

Posterior axillary fold

Axillary fossa

Sternocostal head of pectoralis major

Areola

Nipple

Xiphoid process

Serratus anterior

Linea alba

External oblique

Rectus abdominis

Anterior View

1.1   SURFACE ANATOMY OF MALE PECTORAL REGION

- The subject is adducting the shoulders against resistance to demonstrate the pectoralis major muscle.
- The sternum (breastbone) lies subcutaneously in the anterior median line and is palpable throughout its length.
- The suprasternal notch can be palpated between the prominent medial ends of the clavicle.
- The pectoralis major muscle has two parts, the sternocostal and clavicular heads.
- The inferior border of the sternocostal head of the pectoralis major muscle forms the anterior axillary fold. The axillary fossa ("armpit") is a surface feature overlying a fat-filled space, the axilla, posterior to the anterior fold.
- The male nipple overlies the fourth intercostal space.

Supraclavicular nerves (C3 and C4)

Clavicle

Deltoid

Clavipectoral
(deltopectoral)
triangle

Cephalic vein

Clavicular head

Pectoralis
major

Sternocostal head

Intercostobrachial nerve (T2)

Lateral mammary and posterior branches
of lateral pectoral cutaneous
nerves (T3 to T6)
(from intercostal nerves)

Serratus anterior

External oblique

Platysma

Skin

Pectoral fascia covering
pectoralis major

Subcutaneous tissue

Lateral mammary branches of
lateral pectoral cutaneous branches
of intercostal nerves

Medial mammary branches of
anterior pectoral cutaneous
branches of intercostal nerves

Costal cartilage of
6th rib

Anterior View

1.2   SUPERFICIAL DISSECTION, MALE PECTORAL REGION

- The platysma muscle, which descends to the 2nd or 3rd rib, is cut short on both sides of the specimen; together with the supraclavicular nerves, it is reflected superiorly on the right side.
- The pectoral fascia covers the pectoralis major.
- The clavicle lies deep to the subcutaneous tissue and the platysma muscle.
- The cephalic vein passes deeply in the clavipectoral (deltopectoral) triangle to join the axillary vein.
- Supraclavicular (C3 and C4) and upper thoracic nerves (T2 to T6) supply cutaneous innervation to the pectoral region.
- The clavipectoral (deltopectoral) triangle, bounded by the clavicle superiorly, the deltoid muscle laterally, and the clavicular head of the pectoralis major muscle medially, underlies a surface depression called the infraclavicular fossa.

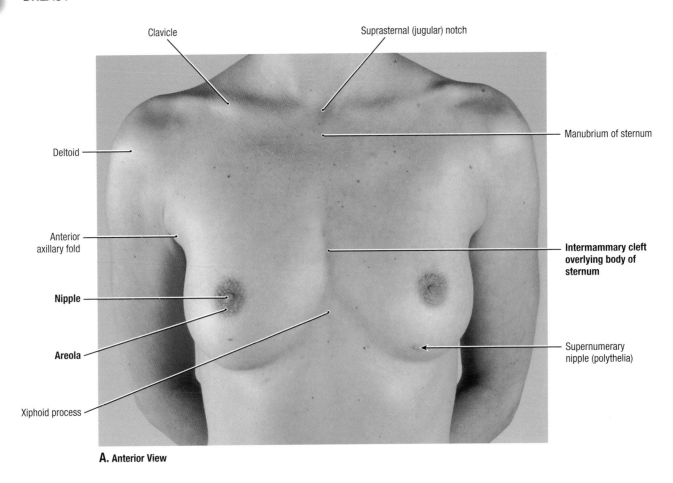

Clavicle

Suprasternal (jugular) notch

Deltoid

Manubrium of sternum

Anterior
axillary fold

**Intermammary cleft
overlying body of
sternum**

Nipple

Areola

Supernumerary
nipple (polythelia)

Xiphoid process

A. Anterior View

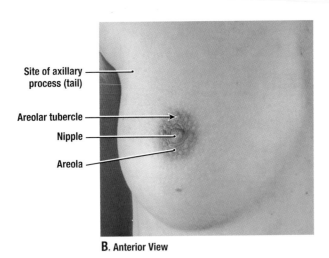

Site of axillary
process (tail)

Areolar tubercle

Nipple

Areola

B. Anterior View

1.3

SURFACE ANATOMY OF FEMALE PECTORAL REGION

A. Overview. **B.** Breast. The roughly circular base of the female breast extends transversely from the lateral border of the sternum to the midaxillary line and vertically from the 2nd to 6th ribs. A small part of the breast may extend along the inferolateral edge of the pectoralis major muscle toward the axillary fossa, forming an axillary process or tail (of Spence).

Polymastia (supernumerary breasts) or **polythelia** (accessory nipples) may occur superior or inferior to the normal pair, occasionally developing in the axillary fossa or anterior abdominal wall. Supernumerary breasts usually consist of only a rudimentary nipple and areola, which may be mistaken for a mole (nevus) until they change pigmentation with the normal nipples during pregnancy.

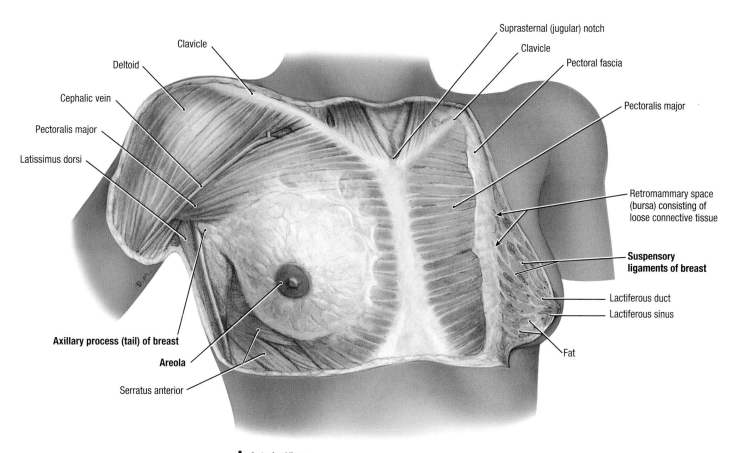

A. Anterior View

SUPERFICIAL DISSECTION, FEMALE
PECTORAL REGION

A. Dissection.
- On the specimen's right side, the skin is removed; on the left side, the breast is sagittally sectioned.
- Two thirds of the breast rests on the pectoral fascia covering the pectoralis major; the other third rests on the fascia covering the serratus anterior muscle.
- The region of loose connective tissue between the pectoral fascia and the deep surface of the breast, the retromammary space (bursa), permits the breast to move on the deep fascia.

Cancer can spread by contiguity (invasion of adjacent tissue). When **breast cancer** cells invade the retromammary space, attach to or invade the pectoral fascia overlying the pectoralis major, or metastasize to the interpectoral nodes (Fig. 1.7), the breast elevates when the muscle contracts. This movement is a clinical sign of advanced cancer of the breast.

    B. Breast Quadrants. For the anatomical location and description of tumors and cysts, the surface of the breast is divided into four quadrants. For example: "A hard irregular mass was felt in the superior medial quadrant of the breast at the 2 o'clock position, approximately 2.5 cm from the margin of the areola."

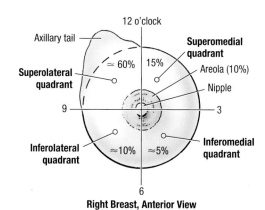

Right Breast, Anterior View

B. Quadrants of Breast: Percentage of Malignant Tumors

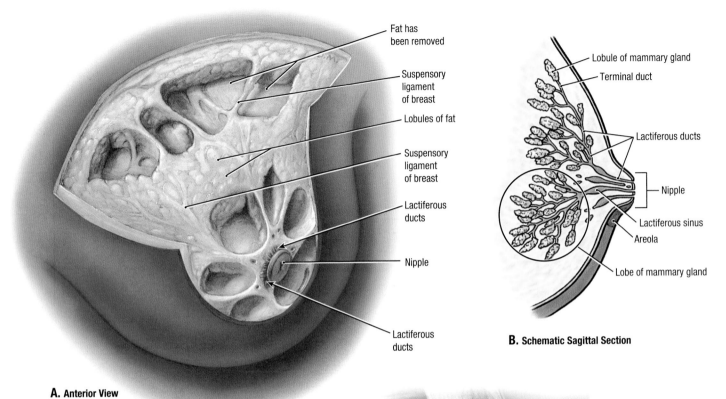

Fat has been removed

Suspensory ligament of breast

Lobules of fat

Suspensory ligament of breast

Lactiferous ducts

Nipple

Lactiferous ducts

A. Anterior View

Lobule of mammary gland

Terminal duct

Lactiferous ducts

Nipple

Lactiferous sinus

Areola

Lobe of mammary gland

B. Schematic Sagittal Section

1.5   FEMALE MAMMARY GLAND

A. Dissection. Areas of subcutaneous fat were removed to show the suspensory ligaments of the breast. The mammary glands are modified sweat glands located in the subcutaneous tissue. They consist of glandular tissue, the parenchyma, and supporting fibrous tissue, the stroma. The mammary glands are attached to the dermis of the skin by suspensory ligaments. **B. and C.** Sagittal sections. The glandular tissue consists of 15 to 20 lobes, each composed of lobules. Each lobe has a lactiferous duct that widens to form the lactiferous sinus before opening on the nipple. **Interference with the lymphatic drainage by cancer** may cause lymphedema (edema, excess fluid in the subcutaneous tissue), which in turn may result in deviation of the nipple and a leathery, thickened appearance of the breast skin. Prominent (puffy) skin between dimpled pores may develop, which gives the skin an orange-peel appearance (*peau d'orange* sign). Larger dimples may form if pulled by cancerous invasion of the suspensory ligaments of the breast.

Pectoral fascia

Subcutaneous tissue

Retromammary space (bursa)

Suspensory ligaments of breast

Glandular tissue (mammary lobule)

Lactiferous duct

Nipple

Lactiferous sinus

Fat

C. Sagittal Section of Breast

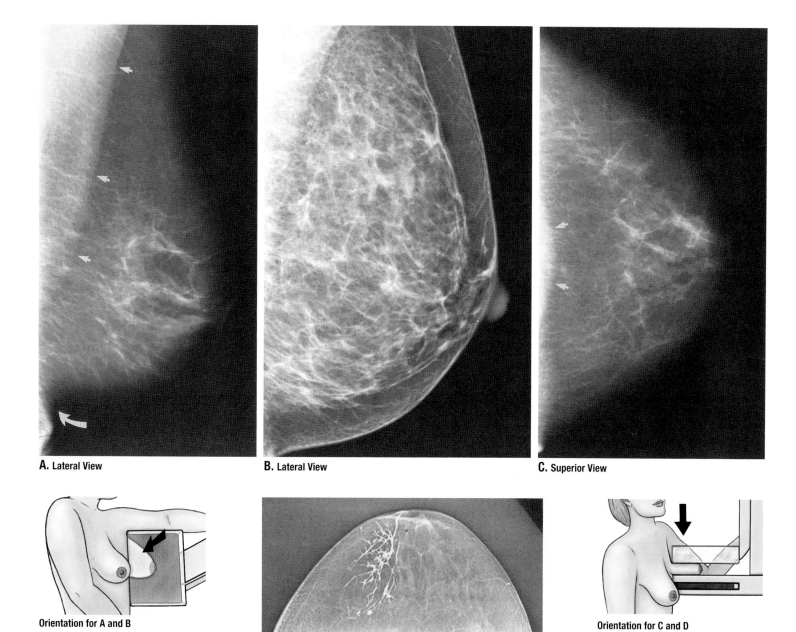

A. Lateral View

B. Lateral View

C. Superior View

Orientation for A and B

Orientation for C and D

D. Superior View

1.6   IMAGING OF BREAST

A. Mediolateral oblique (MLO) mammogram of left breast. The pectoralis major muscle is indicated with *white arrowheads* and the inframammary fold with a *curved white arrow*. The nipple is seen in profile. Observe the connective tissue network of the breast. The stroma is radiopaque and changes with age and during lactation.
B. Digital mammogram. **C.** Craniocaudal (CC) mammogram of left breast. Pectoralis major (*white arrows*).
D. Glactogram. Contrast has been injected into a lactiferous duct, outlining the branching pattern of its tributaries.

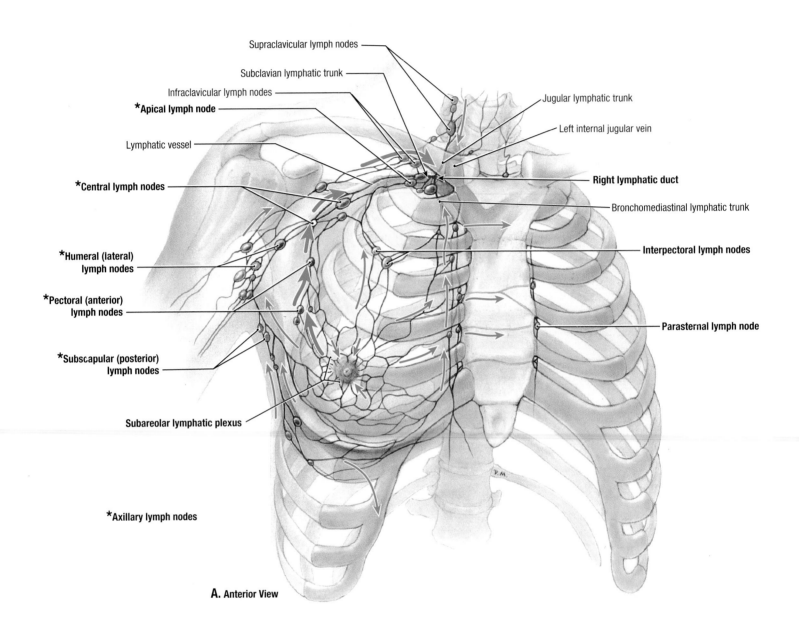

Supraclavicular lymph nodes

Subclavian lymphatic trunk

Infraclavicular lymph nodes

*Apical lymph node

Lymphatic vessel

*Central lymph nodes

*Humeral (lateral) lymph nodes

*Pectoral (anterior) lymph nodes

*Subscapular (posterior) lymph nodes

Subareolar lymphatic plexus

*Axillary lymph nodes

Jugular lymphatic trunk

Left internal jugular vein

Right lymphatic duct

Bronchomediastinal lymphatic trunk

Interpectoral lymph nodes

Parasternal lymph node

A. Anterior View

| 1.7 | LYMPHATIC DRAINAGE OF BREAST |

A. Overview. Lymph drained from the upper limb and breast passes through nodes arranged irregularly in groups of axillary lymph nodes: (1) pectoral, along the inferior border of the pectoralis minor muscle; (2) subscapular, along the subscapular artery and veins; (3) humeral, along the distal part of the axillary vein; (4) central, at the base of the axilla, embedded in axillary fat; and (5) apical, along the axillary vein between the clavicle and the pectoralis minor muscle. Most of the breast drains via the pectoral, central, and apical axillary nodes to the subclavian lymph trunk, which joins the venous system at the junction of the subclavian and internal jugular veins. The medial part of the breast drains to the parasternal nodes, which are located along the internal thoracic vessels.

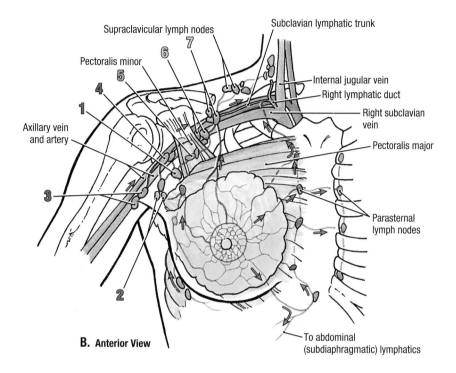

Supraclavicular lymph nodes

Subclavian lymphatic trunk

Pectoralis minor

Internal jugular vein

Right lymphatic duct

Right subclavian vein

Axillary vein and artery

Pectoralis major

Parasternal lymph nodes

B. Anterior View

To abdominal (subdiaphragmatic) lymphatics

Breast	Upper Limb

Axillary lymph nodes
Location: Inferolateral to pectoralis minor (Level I)

1. Pectoral nodes
2. Subscapular nodes
3. Humeral nodes
4. Central nodes

Interpectoral nodes (5)
Location: On pectoralis minor (Level II)

Apical nodes (6)

Infraclavicular (deltopectoral) nodes (7)
Location: Superomedial to pectoralis minor (Level III)

Subclavian lymph trunk

Thoracic duct or right lymphatic duct

Venous angle (junction of internal jugular and subclavian veins)

C. Flow of lymph from the breast and upper limb to the venous angle.

1.7	**LYMPHATIC DRAINAGE OF BREAST** *(CONTINUED)*

B. Pattern of lymphatic drainage. **Breast cancer** typically spreads by means of lymphatic vessels (lymphogenic metastasis), which carry cancer cells from the breast to the lymph nodes, chiefly those in the axilla. The cells lodge in the nodes, producing nests of tumor cells (metastases). Abundant communications among lymphatic pathways and among axillary, cervical, and parasternal nodes may also cause metastases from the breast to develop in the supraclavicular lymph nodes, the opposite breast, or the abdomen. The prognosis of breast cancer has been correlated with the level of metastasis (I, II, or III) and to the number of involved axillary lymph nodes. **C.** Flow of lymph from the breast and upper limb to the venous angle.

Anterior View

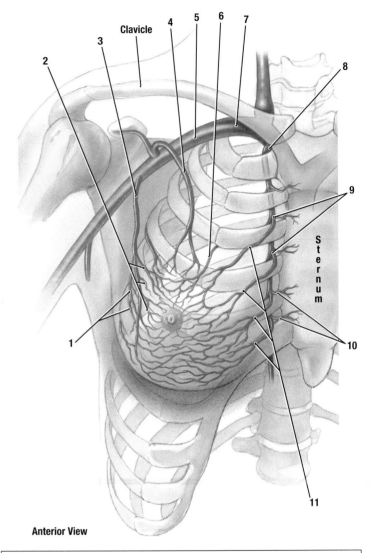

Anterior View

Arteries:
1. Lateral mammary branches of lateral cutaneous branches of posterior intercostal arteries
2. Lateral mammary branches of lateral thoracic artery
3. Lateral thoracic artery
4. Pectoral branch of thoraco-acromial artery
5. Axillary artery
6. Mammary branch of anterior intercostal artery
7. Subclavian artery
8. Internal thoracic artery
9. Perforating branches
10. Sternal branches
11. Medial mammary branches

Veins:
1. Lateral mammary branches of lateral cutaneous branches of posterior intercostal veins
2. Lateral mammary branches of lateral thoracic vein
3. Lateral thoracic vein
4. Pectoral branch of thoraco-acromial vein
5. Axillary vein
6. Mammary branch of anterior intercostal vein
7. Subclavian vein
8. Internal thoracic vein
9. Perforating branches
10. Sternal branches
11. Medial mammary veins

1.8   ARTERIAL SUPPLY AND VENOUS DRAINAGE OF BREAST

Arteries enter and veins drain the breast from its superomedial and superolateral aspects; vessels also penetrate the deep surface of the breast. The vessels branch profusely and anastomose with each other.

Breast incisions are placed in the inferior breast quadrants when possible because these quadrants are less vascular than the superior ones.

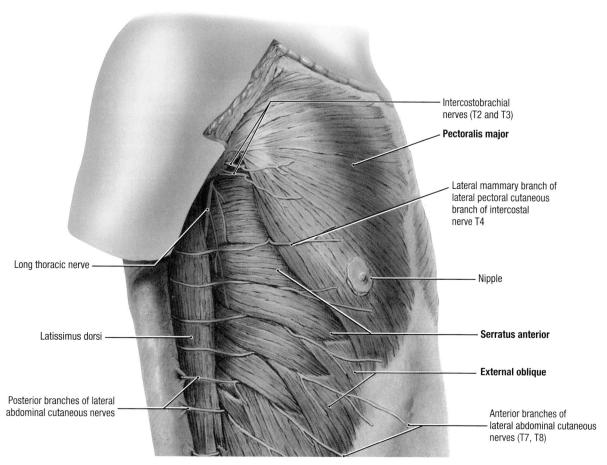

Intercostobrachial
nerves (T2 and T3)

Pectoralis major

Lateral mammary branch of
lateral pectoral cutaneous
branch of intercostal
nerve T4

Long thoracic nerve

Nipple

Latissimus dorsi

Serratus anterior

External oblique

Posterior branches of lateral
abdominal cutaneous nerves

Anterior branches of
lateral abdominal cutaneous
nerves (T7, T8)

A. Anterolateral View (Male)

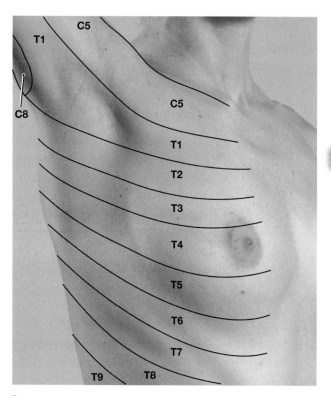

C5
T1
C8
C5
T1
T2
T3
T4
T5
T6
T7
T9   T8

B. Anterolateral View (Female)

1.9   **MUSCLES AND NERVES OF
BED OF BREAST**

A. Muscles comprising bed and cutaneous
nerves. **B.** Dermatomes.

**Local anesthesia of an intercostal
space** (intercostal nerve block) is produced
by injecting a local anesthetic agent around
the intercostal nerves between the paravertebral line and the area of required anesthesia. Because any particular area of skin
usually receives innervation from two adjacent nerves, considerable overlapping of
contiguous dermatomes occurs. Therefore,
complete loss of sensation usually does not
occur unless two or more intercostal nerves
are anesthetized.

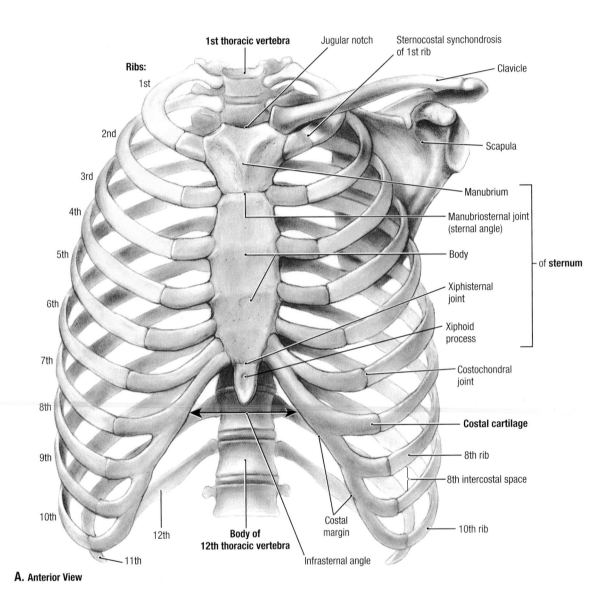

1st thoracic vertebra

Jugular notch

Sternocostal synchondrosis
of 1st rib

Ribs:

1st

Clavicle

2nd

Scapula

3rd

4th

Manubrium

Manubriosternal joint
(sternal angle)

5th

Body

— of **sternum**

Xiphisternal
joint

6th

Xiphoid
process

7th

Costochondral
joint

8th

Costal cartilage

9th

8th rib

8th intercostal space

10th

Costal
margin

10th rib

12th

**Body of
12th thoracic vertebra**

11th

Infrasternal angle

A. Anterior View

1.10   BONY THORAX

- The thoracic cage consists of 12 thoracic vertebrae, 12 pairs of ribs and costal cartilages, and the sternum.
- Anteriorly, the superior seven costal cartilages articulate with the sternum; the 8th, 9th, and 10th cartilages articulate with the cartilage above forming the costal margin; the 11th and 12th are "floating" ribs, that is, their cartilages do not articulate anteriorly.
- The clavicle lies over the 1st rib, making it difficult to palpate. The 2nd rib is easily palpable because its costal cartilage articulates with the sternum

at the sternal angle, located at the junction of the manubrium and body of the sternum.
- The 3rd to 10th ribs can be palpated in sequence inferolaterally from the 2nd rib; the fused costal cartilages of the 7th to 10th ribs form the costal arch (margin), and the tips of the 11th and 12th ribs can be palpated posterolaterally.
- A **rib dislocation** is the displacement of a costal cartilage from the sternum; a **rib separation** refers to dislocation of the costochondral joint.

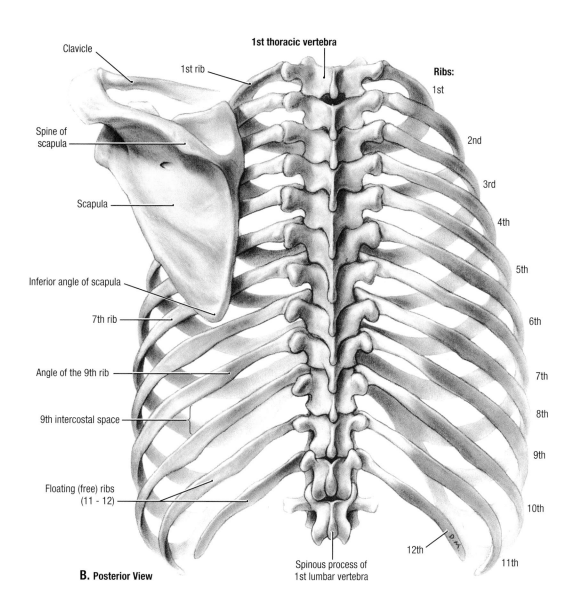

Clavicle

1st rib

1st thoracic vertebra

Ribs:

1st

Spine of
scapula

2nd

3rd

Scapula

4th

5th

Inferior angle of scapula

6th

7th rib

Angle of the 9th rib

7th

8th

9th intercostal space

9th

Floating (free) ribs
(11 - 12)

10th

12th

11th

Spinous process of
1st lumbar vertebra

B. Posterior View

BONY THORAX (*CONTINUED*)

- The superior thoracic aperture (thoracic inlet) is the doorway between the thoracic cavity and the neck region; it is bounded by the 1st thoracic vertebra, the 1st ribs and their cartilages, and the manubrium of the sternum.
- Each rib articulates posteriorly with the vertebral column.
- Posteriorly, all ribs angle inferiorly; anteriorly, the 3rd to 10th costal cartilages angle superiorly.
- The scapula is suspended from the clavicle and extends across the 2nd to 7th ribs posteriorly.

- When clinicians refer to the superior thoracic aperture as the thoracic "outlet," they are emphasizing the important nerves and arteries that pass through this aperture into the lower neck and upper limb. Hence, various types of **thoracic outlet syndromes** exist, such as the costoclavicular syndrome—pallor and coldness of the **skin of the upper limb** and diminished radial pulse—resulting from compression of the subclavian artery between the clavicle and the 1st rib.

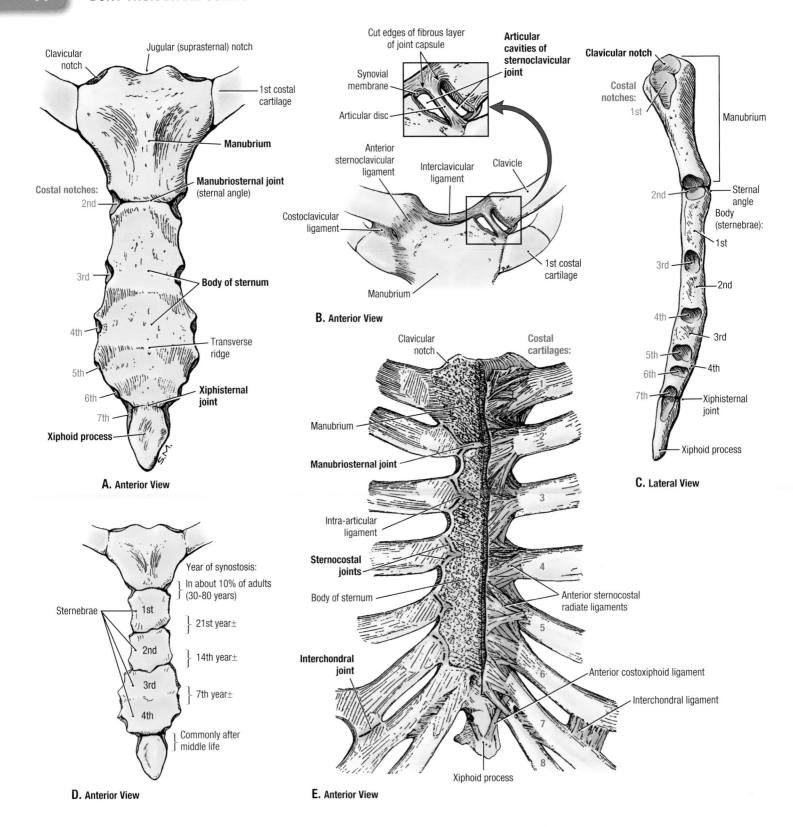

A. Anterior View

B. Anterior View

C. Lateral View

D. Anterior View

E. Anterior View

1.11   STERNUM AND ASSOCIATED JOINTS

A. Parts of sternum. **B.** Sternoclavicular joint. **C.** Features of the lateral aspect of the sternum. **D.** Ages of ossification of sternum. **E.** Sternocostal, manubriosternal, and interchondral joints. On the right side of the specimen, the cortex of the sternum and the external surface of the costal cartilages have been shaved away.

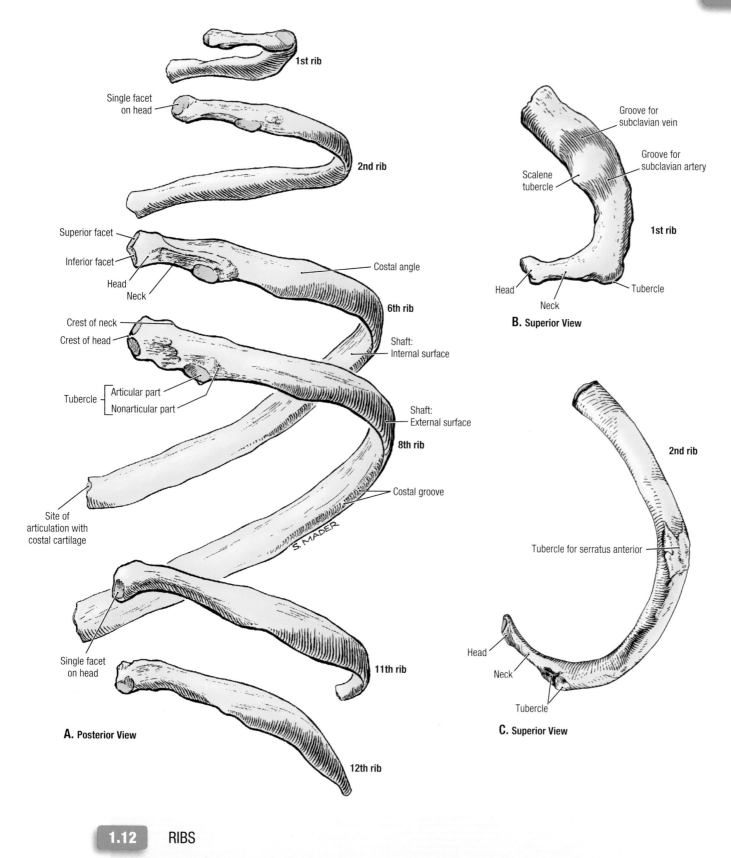

1st rib

Single facet on head

2nd rib

Superior facet

Inferior facet

Head

Neck

Costal angle

6th rib

Crest of neck

Crest of head

Shaft: Internal surface

Tubercle — Articular part

Nonarticular part

Shaft: External surface

8th rib

Site of articulation with costal cartilage

Costal groove

S. MADER

Single facet on head

11th rib

A. Posterior View

12th rib

Groove for subclavian vein

Groove for subclavian artery

Scalene tubercle

1st rib

Head

Tubercle

Neck

B. Superior View

2nd rib

Tubercle for serratus anterior

Head

Neck

Tubercle

C. Superior View

1.12   RIBS

A. "Typical" (6th and 8th) and "atypical" (1st and 2nd and 11th and 12th) ribs. **B.** First rib. **C.** Second rib.
   Rib fractures. The weakest part of a rib is immediately anterior to its angle. The middle ribs are most commonly fractured.

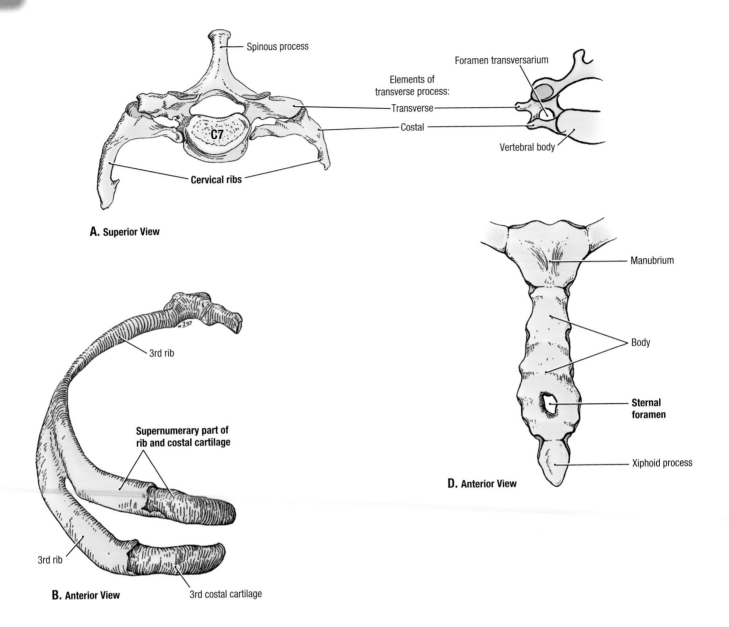

A. Superior View

B. Anterior View

D. Anterior View

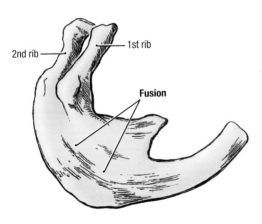

C. Superior View

1.13   RIB AND STERNUM ANOMALIES

A. Cervical ribs. People usually have 12 ribs on each side, but the number may be increased by the presence of cervical and/or lumbar ribs (supernumerary ribs) or decreased by a failure of the 12th pair to form. **Cervical ribs** (present in up to 1% of people) articulate with the C7 vertebra and are clinically significant because they may compress spinal nerves C8 and T1 or the inferior trunk of the brachial plexus supplying the upper limb. Tingling and numbness may occur along the medial border of the forearm. They may also compress the subclavian artery, resulting in **ischemic muscle pain** (caused by poor blood supply) in the upper limb. **Lumbar ribs** are less common than cervical ribs, but have clinical significance in that they may confuse the identity of vertebral levels in diagnostic images. **B.** Bifid rib. The superior component of this 3rd rib is supernumerary and articulated with the lateral aspect of the 1st sternebra. The inferior component articulated at the junction of the 1st and 2nd sternebrae. **C.** Bicipital rib. In this specimen, there has been partial fusion of the first two thoracic ribs. **D.** Sternal foramen.

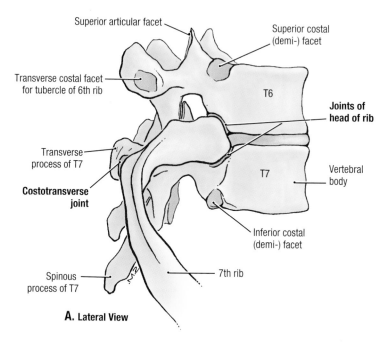

Superior articular facet

Superior costal (demi-) facet

Transverse costal facet for tubercle of 6th rib

T6

Joints of head of rib

Transverse process of T7

Costotransverse joint

Vertebral body

T7

Inferior costal (demi-) facet

Spinous process of T7

7th rib

A. Lateral View

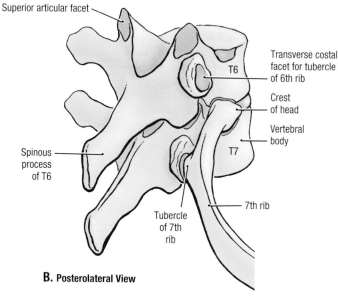

Superior articular facet

T6

Transverse costal facet for tubercle of 6th rib

Crest of head

Vertebral body

T7

Spinous process of T6

7th rib

Tubercle of 7th rib

B. Posterolateral View

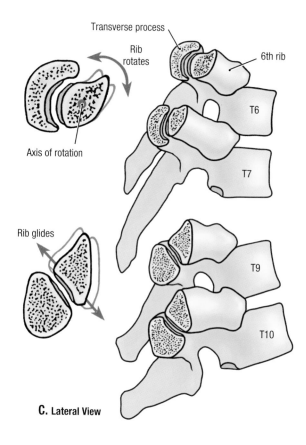

Transverse process

Rib rotates

6th rib

T6

Axis of rotation

T7

Rib glides

T9

T10

C. Lateral View

1.14   COSTOVERTEBRAL ARTICULATIONS

A. and B. Articulating structures.
- There are two articular facets on the head of the rib: a larger, inferior costal facet for articulation with the vertebral body of its own number, and a smaller, superior costal facet for articulation with the vertebral body of the vertebra superior to the rib.
- The crest of the head of the rib separates the superior and inferior costal facets.

- The smooth articular part of the tubercle of the rib, the transverse costal facet, articulates with the transverse process of the same numbered vertebra at the costotransverse joint.

C. Movements at the costotransverse joints. At the 1st to 7th costotransverse joints, the ribs rotate, increasing the anteroposterior diameter of the thorax; at the 8th, 9th, and 10th, they glide, increasing the transverse diameter of the upper abdomen.

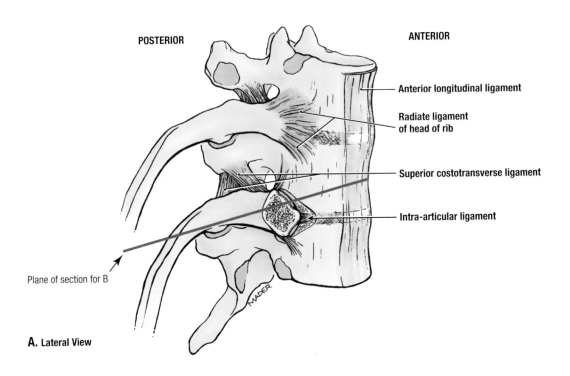

POSTERIOR

ANTERIOR

Anterior longitudinal ligament

Radiate ligament
of head of rib

Superior costotransverse ligament

Intra-articular ligament

Plane of section for B

A. Lateral View

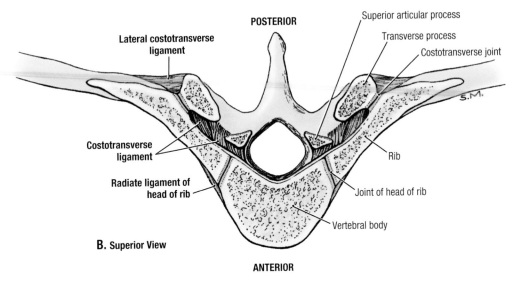

POSTERIOR

Superior articular process

Transverse process

Costotransverse joint

Lateral costotransverse
ligament

Costotransverse
ligament

Radiate ligament of
head of rib

Rib

Joint of head of rib

Vertebral body

B. Superior View

ANTERIOR

| 1.15 | LIGAMENTS OF COSTOVERTEBRAL ARTICULATIONS |

A. External and internal ligaments.
- The radiate ligament joins the head of the rib to two vertebral bodies and the interposed intervertebral disc.
- The superior costotransverse ligament joins the crest of the neck of the rib to the transverse process above.
- The intra-articular ligament joins the crest of the head of the rib to the intervertebral disc.

B. Transverse section.
- The vertebral body, transverse processes, superior articulating processes, and posterior elements of the articulating ribs have been transversely sectioned to visualize the joint surfaces and ligaments.
- The costotransverse ligament joins the posterior aspect of the neck of the rib to the adjacent transverse process.
- The lateral costotransverse ligament joins the nonarticulating part of the tubercle of the rib to the tip (apex) of the transverse process.

Transverse process

Anterior ramus
Posterior ramus } of thoracic nerve

Spinal ganglion

Superior costotransverse ligament

External intercostal

Innermost intercostal

Radiate ligament of head of rib

Subcostales

Internal intercostal membrane

Posterior intercostal [vein / artery]

Intercostal nerve

Anterior longitudinal ligament

Collateral branches of intercostal vessels and nerve

Rami communicantes

Anterior View

Sympathetic trunk

Splanchnic nerve

1.16   VERTEBRAL ENDS OF INTERNAL ASPECT OF INTERCOSTAL SPACES

- Portions of the innermost intercostal muscle that bridge two intercostal spaces are called subcostales muscles.
- The internal intercostal membrane, in the middle space, is continuous medially with the superior costotransverse ligament.
- Note the order of the structures in the most inferior space: posterior intercostal vein and artery, and intercostal nerve; note also their collateral branches.
- The anterior ramus crosses anterior to the superior costotransverse ligament; the posterior ramus is posterior to it.
- The intercostal nerves attach to the sympathetic trunk by rami communicantes; the splanchnic nerve is a visceral branch of the trunk.

Longissimus
Iliocostalis
Levatores costarum
7th rib
Angle of 8th rib
Posterior ramus of thoracic nerve
Posterior intercostal vessels and intercostal nerve,
posterior to transparent parietal pleura covering the lung
Collateral branch of intercostal nerve
Lateral costotransverse ligament
Innermost intercostal
Internal intercostal
External intercostal
Semispinalis
Tip of transverse process
Internal intercostal membrane
of the 10th intercostal space
Posterior View

| 1.17 | VERTEBRAL ENDS OF EXTERNAL ASPECT OF INFERIOR INTERCOSTAL SPACES |

- The iliocostalis and longissimus muscles have been removed, exposing the levatores costarum muscle. Of the five intercostal spaces shown, the superior two (6th and 7th) are intact. In the 8th and 10th spaces, varying portions of the external intercostal muscle have been removed to reveal the underlying internal intercostal membrane, which is continuous with the internal intercostal muscle. In the 9th space, the levatores costarum muscle has been removed to show the posterior intercostal vessels and intercostal nerve.
- The intercostal vessels and nerve disappear laterally between the internal and innermost intercostal muscles.
- The intercostal nerve is the most inferior of the neurovascular trio (posterior intercostal vein and artery and intercostal nerve) and the least sheltered in the intercostal groove; a collateral branch arises near the angle of the rib.
- **Thoracocentesis.** Sometimes it is necessary to insert a hypodermic needle through an intercostal space into the pleural cavity (see Fig. 1.27) to obtain a sample of pleural fluid or to remove blood or pus. To avoid damage to the intercostal nerve and vessels, the needle is inserted superior to the rib, high enough to avoid the collateral branches.

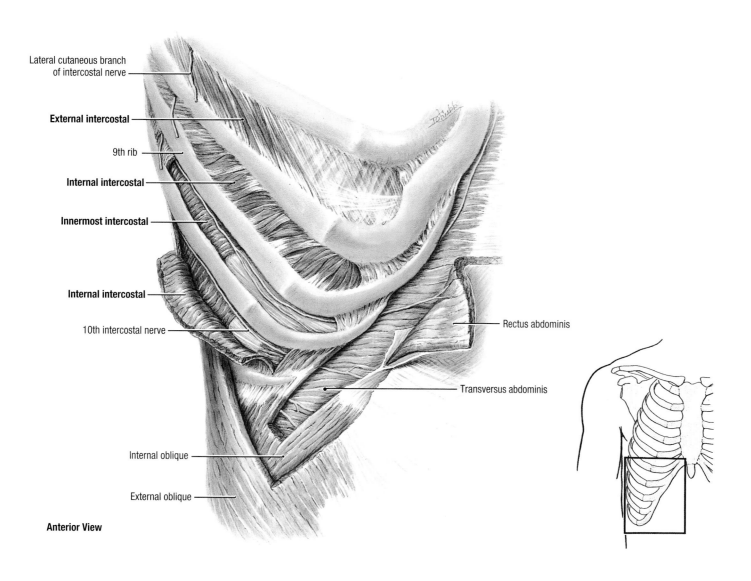

Lateral cutaneous branch of intercostal nerve

External intercostal

9th rib

Internal intercostal

Innermost intercostal

Internal intercostal

10th intercostal nerve

Rectus abdominis

Transversus abdominis

Internal oblique

External oblique

Anterior View

| 1.18 | ANTERIOR ENDS OF INFERIOR INTERCOSTAL SPACES |

- The fibers of the external intercostal and external oblique muscles run inferomedially.
- The internal intercostal and internal oblique muscles are in continuity at the ends of the 9th, 10th, and 11th intercostal spaces.
- The intercostal nerves lie deep to the internal intercostal muscle but superficial to the innermost intercostal muscle; anteriorly, these nerves lie superficial to the transversus thoracis or transversus abdominis muscles.
- Intercostal nerves run parallel to the ribs and costal cartilages; on reaching the abdominal wall, nerves T7 and T8 continue superiorly, T9 continues nearly horizontally, and T10 continues inferomedially toward the umbilicus. These nerves provide cutaneous innervation in overlapping segmental bands.

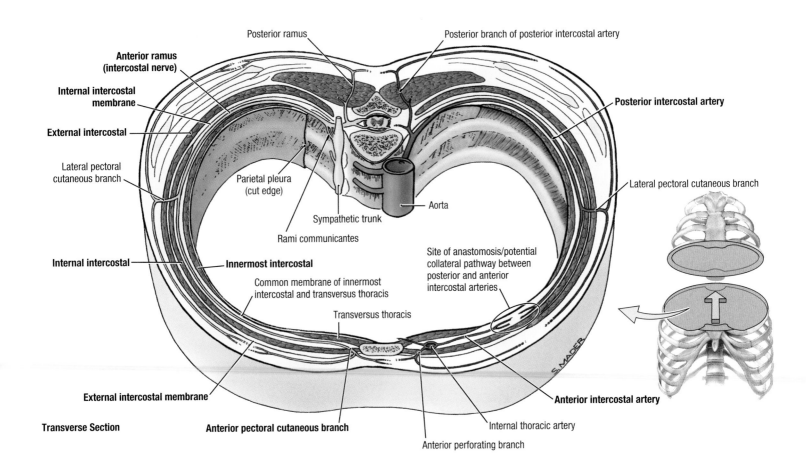

Posterior ramus

Posterior branch of posterior intercostal artery

Anterior ramus (intercostal nerve)

Internal intercostal membrane

External intercostal

Lateral pectoral cutaneous branch

Parietal pleura (cut edge)

Sympathetic trunk

Rami communicantes

Internal intercostal

Innermost intercostal

Common membrane of innermost intercostal and transversus thoracis

Transversus thoracis

Aorta

Posterior intercostal artery

Lateral pectoral cutaneous branch

Site of anastomosis/potential collateral pathway between posterior and anterior intercostal arteries

External intercostal membrane

Transverse Section

Anterior pectoral cutaneous branch

Anterior intercostal artery

Internal thoracic artery

Anterior perforating branch

1.19   CONTENTS OF INTERCOSTAL SPACE, TRANSVERSE SECTION

- The diagram is simplified by showing nerves on the right and arteries on the left.
- The three musculomembranous layers are the external intercostal muscle and membrane, internal intercostal muscle and membrane, and the innermost intercostal muscle, transversus thoracis muscle, and the membrane connecting them.
- The intercostal nerves are the anterior rami of spinal nerves T1 to T11; the anterior ramus of T12 is the subcostal nerve.
- Posterior intercostal arteries are branches of the aorta (the superior two spaces are supplied from the superior intercostal branch of the costocervical trunk); the anterior intercostal arteries are branches of the internal thoracic artery or its branch, the musculophrenic artery.
- The posterior rami innervate the deep back muscles and skin adjacent to the vertebral column.

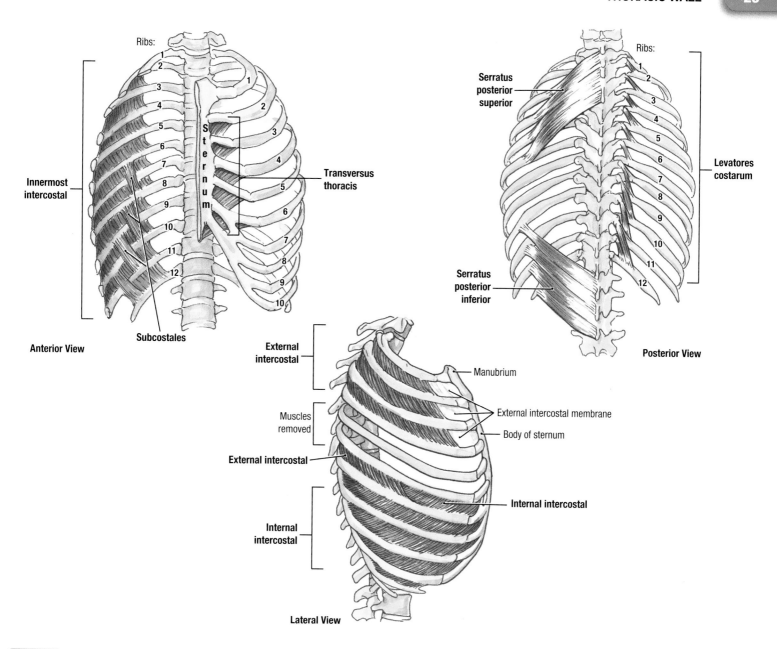

Ribs: 1, 2, 3, 4, 5, 6, 7, 8, 9, 10, 11, 12

Innermost intercostal

Sternum

Transversus thoracis

Subcostales

Anterior View

Serratus posterior superior

Levatores costarum

Serratus posterior inferior

Ribs: 1, 2, 3, 4, 5, 6, 7, 8, 9, 10, 11, 12

Posterior View

External intercostal

Manubrium

External intercostal membrane

Muscles removed

Body of sternum

External intercostal

Internal intercostal

Internal intercostal

Lateral View

1.20   MUSCLES OF THORACIC WALL

TABLE 1.1 MUSCLES OF THORACIC WALL

Muscle	Superior Attachment	Inferior Attachment	Innervation	Action[a]
External intercostal				Elevate ribs
Internal intercostal	Inferior border of ribs	Superior border of rib below		Depress ribs
Innermost intercostal			Intercostal nerve	Probably elevate ribs
Transversus thoracis	Posterior surface of lower sternum	Internal surface of costal cartilages 2–6		Depress ribs
Subcostales	Internal surface of lower ribs near their angles	Superior borders of 2nd or 3rd ribs below		
Levatores costarum	Transverse processes of C7–T11	Subjacent ribs between tubercle and angle	Posterior rami of C8–T11 nerves	Elevate ribs
Serratus posterior superior	Nuchal ligament, spinous processes of C7–T3	Superior borders of 2nd–4th ribs	Second to fifth intercostal nerves	
Serratus posterior inferior	Spinous processes of T11–L2	Inferior borders of 8th–12th ribs near their angles	Anterior rami of T9–T12 nerves	Depress ribs

[a]The tonus of all intercostal muscles keep intercostal spaces rigid, thereby preventing them from bulging out during expiration and from being drawn in during inspiration. Role of individual intercostal muscles and accessory muscles of respiration in moving the ribs is difficult to interpret despite many electromyographic studies. The role of the respiratory muscles depends on which accessory muscles are contracting at the same time.

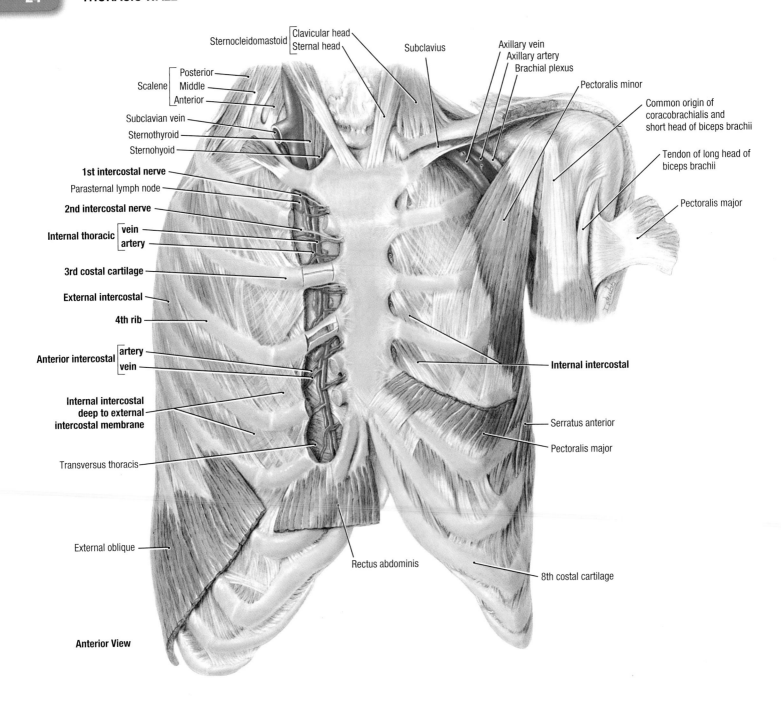

Sternocleidomastoid

Clavicular head
Sternal head

Subclavius

Axillary vein
Axillary artery
Brachial plexus

Pectoralis minor

Scalene — Posterior
Middle
Anterior

Subclavian vein

Sternothyroid

Sternohyoid

Common origin of
coracobrachialis and
short head of biceps brachii

1st intercostal nerve

Parasternal lymph node

2nd intercostal nerve

Internal thoracic — vein
artery

3rd costal cartilage

External intercostal

4th rib

Anterior intercostal — artery
vein

**Internal intercostal
deep to external
intercostal membrane**

Transversus thoracis

Tendon of long head of
biceps brachii

Pectoralis major

Internal intercostal

Serratus anterior

Pectoralis major

External oblique

Rectus abdominis

8th costal cartilage

Anterior View

1.21   EXTERNAL ASPECT OF THORACIC WALL

- H-shaped cuts were made through the perichondrium of the 3rd and 4th costal cartilages to shell out segments of cartilage. During surgery, retaining perichondrium promotes regrowth of removed cartilages.
- The internal thoracic (internal mammary) vessels run inferiorly deep to the costal cartilages and just lateral to the edge of the sternum, providing anterior intercostal branches.
- The parasternal lymph nodes (*green*) receive lymphatic vessels from the anterior parts of intercostal spaces, the costal pleura and diaphragm, and the medial part of the breast.

- The subclavian vessels are "sandwiched" between the 1st rib and clavicle and are "padded" by the subclavius.
- **Surgical access to thorax**. To gain access to the thoracic cavity for surgical procedures, the sternum is divided in the median plane (median sternotomy) and retracted (spread apart). After surgery, the halves of the sternum are held together with wire structures.

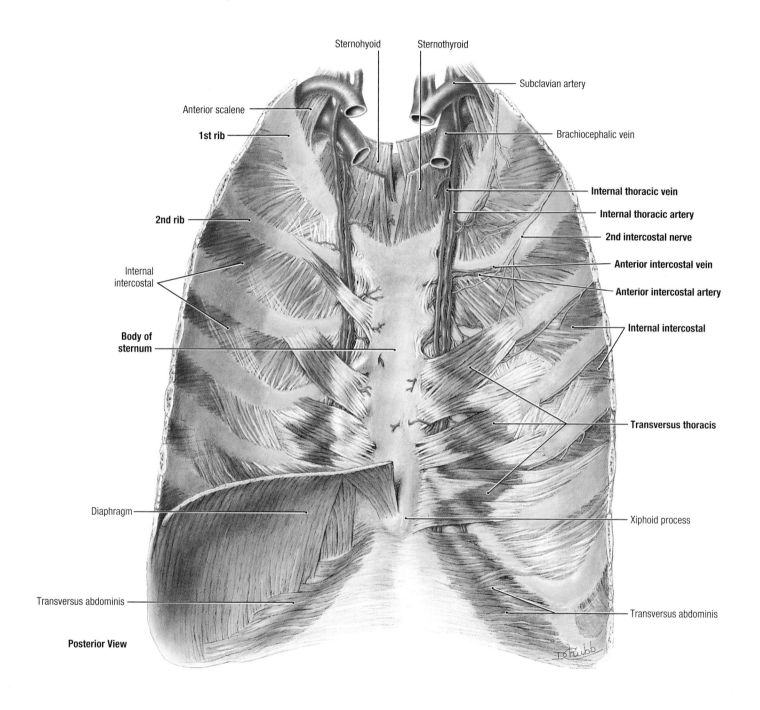

Sternohyoid

Sternothyroid

Subclavian artery

Anterior scalene

1st rib

Brachiocephalic vein

Internal thoracic vein

Internal thoracic artery

2nd rib

2nd intercostal nerve

Internal
intercostal

Anterior intercostal vein

Anterior intercostal artery

Internal intercostal

**Body of
sternum**

Transversus thoracis

Diaphragm

Xiphoid process

Transversus abdominis

Transversus abdominis

Posterior View

| 1.22 | INTERNAL ASPECT OF THE ANTERIOR THORACIC WALL |

- The inferior portions of the internal thoracic vessels are covered posteriorly by the transversus thoracis muscle; the superior portions are in contact with the parietal pleura (removed).
- The transversus thoracis muscle (superior to diaphragm) is continuous with the transversus abdominis muscle (inferior to diaphragm); these form the innermost layer of the three flat muscles of the thoracoabdominal wall.
- The internal thoracic (internal mammary) artery arises from the subclavian artery and is accompanied by two venae comitantes up to the 2nd costal cartilage in this specimen and, superior to this, by the single internal thoracic vein, which drains into the brachiocephalic vein.

Sternal head
Clavicular head] Sternocleidomastoid

Posterior
Scalene Middle
Anterior

1st rib

Clavicle

Manubrium of sternum

2nd rib

External intercostal

Serratus posterior superior

Interchondral part
of internal intercostal

Costal cartilage

Interosseous part
of internal intercostal

Central tendon of diaphragm

Rectus abdominis

Diaphragm

External oblique

Vertebral attachment
of diaphragm

Internal oblique

Costal
margin

Transversus abdominis

1.23   MUSCLES OF RESPIRATION

TABLE 1.2 MUSCLES OF RESPIRATION

		Inspiration	Expiration
Normal (Quiet)	Major	Diaphragm (Active Contraction)	Passive (Elastic) Recoil of Lungs and Thoracic Cage
	Minor	*Tonic contraction* of external intercostals and interchondral portion of internal intercostals to resist negative pressure	*Tonic contraction* of muscles of anterolateral abdominal walls (rectus abdominis, external and internal obliques, transversus abdominis) to antagonize diaphragm by maintaining intra-abdominal pressure
Active (Forced)		In addition to the above, *active contraction* of sternocleido-mastoid, descending (superior) trapezius, pectoralis minor, and scalenes, to elevate and fix upper rib cage	In addition to the above, *active contraction* of muscles of anterolateral abdominal wall (antagonizing diaphragm by increasing intra-abdominal pressure and by pulling inferiorly and fixing inferior costal margin): rectus abdominis, external and internal obliques, and transversus abdominis
		External intercostals, interchondral portion of internal intercostals, subcostales, levatores costarum, and serratus posterior superior[a] to elevate ribs	Internal intercostal (interosseous part) and serratus posterior inferior[a] to depress ribs

[a]Recent studies indicate that the serratus posterior superior and inferior muscles may serve primarily as organs of proprioception rather than motion.

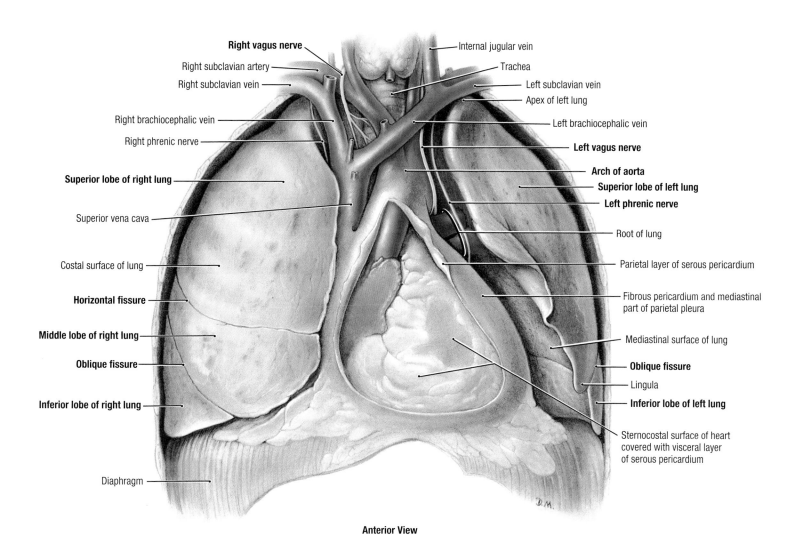

Right vagus nerve — Internal jugular vein
Right subclavian artery — Trachea
Right subclavian vein — Left subclavian vein
— Apex of left lung
Right brachiocephalic vein — Left brachiocephalic vein
Right phrenic nerve — **Left vagus nerve**
Superior lobe of right lung — **Arch of aorta**
Superior lobe of left lung
Left phrenic nerve
Superior vena cava — Root of lung
Costal surface of lung — Parietal layer of serous pericardium
Horizontal fissure — Fibrous pericardium and mediastinal part of parietal pleura
Middle lobe of right lung — Mediastinal surface of lung
Oblique fissure — **Oblique fissure**
— Lingula
Inferior lobe of right lung — **Inferior lobe of left lung**
Sternocostal surface of heart covered with visceral layer of serous pericardium
Diaphragm —

Anterior View

1.24   THORACIC CONTENTS IN SITU

- The fibrous pericardium, lined by the parietal layer of serous pericardium, is removed anteriorly to expose the heart and great vessels.
- The right lung has three lobes; the superior lobe is separated from the middle lobe by the horizontal fissure, and the middle lobe is separated from the inferior lobe by the oblique fissure. The left lung has two lobes, superior and inferior, separated by the oblique fissure.
- The anterior border of the left lung is reflected laterally to visualize the phrenic nerve passing anterior to the root of the lung and the vagus nerve lying anterior to the arch of the aorta and then passing posterior to the root of the lung.
- As the right vagus nerve passes anterior to the right subclavian artery, it gives rise to the recurrent branch and then divides to contribute fibers to the esophageal, cardiac, and pulmonary plexuses.

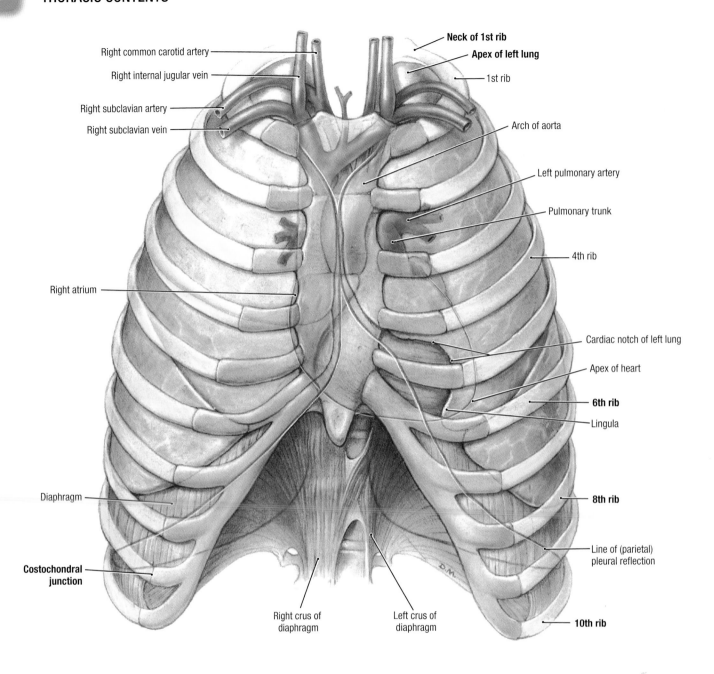

Right common carotid artery

Right internal jugular vein

Right subclavian artery

Right subclavian vein

Neck of 1st rib

Apex of left lung

1st rib

Arch of aorta

Left pulmonary artery

Pulmonary trunk

4th rib

Right atrium

Cardiac notch of left lung

Apex of heart

6th rib

Lingula

8th rib

Diaphragm

Line of (parietal) pleural reflection

Costochondral junction

Right crus of diaphragm

Left crus of diaphragm

10th rib

1.25   TOPOGRAPHY OF THE LUNGS AND MEDIASTINUM

- The mediastinum is located between the pleural cavities and is occupied by the heart and the tissues anterior, posterior, and superior to the heart.
- The apex of the lungs is at the level of the neck of the 1st rib, and the inferior border of the lungs is at the 6th rib in the left midclavicular line and the 8th rib at the lateral aspect of the bony thorax at the midaxillary line.
- The cardiac notch of the left lung and the corresponding deviation of the parietal pleura are away from the median plane toward the left side.
- The inferior reflection of parietal pleura is at the 8th costochondral junction in the midclavicular line, at the 10th rib in the midaxillary line.
- The apex of the heart is in the 5th intercostal space at the left midclavicular line.
- The right atrium forms the right border of the heart and extends just beyond the lateral margin of the sternum.
- The branches of the great vessels pass through the superior thoracic aperture.

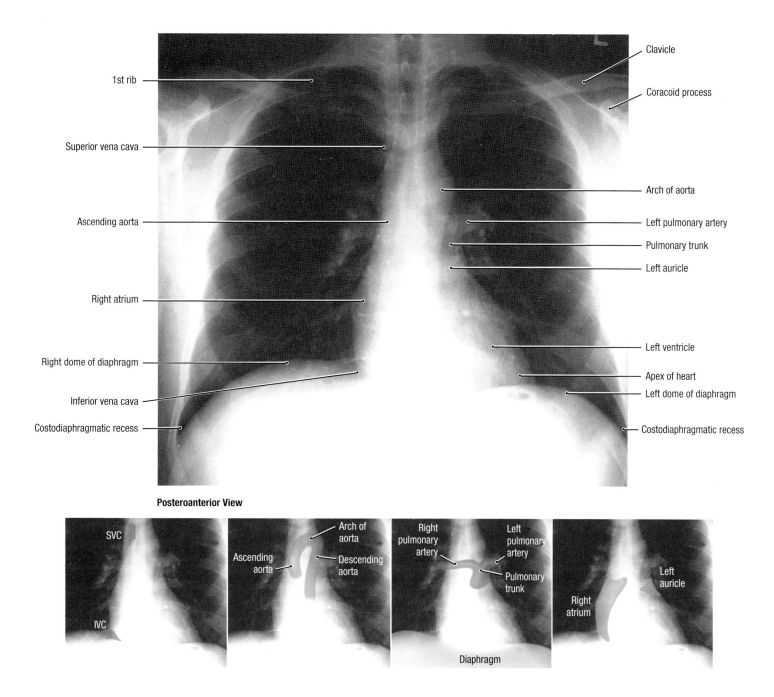

1st rib

Superior vena cava

Ascending aorta

Right atrium

Right dome of diaphragm

Inferior vena cava

Costodiaphragmatic recess

Clavicle

Coracoid process

Arch of aorta

Left pulmonary artery

Pulmonary trunk

Left auricle

Left ventricle

Apex of heart

Left dome of diaphragm

Costodiaphragmatic recess

Posteroanterior View

SVC

IVC

Ascending aorta

Arch of aorta

Descending aorta

Right pulmonary artery

Left pulmonary artery

Pulmonary trunk

Diaphragm

Right atrium

Left auricle

1.26   RADIOGRAPH OF CHEST

- The right dome of the diaphragm is higher than the left dome due primarily to the large underlying liver.
- The convex right mediastinal border of the heart is formed by the right atrium; above this, the superior vena cava and ascending aorta produce less convex borders.
- The left border of the mediastinal silhouette is formed by the arch of the aorta, pulmonary trunk, left auricle (normally not prominent), and left ventricle.

- Follow the 1st rib to where it curves laterally and then medially to cross inferior to the clavicle.
- Any structure in the mediastinum may contribute to **pathological widening of the mediastinal silhouette**, e.g., after trauma that produces hemorrhage into the mediastinum, malignant lymphoma (cancer of lymphatic tissue) that produces massive enlargement of mediastinal lymph nodes, or enlargement (hypertrophy) of the heart occurring with congestive heart failure.

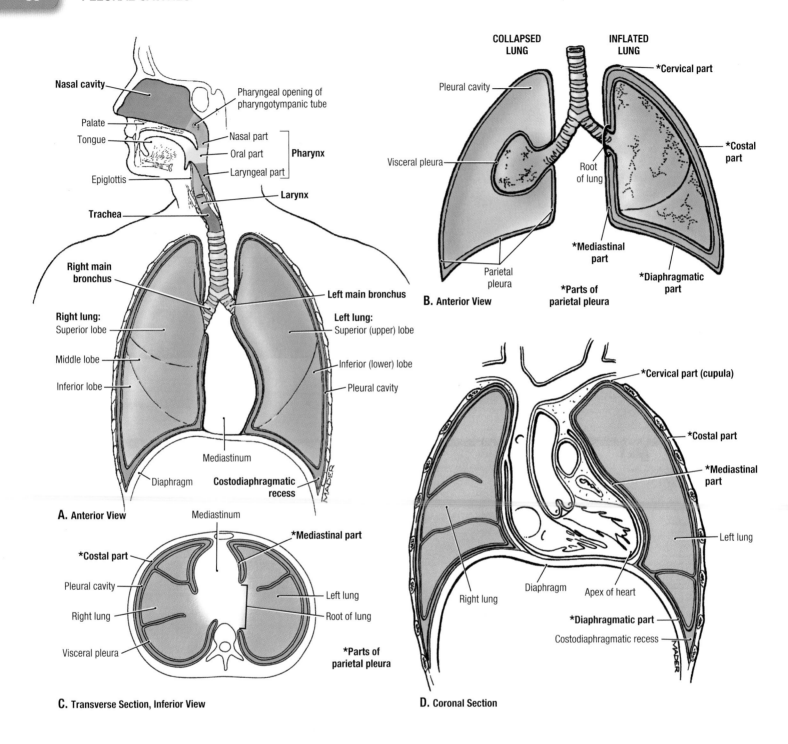

A. Anterior View

Nasal cavity
Pharyngeal opening of pharyngotympanic tube
Palate
Tongue
Nasal part
Oral part — **Pharynx**
Epiglottis
Laryngeal part
Larynx
Trachea
Right main bronchus
Left main bronchus
Right lung:
Superior lobe
Left lung:
Superior (upper) lobe
Middle lobe
Inferior (lower) lobe
Inferior lobe
Pleural cavity
Mediastinum
Diaphragm **Costodiaphragmatic recess**

B. Anterior View

COLLAPSED LUNG
INFLATED LUNG
*Cervical part
Pleural cavity
*Costal part
Visceral pleura
Root of lung
*Mediastinal part
Parietal pleura
*Diaphragmatic part
*Parts of parietal pleura

C. Transverse Section, Inferior View

Mediastinum
*Mediastinal part
*Costal part
Pleural cavity
Left lung
Right lung
Root of lung
Visceral pleura
*Parts of parietal pleura

D. Coronal Section

*Cervical part (cupula)
*Costal part
*Mediastinal part
Left lung
Diaphragm Apex of heart
Right lung
*Diaphragmatic part
Costodiaphragmatic recess

1.27 **RESPIRATORY SYSTEM**

A. Overview. **B.** Pleural cavity and pleura. **C.** Transverse section. **D.** Coronal section through heart and lungs.

- The lungs invaginate a continuous membranous pleural sac; the visceral (pulmonary) pleura covers the lungs, and the parietal pleura lines the thoracic cavity; the visceral and parietal pleurae are continuous around the root of the lung.
- The parietal pleura can be divided regionally into the costal, diaphragmatic, mediastinal, and cervical parts; note the costodiaphragmatic recess.

- The pleural cavity is a potential space between the visceral and parietal pleurae that contains a thin layer of fluid. If a sufficient amount of air enters the pleural cavity, the surface tension adhering visceral to parietal pleura (lung to thoracic wall) is broken, and the lung collapses (**atelectasis**) because of its inherent elasticity (elastic recoil). When a lung collapses, the pleural cavity—normally a potential space—becomes a real space (**B**) and may contain air (**pneumothorax**), blood (**hemothorax**), etc.

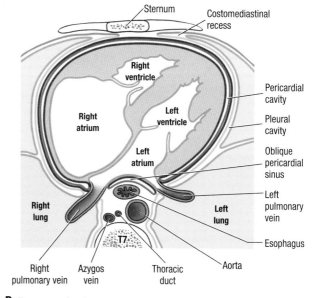

A. Median Section, Left Lateral View

B. Transverse Section, Inferior View

C. Median Section, Right Lateral View

D. Transverse Section, Inferior View

Key for C.

Pericardium
▬▬ Fibrous pericardium
Serous pericardium:
▬▬ Parietal layer of serous pericardium (lines fibrous pericardium)
▬▬ Visceral layer of serous pericardium (outermost layer of heart wall)
Thin film of fluid in pericardial cavity between visceral and parietal layers allows the heart to move freely within the pericardial sac.

Heart
▬▬ Epicardium (visceral layer of serous pericardium)
▬▬ Myocardium
▬▬ Endocardium

Pleurae
▬▬ Visceral pleura
Parietal pleura:
▬▬ Mediastinal
▬▬ Costal

1.28   **MEDIASTINUM AND PERICARDIUM**

A. and B. Subdivisions of mediastinum. **C. and D.** Layers of pericardium and heart.

  Cardiac tamponade (heart compression) is a potentially lethal condition because heart volume is increasingly compromised by the fluid outside the heart but inside the pericardial cavity. The heart is increasingly compressed and circulation fails. Blood in the pericardial cavity, **hemopericardium**, produces cardiac tamponade.

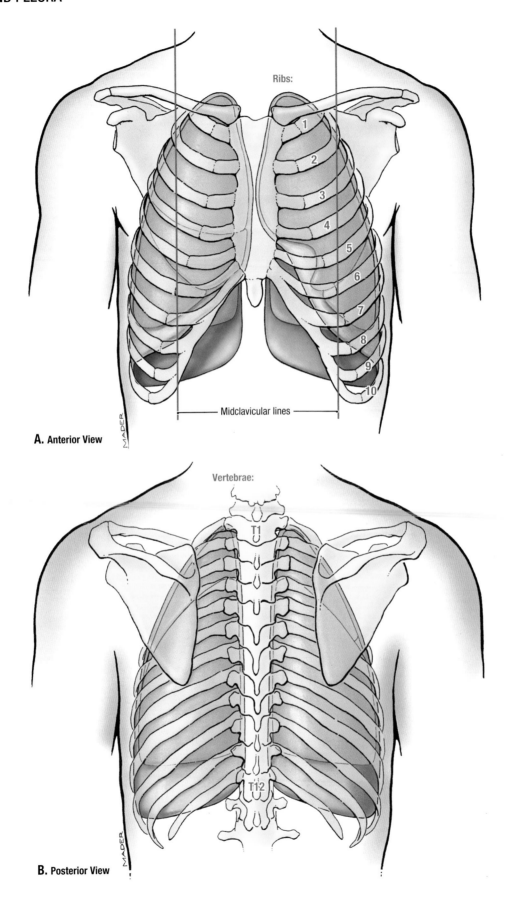

Ribs:

1
2
3
4
5
6
7
8
9
10

Midclavicular lines

A. Anterior View

Vertebrae:

T1

T12

B. Posterior View

1.29 EXTENT OF PARIETAL PLEURA AND LUNGS

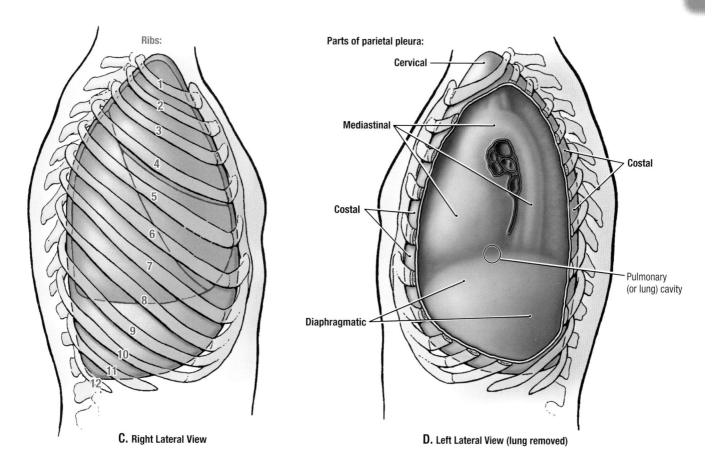

C. Right Lateral View

D. Left Lateral View (lung removed)

Ribs:

Parts of parietal pleura:

Cervical

Mediastinal

Costal

Costal

Pulmonary (or lung) cavity

Diaphragmatic

1.29 EXTENT OF PARIETAL PLEURA AND LUNGS (*CONTINUED*)

TABLE 1.3   SURFACE MARKINGS OF PARIETAL PLEURA (BLUE)

Level	Left Pleura	Right Pleura
Apex	About 4 cm superior to middle of clavicle	About 4 cm superior to middle of clavicle
4th costal cartilage	Midline (anteriorly)	Midline (anteriorly)
6th costal cartilage	Lateral margin of sternum	Midline (anteriorly)
8th costal cartilage	Midclavicular line	Midclavicular line
10th rib	Midaxillary line	Midaxillary line
11th rib	Line of inferior angle of scapula	Line of inferior angle of scapula
12th rib	Lateral border of erector spinae to T12 spinous process (slightly lower level than right pleura)	Lateral border of erector spinae to T12 spinous process

SURFACE MARKINGS OF LUNGS COVERED WITH VISCERAL PLEURA (PINK)

Level	Left Lung	Right Lung
Apex	About 4 cm superior to middle of clavicle	About 4 cm superior to middle of clavicle
2nd costal cartilage	Midline (anteriorly)	Midline (anteriorly)
4th costal cartilage	Lateral margin of sternum	Lateral margin of sternum
6th costal cartilage	Follows 4th costal cartilage, turns inferiorly to 6th costal cartilage in the midclavicular line (cardiac notch)	Midclavicular line
8th rib	Midaxillary line	Midaxillary line
10th rib	Line of inferior angle of scapula to T10 spinous process	Line of inferior angle of scapula to T10 spinous process

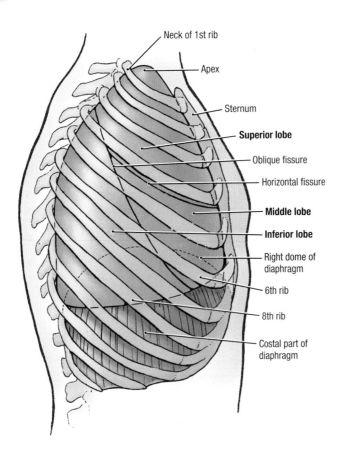

Neck of 1st rib

Apex

Sternum

Superior lobe

Oblique fissure

Horizontal fissure

Middle lobe

Inferior lobe

Right dome of diaphragm

6th rib

8th rib

Costal part of diaphragm

A. Lateral View

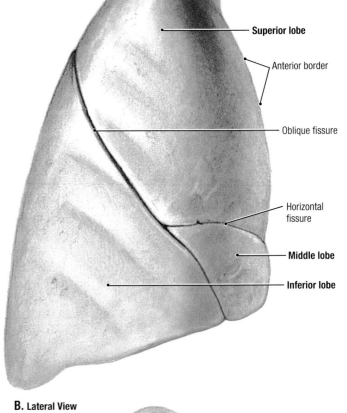

Apex

Superior lobe

Anterior border

Oblique fissure

Horizontal fissure

Middle lobe

Inferior lobe

B. Lateral View

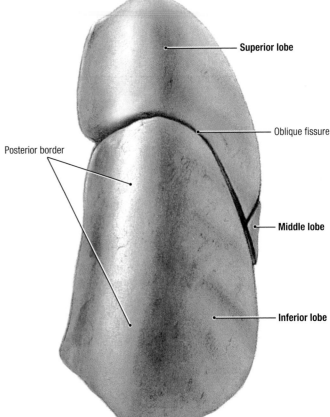

Superior lobe

Oblique fissure

Posterior border

Middle lobe

Inferior lobe

C. Posterior View

1.30 **RIGHT LUNG**

- The oblique and horizontal fissures divide the right lung into three lobes: superior, middle and inferior.
- The right lung is larger and heavier than the left, but is shorter and wider because the right dome of the diaphragm is higher and the heart bulges more to the left.
- Cadaveric lungs may be shrunken, firm and discolored, whereas healthy lungs in living people are normally soft, light and spongy.
- Each lung has an apex and base, three surfaces (costal, mediastinal and diaphragmatic) and three borders (anterior, inferior and posterior).

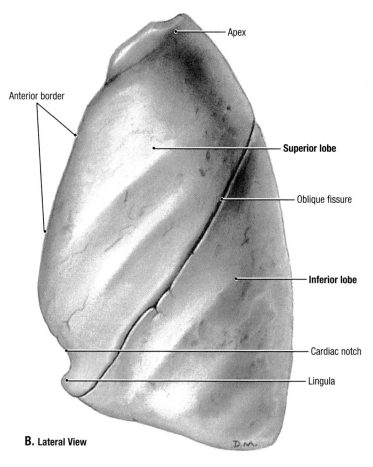

Apex

Anterior border

Superior lobe

Oblique fissure

Inferior lobe

Cardiac notch

Lingula

B. Lateral View

D.M.

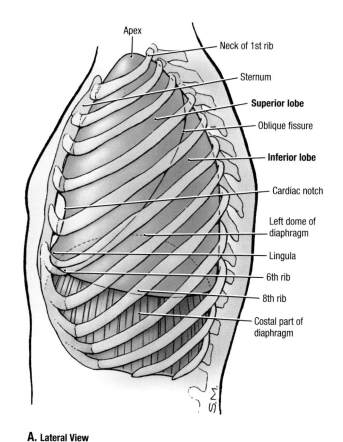

Apex

Neck of 1st rib

Sternum

Superior lobe

Oblique fissure

Inferior lobe

Cardiac notch

Left dome of
diaphragm

Lingula

6th rib

8th rib

Costal part of
diaphragm

A. Lateral View

S.M.

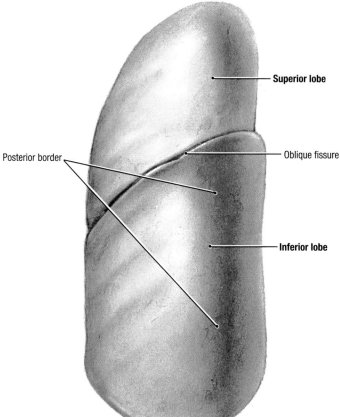

Superior lobe

Oblique fissure

Posterior border

Inferior lobe

C. Posterior View

1.31   LEFT LUNG

- The left lung has two lobes, superior and inferior, separated by the oblique fissure.
- The anterior border has a deep cardiac notch that indents the anteroinferior aspect of the superior lobe.
- The lingula, a tonguelike process of the superior lobe, extends below the cardiac notch and slides in and out of the costomediastinal recess during inspiration and expiration.
- The lungs of an embalmed cadaver usually retain impressions of structures that lie adjacent to them, such as the ribs and heart.

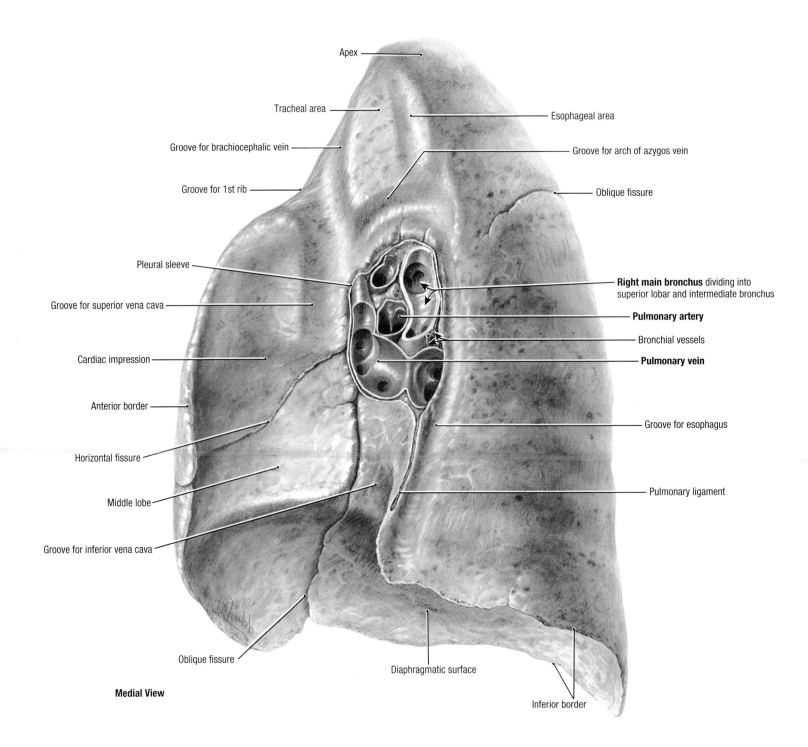

Apex

Tracheal area — — Esophageal area

Groove for brachiocephalic vein — — Groove for arch of azygos vein

Groove for 1st rib — — Oblique fissure

Pleural sleeve — — **Right main bronchus** dividing into superior lobar and intermediate bronchus

Groove for superior vena cava — — **Pulmonary artery**

— Bronchial vessels

Cardiac impression — — **Pulmonary vein**

Anterior border —

Horizontal fissure — — Groove for esophagus

Middle lobe — — Pulmonary ligament

Groove for inferior vena cava —

Oblique fissure — Diaphragmatic surface

Medial View

Inferior border

1.32 MEDIASTINAL (MEDIAL) SURFACE AND HILUM OF RIGHT LUNG

The embalmed lung shows impressions of the structures with which it comes into contact, clearly demarcated as surface features; the base is contoured by the domes of the diaphragm; the costal surface bears the impressions of the ribs; distended vessels leave their mark, but nerves do not. The oblique fissure is incomplete here.

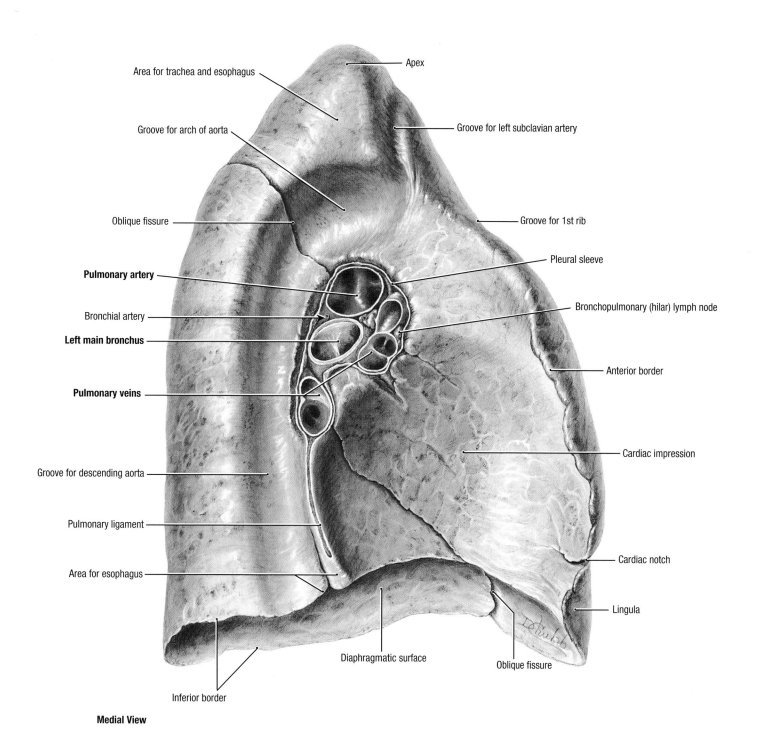

Apex

Area for trachea and esophagus

Groove for arch of aorta

Groove for left subclavian artery

Oblique fissure

Groove for 1st rib

Pleural sleeve

Pulmonary artery

Bronchopulmonary (hilar) lymph node

Bronchial artery

Left main bronchus

Anterior border

Pulmonary veins

Groove for descending aorta

Cardiac impression

Pulmonary ligament

Cardiac notch

Area for esophagus

Lingula

Diaphragmatic surface

Oblique fissure

Inferior border

Medial View

1.33   **MEDIASTINAL (MEDIAL) SURFACE AND HILUM OF LEFT LUNG**

Note the site of contact with esophagus, between the descending aorta and the inferior end of the pulmonary ligament. In the right and left roots, the artery is superior, the bronchus is posterior, one vein is anterior, and the other is inferior; in the right root, the bronchus to the superior lobe (also called the *eparterial bronchus*) is the most superior structure.

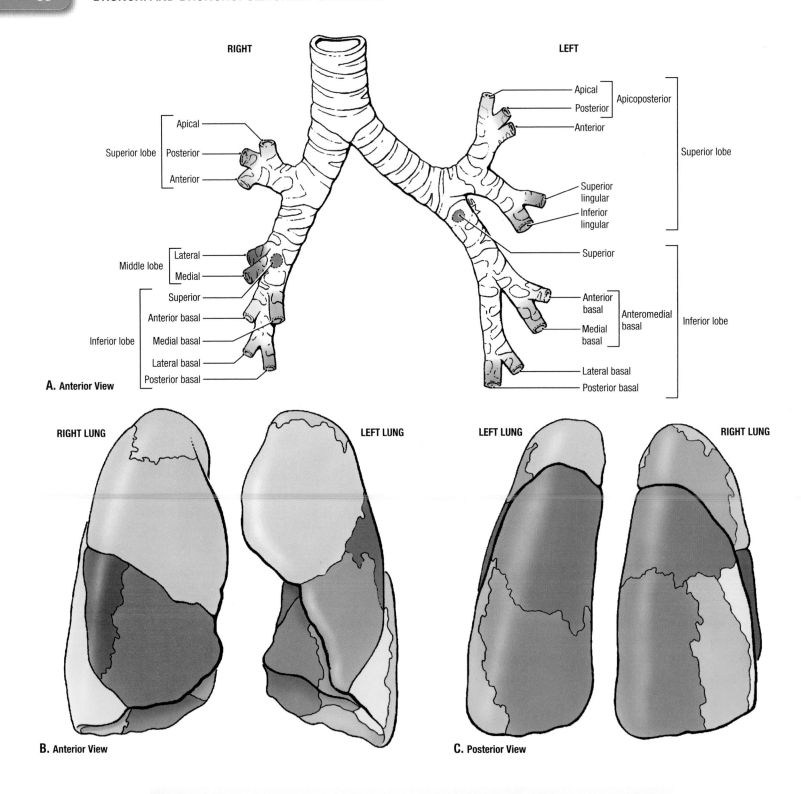

A. Anterior View

B. Anterior View

C. Posterior View

1.34 SEGMENTAL BRONCHI AND BRONCHOPULMONARY SEGMENTS

A. There are 10 tertiary or segmental bronchi on the right, and 8 on the left. Note that on the left, the apical and posterior bronchi arise from a single stem, as do the anterior basal and medial basal. **B.–F.** A broncho-pulmonary segment consists of a tertiary bronchus, pulmonary vein and artery, and the portion of lung they serve. These structures are surgically separable to allow segmental resection of the lung. To prepare these specimens, the tertiary bronchi of fresh lungs were isolated within the hilum and injected with latex of various colors. Minor variations in the branching of the bronchi result in variations in the surface patterns.

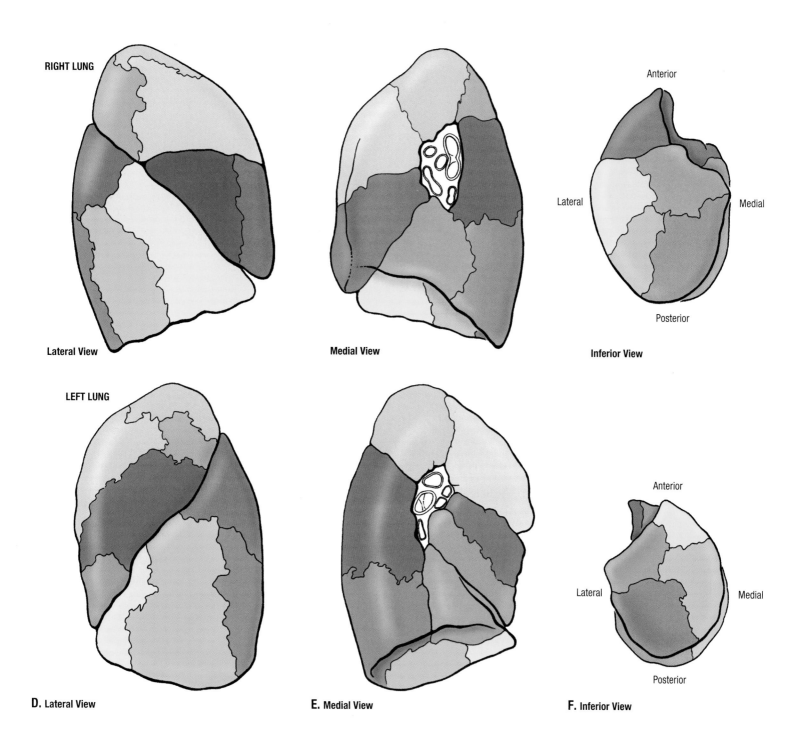

RIGHT LUNG

Lateral View

Medial View

Anterior

Lateral

Medial

Posterior

Inferior View

LEFT LUNG

D. Lateral View

E. Medial View

Anterior

Lateral

Medial

Posterior

F. Inferior View

1.34 SEGMENTAL BRONCHI AND BRONCHOPULMONARY SEGMENTS (*CONTINUED*)

Knowledge of the anatomy of the bronchopulmonary segments is essential for precise interpretations of diagnostic images of the lungs and for surgical resection (removal) of diseased segments. During the treatment of lung cancer, the surgeon may remove a whole lung (**pneumonectomy**), a lobe (**lobectomy**), or one or more bronchopulmonary segments (**segmentectomy**). Knowledge and understanding of the bronchopulmonary segments and their relationship to the bronchial tree are also essential for planning drainage and clearance techniques used in physical therapy for enhancing drainage from specific areas (e.g., in patients with pneumonia or cystic fibrosis).

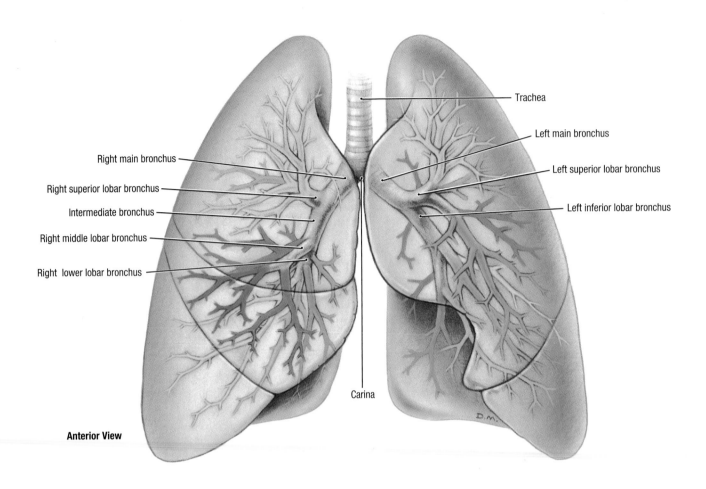

Trachea

Left main bronchus

Right main bronchus

Left superior lobar bronchus

Right superior lobar bronchus

Intermediate bronchus

Left inferior lobar bronchus

Right middle lobar bronchus

Right lower lobar bronchus

Carina

Anterior View

1.35 TRACHEA AND BRONCHI IN SITU

- The segmental (tertiary) bronchi are color coded.
- The trachea bifurcates into right and left main (primary) bronchi; the right main bronchus is shorter, wider, and more vertical than the left. Therefore, it is more likely that **aspirated foreign bodies** will enter and lodge in the right main bronchus or one of its descending branches.
- The right main bronchus gives off the right superior lobe bronchus (eparterial bronchus) before entering the hilum (hilus) of the lung; after entering the hilum, the continuing intermediate bronchus divides into the right middle and inferior lobar bronchi.
- The left main bronchus divides at the hilum into the left superior and left inferior lobar bronchi; the lobar bronchi further divide into segmental (tertiary) bronchi.

Segmental bronchi:

RIGHT LUNG	LEFT LUNG
Superior Lobe	**Superior Lobe**
☐ Apical	☐ Apical ⎫
☐ Posterior	☐ Posterior ⎬ Apicoposterior
☐ Anterior	☐ Anterior ⎭
	☐ Superior lingular
Middle Lobe	☐ Inferior lingular
☐ Lateral	
☐ Medial	**Inferior Lobe**
	☐ Superior
Inferior Lobe	☐ Anterior basal ⎫ Anteromedial
☐ Superior	☐ Medial basal ⎬ basal
☐ Anterior basal	☐ Lateral basal
☐ Medial basal	☐ Posterior basal
☐ Lateral basal	
☐ Posterior basal	

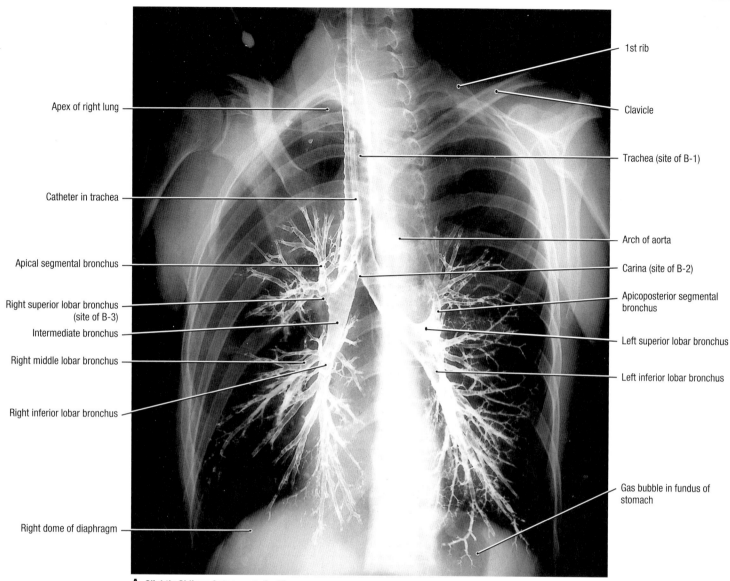

Apex of right lung

Catheter in trachea

Apical segmental bronchus

Right superior lobar bronchus
(site of B-3)

Intermediate bronchus

Right middle lobar bronchus

Right inferior lobar bronchus

Right dome of diaphragm

1st rib

Clavicle

Trachea (site of B-1)

Arch of aorta

Carina (site of B-2)

Apicoposterior segmental
bronchus

Left superior lobar bronchus

Left inferior lobar bronchus

Gas bubble in fundus of
stomach

A. Slightly Oblique Anteroposterior View

Carina

Carina

Right main
bronchus

Left main
bronchus

B-1. Entire trachea
and carina

B-2. Carina

Segmental
bronchi

B-3. Right upper lobe
bronchus

B. Bronchoscopic Views

1.36   **BRONCHOGRAMS**

A. Bronchogram of tracheobronchial tree. **B.** Bronchoscopy.

When examining the bronchi with a *bronchoscope*—an endoscope for inspecting the interior of the tracheobronchial tree for diagnostic purposes—one can observe a ridge, the *carina*, between the orifices of the main bronchi. If the tracheobronchial lymph nodes in the angle between the main bronchi are enlarged because cancer cells have metastasized from a bronchogenic carcinoma, for example, the carina is distorted, widened posteriorly, and immobile.

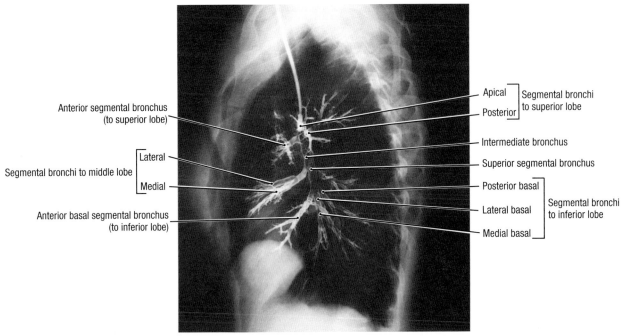

Anterior segmental bronchus (to superior lobe)

Segmental bronchi to middle lobe — Lateral / Medial

Anterior basal segmental bronchus (to inferior lobe)

Apical / Posterior — Segmental bronchi to superior lobe

Intermediate bronchus

Superior segmental bronchus

Posterior basal / Lateral basal / Medial basal — Segmental bronchi to inferior lobe

C. Right Segmental Bronchi, Right Lateral View

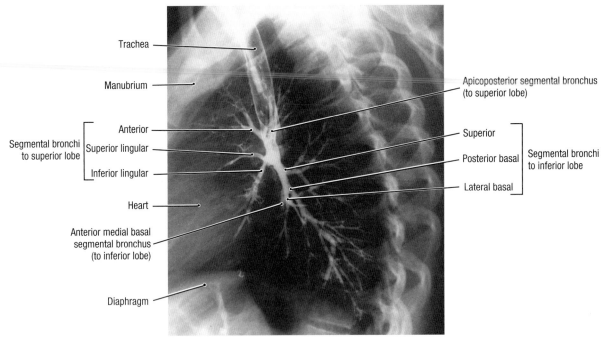

Trachea

Manubrium

Segmental bronchi to superior lobe — Anterior / Superior lingular / Inferior lingular

Heart

Anterior medial basal segmental bronchus (to inferior lobe)

Diaphragm

Apicoposterior segmental bronchus (to superior lobe)

Superior / Posterior basal / Lateral basal — Segmental bronchi to inferior lobe

D. Left Segmental Bronchi, Left Lateral View

1.36   BRONCHOGRAMS (*CONTINUED*)

C. Right lateral bronchogram, showing segmental bronchi. **D.** Left lateral bronchogram, showing segmental bronchi.

Medial views

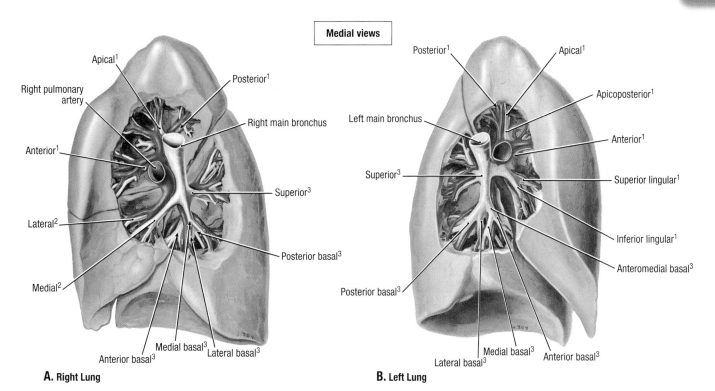

Apical[1]

Posterior[1]

Right pulmonary artery

Anterior[1]

Right main bronchus

Lateral[2]

Superior[3]

Medial[2]

Posterior basal[3]

Medial basal[3]   Lateral basal[3]

Anterior basal[3]

A. Right Lung

Posterior[1]

Apical[1]

Apicoposterior[1]

Left main bronchus

Anterior[1]

Superior[3]

Superior lingular[1]

Inferior lingular[1]

Anteromedial basal[3]

Posterior basal[3]

Medial basal[3]   Anterior basal[3]

Lateral basal[3]

B. Left Lung

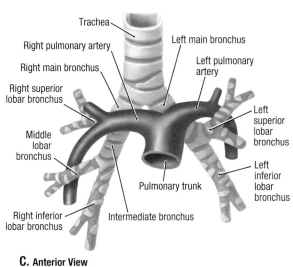

Trachea

Right pulmonary artery

Left main bronchus

Right main bronchus

Left pulmonary artery

Right superior lobar bronchus

Middle lobar bronchus

Left superior lobar bronchus

Left inferior lobar bronchus

Pulmonary trunk

Right inferior lobar bronchus

Intermediate bronchus

C. Anterior View

Aorta   Azygos vein

PT

SVC

LPA   RPA

LSPV

RSPV

LA

LIPV

RIPV

Posterior View

1.37

RELATIONSHIP OF BRONCHI AND PULMONARY ARTERIES

A. Right lung. **B.** Left lung. **C.** Pulmonary arteries and main bronchii. Superscripts indicate segmental bronchi to the [1]superior lobe, [2]middle lobe, and [3]inferior lobe. The pulmonary arteries of fresh lungs were filled with latex, the bronchi were inflated with air. The tissues surrounding the bronchi and vessels were removed.

Obstruction of a pulmonary artery by a blood clot (**pulmonary embolism**) results in partial or complete obstruction of blood flow to the lung.

1.38

3D VOLUME RECONSTRUCTION (3DVR) OF PULMONARY ARTERIES AND VEINS AND LEFT ATRIUM

The pulmonary trunk (*PT*) divides into a longer right pulmonary artery (*RPA*) and shorter left pulmonary artery (*LPA*); the left superior (*LSPV*) and inferior (*LIPV*) and the right superior (*RSPV*) and inferior (*RIPV*) pulmonary veins drain into the left atrium (*LA*). Superior vena cava (*SVC*).

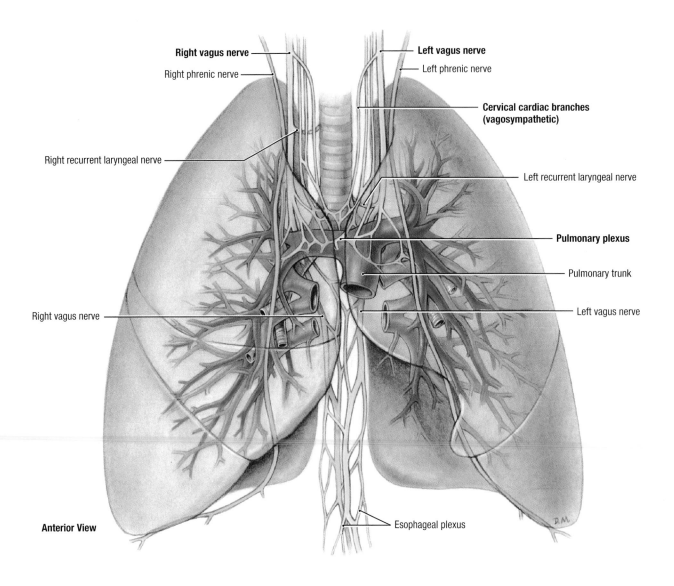

Right vagus nerve

Right phrenic nerve

Right recurrent laryngeal nerve

Right vagus nerve

Left vagus nerve

Left phrenic nerve

Cervical cardiac branches (vagosympathetic)

Left recurrent laryngeal nerve

Pulmonary plexus

Pulmonary trunk

Left vagus nerve

Esophageal plexus

Anterior View

1.39   INNERVATION OF LUNGS

- The pulmonary plexuses, located anterior and posterior to the roots of the lungs, receive sympathetic contributions from the right and left sympathetic trunks (2nd to 5th thoracic ganglia, not shown) and parasympathetic contributions from the right and left vagus nerves; cell bodies of postsynaptic parasympathetic neurons are in the pulmonary plexuses and along the branches of the pulmonary tree.
- The right and left vagus nerves continue inferiorly from the posterior pulmonary plexus to contribute fibers to the esophageal plexus.
- The phrenic nerves pass anterior to the root of the lung on their way to the diaphragm.
- **Pleurisy/pleuritis.** The visceral pleura is insensitive to pain. The autonomic nerves reach the visceral pleura in company with the bronchial vessels. The visceral pleura receives no nerves of general sensation.
- The parietal pleura is sensitive to pain because it is richly supplied by branches of the somatic intercostal and phrenic nerves. Irritation of the parietal pleura produces local pain and referred pain to the areas sharing innervation by the same segments of the spinal cord.

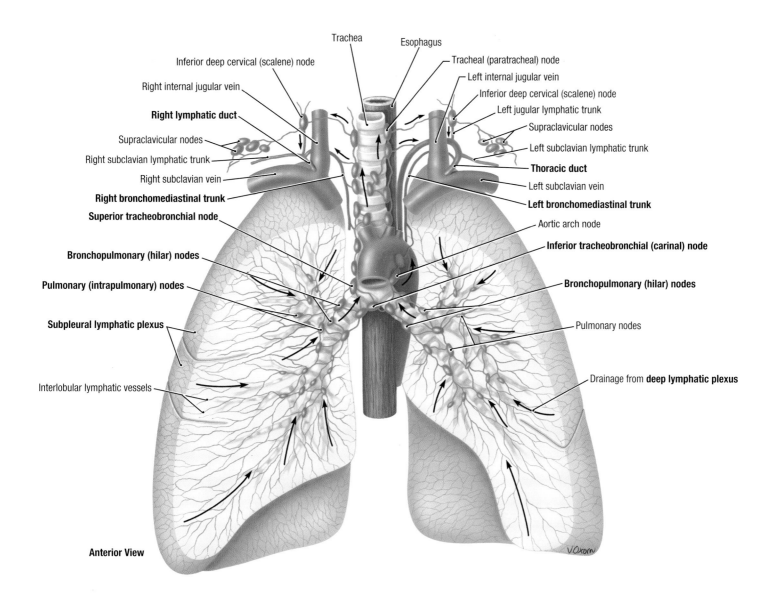

Trachea

Esophagus

Inferior deep cervical (scalene) node

Right internal jugular vein

Right lymphatic duct

Supraclavicular nodes

Right subclavian lymphatic trunk

Right subclavian vein

Right bronchomediastinal trunk

Superior tracheobronchial node

Bronchopulmonary (hilar) nodes

Pulmonary (intrapulmonary) nodes

Subpleural lymphatic plexus

Interlobular lymphatic vessels

Tracheal (paratracheal) node

Left internal jugular vein

Inferior deep cervical (scalene) node

Left jugular lymphatic trunk

Supraclavicular nodes

Left subclavian lymphatic trunk

Thoracic duct

Left subclavian vein

Left bronchomediastinal trunk

Aortic arch node

Inferior tracheobronchial (carinal) node

Bronchopulmonary (hilar) nodes

Pulmonary nodes

Drainage from **deep lymphatic plexus**

Anterior View

V.Oxom

1.40   **LYMPHATIC DRAINAGE OF LUNGS**

- Lymphatic vessels originate in the subpleural (superficial) and deep lymphatic plexuses.
- The subpleural lymphatic plexus is superficial, lying deep to the visceral pleura, and drains lymph from the surface of the lung to the bronchopulmonary (hilar) nodes.
- The deep lymphatic plexus is in the lung and follows the bronchi and pulmonary vessels to the pulmonary, and then bronchopulmonary, nodes located at the root of the lung.
- All lymph from the lungs enters the inferior (carinal) and superior tracheobronchial nodes and then continues to the right and left bronchomediastinal trunks to drain into the venous system via the right lymphatic and thoracic ducts; lymph from the left inferior lobe passes largely to the right side.
- Lymph from the parietal pleura drains into lymph nodes of the thoracic wall (Fig. 1.71).

Lung cancer (carcinoma) metastasizes early to the bronchopulmonary lymph nodes and subsequently to the other thoracic lymph nodes. Common sites of **hematogenous metastases** (spreading through the blood) of cancer cells from a bronchogenic carcinoma are the brain, bones, lungs, and suprarenal glands. Often the lymph nodes superior to the clavicle—the supraclavicular lymph nodes—are enlarged when lung (bronchogenic) carcinoma develops owing to metastasis of cancer cells from the tumor. Consequently, the supraclavicular nodes were once referred to as sentinel lymph nodes. More recently, the term sentinel lymph node has been applied to a node or nodes that first receive lymph drainage from a cancer-containing area, regardless of location, following injection of blue dye containing radioactive tracer (technetium-99).

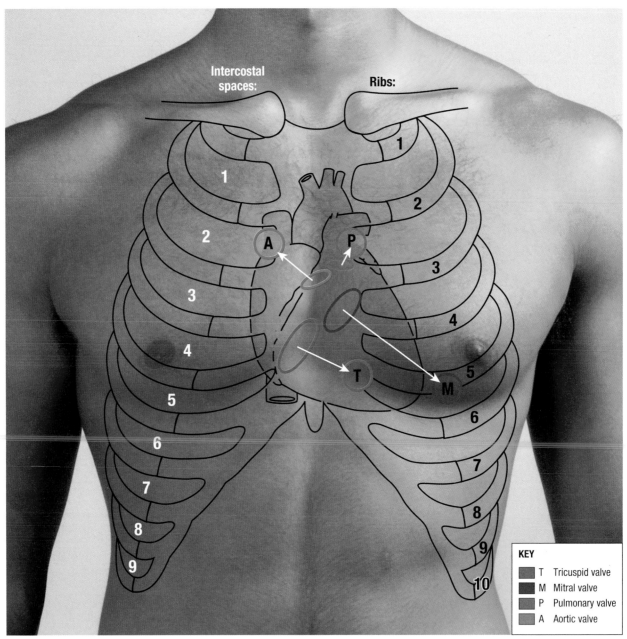

Anterior View

KEY

▮	T	Tricuspid valve
▮	M	Mitral valve
▮	P	Pulmonary valve
▮	A	Aortic valve

1.41   **SURFACE MARKINGS OF THE HEART, HEART VALVES, AND THEIR AUSCULTATION AREAS**

- The location of each heart valve in situ is indicated by a colored oval and the area of auscultation of the valve is indicated as a circle of the same color containing the first letter of the valve name.
- The auscultation areas are sites where the sounds of each of the heart's valves can be heard most distinctly through a stethoscope (*cardiac auscultation*).
- The aortic (*A*) and pulmonary (*P*) auscultation areas are in the 2nd intercostal space to the right and left of the sternal border; the tricuspid area (*T*) is near the left sternal border in the 5th or 6th intercostal space; the mitral valve (*M*) is heard best near the apex of the heart in the 5th intercostal space in the midclavicular line.

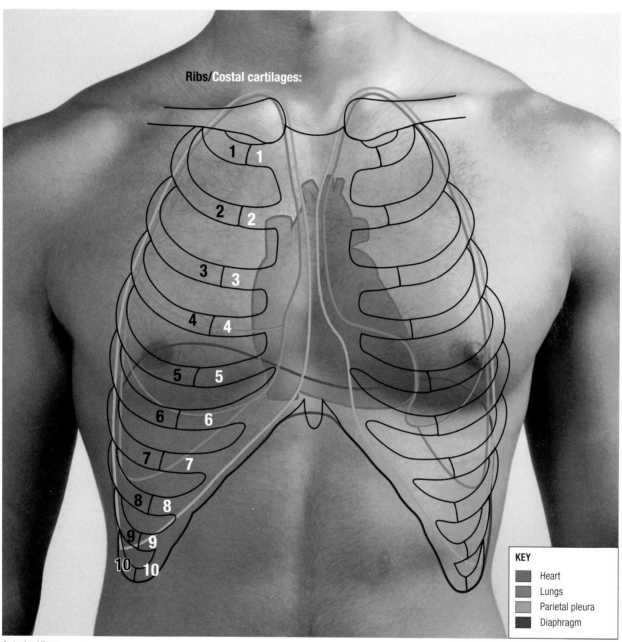

Ribs/Costal cartilages:

KEY
- Heart
- Lungs
- Parietal pleura
- Diaphragm

Anterior View

1.42   SURFACE MARKINGS OF THE HEART, LUNGS, AND DIAPHRAGM

- The superior border of the heart is represented by a slightly oblique line joining the 3rd costal cartilages; the convex right side of the heart projects lateral to the sternum and inferiorly, lying at the 6th or 7th costochondral junction; the inferior border of the heart is lying superior to the central tendon of the diaphragm and sloping slightly inferiorly to the apex at the 5th interspace at the midclavicular line.
- The right dome of the diaphragm is higher than the left because of the large size of the liver inferior to the dome; during expiration the right dome reaches as high as the 5th rib and the left dome ascends to the 5th intercostal space.
- The left pleural cavity is smaller than the right because of the projection of the heart to the left side.

Left common carotid artery

Brachiocephalic trunk

Right brachiocephalic vein

Superior vena cava (1)

Right pulmonary arteries

Ascending aorta (2)

Right pulmonary veins { Superior / Inferior

Right auricle (3)

Right coronary artery (4)

Anterior cardiac veins

Right border of heart ➤

Right atrium (5)

Coronary (atrioventricular) sulcus (6)

Right ventricle (7)

Right marginal artery

Small cardiac vein

Inferior vena cava (8)

Left subclavian artery

Left brachiocephalic vein

Arch of aorta

Ligamentum arteriosum

Left pulmonary artery

Pulmonary trunk (13)

Superior / Inferior] **Left pulmonary veins**

Left coronary artery

Left auricle (12)

Circumflex branch (11)

Great cardiac vein

Left marginal artery

Anterior interventricular artery (10)

Left ventricle (9)

Left border of heart ◀

Apex of heart

A. Anterior View

Inferior border of heart

B. Anterior View

From upper body

To head and upper limbs

KEY for C:
■ ■ Deoxygenated blood
■ ■ Oxygenated blood

Pulmonary trunk

To right lung via right pulmonary artery

SVC

From right lung via right pulmonary veins

Pulmonary valve

Right atrium

IVC

Aorta

To left lung via left pulmonary artery

Left atrium

From left lung via left pulmonary veins

Mitral valve

Left ventricle

Aortic valve

Right ventricle

Tricuspid valve

Descending aorta

C. Schematic Coronal Section

From lower trunk and limbs

To lower trunk and limbs

Left common carotid artery

Left subclavian artery

Brachiocephalic trunk

Arch of aorta

Arch of azygos vein

Ligamentum arteriosum

Superior vena cava

Left pulmonary artery (1)

Right pulmonary artery (15)

Left pulmonary veins — Superior (2) / Inferior (3)

Superior (14) / Inferior (13) — **Right pulmonary veins**

Left auricle (4)

Left atrium (5)

Right atrium (12)

Great cardiac vein

Coronary sinus (11)

Circumflex branch (6)

Oblique vein of left atrium

Inferior vena cava

Left posterior ventricular vein

Small cardiac vein

Right coronary artery (10)

Middle cardiac vein (9)

Posterior interventricular artery (8)

Left ventricle (7)

Right ventricle

Anterior interventricular artery

D. Posteroinferior View

E. Posteroinferior View

1.43   HEART AND GREAT VESSELS (*CONTINUED*)

A. Anatomical specimen
- The right border of the heart, formed by the right atrium, is slightly convex and almost in line with the superior vena cava.
- The inferior border is formed primarily by the right ventricle and part of the left ventricle.
- The left border is formed primarily by the left ventricle and part of the left auricle.

B. 3D volume reconstruction from MRI of heart and coronary vessels (living patient). Numbers refer to structures in **A.**

C. Circulation of blood through the heart

D. Anatomical specimen, posterior view.
- Most of the left atrium and left ventricle are visible in this posteroinferior view.
- The right and left pulmonary veins open into the left atrium.
- The arch of the aorta extends superiorly, posteriorly and to the left, in a nearly sagittal planes.

E. 3D volume reconstruction from MRI of heart and coronary vessels. Numbers refer to structures in **D.**

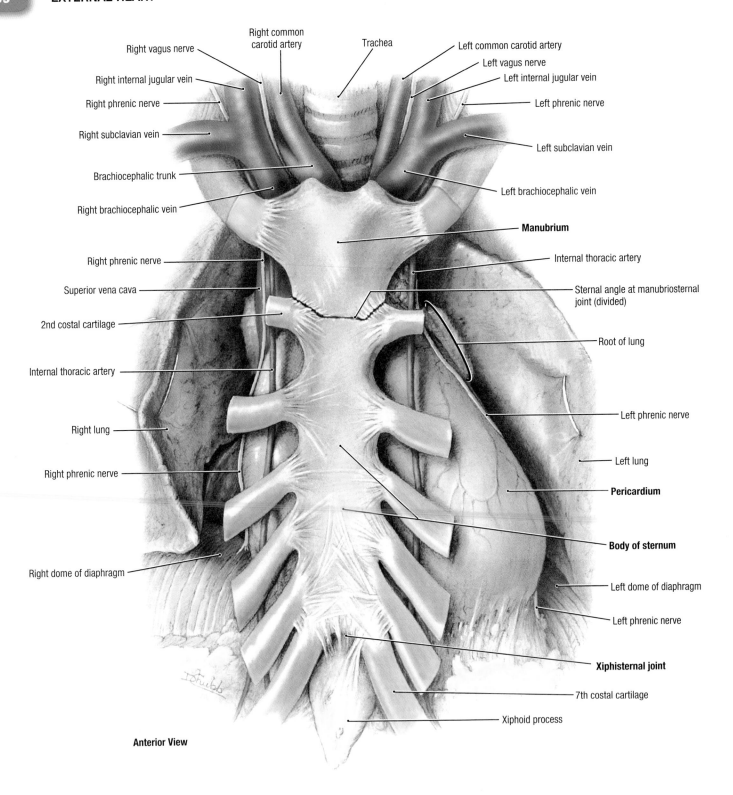

Right vagus nerve
Right common carotid artery
Trachea
Left common carotid artery
Left vagus nerve
Right internal jugular vein
Left internal jugular vein
Right phrenic nerve
Left phrenic nerve
Right subclavian vein
Left subclavian vein
Brachiocephalic trunk
Left brachiocephalic vein
Right brachiocephalic vein
Manubrium
Right phrenic nerve
Internal thoracic artery
Superior vena cava
Sternal angle at manubriosternal joint (divided)
2nd costal cartilage
Root of lung
Internal thoracic artery
Right lung
Left phrenic nerve
Right phrenic nerve
Left lung
Pericardium
Right dome of diaphragm
Body of sternum
Left dome of diaphragm
Left phrenic nerve
Xiphisternal joint
7th costal cartilage
Xiphoid process

Anterior View

1.44 PERICARDIUM IN RELATION TO STERNUM

- The pericardium lies posterior to the body of the sternum, extending from just superior to the sternal angle to the level of the xiphisternal joint; approximately two thirds lies to the left of the median plane.
- The heart lies between the sternum and the anterior mediastinum anteriorly and the vertebral column and the posterior mediastinum posteriorly.

In **cardiac compression**, the sternum is depressed 4 to 5 cm, forcing blood out of the heart and into the great vessels.

- Internal thoracic arteries arise from the subclavian arteries and descend posterior to the costal cartilages, running lateral to the sternum and anterior to the pleura.

Inferior cervical cardiac nerve (sympathetic: from cervicothoracic (stellate) ganglion)

Right brachiocephalic vein

Brachiocephalic trunk

Left common carotid artery

Left vagus nerve

Left subclavian artery

Inferior cervical cardiac branch (CN X)

Arch of aorta

Arch of azygos vein

Superior vena cava

Ascending aorta

Pericardium (cut edge)

Right superior pulmonary vein

Arrow traversing transverse pericardial sinus

Right auricle

Sulcus terminalis (terminal groove)

Right coronary artery

Right atrium

Anterior cardiac vein

Marginal artery

Pericardium (cut edge)

Diaphragm

Anterior View

Left recurrent laryngeal nerve

Ligamentum arteriosum

Left pulmonary artery

Anterior pulmonary plexus

Left superior pulmonary vein

Pulmonary trunk

Arrow traversing transverse pericardial sinus

Left auricle

Anterior interventricular branch of left coronary artery (left anterior descending branch)

Great cardiac vein

Right ventricle

Left ventricle

1.45   STERNOCOSTAL (ANTERIOR) SURFACE OF HEART AND GREAT VESSELS IN SITU

- The right ventricle forms most of the sternocostal surface.
- The entire right auricle and much of the right atrium are visible anteriorly, but only a small portion of the left auricle is visible; the auricles, like a closing claw, grasp the origins of the pulmonary trunk and ascending aorta from a posterior approach.
- The ligamentum arteriosum passes from the origin of the left pulmonary artery to the arch of the aorta.
- The right coronary artery courses in the anterior atrioventricular groove, and the anterior interventricular branch of the left coronary artery (anterior

descending branch) courses in or parallel to the anterior interventricular groove (see Fig. 1.43B).
- The left vagus nerve passes lateral to the arch of the aorta and then posterior to the root of the lung; the left recurrent laryngeal nerve passes inferior to the arch of the aorta posterior to the ligamentum arteriosum.
- The great cardiac vein ascends beside the anterior interventricular branch of the left coronary artery to drain into the coronary sinus posteriorly.

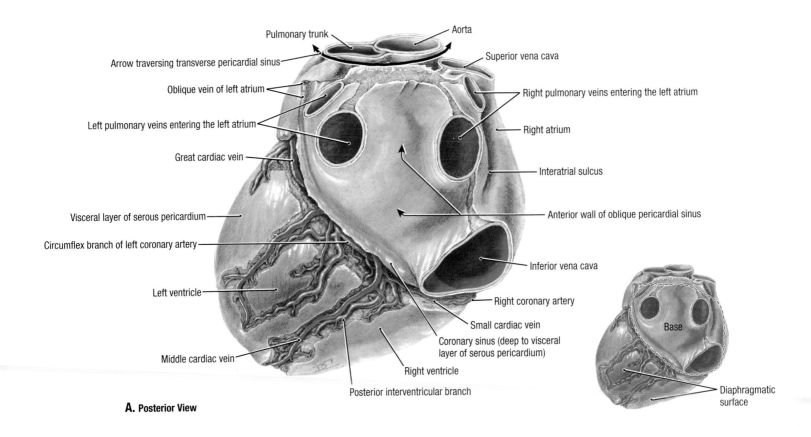

Pulmonary trunk

Aorta

Arrow traversing transverse pericardial sinus

Superior vena cava

Oblique vein of left atrium

Right pulmonary veins entering the left atrium

Left pulmonary veins entering the left atrium

Right atrium

Great cardiac vein

Interatrial sulcus

Visceral layer of serous pericardium

Anterior wall of oblique pericardial sinus

Circumflex branch of left coronary artery

Inferior vena cava

Left ventricle

Right coronary artery

Small cardiac vein

Middle cardiac vein

Coronary sinus (deep to visceral layer of serous pericardium)

Right ventricle

Posterior interventricular branch

Base

Diaphragmatic surface

A. Posterior View

| 1.46 | **HEART AND PERICARDIUM** |

- This heart **(A)** was removed from the interior of the pericardial sac **(B).**
- The entire base, or posterior surface, and part of the diaphragmatic or inferior surface of the heart are in view.
- The superior vena cava and larger inferior vena cava join the superior and inferior aspects of the right atrium.
- The left atrium forms the greater part of the base (posterior surface) of the heart.
- The left coronary artery in this specimen is dominant, since it supplies the posterior interventricular branch.
- Most branches of cardiac veins cross branches of the coronary arteries superficially.
- The visceral layer of serous pericardium (epicardium) covers the surface of the heart and reflects onto the great vessels; from around the great vessels, the serous pericardium reflects to line the internal aspect of the

fibrous pericardium as the parietal layer of serous pericardium. The fibrous pericardium and the parietal layer of serous pericardium form the pericardial sac that encases the heart.

- Note the cut edges of the reflections of serous pericardia around the arterial vessels (the pulmonary trunk and aorta) and venous vessels (the superior and inferior venae cavae and the pulmonary veins).
- **Surgical isolation of cardiac outflow.** The transverse pericardial sinus is especially important to cardiac surgeons. After the pericardial sac has been opened anteriorly, a finger can be passed through the transverse pericardial sinus posterior to the aorta and pulmonary trunk. By passing a surgical clamp or placing a ligature around these vessels, inserting the tubes of a coronary bypass machine, and then tightening the ligature, surgeons can stop or divert the circulation of blood in these large arteries while performing cardiac surgery.

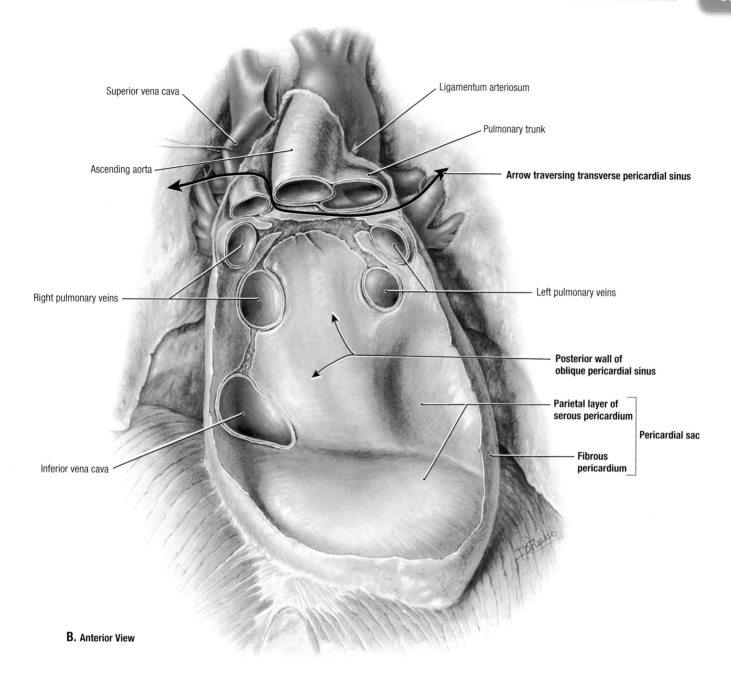

Superior vena cava

Ligamentum arteriosum

Pulmonary trunk

Ascending aorta

Arrow traversing transverse pericardial sinus

Right pulmonary veins

Left pulmonary veins

**Posterior wall of
oblique pericardial sinus**

**Parietal layer of
serous pericardium**

Pericardial sac

Inferior vena cava

**Fibrous
pericardium**

B. Anterior View

1.46   **HEART AND PERICARDIUM (*CONTINUED*)**

- Interior of pericardial sac. Eight vessels were severed to excise the heart: superior and inferior venae cavae, four pulmonary veins, and two pulmonary arteries.
- The oblique sinus is bounded anteriorly by the visceral layer of serous pericardium covering the left atrium **(A)**, posteriorly by the parietal layer of serous pericardium lining the fibrous pericardium, and superiorly and laterally by the reflection of serous pericardium around the four pulmonary veins and the superior and inferior venae cavae **(B)**.
- The transverse sinus is bounded anteriorly by the serous pericardium covering the posterior aspect of the pulmonary trunk and aorta, and posteriorly

by the visceral pericardium reflecting from the atria **(A)** inferiorly and the superior vena cava superiorly on the right.

- Blood in the pericardial cavity, **hemopericardium**, produces *cardiac tamponade*. Hemopericardium may result from perforation of a weakened area of the heart muscle owing to a previous **myocardial infarction (MI)** or heart attack, from bleeding into the pericardial cavity after cardiac operations, or from stab wounds. Heart volume is increasingly compromised and circulation fails.

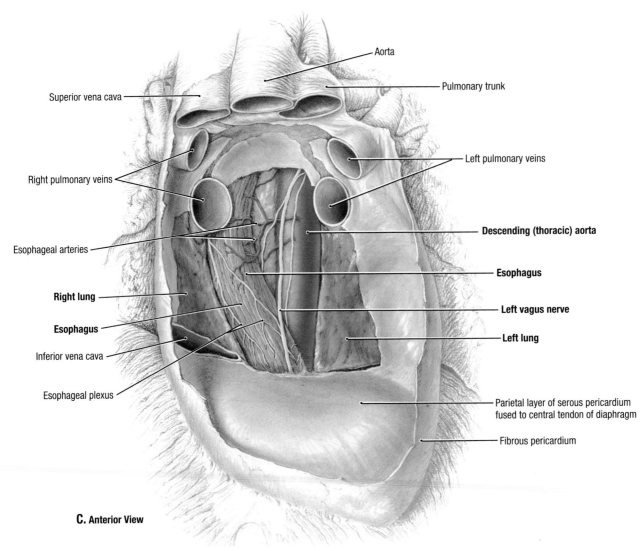

Aorta

Superior vena cava

Pulmonary trunk

Right pulmonary veins

Left pulmonary veins

Esophageal arteries

Descending (thoracic) aorta

Esophagus

Right lung

Left vagus nerve

Esophagus

Left lung

Inferior vena cava

Esophageal plexus

Parietal layer of serous pericardium fused to central tendon of diaphragm

Fibrous pericardium

C. Anterior View

1.46 **HEART AND PERICARDIUM** (*CONTINUED*)

C. Posterior relationships; dissection. The fibrous and parietal layers of serous pericardium have been removed from posterior and lateral to the oblique sinus. The esophagus in this specimen is deflected to the right; it usually lies in contact with the aorta, forming primary posterior relationships of the heart. **D.** Posterior relationships of heart. Axial computed tomographic (CT) scan at level of T9 vertebra. *1*, left lung; *2*, right lung; *3*, descending aorta; *4*, esophagus; *5*, inferior vena cava; *6*, right atrium; *7*, left ventricle.

D. Axial CT Scan, Inferior View

Ductus arteriosus

Ligamentum arteriosum
(obliterated ductus arteriosus)

Right lung

Left lung

Arrow traverses
patent foramen ovale
(white circle)

Ductus venosus

Liver

Umbilical vein

Umbilicus

Umbilical arteries

Placenta

Ligamentum venosum
(obliterated
ductus venosus)

Round ligament of
liver (obliterated
umbilical vein)

Umbilicus

Median umbilical ligament

Medial umbilical ligaments
(obliterated umbilical arteries)

* Location of oval fossa
(closed foramen ovale)
(white asterisk)

| | Oxygenated blood |
| | Deoxygenated blood |

	Oxygenated blood
	Partially oxygenated blood
	Deoxygenated blood

Heart and blood vessels:	**4** Inferior vena cava	**8** Pulmonary arteries	**12** Right ventricle
1 Abdominal aorta	**5** Left atrium	**9** Pulmonary trunk	**13** Superior vena cava
2 Arch of aorta	**6** Left ventricle	**10** Pulmonary veins	**14** Thoracic aorta
3 Ascending aorta	**7** Portal vein	**11** Right atrium	

1.47   PRE- AND POSTNATAL CIRCULATION

At birth two major changes take place: (1) pulmonary respiration starts and (2) after the umbilical cord is ligated, the umbilical arteries (except the most proximal part), umbilical vein, and ductus venosus are occluded and become ligaments.

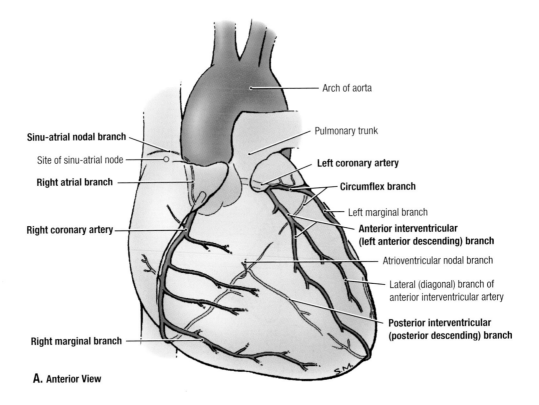

Arch of aorta

Pulmonary trunk

Sinu-atrial nodal branch

Site of sinu-atrial node

Right atrial branch

Left coronary artery

Circumflex branch

Left marginal branch

**Anterior interventricular
(left anterior descending) branch**

Right coronary artery

Atrioventricular nodal branch

Lateral (diagonal) branch of
anterior interventricular artery

**Posterior interventricular
(posterior descending) branch**

Right marginal branch

A. Anterior View

| **1.48** | **CORONARY ARTERIES** |

- In the most common pattern, the right coronary artery travels in the coronary sulcus to reach the posterior surface of the heart, where it anastomoses with the circumflex branch of the left coronary artery. Early in its course, it gives off the right atrial branch, which supplies the sinu-atrial (SA) node via its sinu-atrial nodal branch. Major branches are a marginal branch supplying much of the anterior wall of the right ventricle, an atrioventricular (AV) nodal branch given off near the posterior border of the interventricular septum, and a posterior interventricular branch in the interventricular groove that anastomoses with the anterior interventricular branch of the left coronary artery.

- The left coronary artery divides into a circumflex branch that passes posteriorly to anastomose with the right coronary artery on the posterior aspect of the heart and an anterior descending branch in the interventricular groove; the origin of the SA nodal branch is variable and may be a branch of the left coronary artery.

- The interventricular septum receives its blood supply from septal branches of the two interventricular (descending) branches: typically the anterior two thirds from the left coronary, and the posterior one third from the right (see Fig. 1.51A).

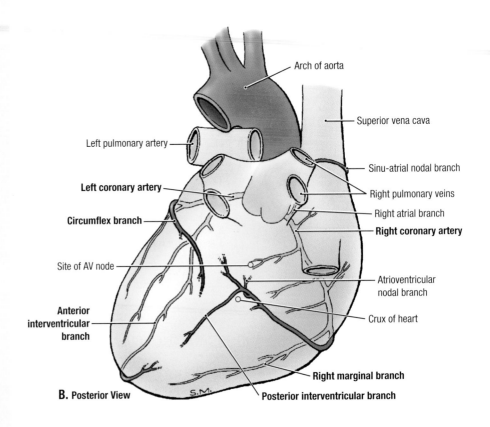

Arch of aorta

Superior vena cava

Left pulmonary artery

Sinu-atrial nodal branch

Left coronary artery

Right pulmonary veins

Circumflex branch

Right atrial branch

Right coronary artery

Site of AV node

Atrioventricular
nodal branch

**Anterior
interventricular
branch**

Crux of heart

Right marginal branch

B. Posterior View

Posterior interventricular branch

A. Anterior View

Oblique vein of
left atrium

Great cardiac
vein

Anterior
cardiac veins

Middle cardiac
vein

Coronary
sinus

Small
cardiac vein

B

Coronary artery

Cardiac vein

Fibrous pericardium

Parietal layer of serous pericardium

Pericardial cavity

Visceral layer of serous
pericardium (epicardium)

Subserous layer
(subendocardial fat)

Myocardium

Endocardium

Smallest cardiac veins
(venae cordis minimae)

C. Posteroinferior View

LA

RA

LV

RV

D. Posteroinferior View

Great cardiac
vein (4)

Left
marginal vein

Posterior vein
of left ventricle

Oblique vein
of left atrium

Coronary sinius (1)

Small cardiac vein (2)

Middle cardiac vein (3)

1.49 **CARDIAC VEINS**

A. Anterior aspect. **B.** Smallest cardiac veins. **C.** 3D volume reconstruction. Numbers refer to veins in **D.** *LA*, left atrium; *RA*, right atrium; *LV*, left ventricle; *RV*, right ventricle. **D.** Posteroinferior aspect.

The coronary sinus is the major venous drainage vessel of the heart; it is located posteriorly in the atrioventricular (coronary) groove and drains into the right atrium. The great, middle, and small cardiac veins; the oblique vein of the left atrium; and the posterior vein of the left ventricle are the principal vessels draining into the coronary sinus. The anterior cardiac veins drain directly into the right atrium. The smallest cardiac veins (venae cordis minimae) drain the myocardium directly into the atria and ventricles **(B).** The cardiac veins accompany the coronary arteries and their branches.

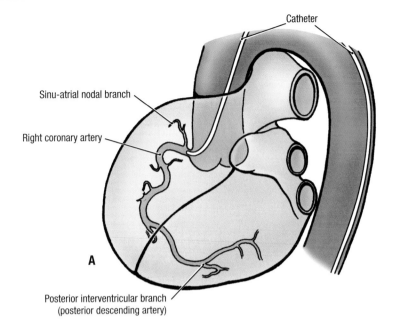

Catheter

Sinu-atrial nodal branch

Right coronary artery

A

Posterior interventricular branch
(posterior descending artery)

B. Left Anterior Oblique View

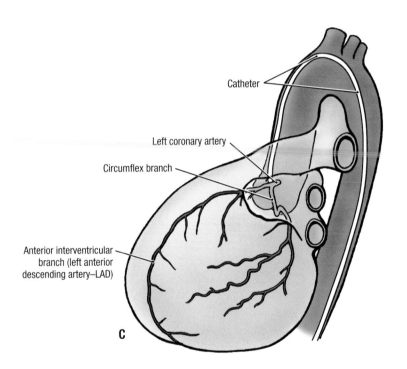

Catheter

Left coronary artery

Circumflex branch

Anterior interventricular
branch (left anterior
descending artery–LAD)

C

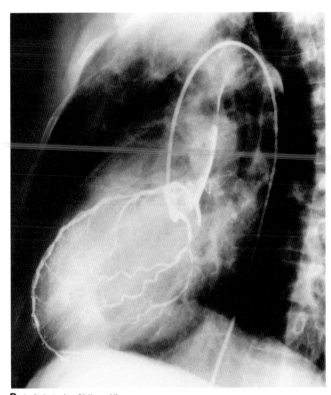

D. Left Anterior Oblique View

1.50   CORONARY ARTERIOGRAMS WITH ORIENTATION DRAWINGS

Right (**A** and **B**) and left (**C** and **D**) coronary arteriograms.

Coronary artery disease (CAD), one of the leading causes of death, results in a reduced blood supply to the vital myocardial tissue. The three most common sites of coronary artery occlusion and the approximate percentage of occlusions involving each artery are the (1) anterior interventricular (clinically referred to as LAD) branch of the left coronary artery (LCA) (40% to 50%); (2) right coronary artery (RCA), (30% to 40%); (3) circumflex branch of the LCA (15% to 20%).

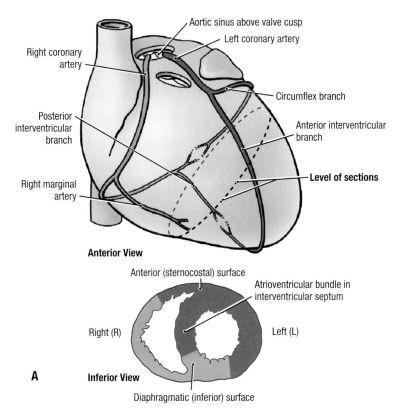

Aortic sinus above valve cusp

Left coronary artery

Right coronary artery

Circumflex branch

Posterior interventricular branch

Anterior interventricular branch

Right marginal artery

Level of sections

Anterior View

Anterior (sternocostal) surface

Atrioventricular bundle in interventricular septum

Right (R)

Left (L)

Diaphragmatic (inferior) surface

A **Inferior View**

A. and B. Most common pattern (67%). Right coronary artery is dominant, giving rise to the posterior interventricular branch.

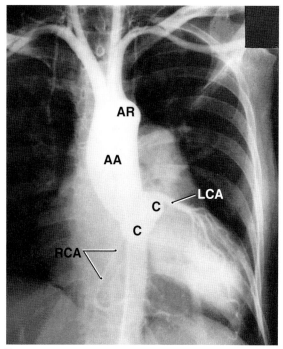

B. Coronary Angiogram, Anteroposterior View

KEY for B:		
AA	Ascending aorta	LCA	Left coronary artery
AR	Arch of aorta	RCA	Right coronary artery
C	Cusp of aortic valve		

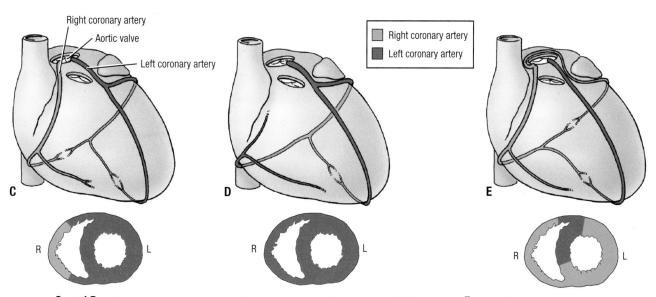

Right coronary artery

Aortic valve

Left coronary artery

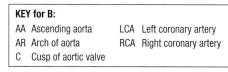
Right coronary artery
Left coronary artery

C R L

D R L

E R L

C. and D. Left coronary artery gives rise to the posterior interventricular branch (15%).

E. Circumflex branch emerging from right coronary sinus.

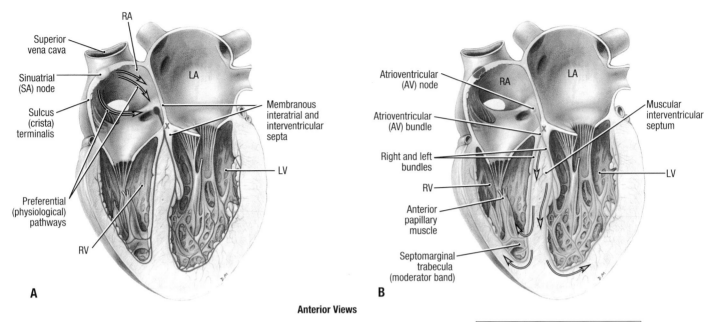

RA

Superior vena cava

Sinuatrial (SA) node

Sulcus (crista) terminalis

Preferential (physiological) pathways

RV

LA

Membranous interatrial and interventricular septa

LV

RV

A

Atrioventricular (AV) node

Atrioventricular (AV) bundle

Right and left bundles

RV

Anterior papillary muscle

Septomarginal trabecula (moderator band)

RA

LA

Muscular interventricular septum

LV

B

Anterior Views

RV	Right ventricle	LV	Left ventricle
	x Crux of heart		
RA	Right atrium	LA	Left atrium

1.52 CONDUCTION SYSTEM OF HEART, CORONAL SECTION

A. Impulses (*arrows*) initiated at the sinu-atrial node. **B.** Atrioventricular (AV) node, AV bundle, and bundle branches. **C.** Echocardiogram, apical four-chamber view.

- The sinu-atrial (SA) node in the wall of the right atrium near the superior end of the sulcus terminalis (internally crista terminalis) extends over the opening of the superior vena cava. The SA node is the "pacemaker" of the heart because it initiates muscle contraction and determines the heart rate. It is supplied by the sinuatrial nodal artery, usually a branch of the right atrial branch of the right coronary artery, but it may arise from the left coronary artery.
- Contraction spreads through the atrial wall (myogenic induction) until it reaches the atrioventricular (AV) node in the interatrial septum superomedial to the opening of the coronary sinus. The AV node is supplied by the atrioventricular nodal artery, usually arising from the right coronary artery posteriorly at the inferior margin of the interatrial septum.
- The AV bundle, usually supplied by the right coronary artery, passes from the AV node in the membranous part of the interventricular septum, dividing into right and left bundle branches on either side of the muscular part of the interventricular septum.
- The right bundle branch travels inferiorly in the interventricular septum to the anterior wall of the ventricle, with part passing via the septomarginal trabecula to the anterior papillary muscle; excitation spreads throughout the right ventricular wall through a network of subendocardial branches from the right bundle (Purkinje fibers).
- The left bundle branch lies beneath the endocardium on the left side of the interventricular septum and branches to enter the anterior and posterior papillary muscles and the wall of the left ventricle; further branching into a plexus of subendocardial branches (Purkinje fibers) allows the impulses to be conveyed throughout the left ventricular wall. The bundle branches are mostly supplied by the left coronary artery except the posterior limb of the left bundle branch, which is supplied by both coronary arteries.
- **Damage to the cardiac conduction system** (often by compromised blood supply as in coronary artery disease) leads to disturbances of muscle contraction. Damage to the AV node results in "heart block" because the atrial excitation wave does not reach the ventricles, which begin to contract independently at their own slower rate. Damage to one of the bundle branches results in "bundle branch block," in which excitation goes down the unaffected branch to cause systole of that ventricle; the impulse then spreads to the other ventricle, producing later asynchronous contraction.

LV

RV

RA

LA

C

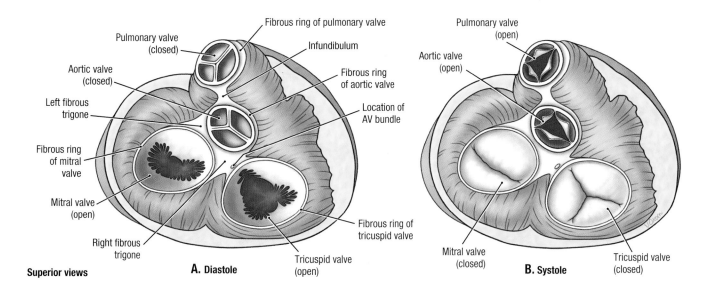

Superior views   **A. Diastole**   **B. Systole**

C.

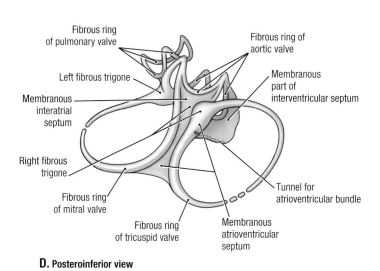

D. Posteroinferior view

1.53   CARDIAC CYCLE AND CARDIAC SKELETON

A. Ventricular diastole. **B.** Ventricular systole. **C.** Correlation of ventricular pressure, electrocardiogram (ECG), and heart sounds. The cardiac cycle describes the complete movement of the heart or heartbeat and includes the period from the beginning of one heartbeat to the beginning of the next one. The cycle consists of diastole (ventricular relaxation and filling) and systole (ventricular contraction and emptying). The right heart is the pump for the pulmonary circuit; the left heart is the pump for the systemic circuit. (see Fig. 1.43C). **D.** Cardiac skeleton. The fibrous framework of dense collagen forms four fibrous rings, which provide attachment for the leaflets and cusps of the valves, and two fibrous trigones that connect the rings, and the membranous parts of the interatrial and interventricular septa. The fibrous skeleton keeps the orifices of the valves patent and separates the myenterically conducted impulses of the atria.

Disorders involving the valves of the heart disturb the pumping efficiency of the heart. **Valvular heart disease** produces either stenosis (narrowing) or insufficiency. **Valvular stenosis** is the failure of a valve to open fully, slowing blood flow from a chamber. **Valvular insufficiency**, or regurgitation, is the failure of the valve to close completely, usually owing to nodule formation on (or scarring and contraction of) the cusps so that the edges do not meet or align. This allows a variable amount of blood (depending on the severity) to flow back into the chamber it was just ejected from. Both stenosis and insufficiency result in an increased workload for the heart. Because valvular diseases are mechanical problems, damaged or defective cardiac valves are often replaced surgically in a procedure called **valvuloplasty**.

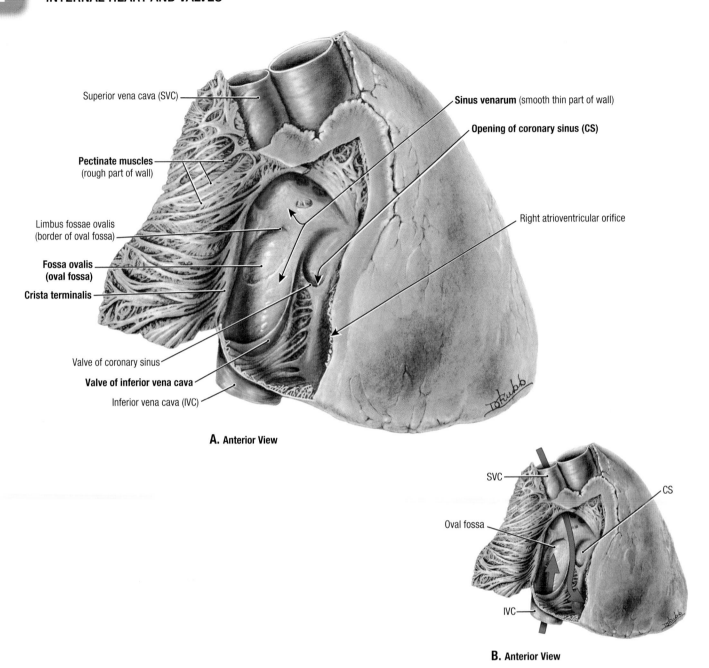

Superior vena cava (SVC)

Pectinate muscles
(rough part of wall)

Limbus fossae ovalis
(border of oval fossa)

Fossa ovalis
(oval fossa)

Crista terminalis

Valve of coronary sinus

Valve of inferior vena cava

Inferior vena cava (IVC)

Sinus venarum (smooth thin part of wall)

Opening of coronary sinus (CS)

Right atrioventricular orifice

A. Anterior View

SVC

Oval fossa

CS

IVC

B. Anterior View

<table>
<tr><td>**1.54**</td><td>**RIGHT ATRIUM**</td></tr>
</table>

A. Interior of right atrium. The anterior wall of the right atrium is reflected. **B.** Blood flow into atrium from the superior and inferior vena cavae.

- The smooth part of the atrial wall is formed by the absorption of the right horn of the sinus venosus, and the rough part is formed from the primitive atrium.
- Crista terminalis, the valve of the inferior vena cava, and the valve of the coronary sinus separate the smooth part from the rough part.
- The pectinate muscle passes anteriorly from the crista terminalis; the crista underlies the sulcus terminalis (not shown), a groove visible externally on the posterolateral surface of the right atrium between the superior and inferior venae cavae.
- The superior and inferior venae cavae and the coronary sinus open onto the smooth part of the right atrium; the anterior cardiac veins and venae cordis minimae (not visible) also open into the atrium.

- The floor of the fossa is the remnant of the fetal septum primum; the crescent-shaped ridge (limbus fossae ovalis) partially surrounding the fossa is the remnant of the septum secundum.
- In **B,** the inflow from the superior vena cava is directed toward the tricuspid orifice, whereas blood from the inferior vena cava is directed toward the fossa ovalis.
- Congenital anomalies of the interatrial septum, most often incomplete closure of the oval foramen (patent foramen ovale), are **atrial septal defects (ASDs)**. A probe-size patency is present in the superior part of the oval fossa in 15% to 25% of adults (Moore and Persaud, 2008). These small openings, by themselves, cause no hemodynamic abnormalities. Large ASDs allow oxygenated blood from the lungs to be shunted from the left atrium through the ASD into the right atrium, causing enlargement of the right atrium and ventricle and dilation of the pulmonary trunk.

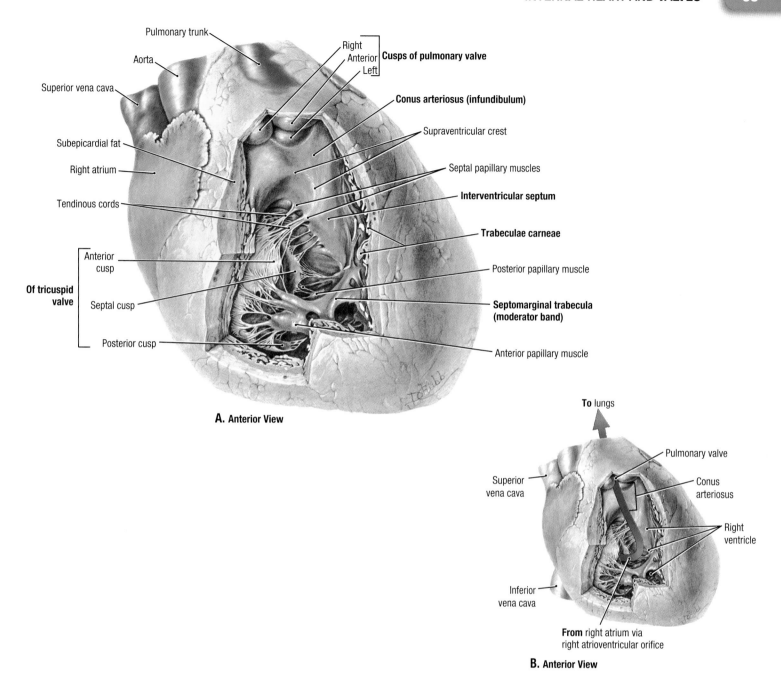

Pulmonary trunk

Aorta

Superior vena cava

Subepicardial fat

Right atrium

Tendinous cords

Of tricuspid valve — Anterior cusp, Septal cusp, Posterior cusp

Right / Anterior / Left — **Cusps of pulmonary valve**

Conus arteriosus (infundibulum)

Supraventricular crest

Septal papillary muscles

Interventricular septum

Trabeculae carneae

Posterior papillary muscle

Septomarginal trabecula (moderator band)

Anterior papillary muscle

A. Anterior View

To lungs

Superior vena cava

Inferior vena cava

Pulmonary valve

Conus arteriosus

Right ventricle

From right atrium via right atrioventricular orifice

B. Anterior View

1.55   **RIGHT VENTRICLE**

A. Interior of right ventricle. **B.** Blood flow through right heart.

- The entrance to this chamber, the right atrioventricular or tricuspid orifice, is situated posteriorly; the exit, the orifice of the pulmonary trunk, is superior.
- The outflow portion of the chamber inferior to the pulmonary orifice (conus arteriosus or infundibulum) has a smooth, funnel-shaped wall; the remainder of the ventricle is rough with fleshy trabeculae.
- There are three types of trabeculae: mere ridges, bridges attached only at each end, and fingerlike projections called papillary muscles. The anterior papillary muscle rises from the anterior wall, the posterior (papillary muscle) from the posterior wall, and a series of small septal papillae from the septal wall.

- The septomarginal trabecula, here thick, extends from the septum to the base of the anterior papillary muscle.
- The membranous part of the interventricular septum develops separately from the muscular part and has a complex embryological origin (Moore and Persaud, 2008). Consequently, this part is the common site of *ventricular septal defects* (VSDs), although defects also occur in the muscular part. VSDs rank first on all lists of cardiac defects. The size of the defect varies from 1 to 25 mm. A VSD causes a left-to-right shunt of blood through the defect. A large shunt increases pulmonary blood flow, which causes severe pulmonary disease (*pulmonary hypertension*, or increased blood pressure) and may cause *cardiac failure*.

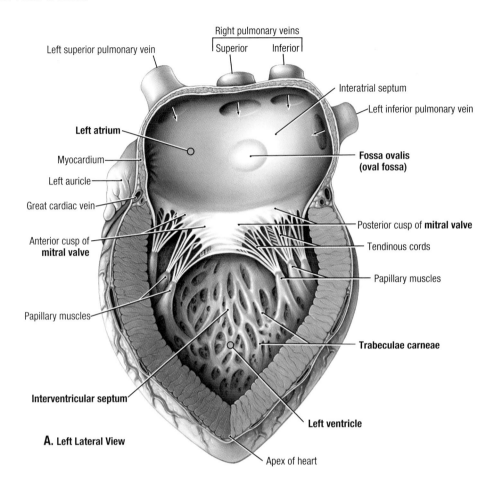

Right pulmonary veins
Superior   Inferior

Left superior pulmonary vein

Interatrial septum

Left inferior pulmonary vein

Left atrium

Myocardium

**Fossa ovalis
(oval fossa)**

Left auricle

Great cardiac vein

Posterior cusp of **mitral valve**

Anterior cusp of
mitral valve

Tendinous cords

Papillary muscles

Papillary muscles

Trabeculae carneae

Interventricular septum

Left ventricle

A. Left Lateral View

Apex of heart

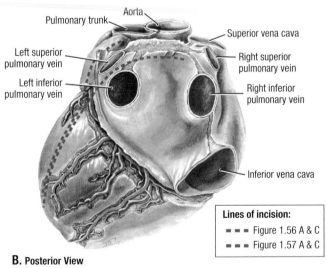

Aorta

Pulmonary trunk

Superior vena cava

Left superior
pulmonary vein

Right superior
pulmonary vein

Left inferior
pulmonary vein

Right inferior
pulmonary vein

Inferior vena cava

Lines of incision:
- - - Figure 1.56 A & C
- - - Figure 1.57 A & C

B. Posterior View

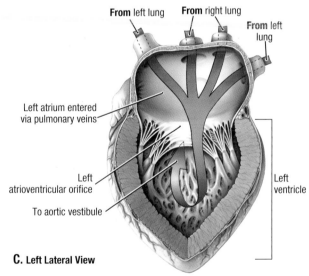

From left lung   **From** right lung

From left
lung

Left atrium entered
via pulmonary veins

Left
atrioventricular orifice

Left
ventricle

To aortic vestibule

C. Left Lateral View

1.56 **LEFT ATRIUM AND LEFT VENTRICLE**

A. Interior of left heart. **B.** Blood flow through the left heart.

- A diagonal cut was made from the base of the heart to the apex, passing between the superior and inferior pulmonary veins and through the posterior cusp of the mitral valve, followed by retraction (spreading) of the left heart wall on each side of the incision.

- The entrances (pulmonary veins) to the left atrium are posterior, and the exit (left atrioventricular or mitral orifice) is anterior.
- The left side of the fossa ovalis is also seen on the left side of the interatrial septum, although the left side is not usually as distinct as the right side is within the right atrium.
- Except for that of the auricle, the atrial wall is smooth.

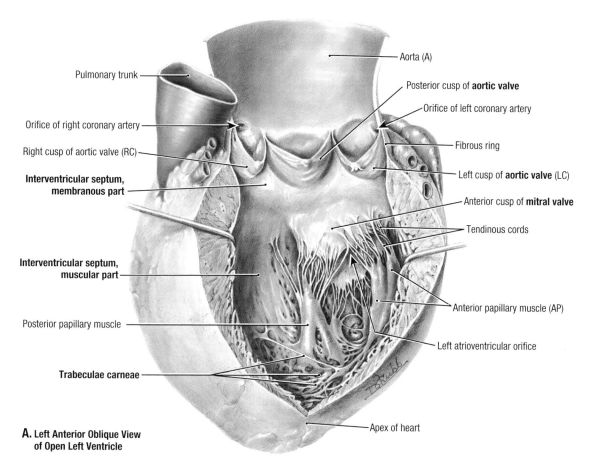

Pulmonary trunk

Orifice of right coronary artery

Right cusp of aortic valve (RC)

**Interventricular septum,
membranous part**

**Interventricular septum,
muscular part**

Posterior papillary muscle

Trabeculae carneae

Aorta (A)

Posterior cusp of **aortic valve**

Orifice of left coronary artery

Fibrous ring

Left cusp of **aortic valve** (LC)

Anterior cusp of **mitral valve**

Tendinous cords

Anterior papillary muscle (AP)

Left atrioventricular orifice

Apex of heart

**A. Left Anterior Oblique View
of Open Left Ventricle**

B. Anterior View

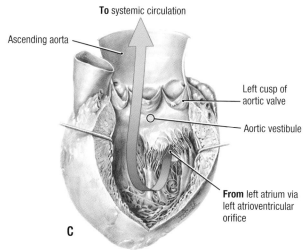

To systemic circulation

Ascending aorta

Left cusp of
aortic valve

Aortic vestibule

From left atrium via
left atrioventricular
orifice

C

1.57   LEFT VENTRICLE

A. Interior of left ventricle. **B.** Coronal CT angiogram. Letters refer to structures in **A. C.** Blood flow through the left ventricle.
- A cut was made from the apex along the left margin of the heart, passing posterior to the pulmonary trunk, to open the aortic vestibule and ascending aorta.
- The chamber has a conical shape.
- The entrance (left atrioventricular, bicuspid, or mitral orifice) is situated posteriorly, and the exit (aortic orifice) is superior.

- The left ventricular wall is thin and muscular near the apex, thick and muscular superiorly, and thin and fibrous (nonelastic) at the aortic orifice.
- Two large papillary muscles, the anterior from the anterior wall and the posterior from the posterior wall, control the adjacent halves of two cusps of the mitral valve with tendinous cords (chordae tendineae).
- The anterior cusp of the mitral valve lies between the inlet (mitral orifice) and the outlet (aortic orifice).

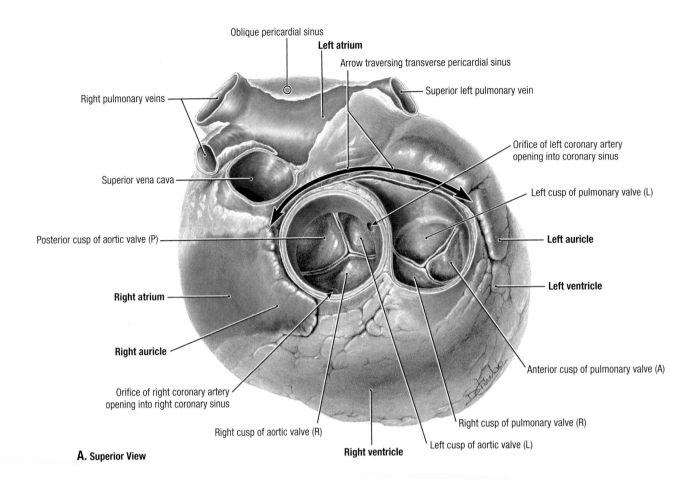

Oblique pericardial sinus

Left atrium

Arrow traversing transverse pericardial sinus

Right pulmonary veins

Superior left pulmonary vein

Orifice of left coronary artery opening into coronary sinus

Superior vena cava

Left cusp of pulmonary valve (L)

Posterior cusp of aortic valve (P)

Left auricle

Right atrium

Left ventricle

Right auricle

Anterior cusp of pulmonary valve (A)

Orifice of right coronary artery opening into right coronary sinus

Right cusp of pulmonary valve (R)

Right cusp of aortic valve (R)

Left cusp of aortic valve (L)

A. Superior View

Right ventricle

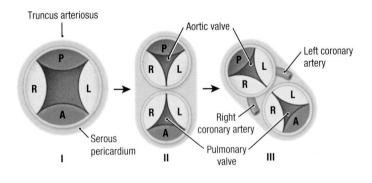

Truncus arteriosus

Aortic valve

Left coronary artery

Right coronary artery

Serous pericardium

Pulmonary valve

I   II   III

Semilunar valves:	
R Right	**A** Anterior
L Left	**P** Posterior

B

1.58 **VALVES OF HEART**

A. Excised heart.

- The ventricles are positioned anteriorly and to the left, the atria posteriorly and to the right.
- The roots of the aorta and pulmonary artery, which conduct blood from the ventricles, are placed anterior to the atria and their incoming blood vessels (the superior and inferior vena cava and pulmonary veins).
- The aorta and pulmonary artery are enclosed within a common tube of serous pericardium and partly embraced by the auricles of the atria.
- The transverse pericardial sinus curves posterior to the enclosed stems of the aorta and pulmonary trunk and anterior to the superior vena cava and upper limits of the atria.
- The three cusps of the aortic and pulmonary valves. Immediately superior to each semilunar cusp, the walls of the origins of the pulmonary trunk and aorta are slightly dilated, forming a sinus. The aortic sinuses and sinuses of the pulmonary trunk (pulmonary sinuses) are the spaces at the origin of the pulmonary trunk and ascending aorta between the dilated wall of the vessel and each cusp of the semilunar valves.

B. Developmental basis for naming of pulmonary and aortic valve cusps.

- The names of these cusps have a developmental origin (**B**) the truncus arteriosus with four cusps (**I**) splits to form two valves, each with three cusps (**II**). The heart undergoes partial rotation to the left on its axis, resulting in the arrangement of cusps shown in (**III**) and in Figure 1.58B.

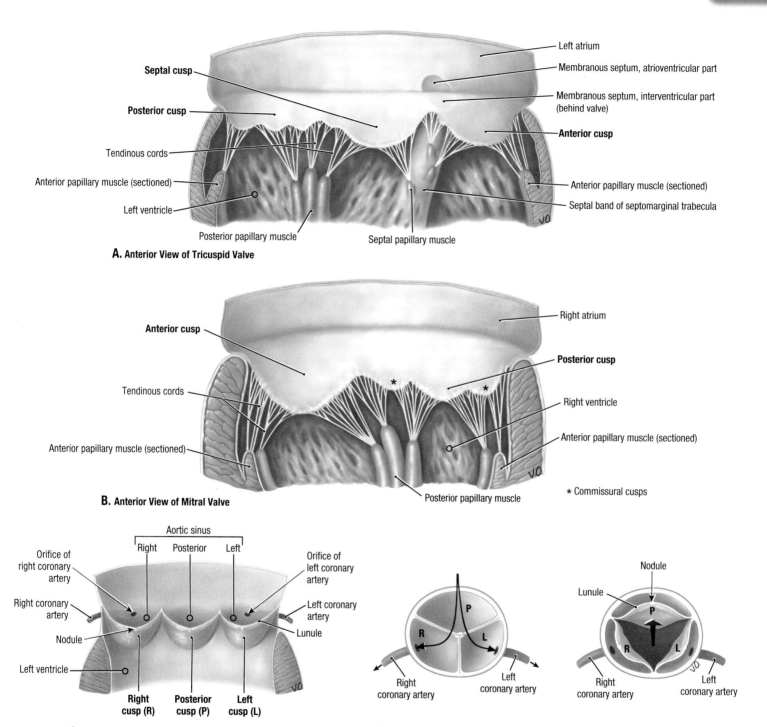

A. Anterior View of Tricuspid Valve

Left atrium
Membranous septum, atrioventricular part
Membranous septum, interventricular part (behind valve)
Anterior cusp
Anterior papillary muscle (sectioned)
Septal band of septomarginal trabecula

Septal cusp
Posterior cusp
Tendinous cords
Anterior papillary muscle (sectioned)
Left ventricle
Posterior papillary muscle
Septal papillary muscle

B. Anterior View of Mitral Valve

Right atrium
Posterior cusp
Right ventricle
Anterior papillary muscle (sectioned)
★ Commissural cusps

Anterior cusp
Tendinous cords
Anterior papillary muscle (sectioned)
Posterior papillary muscle

C. Left Posterior Oblique View of Aortic Valve

Aortic sinus
Right   Posterior   Left
Orifice of right coronary artery
Orifice of left coronary artery
Right coronary artery
Left coronary artery
Nodule
Lunule
Left ventricle
Right cusp (R)   Posterior cusp (P)   Left cusp (L)

D. Superior Views of Aortic Valve (Arrows indicate direction of blood flow)

Nodule
Lunule
P
R   L
Right coronary artery
Left coronary artery
Right coronary artery
Left coronary artery

1.59   VALVES OF THE HEART

A. and B. Atrioventricular valves. **C. and D.** Semilunar valves.

Tendinous cords pass from the tips of the papillary muscles to the free margins and ventricular surfaces of the cusps of the tricuspid **(A)** and mitral **(B)** valves. Each papillary muscle or muscle group controls the adjacent sides of two cusps, resisting valve prolapse during systole. In **(C)**, as in Figure 1.57A, the anulus of the aortic valve has been incised between the right and left cusps and spread open. Each cusp of the semilunar valves bears a nodule in the midpoint of its free edge, flanked by thin connective tissue areas (lunules). When the ventricles relax to fill (diastole), backflow of blood from aortic recoil or pulmonary resistance fills the sinus (space between cusp and dilated part of the aortic or pulmonary wall), causing the nodules and lunules to meet centrally, closing the valve **(D, left)**. Filling of the coronary arteries occurs during diastole (when ventricular walls are relaxed) as backflow "inflates" the cusps to close the valve.

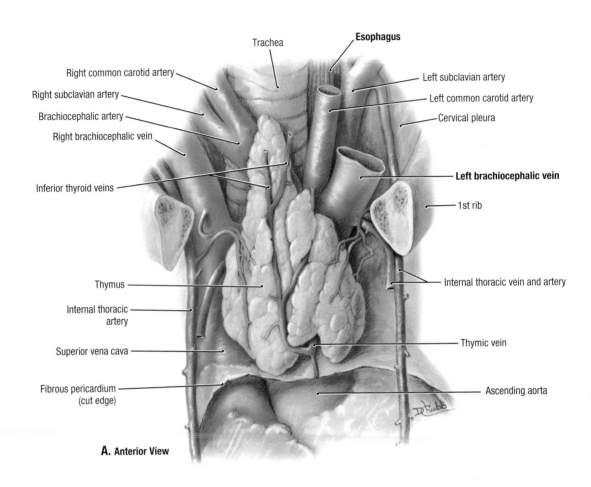

Trachea

Esophagus

Right common carotid artery

Right subclavian artery

Brachiocephalic artery

Right brachiocephalic vein

Inferior thyroid veins

Thymus

Internal thoracic artery

Superior vena cava

Fibrous pericardium (cut edge)

Left subclavian artery

Left common carotid artery

Cervical pleura

Left brachiocephalic vein

1st rib

Internal thoracic vein and artery

Thymic vein

Ascending aorta

A. Anterior View

1.60   SUPERIOR MEDIASTINUM I AND II: SUPERFICIAL DISSECTIONS

A. Thymus in situ. The sternum and ribs have been excised and the pleurae removed. It is unusual in an adult to see such a discrete thymus, which is large during puberty but subsequently regresses and is for the most part replaced by fat and fibrous tissue. **B.** Thymus removed. **C.** Relationship of nerves and vessels. The right vagus nerve (CN X) crosses anterior to the right subclavian artery and gives off the right recurrent laryngeal nerve, which passes medially to reach the trachea and esophagus. The left recurrent laryngeal nerve passes inferior and then posterior to the arch of the aorta and ascends between the trachea and esophagus to the larynx.

The distal part of the ascending aorta receives a strong thrust of blood when the left ventricle contracts. Because its wall is not reinforced by fibrous pericardium (the fibrous pericardium blends with the aortic adventitia at the beginning of the arch), an aneurysm may develop. An **aortic aneurysm** is evident on chest film (radiograph of the thorax) or a magnetic resonance angiogram as an enlarged area of the ascending aorta silhouette. Individuals with an aneurysm usually complain of chest

pain that radiates to the back. The aneurysm may exert pressure on the trachea, esophagus, and recurrent laryngeal nerve, causing difficulty in breathing and swallowing.

The recurrent laryngeal nerves supply all the intrinsic muscles of the larynx, except the cricothyroid. Consequently, any investigative procedure or disease process in the superior mediastinum may involve these nerves and affect the voice. Because the left recurrent laryngeal nerve hooks around the arch of the aorta and ascends between the trachea and the esophagus, it may be involved when there is a bronchial or esophageal carcinoma, enlargement of mediastinal lymph nodes, or an aneurysm of the arch of the aorta.

The thymus is a prominent feature during infancy and childhood. In some infants, the thymus may compress the trachea. The thymus plays an important role in the development and maintenance of the immune system. As puberty is reached, the thymus begins to diminish in relative size. By adulthood, it is replaced by adipose tissue.

Right common carotid artery

Recurrent laryngeal nerves

Esophagus

Right vagus nerve

Left vagus nerve

Right subclavian artery

Left subclavian artery

Trachea

Phrenic nerve

Phrenic nerve

Internal thoracic artery

Left common carotid artery

Brachiocephalic artery

Cervical pleura

Right brachiocephalic vein

Left brachiocephalic vein

Left superior intercostal vein

1st rib

Left vagus nerve

Arch of aorta

Left recurrent laryngeal nerve

Cardiac nerves

Ligamentum arteriosum

Pulmonary plexus

Superior vena cava

Pericardium (cut edge)

Phrenic nerve

Ascending aorta

B. Anterior View

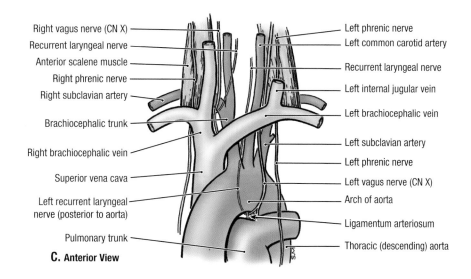

Right vagus nerve (CN X)

Left phrenic nerve

Recurrent laryngeal nerve

Left common carotid artery

Anterior scalene muscle

Right phrenic nerve

Recurrent laryngeal nerve

Right subclavian artery

Left internal jugular vein

Brachiocephalic trunk

Left brachiocephalic vein

Right brachiocephalic vein

Left subclavian artery

Superior vena cava

Left phrenic nerve

Left recurrent laryngeal nerve (posterior to aorta)

Left vagus nerve (CN X)

Arch of aorta

Pulmonary trunk

Ligamentum arteriosum

Thoracic (descending) aorta

C. Anterior View

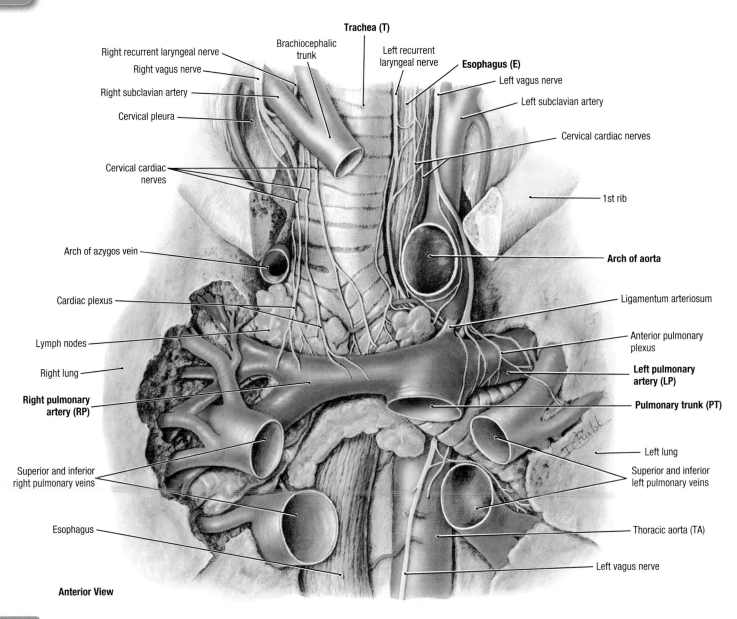

Trachea (T)

Right recurrent laryngeal nerve

Right vagus nerve

Right subclavian artery

Cervical pleura

Brachiocephalic trunk

Left recurrent laryngeal nerve

Esophagus (E)

Left vagus nerve

Left subclavian artery

Cervical cardiac nerves

Cervical cardiac nerves

1st rib

Arch of azygos vein

Cardiac plexus

Lymph nodes

Right lung

Right pulmonary artery (RP)

Superior and inferior right pulmonary veins

Esophagus

Arch of aorta

Ligamentum arteriosum

Anterior pulmonary plexus

Left pulmonary artery (LP)

Pulmonary trunk (PT)

Left lung

Superior and inferior left pulmonary veins

Thoracic aorta (TA)

Left vagus nerve

Anterior View

1.61 SUPERIOR MEDIASTINUM III: CARDIAC PLEXUS AND PULMONARY ARTERIES

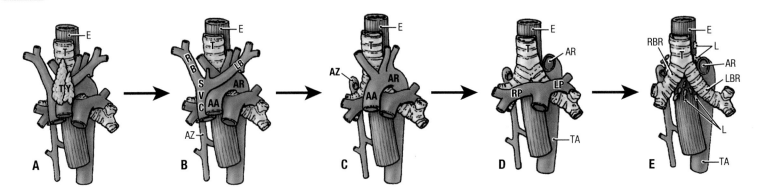

1.62 RELATIONS OF GREAT VESSELS AND TRACHEA

Observe, from superficial to deep: **(A)** Thymus (*TY*); **(B)** the right (*RB*) and left (*LB*) brachiocephalic veins form the superior vena cava (*SVC*) and receive the arch of the azygos vein (*AZ*) posteriorly; **(C)** the ascending aorta (*AA*) and arch of the aorta (*AR*) arch over the right pulmonary artery and left main bronchus; **(D)** the right and left pulmonary arteries (*RP* and *LP*); and **(E)** the tracheobronchial lymph nodes (*L*) at the tracheal bifurcation (*T*).

Longus colli

Cervical pleura

Trachea

Left recurrent
laryngeal nerve

Arch of azygos vein

Left recurrent
laryngeal nerve

**Right main
bronchus**

Right bronchial
artery

Right lung

Esophagus

Esophagus

Thoracic duct

Left vagus nerve

1st rib

Arch of aorta

Ligamentum arteriosum

Left bronchial artery

**Left main
bronchus**

**Intrapulmonary
bronchi**

Left lung

Thoracic (descending)
aorta

A. Anterior View

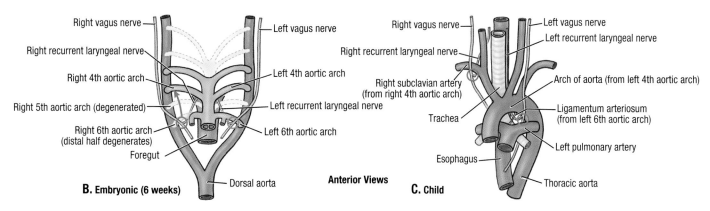

Right vagus nerve

Right recurrent laryngeal nerve

Right 4th aortic arch

Right 5th aortic arch (degenerated)

Right 6th aortic arch
(distal half degenerates)

Foregut

B. Embryonic (6 weeks)

Left vagus nerve

Left 4th aortic arch

Left recurrent laryngeal nerve

Left 6th aortic arch

Dorsal aorta

Anterior Views

Right vagus nerve

Right recurrent laryngeal nerve

Right subclavian artery
(from right 4th aortic arch)

Trachea

Esophagus

Left vagus nerve

Left recurrent laryngeal nerve

Arch of aorta (from left 4th aortic arch)

Ligamentum arteriosum
(from left 6th aortic arch)

Left pulmonary artery

Thoracic aorta

C. Child

| 1.63 | **SUPERIOR MEDIASTINUM IV: TRACHEAL BIFURCATION AND BRONCHI** |

A. Dissection. **B.** Asymmetrical course of right and left recurrent laryngeal nerves. Arch VI disappears on the right, leaving the right recurrent laryngeal nerve to pass under arch IV, which becomes the right subclavian artery. Arch VI becomes part of the ductus arteriosus on the left side, and arch IV "descends" to become the arch of the aorta; thus the left recurrent laryngeal nerve is pulled into the thorax.

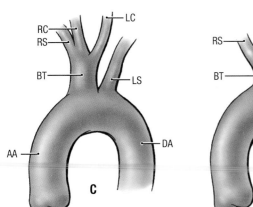

Right common carotid artery (RC)
Left common carotid artery (LC)
Right subclavian artery (RS)
Brachiocephalic trunk (BT)
Left subclavian artery (LS)
Arch of aorta (AR)
Descending aorta (DA)
Ascending aorta (AA)

A

A. and B. Most common pattern (65%)

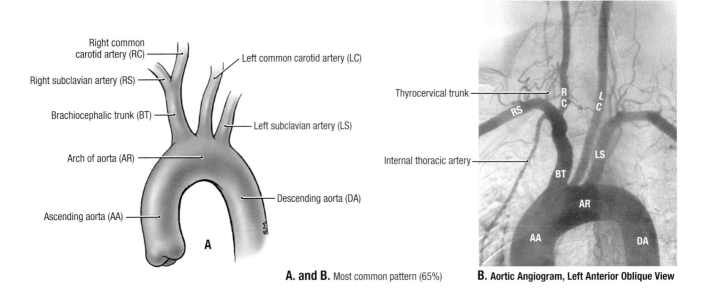

Thyrocervical trunk
Internal thoracic artery

B. Aortic Angiogram, Left Anterior Oblique View

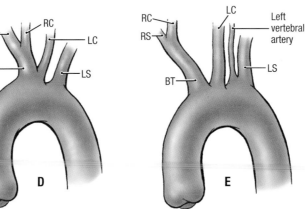

C

D

E
Left vertebral artery

F

C. and D. Left common carotid artery originating from the brachiocephalic trunk (27%)

E. Four arteries originating independently from the arch of the aorta (2.5%)

F. Right and left brachiocephalic trunks originating from the arch of the aorta (1.2%)

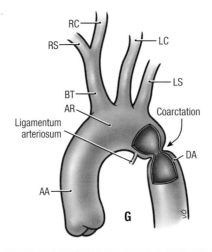

RC
RS
LC
BT
LS
AR
Coarctation
Ligamentum arteriosum
DA
AA

G

KEY
AA   Ascending aorta
AR   Arch of aorta
DA   Descending aorta
BT   Brachiocephalic trunk (artery)
LC   Left common carotid artery
LS   Left subclavian artery
RC   Right common carotid artery
RS   Right subclavian artery

1.64   BRANCHES OF AORTIC ARCH

A. and B. Most common pattern (65%). **C.–F.** Variations. **G. In coarctation of the aorta,** the arch or descending aorta has an abnormal narrowing (stenosis) that diminishes the caliber of the aortic lumen, producing an obstruction to blood flow. The most common site is near the ligamentum arteriosum. When the coarctation is inferior to this site (postductal coarctation), a good collateral circulation usually develops between the proximal and distal parts of the aorta through the intercostal and internal thoracic arteries.

Middle cervical cardiac nerve

Trachea

Middle cervical ganglion

Inferior cervical cardiac nerve

Cervicothoracic (stellate) ganglion (inferior cervical and 1st thoracic ganglia)

3rd thoracic sympathetic ganglion

2nd thoracic sympathetic ganglion

Thoracic cardiac branch

Cardiac plexus

Esophagus

Pulmonary trunk

Thoracic aorta

A

Anterior Views

Right vagus nerve

Trachea

Left vagus nerve

Right recurrent laryngeal nerve

Superior cervical cardiac branch

Left recurrent laryngeal nerve

Recurrent cardiac branch

Inferior cervical cardiac branch

Thoracic cardiac branch

Cardiac plexus

Esophagus

Pulmonary trunk

Thoracic aorta

B

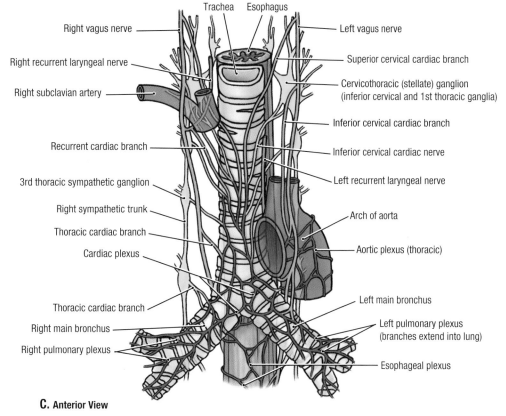

Right vagus nerve

Trachea Esophagus

Left vagus nerve

Right recurrent laryngeal nerve

Superior cervical cardiac branch

Right subclavian artery

Cervicothoracic (stellate) ganglion (inferior cervical and 1st thoracic ganglia)

Inferior cervical cardiac branch

Recurrent cardiac branch

Inferior cervical cardiac nerve

3rd thoracic sympathetic ganglion

Left recurrent laryngeal nerve

Right sympathetic trunk

Arch of aorta

Thoracic cardiac branch

Aortic plexus (thoracic)

Cardiac plexus

Thoracic cardiac branch

Left main bronchus

Right main bronchus

Left pulmonary plexus (branches extend into lung)

Right pulmonary plexus

Esophageal plexus

C. Anterior View

| 1.65 | CARDIAC AND PULMONARY PLEXUSES |

A. Sympathetic contribution. **B.** Parasympathetic contribution. **C.** Overview. *Yellow*, sympathetic; *blue*, parasympathetic; *green*, mixed sympathetic and parasympathetic nerves.

Heart: Sympathetic stimulation increases the heart's rate and the force of its contractions. Parasympathetic stimulation slows the heart rate, reduces the force of contraction, and constricts the coronary arteries, saving energy between periods of increased demand. While the cardiac plexus is shown in relation to the bifurcation of the trachea, note that it lies directly posterior to the superior margin of the heart (see Fig. 1.28C) and in close proximity to the nodal tissue and origins of the coronary arteries.

Lungs: Sympathetic fibers are inhibitory to the bronchial muscle (bronchodilator), motor to pulmonary vessels (vasoconstrictor) and inhibitory to the alveolar glands of the bronchial tree. Parasympathetic fibers from CN X are bronchoconstrictors, secretory to the glands of the bronchial tree (secretomotor).

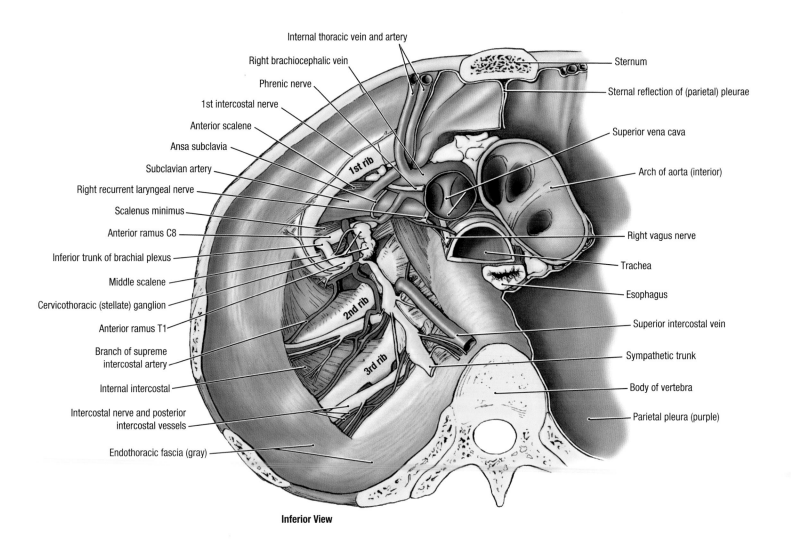

Internal thoracic vein and artery

Right brachiocephalic vein

Phrenic nerve

1st intercostal nerve

Anterior scalene

Ansa subclavia

Subclavian artery

Right recurrent laryngeal nerve

Scalenus minimus

Anterior ramus C8

Inferior trunk of brachial plexus

Middle scalene

Cervicothoracic (stellate) ganglion

Anterior ramus T1

Branch of supreme intercostal artery

Internal intercostal

Intercostal nerve and posterior intercostal vessels

Endothoracic fascia (gray)

1st rib

2nd rib

3rd rib

Sternum

Sternal reflection of (parietal) pleurae

Superior vena cava

Arch of aorta (interior)

Right vagus nerve

Trachea

Esophagus

Superior intercostal vein

Sympathetic trunk

Body of vertebra

Parietal pleura (purple)

Inferior View

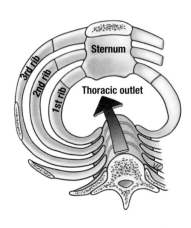

1.66

SUPERIOR MEDIASTINUM AND ROOF OF PLEURAL CAVITY

- The cervical, costal, and mediastinal parietal pleura (*purple*) and portions of the endothoracic fascia (*gray*) have been removed from the right side of the specimen to demonstrate structures traversing the superior thoracic aperture.
- The first part of the subclavian artery disappears as it crosses the first rib anterior to the anterior scalene muscle.
- The ansa subclavia from the sympathetic trunk and right recurrent laryngeal nerve from the vagus are seen looping inferior to the subclavian artery.
- The anterior rami of C8 and T1 merge to form the inferior trunk of the brachial plexus, which crosses the first rib posterior to the anterior scalene muscle.

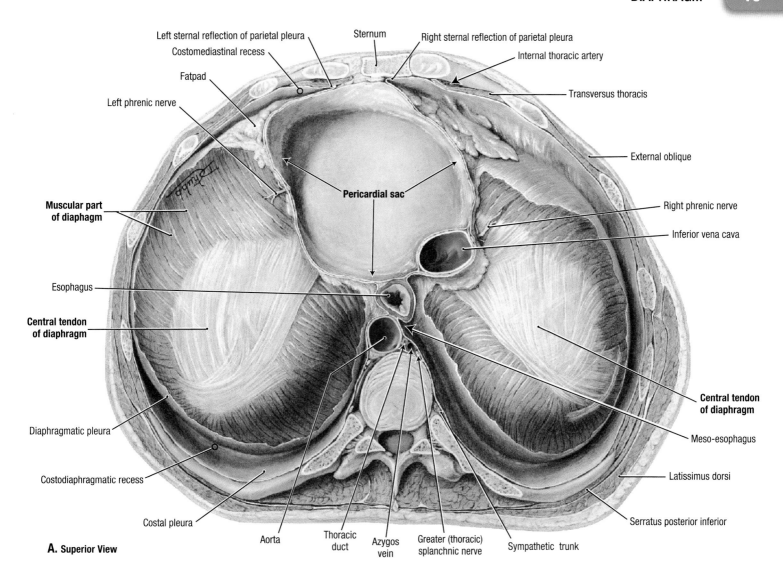

Left sternal reflection of parietal pleura
Costomediastinal recess
Fatpad
Left phrenic nerve
Muscular part of diaphagm
Esophagus
Central tendon of diaphragm
Diaphragmatic pleura
Costodiaphragmatic recess
Costal pleura

Sternum
Right sternal reflection of parietal pleura
Internal thoracic artery
Transversus thoracis
External oblique

Pericardial sac

Right phrenic nerve
Inferior vena cava

Central tendon of diaphragm
Meso-esophagus
Latissimus dorsi
Serratus posterior inferior

Aorta
Thoracic duct
Azygos vein
Greater (thoracic) splanchnic nerve
Sympathetic trunk

A. Superior View

1.67 **DIAPHRAGM AND PERICARDIAL SAC**

A. The diaphragmatic pleura is mostly removed. The pericardial sac is situated on the anterior half of the diaphragm; one third is to the right of the median plane, and two thirds to the left. Note also that anterior to the pericardium, the sternal reflection of the left pleural sac approaches but fails to meet that of the right sac in the median plane; and on reaching the vertebral column, the costal pleura becomes the mediastinal pleura. Irritation of the parietal pleura produces local pain and referred pain to the areas sharing innervation by the same segments of the spinal cord. Irritation of the costal and peripheral parts of the diaphragmatic pleura results in local pain and referred pain along the intercostal nerves to the thoracic and abdominal walls. Irritation of the mediastinal and central diaphragmatic areas of the parietal pleura results in pain that is referred to the root of the neck and over the shoulder (C3–C5 dermatomes). **B.** Between the inferior part of the esophagus and the aorta, the right and left layers of mediastinal pleura form a dorsal meso-esophagus, especially when the body is in the prone position.

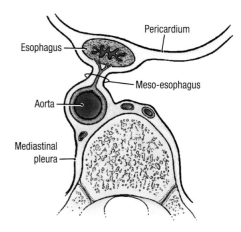

Pericardium
Esophagus
Meso-esophagus
Aorta
Mediastinal pleura

B. Superior View

Trachea Esophagus

Right common carotid artery

Right subclavian artery

Brachiocephalic trunk

Vertebral artery

Costocervical trunk

Thyrocervical trunk

Internal thoracic artery

Left subclavian artery

Left common carotid artery

Arch of aorta

Arch of azygos vein

Tracheobronchial lymph node

Right main bronchus

Right superior lobar bronchus

Intermediate bronchus
(to right inferior and middle lobes)

Left main bronchus

Left superior lobar bronchus

Left inferior lobar bronchus

Thoracic aorta

Esophagus

Thoracic duct

Esophageal hiatus

Diaphragm

Median arcuate ligament

Abdominal aorta

Cisterna chyli

Left crus of diaphragm

Anterior View

Right crus of diaphragm

1.68   ESOPHAGUS, TRACHEA, AND AORTA

- The anterior relations of the thoracic part of the esophagus from superior to inferior are the trachea (from origin at cricoid cartilage to bifurcation), right and left bronchi, inferior tracheobronchial lymph nodes, pericardium (not shown) and, finally, the diaphragm.
- The arch of the aorta passes posterior to the left of these four structures as it arches over the left main bronchus; the arch of the azygos vein passes anterior to their right as it arches over the right main bronchus.

- The impressions produced in the esophagus by adjacent structures (aorta, left main bronchus, and esophageal hiatus) are of clinical interest because of the slower passage of substances at these sites. The impressions indicate where swallowed foreign objects are most likely to lodge and where a stricture may develop after the accidental drinking of a caustic liquid such as lye.

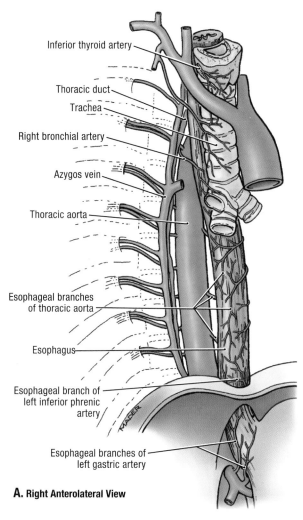

Inferior thyroid artery

Thoracic duct

Trachea

Right bronchial artery

Azygos vein

Thoracic aorta

Esophageal branches
of thoracic aorta

Esophagus

Esophageal branch of
left inferior phrenic
artery

Esophageal branches of
left gastric artery

A. Right Anterolateral View

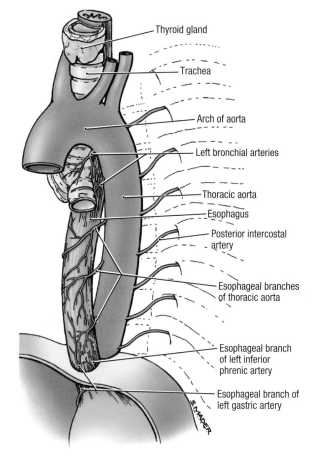

Thyroid gland

Trachea

Arch of aorta

Left bronchial arteries

Thoracic aorta

Esophagus

Posterior intercostal
artery

Esophageal branches
of thoracic aorta

Esophageal branch
of left inferior
phrenic artery

Esophageal branch of
left gastric artery

B. Left Anterolateral View

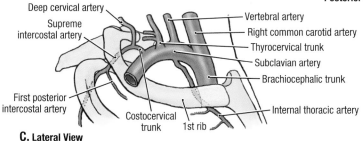

Deep cervical artery

Supreme
intercostal artery

Vertebral artery

Right common carotid artery

Thyrocervical trunk

Subclavian artery

Brachiocephalic trunk

First posterior
intercostal artery

Costocervical
trunk

1st rib

Internal thoracic artery

C. Lateral View

Posterior intercostal
arteries:

1st

2nd

3rd

4th

5th

6th

7th

8th

9th

10th

11th

Subcostal
artery

Deep cervical artery

Costocervical trunk

1st rib

Ligamentum arteriosum

Bronchial arteries

* Coronary arteries

Esophageal branches

Posterior
intercostal arteries

Superior phrenic arteries

Subcostal artery

Diaphragm

Celiac trunk

D. Anterior View

| 1.69 | ARTERIAL SUPPLY TO TRACHEA AND ESOPHAGUS |

A. and B. The continuous anastomotic chain of arteries on the esophagus is formed (1) by branches of the right and left inferior thyroid and right supreme intercostal arteries superiorly, (2) by the unpaired median aortic (bronchial and esophageal) branches, and (3) by branches of the left gastric and left inferior phrenic arteries inferiorly. The right bronchial artery usually arises from the superior left bronchial or 3rd right posterior intercostal artery (here the 5th) or from the aorta directly. The unpaired median aortic branches also supply the trachea and bronchi. **C.** Origin of supreme intercostal artery. **D.** Branches of the thoracic aorta.

Right internal jugular vein

Jugular lymphatic trunk

Right lymphatic duct

Subclavian lymphatic trunk

Right venous angle

Right subclavian vein

Right bronchomediastinal lymphatic trunk

Right brachiocephalic vein

Superior vena cava

Azygos vein

Intercostal lymphatic vessel

Thoracic duct

Posterior mediastinal lymph node

Intercostal lymphatic vessel

Diaphragm

Inferior vena cava

Cisterna chyli (chyle cistern)

Left internal jugular vein

Jugular lymphatic trunk

Thoracic duct

Subclavian lymphatic trunk

Left venous angle

Left subclavian vein

Left brachiocephalic vein

Left bronchomediastinal lymphatic trunk

Left superior intercostal vein

Thoracic aorta

Esophagus

S. MADER AFTER N. JOY

Anterior View

1.70 THORACIC DUCT

- The descending aorta is located to the left, and the azygos vein slightly to the right of the midline.
- The thoracic duct (1) originates from the cisterna chyli at the T12 vertebral level, (2) ascends on the vertebral column between the azygos vein and the descending aorta, (3) passes to the left at the junction of the posterior and superior mediastina, and continues its ascent to the neck, where (4) it arches laterally to enter the venous system near or at the angle of union of the left internal jugular and subclavian veins (left venous angle).
- The thoracic duct is commonly plexiform (resembling a network) in the posterior mediastinum.

- The termination of the thoracic duct typically receives the left jugular, subclavian, and bronchomediastinal trunks.
- The right lymph duct is short and formed by the union of the right jugular, subclavian, and bronchomediastinal trunks.
- Because the thoracic duct is thin walled and may be colorless, it may not be easily identified. Consequently, it is vulnerable to inadvertent injury during investigative and/or surgical procedures in the posterior mediastinum. **Laceration of the thoracic duct** results in chyle escaping into the thoracic cavity. Chyle may also enter the pleural cavity, producing chylothorax.

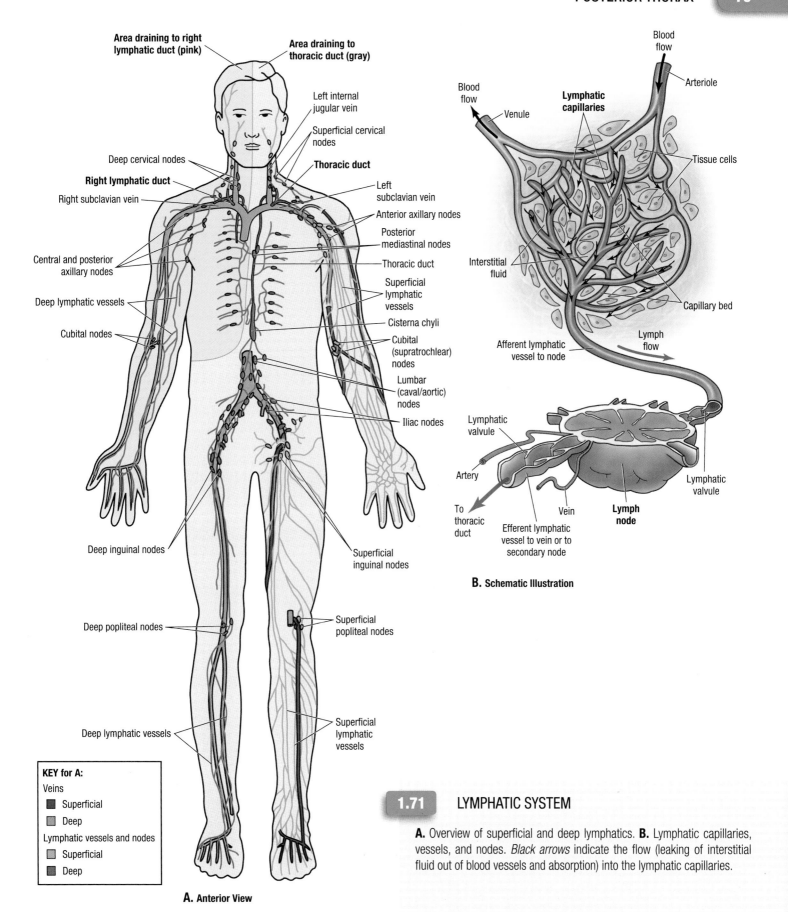

Area draining to right lymphatic duct (pink)

Area draining to thoracic duct (gray)

Left internal jugular vein

Superficial cervical nodes

Deep cervical nodes

Thoracic duct

Right lymphatic duct

Right subclavian vein

Left subclavian vein

Anterior axillary nodes

Posterior mediastinal nodes

Central and posterior axillary nodes

Thoracic duct

Superficial lymphatic vessels

Deep lymphatic vessels

Cisterna chyli

Cubital nodes

Cubital (supratrochlear) nodes

Lumbar (caval/aortic) nodes

Iliac nodes

Deep inguinal nodes

Superficial inguinal nodes

Deep popliteal nodes

Superficial popliteal nodes

Deep lymphatic vessels

Superficial lymphatic vessels

KEY for A:

Veins

- ■ Superficial
- □ Deep

Lymphatic vessels and nodes

- ▦ Superficial
- ▦ Deep

A. Anterior View

Blood flow

Arteriole

Blood flow

Lymphatic capillaries

Venule

Tissue cells

Interstitial fluid

Capillary bed

Lymph flow

Afferent lymphatic vessel to node

Lymphatic valvule

Artery

Lymphatic valvule

To thoracic duct

Vein

Lymph node

Efferent lymphatic vessel to vein or to secondary node

B. Schematic Illustration

1.71   LYMPHATIC SYSTEM

A. Overview of superficial and deep lymphatics. **B.** Lymphatic capillaries, vessels, and nodes. *Black arrows* indicate the flow (leaking of interstitial fluid out of blood vessels and absorption) into the lymphatic capillaries.

Right brachiocephalic vein

Superior vena cava

Azygos vein

Parietal pleura (cut edge)

Right posterior intercostal veins

Vertebral body T11

Diaphragm

Inferior vena cava

Left brachiocephalic vein

Left superior intercostal vein

Arch of aorta

Left posterior intercostal veins

Accessory hemi-azygos vein

Hemi-azygos vein

Parietal pleura (cut edge)

Costodiaphragmatic recess

Celiac artery

Superior mesenteric artery

Left renal vein

Aorta

A. Anterior View

1.72 AZYGOS SYSTEM OF VEINS

The ascending lumbar veins connect the common iliac veins to the lumbar veins and join the subcostal veins to become the lateral roots of the azygos and hemi-azygos veins; the medial roots of the azygos and hemi-azygos veins are usually from the inferior vena cava and left renal vein, if present. Typically the upper four left posterior intercostal veins drain into the left brachiocephalic vein, directly and via the left superior intercostal veins.

In **A,** the hemi-azygos, accessory hemi-azygos, and left superior intercostals veins are continuous here, but commonly they are discontinuous. The hemi-azygos vein crosses the vertebral column at approximately T9, and the accessory hemi-azygos vein crosses at T8, to enter the azygos vein. In **A,** there are four cross-connecting channels between the azygos and hemi-azygos systems. The azygos vein arches superior to the root of the right lung at T4 to drain into the superior vena cava.

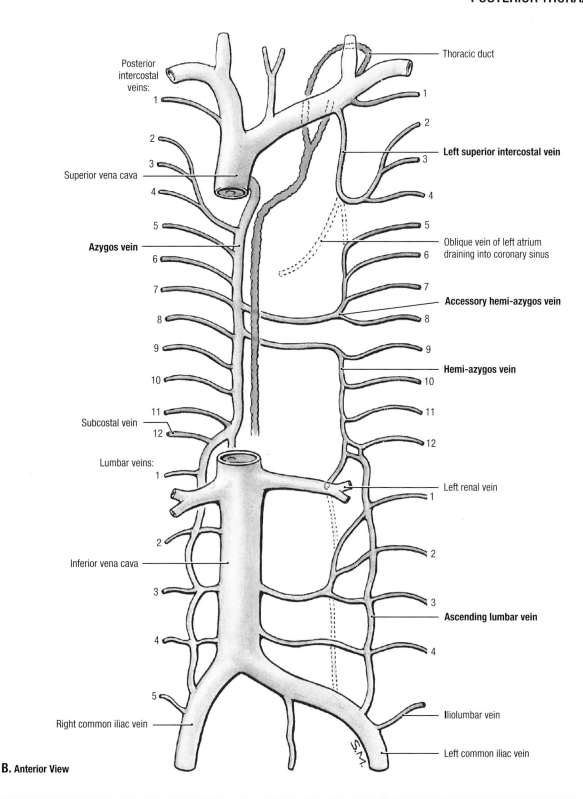

Posterior intercostal veins:
1
2
3
4
5
6
7
8
9
10
11
12

Superior vena cava

Azygos vein

Subcostal vein

Lumbar veins:
1
2

Inferior vena cava

3

4

5

Right common iliac vein

B. Anterior View

Thoracic duct

1
2
3   **Left superior intercostal vein**
4
5
Oblique vein of left atrium
6   draining into coronary sinus
7
Accessory hemi-azygos vein
8
9
Hemi-azygos vein
10
11
12

Left renal vein
1

2

3   **Ascending lumbar vein**

4

Iliolumbar vein

Left common iliac vein

| **1.72** | **AZYGOS SYSTEM OF VEINS** (*CONTINUED*) |

The azygos, hemi-azygos, and accessory hemi-azygos veins offer alternate means of venous drainage from the thoracic, abdominal, and back regions when **obstruction of the IVC** occurs. In some people, an accessory azygos vein parallels the main azygos vein on the right side. Other people have no hemi-azygos system of veins. A clinically important variation, although uncommon, is when the azygos system receives all the blood from the IVC, except that from the liver. In these people, the azygos system drains nearly all the blood inferior to the diaphragm, except that from the digestive tract. When **obstruction of the SVC** occurs superior to the entrance of the azygos vein, blood can drain inferiorly into the veins of the abdominal wall and return to the right atrium through the IVC and azygos system of veins.

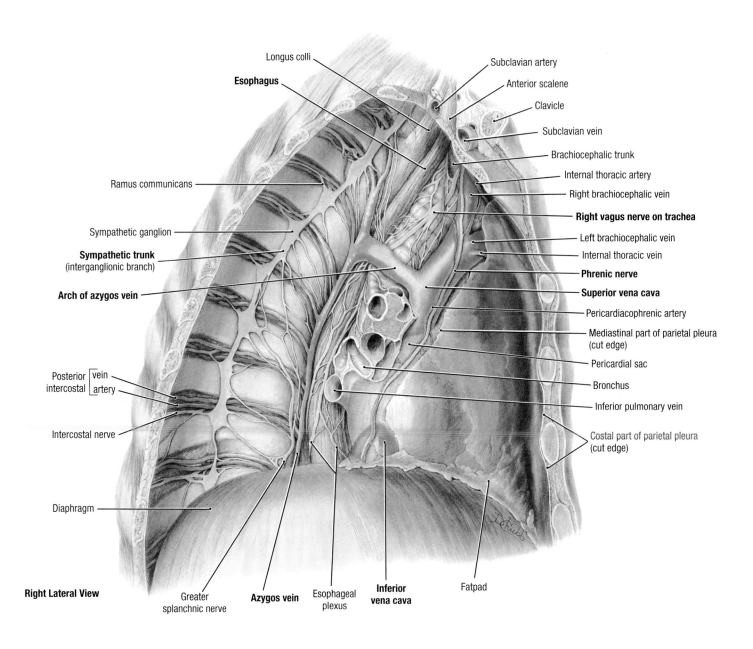

Longus colli

Esophagus

Subclavian artery

Anterior scalene

Clavicle

Subclavian vein

Brachiocephalic trunk

Internal thoracic artery

Ramus communicans

Right brachiocephalic vein

Right vagus nerve on trachea

Sympathetic ganglion

Left brachiocephalic vein

Internal thoracic vein

Sympathetic trunk
(interganglionic branch)

Phrenic nerve

Superior vena cava

Arch of azygos vein

Pericardiacophrenic artery

Mediastinal part of parietal pleura
(cut edge)

Pericardial sac

Posterior ⌐vein
intercostal ⌐artery

Bronchus

Intercostal nerve

Inferior pulmonary vein

Costal part of parietal pleura
(cut edge)

Diaphragm

Right Lateral View

Greater
splanchnic nerve

Azygos vein

Esophageal
plexus

**Inferior
vena cava**

Fatpad

1.73 MEDIASTINUM, RIGHT SIDE

- The costal and mediastinal pleurae have mostly been removed, exposing the underlying structures. Compare with the mediastinal surface of the right lung in Figure 1.32.
- The right side of the mediastinum is the "blue side," dominated by the arch of the azygos vein and the superior vena cava.
- Both the trachea and the esophagus are visible from the right side.
- The right vagus nerve descends on the medial surface of the trachea, passes medial to the arch of the azygos vein, posterior to the root of the lung, and then enters the esophageal plexus.
- The right phrenic nerve passes anterior to the root of the lung lateral to both venae cavae.

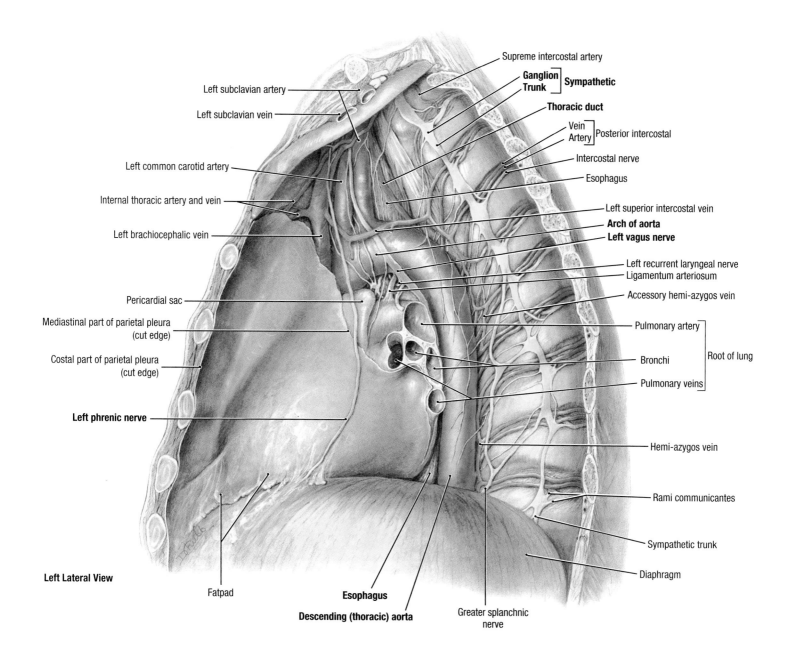

Supreme intercostal artery

Ganglion Trunk | **Sympathetic**

Left subclavian artery

Thoracic duct

Left subclavian vein

Vein
Artery | Posterior intercostal

Intercostal nerve

Left common carotid artery

Esophagus

Internal thoracic artery and vein

Left superior intercostal vein

Arch of aorta

Left brachiocephalic vein

Left vagus nerve

Left recurrent laryngeal nerve
Ligamentum arteriosum

Pericardial sac

Accessory hemi-azygos vein

Mediastinal part of parietal pleura (cut edge)

Pulmonary artery ⎤

Costal part of parietal pleura (cut edge)

Bronchi | Root of lung

Pulmonary veins ⎦

Left phrenic nerve

Hemi-azygos vein

Rami communicantes

Sympathetic trunk

Left Lateral View

Diaphragm

Fatpad

Esophagus

Descending (thoracic) aorta

Greater splanchnic nerve

1.74   MEDIASTINUM, LEFT SIDE

- Compare with the mediastinal surface of the left lung in Figure 1.33.
- The left side of the mediastinum is the "red side," dominated by the arch and descending portion of the aorta, the left common carotid and subclavian arteries; the latter obscure the trachea from view.
- The thoracic duct can be seen on the left side of the esophagus.
- The left vagus nerve passes posterior to the root of the lung, sending its recurrent laryngeal branch around the ligamentum arteriosum inferior and then medial to the aortic arch.
- The phrenic nerve passes anterior to the root of the lung and penetrates the diaphragm more anteriorly than on the right side.

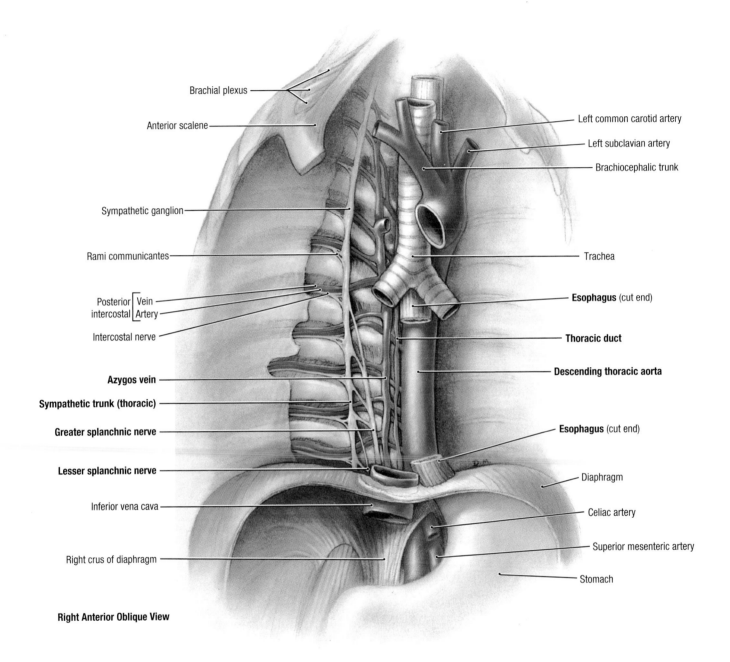

Brachial plexus

Anterior scalene

Left common carotid artery

Left subclavian artery

Brachiocephalic trunk

Sympathetic ganglion

Rami communicantes

Trachea

Posterior intercostal — Vein / Artery

Intercostal nerve

Esophagus (cut end)

Thoracic duct

Azygos vein

Descending thoracic aorta

Sympathetic trunk (thoracic)

Greater splanchnic nerve

Esophagus (cut end)

Lesser splanchnic nerve

Diaphragm

Inferior vena cava

Celiac artery

Superior mesenteric artery

Right crus of diaphragm

Stomach

Right Anterior Oblique View

1.75   STRUCTURES OF POSTERIOR MEDIASTINUM I

- In this specimen, the parietal pleura is intact on the left side and partially removed on the right side. A portion of the esophagus, between the bifurcation of the trachea and the diaphragm, is also removed.
- The thoracic sympathetic trunk is connected to each intercostal nerve by rami communicantes.
- The greater splanchnic nerve is formed by fibers from the 5th to 10th thoracic sympathetic ganglia, and the lesser splanchnic nerve receives fibers from the 10th and 11th thoracic ganglia. Both nerves contain presynaptic and visceral afferent fibers.
- The azygos vein ascends anterior to the intercostal vessels and to the right of the thoracic duct and aorta and drains into the superior vena cava.

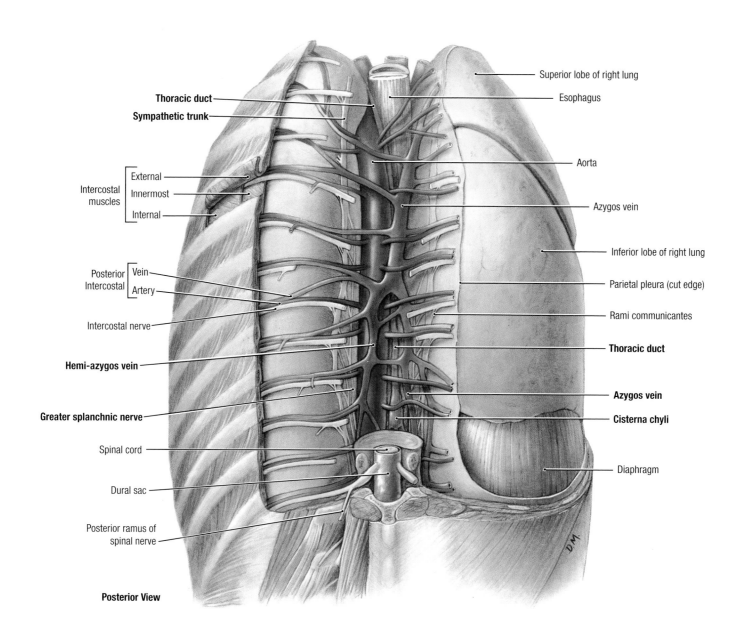

Thoracic duct

Sympathetic trunk

Intercostal muscles
- External
- Innermost
- Internal

Posterior Intercostal
- Vein
- Artery

Intercostal nerve

Hemi-azygos vein

Greater splanchnic nerve

Spinal cord

Dural sac

Posterior ramus of spinal nerve

Posterior View

Superior lobe of right lung

Esophagus

Aorta

Azygos vein

Inferior lobe of right lung

Parietal pleura (cut edge)

Rami communicantes

Thoracic duct

Azygos vein

Cisterna chyli

Diaphragm

1.76   STRUCTURES OF POSTERIOR MEDIASTINUM II

- The thoracic vertebral column and thoracic cage are removed on the right. On the left, the ribs and intercostal musculature are removed posteriorly as far laterally as the angles of the ribs. The parietal pleura is intact on the left side but partially removed on the right to reveal the visceral pleura covering the right lung.
- The azygos vein is on the right side, and the hemi-azygos vein is on the left, crossing the midline (usually at T9, but higher in this specimen) to join the azygos vein. The accessory hemi-azygos vein is absent in this specimen; instead, three most superior posterior intercostal veins drain directly into the azygos vein.

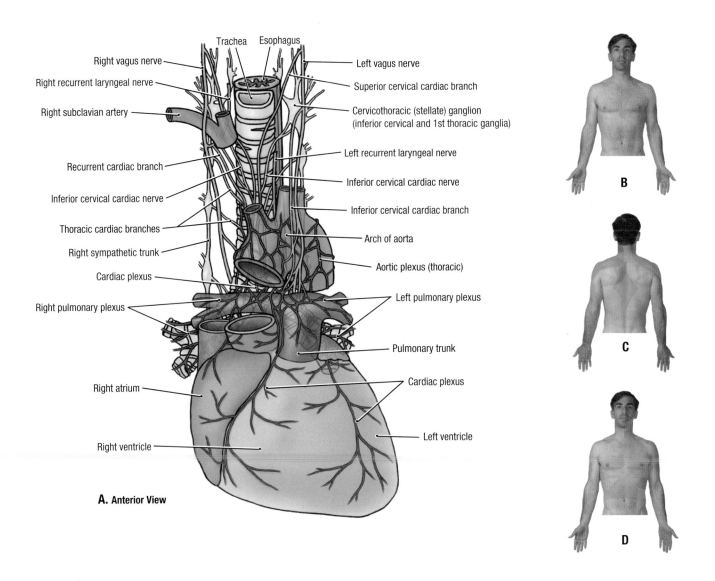

Trachea Esophagus

Right vagus nerve

Right recurrent laryngeal nerve

Right subclavian artery

Recurrent cardiac branch

Inferior cervical cardiac nerve

Thoracic cardiac branches

Right sympathetic trunk

Cardiac plexus

Right pulmonary plexus

Right atrium

Right ventricle

Left vagus nerve

Superior cervical cardiac branch

Cervicothoracic (stellate) ganglion
(inferior cervical and 1st thoracic ganglia)

Left recurrent laryngeal nerve

Inferior cervical cardiac nerve

Inferior cervical cardiac branch

Arch of aorta

Aortic plexus (thoracic)

Left pulmonary plexus

Pulmonary trunk

Cardiac plexus

Left ventricle

A. Anterior View

B

C

D

1.77   OVERVIEW OF AUTONOMIC AND VISCERAL AFFERENT INNERVATION OF THORAX

A. Innervation of heart. **B.–D.** Areas of cardiac referred pain (*red*). **E.** Innervation of posterior and superior mediastina.

The heart is insensitive to touch, cutting, cold, and heat; however, ischemia and the accumulation of metabolic products stimulate pain endings in the myocardium. The afferent pain fibers run centrally in the middle and inferior cervical branches and especially in the thoracic cardiac branches of the sympathetic trunk. The axons of these primary sensory neurons enter spinal cord segments T1 through T4 or T5, especially on the left side.

Cardiac referred pain is a phenomenon whereby noxious stimuli originating in the heart are perceived by a person as pain arising from a superficial part of the body—the skin on the left upper limb, for example. Visceral referred pain is transmitted by visceral afferent fibers accompanying sympathetic fibers and is typically referred to somatic structures or areas such as a limb having afferent fibers with cell bodies in the same

spinal ganglion, and central processes that enter the spinal cord through the same posterior roots (Hardy and Naftel, 2001).

Anginal pain is commonly felt as radiating from the substernal and left pectoral regions to the left shoulder and the medial aspect of the left upper limb (**B**). This part of the limb is supplied by the medial cutaneous nerve of the arm. Often the lateral cutaneous branches of the 2nd and 3rd intercostal nerves (the intercostobrachial nerves) join or overlap in their distribution with the medial cutaneous nerve of the arm. Consequently, cardiac pain is referred to the upper limb because the spinal cord segments of these cutaneous nerves (T1–T3) are also common to the visceral afferent terminations for the coronary arteries. Synaptic contacts may also be made with commissural (connector) neurons, which conduct impulses to neurons on the right side of comparable areas of the spinal cord. This occurrence explains why pain of cardiac origin, although usually referred to the left side, may be referred to the right side, both sides, or the back (**C and D**).

Right sympathetic trunk (cervical)

Right recurrent laryngeal nerve

Right vagus nerve

Esophageal branch

5th thoracic sympathetic ganglion

Greater splanchnic nerve

Intercostal nerves

Diaphragm

Thoracic aorta

Splanchnic nerves
- Greater
- Lesser
- Least

Right sympathetic trunk (lumbar)

Right crus of diaphragm

Cervicothoracic (stellate) ganglion (inferior cervical and 1st thoracic ganglia)

Left vagus nerve

Left recurrent laryngeal nerve

Arch of aorta

Aortic plexus (thoracic)

Esophagus

Esophageal plexus

Left sympathetic trunk (thoracic)

Anterior vagal trunk

Posterior vagal trunk

Celiac ganglion

Celiac trunk

Subcostal nerve

Abdominal aorta

E. Anterior View

	Sympathetic
	Parasympathetic
	Mixed sympathetic and parasympathetic
	Somatic

1.77 OVERVIEW OF AUTONOMIC INNERVATION OF THE THORAX (*CONTINUED*)

Areas of thorax (superficial and deep):

☐ Drained by right lymphatic duct

☐ Drained by thoracic duct

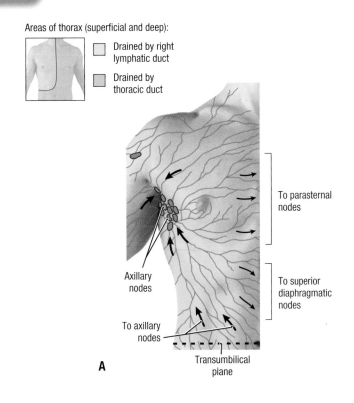

To parasternal nodes

Axillary nodes

To superior diaphragmatic nodes

To axillary nodes

Transumbilical plane

A

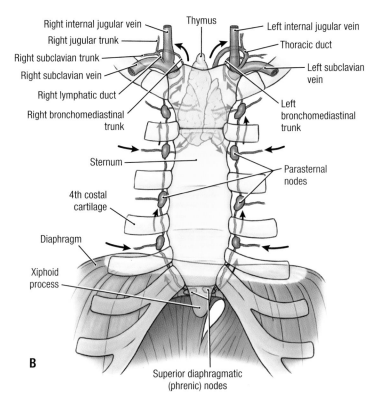

Right internal jugular vein

Right jugular trunk

Right subclavian trunk

Right subclavian vein

Right lymphatic duct

Right bronchomediastinal trunk

Thymus

Left internal jugular vein

Thoracic duct

Left subclavian vein

Left bronchomediastinal trunk

Sternum

4th costal cartilage

Diaphragm

Xiphoid process

Parasternal nodes

Superior diaphragmatic (phrenic) nodes

B

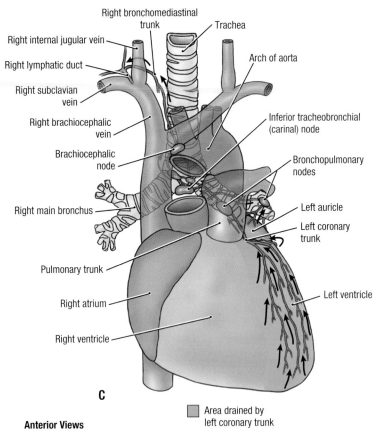

Right bronchomediastinal trunk

Right internal jugular vein

Right lymphatic duct

Right subclavian vein

Right brachiocephalic vein

Brachiocephalic node

Right main bronchus

Pulmonary trunk

Right atrium

Right ventricle

Trachea

Arch of aorta

Inferior tracheobronchial (carinal) node

Bronchopulmonary nodes

Left auricle

Left coronary trunk

Left ventricle

☐ Area drained by left coronary trunk

Anterior Views

C

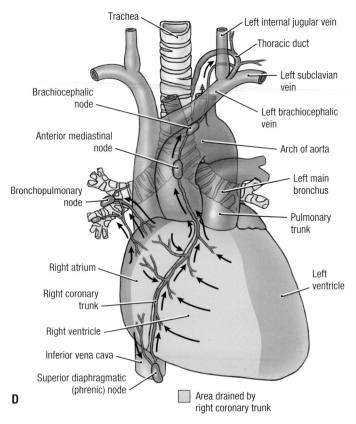

Trachea

Brachiocephalic node

Anterior mediastinal node

Bronchopulmonary node

Right atrium

Right coronary trunk

Right ventricle

Inferior vena cava

Superior diaphragmatic (phrenic) node

Left internal jugular vein

Thoracic duct

Left subclavian vein

Left brachiocephalic vein

Arch of aorta

Left main bronchus

Pulmonary trunk

Left ventricle

☐ Area drained by right coronary trunk

D

1.78   OVERVIEW OF LYMPHATIC DRAINAGE OF THORAX

A. Superficial lymphatic drainage. **B.** Deep lymphatic drainage of parasternal nodes. **C.** Lymphatic drainage of left side of heart. **D.** Lymphatic drainage of right side of heart.

E. Anterior View

Trachea
Esophagus
Left internal jugular vein
Paraesophageal node
Deep cervical node
Right internal jugular vein
Right jugular trunk
Left jugular trunk
Right subclavian trunk
Deep cervical node
Right lymphatic duct
Thoracic duct
Right subclavian vein
Left bronchomediastinal trunk
Right bronchomediastinal trunk
Left subclavian vein
Paratracheal nodes
Node of ligamentum arteriosum
Superior tracheobronchial node
Intrapulmonary nodes
Inferior tracheobronchial (carinal) node
Bronchopulmonary (hilar) node
Bronchopulmonary (hilar) nodes
Azygos vein
Intrapulmonary node
Pulmonary ligament
Paraesophageal node
Inferior vena cava
Descending aorta
Right phrenic nerve
To superior diaphragmatic (phrenic) nodes
Superior diaphragmatic (phrenic) nodes
Left phrenic nerve
Superior diaphragmatic (phrenic) node
Fibrous pericardium (cut edge)

Lymphatic drainage of esophagus to:
- Jugular trunks
- Bronchomediastinal trunks
- Superior diaphragmatic nodes
- Celiac (abdominal) nodes

F. Posteroinferior View

Left internal jugular vein
Right bronchomediastinal trunk
Trachea
Right internal jugular vein
Right subclavian vein
Left subclavian vein
Left bronchomediastinal trunk
Paratracheal node
Arch of aorta
Superior vena cava
Inferior tracheobronchial (carinal) nodes
Bronchopulmonary nodes
Bronchopulmonary node
Left pulmonary veins
Left atrium
Left coronary trunk
Right atrium
Superior diaphragmatic (phrenic) node
Left ventricle
Inferior vena cava
Right ventricle
Right coronary trunk

- Area drained by left coronary trunk
- Area drained by right coronary trunk

G. Anterior View

Right lymphatic duct
Left broncho-mediastinal trunk
Right bronchomediastinal trunk
Thoracic duct
Superior vena cava
Intercostal nodes
Azygos vein
Posterior intercostal vein
Prevertebral nodes
Prevertebral nodes
Intercostal node
Hemi-azygos vein
Diaphragm
Superior diaphragmatic (phrenic) node
Superior diaphragmatic (phrenic) node
Subcostal vein
Chyle cistern
Lymphatic drainage from abdomen and lower limbs

1.78 OVERVIEW OF LYMPHATIC DRAINAGE OF THORAX (*CONTINUED*)

E. Lymphatic drainage of lungs, esophagus, and superior surface of diaphragm. **F.** Lymphatic drainage of posterior and inferior surfaces of heart. **G.** Lymphatic drainage of posterior mediastinum.

AA	Ascending aorta
AI	Anterior interventricular artery
AZ	Azygos vein
CA	Cusp of aortic valve
CI	Confluence of internal jugular vein
DA	Descending aorta
DM	Deep back muscles
E	Esophagus
HR	Head of rib
HZ	Hemi-azygos vein
IT	Internal thoracic vessels
IVS	Interventricular septum
LA	Left atrium
LC	Left coronary artery
LCC	Left common carotid artery
LIJ	Left internal jugular vein
LL	Left lung
LM	Left main bronchus
LPA	Left pulmonary artery
LPV	Left pulmonary vein
LS	Left subclavian artery
LV	Left vertebral artery
M	Manubrium
P	Pericardium
PC	Pectoralis major
PI	Pulmonary infundibulum
PM	Papillary muscle
PT	Pulmonary trunk
RA	Right atrium
RBC	Right brachiocephalic vein
RCC	Right common carotid artery
RL	Right lung
RM	Right middle lobar bronchus
RPA	Right pulmonary artery
RPV	Right pulmonary vein
RSV	Right subclavian vein
RV	Right vertebral artery
S	Sternum
SC	Spinal cord
SP	Spinous process
ST	Sternoclavicular joint
SVC	Superior vena cava
T3-T10	Vertebral body
T	Trachea
TH	Thymus
VA	Vertebral artery

1.79

TRANSVERSE (AXIAL) MRIs
OF THORAX (A–F)

1.79   TRANSVERSE (AXIAL) MRIs OF THORAX (*CONTINUED*)

A

B

C

AA	Ascending aorta	IVC	Inferior vena cava	LU	Left auricle	RD	Right dome of diaphragm
AR	Arch of aorta	LA	Left atrium	LV	Left ventricle	RL	Right lung
AZ	Azygos vein	LCC	Left common carotid artery	PT	Pulmonary trunk	RV	Right ventricle
BT	Brachiocephalic trunk	LD	Left dome of diaphragm	RA	Right atrium	SVC	Superior vena cava
CD	Costodiaphragmatic recess	LL	Left lung	RBC	Right brachiocephalic vein	T	Trachea
DA	Descending aorta	LPA	Left pulmonary artery	RCC	Right common carotid artery	V	Vertebral body

1.80   CORONAL MRIs OF THORAX

A

AR	Arch of aorta
AA	Ascending aorta
DA	Descending aorta
F	Fat
IVC	Inferior vena cava
LA	Left atrium
LBC	Left brachiocephalic vein
LCC	Left common carotid artery
LL	Left lung
LM	Left main bronchus
LS	Left subclavian artery
LV	Left ventricle
P	Pericardium
RA	Right atrium
RL	Right lung
RM	Right main bronchus
RPA	Right pulmonary artery
RV	Right ventricle
SVC	Superior vena cava

B

1.81   SAGITTAL MRIs OF THORAX

A

B

AA	Ascending aorta
AZ	Azygos vein
DA	Descending aorta
E	Esophagus
ILPV	Inferior left pulmonary vein
IRPV	Inferior right pulmonary vein
IS	Interventricular septum
LA	Left atrium
LCA	Left coronary artery
LPA	Left pulmonary artery
LPV	Left pulmonary vein
LV	Left ventricle
MV	Mitral valve
PT	Pulmonary trunk
RA	Right atrium
RCA	Right coronary artery
RPA	Right pulmonary artery
RPV	Right pulmonary vein
RV	Right ventricle
SLPV	Superior left pulmonary vein
SRPV	Superior right pulmonary vein
SVC	Superior vena cava
V	Vertebra
ST	Sternum

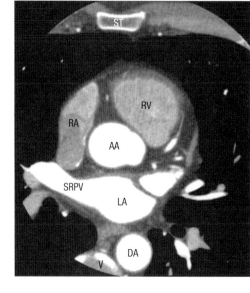

C

1.82   TRANSVERSE OR HORIZONTAL (AXIAL) 3D VOLUME RECONSTRUCTIONS (ON LEFT SIDE OF PAGE) AND CT ANGIOGRAMS OF THORAX (A–F)

TRANSVERSE OR HORIZONTAL (AXIAL) 3D VOLUME RECONSTRUCTIONS (ON LEFT SIDE OF PAGE) AND CT ANGIOGRAMS OF THORAX (A–F) (*CONTINUED*)

Abdomen

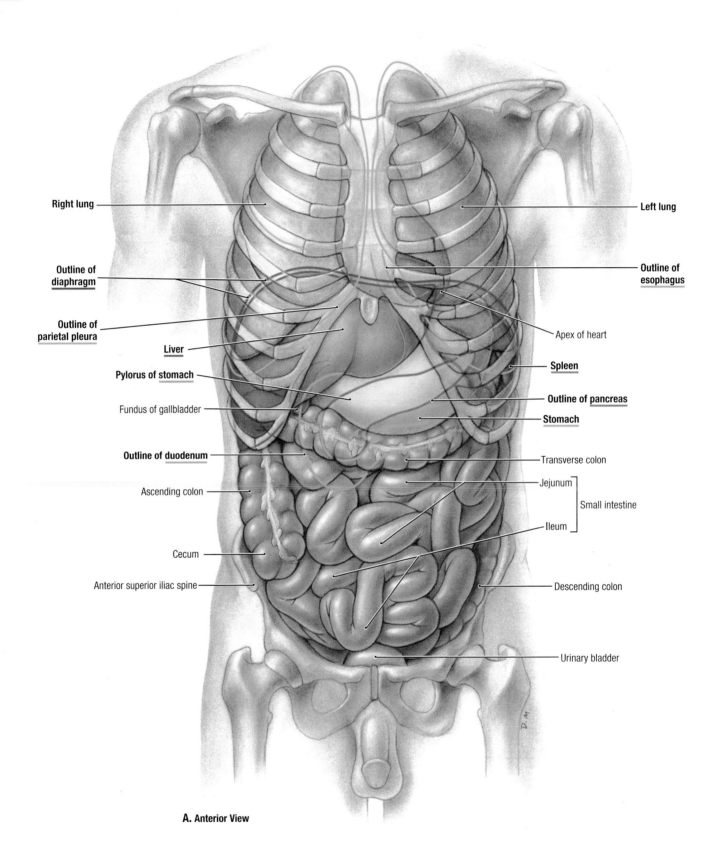

Right lung

Left lung

Outline of
diaphragm

Outline of
esophagus

Outline of
parietal pleura

Apex of heart

Liver

Spleen

Pylorus of stomach

Outline of pancreas

Fundus of gallbladder

Stomach

Outline of duodenum

Transverse colon

Ascending colon

Jejunum

Small intestine

Ileum

Cecum

Anterior superior iliac spine

Descending colon

Urinary bladder

A. Anterior View

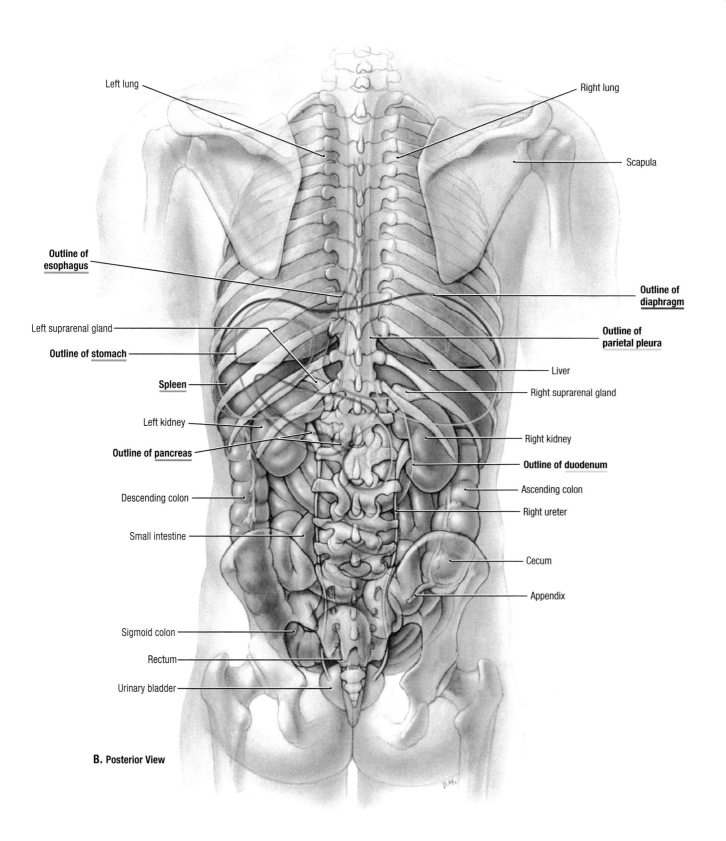

Left lung

Right lung

Scapula

Outline of esophagus

Outline of diaphragm

Left suprarenal gland

Outline of parietal pleura

Outline of stomach

Liver

Spleen

Right suprarenal gland

Left kidney

Right kidney

Outline of pancreas

Outline of duodenum

Descending colon

Ascending colon

Right ureter

Small intestine

Cecum

Appendix

Sigmoid colon

Rectum

Urinary bladder

B. Posterior View

2.1 ABDOMINAL VISCERA IN SITU (*CONTINUED*)

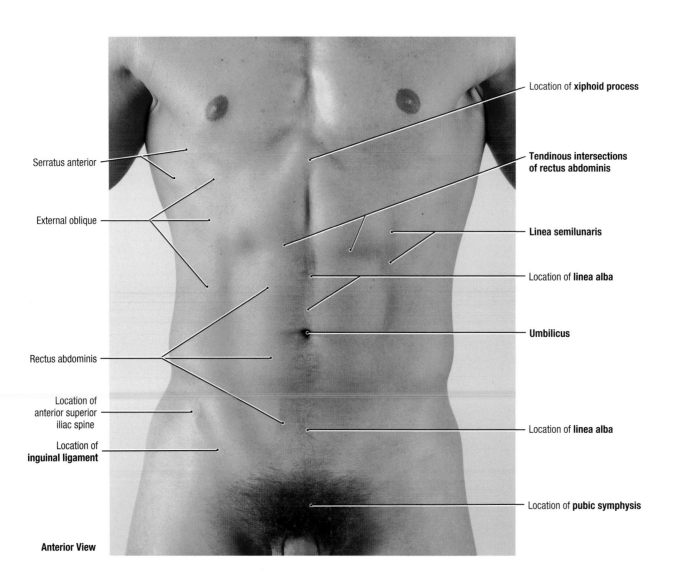

Location of **xiphoid process**

Serratus anterior

Tendinous intersections of rectus abdominis

External oblique

Linea semilunaris

Location of **linea alba**

Rectus abdominis

Umbilicus

Location of anterior superior iliac spine

Location of **linea alba**

Location of **inguinal ligament**

Location of **pubic symphysis**

Anterior View

2.2 SURFACE ANATOMY

A. Surface features.
- The umbilicus is where the umbilical cord entered the fetus and indicates the anterior level of the T10 dermatome, typically at the level of the IV disc between the L3 and L4 vertebrae.
- The linea alba is a fibrous band extending from the xiphoid process to the pubic symphysis that is demarcated superficially by a midline vertical skin groove as far inferiorly as the umbilicus.

- Curved skin grooves, the linea semilunaris, demarcate the lateral borders of the rectus abdominis muscle and rectus sheath.
- In lean individuals with good muscle development, three transverse skin grooves overlie the tendinous intersections of the rectus abdominis muscle.
- The site of the inguinal ligament is indicated by a skin crease, the inguinal groove, just inferior and parallel to the ligament, marking the division between the anterolateral abdominal wall and the thigh.

Abdominal Quadrants:

RUQ Right upper quadrant ⎯⎯⎯ Median plane
LUQ Left upper quadrant ⎯⎯⎯ Transumbilical plane
RLQ Right lower quadrant
LLQ Left lower quadrant

Abdominal Regions:

RH Right hypochondrium   LH Left hypochondrium
RL Right flank (lateral region)   LL Left flank (lateral region)
RI Right inguinal (groin)   LI Left inguinal (groin)

E Epigastric   ⎯⎯⎯ Midclavicular plane
U Umbilical   ⎯⎯⎯ Transtubercular plane
P Pubic   ⎯⎯⎯ Subcostal plane

Right upper quadrant (RUQ)	Left upper quadrant (LUQ)
Liver: right lobe	Liver: left lobe
Gallbladder	Spleen
Stomach: pylorus	Stomach
Duodenum: parts 1-3	Jejunum and proximal ileum
Pancreas: head	Pancreas: body and tail
Right suprarenal gland	Left kidney
Right kidney	Left suprarenal gland
Right colic (hepatic) flexure	Left colic (splenic) flexure
Ascending colon: superior part	Transverse colon: left half
Transverse colon: right half	Descending colon: superior part

Right lower quadrant (RLQ)	Left lower quadrant (LLQ)
Cecum	Sigmoid colon
Appendix	Descending colon: inferior part
Most of ileum	Left ovary
Ascending colon: inferior part	Left uterine tube
Right ovary	Left ureter: abdominal part
Right uterine tube	Left spermatic cord:
Right ureter: abdominal part	abdominal part
Right spermatic cord:	Uterus (if enlarged)
abdominal part	Urinary bladder (if very full)
Uterus (if enlarged)	
Urinary bladder (if very full)	

2.3 **ABDOMINAL REGIONS AND QUADRANTS**

A. Quadrants. **B.** Regions. It is important to know what organs are located in each abdominal region or quadrant so that one knows where to auscultate, percuss, and palpate them and to record the locations of findings during a physical exam.

The six common causes of **abdominal protrusion** begin with the letter F: food, fluid, fat, feces, flatus, and fetus. Eversion of the umbilicus may be a sign of increased intra-abdominal pressure, usually resulting from ascites (abdominal accumulation of serous fluid in the peritoneal cavity), or a large mass (e.g., a tumor, fetus, or enlarged organ such as the liver [hepatomegaly]).

Warm hands are important when palpating the abdominal wall because cold hands make the anterolateral abdominal muscles tense, producing involuntary muscle spasms known as guarding. Intense guarding, boardlike reflexive muscular rigidity that cannot be willfully suppressed, occurs during palpation when an organ (such as the appendix) is inflamed and in itself constitutes a clinically significant sign of **acute abdomen.** The involuntary muscular spasms attempt to protect the viscera from pressure, which is painful when an abdominal infection is present. The common nerve supply of the skin and muscles of the wall explains why these spasms occur.

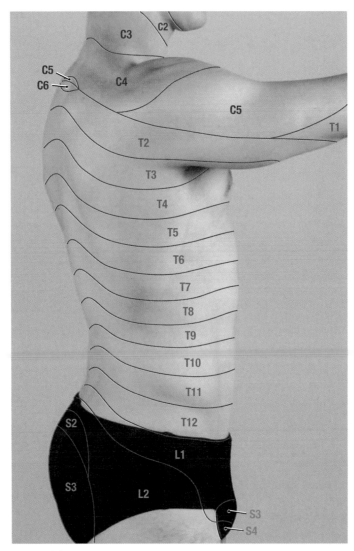

Lateral View

2.4   DERMATOMES

The thoraco-abdominal (T7–T11) nerves run between the external and internal oblique muscles to supply sensory innervation to the overlying skin. The T10 nerve supplies the region of the umbilicus. The subcostal nerve (T12) runs along the inferior border of the 12th rib to supply the skin over the anterior superior iliac spine and hip. The iliohypogastric nerve (L1) innervates the skin over the iliac crest and hypogastric region and the ilio-inguinal nerve (L1) the skin of the medial aspect of the thigh, the scrotum or labium majus, and mons pubis.

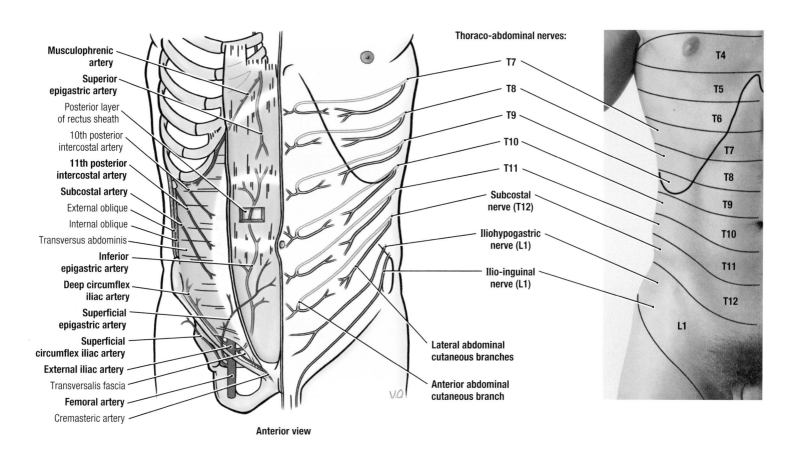

Musculophrenic artery

Superior epigastric artery

Posterior layer of rectus sheath

10th posterior intercostal artery

11th posterior intercostal artery

Subcostal artery

External oblique

Internal oblique

Transversus abdominis

Inferior epigastric artery

Deep circumflex iliac artery

Superficial epigastric artery

Superficial circumflex iliac artery

External iliac artery

Transversalis fascia

Femoral artery

Cremasteric artery

Anterior view

Thoraco-abdominal nerves:

T7

T8

T9

T10

T11

Subcostal nerve (T12)

Iliohypogastric nerve (L1)

Ilio-inguinal nerve (L1)

Lateral abdominal cutaneous branches

Anterior abdominal cutaneous branch

T4, T5, T6, T7, T8, T9, T10, T11, T12, L1

2.5   ARTERIES AND NERVES OF ANTEROLATERAL ABDOMINAL WALL

The skin and muscles of the anterolateral abdominal wall are supplied mainly by the:

- Thoraco-abdominal nerves: distal, abdominal parts of the anterior rami of the inferior six thoracic spinal nerves (T7–T11), which have muscular branches and anterior and lateral abdominal cutaneous branches. The anterior abdominal cutaneous branches pierce the rectus sheath a short distance from the median plane, after the rectus abdominis muscle has been supplied. Spinal nerves T7–T9 supply the skin superior to the umbilicus; T10 innervates the skin around the umbilicus.
- Subcostal nerve: large anterior ramus of spinal nerve T12.
- Iliohypogastric and ilio-inguinal nerves: terminal branches of the anterior ramus of spinal nerve L1.
- Spinal nerve T11, plus the cutaneous branches of the subcostal (T12), iliohypogastric, and ilio-inguinal (L1) nerves: supply the skin inferior to the umbilicus.

The blood vessels of the anterolateral abdominal wall are the:
- Superior epigastric vessels and branches of the musculophrenic vessels from the internal thoracic vessels.

- Inferior epigastric and deep circumflex iliac vessels from the external iliac vessels.
- Superficial circumflex iliac and superficial epigastric vessels from the femoral artery and great saphenous vein.
- Posterior intercostal vessels in the 11th intercostal space and anterior branches of subcostal vessels.

Incisional nerve injury. The inferior thoracic spinal nerves (T7–T12) and the iliohypogastric and ilio-inguinal nerves (L1) approach the abdominal musculature separately to provide the multisegmental innervation of the abdominal muscles. Thus they are distributed across the anterolateral abdominal wall, where they run oblique but mostly horizontal courses. They are susceptible to injury in surgical incisions or from trauma at any level of the abdominal wall. Injury to them may result in weakening of the muscles. In the inguinal region, such a weakness may predispose an individual to development of an inguinal hernia.

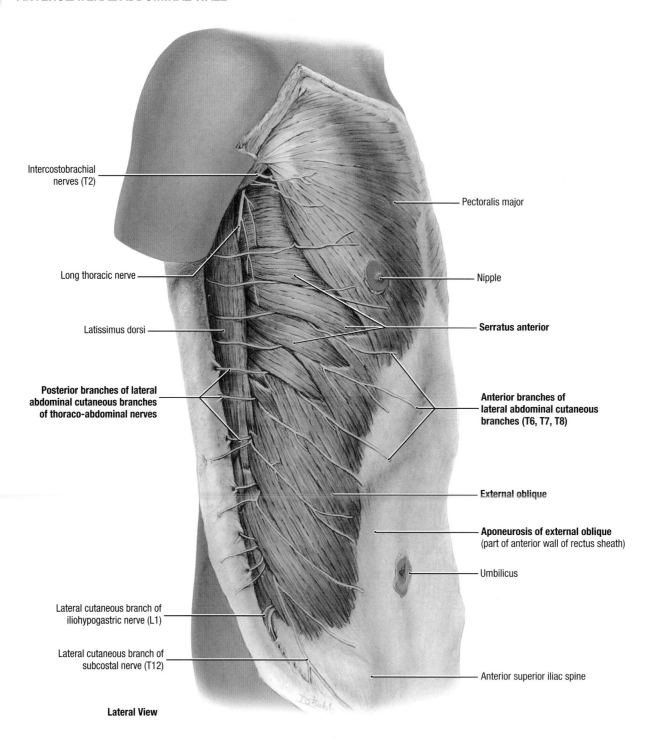

Intercostobrachial nerves (T2)

Pectoralis major

Long thoracic nerve

Nipple

Latissimus dorsi

Serratus anterior

Posterior branches of lateral abdominal cutaneous branches of thoraco-abdominal nerves

Anterior branches of lateral abdominal cutaneous branches (T6, T7, T8)

External oblique

Aponeurosis of external oblique (part of anterior wall of rectus sheath)

Umbilicus

Lateral cutaneous branch of iliohypogastric nerve (L1)

Lateral cutaneous branch of subcostal nerve (T12)

Anterior superior iliac spine

Lateral View

2.6   **ANTEROLATERAL ABDOMINAL WALL, SUPERFICIAL DISSECTION**

The muscular portion of the external oblique muscle interdigitates with slips of the serratus anterior muscle, and the aponeurotic portion contributes to the anterior wall of the rectus sheath. The anterior and posterior branches of the lateral abdominal cutaneous branches of the thoraco-abdominal nerves course superficially in the subcutaneous tissue.

- **Umbilical hernias** are usually small protrusions of extraperitoneal fat and/or peritoneum and omentum and sometimes bowel. They result from increased intra-abdominal pressure in the presence of weakness

or incomplete closure of the anterior abdominal wall after ligation of the umbilical cord at birth, or may be acquired later, most commonly in women and obese people.

- The lines along which the fibers of the abdominal aponeurosis interlace (see Fig. 2.10A,B,D) are also potential sites of herniation. These gaps may be congenital, the result of the stresses of obesity and aging, or the consequence of surgical or traumatic wounds.

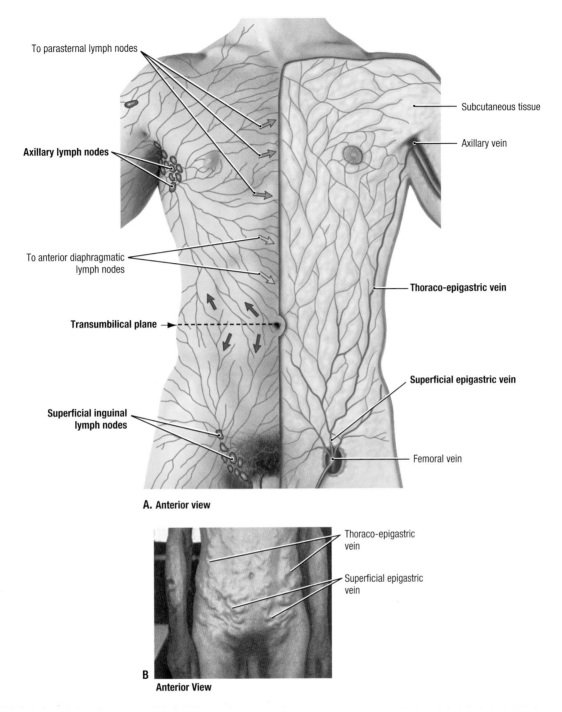

To parasternal lymph nodes

Axillary lymph nodes

To anterior diaphragmatic
lymph nodes

Transumbilical plane →

**Superficial inguinal
lymph nodes**

Subcutaneous tissue

Axillary vein

Thoraco-epigastric vein

Superficial epigastric vein

Femoral vein

A. Anterior view

Thoraco-epigastric
vein

Superficial epigastric
vein

B

Anterior View

2.7   LYMPHATIC DRAINAGE AND SUBCUTANEOUS (SUPERFICIAL) VENOUS DRAINAGE OF ANTEROLATERAL ABDOMINAL WALL

A. Overview.

- The skin and subcutaneous tissue of the abdominal wall are served by an intricate subcutaneous venous plexus, draining superiorly to the internal thoracic vein medially and the lateral thoracic vein laterally and inferiorly to the superficial and inferior epigastric veins, tributaries of the femoral and external iliac veins, respectively.
- Superficial lymphatic vessels accompany the subcutaneous veins; those superior to the transumbilical plane drain mainly to the axillary lymph nodes; however, a few drain to the parasternal lymph nodes. Superficial lymphatic vessels inferior to the transumbilical plane drain to the superficial inguinal lymph nodes.

B. Enlargement of subcutaneous veins.

- **Liposuction** is a surgical method for removing unwanted subcutaneous fat using a percutaneously placed suction tube and high vacuum pressure. The tubes are inserted subdermally through small skin incisions.
- When flow in the superior or inferior vena cava is obstructed, anastomoses between the tributaries of these systemic veins, such as the thoraco-epigastric vein, may provide **collateral pathways** by which the obstruction may be bypassed, allowing blood to return to the heart. The veins become enlarged and tortuous **(B).**

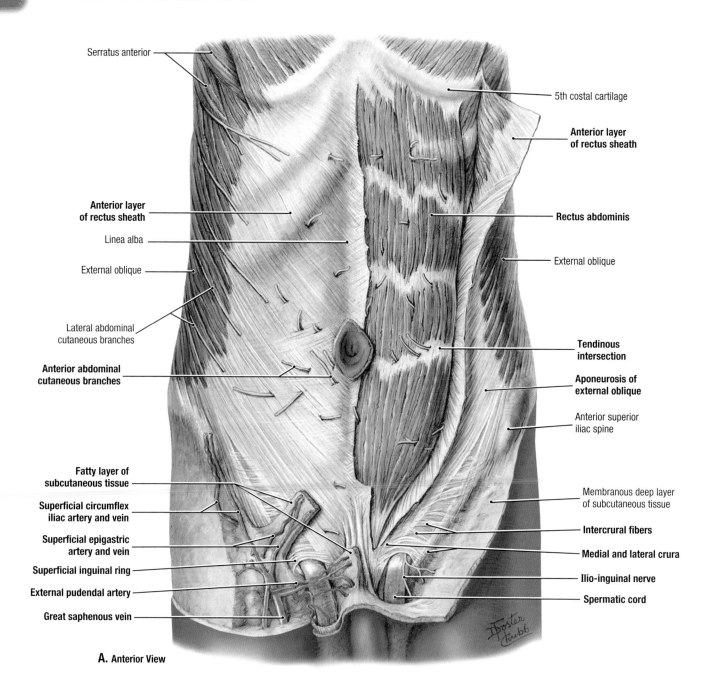

Serratus anterior

5th costal cartilage

Anterior layer of rectus sheath

Anterior layer of rectus sheath

Linea alba

External oblique

Rectus abdominis

External oblique

Lateral abdominal cutaneous branches

Anterior abdominal cutaneous branches

Tendinous intersection

Aponeurosis of external oblique

Anterior superior iliac spine

Fatty layer of subcutaneous tissue

Membranous deep layer of subcutaneous tissue

Superficial circumflex iliac artery and vein

Intercrural fibers

Superficial epigastric artery and vein

Medial and lateral crura

Superficial inguinal ring

Ilio-inguinal nerve

External pudendal artery

Spermatic cord

Great saphenous vein

A. Anterior View

2.8 ANTERIOR ABDOMINAL WALL

A. Superficial dissection demonstrating the relationship of the cutaneous nerves and superficial vessels to the musculoaponeurotic structures. The anterior wall of the left rectus sheath is reflected, revealing the rectus abdominis muscle, segmented by tendinous intersections.

- After the T7 to T12 spinal nerves supply the muscles, their anterior abdominal cutaneous branches emerge from the rectus abdominis muscle and pierce the anterior wall of its sheath.
- The three superficial inguinal branches of the femoral artery (superficial circumflex iliac artery, superficial epigastric artery, and external pudendal

artery) and the great saphenous vein lie in the fatty layer of subcutaneous tissue.

- The fibers of the external oblique aponeurosis separate into medial and lateral crura, which, with the intercrural fibers that unite them, form the superficial inguinal ring. The spermatic cord of the male (shown here), or round ligament of the female, exits the inguinal canal through the superficial inguinal ring along with the ilio-inguinal nerve.

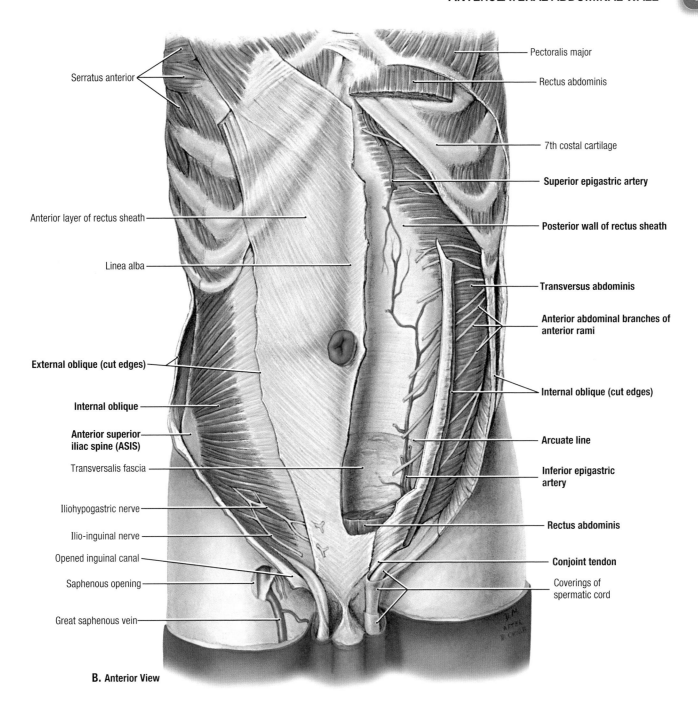

Serratus anterior

Anterior layer of rectus sheath

Linea alba

External oblique (cut edges)

Internal oblique

Anterior superior iliac spine (ASIS)

Transversalis fascia

Iliohypogastric nerve

Ilio-inguinal nerve

Opened inguinal canal

Saphenous opening

Great saphenous vein

Pectoralis major

Rectus abdominis

7th costal cartilage

Superior epigastric artery

Posterior wall of rectus sheath

Transversus abdominis

Anterior abdominal branches of anterior rami

Internal oblique (cut edges)

Arcuate line

Inferior epigastric artery

Rectus abdominis

Conjoint tendon

Coverings of spermatic cord

B. Anterior View

2.8   ANTERIOR ABDOMINAL WALL (*CONTINUED*)

B. Deep dissection. On the right side of the specimen, most of the external oblique muscle is excised. On the left, the internal oblique muscle is divided and the rectus abdominis muscle is excised, revealing the posterior wall of the rectus sheath.

- The fibers of the internal oblique muscle run horizontally at the level of the anterior superior iliac spine (ASIS), obliquely upward superior to the ASIS, and obliquely downward inferior to the ASIS.
- The arcuate line is at the level of the ASIS; inferior to the line, only transversalis fascia lies posterior to the rectus abdominis muscle.

- Initially, the anterior abdominal branches of the anterior rami course between the internal oblique and transversus abdominis muscles.
- The anastomosis between the superior and inferior epigastric arteries indirectly unites the subclavian artery of the upper limb to the external iliac arteries of the lower limb. The anastomosis can become functionally patent in response to **slowly developing occlusion of the aorta.**

A. Lateral View

B. Lateral View

C. Lateral View

D. Anterior View

E. Lateral View

2.9   MUSCLES OF ANTEROLATERAL ABDOMINAL WALL

A. External oblique. **B.** Internal oblique. **C.** Transversus abdominis. **D. and E.** Rectus abdominis and pyramidalis.

TABLE 2.1 PRINCIPAL MUSCLES OF ANTEROLATERAL ABDOMINAL WALL

Muscles[a]	Origin	Insertion	Innervation	Action(s)
External oblique **(A)**	External surfaces of 5th–12th ribs	Linea alba, pubic tubercle, and anterior half of iliac crest	Thoraco-abdominal nerves (anterior rami of T7–T11) and subcostal nerve	Compresses and supports abdominal viscera; flexes and rotates trunk
Internal oblique **(B)**	Thoracolumbar fascia, anterior two thirds of iliac crest, and connective tissue deep to inguinal ligament	Inferior borders of 10th–12th ribs, linea alba, and pubis via conjoint tendon	Thoraco-abdominal nerves (anterior rami of T7–T11), subcostal nerve, and first lumbar nerve	
Transversus abdominis **(C)**	Internal surfaces of 7th–12th costal cartilages, thoracolumbar fascia, iliac crest, and connective tissue deep to inguinal ligament (iliopsoas fascia)	Linea alba with aponeurosis of internal oblique, pubic crest, and pectin pubis via conjoint tendon		Compresses and supports abdominal viscera (external oblique ipsilaterally, internal oblique contralaterally)
Rectus abdominis **(D)**	Pubic symphysis and pubic crest	Xiphoid process and 5th–7th costal cartilages	Thoraco-abdominal nerves (T7–T11) and subcostal nerve	Flexes trunk (lumbar vertebrae) and compresses abdominal viscera;[b] stabilizes and controls tilt of pelvis (antilordosis)

[a]Approximately 80% of people have a *pyramidalis muscle,* which is located in the rectus sheath anterior to the most inferior part of the rectus abdominis. It extends from the pubic crest of the hip bone to the linea alba. This small muscle tenses the linea alba.
[b]In so doing, these muscles act as antagonists of the diaphragm to produce expiration.

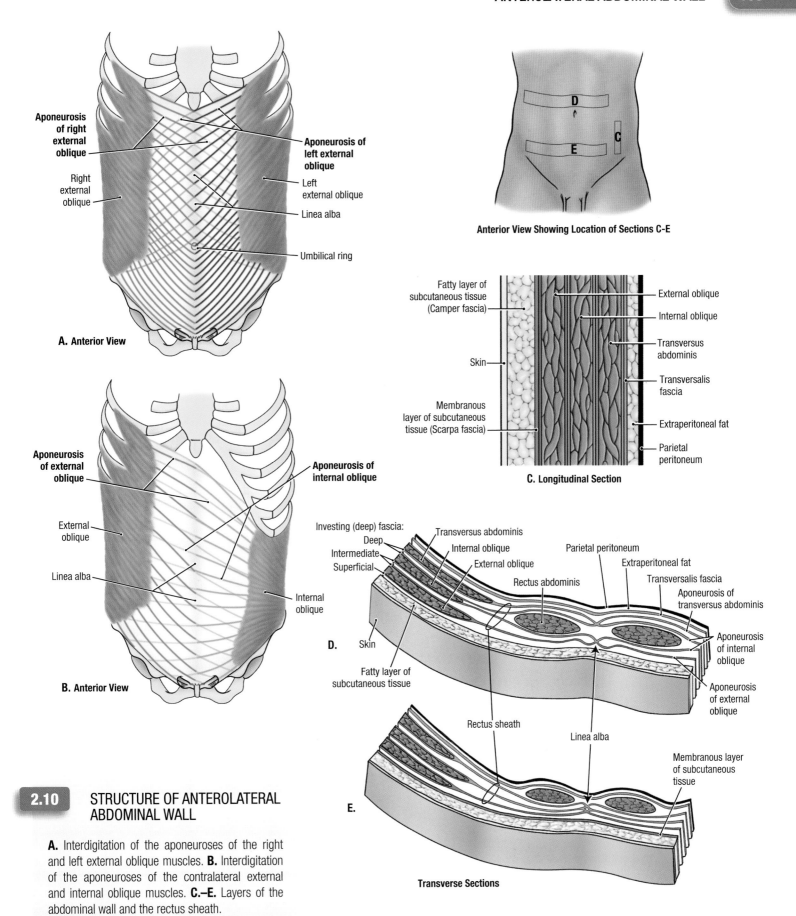

A. Anterior View

Aponeurosis of right external oblique

Right external oblique

Aponeurosis of left external oblique

Left external oblique

Linea alba

Umbilical ring

B. Anterior View

Aponeurosis of external oblique

External oblique

Linea alba

Aponeurosis of internal oblique

Internal oblique

Anterior View Showing Location of Sections C-E

C. Longitudinal Section

Fatty layer of subcutaneous tissue (Camper fascia)

Skin

Membranous layer of subcutaneous tissue (Scarpa fascia)

External oblique

Internal oblique

Transversus abdominis

Transversalis fascia

Extraperitoneal fat

Parietal peritoneum

D.

Investing (deep) fascia:
Deep
Intermediate
Superficial

Skin

Fatty layer of subcutaneous tissue

Transversus abdominis

Internal oblique

External oblique

Rectus abdominis

Rectus sheath

Parietal peritoneum

Extraperitoneal fat

Transversalis fascia

Aponeurosis of transversus abdominis

Aponeurosis of internal oblique

Aponeurosis of external oblique

Linea alba

E.

Membranous layer of subcutaneous tissue

Transverse Sections

2.10

STRUCTURE OF ANTEROLATERAL ABDOMINAL WALL

A. Interdigitation of the aponeuroses of the right and left external oblique muscles. **B.** Interdigitation of the aponeuroses of the contralateral external and internal oblique muscles. **C.–E.** Layers of the abdominal wall and the rectus sheath.

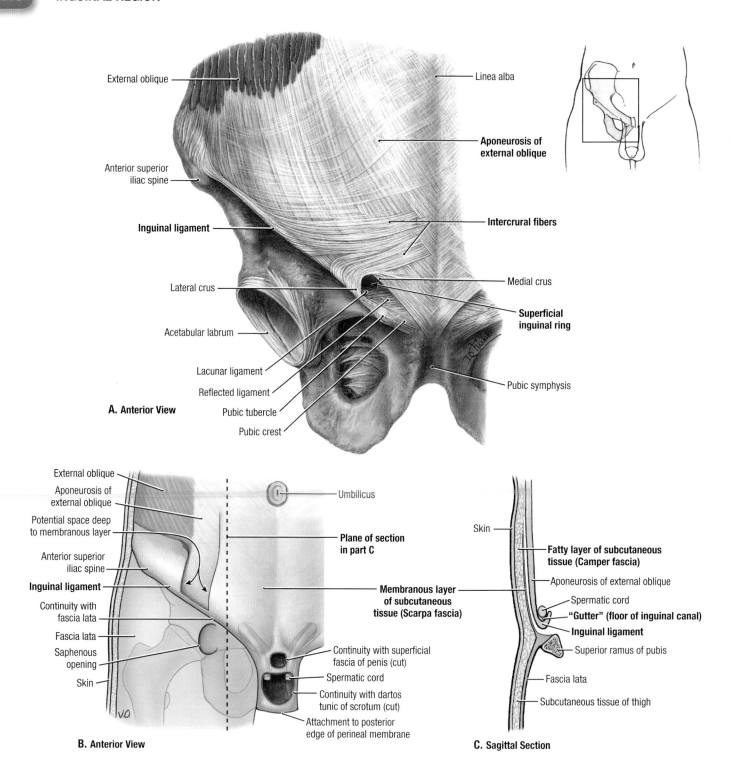

A. Anterior View

External oblique

Anterior superior iliac spine

Inguinal ligament

Lateral crus

Acetabular labrum

Lacunar ligament

Reflected ligament

Pubic tubercle

Pubic crest

Linea alba

Aponeurosis of external oblique

Intercrural fibers

Medial crus

Superficial inguinal ring

Pubic symphysis

B. Anterior View

External oblique

Aponeurosis of external oblique

Potential space deep to membranous layer

Anterior superior iliac spine

Inguinal ligament

Continuity with fascia lata

Fascia lata

Saphenous opening

Skin

Umbilicus

Plane of section in part C

Membranous layer of subcutaneous tissue (Scarpa fascia)

Continuity with superficial fascia of penis (cut)

Spermatic cord

Continuity with dartos tunic of scrotum (cut)

Attachment to posterior edge of perineal membrane

C. Sagittal Section

Skin

Fatty layer of subcutaneous tissue (Camper fascia)

Aponeurosis of external oblique

Spermatic cord

"Gutter" (floor of inguinal canal)

Inguinal ligament

Superior ramus of pubis

Fascia lata

Subcutaneous tissue of thigh

2.11   **INGUINAL REGION OF MALE I**

A. Formations of the aponeurosis of the external oblique muscle. **B. and C.** Membranous (deep) layer of subcutaneous tissue. Inferior to the umbilicus, the subcutaneous tissue is composed of two layers: a superficial fatty layer and a deep membranous layer. Laterally, the membranous layer fuses with the fascia lata of the thigh about a finger's breadth inferior to the inguinal ligament. Medially, it fuses with the linea alba and pubic symphysis in the midline, and inferiorly, it continues as the membranous layer of the subcutaneous tissue of the perineum and penis and the dartos fascia of the scrotum. The inferior margin of the external oblique aponeurosis is thickened and turned internally forming the inguinal ligament. The superior surface of the in-turning inguinal ligament forms a shallow trough or "gutter" that is the floor of the inguinal canal.

External oblique

Internal oblique

Iliohypogastric nerve

Ilio-inguinal nerve

Aponeurosis of external oblique

Inguinal ligament

Cremaster muscle

Saphenous opening (falciform margin)

Inguinal lymph nodes

Linea alba

Anterior layer of rectus sheath

Conjoint tendon

Fundiform ligament of penis

Reflected ligament

Medial crus
Intercrural fibers — Of aponeurosis of external oblique
Lateral crus

Superficial inguinal ring

A. Anterior View

Spermatic cord (cut ends)

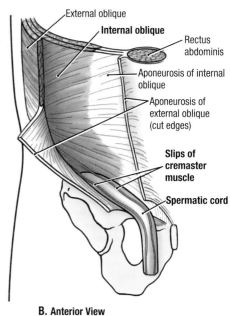

External oblique
Internal oblique
Rectus abdominis
Aponeurosis of internal oblique
Aponeurosis of external oblique (cut edges)
Slips of cremaster muscle
Spermatic cord

B. Anterior View

2.12 INGUINAL REGION OF MALE II

A. Internal oblique and cremaster muscle. Part of the aponeurosis of the external oblique muscle is cut away, and the spermatic cord is cut short. **B.** Schematic illustration.

- The cremaster muscle covers the spermatic cord.
- The reflected ligament is formed by aponeurotic fibers of the external oblique muscle and lies anterior to the conjoint tendon. The conjoint tendon is formed by the fusion of the aponeurosis of the internal oblique and transversus abdominis muscles.
- The cutaneous branches of the iliohypogastric and ilio-inguinal nerves (L1) course between the internal and external oblique muscles and must be avoided when an **appendectomy (gridiron) incision** is made in this region.

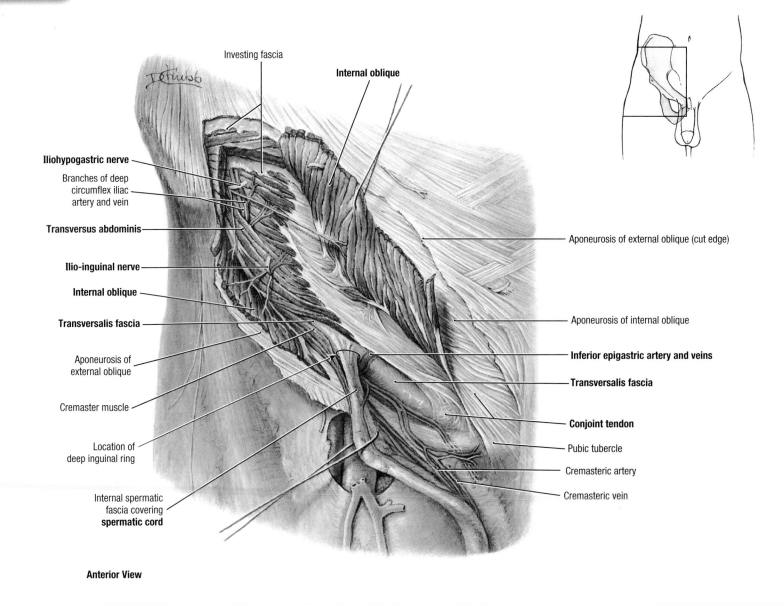

Investing fascia

Internal oblique

Iliohypogastric nerve

Branches of deep
circumflex iliac
artery and vein

Transversus abdominis

Ilio-inguinal nerve

Internal oblique

Transversalis fascia

Aponeurosis of
external oblique

Cremaster muscle

Location of
deep inguinal ring

Internal spermatic
fascia covering
spermatic cord

Aponeurosis of external oblique (cut edge)

Aponeurosis of internal oblique

Inferior epigastric artery and veins

Transversalis fascia

Conjoint tendon

Pubic tubercle

Cremasteric artery

Cremasteric vein

Anterior View

2.13   INGUINAL REGION OF MALE III

The internal oblique muscle is reflected, and the spermatic cord is retracted.
- The internal oblique muscle portion of the conjoint tendon is attached to the pubic crest, and the transversus abdominis portion to the pectineal line.
- The iliohypogastric and ilio-inguinal nerves (L1) supply the internal oblique and transversus abdominis muscles.

- The transversalis fascia is evaginated to form the tubular internal spermatic fascia. The mouth of the tube, called the deep inguinal ring, is situated lateral to the inferior epigastric vessels.

TABLE 2.2 BOUNDARIES OF INGUINAL CANAL

Boundary	Deep Ring/Lateral Third	Middle Third	Lateral Third/Superficial Ring
Posterior wall	Transversalis fascia	Transversalis fascia	Inguinal falx (conjoint tendon) plus reflected inguinal ligament
Anterior wall	Internal oblique plus lateral crus of aponeurosis of external oblique	Aponeurosis of external oblique (lateral crus and intercrural fibers)	Aponeurosis of external oblique (intercrural fibers), with fascia of external oblique continuing onto cord as external spermatic fascia
Roof	Transversalis fascia	Musculoa-poneurotic arches of internal oblique and transversus abdominis	Medial crus of aponeurosis of external oblique
Floor	Iliopubic tract	Inguinal ligament	Lacunar ligament

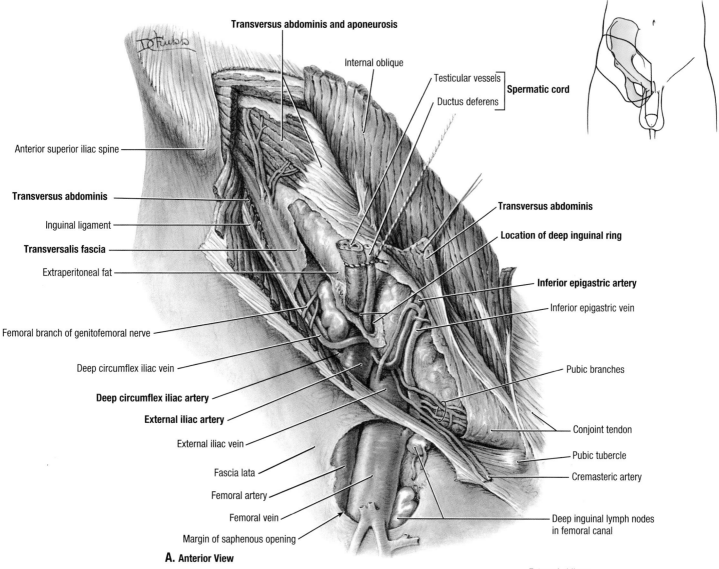

Transversus abdominis and aponeurosis

Internal oblique

Testicular vessels ⎤
Ductus deferens ⎦ **Spermatic cord**

Anterior superior iliac spine

Transversus abdominis

Inguinal ligament

Transversalis fascia

Extraperitoneal fat

Femoral branch of genitofemoral nerve

Deep circumflex iliac vein

Deep circumflex iliac artery

External iliac artery

External iliac vein

Fascia lata

Femoral artery

Femoral vein

Margin of saphenous opening

Transversus abdominis

Location of deep inguinal ring

Inferior epigastric artery

Inferior epigastric vein

Pubic branches

Conjoint tendon

Pubic tubercle

Cremasteric artery

Deep inguinal lymph nodes in femoral canal

A. Anterior View

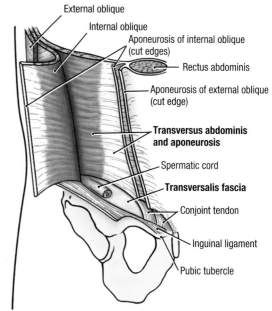

External oblique

Internal oblique

Aponeurosis of internal oblique (cut edges)

Rectus abdominis

Aponeurosis of external oblique (cut edge)

Transversus abdominis and aponeurosis

Spermatic cord

Transversalis fascia

Conjoint tendon

Inguinal ligament

Pubic tubercle

B. Anterior View

2.14   ## INGUINAL REGION OF MALE IV

A. The inguinal part of the transversus abdominis muscle and transversalis fascia is partially cut away, the spermatic cord is excised, and the ductus deferens is retracted.
B. Schematic illustration.
- The deep inguinal ring is located superior to the inguinal ligament at the midpoint between the anterior superior iliac spine and pubic tubercle.
- The external iliac artery has two branches, the deep circumflex iliac and inferior epigastric arteries. Note also the cremasteric artery and pubic branch arising from the latter.

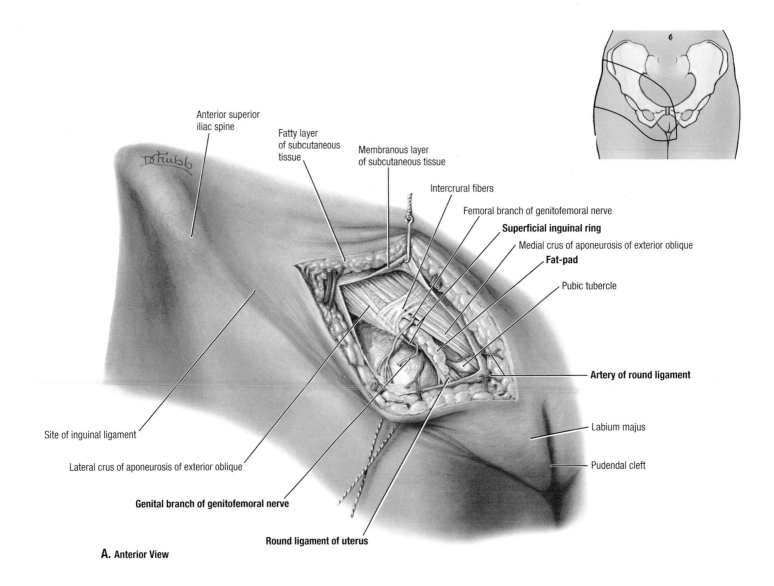

Anterior superior
iliac spine

Fatty layer
of subcutaneous
tissue

Membranous layer
of subcutaneous tissue

Intercrural fibers

Femoral branch of genitofemoral nerve

Superficial inguinal ring

Medial crus of aponeurosis of exterior oblique

Fat-pad

Pubic tubercle

Artery of round ligament

Labium majus

Pudendal cleft

Site of inguinal ligament

Lateral crus of aponeurosis of exterior oblique

Genital branch of genitofemoral nerve

Round ligament of uterus

A. Anterior View

2.15 INGUINAL CANAL OF FEMALE

Progressive dissections of the female inguinal canal **(A.–D)**.

- In **A,** the superficial inguinal ring is small. Passing through the superficial inguinal ring are the round ligament of the uterus, a closely applied fat pad, the genital branch of the genitofemoral nerve, and the artery of the round ligament of the uterus. The ilio-inguinal nerve may also pass through the ring.
- The round ligament breaks up into strands as it leaves the inguinal canal and approaches the labium majus **(C)**.
- The external iliac artery and vein are exposed deep to the inguinal canal by excising the transversalis fascia **(D)**.

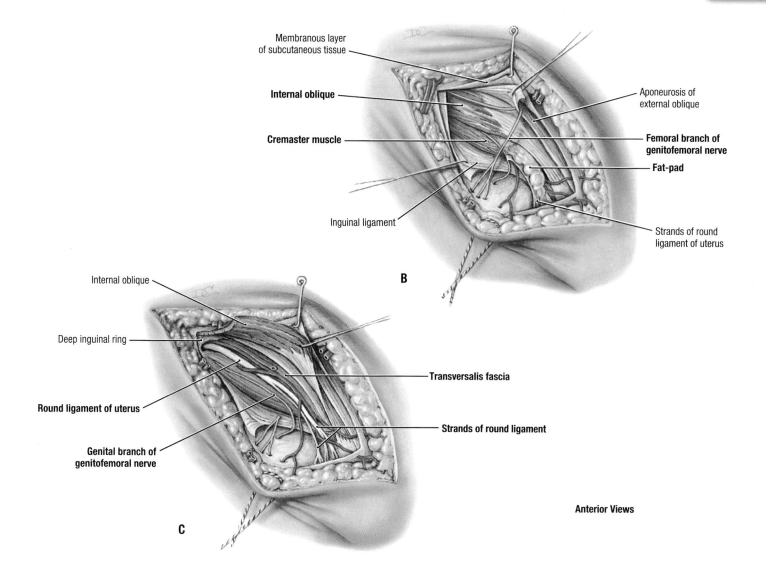

Membranous layer
of subcutaneous tissue

Internal oblique

Aponeurosis of
external oblique

Cremaster muscle

**Femoral branch of
genitofemoral nerve**

Fat-pad

Inguinal ligament

Strands of round
ligament of uterus

B

Internal oblique

Deep inguinal ring

Transversalis fascia

Round ligament of uterus

Strands of round ligament

**Genital branch of
genitofemoral nerve**

Anterior Views

C

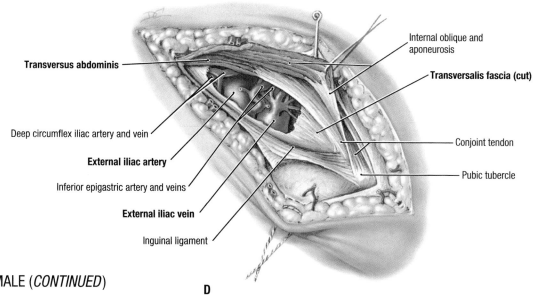

Transversus abdominis

Internal oblique and
aponeurosis

Transversalis fascia (cut)

Deep circumflex iliac artery and vein

External iliac artery

Conjoint tendon

Inferior epigastric artery and veins

Pubic tubercle

External iliac vein

Inguinal ligament

2.15   INGUINAL CANAL OF FEMALE (*CONTINUED*)   D

External oblique (cut edges)

Internal oblique

Posterior layer of rectus sheath

Iliohypogastric nerve

Ilio-inguinal nerve

Fascia lata

Femoral branches of genitofemoral nerve

Edge of saphenous opening

Femoral sheath

Genital branch of genitofemoral nerve to scrotal wall

Great saphenous vein

12th thoracic nerve

Inferior epigastric artery

Iliohypogastric nerve

Internal oblique

Transversus abdominis

Ascending branch of deep circumflex iliac artery

Femoral branch of genitofemoral nerve

Deep inguinal ring

Inferior epigastric artery

Genital branch of genitofemoral nerve to cremaster

Cremasteric artery

Conjoint tendon

Internal spermatic fascia

Cremaster

External spermatic fascia

A. Anterior View

Aponeurosis of external oblique (cut edge)

Internal oblique and aponeurosis

Conjoint tendon

Cremaster

Suspensory ligament of penis

Internal oblique (reflected)

Transversus abdominis

Arch of transversus abdominis

Transversalis fascia

Internal spermatic fascia

Cremaster muscle and fascia

Conjoint tendon

External spermatic fascia

Cremaster and fascia

Internal spermatic fascia

Tunica vaginalis (parietal layer)

Epididymis (head)

Tunica vaginalis (visceral layer) covering testis

B. Anterior View

2.16 INGUINAL CANAL, SPERMATIC CORD, AND TESTIS

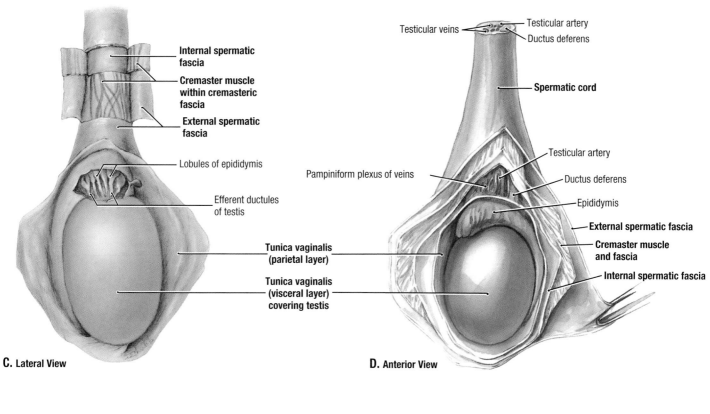

C. Lateral View

Internal spermatic fascia

Cremaster muscle within cremasteric fascia

External spermatic fascia

Lobules of epididymis

Efferent ductules of testis

Tunica vaginalis (parietal layer)

Tunica vaginalis (visceral layer) covering testis

D. Anterior View

Testicular veins

Testicular artery

Ductus deferens

Spermatic cord

Testicular artery

Pampiniform plexus of veins

Ductus deferens

Epididymis

External spermatic fascia

Cremaster muscle and fascia

Internal spermatic fascia

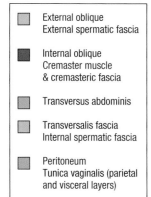

External oblique
External spermatic fascia

Internal oblique
Cremaster muscle & cremasteric fascia

Transversus abdominis

Transversalis fascia
Internal spermatic fascia

Peritoneum
Tunica vaginalis (parietal and visceral layers)

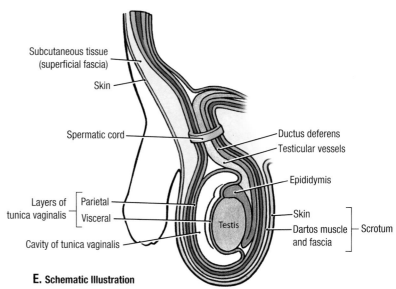

Subcutaneous tissue (superficial fascia)

Skin

Spermatic cord

Ductus deferens

Testicular vessels

Epididymis

Layers of tunica vaginalis
Parietal
Visceral

Skin

Testis

Dartos muscle and fascia — Scrotum

Cavity of tunica vaginalis

E. Schematic Illustration

2.16 INGUINAL CANAL, SPERMATIC CORD, AND TESTIS (*CONTINUED*)

A. Dissection of inguinal canal. **B.** Dissection of inguinal region and coverings of the spermatic cord and testis.
C.–E. Coverings of spermatic cord and testis.

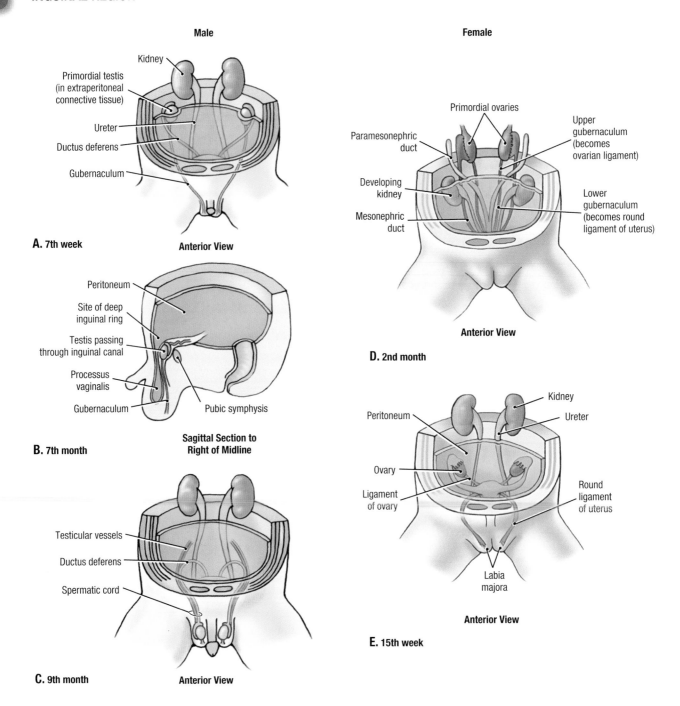

Male

Kidney

Primordial testis (in extraperitoneal connective tissue)

Ureter

Ductus deferens

Gubernaculum

A. 7th week   Anterior View

Peritoneum

Site of deep inguinal ring

Testis passing through inguinal canal

Processus vaginalis

Gubernaculum

Pubic symphysis

B. 7th month   Sagittal Section to Right of Midline

Testicular vessels

Ductus deferens

Spermatic cord

C. 9th month   Anterior View

Female

Primordial ovaries

Paramesonephric duct

Upper gubernaculum (becomes ovarian ligament)

Developing kidney

Mesonephric duct

Lower gubernaculum (becomes round ligament of uterus)

Anterior View

D. 2nd month

Kidney

Peritoneum

Ureter

Ovary

Ligament of ovary

Round ligament of uterus

Labia majora

Anterior View

E. 15th week

2.17   DESCENT OF GONADS

The inguinal canals in females are narrower than those in males, and the canals in infants of both sexes are shorter and much less oblique than in adults. For a complete description of the embryology of the inguinal region, see Moore and Persaud (2008).

The fetal testes descend from the dorsal abdominal wall in the superior lumbar region to the deep inguinal rings during the 9th to 12th fetal weeks. This movement probably results from the growth of the vertebral column and pelvis. The male gubernaculum, attached to the caudal pole of the testis and accompanied by an outpouching of peritoneum, the processus vaginalis, projects into the scrotum. The testis descends posterior to the processus vaginalis. The inferior remnant of the processus vaginalis forms the tunica vaginalis covering the testis. The ductus deferens, testicular vessels, nerves,

and lymphatics accompany the testis. The final descent of the testis usually occurs before or shortly after birth.

The fetal ovaries also descend from the dorsal abdominal wall in the superior lumbar region during the 12th week but pass into the lesser pelvis. The female gubernaculum attaches to the caudal pole of the ovary and projects into the labia majora, attaching en route to the uterus; the part passing from the uterus to the ovary forms the ovarian ligament, and the remainder of it becomes the round ligament of the uterus. Because of the attachment of the ovarian ligaments to the uterus, the ovaries do not descend to the inguinal region; however, the round ligament passes through the inguinal canal and attaches to the subcutaneous tissue of the labium majus.

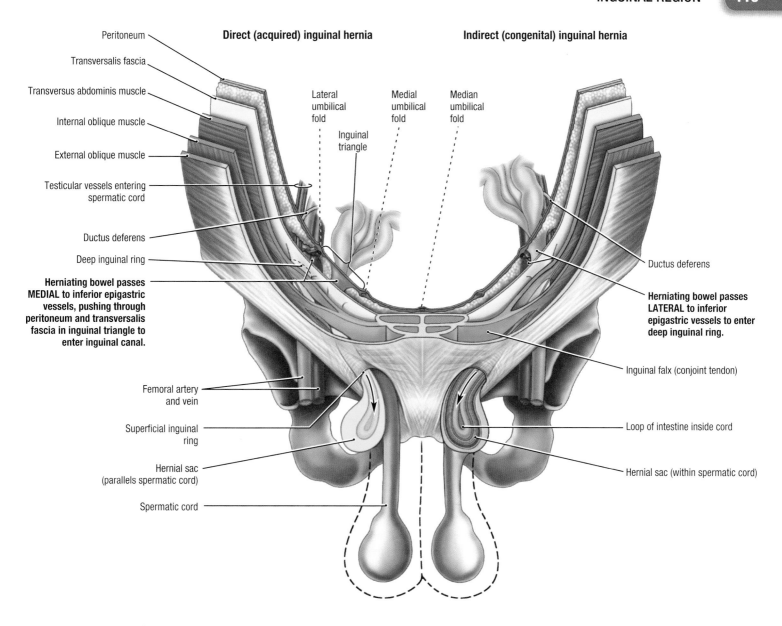

Direct (acquired) inguinal hernia   **Indirect (congenital) inguinal hernia**

Peritoneum

Transversalis fascia

Transversus abdominis muscle

Internal oblique muscle

External oblique muscle

Testicular vessels entering spermatic cord

Ductus deferens

Deep inguinal ring

Herniating bowel passes MEDIAL to inferior epigastric vessels, pushing through peritoneum and transversalis fascia in inguinal triangle to enter inguinal canal.

Femoral artery and vein

Superficial inguinal ring

Hernial sac (parallels spermatic cord)

Spermatic cord

Lateral umbilical fold

Medial umbilical fold

Median umbilical fold

Inguinal triangle

Ductus deferens

Herniating bowel passes LATERAL to inferior epigastric vessels to enter deep inguinal ring.

Inguinal falx (conjoint tendon)

Loop of intestine inside cord

Hernial sac (within spermatic cord)

2.18   COURSE OF DIRECT AND INDIRECT INGUINAL HERNIAS

An **inguinal hernia** is a protrusion of parietal peritoneum and viscera, such as the small intestine, through the abdominal wall in the inguinal region. There are two major categories of inguinal hernia: indirect and direct. More than two thirds are indirect hernias, most commonly occurring in males.

TABLE 2.3 CHARACTERISTICS OF INGUINAL HERNIAS

Characteristics[a]	Direct (Acquired)	Indirect (Congenital)
Predisposing factors	Weakness of anterior abdominal wall in inguinal triangle (e.g., owing to distended superficial ring, narrow conjoint tendon, or attenuation of aponeurosis in males >40 years of age)	Patency of processus vaginalis (complete or at least of superior part) in younger persons, the great majority of whom are males
Frequency	Less common (one third to one fourth of inguinal hernias)	More common (two third to three fourth of inguinal hernias)
Coverings at exit from abdominal cavity (**A** and **B**)	Peritoneum plus transversalis fascia (lies outside inner one or two fascial coverings of cord)	Peritoneum of persistent processus vaginalis plus all three fascial coverings of cord/round ligament
Course (**C**)	Usually traverses only medial third of inguinal canal, external and parallel to vestige of processus vaginalis	Traverses inguinal canal (entire canal if it is sufficient size) within processus vaginalis
Exit from anterior abdominal wall	Via superficial ring, lateral to cord; rarely enters scrotum	Via superficial ring inside cord, commonly passing into scrotum/labium majus

[a]Letters in parentheses refer to the figure parts.

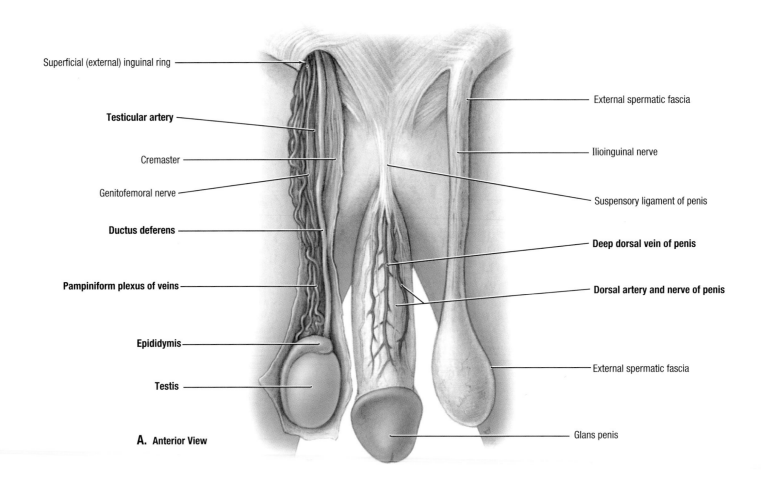

Superficial (external) inguinal ring

Testicular artery

Cremaster

Genitofemoral nerve

Ductus deferens

Pampiniform plexus of veins

Epididymis

Testis

External spermatic fascia

Ilioinguinal nerve

Suspensory ligament of penis

Deep dorsal vein of penis

Dorsal artery and nerve of penis

External spermatic fascia

Glans penis

A. Anterior View

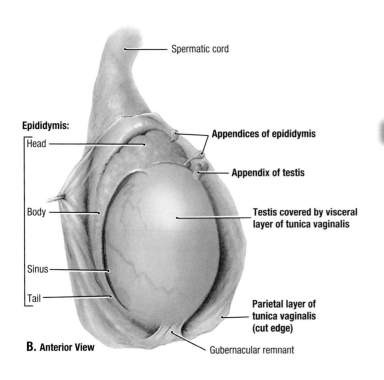

Spermatic cord

Epididymis:

Head

Body

Sinus

Tail

Appendices of epididymis

Appendix of testis

Testis covered by visceral layer of tunica vaginalis

Parietal layer of tunica vaginalis (cut edge)

Gubernacular remnant

B. Anterior View

2.19   SPERMATIC CORD, TESTIS, AND EPIDIDYMIS

A. Dissection of spermatic cord. The subcutaneous tissue (dartos fascia) covering the penis has been removed and the deep fascia rendered transparent to demonstrate the median deep dorsal vein and the bilateral dorsal arteries and nerves of the penis. On the specimen's right, the coverings of the spermatic cord and testis are reflected, and the contents of the cord are separated. The testicular artery has been separated from the pampiniform plexus of veins that surrounds it as it courses parallel to the ductus deferens. Lymphatic vessels and autonomic nerve fibers (not shown) are also present. **B.** The tunica vaginalis has been incised longitudinally to expose its cavity, surrounding the testis anteriorly and laterally, and extending between the testis and epididymis at the sinus of the epididymis. The epididymis is located posterolateral to the left testis, that is, on the right side of the right testis and on the left side of the left testis. The appendices of the testis and epididymis may be observed in some specimens. These structures are small remnants of the embryonic genital (paramesonephric) duct.

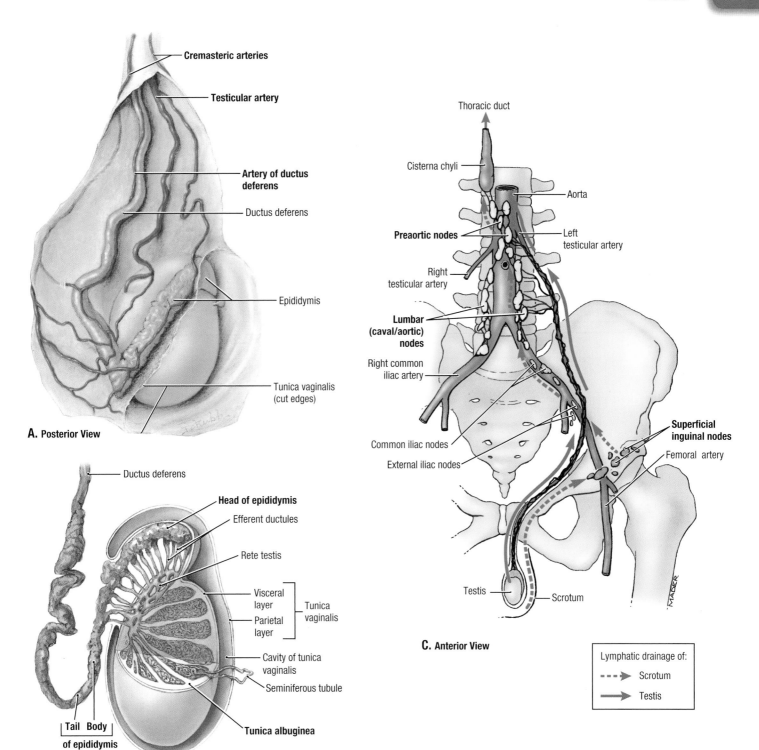

A. Posterior View

Cremasteric arteries

Testicular artery

Artery of ductus deferens

Ductus deferens

Epididymis

Tunica vaginalis (cut edges)

B. Longitinal Section of Tunica Vaginalis; Testis Sectioned in Sagittal and Transverse Planes

Ductus deferens

Head of epididymis

Efferent ductules

Rete testis

Visceral layer
Parietal layer
} Tunica vaginalis

Cavity of tunica vaginalis

Seminiferous tubule

Tail Body of epididymis

Tunica albuginea

C. Anterior View

Thoracic duct

Cisterna chyli

Aorta

Preaortic nodes

Left testicular artery

Right testicular artery

Lumbar (caval/aortic) nodes

Right common iliac artery

Common iliac nodes

External iliac nodes

Superficial inguinal nodes

Femoral artery

Testis

Scrotum

Lymphatic drainage of:
- - - ▶ Scrotum
——▶ Testis

2.20   BLOOD SUPPLY AND LYMPHATIC DRAINAGE OF TESTIS

A. Blood supply. **B.** Internal structure. **C.** Lymphatic drainage. Because the testes descend from the posterior abdominal wall into the scrotum during fetal development, their lymphatic drainage differs from that of the scrotum, which is an outpouching of the abdominal skin. Consequently, **cancer of the testis** metastasizes initially to the lumbar lymph nodes, and **cancer of the scrotum** metastasizes initially to the superficial inguinal lymph nodes.

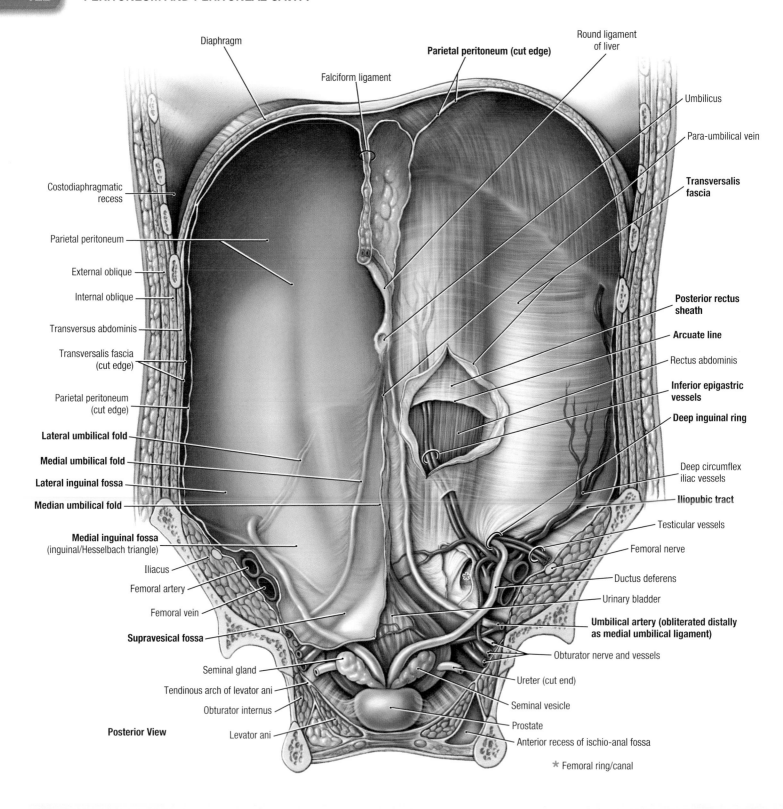

Diaphragm

Round ligament of liver

Parietal peritoneum (cut edge)

Falciform ligament

Umbilicus

Para-umbilical vein

Transversalis fascia

Costodiaphragmatic recess

Parietal peritoneum

External oblique

Internal oblique

Transversus abdominis

Transversalis fascia (cut edge)

Parietal peritoneum (cut edge)

Lateral umbilical fold

Medial umbilical fold

Lateral inguinal fossa

Median umbilical fold

Medial inguinal fossa
(inguinal/Hesselbach triangle)

Iliacus

Femoral artery

Femoral vein

Supravesical fossa

Posterior View

Seminal gland

Tendinous arch of levator ani

Obturator internus

Levator ani

Posterior rectus sheath

Arcuate line

Rectus abdominis

Inferior epigastric vessels

Deep inguinal ring

Deep circumflex iliac vessels

Iliopubic tract

Testicular vessels

Femoral nerve

Ductus deferens

Urinary bladder

Umbilical artery (obliterated distally as medial umbilical ligament)

Obturator nerve and vessels

Ureter (cut end)

Seminal vesicle

Prostate

Anterior recess of ischio-anal fossa

✱ Femoral ring/canal

2.21   POSTERIOR ASPECT OF THE ANTEROLATERAL ABDOMINAL WALL

Umbilical folds (median, medial, and lateral) are reflections of the parietal peritoneum that are raised from the body wall by underlying structures. The median umbilical fold extends from the urinary bladder to the umbilicus and covers the median umbilical ligament (the remnant of the urachus). The two medial umbilical folds cover the medial umbilical ligaments (occluded remnants of the fetal umbilical arteries). Two lateral umbilical folds cover the inferior epigastric vessels. The supravesical fossae are between the median and medial umbilical folds, the medial inguinal fossae (inguinal triangles) are between the medial and lateral umbilical folds, and the lateral inguinal fossae and deep inguinal rings are lateral to the lateral umbilical folds.

Thoracic duct

Azygos vein

Inferior vena cava

Diaphragm

Falciform ligament

Costodiaphragmatic recess

Right lobe of liver

**Round ligament of liver
(ligamentum teres)**

Fundus of gallbladder
(more inferiorly placed
here due to "tall"
variation of liver)

External oblique

Internal oblique

Transversus abdominis

Rectus abdominis

Descending (thoracic) aorta

Esophagus

Pericardial sac

Left lobe of liver

Gastrosplenic ligament

Stomach

Gastrocolic ligament

*The term greater omentum
is often used as a synonym
for the gastrocolic ligament,
but it actually also includes
the gastrosplenic and
gastrosphrenic ligaments, all
of which have a continuous
attachment to the greater
curvature of the stomach.

A. Anterior View

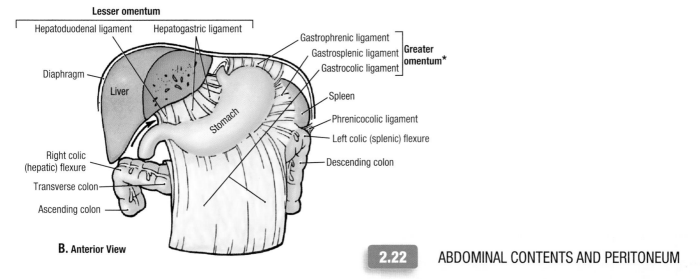

Lesser omentum

Hepatoduodenal ligament   Hepatogastric ligament

Diaphragm

Liver

Right colic
(hepatic) flexure

Transverse colon

Ascending colon

Stomach

Gastrophrenic ligament

Gastrosplenic ligament   **Greater
omentum***

Gastrocolic ligament

Spleen

Phrenicocolic ligament

Left colic (splenic) flexure

Descending colon

B. Anterior View

2.22   ABDOMINAL CONTENTS AND PERITONEUM

A. Dissection. **B.** Components of greater and lesser omentum.
Arrow, site of omental (epiploic) foramen.

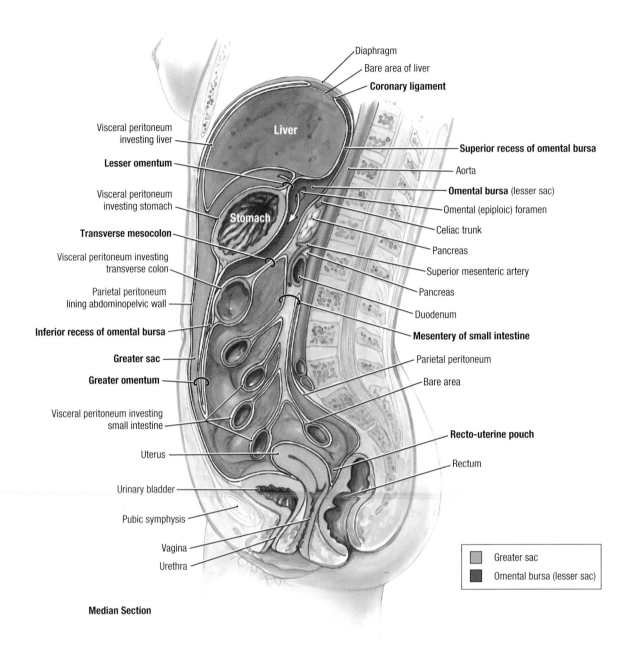

Diaphragm

Bare area of liver

Coronary ligament

Visceral peritoneum investing liver

Liver

Superior recess of omental bursa

Aorta

Lesser omentum

Omental bursa (lesser sac)

Visceral peritoneum investing stomach

Omental (epiploic) foramen

Stomach

Celiac trunk

Transverse mesocolon

Pancreas

Visceral peritoneum investing transverse colon

Superior mesenteric artery

Pancreas

Parietal peritoneum lining abdominopelvic wall

Duodenum

Inferior recess of omental bursa

Mesentery of small intestine

Greater sac

Parietal peritoneum

Greater omentum

Bare area

Visceral peritoneum investing small intestine

Recto-uterine pouch

Uterus

Rectum

Urinary bladder

Pubic symphysis

Vagina

Urethra

| | Greater sac |
| | Omental bursa (lesser sac) |

Median Section

2.23 PERITONEAL FORMATIONS AND BARE AREAS

Various terms are used to describe the parts of the peritoneum that connect organs with other organs or to the abdominal wall and to describe the compartments and recesses that are formed as a consequence. The *arrow* passes through the omental (epiploic) foramen.

TABLE 2.4 *TERMS USED TO DESCRIBE PARTS OF PERITONEUM*

Term	Definition
Peritoneal ligament	Double layer of peritoneum that connects an organ with another organ or to the abdominal wall.
Mesentery	Double layer of peritoneum that occurs as a result of the invagination of the peritoneum by an organ and constitutes a continuity of the visceral and parietal peritoneum.
Omentum	Double-layered extension of peritoneum passing from the stomach and proximal part of the duodenum to adjacent organs. The greater omentum extends from the greater curvature of the stomach and the proximal duodenum; the lesser omentum from the lesser curvature.
Bare area	Every organ must have an area, the bare area, that is not covered with visceral peritoneum, to allow the entrance and exit of neurovascular structures. Bare areas are formed in relation to the attachments of mesenteries, omenta, and ligaments. Named bare areas, e.g., bare area of liver, are especially extensive in area.

A. Right Lateral View

B. Infant   **C.** Adult

Schematic Sagittal Sections, Lateral View

2.24   SUBDIVISIONS OF PERITONEAL CAVITY

A. Sagittal section. **B.** In an infant, the omental bursa (lesser sac) is an isolated part of the peritoneal cavity, lying dorsal to the stomach and extending superiorly to the liver and diaphragm (superior recess of the omental bursa) and inferiorly between the layers of the greater omentum (inferior recess of the omental bursa). **C.** In an adult, after fusion of the layers of the greater omentum, the inferior recess of the omental bursa now extends inferiorly only as far as the transverse colon. The *red arrows* pass from the greater sac through the omental (epiploic) foramen into the omental bursa.

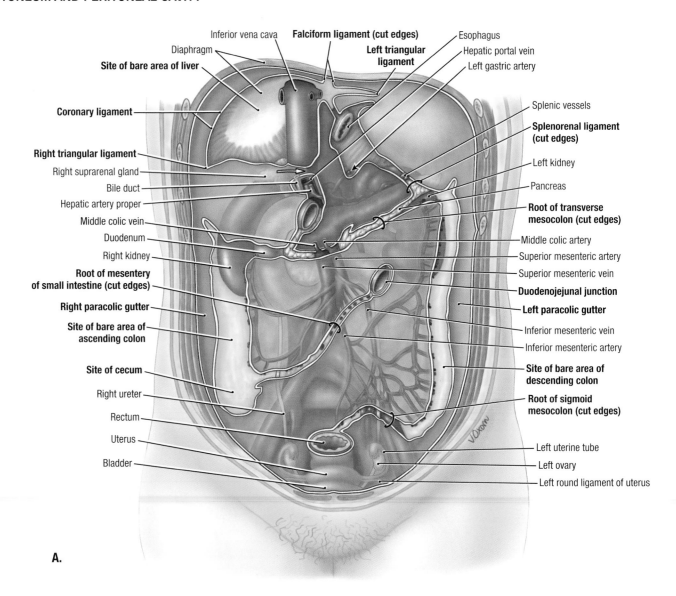

Inferior vena cava
Diaphragm
Site of bare area of liver
Coronary ligament
Right triangular ligament
Right suprarenal gland
Bile duct
Hepatic artery proper
Middle colic vein
Duodenum
Right kidney
Root of mesentery of small intestine (cut edges)
Right paracolic gutter
Site of bare area of ascending colon
Site of cecum
Right ureter
Rectum
Uterus
Bladder

Falciform ligament (cut edges)
Left triangular ligament
Esophagus
Hepatic portal vein
Left gastric artery
Splenic vessels
Splenorenal ligament (cut edges)
Left kidney
Pancreas
Root of transverse mesocolon (cut edges)
Middle colic artery
Superior mesenteric artery
Superior mesenteric vein
Duodenojejunal junction
Left paracolic gutter
Inferior mesenteric vein
Inferior mesenteric artery
Site of bare area of descending colon
Root of sigmoid mesocolon (cut edges)
Left uterine tube
Left ovary
Left round ligament of uterus

A.

Anterior Views

Transverse colon
Right colic (hepatic) flexure
Ascending colon

Supracolic compartment
Transverse mesocolon
Phrenicocolic ligament
Left colic (splenic) flexure
Tenia coli
Root of mesentery of small intestine
Descending colon

Right paracolic gutter   **Right infracolic space**   **Left infracolic space**   **Left paracolic gutter**

Infracolic compartment

B.

2.25   POSTERIOR WALL OF PERITONEAL CAVITY

A. Roots of the peritoneal reflections. The peritoneal reflections from the posterior abdominal wall (mesenteries and reflections surrounding bare areas of liver and secondarily retroperitoneal organs) have been cut at their roots, and the intraperitoneal and secondarily retroperitoneal viscera have been removed. The *white arrow* passes through the omental (epiploic) foramen. **B.** Supracolic and infracolic compartments of the greater sac. The infracolic spaces and paracolic gutters are of clinical importance because they determine the paths (*black arrows*) for the **flow of ascitic fluid with changes in position**, and the spread of intraperitoneal infections.

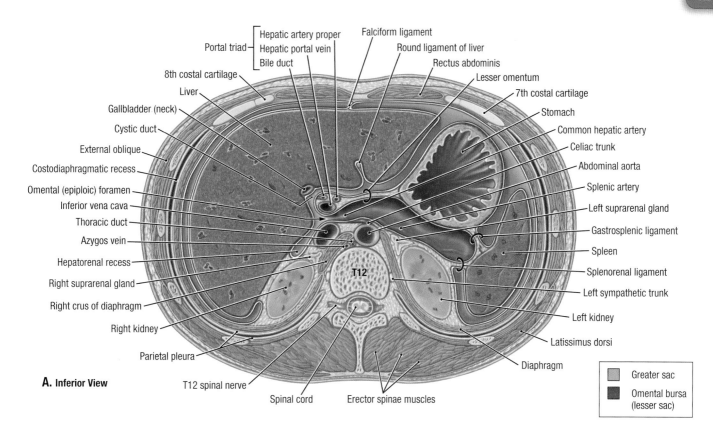

A. Inferior View

Portal triad — Hepatic artery proper
Hepatic portal vein
Bile duct
8th costal cartilage
Liver
Gallbladder (neck)
Cystic duct
External oblique
Costodiaphragmatic recess
Omental (epiploic) foramen
Inferior vena cava
Thoracic duct
Azygos vein
Hepatorenal recess
Right suprarenal gland
Right crus of diaphragm
Right kidney
Parietal pleura
T12 spinal nerve
Spinal cord
Erector spinae muscles

Falciform ligament
Round ligament of liver
Rectus abdominis
Lesser omentum
7th costal cartilage
Stomach
Common hepatic artery
Celiac trunk
Abdominal aorta
Splenic artery
Left suprarenal gland
Gastrosplenic ligament
Spleen
Splenorenal ligament
Left sympathetic trunk
Left kidney
Latissimus dorsi
Diaphragm

T12

Greater sac
Omental bursa
(lesser sac)

B. CT Scan Inferior View

Left lobe of liver
Falciform ligament
Gallbladder
Common hepatic duct
Right suprarenal gland
Right crus of diaphragm
Right kidney
Right lobe of liver
Deep back muscles

7th costal cartilage
Stomach (filled with contrast medium)
Hepatic artery proper
Hepatic portal vein
Rib
Caudate lobe of liver
Inferior vena cava
Azygos vein
Abdominal aorta
Spleen
Left crus of diaphragm
Renal fat
Spinous process of T12 vertebra

T12

Plane of section
(T12 vertebra)
in A & B

2.26   TRANSVERSE SECTIONS THROUGH GREATER SAC AND OMENTAL BURSA

- When bacterial contamination occurs or when the gut is traumatically penetrated or ruptured as the result of infection and inflammation, gas, fecal matter, and bacteria enter the peritoneal cavity. The result is infection and inflammation of the peritoneum, called **peritonitis**.
- Under certain pathological conditions such as peritonitis, the peritoneal cavity may be distended with abnormal fluid, **ascites**. Widespread

metastases (spread) of cancer cells to the abdominal viscera cause exudation (escape) of fluid that is often blood stained. Thus the peritoneal cavity may be distended with several liters of abnormal fluid. Surgical puncture of the peritoneal cavity for the aspiration of drainage of fluid is called **paracentesis**.

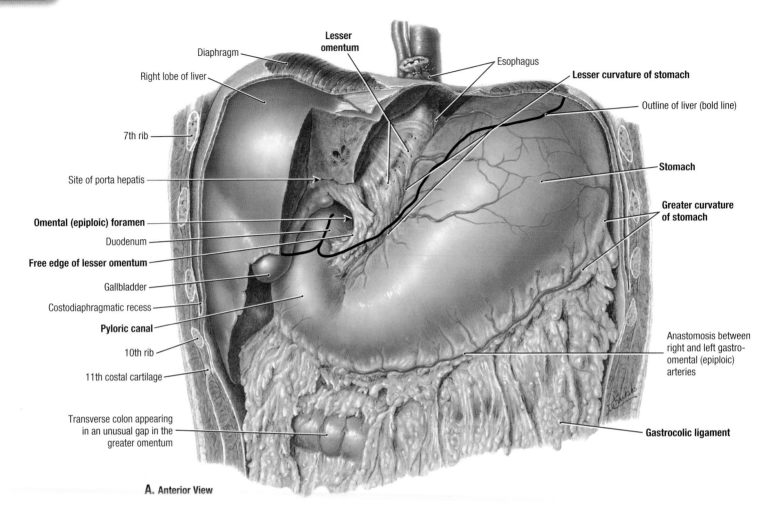

Lesser omentum

Diaphragm

Right lobe of liver

Esophagus

Lesser curvature of stomach

Outline of liver (bold line)

7th rib

Site of porta hepatis

Stomach

Omental (epiploic) foramen

Greater curvature of stomach

Duodenum

Free edge of lesser omentum

Gallbladder

Costodiaphragmatic recess

Pyloric canal

Anastomosis between right and left gastro-omental (epiploic) arteries

10th rib

11th costal cartilage

Transverse colon appearing in an unusual gap in the greater omentum

Gastrocolic ligament

A. Anterior View

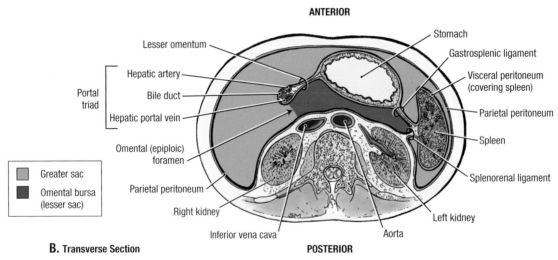

ANTERIOR

Lesser omentum

Stomach

Gastrosplenic ligament

Hepatic artery

Portal triad

Bile duct

Hepatic portal vein

Visceral peritoneum (covering spleen)

Parietal peritoneum

Spleen

Omental (epiploic) foramen

Parietal peritoneum

Splenorenal ligament

Right kidney

Left kidney

Greater sac

Omental bursa (lesser sac)

Inferior vena cava

Aorta

B. Transverse Section

POSTERIOR

2.27   STOMACH AND OMENTA

A. Lesser and greater omenta. The stomach is inflated with air, and the left part of the liver is cut away. The gallbladder, followed superiorly, leads to the free margin of the lesser omentum and serves as a guide to the omental (epiploic) foramen, which lies posterior to that free margin. **B.** Omental bursa (lesser sac), schematic transverse section.

A. Anterior View

B. Anterior View

2.28   POSTERIOR RELATIONSHIPS OF OMENTAL BURSA (LESSER SAC)

A. Opened omental bursa. The greater omentum has been cut along the greater curvature of the stomach; the stomach is reflected superiorly. Peritoneum of the stomach bed is partially removed. **B.** Stomach bed. The stomach is excised. Peritoneum covering the stomach bed and inferior part of the kidney and pancreas is largely removed. **Adhesions** binding the spleen to the diaphragm are pathological, but not unusual.

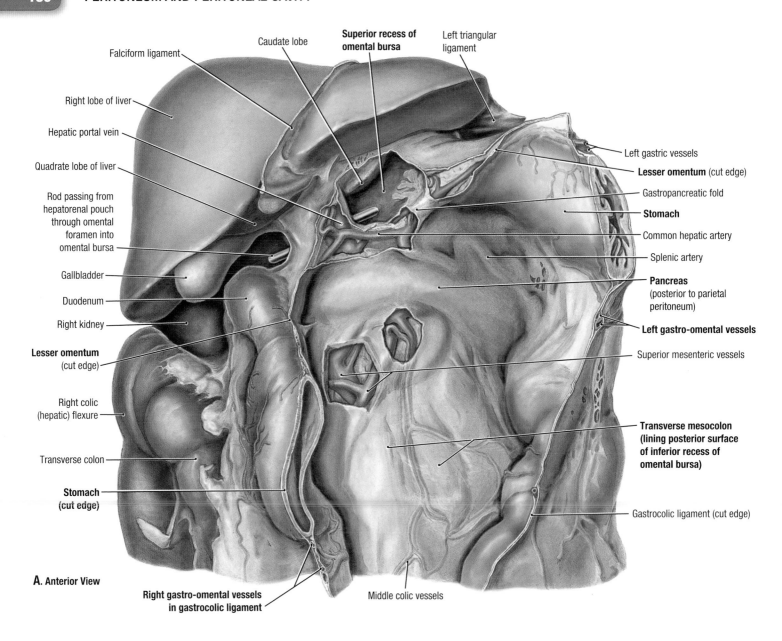

Falciform ligament

Caudate lobe

Superior recess of omental bursa

Left triangular ligament

Right lobe of liver

Left gastric vessels

Hepatic portal vein

Lesser omentum (cut edge)

Quadrate lobe of liver

Gastropancreatic fold

Rod passing from hepatorenal pouch through omental foramen into omental bursa

Stomach

Common hepatic artery

Splenic artery

Gallbladder

Pancreas (posterior to parietal peritoneum)

Duodenum

Right kidney

Left gastro-omental vessels

Lesser omentum (cut edge)

Superior mesenteric vessels

Right colic (hepatic) flexure

Transverse mesocolon (lining posterior surface of inferior recess of omental bursa)

Transverse colon

Stomach (cut edge)

Gastrocolic ligament (cut edge)

A. Anterior View

Right gastro-omental vessels in gastrocolic ligament

Middle colic vessels

2.29   OMENTAL BURSA (LESSER SAC), OPENED

A. Dissection. **B.** Line of incision in **A.** The anterior wall of the omental bursa, consisting of the stomach, lesser omentum, anterior layer of the greater omentum, and vessels along the curvatures of the stomach, has been sectioned sagittally. The two halves have been retracted to the left and right: the body of the stomach on the left side, and the pyloric part of the stomach and first part of the duodenum on the right. The right kidney forms the posterior wall of the hepatorenal pouch (part of greater sac), and the pancreas lies horizontally on the posterior wall of the main compartment of the omental bursa (lesser sac). The gastrocolic ligament forms the anterior wall and the lower part of the posterior wall of the inferior recess of the omental bursa. The transverse mesocolon forms the upper part of the posterior wall of the inferior recess of the omental bursa.

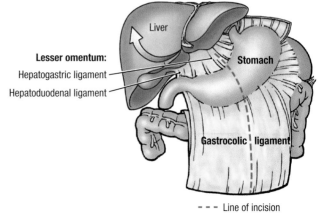

Liver

Lesser omentum:

Hepatogastric ligament

Hepatoduodenal ligament

Stomach

Gastrocolic ligament

- - - Line of incision

B. Anterior View

Superior recess of omental bursa

Liver   Caudate lobe   Esophagus   Left triangular ligament   Esophageal branches

Left gastric vein and artery

Celiac trunk

Spleen

Common hepatic artery

Stomach

Hepatic portal vein

Omental bursa

Right gastric artery and vein

Splenic artery and vein in splenorenal ligament

Gallbladder

Splenic artery

Gastrocolic ligament

Stomach (reflected to right)

Left gastro-omental vessels

Splenic vein

Pancreas

Left renal vein

Neck of pancreas

Inferior mesenteric vein

Left testicular vein

Superior mesenteric vein

Right gastro-omental vessels

Superior mesenteric artery

Uncinate process of pancreas

Right colic vessels

Middle colic artery and vein

Head of pancreas   Accessory middle colic artery   Ileocolic vein

Anterior View

| 2.30 | **POSTERIOR WALL OF OMENTAL BURSA** |

The parietal peritoneum of the posterior wall of the omental bursa has been mostly removed, and a section of the pancreas has been excised. The rod passes through the omental foramen.

- The celiac trunk gives rise to the left gastric artery, the splenic artery that runs tortuously to the left, and the common hepatic artery that runs to the right, passing anterior to the hepatic portal vein.
- The hepatic portal vein is formed posterior to the neck of the pancreas by the union of the superior mesenteric and splenic veins, with the inferior mesenteric vein joining at or near the angle of union.

- The left testicular vein usually drains into the left renal vein. Both are systemic veins.
- **Inflammation of the parietal peritoneum** can occur due to an enlarged organ or by the escape of fluid from an organ. The area becomes inflamed and causes pain over the affected region.
- **Rebound tenderness** is a pain that is elicited after pressure over the inflamed area is released.

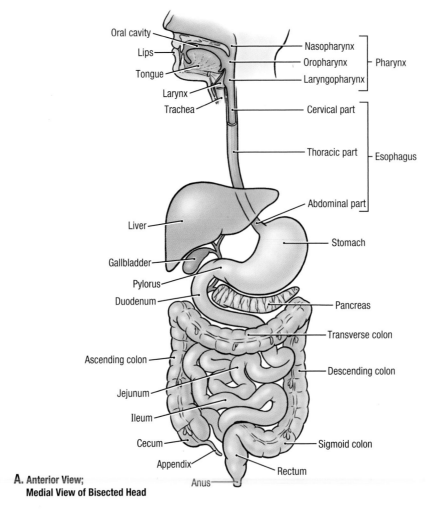

Oral cavity
Lips
Tongue
Larynx
Trachea

Nasopharynx
Oropharynx — Pharynx
Laryngopharynx

Cervical part

Thoracic part — Esophagus

Abdominal part

Liver

Stomach

Gallbladder
Pylorus
Duodenum

Pancreas

Transverse colon

Ascending colon

Descending colon

Jejunum

Ileum

Cecum

Sigmoid colon

Appendix

Rectum

Anus

A. Anterior View;
Medial View of Bisected Head

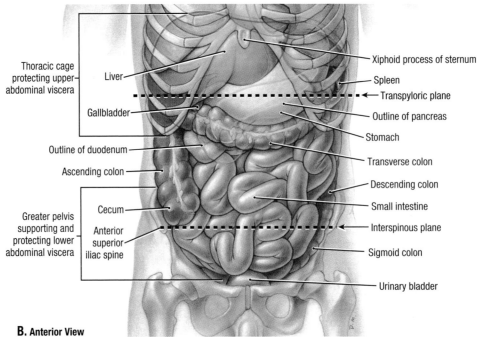

Thoracic cage
protecting upper
abdominal viscera

Liver

Xiphoid process of sternum

Spleen

Transpyloric plane

Gallbladder

Outline of pancreas

Stomach

Outline of duodenum

Transverse colon

Ascending colon

Descending colon

Greater pelvis
supporting and
protecting lower
abdominal viscera

Cecum

Small intestine

Anterior
superior
iliac spine

Interspinous plane

Sigmoid colon

Urinary bladder

B. Anterior View

2.31   DIGESTIVE SYSTEM

A. Schematic illustration. **B.** Abdominal portion. The digestive system extends from the lips to the anus.
Associated organs include the liver, gallbladder, and pancreas.

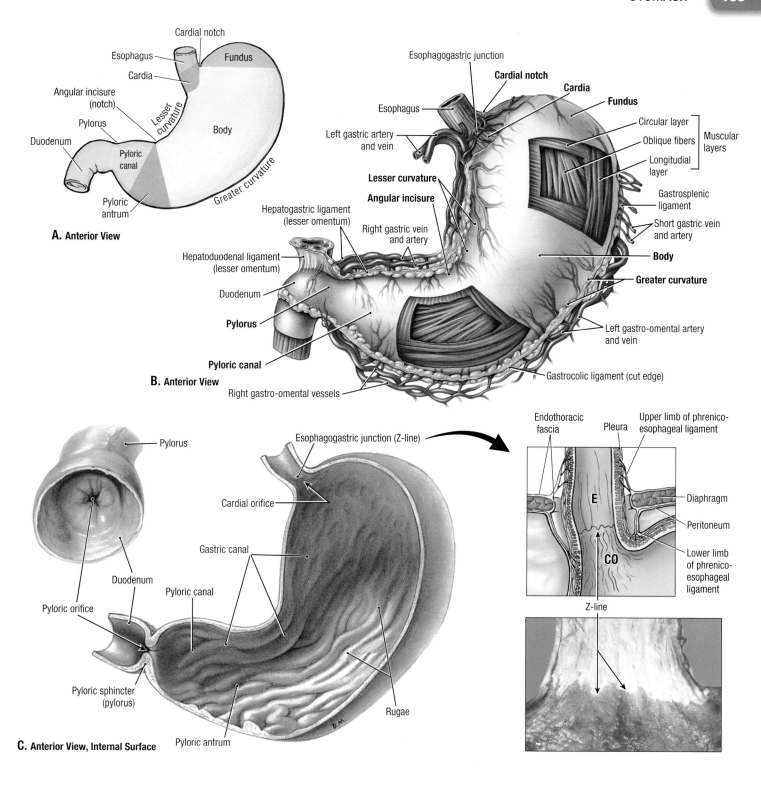

A. Anterior View

B. Anterior View

C. Anterior View, Internal Surface

2.32 STOMACH

A. Parts. **B.** External surface. **C.** Internal surface (mucous membrane), anterior wall removed. Insets: Left side of page—pylorus, viewed from the duodenum. Right side of page—details of the esophagogastric junction. The Z-line is where the stratified squamous epithelium of the esophagus (white portion in photograph) to the simple columnar epithelium of the stomach (dark portion).

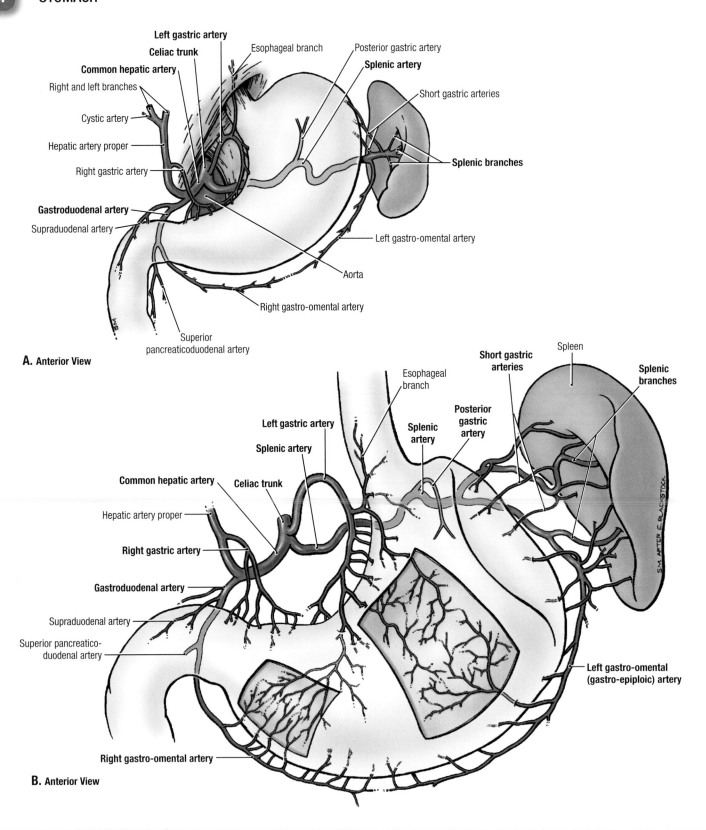

A. Anterior View

B. Anterior View

Labels in part A:
Left gastric artery
Celiac trunk
Common hepatic artery
Right and left branches
Cystic artery
Hepatic artery proper
Right gastric artery
Gastroduodenal artery
Supraduodenal artery
Esophageal branch
Posterior gastric artery
Splenic artery
Short gastric arteries
Splenic branches
Left gastro-omental artery
Aorta
Right gastro-omental artery
Superior pancreaticoduodenal artery

Labels in part B:
Common hepatic artery
Hepatic artery proper
Right gastric artery
Gastroduodenal artery
Supraduodenal artery
Superior pancreatico-duodenal artery
Right gastro-omental artery
Left gastric artery
Splenic artery
Celiac trunk
Esophageal branch
Splenic artery
Posterior gastric artery
Short gastric arteries
Spleen
Splenic branches
Left gastro-omental (gastro-epiploic) artery

2.33 CELIAC ARTERY

A. Branches of celiac trunk. The celiac trunk is a branch of the abdominal aorta, arising immediately inferior to the aortic hiatus of the diaphragm (T12 vertebral level). The vessel is usually 1 to 2 cm long and divides into the left gastric, common hepatic, and splenic arteries. The celiac trunk supplies the liver, gall bladder, inferior esophagus, stomach, pancreas, spleen, and duodenum. **B.** Arteries of stomach and spleen. The serous and muscular coats are removed from two areas of the stomach, revealing anastomotic networks in the submucous coat.

Five main sites where
esophagus is constricted:

1. Junction of pharynx
and esophagus
(in neck)

2. Aortic arch

3. Left main bronchus
(at tracheal bifurcation)

4. Left atrium

5. Esophageal hiatus

A. Lateral View

Gallbladder

Duodenal cap

Pylorus

Pyloric antrum

Jejunum

Fundus of stomach

Peristaltic wave

Gastric folds (rugae)

Greater curvature

B

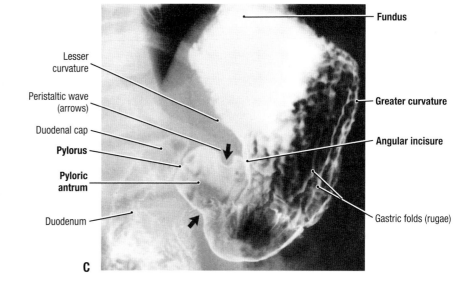

Fundus

Lesser
curvature

Peristaltic wave
(arrows)

Duodenal cap

Pylorus

**Pyloric
antrum**

Duodenum

Greater curvature

Angular incisure

Gastric folds (rugae)

C

2.34 RADIOGRAPHS OF ESOPHAGUS,
STOMACH, DUODENUM (BARIUM
SWALLOW)

A. Five sites of normal esophageal constriction. **B.** Stomach,
small intestine, and gallbladder. Note additional contrast
medium in gallbladder. **C.** Stomach and duodenum. **D.** Pyloric
antrum and duodenal cap.

   Blockage of esophagus. The impressions produced
in the esophagus by adjacent structures are of clinical
interest because of the slower passage of substances at
these sites. The impressions indicate where swallowed
foreign objects are most likely to lodge and where a stricture may develop, for example, after the accidental drinking of a caustic liquid, such as lye.

   A **hiatal (hiatus) hernia** is a protrusion of a part of
the stomach into the mediastinum through the esophageal
hiatus of the diaphragm. The hernias occur most often in
people after middle age, possibly because of weakening
of the muscular part of the diaphragm and widening of the
esophageal hiatus.

Peristaltic wave
(arrows)

Duodenal
cap

Pylorus

**Pyloric
antrum**

Duodenum

D

Anterior Views (B–D)

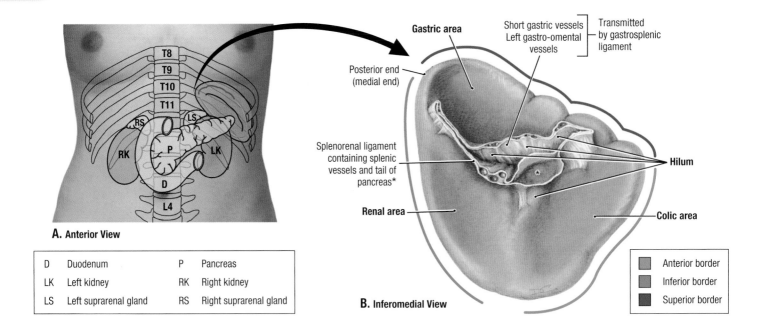

A. Anterior View

D	Duodenum	P	Pancreas
LK	Left kidney	RK	Right kidney
LS	Left suprarenal gland	RS	Right suprarenal gland

B. Inferomedial View

Anterior border
Inferior border
Superior border

2.35   SPLEEN

A. The surface anatomy of the spleen. The spleen lies superficially in the left upper abdominal quadrant between the 9th and 11th ribs. **B.** Note the impressions (colic, renal, and gastric areas) made by structures in contact with its visceral surface. The superior border is notched.

2.36   CELIAC ARTERIOGRAM

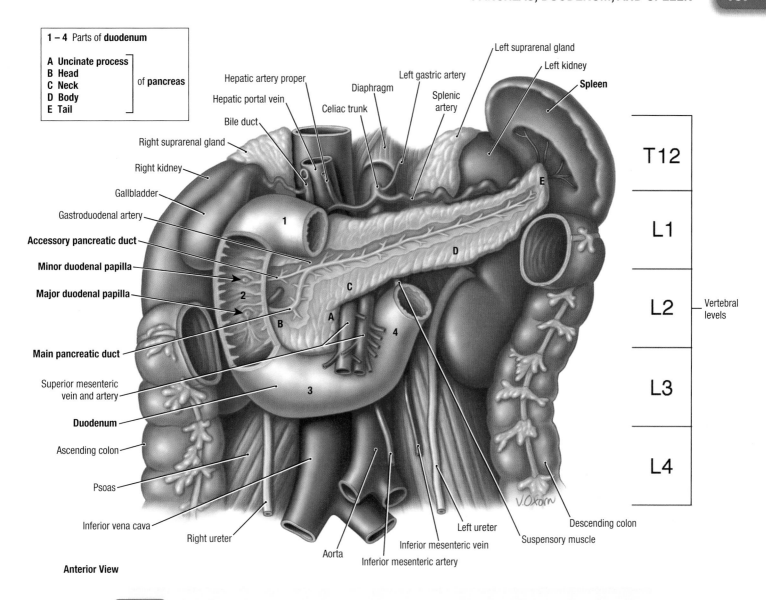

1 – 4 Parts of duodenum

A Uncinate process
B Head
C Neck   } of **pancreas**
D Body
E Tail

Left suprarenal gland
Left kidney
Spleen
Hepatic artery proper
Left gastric artery
Diaphragm
Hepatic portal vein
Splenic artery
Celiac trunk
Bile duct
Right suprarenal gland
Right kidney
Gallbladder
Gastroduodenal artery
Accessory pancreatic duct
Minor duodenal papilla
Major duodenal papilla
Main pancreatic duct
Superior mesenteric vein and artery
Duodenum
Ascending colon
Psoas
Inferior vena cava
Right ureter
Aorta
Inferior mesenteric artery
Inferior mesenteric vein
Left ureter
Suspensory muscle
Descending colon

V.Oxorn

T12
L1
L2   Vertebral levels
L3
L4

Anterior View

2.37   PARTS AND RELATIONSHIPS OF PANCREAS AND DUODENUM

Pancreas and duodenum in situ.

TABLE 2.5 PARTS AND RELATIONSHIPS OF DUODENUM

Part of Duodenum	Anterior	Posterior	Medial	Superior	Inferior	Vertebral Level
Superior (1st part)	Peritoneum Gallbladder Quadrate lobe of liver	Bile duct Gastroduodenal artery Hepatic portal vein IVC		Neck of gallbladder	Neck of pancreas	Anterolateral to L1 vertebra
Descending (2nd part)	Transverse colon Transverse mesocolon Coils of small intestine	Hilum of right kidney Renal vessels Ureter Psoas major	Head of pancreas Pancreatic duct Bile duct			Right of L2–L3 vertebrae
Inferior (horizontal or 3rd part)	Superior mesenteric artery Superior mesenteric vein Coils of small intestine	Right psoas major IVC Aorta Right ureter		Head and uncinate process of pancreas Superior mesenteric artery and vein		Anterior to L3 vertebra
Ascending (4th part)	Beginning of root of mesentery Coils of jejunum	Left psoas major Left margin of aorta	Superior mesenteric artery and vein	Body of pancreas		Left of L3 vertebra

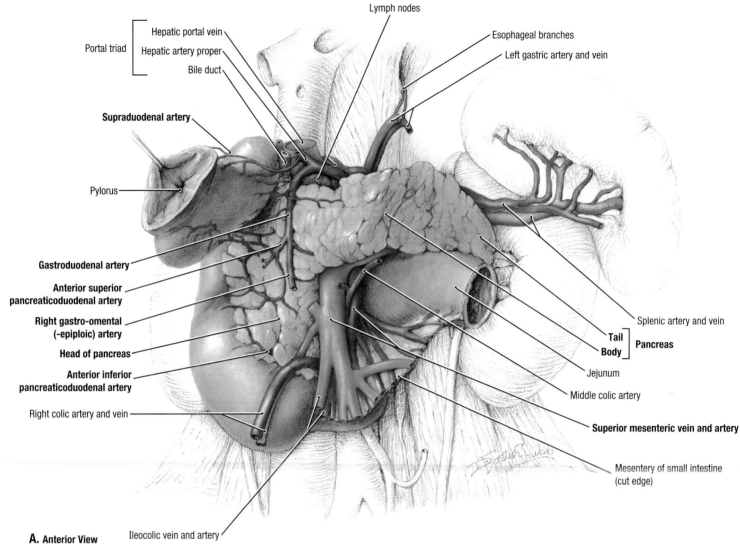

Lymph nodes

Portal triad
- Hepatic portal vein
- Hepatic artery proper
- Bile duct

Esophageal branches

Left gastric artery and vein

Supraduodenal artery

Pylorus

Gastroduodenal artery

Anterior superior pancreaticoduodenal artery

Right gastro-omental (-epiploic) artery

Head of pancreas

Anterior inferior pancreaticoduodenal artery

Right colic artery and vein

Splenic artery and vein

Tail | **Pancreas**
Body |

Jejunum

Middle colic artery

Superior mesenteric vein and artery

Mesentery of small intestine (cut edge)

A. Anterior View

Ileocolic vein and artery

PARTS AND RELATIONSHIPS OF PANCREAS AND DUODENUM (*CONTINUED*)

A. Anterior relationships. The gastroduodenal artery descends anterior to the neck of the pancreas. **B.** Posterior relationships. The splenic artery and vein course on the posterior aspect of the pancreatic tail, which usually extends to the spleen. The pancreas "loops" around the right side of the superior mesenteric vessels so that its neck is anterior, its head is to the right, and its uncinate process is posterior to the vessels. The splenic and superior mesenteric veins unite posterior to the neck to form the hepatic portal vein. The bile duct descends in a fissure (opened up) in the posterior part of the head of the pancreas. Most inflammatory erosions of the duodenal wall, **duodenal (peptic) ulcers**, are in the posterior wall of the superior (1st) part of the duodenum within 3 cm of the pylorus.

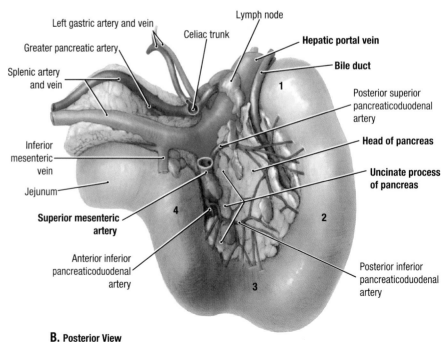

Left gastric artery and vein

Greater pancreatic artery

Splenic artery and vein

Inferior mesenteric vein

Jejunum

Superior mesenteric artery

Anterior inferior pancreaticoduodenal artery

Celiac trunk

Lymph node

Hepatic portal vein

Bile duct

Posterior superior pancreaticoduodenal artery

Head of pancreas

Uncinate process of pancreas

Posterior inferior pancreaticoduodenal artery

B. Posterior View

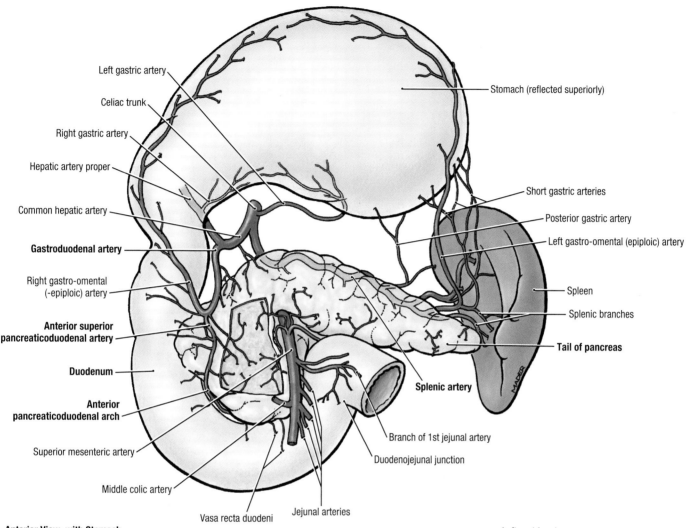

A. Anterior View, with Stomach Reflected Superiorly

2.39 BLOOD SUPPLY TO THE PANCREAS, DUODENUM, AND SPLEEN

A. Celiac trunk and superior mesenteric artery. **B.** Pancreatic and pancreaticoduodenal arteries.

- The anterior superior pancreaticoduodenal artery from the gastroduodenal artery and the anterior inferior pancreaticoduodenal artery of the superior mesenteric artery form the anterior pancreaticoduodenal arch anterior to the head of the pancreas. The posterior superior and posterior inferior branches of the same two arteries form the posterior pancreaticoduodenal arch posterior to the pancreas. The anterior and posterior inferior arteries often arise from a common stem.
- Arteries supplying the pancreas are derived from the common hepatic artery, gastroduodenal artery, pancreaticoduodenal arches, splenic artery, and superior mesenteric artery.

B. Anterior View

A. Proximal Jejunum

B. Proximal Ileum

C. Distal Ileum

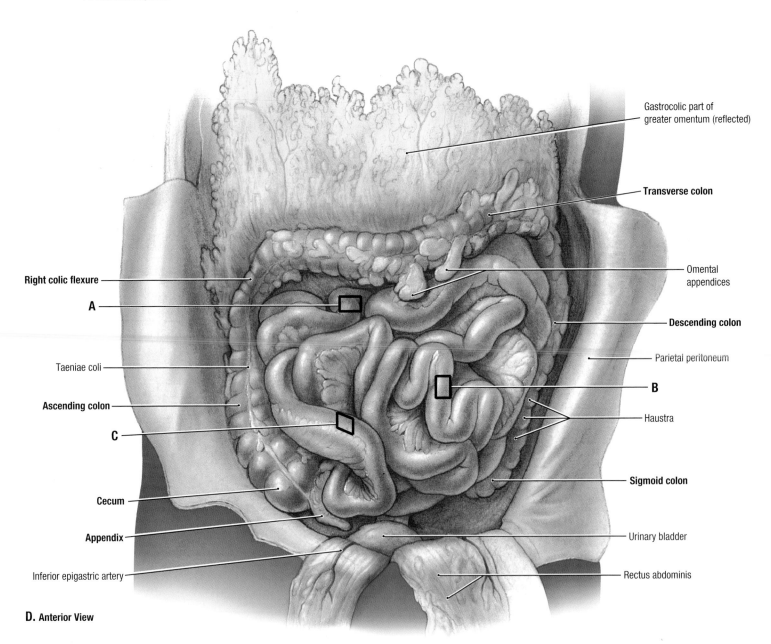

Gastrocolic part of greater omentum (reflected)

Transverse colon

Omental appendices

Right colic flexure

A

Descending colon

Parietal peritoneum

Taeniae coli

B

Ascending colon

Haustra

C

Sigmoid colon

Cecum

Appendix

Urinary bladder

Inferior epigastric artery

Rectus abdominis

D. Anterior View

2.40   INTESTINES IN SITU, INTERIOR OF SMALL INTESTINE

A. Proximal jejunum. The circular folds are tall, closely packed, and commonly branched. **B.** Proximal ileum. The circular folds are low and becoming sparse. The caliber of the gut is reduced, and the wall is thinner. **C.** Distal ileum. Circular folds are absent, and solitary lymph nodules stud the wall.

D. Intestines in situ, greater omentum reflected. The ileum is reflected to expose the appendix. The appendix usually lies posterior to the cecum (retrocecal) or, as in this case, projects over the pelvic brim. The features of the large intestines are the taeniae coli, haustra, and omental appendices.

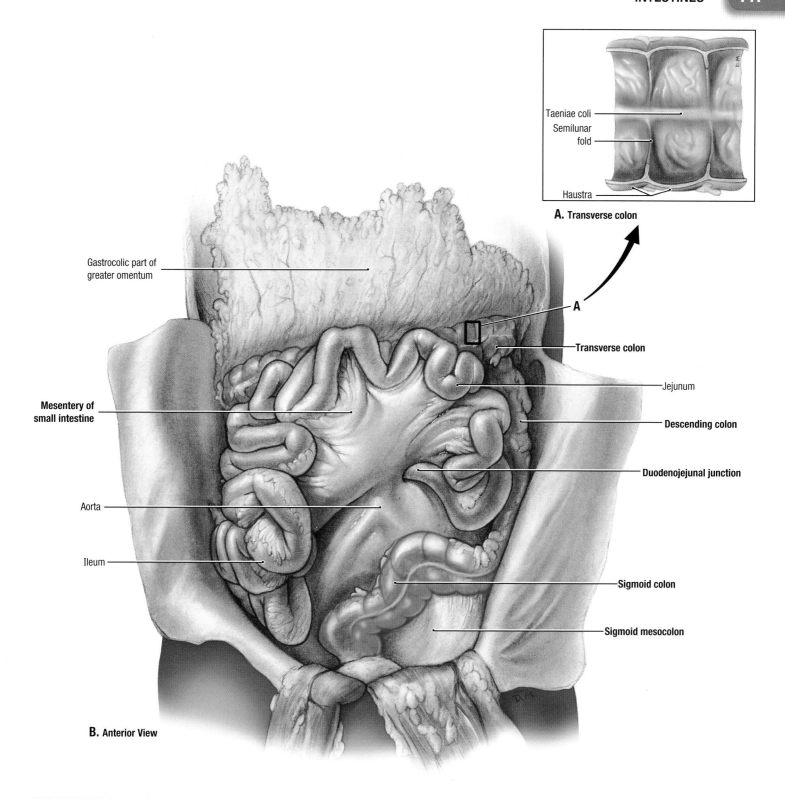

Taeniae coli
Semilunar fold
Haustra

A. Transverse colon

Gastrocolic part of greater omentum

A

Mesentery of small intestine

Transverse colon

Jejunum

Descending colon

Duodenojejunal junction

Aorta

Ileum

Sigmoid colon

Sigmoid mesocolon

B. Anterior View

2.41   SIGMOID MESOCOLON AND MESENTERY OF SMALL INTESTINE, INTERIOR OF TRANSVERSE COLON

A. Transverse colon. The semilunar folds and taeniae coli form prominent features on the smooth-surfaced wall. **B.** Sigmoid mesocolon and mesentery of the small intestine.

- The duodenojejunal junction is situated to the left of the median plane.
- The mesentery of the small intestine fans out extensively from its short root to accommodate the length of jejunum and ileum (~6 m).

- The descending colon is the narrowest part of the large intestine and is retroperitoneal. The sigmoid colon has a mesentery, the sigmoid mesocolon; the sigmoid colon is continuous with the rectum at the point at which the sigmoid mesocolon ends.

A Postero-anterior Radiographs

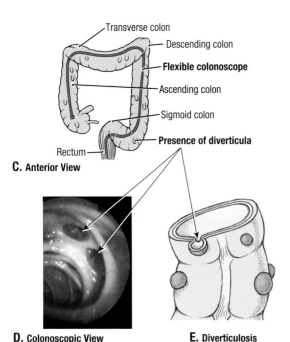

C. **Anterior View**
- Transverse colon
- Descending colon
- **Flexible colonoscope**
- Ascending colon
- Sigmoid colon
- **Presence of diverticula**
- Rectum

D. **Colonoscopic View**

E. **Diverticulosis**

A	Ascending colon	G	Sigmoid colon	S	Splenic flexure
C	Cecum	H	Hepatic flexure	T	Transverse colon
D	Descending colon	R	Rectum	U	Haustra

2.42 BARIUM ENEMA AND COLONOSCOPY OF COLON

A. Single-contrast study. A barium enema has filled the colon. **B. Double-contrast study.** Barium can be seen coating the walls of the colon, which is distended with air, providing a vivid view of the mucosal relief and haustra. C. The interior of the colon can be observed with an elongated endoscope, usually a fiberoptic **flexible colonoscope.** The endoscope is a tube that inserts into the colon through the anus and rectum. **D. Diverticulosis of the colon** can be photographed through a colonoscope. **E. Diverticulosis** is a disorder in which multiple false diverticula (external evaginations or outpocketings of the mucosa of the colon) develop along the intestine. It primarily affects middle-aged and elderly people. Diverticulosis is commonly (60%) found in the sigmoid colon. Diverticula are subject to infection and rupture, leading to **diverticulitis,** and they can distort and erode the nutrient arteries, leading to hemorrhage.

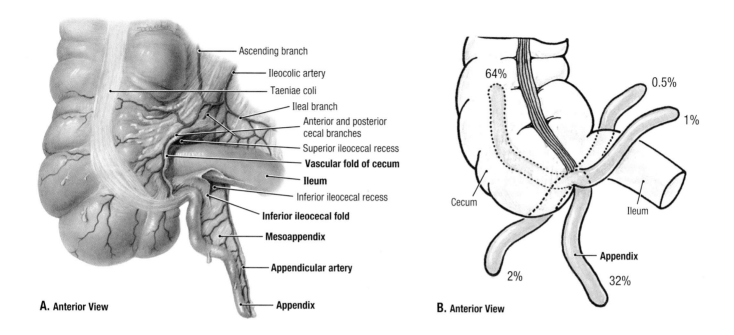

Ascending branch
Ileocolic artery
Taeniae coli
Ileal branch
Anterior and posterior cecal branches
Superior ileocecal recess
Vascular fold of cecum
Ileum
Inferior ileocecal recess
Inferior ileocecal fold
Mesoappendix
Appendicular artery
Appendix

A. Anterior View

64%
0.5%
1%
Cecum
Ileum
Appendix
2%
32%

B. Anterior View

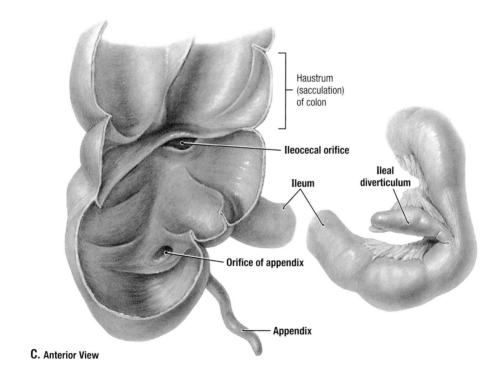

Haustrum (sacculation) of colon
Ileocecal orifice
Ileum
Orifice of appendix
Appendix
Ileal diverticulum

C. Anterior View

2.43   ILEOCECAL REGION AND APPENDIX

A. Blood supply. The appendicular artery is located in the free edge of the mesoappendix. The inferior ileocecal fold is bloodless, whereas the superior ileocecal fold is called the vascular fold of the cecum. **B.** The approximate incidence of various positions of the appendix. **C.** Interior of a dried cecum and ileal diverticulum (of Meckel). This cecum was filled with air until dry, opened, and varnished. **Ileal diverticulum** is a congenital anomaly that occurs in 1% to 2% of persons. It is a pouchlike remnant (3 to 6 cm long) of the proximal part of the yolk stalk, typically within 50 cm of the ileocecal junction. It sometimes becomes inflamed and produces pain that may mimic that produced by appendicitis.

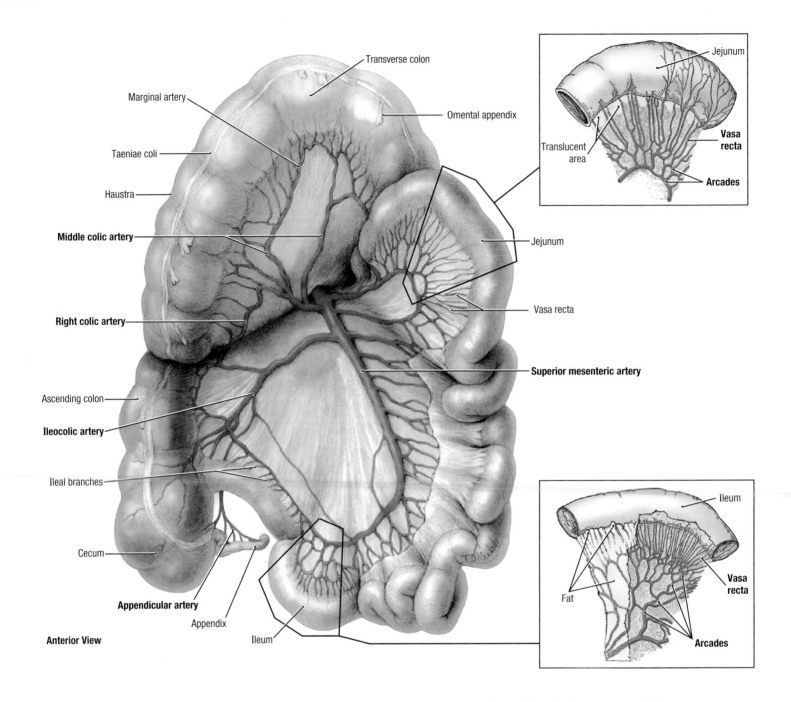

Transverse colon

Marginal artery

Omental appendix

Taeniae coli

Haustra

Jejunum

Translucent area

Vasa recta

Arcades

Middle colic artery

Jejunum

Right colic artery

Vasa recta

Superior mesenteric artery

Ascending colon

Ileocolic artery

Ileal branches

Ileum

Fat

Vasa recta

Cecum

Appendicular artery

Appendix

Arcades

Anterior View

Ileum

2.44 SUPERIOR MESENTERIC ARTERY AND ARTERIAL ARCADES

The peritoneum is partially stripped off.

- The superior mesenteric artery ends by anastomosing with one of its own branches, the ileal branch of the ileocolic artery.
- On the inset drawings of jejunum and ileum compare the diameter, thickness of wall, number of arterial arcades, long or short vasa recta, presence of translucent (fat-free) areas at the mesenteric border, and fat encroaching on the wall of the gut between the jejunum and ileum.
- **Acute inflammation of the appendix** is a common cause of an acute abdomen (severe abdominal pain arising suddenly). The pain of appendicitis usually commences as a vague pain in the periumbilical region because afferent pain fibers enter the spinal cord at the T10 level. Later, severe pain in the right lower quadrant results from irritation of the parietal peritoneum lining the posterior abdominal wall.

Gas in transverse colon

Marginal artery

Gas in ascending colon

Right colic artery

Ileocolic artery

Ileocecal junction

Superior mesenteric artery

Middle colic artery

Jejunal arteries

Ileal arteries

Catheter

A

Anteroposterior Arteriograms

Vasa recta

Superior mesenteric artery

Arterial arcades

Jejunal arteries

B

2.45   SUPERIOR MESENTERIC ARTERIOGRAMS

A. Branches of superior mesenteric artery. Consult Figure 2.44 to identify the branches. **B.** Enlargement to show the jejunal arteries, arterial arcades, and vasa recta.

- The branches of the superior mesenteric artery include, from its left side, 12 or more jejunal and ileal arteries that anastomose to form arcades from which vasa recta pass to the small intestine and, from its right side, the middle colic, ileocolic, and commonly (but not here) an independent right colic artery that anastomose to form a marginal artery that parallels the mesenteric border at the colon and from which vasa recta pass to the large intestine. **Occlusion of the vasa recta** by emboli results in ischemia of the part of the intestine concerned. If the ischemia is severe, necrosis of the involved segment results and **ileus** (obstruction of the intestine) of the paralytic type occurs. Ileus is accompanied by a severe colicky pain, along with abdominal distension, vomiting, and often fever and dehydration. If the condition is diagnosed early (e.g., using a superior mesenteric arteriogram), the obstructed part of the vessel may be cleared surgically.

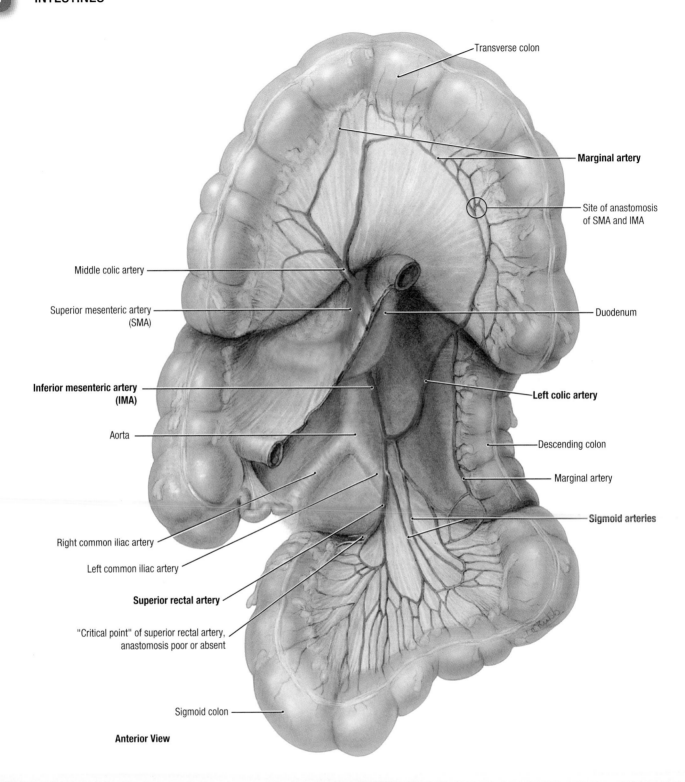

Transverse colon

Marginal artery

Site of anastomosis of SMA and IMA

Middle colic artery

Superior mesenteric artery (SMA)

Duodenum

Inferior mesenteric artery (IMA)

Left colic artery

Aorta

Descending colon

Marginal artery

Sigmoid arteries

Right common iliac artery

Left common iliac artery

Superior rectal artery

"Critical point" of superior rectal artery, anastomosis poor or absent

Sigmoid colon

Anterior View

| **2.46** | **INFERIOR MESENTERIC ARTERY** |

The mesentery of the small intestine has been cut at its root.

- The inferior mesenteric artery arises posterior to the ascending part of the duodenum, about 4 cm superior to the bifurcation of the aorta; on crossing the left common iliac artery, it becomes the superior rectal artery.
- The branches of the inferior mesenteric artery include the left colic artery and several sigmoid arteries; the inferior two sigmoid arteries branch from the superior rectal artery.

- The point at which the last artery to the colon branches from the superior rectal artery is known as the "critical point" of the superior rectal artery; distal to this point, there are poor or no anastomotic connections with the superior rectal artery.

Right renal pelvis

Right ureter

Gas in
ascending colon

Catheter

**Superior
rectal artery**

**Ascending branch
of left colic artery**

**Inferior mesenteric
artery**

Marginal artery

Left colic artery

**Descending branch
of left colic artery**

Descending colon

Sigmoid arteries

Gonadal radiation shield

Postero-anterior Arteriogram

2.47 **INFERIOR MESENTERIC ARTERIOGRAM**

- The left colic artery courses to the left toward the descending colon and splits into ascending and descending branches.
- The sigmoid arteries, two to four in number, supply the sigmoid colon.

- The superior rectal artery, which is the continuation of the inferior mesenteric artery, supplies the rectum; the superior rectal anastomoses are formed by branches of the middle and inferior rectal arteries (from the internal iliac artery).

Transverse colon

Gastrocolic ligament
(part of greater omentum)

Duodenojejunal junction

Middle colic artery in
transverse mesocolon

Jejunum

Root of mesentery of
small intestine (cut)

Right colic flexure

Descending colon

Duodenum

Aorta

Inferior mesenteric artery

Ascending colon

Psoas

Appendices epiploicae

Taenia coli

Sigmoid colon

Sigmoid mesocolon

Cecum

Inferior epigastric artery

Ileum

Obliterated umbilical artery

Anterior View

2.48   PERITONEUM OF POSTERIOR ABDOMINAL CAVITY

The gastrocolic ligament is retracted superiorly, along with the transverse colon and transverse mesocolon. The appendix had been surgically removed. This dissection is continued in Figure 2.49.

- The root of the mesentery of the small intestine, approximately 15 to 20 cm in length, extends between the duodenojejunal junction and ileocecal junction.
- The large intestine forms 3½ sides of a square around the jejunum and ileum. On the right are the cecum and ascending colon, superior is the transverse colon, on the left is the descending and sigmoid colon, and inferiorly is the sigmoid colon.

- **Chronic inflammation of the colon (ulcerative colitis, Crohn disease)** is characterized by severe inflammation and ulceration of the colon and rectum. In some patients, a colectomy is performed, during which the terminal ileum and colon as well as the rectum and anal canal are removed. An ileostomy is then constructed to establish an artificial cutaneous opening between the ileum and the skin of the anterolateral abdominal wall.

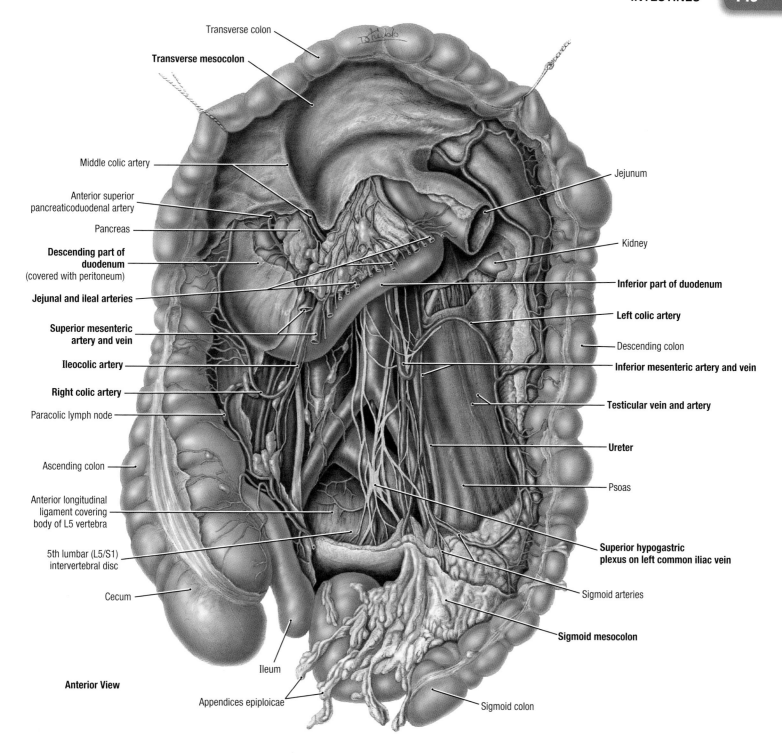

Transverse colon

Transverse mesocolon

Middle colic artery

Anterior superior pancreaticoduodenal artery

Pancreas

Descending part of duodenum (covered with peritoneum)

Jejunal and ileal arteries

Superior mesenteric artery and vein

Ileocolic artery

Right colic artery

Paracolic lymph node

Ascending colon

Anterior longitudinal ligament covering body of L5 vertebra

5th lumbar (L5/S1) intervertebral disc

Cecum

Ileum

Anterior View

Appendices epiploicae

Jejunum

Kidney

Inferior part of duodenum

Left colic artery

Descending colon

Inferior mesenteric artery and vein

Testicular vein and artery

Ureter

Psoas

Superior hypogastric plexus on left common iliac vein

Sigmoid arteries

Sigmoid mesocolon

Sigmoid colon

2.49 POSTERIOR ABDOMINAL CAVITY WITH PERITONEUM REMOVED

The jejunal and ileal branches (cut) pass from the left side of the superior mesenteric artery. The right colic artery here is a branch of the ileocolic artery. This is the same specimen as in Figure 2.48.

- The duodenum is large in diameter before crossing the superior mesenteric vessels and narrow afterward.
- On the right side, there are lymph nodes on the colon, paracolic nodes beside the colon, and nodes along the ileocolic artery, which drain into nodes anterior to the pancreas.

- The intestines and intestinal vessels lie on a resectable plane anterior to that of the testicular vessels; these in turn lie anterior to the plane of the kidney, its vessels, and the ureter.
- The superior hypogastric plexus lie inferior to the bifurcation of the aorta and anterior to the left common iliac vein, the body of the 5th lumbar vertebra, and the 5th intervertebral disc.

A. Anterior View

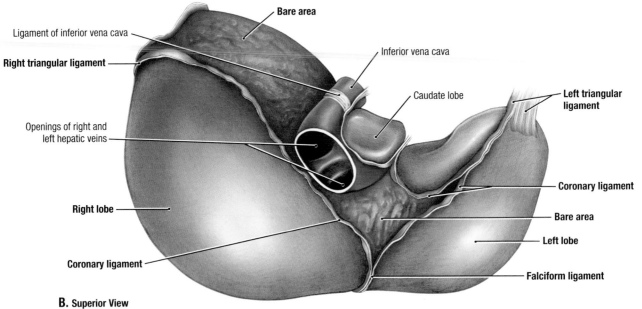

B. Superior View

2.50   DIAPHRAGMATIC (ANTERIOR AND SUPERIOR) SURFACE OF LIVER

A. The falciform ligament has been severed close to its attachment to the diaphragm and anterior abdominal wall and demarcates the right and left lobes of the liver. The round ligament of the liver (ligamentum teres) lies within the free edge of the falciform ligament.

B. The two layers of peritoneum that form the falciform ligament separate over the superior aspect (surrounding the bare area) of the liver to form the superior layer of the coronary ligament and the right and left triangular ligaments.

A. Postero-inferior View

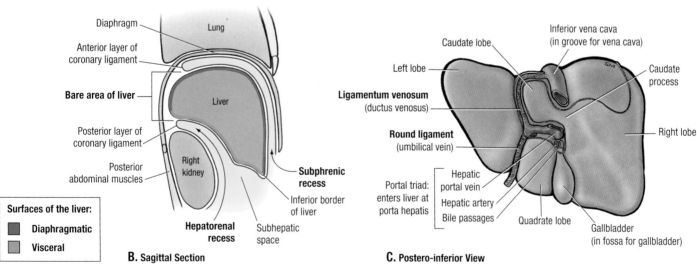

B. Sagittal Section

C. Postero-inferior View

2.51 VISCERAL (POSTERO-INFERIOR) SURFACE OF LIVER

A. Isolated specimen demonstrating lobes, and impressions of adjacent viscera. **B.** Hepatic surfaces and peritoneal recesses. **C.** Round ligament of liver and ligamentum venosum. The round ligament of liver includes the obliterated remains of the umbilical vein that carried well-oxygenated blood from the placenta to the fetus. The ligamentum venosum is the fibrous remnant of the fetal ductus venosus that shunted blood from the umbilical vein to the inferior vena cava, short circuiting the liver. Hepatic tissue may be obtained for diagnostic purposes by **liver biopsy.** The needle puncture is commonly made through the right 10th intercostal space in the midaxillary line. Before the physician takes the biopsy, the person is asked to hold his or her breath in full expiration to reduce the costodiaphragmatic recess and to lessen the possibility of damaging the lung and contaminating the pleural cavity.

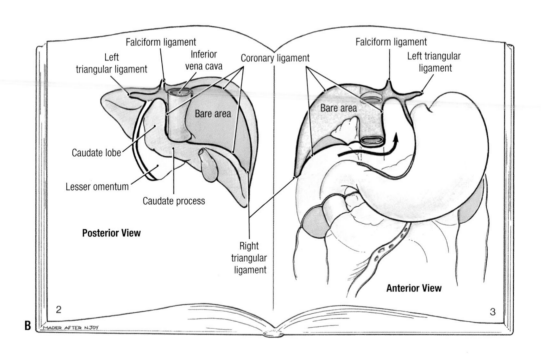

LIVER AND ITS POSTERIOR RELATIONS, SCHEMATIC ILLUSTRATION

A. Liver in situ. The jejunum, ileum, and the ascending, transverse, and descending colons have been removed. **B.** The liver is drawn schematically on a page in a book, so that as the page is turned (*arrow in A*), the liver is reflected to the right to reveal its posterior surface, and on the facing page, the posterior relations that compose the bed of the liver are viewed. The *arrow in B*

traverses the omental (epiploic) foramen to enter the omental bursa and its superior recess (*arrowhead*). The bare area is triangular, hence the coronary ligament that surrounds it is three-sided; its left side, or base, is between the inferior vena cava and caudate lobe, and its apex is at the right triangular ligament, where the superior and inferior layers of the coronary ligament meet.

A. Superior View

Inferior vena cava

Right
Intermediate (middle)
Left

} Hepatic veins

Hepatic artery
Hepatic portal vein
Bile duct

} Portal triad

Round ligament of liver

Removed portion of liver

Plane of section

B. Inferior View

Liver tissue

Right hepatic vein

Diaphragm

Hepatic portal vein (portal triad)

Intermediate (middle) hepatic vein

Left hepatic vein

2.53 HEPATIC VEINS

A. Approximately horizontal section of liver with the posterior aspect at the top of page. Note the multiple perivascular fibrous capsules sectioned throughout the cut surface, each containing a portal triad (the hepatic portal vein, hepatic artery, bile ductules) plus lymph vessels. Interdigitating with these are branches of the three main hepatic veins (right, intermediate, and left), which, unaccompanied and lacking capsules, converge on the inferior vena cava. **B.** Ultrasound scan. The transducer was placed under the costal margin and directed posteriorly, producing an inverted image corresponding to **A.**

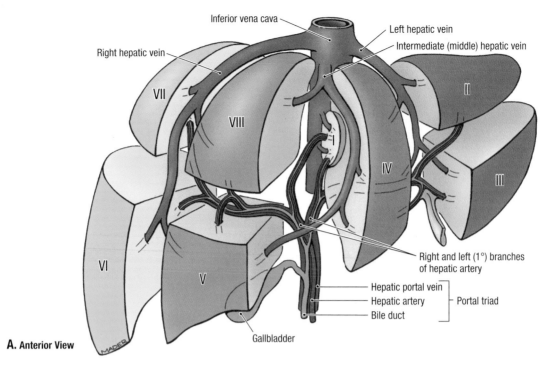

Inferior vena cava
Left hepatic vein
Intermediate (middle) hepatic vein
Right hepatic vein
VII
VIII
II
I
IV
III
VI
V
Right and left (1°) branches of hepatic artery
Hepatic portal vein
Hepatic artery — Portal triad
Bile duct
Gallbladder

A. Anterior View

MADER

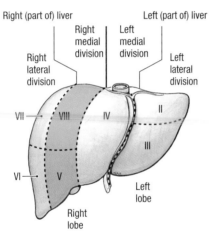

Right (part of) liver
Left (part of) liver
Right medial division
Left medial division
Right lateral division
Left lateral division
VII
VIII
IV
II
III
VI
V
Left lobe
Right lobe

B

Posterior (part of) liver (caudate lobe)
II
VII
I
III
IV
V
VI
Division between right and left (parts of) liver (right sagittal fissure)

C

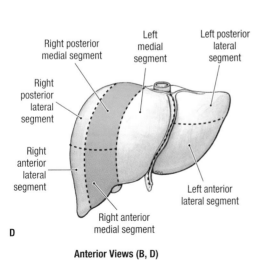

Right posterior medial segment
Left medial segment
Left posterior lateral segment
Right posterior lateral segment
Right anterior lateral segment
Left anterior lateral segment
Right anterior medial segment

D

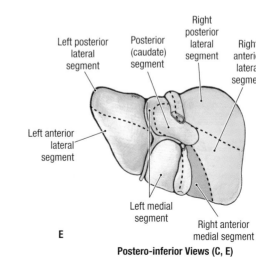

Left posterior lateral segment
Posterior (caudate) segment
Right posterior lateral segment
Right anterior lateral segment
Left anterior lateral segment
Left medial segment
Right anterior medial segment

E

Anterior Views (B, D)

Postero-inferior Views (C, E)

2.54   HEPATIC SEGMENTATION

2.54   HEPATIC SEGMENTATION *(CONTINUED)*

Each segment is supplied by a secondary or tertiary branch of the hepatic artery, bile duct, and portal vein. The hepatic veins interdigitate between the structures of the portal triad and are intersegmental in that they drain adjacent segments. Since the right and left hepatic arteries and ducts and branches of the right and left portal veins do not communicate, it is possible to perform **hepatic lobectomies** (removal of the right or left part of the liver) and **segmentectomies.** Each segment can be identified numerically or by name (Table 2.6).

TABLE 2.6 *SCHEMA OF TERMINOLOGY FOR SUBDIVISIONS OF THE LIVER*

Anatomical Term	Right Lobe		Left Lobe		Caudate Lobe	
Functional/surgical term[a]	Right (part of) liver [Right portal lobe[b]]		Left (part of) liver [Left portal lobe[c]]		Posterior (part of) liver	
	Right lateral division	Right medial division	Left medial division	Left lateral division	[Right caudate lobe[b]]	[Left caudate lobe[c]]
	Posterior lateral segment **Segment VII** [Posterior superior area]	Posterior medial segment **Segment VIII** [Anterior superior area]	[Medial superior area] Left medial segment **Segment IV**	Lateral segment **Segment II** [Lateral superior area]	Posterior segment **Segment I**	
	Right anterior lateral segment **Segment VI** [Posterior inferior area]	Anterior medial segment **Segment V** [Anterior inferior area]	[Medial inferior area = quadrate lobe]	Left anterior lateral segment **Segment III** [Lateral inferior area]		

[a]The labels in the table and figure above reflect the Terminologia *Anatomica: International Anatomical Terminology.* Previous terminology is in brackets.
[b,c]Under the schema of the previous terminology, the caudate lobe was divided into right and left halves, and [b] the right half of the caudate lobe was considered a subdivision of the right portal lobe; [c] the left half of the caudate lobe was considered a subdivision of the left portal lobe.

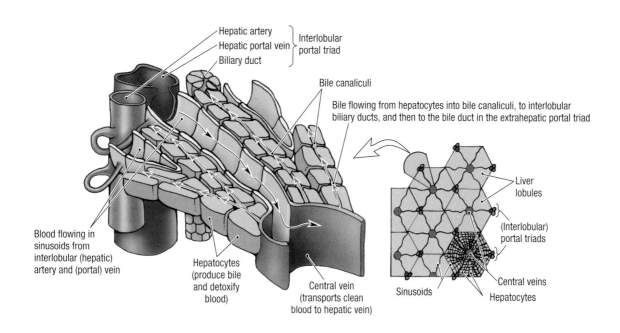

2.55   FLOW OF BLOOD AND BILE IN THE LIVER

This small part of a liver lobule shows the components of the interlobular portal triad and the positioning of the sinusoids and bile canaliculi. **Right.** The cut surface of the liver shows the hexagonal pattern of the lobules.

- With the exception of lipids, every substance absorbed by the alimentary tract is received first by the liver, via the hepatic portal vein. In addition to its many metabolic activities, the liver stores glycogen and secretes bile.

- There is progressive destruction of hepatocytes in **cirrhosis of the liver** and replacement of them by fibrous tissue. This tissue surrounds the intrahepatic blood vessels and biliary ducts, making the liver firm and impeding circulation of blood through it.

Falciform ligament

Liver

Caudate lobe

Left (hepatic) branch

Round ligament
of liver

Common hepatic duct

Hepatic portal vein

Right (hepatic) branch

Gallbladder

Bile duct

Cystic duct

Peritoneum

Duodenum
(retracted anteriorly)

Peritoneum (cut edge)

Areolar membrane
(fusion fascia)

Hepatorenal
recess

Bare area for colon

Perirenal fat

Pancreas

Right kidney

Ureter

Testicular vein and artery

Aorta

Inferior vena cava

A. Anterior View

Diaphragm

Liver

Gallbladder

Bile duct

Transverse
colon

Duodenum

Anterior abdominal wall

B. Schematic Sagittal Section,
in Right Midclavicular Plane

2.56   EXPOSURE OF THE PORTAL TRIAD

A. The portal triad typically consists of the hepatic portal vein (posteriorly), the hepatic artery proper (ascending from the left), and the bile passages (descending to the right). Here, the hepatic artery proper is replaced by a left hepatic branch, arising directly from the common hepatic artery, and a right hepatic branch, arising from the superior mesenteric artery (a common variation). A rod traverses the omental (epiploic) foramen. The lesser omentum and transverse colon are removed, and the peritoneum is cut along the right border of the duodenum; this part of the duodenum is retracted anteriorly. The space opened up reveals two smooth areolar membranes (fusion fascia) normally applied to each other that are vestiges of the embryonic peritoneum originally covering these surfaces. **B.** Typical relations of gallbladder, cystic duct, and bile duct to the duodenum.

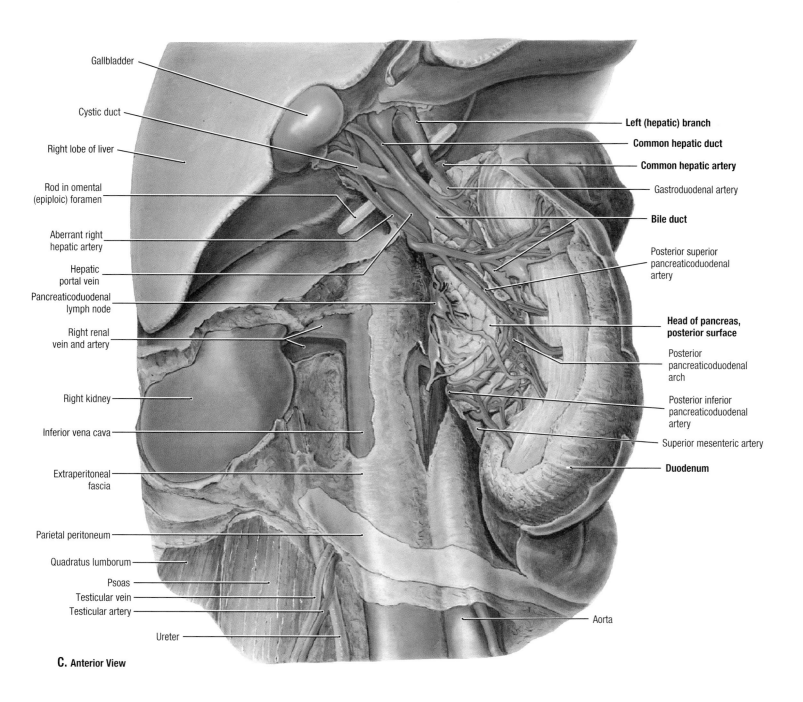

Gallbladder

Cystic duct

Right lobe of liver

Rod in omental
(epiploic) foramen

Aberrant right
hepatic artery

Hepatic
portal vein

Pancreaticoduodenal
lymph node

Right renal
vein and artery

Right kidney

Inferior vena cava

Extraperitoneal
fascia

Parietal peritoneum

Quadratus lumborum

Psoas

Testicular vein

Testicular artery

Ureter

Left (hepatic) branch

Common hepatic duct

Common hepatic artery

Gastroduodenal artery

Bile duct

Posterior superior
pancreaticoduodenal
artery

**Head of pancreas,
posterior surface**

Posterior
pancreaticoduodenal
arch

Posterior inferior
pancreaticoduodenal
artery

Superior mesenteric artery

Duodenum

Aorta

C. Anterior View

| 2.56 | **EXPOSURE OF THE PORTAL TRIAD (*CONTINUED*)** |

C. Continuing the dissection in **A**, the secondarily retroperitoneal viscera (duodenum and head of the pancreas) are retracted anteriorly and to the left. The areolar membrane (fusion fascia) covering the posterior aspect of the pancreas and duodenum is largely removed, and that covering the anterior aspect of the great vessels is partly removed. A common method for

reducing portal hypertension is to divert blood from the portal venous system to the systemic venous system by creating a communication between the portal vein and the IVC. This **portacaval anastomosis or portosystemic shunt** may be created where these vessels lie close to each other posterior to the liver.

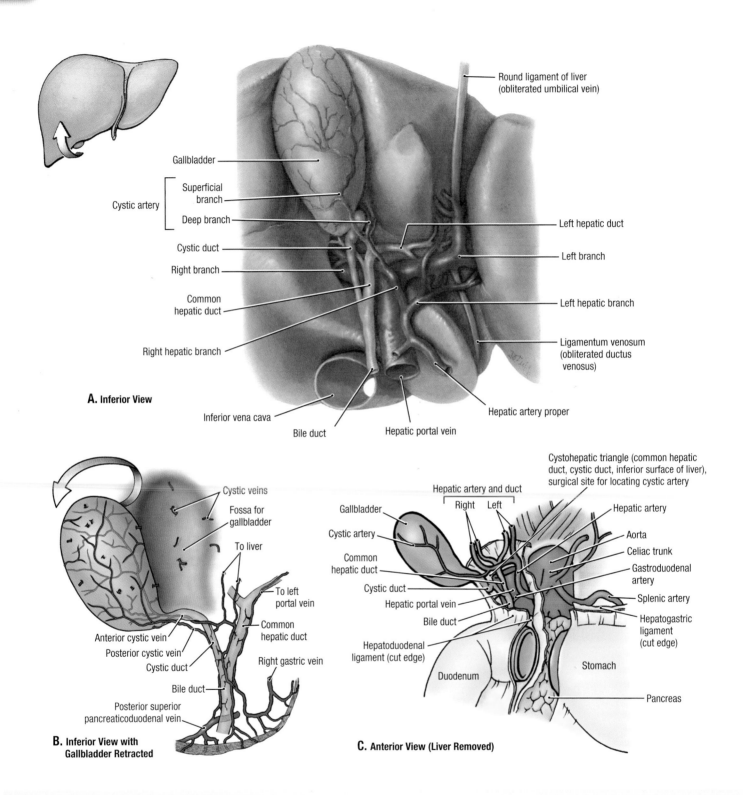

Round ligament of liver
(obliterated umbilical vein)

Gallbladder

Cystic artery
  Superficial branch
  Deep branch

Cystic duct

Right branch

Common hepatic duct

Right hepatic branch

Left hepatic duct

Left branch

Left hepatic branch

Ligamentum venosum
(obliterated ductus venosus)

A. Inferior View

Inferior vena cava

Bile duct

Hepatic portal vein

Hepatic artery proper

Cystic veins

Fossa for gallbladder

To liver

To left portal vein

Common hepatic duct

Anterior cystic vein

Posterior cystic vein

Cystic duct

Right gastric vein

Bile duct

Posterior superior pancreaticoduodenal vein

B. Inferior View with Gallbladder Retracted

Cystohepatic triangle (common hepatic duct, cystic duct, inferior surface of liver), surgical site for locating cystic artery

Hepatic artery and duct
  Right   Left

Gallbladder

Cystic artery

Common hepatic duct

Cystic duct

Hepatic portal vein

Bile duct

Hepatoduodenal ligament (cut edge)

Duodenum

Hepatic artery

Aorta

Celiac trunk

Gastroduodenal artery

Splenic artery

Hepatogastric ligament (cut edge)

Stomach

Pancreas

C. Anterior View (Liver Removed)

2.57   GALLBLADDER AND STRUCTURES OF PORTA HEPATIS

A. Gallbladder, cystic artery, and extrahepatic bile ducts. The inferior border of the liver is elevated to demonstrate its visceral surface (as in orientation figure). **B.** Venous drainage of the gall bladder and extrahepatic ducts. Most veins are tributaries of the hepatic portal vein, but some drain directly to the liver. **C.** Portal triad within the hepatoduodenal ligament (free edge of lesser omentum). **Gallstones** are concretions, in the gallbladder or extrahepatic biliary ducts. The cystohepatic (hepatobiliary) triangle (Calot), between the common hepatic duct, cystic duct, and liver, is an important endoscopic landmark for locating the cystic artery during **cholecystectomy.**

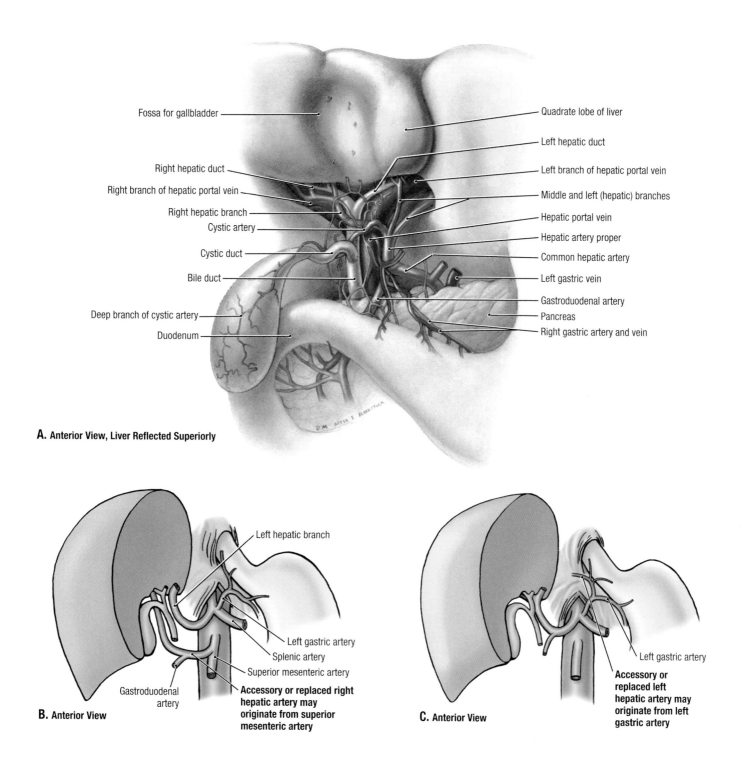

Fossa for gallbladder

Right hepatic duct

Right branch of hepatic portal vein

Right hepatic branch

Cystic artery

Cystic duct

Bile duct

Deep branch of cystic artery

Duodenum

Quadrate lobe of liver

Left hepatic duct

Left branch of hepatic portal vein

Middle and left (hepatic) branches

Hepatic portal vein

Hepatic artery proper

Common hepatic artery

Left gastric vein

Gastroduodenal artery

Pancreas

Right gastric artery and vein

A. Anterior View, Liver Reflected Superiorly

Left hepatic branch

Left gastric artery

Splenic artery

Superior mesenteric artery

Gastroduodenal artery

Accessory or replaced right hepatic artery may originate from superior mesenteric artery

B. Anterior View

Left gastric artery

Accessory or replaced left hepatic artery may originate from left gastric artery

C. Anterior View

| **2.58** | **VESSELS IN PORTA HEPATIS** |

A. Hepatic and cystic vessels. The liver is reflected superiorly. The gallbladder, freed from its bed or fossa, has remained nearly in its anatomical position, pulled slightly to the right. The deep branch of the cystic artery on the deep, or attached, surface of the gallbladder anastomoses with branches of the superficial branch of the cystic artery and sends twigs into the bed of the gallbladder. Veins (not all shown) accompany most arteries. **B.** Aberrant (accessory or replaced) right hepatic artery. **C.** Aberrant left hepatic artery. Awareness of the variations in arteries and bile duct formation is important for surgeons when they ligate the cystic duct during **cholecystectomy** (removal of the gallbladder).

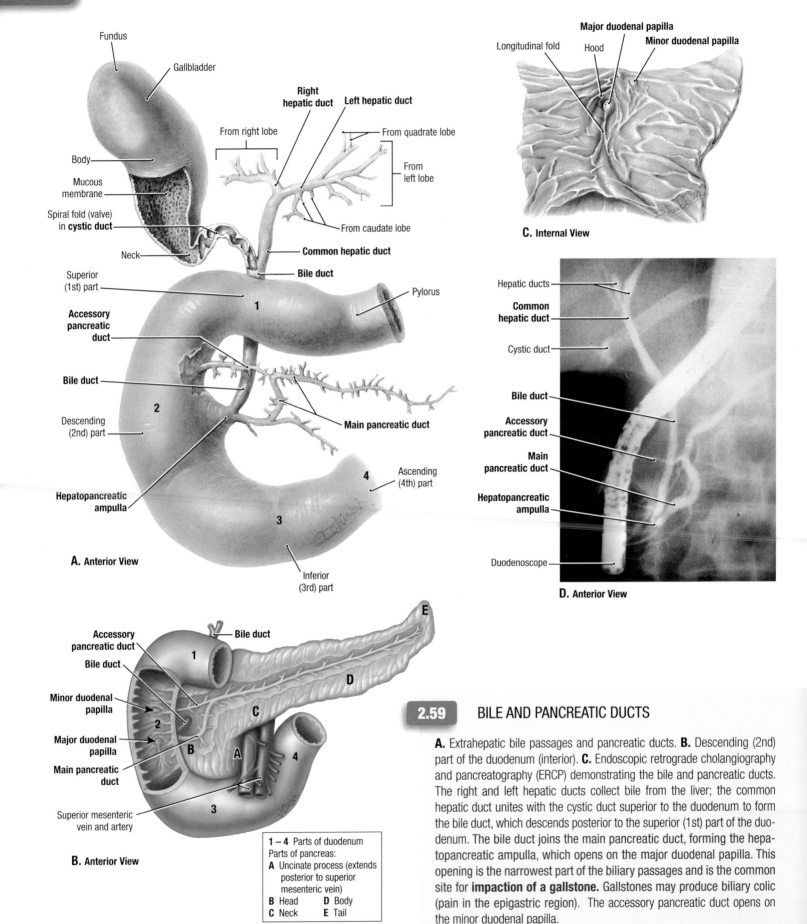

A. Anterior View

Fundus
Gallbladder
Right hepatic duct
Left hepatic duct
From right lobe
From quadrate lobe
From left lobe
Body
Mucous membrane
Spiral fold (valve) in **cystic duct**
From caudate lobe
Neck
Common hepatic duct
Bile duct
Superior (1st) part
Pylorus
Accessory pancreatic duct
Bile duct
Descending (2nd) part
Main pancreatic duct
Hepatopancreatic ampulla
Ascending (4th) part
Inferior (3rd) part
1 2 3 4

B. Anterior View

Accessory pancreatic duct
Bile duct
Bile duct
Minor duodenal papilla
Major duodenal papilla
Main pancreatic duct
Superior mesenteric vein and artery
A B C D E
1 2 3 4

1–4 Parts of duodenum
Parts of pancreas:
A Uncinate process (extends posterior to superior mesenteric vein)
B Head   **D** Body
C Neck   **E** Tail

C. Internal View

Longitudinal fold
Hood
Major duodenal papilla
Minor duodenal papilla

D. Anterior View

Hepatic ducts
Common hepatic duct
Cystic duct
Bile duct
Accessory pancreatic duct
Main pancreatic duct
Hepatopancreatic ampulla
Duodenoscope

2.59 BILE AND PANCREATIC DUCTS

A. Extrahepatic bile passages and pancreatic ducts. **B.** Descending (2nd) part of the duodenum (interior). **C.** Endoscopic retrograde cholangiography and pancreatography (ERCP) demonstrating the bile and pancreatic ducts. The right and left hepatic ducts collect bile from the liver; the common hepatic duct unites with the cystic duct superior to the duodenum to form the bile duct, which descends posterior to the superior (1st) part of the duodenum. The bile duct joins the main pancreatic duct, forming the hepatopancreatic ampulla, which opens on the major duodenal papilla. This opening is the narrowest part of the biliary passages and is the common site for **impaction of a gallstone.** Gallstones may produce biliary colic (pain in the epigastric region). The accessory pancreatic duct opens on the minor duodenal papilla.

Anterior Views

Transverse Sections

Anterior Views

2.60   DEVELOPMENT AND VARIABILITY OF THE PANCREATIC DUCTS

A.–C. Anterior views (*top*) and transverse sections (*bottom*) of the stages in the development of the pancreas. **A.** The small, primitive ventral bud arises in common with the bile duct, and a larger, primitive dorsal bud arises independently from the duodenum. **B.** The 2nd, or descending, part of the duodenum rotates on its long axis, which brings the ventral bud and bile duct posterior to the dorsal bud. **C.** A connecting segment unites the dorsal duct to the ventral duct, whereupon the duodenal end of the dorsal duct atrophies, and the direction of flow within it is reversed. **D.–G.** Common variations of the pancreatic duct. **D.** An accessory duct that has lost its connection with the duodenum. **E.** An accessory duct that is large enough to relieve an obstructed main duct. **F.** An accessory duct that could probably substitute for the main duct. **G.** A persisting primitive dorsal duct unconnected to the primitive ventral duct.

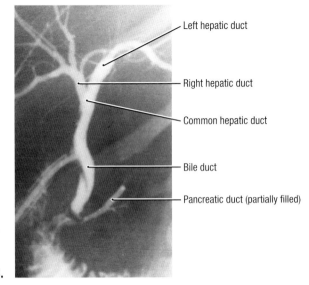

A.

Left hepatic duct
Right hepatic duct
Common hepatic duct
Bile duct (common bile duct)
Pancreatic duct
T tube
Duodenum

B.

Left hepatic duct
Right hepatic duct
Common hepatic duct
Bile duct
Pancreatic duct (partially filled)

2.61   RADIOGRAPHS OF BILIARY PASSAGES

After a cholecystectomy (removal of the gallbladder), contrast medium was injected with a T tube inserted into the bile passages. The biliary passages are visualized in the superior abdomen in **A** and are more localized in **B**.

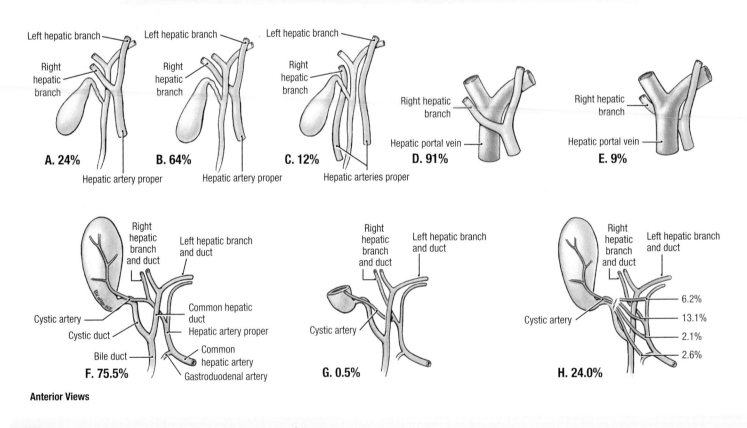

Anterior Views

2.62   VARIATIONS IN HEPATIC AND CYSTIC ARTERIES

In a study of 165 cadavers in Dr. Grant's laboratory, five patterns were observed. **A.** Right hepatic artery crossing anterior to bile passages, 24%. **B.** Right hepatic artery crossing posterior to bile passages, 64%. **C.** Aberrant artery arising from the superior mesenteric artery, 12%. The artery crossed anterior **(D)** to the portal vein in 91% and posterior **(E)** in 9%. The cystic artery usually arises from the right hepatic artery in the angle between the common hepatic duct and cystic duct (see cystohepatic triangle, Fig. 2.57A), without crossing the common hepatic duct **(F. and G)**. However, when it arises on the left of the bile passages, it almost always crosses anterior to the passages **(H)**.

A. Anterior View

- Right hepatic duct
- Left hepatic duct
- Common hepatic duct
- Neck of gallbladder
- Cystic duct
- Bile duct
- Duodenum

Parts of gallbladder:
- Neck
- Body
- Fundus

B. Anterior View

2.63 ENDOSCOPIC RETROGRADE CHOLANGIOGRAPHY OF GALLBLADDER AND BILIARY PASSAGES

A. Cystic duct. **B.** Parts of gallbladder.

Endoscopic retrograde cholangiography (ERCP) is done by first passing a fiberoptic endoscope through the mouth, esophagus, and stomach. Then the duodenum is entered, and a cannula is inserted into the major duodenal papilla and advanced under fluoroscopic control into the duct of choice (bile duct or pancreatic duct) for injection of radiographic contrast medium.

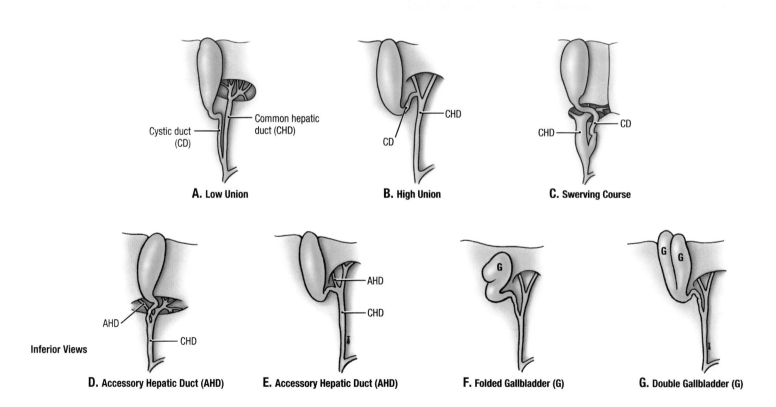

Cystic duct (CD) — Common hepatic duct (CHD)

A. Low Union

CHD — CD

B. High Union

CHD — CD

C. Swerving Course

Inferior Views

AHD — CHD

D. Accessory Hepatic Duct (AHD)

AHD — CHD

E. Accessory Hepatic Duct (AHD)

G

F. Folded Gallbladder (G)

G G

G. Double Gallbladder (G)

2.64 VARIATIONS OF CYSTIC AND HEPATIC DUCTS AND GALLBLADDER

The cystic duct usually lies on the right side of the common hepatic duct, joining it just above the superior (1st) part of the duodenum, but this varies as in **A.–C.** Of 95 gallbladders and bile passages studied in Dr. Grant's laboratory, 7 had accessory ducts. Of these, four joined the common hepatic duct near the cystic duct **(D)**, two joined the cystic duct **(E)**, and one was an anastomosing duct connecting the cystic with the common hepatic duct. **F.** Folded gallbladder. **G.** Double gallbladder.

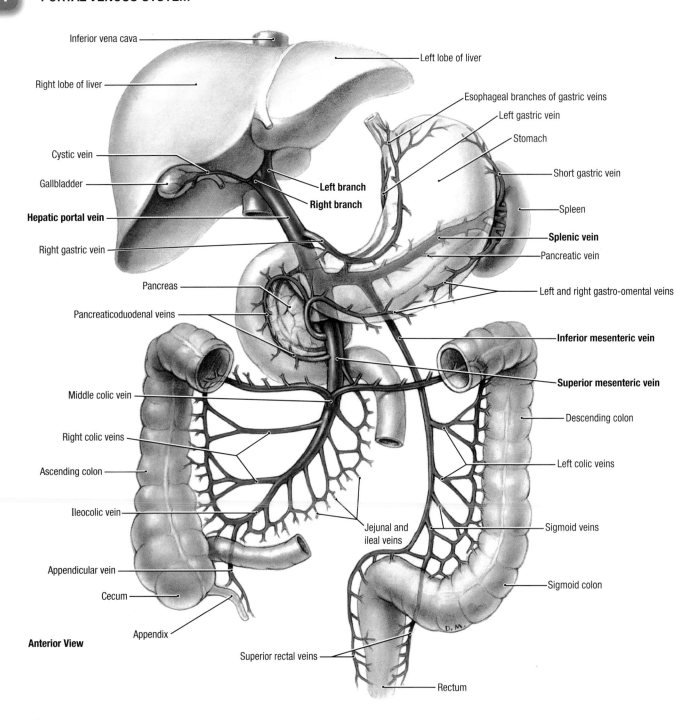

Inferior vena cava

Right lobe of liver

Cystic vein

Gallbladder

Hepatic portal vein

Right gastric vein

Pancreas

Pancreaticoduodenal veins

Middle colic vein

Right colic veins

Ascending colon

Ileocolic vein

Appendicular vein

Cecum

Appendix

Anterior View

Left lobe of liver

Esophageal branches of gastric veins

Left gastric vein

Stomach

Short gastric vein

Left branch

Right branch

Spleen

Splenic vein

Pancreatic vein

Left and right gastro-omental veins

Inferior mesenteric vein

Superior mesenteric vein

Descending colon

Left colic veins

Jejunal and ileal veins

Sigmoid veins

Sigmoid colon

Superior rectal veins

Rectum

D. M.

2.65   PORTAL VENOUS SYSTEM

- The hepatic portal vein drains venous blood from the gastrointestinal tract, spleen, pancreas, and gallbladder to the sinusoids of the liver; from here, the blood is conveyed to the systemic venous system by the hepatic veins that drain directly to the inferior vena cava.
- The hepatic portal vein forms posterior to the neck of the pancreas by the union of the superior mesenteric and splenic veins, with the inferior mesenteric vein joining at or near the angle of union.
- The splenic vein drains blood from the inferior mesenteric, left gastro-omental (epiploic), short gastric, and pancreatic veins.

- The right gastro-omental, pancreaticoduodenal, jejunal, ileal, right, and middle colic veins drain into the superior mesenteric vein.
- The inferior mesenteric vein commences in the rectal plexus as the superior rectal vein and, after crossing the common iliac vessels, becomes the inferior mesenteric vein; branches include the sigmoid and left colic veins.
- The hepatic portal vein divides into right and left branches at the porta hepatis. The left branch carries mainly, but not exclusively, blood from the inferior mesenteric, gastric, and splenic veins, and the right branch carries blood mainly from the superior mesenteric vein.

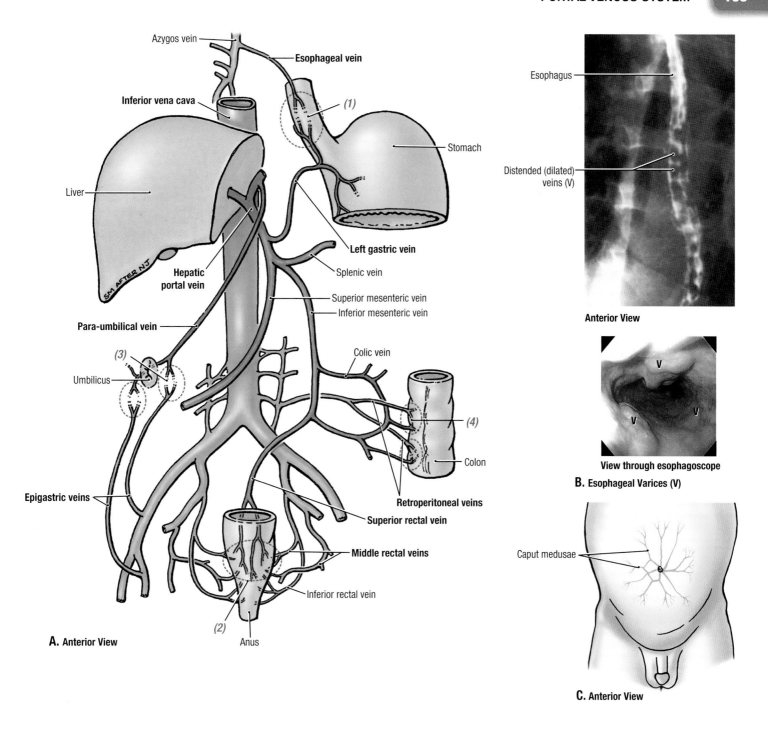

Anterior View

B. Esophageal Varices (V)

C. Anterior View

A. Anterior View

2.66 PORTACAVAL SYSTEM

A. Portacaval system. In this diagram, portal tributaries are *dark blue*, and systemic tributaries and communicating veins are *light blue*. In **portal hypertension** (as in hepatic cirrhosis), the portal blood cannot pass freely through the liver, and the portocaval anastomoses become engorged, dilated, or even varicose; as a consequence, these veins may rupture. The sites of the portocaval anastomosis shown are between *(1)* esophageal veins draining into the azygos vein (systemic) and left gastric vein (portal), which when dilated are esophageal varices; *(2)* the inferior and middle rectal veins, draining into the inferior vena cava (systemic) and the superior rectal vein continuing as the inferior mesenteric vein (portal) (hemorrhoids result if the vessels are dilated); *(3)* paraumbilical veins (portal) and small epigastric veins of the anterior abdominal wall (systemic), which when varicose form "caput medusae" (so named because of the resemblance of the radiating veins to the serpents on the head of Medusa, a character in Greek mythology); and *(4)* twigs of colic veins (portal) anastomosing with systemic retroperitoneal veins. **B.** Esophageal varices. **C.** Caput medusae.

For bare area of liver

For caudate lobe of liver

IVC

Esophagus and left gastric artery

Right suprarenal gland

For stomach

Omental (epiploic) foramen (arrow)

For spleen

Root of transverse mesocolon

For right lobe of liver

Pancreas

Left kidney

Duodenum

For bare area of descending colon

Right kidney

For bare area of ascending colon

For small intestine

For small intestine

Root of mesentery of small intestine

A. Anterior View

Superior mesenteric artery and vein

Ureter

Coronary ligament

Left

Superior

Inferior

Falciform ligament

Left triangular ligament

Superior recess of omental bursa (lesser sac)

IVC

SG

K

Splenorenal ligament

Right triangular ligament

Portal triad (Hepatoduodenal ligament)

Tail of pancreas

Right renal vein

Left suprarenal gland

Jejunum

Right ureter

Left renal vein

Duodenum

Intestinal vessels

Right gonadal (ovarian/testicular) vein and artery

Left gonadal (ovarian/testicular) artery and vein

C. Anterior View

B. Anterior View

2.67   POSTERIOR ABDOMINAL VISCERA AND THEIR ANTERIOR RELATIONS

The peritoneal coverings are yellow. **A.** Duodenum and pancreas in situ. Note the line of attachment of the root of the transverse mesocolon is to the body and tail of the pancreas. The viscera contacting specific regions are indicated by the term "for." The omental (epiploic) foramen is traversed by an arrow. **B.**

After removal of duodenum and pancreas. The three parts of the coronary ligament are attached to the diaphragm, except where the inferior vena cava (IVC), suprarenal gland (SG), and kidney (K) intervene. **C.** Pancreas and duodenum removed from **A.**

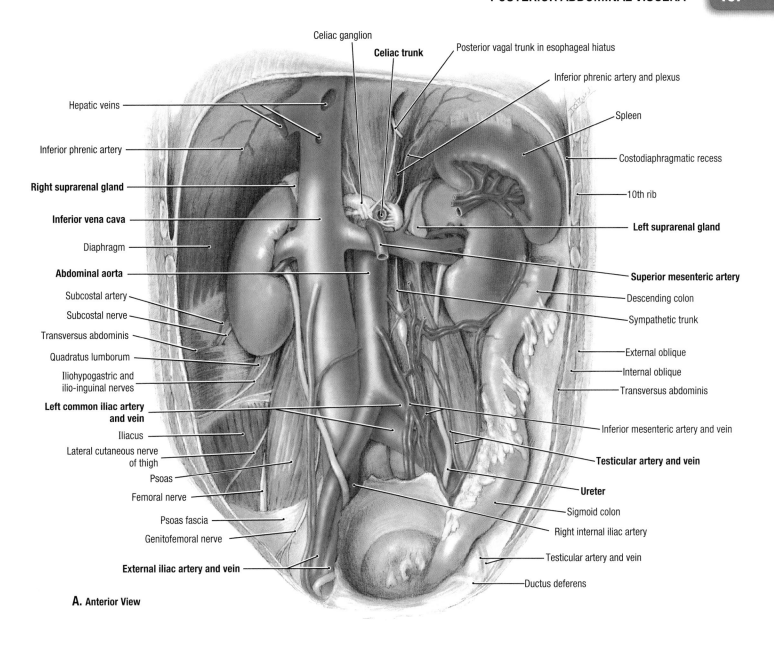

Celiac ganglion
Celiac trunk
Posterior vagal trunk in esophageal hiatus
Inferior phrenic artery and plexus
Hepatic veins
Spleen
Inferior phrenic artery
Costodiaphragmatic recess
Right suprarenal gland
10th rib
Inferior vena cava
Left suprarenal gland
Diaphragm
Abdominal aorta
Superior mesenteric artery
Subcostal artery
Descending colon
Subcostal nerve
Sympathetic trunk
Transversus abdominis
Quadratus lumborum
External oblique
Iliohypogastric and ilio-inguinal nerves
Internal oblique
Transversus abdominis
Left common iliac artery and vein
Inferior mesenteric artery and vein
Iliacus
Lateral cutaneous nerve of thigh
Testicular artery and vein
Psoas
Ureter
Femoral nerve
Sigmoid colon
Psoas fascia
Right internal iliac artery
Genitofemoral nerve
Testicular artery and vein
External iliac artery and vein
Ductus deferens

A. Anterior View

2.68

VISCERA AND VESSELS OF POSTERIOR ABDOMINAL WALL

A. Great vessels, kidneys, and suprarenal glands. **B.** Relationships of left renal vein and inferior (3rd) part of duodenum to aorta and superior mesenteric artery.

- The abdominal aorta is shorter and smaller in caliber than the inferior vena cava.
- The inferior mesenteric artery arises about 4 cm superior to the aortic bifurcation and crosses the left common iliac vessels to become the superior rectal artery.
- The left renal vein drains the left testis, left suprarenal gland, and left kidney; the renal arteries are posterior to the renal veins.
- The ureter crosses the external iliac artery just beyond the common iliac bifurcation.
- The testicular vessels cross anterior to the ureter and join the ductus deferens at the deep inguinal ring.
- In **B**, the left renal vein and duodenum (and uncinate process of pancreas—not shown) pass between the aorta posteriorly and the superior mesenteric artery anteriorly; they may be compressed like nuts in a nutcracker.

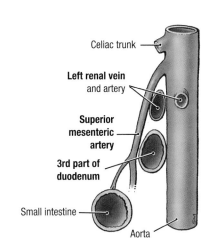

Celiac trunk
Left renal vein and artery
Superior mesenteric artery
3rd part of duodenum
Small intestine
Aorta

B. Lateral View (from left)

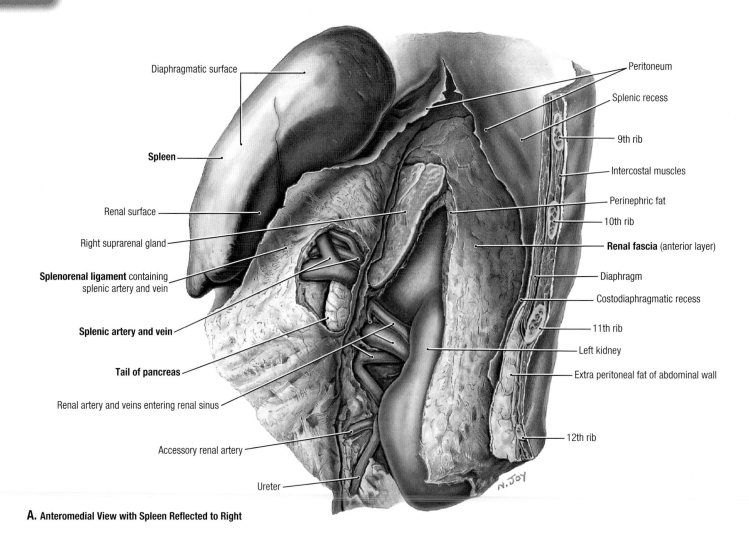

Diaphragmatic surface

Peritoneum

Splenic recess

9th rib

Spleen

Intercostal muscles

Renal surface

Perinephric fat

10th rib

Right suprarenal gland

Renal fascia (anterior layer)

Splenorenal ligament containing splenic artery and vein

Diaphragm

Costodiaphragmatic recess

Splenic artery and vein

11th rib

Left kidney

Tail of pancreas

Extra peritoneal fat of abdominal wall

Renal artery and veins entering renal sinus

Accessory renal artery

12th rib

Ureter

A. Anteromedial View with Spleen Reflected to Right

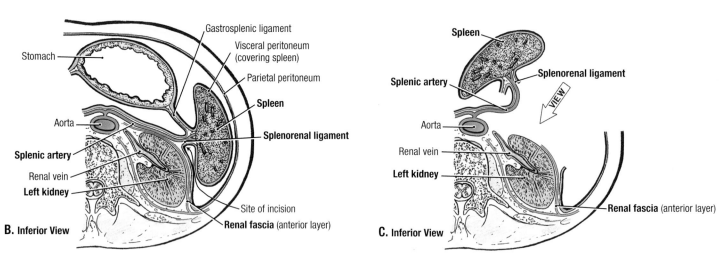

Gastrosplenic ligament

Stomach

Visceral peritoneum (covering spleen)

Parietal peritoneum

Spleen

Aorta

Splenorenal ligament

Splenic artery

Renal vein

Left kidney

Site of incision

B. Inferior View

Renal fascia (anterior layer)

Spleen

Splenic artery

Splenorenal ligament

Aorta

Renal vein

Left kidney

Renal fascia (anterior layer)

C. Inferior View

2.69 | EXPOSURE OF THE LEFT KIDNEY AND SUPRARENAL GLAND

A. Dissection. **B.** Schematic section with spleen and splenorenal ligament intact. **C.** Procedure used in **A** to expose the kidney. The spleen and splenorenal ligament are reflected anteriorly, with the splenic vessels and tail of the pancreas. Part of the renal fascia of the kidney is removed. Note the proximity of the splenic vein and left renal vein, enabling a **splenorenal shunt** to be established surgically to relieve portal hypertension.

A. Anterior View

Labels (top to bottom):
- Left suprarenal gland
- **Left kidney**
- 11th rib
- 12th rib
- Inferior vena cava
- Aorta
- L5
- Ureter
- Urinary bladder
- Urethra

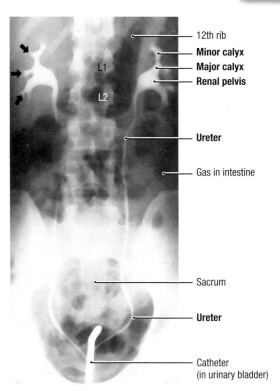

B. Anteroposterior Pyelogram

Labels (top to bottom):
- 12th rib
- **Minor calyx**
- **Major calyx**
- **Renal pelvis**
- L1
- L2
- **Ureter**
- Gas in intestine
- Sacrum
- **Ureter**
- Catheter (in urinary bladder)

C. Anterior View

Labels:
- Aortic hiatus in diaphragm
- **Left inferior phrenic artery**
- **Left superior suprarenal arteries**
- Left suprarenal gland
- Left kidney
- **Left middle suprarenal artery**
- **Left inferior suprarenal artery**
- **Left renal artery**
- Left ureter
- Aorta
- **Left gonadal artery** (testicular or ovarian)
- **Left common iliac artery**
- **Left internal iliac artery**

2.70   KIDNEYS AND SUPRARENAL GLANDS

A. Overview of urinary system. **B.** Pyelogram. Radiopaque material occupies the cavities that normally conduct urine. Note the papillae (indicated with *arrows*) bulging into the minor calices, which empty into a major calyx that opens, in turn, into the renal pelvis drained by the ureter. **C.** Arterial supply of the suprarenal glands, kidneys, and ureters.

Renal transplantation is now an established operation for the treatment of selected cases of chronic renal failure. The kidney can be removed from the donor without damaging the suprarenal gland because of the weak septum of renal fascia that separates the kidney from this gland. The site for transplanting a kidney is in the iliac fossa of the greater pelvis. The renal artery and vein are joined to the external iliac artery and vein, respectively, and the ureter is sutured into the urinary bladder.

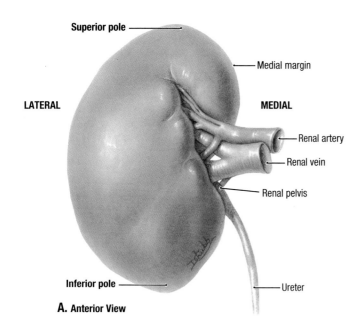

A. Anterior View

Superior pole

Medial margin

LATERAL

MEDIAL

Renal artery

Renal vein

Renal pelvis

Inferior pole

Ureter

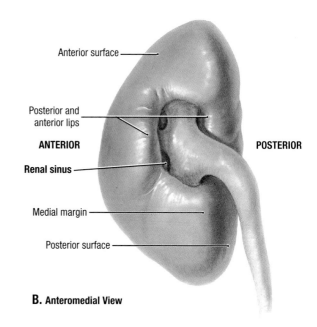

B. Anteromedial View

Anterior surface

Posterior and anterior lips

ANTERIOR

POSTERIOR

Renal sinus

Medial margin

Posterior surface

C. Anterior View

Fibrous capsule

Renal cortex

Renal medulla

Renal column

Renal papilla

Renal pyramid

Minor calyx

Major calyx

Renal sinus

Renal pelvis

Ureter

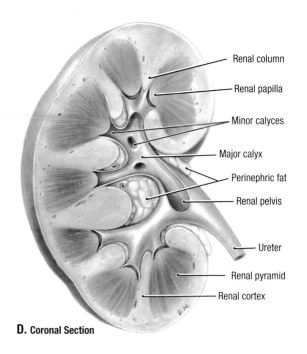

D. Coronal Section

Renal column

Renal papilla

Minor calyces

Major calyx

Perinephric fat

Renal pelvis

Ureter

Renal pyramid

Renal cortex

2.71 STRUCTURE OF KIDNEY

A. External features. The superior pole of the kidney is closer to the median plane than the inferior pole. Approximately 25% of kidneys may have a 2nd, 3rd, and even 4th accessory renal artery branching from the aorta. These multiple vessels enter through the renal sinus or at the superior or inferior pole. **B.** Renal sinus. The renal sinus is a vertical "pocket" opening on the medial side of the kidney. Tucked into the pocket are the renal pelvis and renal vessels in a matrix of perinephric fat. **C.** Renal calices. The anterior wall of the renal sinus has been cut away to expose the renal pelvis and the calices. **D.** Internal features. **Cysts in the kidney**, multiple or solitary, are common and usually benign findings during ultrasound examinations and dissection of cadavers. **Adult polycystic disease** of the kidneys, however, is an important cause of renal failure.

A. Segmental arteries. Right Kidney, Anterior View. Right Kidney, Posterior View.

Labels on A: Superior segmental artery; Anterosuperior segmental artery; Antero-inferior segmental artery; Posterior segmental artery; Inferior segmental artery

Segments: Apical, Anterosuperior, Antero-inferior, Posterior, Inferior

B. Anteroposterior Arteriogram

Labels on B: 11th and 12th ribs; Superior pole; Inferior suprarenal artery; Renal artery; Interlobar artery; Inferior pole

C. Anterior View

Labels on C: Interlobular; Arcuate; Interlobar; Lobar; Posterior segmental; Interlobar

D. Schematic Diagram

Labels on D: Renal corpuscle (Glomerular capsule, Glomerulus); Proximal convoluted tubule; Distal convoluted tubule; Peritubular capillaries; Collecting duct; Papillary duct; Renal papilla; Minor calyx; Efferent glomerular arteriole; Afferent glomerular arteriole; Interlobular artery; Interlobular vein; Renal cortex; Interlobar artery and vein; Arcuate vein and artery; Collecting duct; Renal medulla; Nephron loop (Loop of Henle) [Descending limb, Ascending limb]; Vasa recta; Papillary duct

2.72   SEGMENTS OF THE KIDNEYS

A. Segmental arteries. Segmental arteries do not anastomose significantly with other segmental arteries; they are end arteries. The area supplied by each segmented artery is an independent, surgically respectable unit or **renal segment. B.** Renal arteriogram. **C.** Corrosion cast of posterior segmental artery of kidney. **D.** The nephron is the functional unit of the kidney consisting of a renal corpuscle, proximal tubule, nephron loop, and distal tubule. Papillary ducts open onto renal papillae, emptying into minor calices.

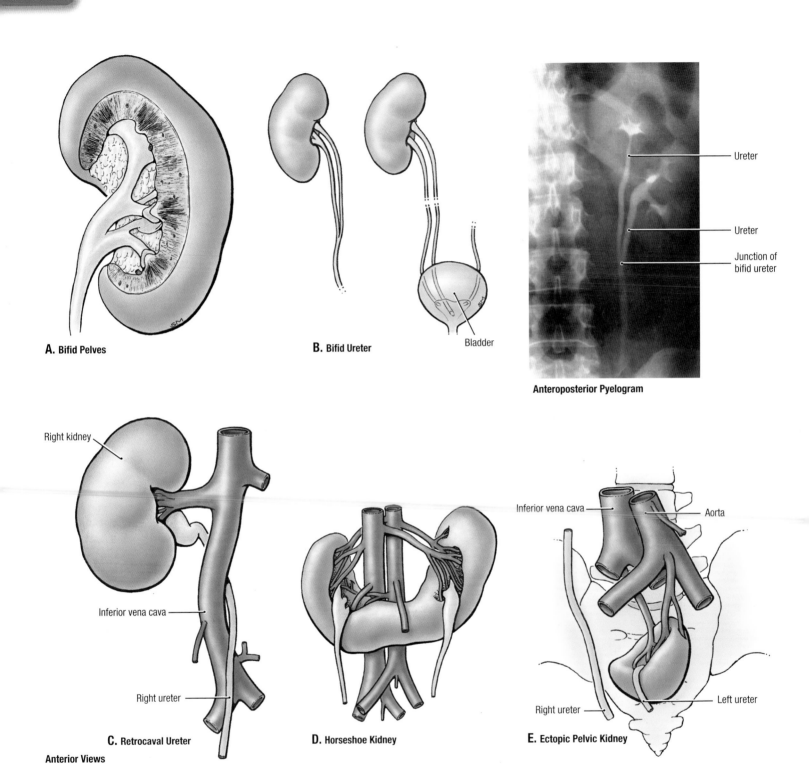

A. Bifid Pelves

B. Bifid Ureter

Bladder

Ureter

Ureter

Junction of bifid ureter

Anteroposterior Pyelogram

Right kidney

Inferior vena cava

Right ureter

C. Retrocaval Ureter

Anterior Views

D. Horseshoe Kidney

Inferior vena cava

Aorta

Right ureter

Left ureter

E. Ectopic Pelvic Kidney

2.73   ANOMALIES OF KIDNEY AND URETER

A. Bifid pelves. The pelves are almost replaced by two long major calices, which extend outside the sinus. **B. Duplicated, or bifid, ureters.** These can be unilateral or bilateral and complete or incomplete. **C. Retrocaval ureter.** The ureter courses posterior and then anterior to the inferior vena cava. **D. Horseshoe kidney.** The right and left kidneys are fused in the midline. **E. Ectopic pelvic kidney.** Pelvic kidneys have no fatty capsule and can be unilateral or bilateral. During childbirth, they may cause obstruction and suffer injury.

Latissimus dorsi

Serratus posterior inferior

12th rib

External oblique

Internal oblique

Thoracolumbar fascia

Lateral cutaneous branch of T12 nerve

Iliac crest

Lateral cutaneous branch of L1 nerve

Cutaneous branches of posterior rami
of nerves L1, L2, L3

Posterolateral View

2.74   POSTEROLATERAL ABDOMINAL WALL: EXPOSURE OF KIDNEY I

The latissimus dorsi is partially reflected.
- The external oblique muscle has an oblique, free posterior border that extends from the tip of the 12th rib to the midpoint of the iliac crest.

- The internal oblique muscle extends posteriorly beyond the border of the external oblique muscle.

Latissimus dorsi

Serratus posterior inferior

12th rib

Subcostal nerve (T12)

External oblique

Internal oblique

Aponeurosis of transversus abdominis and aponeurosis

Iliohypogastric nerve (L1)

Posterolateral View

2.75 POSTEROLATERAL ABDOMINAL WALL: EXPOSURE OF KIDNEY II

The external oblique muscle is incised and reflected laterally, and the internal oblique muscle is incised and reflected medially; the transversus abdominis muscle and its posterior aponeurosis are exposed where pierced by the subcostal (T12) and iliohypogastric (L1) nerves. These nerves give off motor twigs and lateral cutaneous branches and continue anteriorly between the internal oblique and transversus abdominis muscles.

2.76 POSTEROLATERAL ABDOMINAL WALL: EXPOSURE OF KIDNEY III AND RENAL FASCIA ⟶

A. The posterior aponeurosis of the transversus abdominis muscle is divided between the subcostal and iliohypogastric nerves and lateral to the oblique lateral border of the quadratus lumborum muscle; the retroperitoneal fat surrounding the kidney is exposed. **B.** Renal fascia and retroperitoneal fat, schematic transverse section. The renal fascia is within this fat; the portion of fat internal to the renal fascia is termed perinephric fat (perirenal fat capsule), and the fat immediately external is paranephric fat (pararenal fat body).

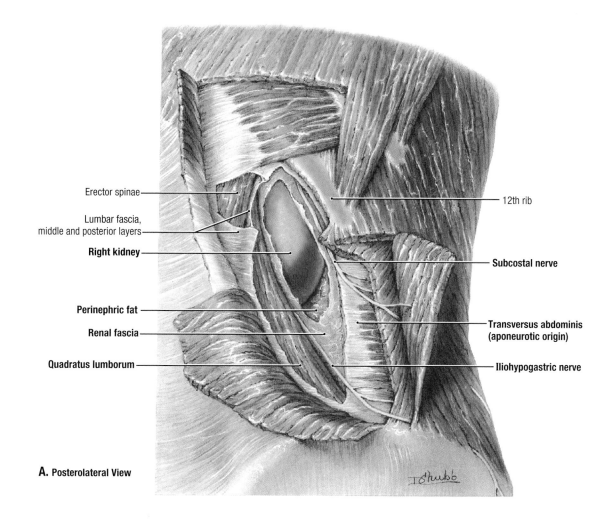

Erector spinae

Lumbar fascia, middle and posterior layers

Right kidney

Perinephric fat

Renal fascia

Quadratus lumborum

12th rib

Subcostal nerve

Transversus abdominis (aponeurotic origin)

Iliohypogastric nerve

A. Posterolateral View

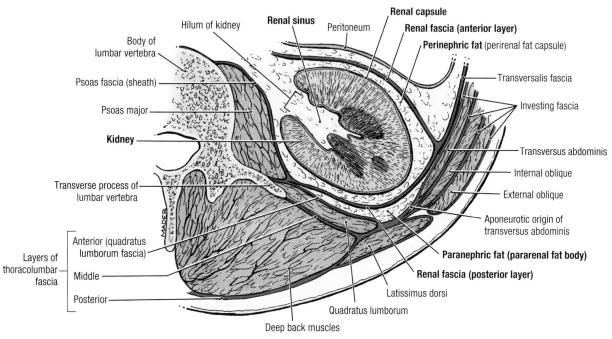

Hilum of kidney

Body of lumbar vertebra

Psoas fascia (sheath)

Psoas major

Kidney

Transverse process of lumbar vertebra

Anterior (quadratus lumborum fascia)

Layers of thoracolumbar fascia

Middle

Posterior

Renal sinus

Peritoneum

Renal capsule

Renal fascia (anterior layer)

Perinephric fat (perirenal fat capsule)

Transversalis fascia

Investing fascia

Transversus abdominis

Internal oblique

External oblique

Aponeurotic origin of transversus abdominis

Paranephric fat (pararenal fat body)

Renal fascia (posterior layer)

Latissimus dorsi

Quadratus lumborum

Deep back muscles

B. Transverse Section

2.76

POSTEROLATERAL ABDOMINAL WALL: EXPOSURE OF KIDNEY III AND RENAL FASCIA (*CONTINUED*)

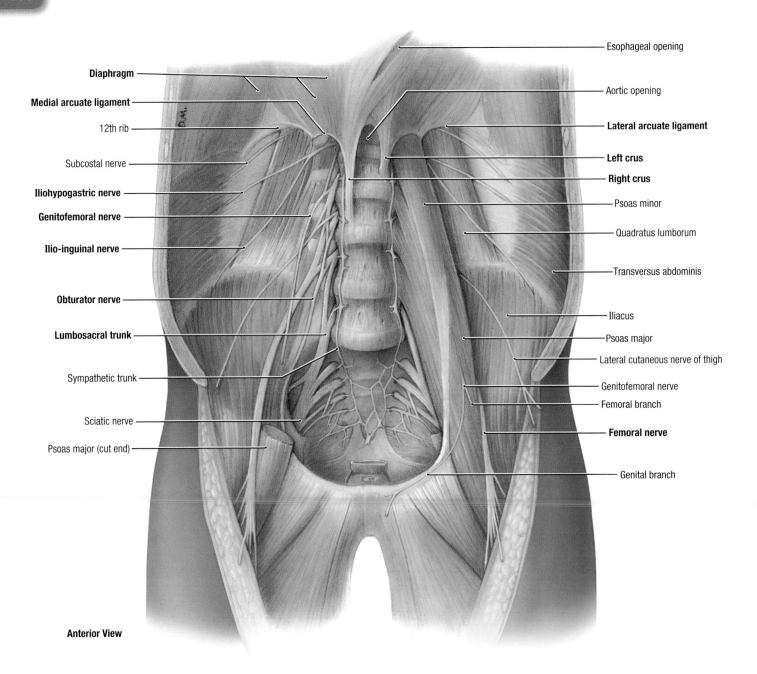

Diaphragm

Medial arcuate ligament

12th rib

Subcostal nerve

Iliohypogastric nerve

Genitofemoral nerve

Ilio-inguinal nerve

Obturator nerve

Lumbosacral trunk

Sympathetic trunk

Sciatic nerve

Psoas major (cut end)

Esophageal opening

Aortic opening

Lateral arcuate ligament

Left crus

Right crus

Psoas minor

Quadratus lumborum

Transversus abdominis

Iliacus

Psoas major

Lateral cutaneous nerve of thigh

Genitofemoral nerve

Femoral branch

Femoral nerve

Genital branch

Anterior View

| **2.77** | LUMBAR PLEXUS AND VERTEBRAL ATTACHMENT OF DIAPHRAGM |

TABLE 2.7 PRINCIPAL MUSCLES OF POSTERIOR ABDOMINAL WALL

Muscle	Superior Attachments	Inferior Attachments	Innervation	Actions
Psoas major[a,b]	Transverse processes of lumbar vertebrae; sides of bodies of T12–L5 vertebrae and intervening intervertebral discs	By a strong tendon to lesser trochanter of femur	Anterior rami of lumbar nerves (**L1, L2**, L3)	Acting inferiorly with iliacus, it flexes thigh at hip; acting superiorly, it flexes vertebral column laterally; it is used to balance the trunk; during sitting it acts inferiorly with iliacus to flex trunk
Iliacus[a]	Superior two thirds of iliac fossa, ala of sacrum, and anterior sacro-iliac ligaments	Lesser trochanter of femur and shaft inferior to it, and to psoas major tendon	Femoral nerve (**L2**, L3, L4)	Flexes thigh and stabilizes hip joint; acts with psoas major
Quadratus lumborum	Medial half of inferior border of 12th rib and tips of lumbar transverse processes	Iliolumbar ligament and internal lip of iliac crest	Anterior rami of T12 and L1–L4 nerves	Extends and laterally flexes vertebral column; fixes 12th rib during inspiration

[a]Psoas major and iliacus muscles are often described together as the iliopsoas muscle when flexion of the thigh is discussed.
[b]Psoas minor attaches proximally to the sides of bodies of T12–L1 vertebrae and intervertebral disc and distally to the pectineal line and iliopectineal eminence via the iliopectineal arch; it does not cross the hip joint. It is used to balance the trunk, in conjunction with psoas major. Innervation is from the anterior rami of lumbar nerves (L1, L2).

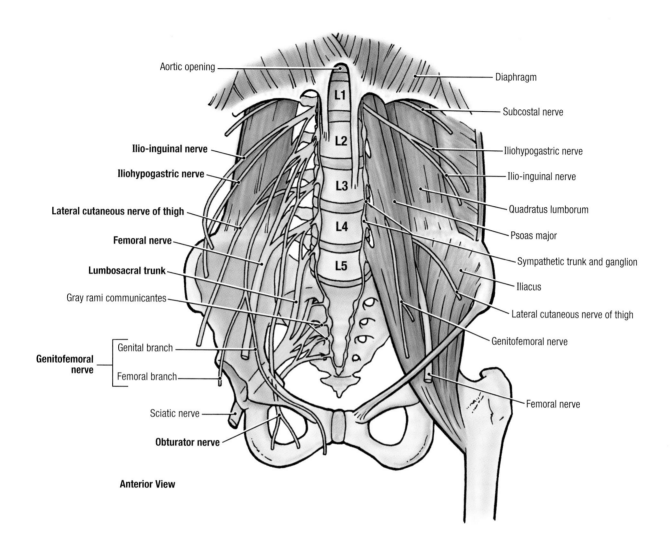

Aortic opening
Diaphragm
Subcostal nerve
Ilio-inguinal nerve
Iliohypogastric nerve
Iliohypogastric nerve
Ilio-inguinal nerve
Quadratus lumborum
Lateral cutaneous nerve of thigh
Psoas major
Femoral nerve
Sympathetic trunk and ganglion
Lumbosacral trunk
Iliacus
Gray rami communicantes
Lateral cutaneous nerve of thigh
Genitofemoral nerve
Genital branch
Genitofemoral nerve
Femoral branch
Sciatic nerve
Femoral nerve
Obturator nerve

Anterior View

2.78   NERVES OF LUMBAR PLEXUS

The lumbar plexus of nerves is in the posterior part of the psoas major, anterior to the lumbar transverse processes. This nerve network is composed of the anterior rami of L1–L4 nerves. All rami receive gray rami communicates from the sympathetic trunks. The following nerves are branches of the lumbar plexus:

- Ilio-inguinal and iliohypogastric nerves (L1) arise from the anterior ramus of L1 and enter the abdomen posterior to the medial arcuate ligaments and pass inferolaterally, anterior to the quadratus lumborum muscle; they pierce the transversus abdominis muscle near the anterior superior iliac spine and pass through the internal and external oblique muscles to supply the skin of the suprapubic and inguinal regions.
- Lateral cutaneous nerve of thigh (L2, L3) runs inferolaterally on the iliacus muscle and enters the thigh posterior to the inguinal ligament, just medial

to the anterior superior iliac spine; it supplies the skin on the anterolateral surface of the thigh.
- Femoral nerve (L2–L4) emerges from the lateral border of the psoas and innervates the iliacus muscle and the extensor muscles of the knee.
- Genitofemoral nerve (L1, L2) pierces the anterior surface of the psoas major muscle and runs inferiorly on it deep to the psoas fascia; it divides lateral to the common and external iliac arteries into femoral and genital branches.
- Obturator nerve (L2–L4) emerges from the medial border of the psoas to supply the adductor muscles of the thigh.
- Lumbosacral trunk (L4, L5) passes over the ala (wing) of the sacrum and descends into the pelvis to take part in the formation of the sacral plexus along with the anterior rami of S1–S4 nerves.

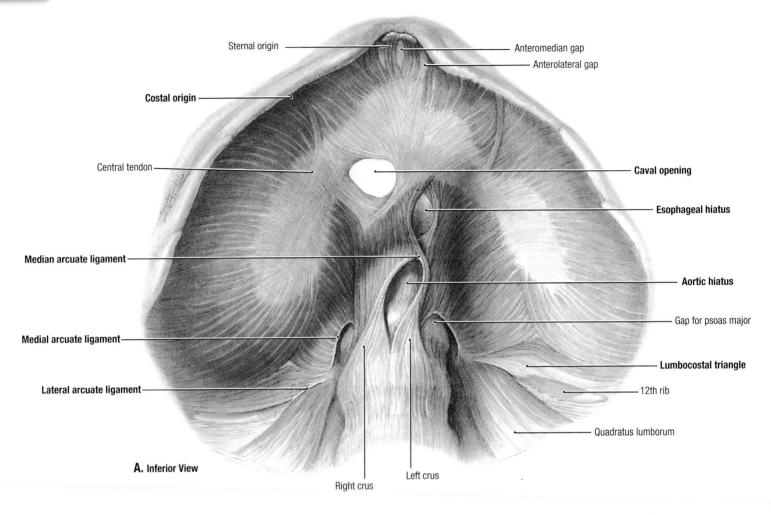

Sternal origin — — Anteromedian gap
— Anterolateral gap
Costal origin —
Central tendon — **Caval opening**
Esophageal hiatus
Median arcuate ligament — **Aortic hiatus**
Gap for psoas major
Medial arcuate ligament — **Lumbocostal triangle**
12th rib
Lateral arcuate ligament — Quadratus lumborum

A. Inferior View

Left crus
Right crus

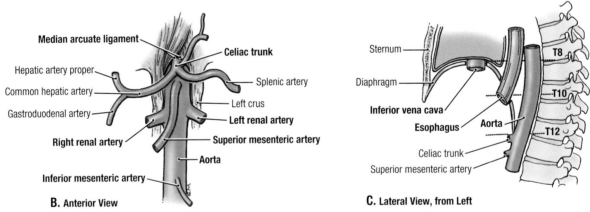

Median arcuate ligament —
Hepatic artery proper — **Celiac trunk**
Common hepatic artery — — Splenic artery
Gastroduodenal artery — — Left crus
— **Left renal artery**
Right renal artery — **Superior mesenteric artery**
— **Aorta**
Inferior mesenteric artery —
B. Anterior View

Sternum — T8
Diaphragm — T10
Inferior vena cava —
Esophagus   **Aorta** — T12
Celiac trunk —
Superior mesenteric artery —
C. Lateral View, from Left

2.79   DIAPHRAGM

A. Dissection. The clover-shaped central tendon is the aponeurotic insertion of the muscle. **Diaphragmatic hernia.** The diaphragm in this specimen fails to arise from the left lateral arcuate ligament, leaving a potential opening, the lumbocostal triangle, through which abdominal contents may be herniated into the thoracic cavity following a sudden increase in intra-thoracic or intra-abdominal pressure. A **hiatal hernia** is a protrusion of part of the stomach into the thorax through the esophageal hiatus.

B. Median arcuate ligament and branches of the aorta. **C.** Openings of the diaphragm. There are three major openings: (1) the caval opening for the inferior vena cava, most anterior, at the T8 vertebral level to the right of the midline; (2) the esophageal hiatus, intermediate, at T10 level and to the left; and (3) the aortic hiatus, which allows the aorta to pass posterior to the vertebral attachment of the diaphragm in the midline at T12.

A. Anterior View

B. Anterior View

Three Vascular Planes

	Origin from Aorta	Class	Distribution	Abdominal Branches (Arteries)	Vertebral Level
1	Anterior midline	Unpaired visceral	Alimentary tract	Celiac	T12
				Superior mesenteric (SMA)	L1
				Inferior mesenteric (IMA)	L3
2	Lateral	Paired visceral	Urogenital and endocrine organs	Suprarenal	L1
				Renal	L1
				Gonadal (testicular or ovarian)	L2
3	Postero-lateral	Paired parietal (segmental)	Diaphragm Body Wall	Subcostal	T12
				Inferior phrenic	T12
				Lumbar	L1–L4

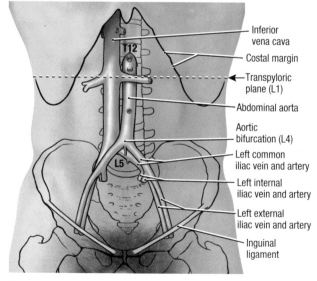

C. Anterior View

2.80   ABDOMINAL AORTA AND INFERIOR VENA CAVA AND THEIR BRANCHES

A. Branches of abdominal aorta. **B.** Tributaries of the inferior vena cava (IVC). **C.** Surface anatomy.

Rupture of an **aortic aneurysm** (localized enlargement of the abdominal aorta) causes severe pain in the abdomen or back. If unrecognized, a ruptured aneurysm has a mortality of nearly 90%

because of heavy blood loss. Surgeons can repair an aneurysm by opening it, inserting a prosthetic graft (such as one made of Dacron), and sewing the wall of the aneurysmal aorta over the graft to protect it. Aneurysms may also be treated by endovascular catheterization procedures.

Fibers from anterior vagal trunk

Diaphragm

Stomach (cut edge)

Fibers from posterior vagal trunk

Splanchnic nerves
Greater
Lesser
Least

Sympathetic fibers to stomach

Celiac ganglion and trunk

Celiac plexus

Superior mesenteric ganglion and artery

Aorticorenal ganglion

Suprarenal plexus

Renal plexus

Abdominal aorta

Intermesenteric plexus

Inferior mesenteric ganglion

Inferior mesenteric artery and plexus

Sympathetic trunk and ganglion

Lumbar splanchnic nerves

Superior hypogastric plexus

Common iliac artery

Hypogastric nerve

Sacral splanchnic nerve

Nerves to descending and sigmoid colon

Internal iliac artery

Inferior hypogastric (pelvic) plexus

Pelvic splanchnic nerves (S2, S3, S4)

External iliac artery

Pelvic splanchnic nerve (S4)

Sciatic nerve

Pudendal nerve

Anterior View

Sympathetic

Parasympathetic

Mixed sympathetic and parasympathetic

Somatic (sacral plexus)

2.81 ABDOMINOPELVIC NERVE PLEXUSES AND GANGLIA

Celiac ganglion

Sympathetic fibers to stomach

Fibers from posterior vagal trunk

Fibers from anterior vagal trunk

Splanchnic nerves
- Greater
- Lesser
- Least

Superior mesenteric ganglion

Aorticorenal ganglion

Inferior mesenteric ganglion

Sympathetic trunk and ganglion

Lumbar splanchnic nerves

Hypogastric nerve

Inferior hypogastric (pelvic) plexus

Sacral splanchnic nerves

Celiac plexus

Suprarenal plexus

Renal plexus

Intermesenteric plexus

Inferior mesenteric plexus

Superior hypogastric plexus

✱ Nerves to descending and sigmoid colon

Inferior hypogastric (pelvic) plexus

Pelvic splanchnic nerves:
- S2
- S3
- S4

Anterior Views

Sympathetic
Somatic (sacral plexus)
Parasympathetic

Parasympathetic
Somatic (sacral plexus)
Sympathetic

A. Sympathetic Innervation

B. Parasympathetic Innervation

2.82   OVERVIEW OF AUTONOMIC NERVOUS SYSTEM

A. Sympathetic. **B.** Parasympathetic.

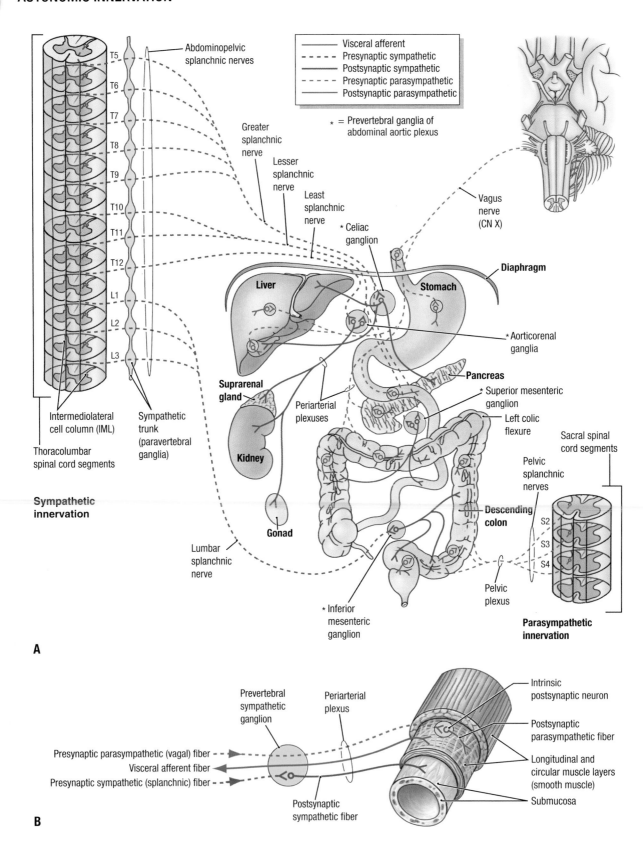

Legend:
- ——— Visceral afferent
- - - - Presynaptic sympathetic
- ——— Postsynaptic sympathetic
- - - - Presynaptic parasympathetic
- ——— Postsynaptic parasympathetic

* = Prevertebral ganglia of abdominal aortic plexus

T5, T6, T7, T8, T9, T10, T11, T12, L1, L2, L3

Abdominopelvic splanchnic nerves

Greater splanchnic nerve
Lesser splanchnic nerve
Least splanchnic nerve

* Celiac ganglion

Vagus nerve (CN X)

Diaphragm

Liver

Stomach

* Aorticorenal ganglia

Pancreas

* Superior mesenteric ganglion

Left colic flexure

Suprarenal gland

Periarterial plexuses

Kidney

Gonad

Intermediolateral cell column (IML)

Sympathetic trunk (paravertebral ganglia)

Thoracolumbar spinal cord segments

Sympathetic innervation

Lumbar splanchnic nerve

* Inferior mesenteric ganglion

Descending colon

Pelvic splanchnic nerves

Sacral spinal cord segments

S2, S3, S4

Pelvic plexus

Parasympathetic innervation

A

Prevertebral sympathetic ganglion

Periarterial plexus

Intrinsic postsynaptic neuron

Presynaptic parasympathetic (vagal) fiber
Visceral afferent fiber
Presynaptic sympathetic (splanchnic) fiber

Postsynaptic parasympathetic fiber

Longitudinal and circular muscle layers (smooth muscle)

Postsynaptic sympathetic fiber

Submucosa

B

2.83

ORIGIN AND DISTRIBUTION OF PRESYNAPTIC AND POSTSYNAPTIC SYMPATHETIC AND PARASYMPATHETIC FIBERS, AND GANGLIA INVOLVED IN SUPPLYING ABDOMINAL VISCERA

A. Overview. **B.** Fibers supplying the intrinsic plexuses of abdominal viscera.

TABLE 2.8 *AUTONOMIC INNERVATION OF ABDOMINAL VISCERA (SPLANCHNIC NERVES)*

Splanchnic Nerves	Autonomic Fiber Type[a]	System	Origin	Destination
A. **Cardiopulmonary** (Cervical and upper thoracic)	Postsynaptic	Sympathetic	Cervical and upper thoracic sympathetic trunk	Thoracic cavity (viscera superior to the level of diaphragm)

B. **Abdominopelvic**
  1. Lower thoracic
    a. Greater
    b. Lesser
    c. Least
  2. Lumbar
  3. Sacral
	Presynaptic		Lower thoracic and abdominopelvic sympathetic trunk:
			1. Thoracic sympathetic trunk:
			  a. T5–T9 or T10 level
			  b. T10–T11 level
			  c. T12 level
			2. Abdominal sympathetic trunk
			3. Pelvic (sacral) sympathetic trunk
				Abdominopelvic cavity (prevertebral ganglia serving viscera and suprarenal glands inferior to the level of diaphragm)
				1. Abdominal prevertebral ganglia:
				  a. Celiac ganglia
				  b. Aorticorenal ganglia
				  c. & 2. Other abdominal prevertebral ganglia (superior and inferior mesenteric and of intermesenteric/hypogastric plexuses)
				3. Pelvic prevertebral ganglia

C. **Pelvic**	Presynaptic	Parasympathetic	Anterior rami of S2–S4 spinal nerves	Intrinsic ganglia of descending and sigmoid colon, rectum, and pelvic viscera

[a]Splanchnic nerves also convey visceral afferent fibers, which are not part of the autonomic nervous system.

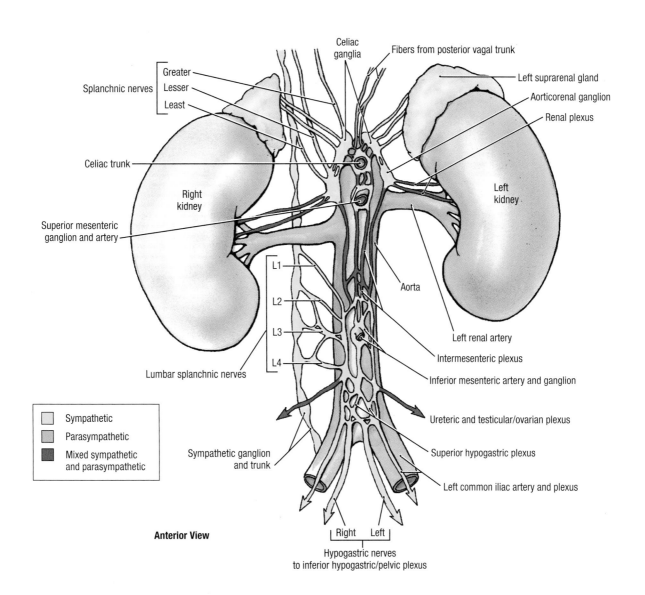

Anterior View

2.84   ABDOMINAL NERVE PLEXUSES AND GANGLIA

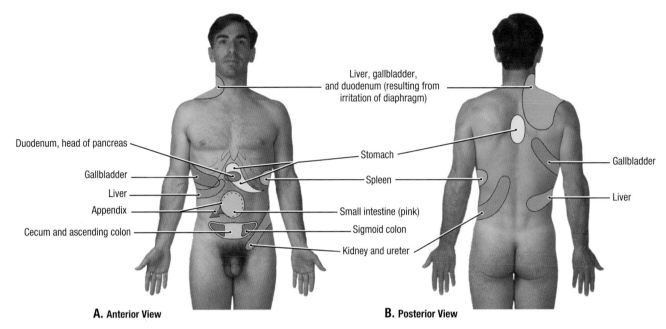

Liver, gallbladder, and duodenum (resulting from irritation of diaphragm)

Duodenum, head of pancreas

Gallbladder

Liver

Appendix

Cecum and ascending colon

Stomach

Spleen

Small intestine (pink)

Sigmoid colon

Kidney and ureter

A. Anterior View

Gallbladder

Liver

B. Posterior View

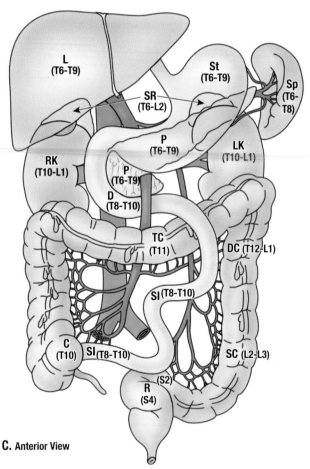

L (T6-T9)

St (T6-T9)

Sp (T6-T8)

SR (T6-L2)

P (T6-T9)

LK (T10-L1)

RK (T10-L1)

P (T6-T9)

D (T8-T10)

TC (T11)

DC (T12-L1)

SI (T8-T10)

C (T10)

SI (T8-T10)

SC (L2-L3)

R (S2) (S4)

C. Anterior View

C	Cecum	P	Pancreas	Sp	Spleen
D	Duodenum	R	Rectum	SR	Suprarenal gands
DC	Descending colon	RK	Right kidney	St	Stomach
L	Liver	SC	Sigmoid colon	TC	Transverse colon
LK	Left kidney	SI	Small intestine		

2.85   SURFACE PROJECTIONS OF VISCERAL PAIN

A. and B. Sites of visceral referred pain. **C.** Approximate spinal cord segments and spinal sensory ganglia involved in sympathetic and visceral afferent (pain) innervation of abdominal viscera.

Pain is an unpleasant sensation associated with actual or potential tissue damage, mediated by specific nerve fibers to the brain, where its conscious appreciation may be modified. Organic pain arising from an organ such as the stomach varies from dull to severe; however, the pain is poorly localized. It radiates to the dermatome level served by the corresponding sensory ganglion, which receives the visceral afferent fibers from the organ concerned. **Visceral referred pain** from a gastric ulcer, for example, is referred to the epigastric region because the stomach is supplied by pain afferents that reach the T7 and T8 spinal sensory ganglia and spinal cord segments through the greater splanchnic nerve. The brain interprets the pain as though the irritation occurred in the skin of the epigastric region, which is also supplied by the same sensory ganglia and spinal cord segments.

Pain arising from the parietal peritoneum is of the somatic type and is usually severe. The site of its origin can be localized. The anatomical basis for this localization of pain is that the parietal peritoneum is supplied by somatic sensory fibers through thoracic nerves, whereas a viscus such as the appendix is supplied by visceral afferent fibers in the lesser splanchnic nerve. Inflamed parietal peritoneum is extremely sensitive to stretching. When digital pressure is applied to the anterolateral abdominal wall over the site of inflammation, the parietal peritoneum is stretched. When the fingers are suddenly removed, extreme localized pain is usually felt, known as **rebound tenderness.**

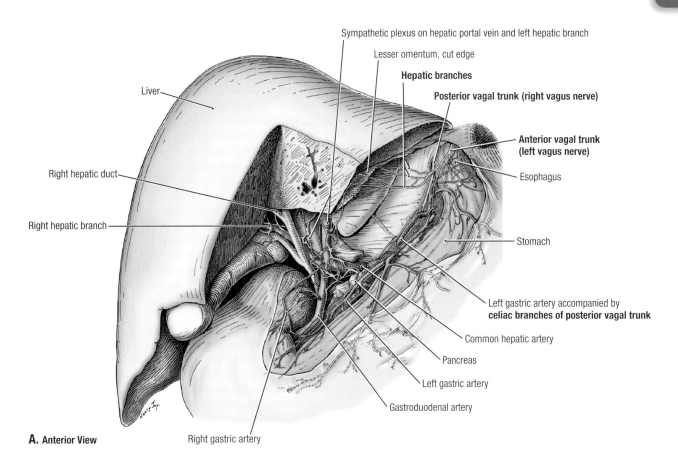

A. Anterior View

Sympathetic plexus on hepatic portal vein and left hepatic branch

Lesser omentum, cut edge

Hepatic branches

Posterior vagal trunk (right vagus nerve)

Anterior vagal trunk (left vagus nerve)

Esophagus

Stomach

Left gastric artery accompanied by **celiac branches of posterior vagal trunk**

Common hepatic artery

Pancreas

Left gastric artery

Gastroduodenal artery

Liver

Right hepatic duct

Right hepatic branch

Right gastric artery

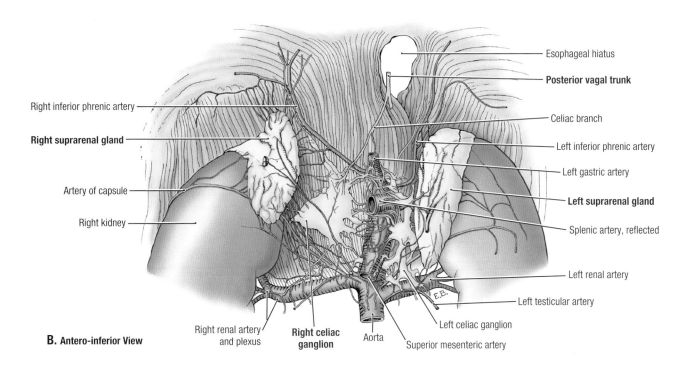

B. Antero-inferior View

Esophageal hiatus

Posterior vagal trunk

Celiac branch

Left inferior phrenic artery

Left gastric artery

Left suprarenal gland

Splenic artery, reflected

Left renal artery

Left testicular artery

Left celiac ganglion

Superior mesenteric artery

Right inferior phrenic artery

Right suprarenal gland

Artery of capsule

Right kidney

Right renal artery and plexus

Right celiac ganglion

Aorta

2.86   VAGUS NERVES IN ABDOMEN

A. Anterior and posterior vagal trunks. **B.** Celiac plexus and ganglia and suprarenal glands.

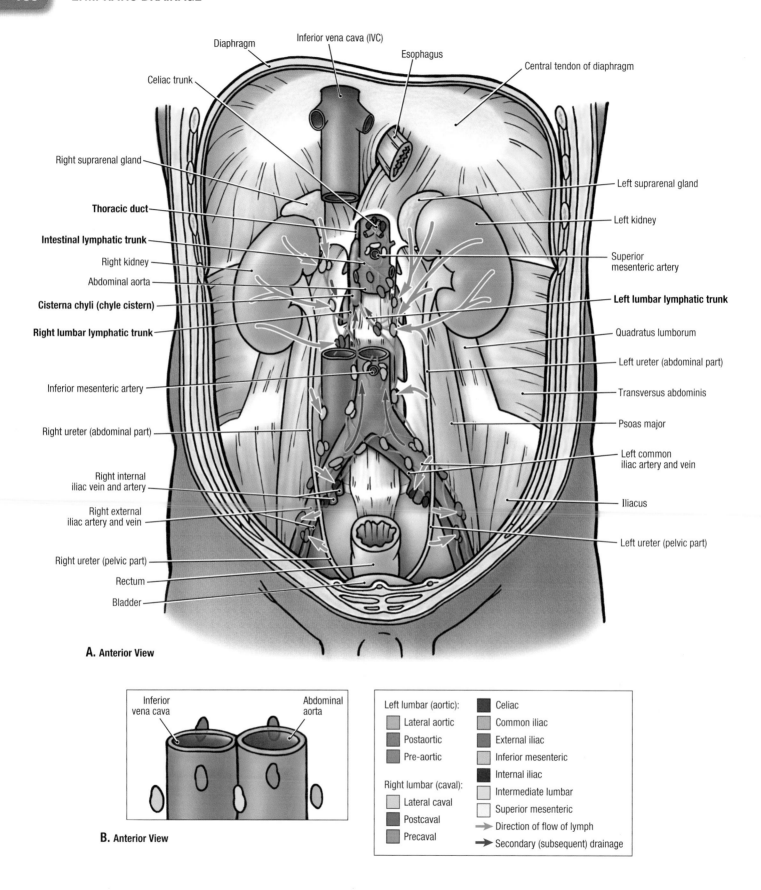

Diaphragm

Inferior vena cava (IVC)

Esophagus

Celiac trunk

Central tendon of diaphragm

Right suprarenal gland

Left suprarenal gland

Thoracic duct

Left kidney

Intestinal lymphatic trunk

Right kidney

Superior mesenteric artery

Abdominal aorta

Cisterna chyli (chyle cistern)

Left lumbar lymphatic trunk

Right lumbar lymphatic trunk

Quadratus lumborum

Left ureter (abdominal part)

Inferior mesenteric artery

Transversus abdominis

Right ureter (abdominal part)

Psoas major

Left common iliac artery and vein

Right internal iliac vein and artery

Iliacus

Right external iliac artery and vein

Left ureter (pelvic part)

Right ureter (pelvic part)

Rectum

Bladder

A. Anterior View

Inferior vena cava

Abdominal aorta

Left lumbar (aortic):
- Lateral aortic
- Postaortic
- Pre-aortic

Right lumbar (caval):
- Lateral caval
- Postcaval
- Precaval

Celiac

Common iliac

External iliac

Inferior mesenteric

Internal iliac

Intermediate lumbar

Superior mesenteric

→ Direction of flow of lymph

➡ Secondary (subsequent) drainage

B. Anterior View

2.87   LYMPHATIC DRAINAGE OF SUPRARENAL GLANDS, KIDNEYS, AND URETERS

Inferior phrenic artery

Diaphragm

Greater and lesser splanchnic nerves

Vein uniting inferior vena cava
to azygos vein

Medial arcuate ligament

Cisterna chyli

Aorta

Rami communicantes

Sympathetic ganglion

Transverse process (L3)

Lumbar splanchnic nerve

Transverse process (L4)

Psoas major

Iliac crest

Common iliac lymph node

Tendon of psoas minor

Anterior View

Ligature retracting **suprarenal gland**

Celiac ganglion

Right kidney (posterior aspect)

Right crus of diaphragm

Probe retracting
inferior vena cava

Right lumbar lymphatic trunk

Right lumbar (caval) lymph nodes

Transversalis fascia

Ascending colon
(posterior aspect)

Ureter

Inferior vena cava

Common iliac artery

Lymph vessels

N. Joy

2.88   LUMBAR LYMPH NODES, SYMPATHETIC TRUNK, NERVES, AND GANGLIA

The right suprarenal gland, kidney, ureter, and colon are reflected to the left; the inferior vena cava is pulled medially, and the third and fourth lumbar veins are removed. In this specimen, the greater and lesser splanchnic nerves, the sympathetic trunk, and a communicating vein pass through an unusually wide cleft in the right crus. The splanchnic nerves convey preganglionic fibers arising from the cell bodies in the (thoracolumbar) sympathetic trunk. The greater splanchnic nerve is from thoracic ganglia 5 to 9, and the lesser from thoracic ganglia 10 to 11.

A. Stomach and small intestine. Left gastric artery. Stomach. Splenic artery. Celiac trunk. Superior mesenteric artery. Duodenum. A. Anterior View. From ileum. From jejunum.

B. Anterior View. Spleen. Celiac trunk. Splenic artery. Superior mesenteric artery. Pancreas. Aorta.

C. Anterior View. Right lymphatic duct. Left internal jugular vein. Thoracic duct. Left subclavian vein. Thoracic aorta. Diaphragm. Thoracic duct. Aortic hiatus. Abdominal aorta. Cisterna chyli (chyle cistern). Intestinal lymphatic trunk. Right lumbar lymphatic trunk. Left lumbar lymphatic trunk.

Celiac	Splenic
Left gastric	Subpyloric
Left gastro-omental	Superior mesenteric
Pancreatic (Superior)	Suprapyloric
Pancreatic (Inferior)	→ Initial drainage
Pancreaticoduodenal	→ Secondary
Right gastro-omental	(subsequent) drainage

2.89   LYMPHATIC DRAINAGE

A. Stomach and small intestine. **B.** Spleen and pancreas. **C.** Drainage from lumbar and intestinal lymphatic trunks. The *arrows* indicate the direction of lymph flow; each group of lymph nodes is color coded. Lymph from the abdominal nodes drains into the cisterna chyli, origin of the inferior end of the thoracic duct. The thoracic duct receives all lymph that forms inferior to the diaphragm and left upper quadrant (thorax and left upper limb) and empties into the junction of the left subclavian and left internal jugular veins.

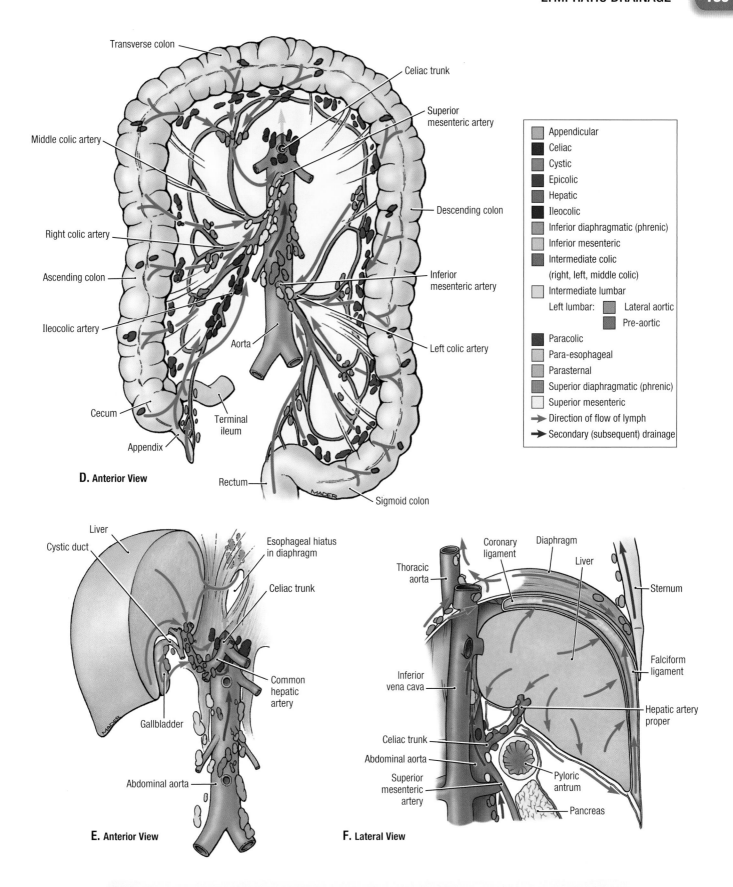

D. Anterior View

Legend:
- Appendicular
- Celiac
- Cystic
- Epicolic
- Hepatic
- Ileocolic
- Inferior diaphragmatic (phrenic)
- Inferior mesenteric
- Intermediate colic (right, left, middle colic)
- Intermediate lumbar
- Left lumbar: Lateral aortic / Pre-aortic
- Paracolic
- Para-esophageal
- Parasternal
- Superior diaphragmatic (phrenic)
- Superior mesenteric
- → Direction of flow of lymph
- → Secondary (subsequent) drainage

E. Anterior View

F. Lateral View

2.89 **LYMPHATIC DRAINAGE (CONTINUED)**

D. Large intestine. **E.** Liver and gallbladder. **F.** Liver.

A

B

C

D

Ac	Ascending colon	Dc	Descending colon	LHV	Left hepatic vein
AF	Air-fluid level of stomach	D2	Descending part of duodenum	LIL	Left inferior lobe of lung
Ao	Aorta	D3	Inferior part of duodenum	LK	Left kidney
Az	Azygos vein	E	Esophagus	LL	Left lobe of liver
CA	Celiac artery	FL	Falciform ligament	LRV	Left renal vein
CHA	Common hepatic artery	GB	Gallbladder	LU	Left ureter
cc	Costal cartilage	HA	Hepatic artery	IHV	Intermediate hepatic vein
CD	Cystic duct	Hz	Hemi-azygos vein	P	Pancreas
CHD	Common hepatic duct	IMV	Inferior mesenteric vein	PA	Pyloric antrum of stomach
CL	Caudate lobe of liver	IVC	Inferior vena cava	PB	Body of pancreas
D	Diaphragm	LC	Left crus of diaphragm	PC	Portal confluence
DBM	Deep back muscles	LG	Left suprarenal gland		

2.90   TRANSVERSE OR HORIZONTAL (AXIAL) MRIs OF ABDOMEN

E

F

G

H

PF	Perinephric fat	RC	Right crus of diaphragm	RRV	Right renal vein	Sp	Spleen
PH	Head of pancreas	RF	Retroperitoneal fat	RU	Right ureter	St	Stomach
PS	Psoas muscle	RG	Right suprarenal gland	S	Spinous process	SV	Splenic vein
PT	Tail of pancreas	RHV	Right hepatic vein	SA	Splenic artery	Tc	Transverse colon
PU	Uncinate process of pancreas	RIL	Right inferior lobe of lung	SC	Spinal cord	TVP	Transverse process
PV	Hepatic portal vein	RK	Right kidney	SF	Splenic flexure	Xp	Xiphoid process
QL	Quadratus lumborum	RL	Right lobe of liver	SI	Small intestine		
R	Rib	RP	Renal pelvis	SMA	Superior mesenteric artery		
RA	Rectus abdominis	RRA	Right renal artery	SMV	Superior mesenteric vein		

2.90 TRANSVERSE OR HORIZONTAL (AXIAL) MRIs OF ABDOMEN (*CONTINUED*)

AB	Aortic bifurcation	IO	Internal oblique	P	Pancreas	SA	Splenic artery
Ac	Ascending colon	IVC	Inferior vena cava	PV	Portal vein	SI	Small intestine
Ao	Aorta	LDD	Left dome of diaphragm	PS	Psoas	SMA	Superior mesenteric artery
CA	Celiac artery	LIL	Left lung (inferior lobe)	RCV	Right colic vein	SMV	Superior mesenteric vein
CIA	Common iliac artery	LK	Left kidney	RDD	Right dome of diaphragm	Sp	Spleen
D	Duodenum	LL	Left lobe of liver	RIL	Right lung (inferior lobe)	St	Stomach
Dc	Descending colon	LRA	Left renal artery	RK	Right kidney	SV	Splenic vein
E	Esophagus	LRV	Left renal vein	RL	Right lobe of liver	TA	Transversus abdominis
EO	External oblique	MHV	Middle hepatic vein	RRA	Right renal artery		

Ao	Aorta	IVC	Inferior vena cava	PH	Head of pancreas	RRA	Right renal artery
ABo	Bifurcation of aorta	LIL	Inferior lobe of left lung	PT	Tail of pancreas	SA	Splenic artery
CA	Celiac artery	LK	Left kidney	PV	Portal vein	SI	Small intestine
D	Diaphragm	LL	Left lobe of liver	PU	Uncinate process of pancreas	SMA	Superior mesenteric artery
DB	Bulb of duodenum	LRV	Left renal vein	Py	Pylorus of stomach	SMV	Superior mesenteric vein
Dc	Descending colon	MHV	Middle hepatic vein	RA	Rectus abdominus	Sp	Spleen
Do	Duodenum	P	Pancreas	RC	Right crus	St	Stomach
DBM	Deep back muscles	Pa	Pyloric antrum	RIL	Inferior lobe of right lung	SV	Splenic vein
GE	Gastroesophageal junction	PC	Portal confluence	RL	Right lobe of right liver	Tc	Transverse colon

A. Transverse Section, Inferior View

B. Transverse Section, Inferior View

C. Median Section, Right Lateral View

2.93   ULTRASOUND SCANS AND MR ANGIOGRAM OF ABDOMEN

A. Transverse ultrasound scan through celiac trunk. **B.** Transverse ultrasound scan through pancreas. **C. and D.** Sagittal ultrasound scans through the aorta, celiac trunk, and superior mesenteric artery. (**D.** with Doppler.) **E.** MR angiogram of abdominal aorta and branches. **F.** Transverse ultrasound scan at hilum of left kidney with the left renal artery and vein (with Doppler). **G.** Sagittal ultrasound scan of the right kidney.

A major advantage of ultrasonography is its ability to produce real-time images, demonstrating motion of structures and flow within blood vessels. In Doppler ultrasonography (**D** and **F**) the shifts in frequency between emitted ultrasonic waves and their echoes are used to measure the velocities of moving objects. This technique is based on the principle of the Doppler effect. Blood flow through vessels is displayed in color, superimposed on the two-dimensional cross-sectional image (slow flow: *blue*, fast flow: *orange*).

D. Median Section, Right Lateral View

E. Anterior View

F. Transverse Section

G. Sagittal Section, Right Lateral View

Ao	Aorta	H	Hilum of kidney	LRV	Left renal vein	SMA	Superior mesenteric artery
BD	Bile duct	HA	Hepatic artery	P	Pancreas	SMV	Superior mesenteric vein
CA	Celiac artery	IR	Perirenal fat in renal sinus	PS	Psoas	ST	Stomach
Cr	Crus of diaphragm	IVC	Inferior vena cava	Pu	Uncinate process of pancreas	SV	Splenic vein
D	Duodenum	K	Cortex of kidney	PV	Portal vein	V	Vertebra
FL	Falciform ligament	L	Liver	PVC	Portal venous confluence		
GDA	Gastroduodenal artery	LGA	Left gastric artery	RRA	Right renal artery		
GE	Gastro-esophageal junction	LRA	Left renal artery	SA	Splenic artery		

2.93 ULTRASOUND SCANS AND MR ANGIOGRAM OF ABDOMEN (*CONTINUED*)

Pelvis and Perineum

A. Anterior View

Labels: Sacrum, Right hip bone, Coccyx, Iliac crest, Anterior superior iliac spine (ASIS), Inguinal fold (dashed line), Pubic tubercle, Pubic symphysis

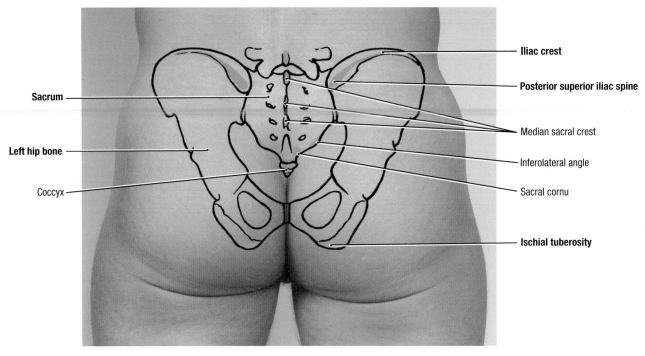

B. Posterior View

Labels: Sacrum, Left hip bone, Coccyx, Iliac crest, Posterior superior iliac spine, Median sacral crest, Inferolateral angle, Sacral cornu, Ischial tuberosity

3.1   SURFACE ANATOMY OF MALE PELVIC GIRDLE

The pelvic girdle (bony pelvis) is a basin-shaped ring of three bones (right and left hip bones and sacrum) that connects the vertebral column to the femora. **Palpable features** (*green*) should be symmetrical across the midline. **A.** The anterior third of the iliac crests are subcutaneous and usually easily palpable. The remainder of the crests may also be palpable, depending on the thickness of the overlying subcutaneous tissue (fat).

The inguinal ligament spans between the palpable anterior superior iliac spine (ASIS) and pubic tubercle, located superior to the lateral and medial ends of the inguinal fold. **B.** The posterior superior iliac spine (PSIS) is usually palpable and often lies deep to a visible dimple, indicating the S2 vertebral level. The ischial tuberosities may be palpated when the hip joint is flexed.

A. Anterior View

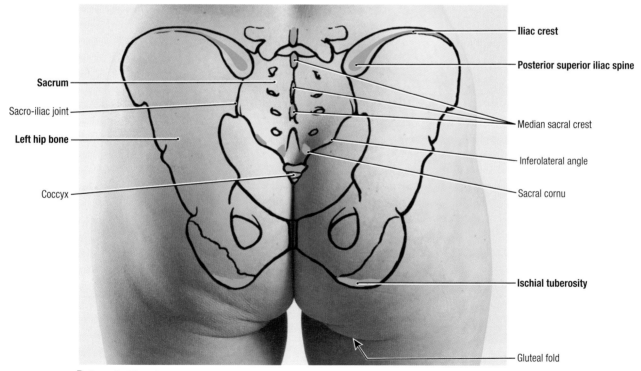

B. Posterior View

| 3.2 | SURFACE ANATOMY OF FEMALE PELVIC GIRDLE |

The female pelvic girdle is relatively wider and shallower than that of the male, related to its additional roles of bearing the weight of the gravid uterus in late **pregnancy** and allowing passage of the fetus through the pelvic outlet during childbirth **(parturition). A.** Palpable features (*green*): The hip bones are joined anteriorly at the pubic symphysis. The presence of a thick overlying pubic fat pad forming the mons pubis may interfere with palpation of the pubic tubercles and symphysis. **B.** Posteriorly the hip bones are joined to the sacrum at the sacro-iliac joints.

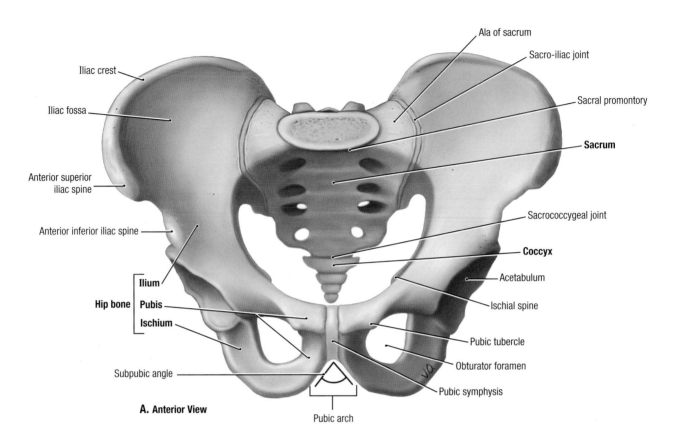

A. Anterior View

- Ala of sacrum
- Sacro-iliac joint
- Sacral promontory
- **Sacrum**
- Sacrococcygeal joint
- **Coccyx**
- Acetabulum
- Ischial spine
- Pubic tubercle
- Obturator foramen
- Pubic symphysis
- Pubic arch
- Iliac crest
- Iliac fossa
- Anterior superior iliac spine
- Anterior inferior iliac spine
- Hip bone { Ilium, Pubis, Ischium }
- Subpubic angle

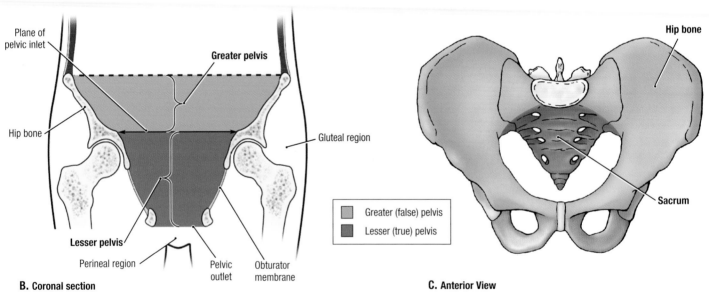

B. Coronal section

- Plane of pelvic inlet
- **Greater pelvis**
- Hip bone
- Gluteal region
- **Lesser pelvis**
- Perineal region
- Pelvic outlet
- Obturator membrane

C. Anterior View

- **Hip bone**
- **Sacrum**
- Greater (false) pelvis
- Lesser (true) pelvis

3.3   BONES AND DIVISIONS OF PELVIS

A. Bones of pelvis. The three bones composing the pelvis are the pubis, ischium, and ilium. **B. and C.** Lesser and greater pelvis, schematic illustrations. The plane of the pelvic inlet (*double-headed arrow* in *B*) separates the greater pelvis (part of the abdominal cavity) from the lesser pelvis (pelvic cavity).

A. Anterosuperior View

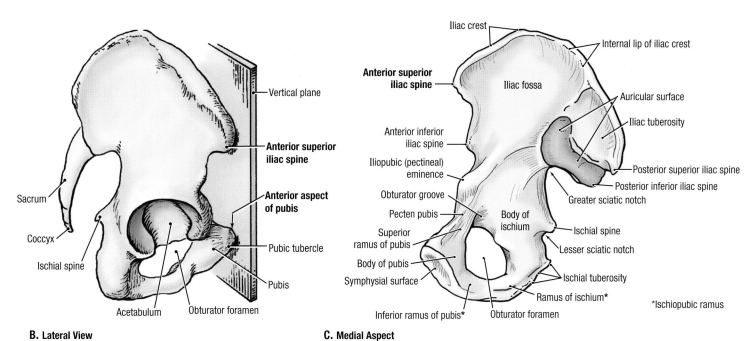

B. Lateral View

C. Medial Aspect

*Ischiopubic ramus

3.4   PELVIS, ANATOMICAL POSITION

A. Pelvic girdle. **B.** Placement of hip bone in anatomical position. In the anatomical position, (1) the anterior superior iliac spine and the anterior aspect of the pubis lie in the same vertical plane and (2) the sacrum is located superiorly, the coccyx posteriorly, and the pubic symphysis antero-inferiorly. **C.** Features of hip bone.

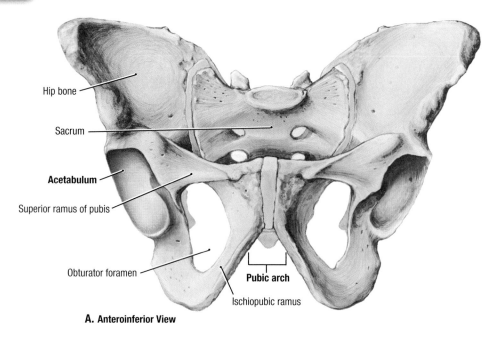

Hip bone

Sacrum

Acetabulum

Superior ramus of pubis

Obturator foramen

Pubic arch

Ischiopubic ramus

A. Anteroinferior View

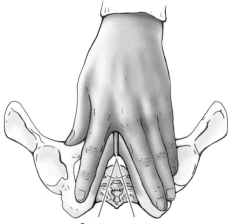

C. Subpubic angle
"V" shaped

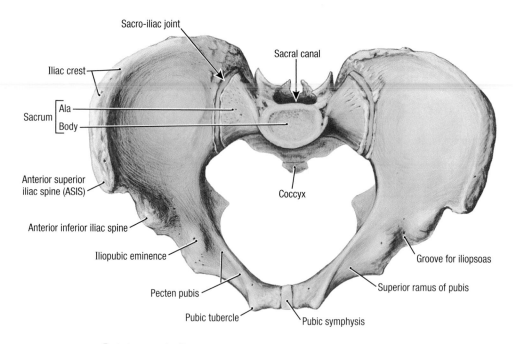

Sacro-iliac joint

Sacral canal

Iliac crest

Sacrum { Ala / Body }

Anterior superior iliac spine (ASIS)

Anterior inferior iliac spine

Iliopubic eminence

Pecten pubis

Pubic tubercle

Coccyx

Groove for iliopsoas

Superior ramus of pubis

Pubic symphysis

B. Anterosuperior View

3.5   MALE PELVIC GIRDLE

TABLE 3.1 DIFFERENCES BETWEEN MALE AND FEMALE PELVES

Bony Pelvis	Male	Female
General structure	Thicker and heavier	Thinner and lighter
Greater pelvis (pelvis major)	Deeper	Shallower
Lesser pelvis (pelvis minor)	Narrower and deeper, tapering	Wider and shallower, cylindrical
Pelvic inlet (superior pelvic aperture)	Heart shaped, narrower	More oval or rounded, wider

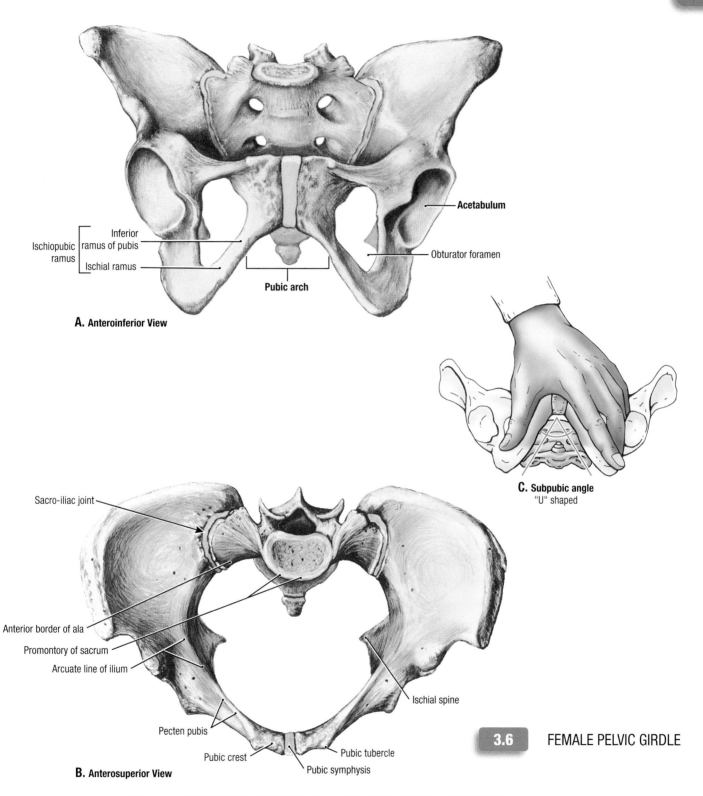

Acetabulum

Ischiopubic ramus {
Inferior ramus of pubis
Ischial ramus }

Pubic arch

Obturator foramen

A. Anteroinferior View

C. Subpubic angle
"U" shaped

Sacro-iliac joint

Anterior border of ala

Promontory of sacrum

Arcuate line of ilium

Ischial spine

Pecten pubis

Pubic crest

Pubic tubercle

Pubic symphysis

3.6   FEMALE PELVIC GIRDLE

B. Anterosuperior View

TABLE 3.1 *DIFFERENCES BETWEEN MALE AND FEMALE PELVES (CONTINUED)*

Bony Pelvis	Male	Female
Sacrum/coccyx	More curved	Less curved
Pelvic outlet (inferior pelvic aperture)	Comparatively small	Comparatively large
Pubic arch and subpubic angle	Narrower	Wider
Obturator foramen	Round	Oval
Acetabulum	Large	Small

A. Anteroposterior View, Male Pelvis

B. Anteroposterior View, Female Pelvis

3.7 **RADIOGRAPHS OF PELVIS**

A. Male. **B.** Female. Some of the main differences of male and female pelves are listed in Table 3.1. The radiographs highlight some of these differences. *A*, acetabulum; *ASIS*, anterior superior iliac spine; *O*, obturator foramen; *PA*, pubic arch.

Transverse process of L5 vertebra

Iliac crest

Iliac fossa

Anterior superior iliac spine

Greater sciatic foramen

Sacrotuberous ligament

Sacrospinous ligament

Head of femur

Inguinal ligament

Femur

Obturator membrane

Pubic symphysis

Anterior longitudinal ligament

Iliolumbar ligament

Anterior sacro-iliac ligament

Anterior sacral foramina

Anterior inferior iliac spine

Pelvic brim (linea terminalis)

Iliofemoral ligament

Pubofemoral ligament

Pubic tubercle

Anterior sacrococcygeal ligament

A. Anterior View

Supraspinous ligament

Posterior superior iliac spine

Posterior sacral foramen

Greater sciatic foramen

Ischiofemoral ligament

Sacrotuberous ligament

Iliolumbar ligament

Posterior sacro-iliac ligament

Posterior sacrococcygeal ligaments

Sacrospinous ligament

Lesser sciatic foramen

Femur

Ischial tuberosity

B. Posterior View

3.8   PELVIS AND PELVIC LIGAMENTS

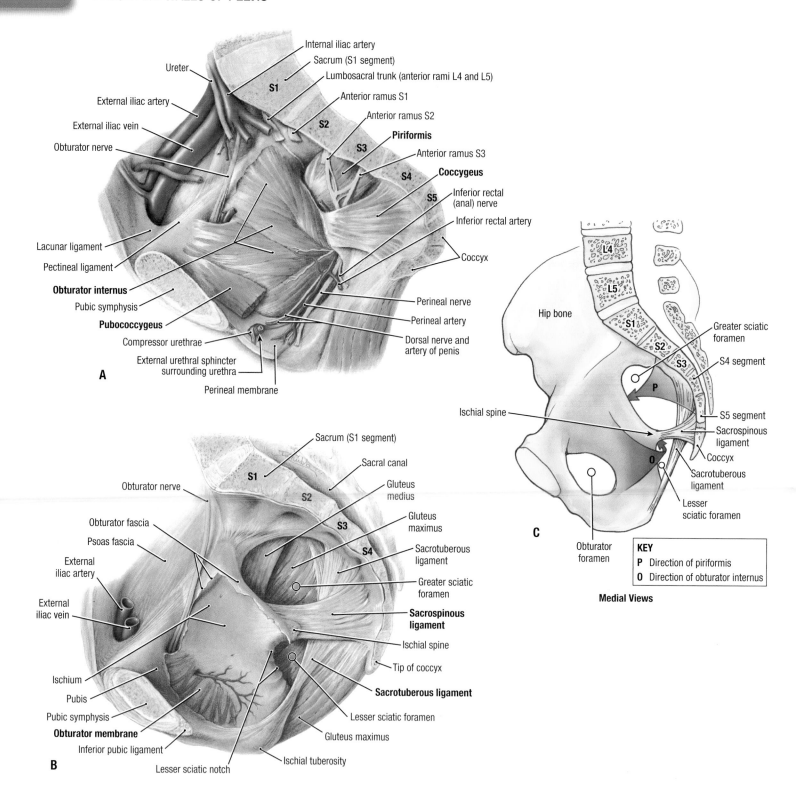

A

- Internal iliac artery
- Ureter
- Sacrum (S1 segment)
- Lumbosacral trunk (anterior rami L4 and L5)
- S1
- External iliac artery
- Anterior ramus S1
- External iliac vein
- S2
- Anterior ramus S2
- Obturator nerve
- **Piriformis**
- S3
- Anterior ramus S3
- S4
- **Coccygeus**
- S5
- Inferior rectal (anal) nerve
- Inferior rectal artery
- Lacunar ligament
- Pectineal ligament
- Coccyx
- **Obturator internus**
- Pubic symphysis
- Perineal nerve
- **Pubococcygeus**
- Perineal artery
- Compressor urethrae
- Dorsal nerve and artery of penis
- External urethral sphincter surrounding urethra
- Perineal membrane

B

- Sacrum (S1 segment)
- Obturator nerve
- Sacral canal
- S1
- Gluteus medius
- S2
- Obturator fascia
- Gluteus maximus
- Psoas fascia
- S3
- External iliac artery
- S4
- Sacrotuberous ligament
- External iliac vein
- Greater sciatic foramen
- **Sacrospinous ligament**
- Ischial spine
- Ischium
- Tip of coccyx
- Pubis
- **Sacrotuberous ligament**
- Pubic symphysis
- **Obturator membrane**
- Lesser sciatic foramen
- Inferior pubic ligament
- Gluteus maximus
- Lesser sciatic notch
- Ischial tuberosity

C

- L4
- L5
- S1
- Hip bone
- S2
- Greater sciatic foramen
- S3
- S4 segment
- Ischial spine
- P
- S5 segment
- Sacrospinous ligament
- Coccyx
- O
- Sacrotuberous ligament
- Lesser sciatic foramen
- Obturator foramen

KEY
P Direction of piriformis
O Direction of obturator internus

Medial Views

3.9   OBTURATOR INTERNUS AND PIRIFORMIS

- On the lateral pelvic wall, the obturator foramen is closed by the obturator membrane; the obturator internus muscle attaches to the obturator membrane and surrounding bone and exits the lesser pelvis through the lesser sciatic foramen; obturator fascia lies on the medial surface of the muscle.

- Piriformis lies on the posterolateral pelvic wall and leaves the lesser pelvis through the greater sciatic foramen.

Internal iliac artery
Ureter
External iliac artery
External iliac vein
Obturator nerve
Ductus deferens
Site of deep inguinal ring
Inferior epigastric artery and vein
Obturator artery and vein
Obturator fascia covering obturator internus
Tendinous arch of levator ani
Pubic symphysis
Urogenital hiatus (edge)
A. Medial View
Rectum

S1
S2
S3
S4
S5
L4
L5
S1
S2 } Anterior rami
Piriformis
Ischial spine
Coccygeus (C)
Coccyx
Iliococcygeus (IC)
Pubococcygeus (PC)
Puborectalis

Muscles of floor of pelvis*:

Pelvic diaphragm (PD) = Levator ani (LA) + Coccygeus (C)
(PD = LA + C)

Levator ani (LA) = Pubococcygeus (PC) + Iliococcygeus (IC)
(LA = PC + IC)

Pubococcygeus (PC ♀) = Puborectalis (PR) + Pubovaginalis (PV)
(PC = PR + PV ♀)

Pubococcygeus (PC ♂) = Puborectalis (PR) + Puboprostaticus (PP)
(PC = PR + PP ♂)   (Levator prostatae)

*Formulas: Dr. Larry M. Ross.
The Univesity of Texas Medical School at Houston

Sacrum
Greater sciatic foramen
Anococcygeal body
Tendinous arch of levator ani
Obturator fascia covering obturator internus
Rectum
Perineal body
B. Anterosuperior View

Coccygeus (C)
Puborectalis
Iliococcygeus (IC)
Pubococcygeus (PC)
Pubovaginalis (PV) (♀)
Puboprostaticus (PP) (♂)
Urogenital hiatus
Pubic symphysis

3.10   MUSCLES OF PELVIC DIAPHRAGM

A. The pelvic floor is formed by the funnel- or bowl-shaped pelvic diaphragm. The funnel shape can be seen in a medial view of a median section. **B.** The bowl shape from a superior view.

TABLE 3.2 MUSCLES OF PELVIC WALLS AND FLOOR

Boundary	Muscle	Proximal Attachment	Distal Attachment	Innervation	Main Action
Lateral wall	Obturator internus	Pelvic surfaces of ilium and ischium, obturator membrane	Greater trochanter of femur	Nerve to obturator internus (L5, S1, S2)	Rotates hip joint laterally; assists in holding head of femur in acetabulum
Posterolateral wall	Piriformis	Pelvic surface of S2–S4 segments, superior margin of greater sciatic notch, sacrotuberous ligament		Anterior rami of S1 and S2	Rotates hip joint laterally; abducts hip joint; assists in holding head of femur in acetabulum
Floor	Levator ani (pubococcygeus, puborectalis, and iliococcygeus)	Body of pubis, tendinous arch of obturator fascia, ischial spine	Perineal body, coccyx, anococcygeal ligament, walls of prostate or vagina, rectum, and anal canal	Nerve to levator ani (branches of S4), inferior anal (rectal) nerve, and coccygeal plexus	Forms most of pelvic diaphragm that helps support pelvic viscera and resists increases in intra-abdominal pressure
	Coccygeus (ischiococcygeus)	Ischial spine	Inferior end of sacrum and coccyx	Branches of S4 and S5 spinal nerves	Forms small part of pelvic diaphragm that supports pelvic viscera; flexes sacrococcygeal joints

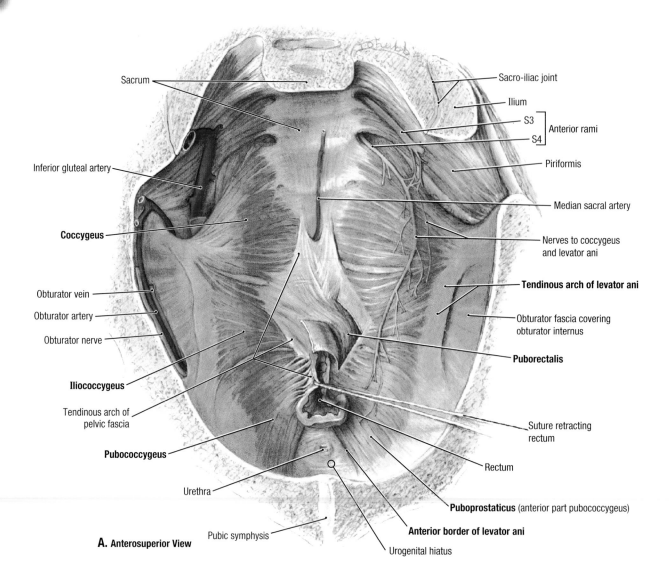

Sacrum

Sacro-iliac joint

Ilium

S3
S4 } Anterior rami

Inferior gluteal artery

Piriformis

Coccygeus

Median sacral artery

Nerves to coccygeus
and levator ani

Tendinous arch of levator ani

Obturator vein

Obturator artery

Obturator nerve

Obturator fascia covering
obturator internus

Puborectalis

Iliococcygeus

Tendinous arch of
pelvic fascia

Suture retracting
rectum

Pubococcygeus

Rectum

Urethra

Puboprostaticus (anterior part pubococcygeus)

Anterior border of levator ani

A. Anterosuperior View

Pubic symphysis

Urogenital hiatus

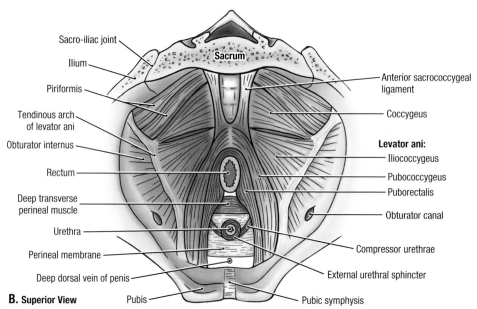

Sacro-iliac joint

Ilium

Piriformis

Sacrum

Anterior sacrococcygeal
ligament

Coccygeus

Tendinous arch
of levator ani

Obturator internus

Levator ani:

Iliococcygeus

Pubococcygeus

Puborectalis

Rectum

Deep transverse
perineal muscle

Obturator canal

Urethra

Perineal membrane

Compressor urethrae

Deep dorsal vein of penis

External urethral sphincter

B. Superior View

Pubis

Pubic symphysis

3.11 FLOOR AND WALLS OF MALE PELVIS, PELVIC DIAPHRAGM

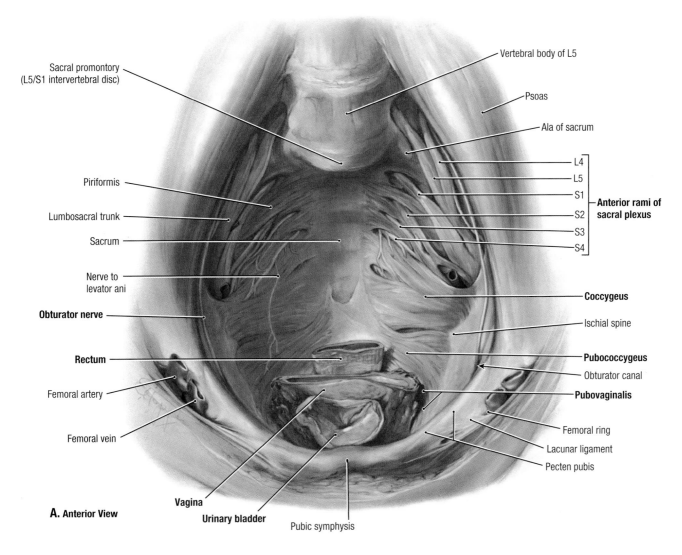

Sacral promontory
(L5/S1 intervertebral disc)

Vertebral body of L5

Psoas

Ala of sacrum

Piriformis

Lumbosacral trunk

Sacrum

Nerve to
levator ani

Obturator nerve

Rectum

Femoral artery

Femoral vein

L4
L5
S1
S2
S3
S4

**Anterior rami of
sacral plexus**

Coccygeus

Ischial spine

Pubococcygeus

Obturator canal

Pubovaginalis

Femoral ring

Lacunar ligament

Pecten pubis

Vagina

Urinary bladder   Pubic symphysis

A. Anterior View

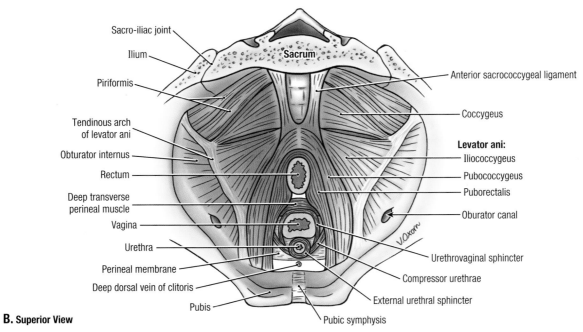

Sacro-iliac joint

Ilium

Piriformis

Tendinous arch
of levator ani

Obturator internus

Rectum

Deep transverse
perineal muscle

Vagina

Urethra

Perineal membrane

Deep dorsal vein of clitoris

Pubis

Sacrum

Anterior sacrococcygeal ligament

Coccygeus

Levator ani:
Iliococcygeus

Pubococcygeus

Puborectalis

Oburator canal

Urethrovaginal sphincter

Compressor urethrae

External urethral sphincter

Pubic symphysis

B. Superior View

3.12   FLOOR AND WALLS OF FEMALE PELVIS

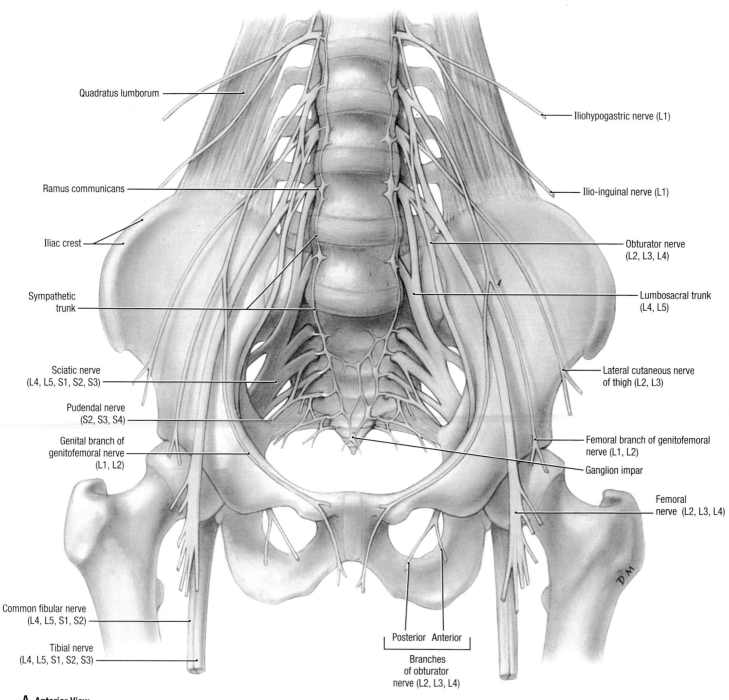

Quadratus lumborum

Ramus communicans

Iliac crest

Sympathetic trunk

Sciatic nerve (L4, L5, S1, S2, S3)

Pudendal nerve (S2, S3, S4)

Genital branch of genitofemoral nerve (L1, L2)

Common fibular nerve (L4, L5, S1, S2)

Tibial nerve (L4, L5, S1, S2, S3)

Iliohypogastric nerve (L1)

Ilio-inguinal nerve (L1)

Obturator nerve (L2, L3, L4)

Lumbosacral trunk (L4, L5)

Lateral cutaneous nerve of thigh (L2, L3)

Femoral branch of genitofemoral nerve (L1, L2)

Ganglion impar

Femoral nerve (L2, L3, L4)

Posterior   Anterior
Branches of obturator nerve (L2, L3, L4)

A. Anterior View

3.13   SACRAL AND COCCYGEAL NERVE PLEXUSES

A. Dissection
- The sympathetic trunk or its ganglia send rami communicantes to each sacral and coccygeal nerve.
- The anterior ramus from L4 joins that of L5 to form the lumbosacral trunk.

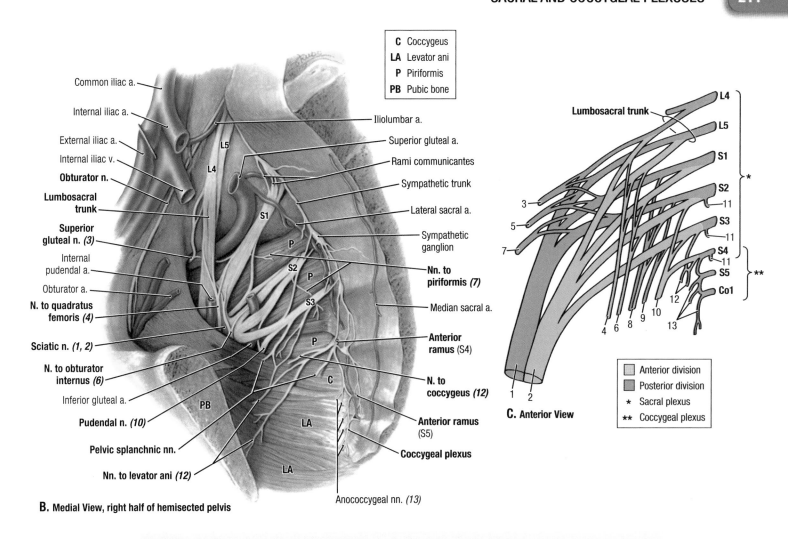

C Coccygeus
LA Levator ani
P Piriformis
PB Pubic bone

Common iliac a.
Internal iliac a.
External iliac a.
Internal iliac v.
Obturator n.
Lumbosacral trunk
Superior gluteal n. (3)
Internal pudendal a.
Obturator a.
N. to quadratus femoris (4)
Sciatic n. (1, 2)
N. to obturator internus (6)
Inferior gluteal a.
Pudendal n. (10)
Pelvic splanchnic nn.
Nn. to levator ani (12)

Iliolumbar a.
Superior gluteal a.
Rami communicantes
Sympathetic trunk
Lateral sacral a.
Sympathetic ganglion
Nn. to piriformis (7)
Median sacral a.
Anterior ramus (S4)
N. to coccygeus (12)
Anterior ramus (S5)
Coccygeal plexus

Anococcygeal nn. (13)

B. Medial View, right half of hemisected pelvis

Lumbosacral trunk

L4
L5
S1
S2
S3
S4
S5
Co1

*
**

Anterior division
Posterior division
* Sacral plexus
** Coccygeal plexus

C. Anterior View

3.13   SACRAL AND COCCYGEAL NERVE PLEXUSES *(CONTINUED)*

B. and C. Schematic illustrations.

TABLE 3.3 NERVES OF SACRAL AND COCCYGEAL PLEXUSES

Nerve	Origin	Distribution
Sciatic:		
1. Common fibular	L4, L5, S1, S2	Articular branches to hip joint and muscular branches to flexors of knee joint in thigh and all muscles in leg and foot
2. Tibial	L4, L5, S1, S2, S3	
3. Superior gluteal	L4, L5, S1	Gluteus medius and gluteus minimus muscles
4. Nerve to quadratus femoris and inferior gemellus	L4, L5, S1	Quadratus femoris and inferior gemellus muscles
5. Inferior gluteal	L5, S1, S2	Gluteus maximus muscle
6. Nerve to obturator internus and superior gemellus	L5, S1, S2	Obturator internus and superior gemellus muscles
7. Nerve to piriformis	S1, S2	Piriformis muscle
8. Posterior cutaneous nerve of thigh	S1, S2, S3	Cutaneous branches to buttock and uppermost medial and posterior surfaces of thigh
9. Perforating cutaneous	S2, S3	Cutaneous branches to medial part of buttock
10. Pudendal	S2, S3, S4	Structures in perineum, sensory to genitalia, muscular branches to perineal muscles, external urethral sphincter, and external anal sphincter
11. Pelvic splanchnic	S2, S3, S4	Pelvic viscera via inferior hypogastric and pelvic plexuses
12. Nerves to levator ani and coccygeus	S3, S4	Levator ani and coccygeus muscles
13. Anococcygeal nerves	S4, S5, Co1	Penetrate coccygeal attachments of sacrospinous/sacrotuberous ligaments to supply overlying skin

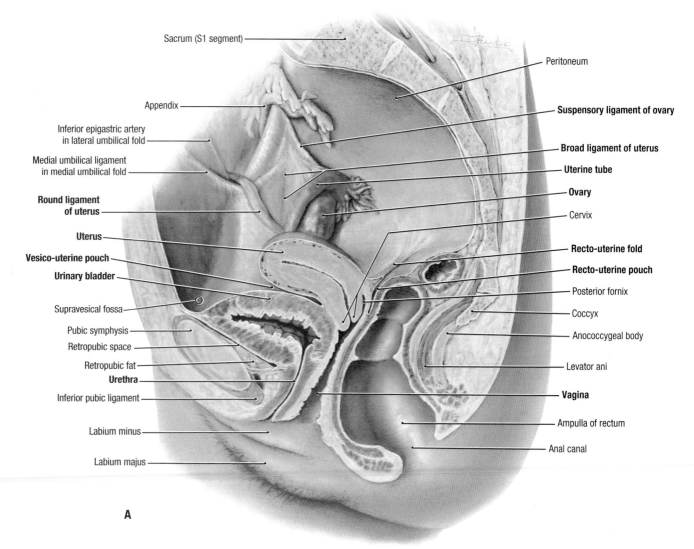

Sacrum (S1 segment)

Appendix

Inferior epigastric artery
in lateral umbilical fold

Medial umbilical ligament
in medial umbilical fold

**Round ligament
of uterus**

Uterus

Vesico-uterine pouch

Urinary bladder

Supravesical fossa

Pubic symphysis

Retropubic space

Retropubic fat

Urethra

Inferior pubic ligament

Labium minus

Labium majus

Peritoneum

Suspensory ligament of ovary

Broad ligament of uterus

Uterine tube

Ovary

Cervix

Recto-uterine fold

Recto-uterine pouch

Posterior fornix

Coccyx

Anococcygeal body

Levator ani

Vagina

Ampulla of rectum

Anal canal

A

**Medial Views of Right Half of
Hemisected Female Pelvis**

Retropubic
space

Urinary bladder

Vagina

Uterus

Rectum

Female:

Peritoneum passes:

- From the anteiror abdominal wall *(1)*
- Superior to the pubic bone *(2)*, forming supravesical fossa
- On the superior surface of the urinary bladder *(3)*
- From the bladder to mid-uterus, forming the vesico-uterine pouch *(4)*
- On the fundus and body of the uterus, and posterior fornix of the vagina *(5)*
- Between the rectum and uterus, forming the recto-uterine pouch *(6)*
- On the anterior and lateral sides of the rectum *(7)*
- Posteriorly to become the sigmoid mesocolon *(8)*

B

3.14   **PERITONEUM COVERING FEMALE PELVIC ORGANS**

A. Organs in situ with peritoneal reflections. **B.** Schematic illustration. The level of the supravesical fossa changes with filling and emptying of bladder.

Medial Views

A. Labels (top to bottom, left side):
Peritoneal cavity
Rectus abdominis
Peritoneum
Supravesical fossa
Retropubic space
Fat pad
Pubic symphysis
Prostate
Puboprostatic ligament
Intermediate (membranous) urethra
Intrabulbar fossa
Spongy urethra

A. Labels (right side):
Sacrum (S1 segment)
Urinary bladder
Rectovesical pouch
Internal urethral sphincter
Rectovesical fascia
Coccyx (Co1 segment)
Prostatic urethra
Levator ani
Rectum
Puborectalis
Deep transverse perineal
External urethral sphincter (sphincter urethrae)
Internal anal sphincter
Anal columns
Subcutaneous
Superficial
Deep } Parts of external anal sphincter

A. Labels (bottom):
Testis
Bulb of penis
Bulbospongiosus
Perineal membrane

A

B labels:
Urinary bladder
Puboprostatic ligament
Rectum
Seminal gland
Prostate

Male:

Peritoneum passes:

- From the anterior abdominal wall *(1)*
- Superior to the pubic bone *(2)*, forming supravesical fossa
- On the superior surface of the urinary bladder *(3)*
- 2 cm inferiorly on the posterior surface of the urinary bladder *(4)*
- On the superior ends of the seminal glands *(5)*
- Posteriorly to line the rectovesical pouch *(6)*
- To cover the rectum *(7)*
- Posteriorly to become the sigmoid mesocolon *(8)*

3.15   PERITONEUM COVERING MALE PELVIC ORGANS

A. Organs in situ. The urinary bladder is distended and displaced posteriorly in this specimen, not anteriorly as is usual, forming a broad and deep supravesical fossa even when the bladder is full. **B.** Peritoneum covering male pelvic organs. Typically, the location of supravesical fossa changes with filling and emptying of bladder.

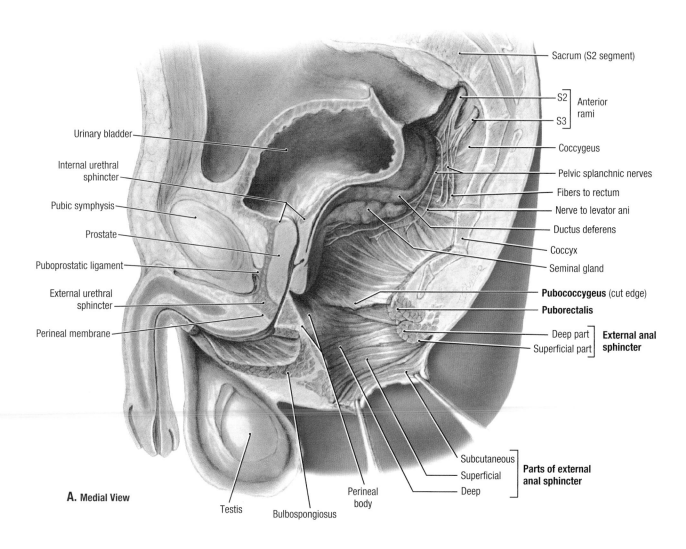

A. Medial View

Sacrum (S2 segment)

S2
S3 } Anterior rami

Coccygeus

Pelvic splanchnic nerves

Fibers to rectum

Nerve to levator ani

Ductus deferens

Coccyx

Seminal gland

Pubococcygeus (cut edge)

Puborectalis

Deep part
Superficial part } **External anal sphincter**

Subcutaneous
Superficial
Deep } **Parts of external anal sphincter**

Urinary bladder

Internal urethral sphincter

Pubic symphysis

Prostate

Puboprostatic ligament

External urethral sphincter

Perineal membrane

Testis

Bulbospongiosus

Perineal body

3.16   ANAL SPHINCTERS AND ANAL CANAL

A. Levator ani, in right half of hemisected pelvis.

- The subcutaneous fibers of the external anal sphincter and overlying skin are reflected with forceps. The pubococcygeus muscle is cut to reveal the anal canal, to which it is, in part, attached.

B. Puborectalis.

- The innermost part of the pubococcygeus muscle, the puborectalis, forms a U-shaped muscular "sling" around the anorectal junction, which maintains the anorectal (perineal) flexure.

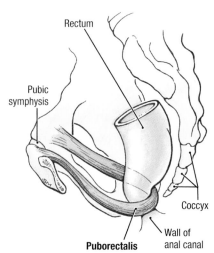

Rectum

Pubic symphysis

Coccyx

Wall of anal canal

Puborectalis

B. Lateral View

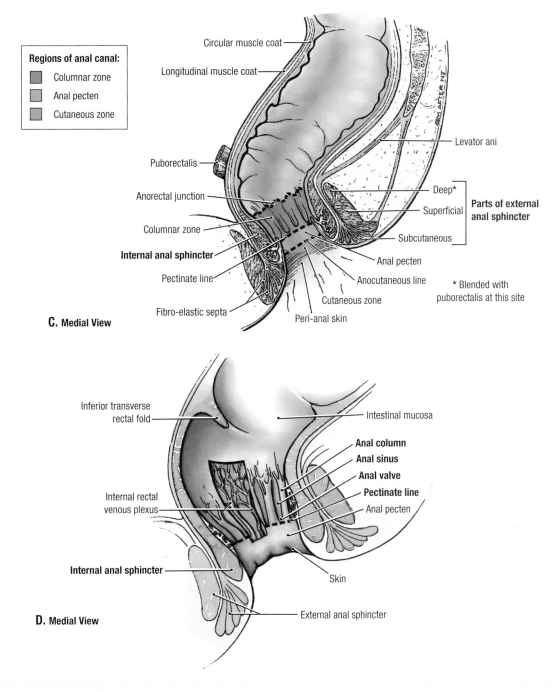

Regions of anal canal:

- Columnar zone
- Anal pecten
- Cutaneous zone

Circular muscle coat

Longitudinal muscle coat

Levator ani

Puborectalis

Deep*

Superficial — **Parts of external anal sphincter**

Anorectal junction

Columnar zone

Subcutaneous

Internal anal sphincter

Anal pecten

Anocutaneous line

Pectinate line

* Blended with puborectalis at this site

Fibro-elastic septa

Cutaneous zone

Peri-anal skin

C. Medial View

Inferior transverse rectal fold

Intestinal mucosa

Anal column

Anal sinus

Anal valve

Internal rectal venous plexus

Pectinate line

Anal pecten

Internal anal sphincter

Skin

External anal sphincter

D. Medial View

3.16 **ANAL SPHINCTERS AND ANAL CANAL** *(CONTINUED)*

C. External and internal anal sphincters.
- The internal anal sphincter is a thickening of the inner, circular muscular coat of the anal canal.
- The external anal sphincter has three often indistinct continuous zones: deep, superficial, and subcutaneous; the deep part intermingles with the puborectalis muscle posteriorly.
- The longitudinal muscle layer of the rectum separates the internal and external anal sphincters and terminates in the subcutaneous tissue and skin around the anus.

D. Features of the anal canal.
- The anal columns are 5 to 10 vertical folds of mucosa separated by anal sinuses and valves; they contain portions of the rectal venous plexus.

- The pecten is a smooth area of hairless stratified epithelium that lies between the anal valves superiorly and the inferior border of the internal anal sphincter inferiorly.
- The pectinate line is an irregular line at the base of the anal valves where the intestinal mucosa is continuous with the pecten; this indicates the junction of the superior part of the anal canal (derived from embryonic hindgut) and the inferior part of the anal canal (derived from the anal pit [proctodeum]). Innervation is visceral proximal to the line and somatic distally; lymphatic drainage is to the pararectal nodes proximally and to the superficial inguinal nodes distally.

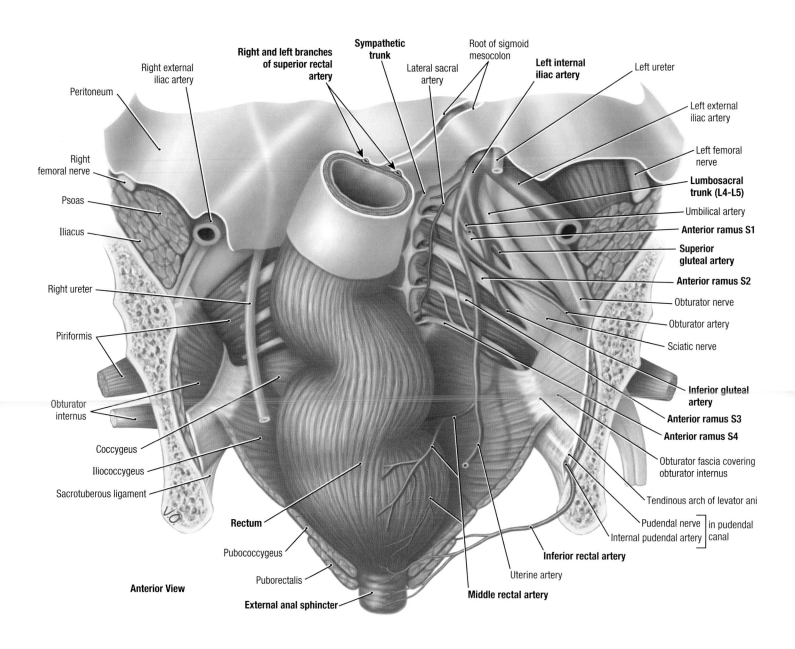

Right external
iliac artery

Right and left branches
of superior rectal
artery

Sympathetic
trunk

Root of sigmoid
mesocolon

Lateral sacral
artery

Left internal
iliac artery

Left ureter

Peritoneum

Right
femoral nerve

Psoas

Iliacus

Right ureter

Piriformis

Obturator
internus

Coccygeus

Iliococcygeus

Sacrotuberous ligament

Rectum

Pubococcygeus

Puborectalis

Anterior View

External anal sphincter

Left external
iliac artery

Left femoral
nerve

Lumbosacral
trunk (L4-L5)

Umbilical artery

Anterior ramus S1

Superior
gluteal artery

Anterior ramus S2

Obturator nerve

Obturator artery

Sciatic nerve

Inferior gluteal
artery

Anterior ramus S3

Anterior ramus S4

Obturator fascia covering
obturator internus

Tendinous arch of levator ani

Pudendal nerve ⎫ in pudendal
Internal pudendal artery ⎭ canal

Inferior rectal artery

Uterine artery

Middle rectal artery

**3.17 RECTUM, ANAL CANAL, AND NEUROVASCULAR STRUCTURES OF POSTERIOR
PELVIS**

The pelvis is coronally bisected anterior to the rectum and anal canal. The superior gluteal artery often passes
posteriorly between the anterior rami of L5 and S1, and the inferior gluteal artery between S2 and S3.

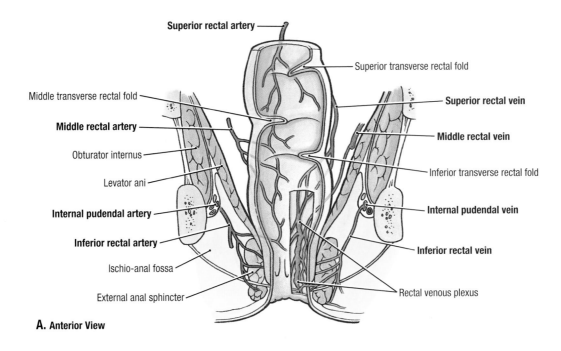

Superior rectal artery

Middle transverse rectal fold

Middle rectal artery

Obturator internus

Levator ani

Internal pudendal artery

Inferior rectal artery

Ischio-anal fossa

External anal sphincter

Superior transverse rectal fold

Superior rectal vein

Middle rectal vein

Inferior transverse rectal fold

Internal pudendal vein

Inferior rectal vein

Rectal venous plexus

A. Anterior View

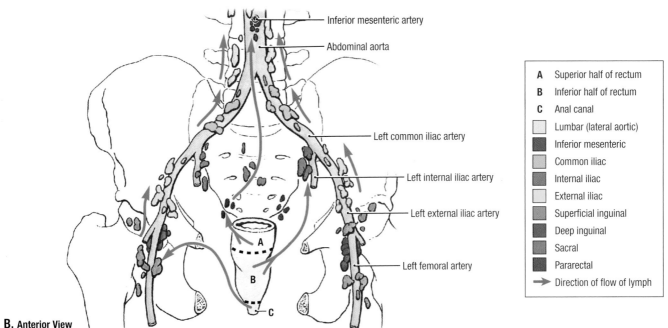

Inferior mesenteric artery

Abdominal aorta

Left common iliac artery

Left internal iliac artery

Left external iliac artery

Left femoral artery

A	Superior half of rectum
B	Inferior half of rectum
C	Anal canal
	Lumbar (lateral aortic)
	Inferior mesenteric
	Common iliac
	Internal iliac
	External iliac
	Superficial inguinal
	Deep inguinal
	Sacral
	Pararectal
→	Direction of flow of lymph

B. Anterior View

3.18   VASCULATURE OF RECTUM

A. Arterial and venous drainage.
- The continuation of the inferior mesenteric artery, the superior rectal artery, supplies the proximal part of rectum.
- Right and left middle rectal arteries, usually arising from the inferior vesical (male) or uterine (female) arteries, supply the middle and inferior parts of the rectum.
- Inferior rectal arteries, arising from the internal pudendal arteries, supply the anorectal junction and the anal canal.
- The rectal venous plexus surrounds the distal rectum and anal canal and consists of an internal rectal plexus deep to the epithelium of the anal

canal and an external rectal plexus external to the muscular coats of the wall of the anal canal.
- The superior rectal vein drains into the portal system, and the middle and inferior veins drain into the systemic system; thus, this is an important area of **portacaval anastomosis** (see information on Hemorrhoids with Fig. 3.30).

B. Lymphatic drainage.
- The superior, middle, and inferior rectal veins drain the rectum and anal canal; there are anastomoses between the plexuses formed by all three veins.

Innervation:
- ···· Presynaptic sympathetic
- —— Postsynaptic sympathetic
- ···· Presynaptic parasympathetic
- —— Postsynaptic parasympathetic
- —— Visceral afferent running with sympathetic and parasympathetic fibers
- —— Somatic sensory
- —— Somatic motor

Spinal ganglion

Spinal cord

T12

L1

L2

L3

L4

L5

Upper lumbar sympathetic trunk

Lumbar splanchnic nerves

Spinal ganglia

Pelvic splanchnic nerves

S1

S2

S3

S4

Pelvic plexus

Prevertebral ganglia

Aortic plexus

Sacral plexus

Superior rectal nerves

Superior hypogastric plexus

Inferior hypogastric plexuses

Pudendal nerve

Pelvic plexus

Internal anal sphincter

External anal sphincter

Inferior anal (rectal) nerve

3.19   INNERVATION OF RECTUM AND ANAL CANAL

The lumbar and pelvic spinal nerves and hypogastric plexuses have been retracted laterally for clarity.

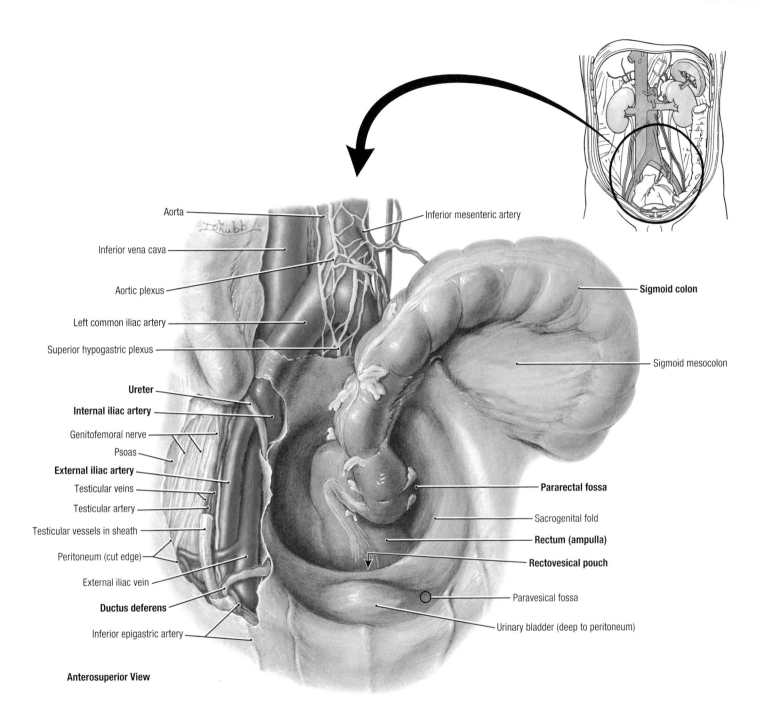

Aorta

Inferior vena cava

Aortic plexus

Left common iliac artery

Superior hypogastric plexus

Ureter

Internal iliac artery

Genitofemoral nerve

Psoas

External iliac artery

Testicular veins

Testicular artery

Testicular vessels in sheath

Peritoneum (cut edge)

External iliac vein

Ductus deferens

Inferior epigastric artery

Inferior mesenteric artery

Sigmoid colon

Sigmoid mesocolon

Pararectal fossa

Sacrogenital fold

Rectum (ampulla)

Rectovesical pouch

Paravesical fossa

Urinary bladder (deep to peritoneum)

Anterosuperior View

| 3.20 | RECTUM IN SITU |

- The sigmoid colon begins at the left pelvic brim and becomes the rectum anterior to the third sacral segment in the midline.
- The superior hypogastric plexus lies inferior to the bifurcation of the aorta and anterior to the left common iliac vein.
- The ureter adheres to the external aspect of the peritoneum, crosses the external iliac vessels, and descends anterior to the internal iliac artery. The ductus deferens and its artery also adhere to the peritoneum, cross the external iliac vessels, and then hook around the inferior epigastric artery to join the other components of the spermatic cord.
- The genitofemoral nerve lies on the psoas.

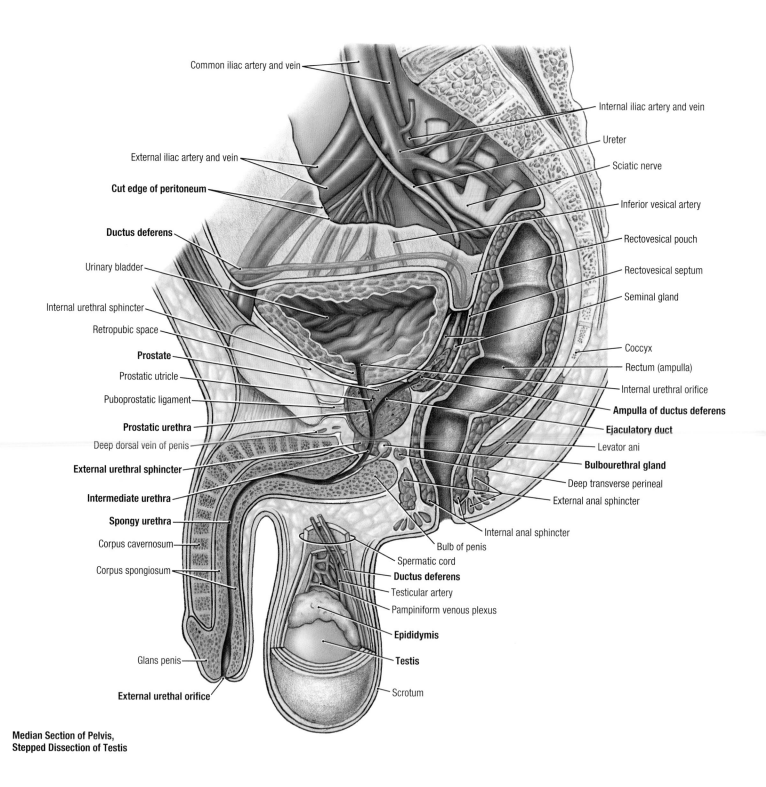

Common iliac artery and vein

External iliac artery and vein

Cut edge of peritoneum

Ductus deferens

Urinary bladder

Internal urethral sphincter

Retropubic space

Prostate

Prostatic utricle

Puboprostatic ligament

Prostatic urethra

Deep dorsal vein of penis

External urethral sphincter

Intermediate urethra

Spongy urethra

Corpus cavernosum

Corpus spongiosum

Glans penis

External urethal orifice

Internal iliac artery and vein

Ureter

Sciatic nerve

Inferior vesical artery

Rectovesical pouch

Rectovesical septum

Seminal gland

Coccyx

Rectum (ampulla)

Internal urethral orifice

Ampulla of ductus deferens

Ejaculatory duct

Levator ani

Bulbourethral gland

Deep transverse perineal

External anal sphincter

Internal anal sphincter

Bulb of penis

Spermatic cord

Ductus deferens

Testicular artery

Pampiniform venous plexus

Epididymis

Testis

Scrotum

**Median Section of Pelvis,
Stepped Dissection of Testis**

3.21   MALE PELVIC ORGANS AND EXTERNAL GENITALIA

- Pelvic viscera are subperitoneal, mostly embedded in a matrix of fatty endopelvic fascia.

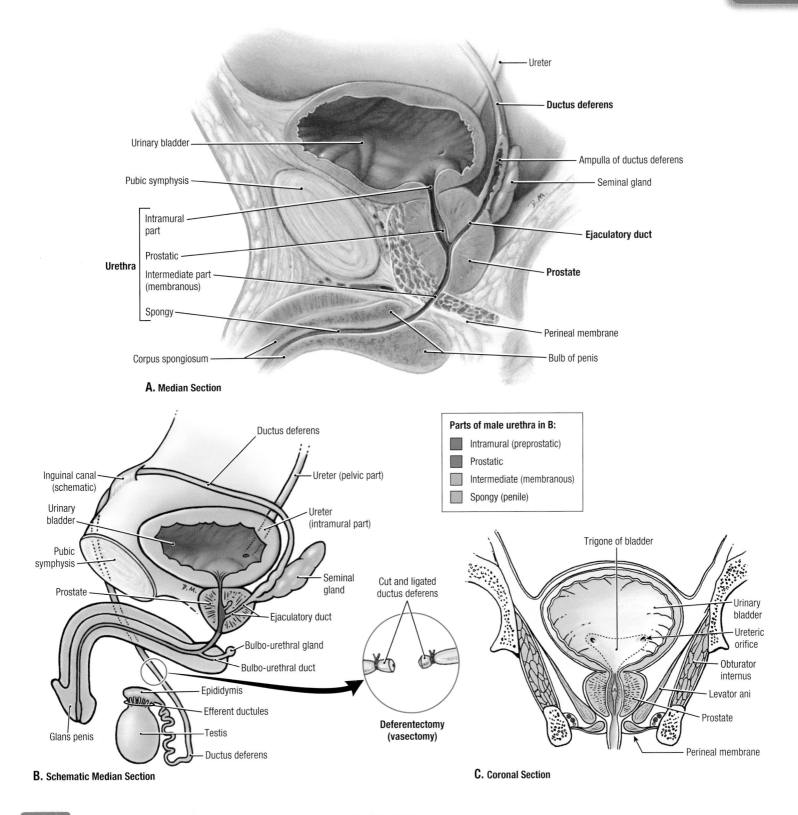

A. Median Section

Parts of male urethra in B:

- Intramural (preprostatic)
- Prostatic
- Intermediate (membranous)
- Spongy (penile)

B. Schematic Median Section

Deferentectomy (vasectomy)

C. Coronal Section

3.22   URINARY BLADDER, PROSTATE, AND DUCTUS DEFERENS

A. Dissection. The ejaculatory duct (~2 cm in length) is formed by the union of the ductus deferens and duct of the seminal gland; it passes anteriorly and inferiorly through the substance of the prostate to enter the prostatic urethra on the seminal colliculus. **B.** Overview of urogenital system, schematic illustration. **C.** Coronal section through urinary bladder, prostate, and proximal urethra.

The common method of sterilizing males is a **deferentectomy**, popularly called **vasectomy**. During this procedure, part of the ductus deferens is ligated and/or excised through an incision in the superior part of the scrotum. Hence, the subsequent ejaculated fluid contains no sperms.

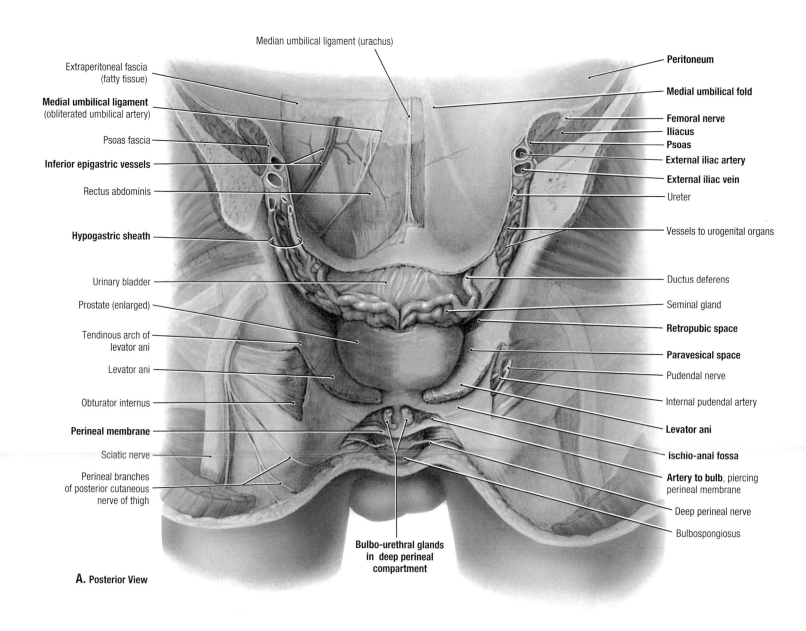

Median umbilical ligament (urachus)

Extraperitoneal fascia (fatty tissue)

Medial umbilical ligament (obliterated umbilical artery)

Psoas fascia

Inferior epigastric vessels

Rectus abdominis

Hypogastric sheath

Urinary bladder

Prostate (enlarged)

Tendinous arch of levator ani

Levator ani

Obturator internus

Perineal membrane

Sciatic nerve

Perineal branches of posterior cutaneous nerve of thigh

A. Posterior View

Bulbo-urethral glands in deep perineal compartment

Peritoneum

Medial umbilical fold

Femoral nerve
Iliacus
Psoas

External iliac artery

External iliac vein

Ureter

Vessels to urogenital organs

Ductus deferens

Seminal gland

Retropubic space

Paravesical space

Pudendal nerve

Internal pudendal artery

Levator ani

Ischio-anal fossa

Artery to bulb, piercing perineal membrane

Deep perineal nerve

Bulbospongiosus

3.23 POSTERIOR APPROACH TO ANTERIOR PELVIC AND PERINEAL STRUCTURES AND SPACES

A. Dissection. The rectovesical septum and all pelvic and perineal structures posterior to it have been removed. **B.** Posterior surface of inferior part of anterior abdominal wall with umbilical folds and ligaments and anterior pelvic viscera. **C.** Schematic coronal section through the anterior pelvis (plane of urinary bladder and prostate) demonstrating pelvic fascia.

- In **A** and **B**, the inferior epigastric artery and accompanying veins enter the rectus sheath, covered posteriorly with peritoneum to form the lateral umbilical fold. The medial umbilical fold is formed by peritoneum overlying the medial umbilical ligament (obliterated umbilical artery), and the median umbilical fold is formed by the median umbilical ligament (urachus).

- In **A**, the femoral nerve lies between the psoas and iliacus muscles, covered on their internal aspects with psoas (membranous parietal) fascia; the external iliac artery and vein lie within the areolar extraperitoneal fascia.
- The pelvic genito-urinary organs are subperitoneal. Near the bladder, the ureter accompanies a "leash" of internal iliac vessels and derivatives within the fibro-areolar hypogastric sheath.
- The levator ani and its fascial coverings separate the retropubic and paravesical spaces of the pelvis from the ischio-anal fossae of the perineum. The fat that occupies these spaces has been removed.
- The bulbo-urethral glands and the initial part of the artery to the bulb lie superior to the perineal membrane in the deep perineal compartment.

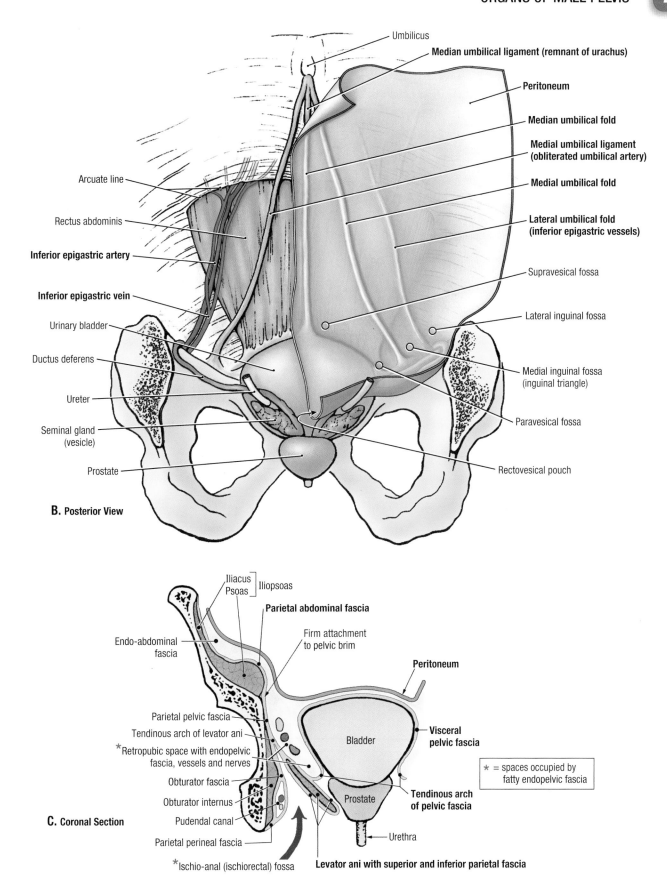

Umbilicus

Median umbilical ligament (remnant of urachus)

Peritoneum

Median umbilical fold

Medial umbilical ligament (obliterated umbilical artery)

Medial umbilical fold

Lateral umbilical fold (inferior epigastric vessels)

Supravesical fossa

Lateral inguinal fossa

Medial inguinal fossa (inguinal triangle)

Paravesical fossa

Rectovesical pouch

Arcuate line

Rectus abdominis

Inferior epigastric artery

Inferior epigastric vein

Urinary bladder

Ductus deferens

Ureter

Seminal gland (vesicle)

Prostate

B. Posterior View

Iliacus
Psoas] Iliopsoas

Parietal abdominal fascia

Firm attachment to pelvic brim

Endo-abdominal fascia

Peritoneum

Parietal pelvic fascia

Tendinous arch of levator ani

Bladder

Visceral pelvic fascia

*Retropubic space with endopelvic fascia, vessels and nerves

Obturator fascia

Obturator internus

Pudendal canal

Prostate

Tendinous arch of pelvic fascia

★ = spaces occupied by fatty endopelvic fascia

C. Coronal Section

Parietal perineal fascia

Urethra

*Ischio-anal (ischiorectal) fossa

Levator ani with superior and inferior parietal fascia

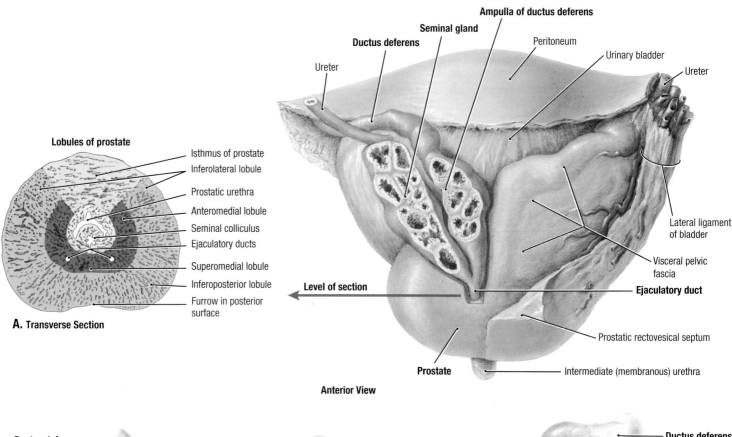

Lobules of prostate

Isthmus of prostate
Inferolateral lobule
Prostatic urethra
Anteromedial lobule
Seminal colliculus
Ejaculatory ducts
Superomedial lobule
Inferoposterior lobule
Furrow in posterior surface

A. Transverse Section

Ureter
Ductus deferens
Seminal gland
Ampulla of ductus deferens
Peritoneum
Urinary bladder
Ureter
Lateral ligament of bladder
Visceral pelvic fascia
Ejaculatory duct
Prostatic rectovesical septum
Intermediate (membranous) urethra
Prostate

Level of section

Anterior View

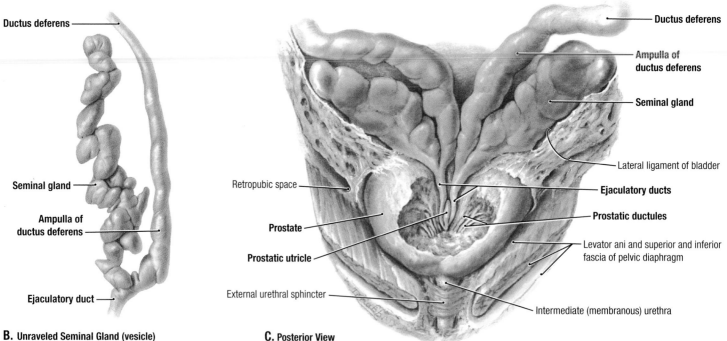

Ductus deferens

Seminal gland

Ampulla of ductus deferens

Ejaculatory duct

B. Unraveled Seminal Gland (vesicle)

Ductus deferens
Ampulla of ductus deferens
Seminal gland
Lateral ligament of bladder
Ejaculatory ducts
Prostatic ductules
Levator ani and superior and inferior fascia of pelvic diaphragm
Intermediate (membranous) urethra

Retropubic space
Prostate
Prostatic utricle
External urethral sphincter

C. Posterior View

| 3.24 | SEMINAL GLANDS AND PROSTATE |

A. Bladder, ductus deferens, seminal glands (vesicles), and lobules of prostate. The left seminal gland and ampulla of the ductus deferens are dissected and opened; part of the prostate is cut away to expose the ejaculatory duct. **B.** Seminal gland unraveled. The gland is a tortuous tube with numerous dilatations. The ampulla of the ductus deferens has similar dilatations. **C.** Prostate, dissected posteriorly. The ejaculatory duct (~2 cm in length) is formed by the union of the ductus deferens and the duct of the seminal gland; it passes anteriorly and inferiorly through the substance of the prostate to enter the prostatic urethra on the seminal colliculus. The prostatic utricle lies between the ends of the two ejaculatory ducts. The prostatic ductules mostly open onto the prostatic sinus.

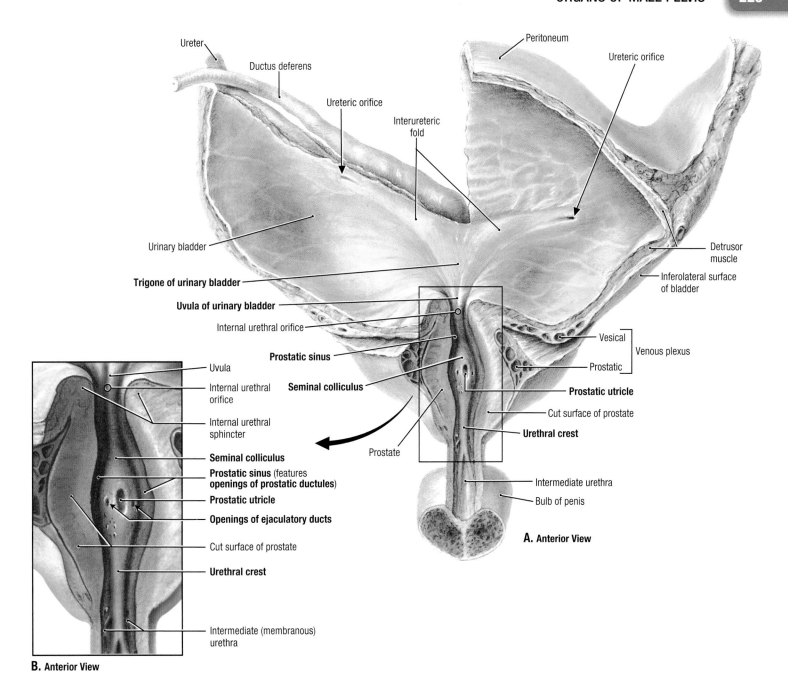

A. Anterior View

B. Anterior View

3.25   INTERIOR OF MALE URINARY BLADDER AND PROSTATIC URETHRA

A. Dissection. The anterior walls of the bladder, prostate, and urethra were cut away. **B.** Features of the prostatic urethra.

- The mucous membrane is smooth over the trigone of the urinary bladder (triangular region demarcated by ureteric and internal urethral orifices) but folded elsewhere, especially when the bladder is empty.
- The opening of the vestigial prostatic utricle is in the seminal colliculus on the urethral crest; there is an orifice of an ejaculatory duct on each side of the prostatic utricle. The prostatic fascia encloses a venous plexus.

The prostate is of considerable medical interest because enlargement or **benign hypertrophy of the prostate (BHP)** is common after middle age,

affecting virtually every male who lives long enough. An enlarged prostate projects into the urinary bladder and impedes urination by distorting the prostatic urethra. The middle lobule usually enlarges the most and obstructs the internal urethral orifice. The more the person strains, the more the valvelike prostatic mass occludes the urethra.

BHP is a common cause of urethral obstruction, leading to **nocturia** (needing to void during the night), **dysuria** (difficulty and/or pain during urination), and **urgency** (sudden desire to void). BHP also increases the risk of bladder infections (**cystitis**) as well as kidney damage.

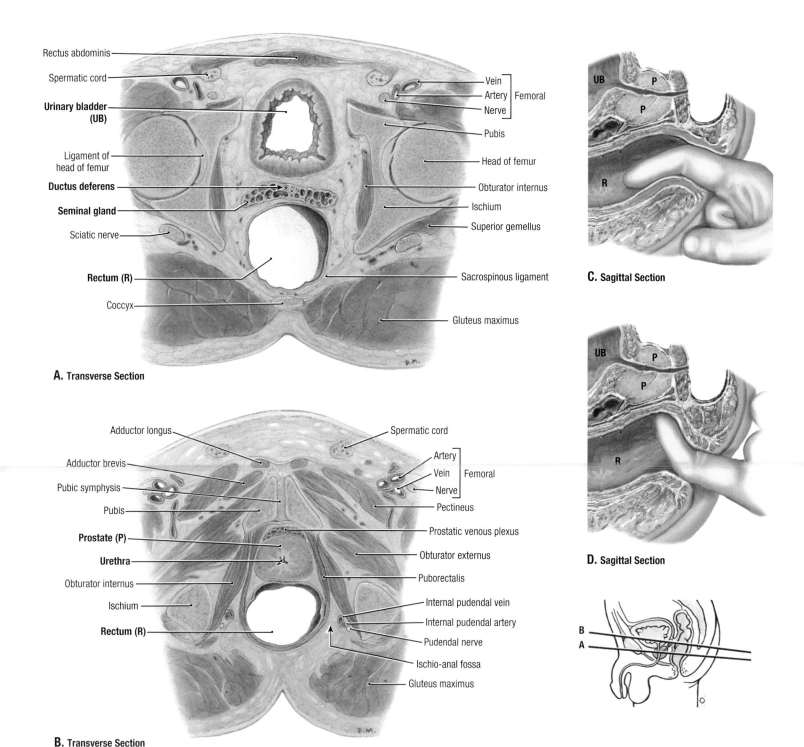

Rectus abdominis
Spermatic cord
Urinary bladder (UB)
Ligament of head of femur
Ductus deferens
Seminal gland
Sciatic nerve
Rectum (R)
Coccyx

Vein
Artery   Femoral
Nerve
Pubis
Head of femur
Obturator internus
Ischium
Superior gemellus
Sacrospinous ligament
Gluteus maximus

A. Transverse Section

C. Sagittal Section
UB   P
P
R

Adductor longus
Adductor brevis
Pubic symphysis
Pubis
Prostate (P)
Urethra
Obturator internus
Ischium
Rectum (R)

Spermatic cord
Artery
Vein   Femoral
Nerve
Pectineus
Prostatic venous plexus
Obturator externus
Puborectalis
Internal pudendal vein
Internal pudendal artery
Pudendal nerve
Ischio-anal fossa
Gluteus maximus

B. Transverse Section

D. Sagittal Section
UB   P
P
R

B
A

3.26   MALE PELVIS, TRANSVERSE SECTIONS

A. Section through prostate and puborectalis. **B.** Section through urinary bladder and seminal gland. **C. and D.** The prostate *(P)* is examined for enlargement and tumors (focal masses or asymmetry) by **digital rectal examination**. A full bladder offers resistance, holding the gland in place and making it more readily palpable. The malignant prostate feels hard and often irregular. (*R, rectum*).

Pubic symphysis (1)
Prostatic urethra (2)
Isthmus (AMZ) of prostate (3)
Intermediate (membranous) urethra (4)
External urethral sphincter (5)

Urinary bladder (6)
Prostate (7)
Ampulla of ductus deferens (8)
Seminal gland (9)
Ejaculatory duct (10)
Rectal wall (11)
Rectum (12)

A. Median Section

Key for US scan:
12 Site of transducer in rectum
13 Concretions surrounding distended and collapsed urethra
14 Calcification in seminal colliculus

Longitudinal (Median) Scan

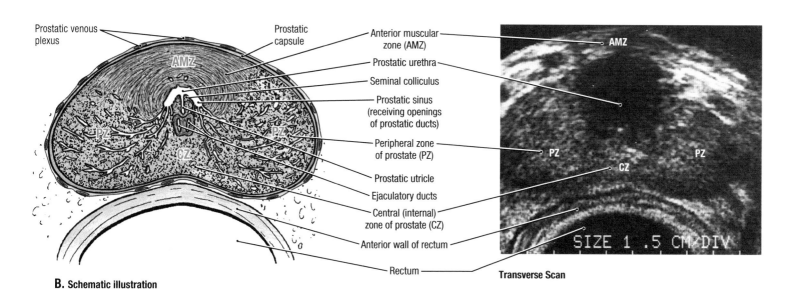

Prostatic venous plexus
Prostatic capsule
AMZ
PZ
PZ
CZ

Anterior muscular zone (AMZ)
Prostatic urethra
Seminal colliculus
Prostatic sinus (receiving openings of prostatic ducts)
Peripheral zone of prostate (PZ)
Prostatic utricle
Ejaculatory ducts
Central (internal) zone of prostate (CZ)
Anterior wall of rectum
Rectum

B. Schematic illustration

AMZ
PZ
CZ
PZ
SIZE 1.5 CM/DIV

Transverse Scan

3.27 TRANSRECTAL ULTRASOUND SCANS OF MALE PELVIS

A. Longitudinal scan. **B.** Transverse scan. The probe was inserted into the rectum to scan the anteriorly located prostate. The ducts of the glands in the peripheral zone open into the prostatic sinuses, whereas the ducts of the glands in the central (internal) zone open into the prostatic sinuses and onto the seminal colliculus.

Because of the close relationship of the prostate to the prostatic urethra, obstructions of the urethra may be relieved endoscopically. The instrument is inserted transurethrally through the external urethral orifice and spongy urethra into the prostatic urethra. All or part of the prostate, or just the hypertrophied part, is removed by **transurethral resection of the prostate (TURP)**. In more serious cases, the entire prostate is removed along with the seminal glands, ejaculatory ducts, and terminal parts of the deferent ducts **(radical prostatectomy)**.

TURP and improved operative techniques (laparoscopic or robotic surgery) attempt to preserve the nerves and blood vessels associated with the capsule of the prostate and adjacent to the seminal vesicles as they pass to and from the penis, increasing the possibility for patients to retain sexual function after surgery, as well as restoring normal urinary control.

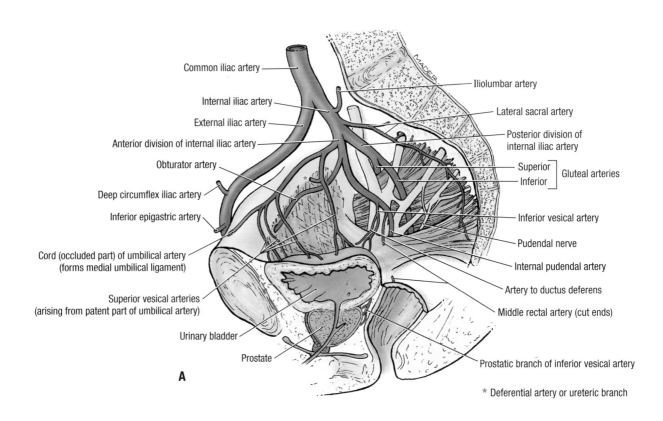

Common iliac artery

Internal iliac artery

External iliac artery

Anterior division of internal iliac artery

Obturator artery

Deep circumflex iliac artery

Inferior epigastric artery

Cord (occluded part) of umbilical artery
(forms medial umbilical ligament)

Superior vesical arteries
(arising from patent part of umbilical artery)

Urinary bladder

Prostate

Iliolumbar artery

Lateral sacral artery

Posterior division of
internal iliac artery

Superior ⎤
Inferior ⎦ Gluteal arteries

Inferior vesical artery

Pudendal nerve

Internal pudendal artery

Artery to ductus deferens

Middle rectal artery (cut ends)

Prostatic branch of inferior vesical artery

* Deferential artery or ureteric branch

A

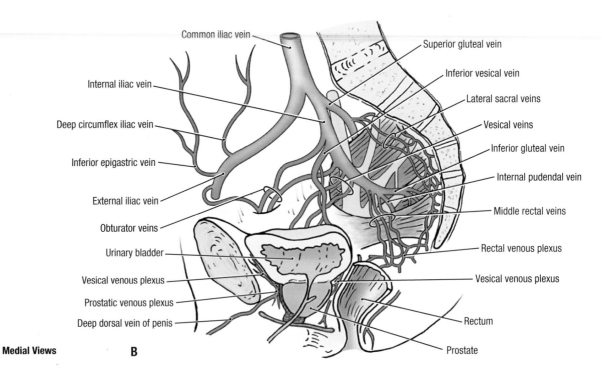

Common iliac vein

Internal iliac vein

Deep circumflex iliac vein

Inferior epigastric vein

External iliac vein

Obturator veins

Urinary bladder

Vesical venous plexus

Prostatic venous plexus

Deep dorsal vein of penis

Superior gluteal vein

Inferior vesical vein

Lateral sacral veins

Vesical veins

Inferior gluteal vein

Internal pudendal vein

Middle rectal veins

Rectal venous plexus

Vesical venous plexus

Rectum

Prostate

Medial Views   **B**

3.28   ARTERIES AND VEINS OF MALE PELVIS

A. Arteries. **B.** Pelvic veins and venous plexuses.

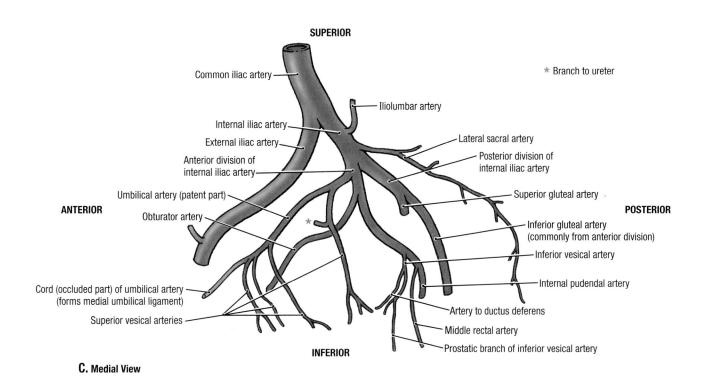

C. Medial View

3.28 ARTERIES AND VEINS OF MALE PELVIS *(CONTINUED)*

C. Arteries, isolated from A.

TABLE 3.4 ARTERIES OF MALE PELVIS

Artery	Origin	Course	Distribution
Internal iliac	Common iliac artery	Passes medially over pelvic brim and descends into pelvic cavity; often forms anterior and posterior divisions	Main blood supply to pelvic organs, gluteal muscles, and perineum
Anterior division of internal iliac artery	Internal iliac artery	Passes laterally along lateral wall of pelvis, dividing into visceral, obturator, and internal pudendal arteries	Pelvic viscera, perineum, and muscles of superior medial thigh
Umbilical	Anterior division of internal iliac artery	Short pelvic course; gives off superior vesical arteries, then obliterates, becoming medial umbilical ligament	Urinary bladder and, in some males, ductus deferens
Superior vesical	Patent part of umbilical artery	Usually multiple; pass to superior aspect of urinary bladder	Superior aspect of urinary bladder and distal ureter
Artery to ductus deferens	Superior or inferior vesical artery	Runs subperitoneally to ductus deferens	Ductus deferens
Obturator	Anterior division of internal iliac artery	Runs antero-inferiorly on lateral pelvic wall	Pelvic muscles, nutrient artery to head of femur and medial compartment of thigh
Inferior vesical		Passes subperitoneally giving rise to prostatic artery and occasionally the artery to the ductus deferens	Inferior aspect of urinary bladder, pelvic ureter, seminal glands, and prostate
Middle rectal		Descends in pelvis to rectum	Seminal glands, prostate, and inferior part of rectum
Internal pudendal		Exits pelvis through greater sciatic foramen and enters perineum via lesser sciatic foramen	Main artery to perineum, including muscles and skin of anal and urogenital triangles; erectile bodies
Posterior division of internal iliac artery	Internal iliac artery	Passes posteriorly and gives rise to parietal branches	Pelvic wall and gluteal region iliac artery
Iliolumbar	Posterior division of internal iliac artery	Ascends anterior to sacro-iliac joint and posterior to common iliac vessels and psoas major	Iliacus, psoas major, quadratus lumborum muscles, and cauda equina in vertebral canal
Lateral sacral (superior and inferior)		Run on anteromedial aspect of piriformis to send branches into pelvic sacral foramina	Piriformis muscle, structures in sacral canal and erector spinae muscles
Testicular (gonadal) [see Fig. 3.28A]	Abdominal aorta	Descends retroperitoneally; traverses inguinal canal and enters scrotum	Abdominal ureter, testis and epididymis

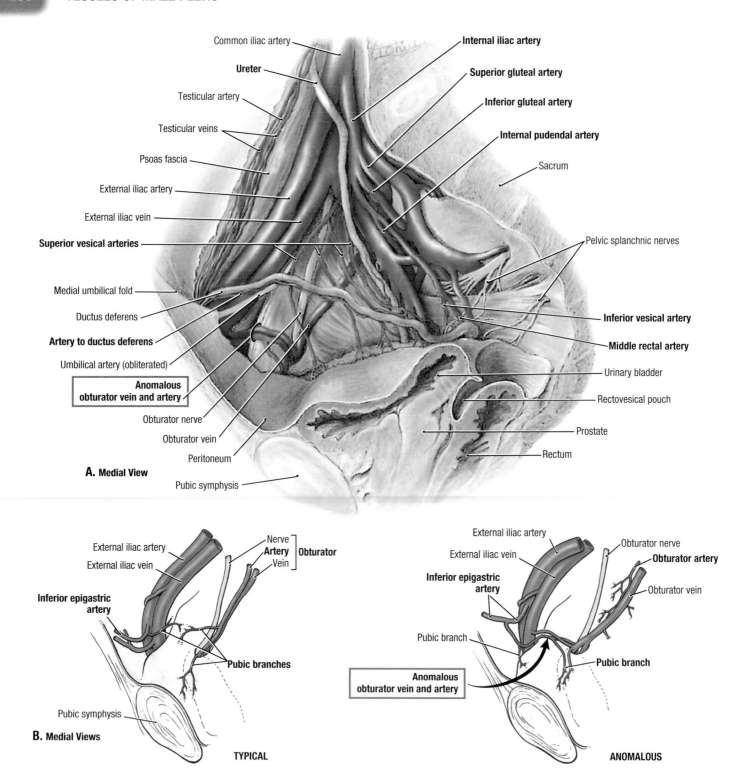

Common iliac artery

Internal iliac artery

Ureter

Superior gluteal artery

Testicular artery

Inferior gluteal artery

Testicular veins

Internal pudendal artery

Psoas fascia

Sacrum

External iliac artery

External iliac vein

Superior vesical arteries

Pelvic splanchnic nerves

Medial umbilical fold

Ductus deferens

Inferior vesical artery

Artery to ductus deferens

Middle rectal artery

Umbilical artery (obliterated)

Anomalous obturator vein and artery

Urinary bladder

Rectovesical pouch

Obturator nerve

Prostate

Obturator vein

Rectum

Peritoneum

A. Medial View

Pubic symphysis

External iliac artery

Nerve
Artery } **Obturator**
Vein

External iliac artery

Obturator nerve

External iliac vein

Obturator artery

External iliac vein

Inferior epigastric artery

Obturator vein

Inferior epigastric artery

Pubic branch

Pubic branches

Pubic branch

Pubic symphysis

Anomalous obturator vein and artery

Pubic branch

B. Medial Views

TYPICAL

ANOMALOUS

3.29   PELVIC VESSELS IN SITU; LATERAL PELVIC WALL

A. Dissection. The ureter crosses the external iliac artery at its origin (common iliac bifurcation), and the ductus deferens crosses the external iliac artery at its termination (deep inguinal ring). The ureter crosses the external iliac artery at its origin (common iliac bifurcation), and the ductus deferens crosses the external iliac artery at its termination (deep inguinal ring). In this speciman, an anomalous (replaced) obturator artery branches from the inferior epigastric artery. **B.** Typical and anomalous obturator arteries.

Anterior View

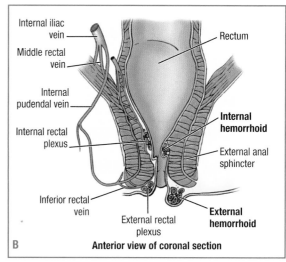

Anterior view of coronal section

PORTAL–SYSTEMIC (PORTACAVAL) ANASTOMOSES

A. The portal tributaries are *purple,* and systemic tributaries are *blue. A–D* indicate sites of portal–systemic anastomoses. *A,* between portal and systemic esophageal veins; *B,* between portal and systemic rectal veins; *C,* para-umbilical veins (portal) anastomosing with small epigastric veins of the anterior abdominal wall (systemic); *D,* twigs of colic veins (portal) anastomosing with retroperitoneal veins (systemic).

B. Hemorrhoids. Internal hemorrhoids (piles) are prolapses of rectal mucosa containing the normally dilated veins of the internal rectal venous plexus. Internal hemorrhoids are thought to result from a breakdown of the muscularis mucosae, a smooth muscle layer deep to the mucosa. Internal hemorrhoids that prolapse through the anal canal are often compressed by the contracted sphincters, impeding blood flow. As a result, they tend to strangulate and ulcerate. Because of the presence of abundant arteriovenous anastomoses, bleeding from internal hemorrhoids is characteristically bright red. The current practice is to treat only prolapsed, ulcerated internal hemorrhoids.

External hemorrhoids are thromboses (blood clots) in the veins of the external rectal venous plexus and are covered by skin. Predisposing factors for hemorrhoids include pregnancy, chronic constipation, and any disorder that impedes venous return including increased intra-abdominal pressure. The superior rectal vein drains into the inferior mesenteric vein, whereas the middle and inferior rectal veins drain through the systemic system into the inferior vena cava. Any abnormal increase in pressure in the valveless portal system or veins of the trunk may cause enlargement of the superior rectal veins, resulting in an increase in blood flow or stasis in the internal rectal venous plexus. In **portal hypertension** that occurs in relation to *hepatic cirrhosis,* the portacaval anastomosis (e.g., esophageal) may become varicose and rupture. It is important to note, however, that the veins of the rectal plexuses normally appear varicose (dilated and tortuous), even in newborns, and that internal hemorrhoids occur most commonly in the absence of portal hypertension.

Regarding pain from and the treatment of hemorrhoids, it is important to note that the anal canal superior to the pectinate line is visceral; thus, it is innervated by visceral afferent pain fibers, so that an incision or needle insertion into this region is painless. Internal hemorrhoids are not painful and can be treated without anesthesia. Inferior to the pectinate line, the anal canal is somatic, supplied by the inferior anal (rectal) nerves containing somatic sensory fibers. Therefore, it is sensitive to painful stimuli (e.g., to the prick of a hypodermic needle). External hemorrhoids can be painful, but often resolve in a few days.

Inferior mesenteric artery

Abdominal aorta

Left testicular artery

Left common iliac artery

Left internal iliac artery

Left external iliac artery

Urinary bladder

Left femoral artery

Prostatic
urethra

Intermediate
(membranous)
part of urethra

Spongy urethra

Lumbar (caval/aortic)
Inferior mesenteric
Common iliac
Internal iliac
External iliac
Superficial inguinal
Deep inguinal
Sacral
Direction of flow

Anterior Views

A

Prostate
Ductus
deferens
Seminal
gland
Testis

B

Penis
Glans
penis
Spongy urethra
Scrotum

C

3.31   LYMPHATIC DRAINAGE OF MALE PELVIS AND PERINEUM

A. Pelvic urinary system. **B.** Internal genital organs. **C.** Penis, spongy urethra, scrotum and testis.

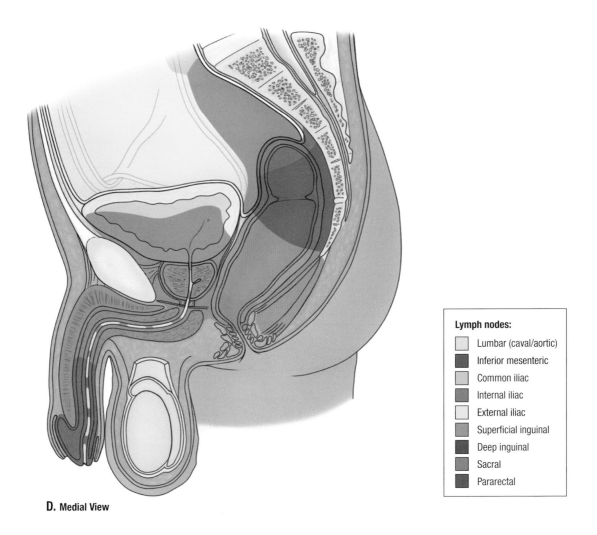

Lymph nodes:

- Lumbar (caval/aortic)
- Inferior mesenteric
- Common iliac
- Internal iliac
- External iliac
- Superficial inguinal
- Deep inguinal
- Sacral
- Pararectal

D. Medial View

3.31 LYMPHATIC DRAINAGE OF MALE PELVIS AND PERINEUM *(CONTINUED)*

D. Zones of pelvis and perineum initially draining into specific groups of lymph nodes.

TABLE 3.5 LYMPHATIC DRAINAGE OF MALE PELVIS AND PERINEUM

Lymph Node Group	Structures Typically Draining to Lymph Node Group
Lumbar	Gonads and associated structures (including testicular vessels), urethra, testis, epididymis, common iliac nodes
Inferior mesenteric nodes	Superiormost rectum, sigmoid colon, descending colon, pararectal nodes
Common iliac nodes	External and internal iliac lymph nodes
Internal iliac nodes	Inferior pelvic structures, deep perineal structures, sacral nodes, prostatic urethra, prostate, base of bladder, inferior part of pelvic ureter, inferior part of seminal glands, cavernous bodies, anal canal (above pectinate line), inferior rectum
External iliac nodes	Anterosuperior pelvic structures, deep inguinal nodes, superior aspect of bladder, superior part of pelvic ureter, upper part of seminal gland, pelvic part of ductus deferens, intermediate and spongy urethra
Superficial inguinal nodes	Lower limb, superficial drainage of inferolateral quadrant of trunk, including anterior abdominal wall inferior to umbilicus, gluteal region, superficial perineal structures, skin of perineum including skin and prepuce of penis, scrotum, perianal skin, anal canal inferior to pectinate line
Deep inguinal nodes	Glans of penis, distal spongy urethra, superficial inguinal nodes
Sacral nodes	Posteroinferior pelvic structures, inferior rectum
Pararectal nodes	Superior rectum

White rami communicans

Presynaptic sympathetic fiber (lumbar splanchnic nerve)

Postsynaptic sympathetic ganglion

Postsynaptic sympathetic fiber entering superior hypogastric plexus

Aortic plexus

Lumbar splanchnic nerves

Right common iliac artery

Right hypogastric nerve

Lumbosacral trunk (L4–L5)

Pelvic splanchnic nerves arising from anterior rami of S2–S4 spinal nerves

Inferior hypogastric plexus

Vesical (pelvic) nerve plexus

Sympathetic fiber to internal urethral sphincter

Presynaptic parasympathetic fiber from inferior hypogastric plexus

Intrinsic postsynaptic parasympathetic ganglion

A. Anterior View   Postsynaptic parasympathetic fiber

Aorta

Sympathetic trunk

Inferior mesenteric ganglion

Sympathetic ganglion

Superior hypogastric plexus

Left hypogastric nerve (cut end)

Left common iliac artery

Gray rami communicantes (postsynaptic fibers to lower limb)

Sciatic nerve

Urinary bladder

Pelvic pain line (inferior extent of peritoneum)

Pudendal nerve (S2–S4)

Internal urethral sphincter

Prostate and prostatic nerve plexus

Somatic motor fibers of pudendal nerve

Somatic sensory fibers of pudendal nerve

External urethral sphincter

Urethra

External urethral orifice

Legend:
- Sympathetic
- Parasympathetic
- Mixed sympathetic and parasympathetic
- Somatic

L1
L2
L3

3.32   INNERVATION OF MALE PELVIS AND PERINEUM

TABLE 3.6 EFFECT OF SYMPATHETIC AND PARASYMPATHETIC STIMULATION ON URINARY TRACT, GENITAL SYSTEM, AND RECTUM

Organ, Tract, or System	Effect of Sympathetic Stimulation	Effect of Parasympathetic Stimulation
Urinary tract	Vasoconstriction of renal vessels slows urine formation; internal sphincter of male bladder contracted to prevent retrograde ejaculation and maintain urinary continence	Inhibits contraction of internal sphincter of bladder in males; contracts detrusor muscle of the bladder wall causing urination
Genital system	Causes ejaculation and vasoconstriction resulting in remission of erection	Produces engorgement (erection) of erectile tissues of the external genitals
Rectum	Maintains tonus of internal anal sphincter; inhibits peristalsis of rectum	Rectal contraction (peristalsis) for defecation; inhibition of contraction of internal anal sphincter

The parasympathetic system is restricted in its distribution to the head, neck, and body cavities (except for erectile tissues of genitalia); otherwise, parasympathetic fibers are never found in the body wall and limbs. Sympathetic fibers, by comparison, are distributed to all vascularized portions of the body.

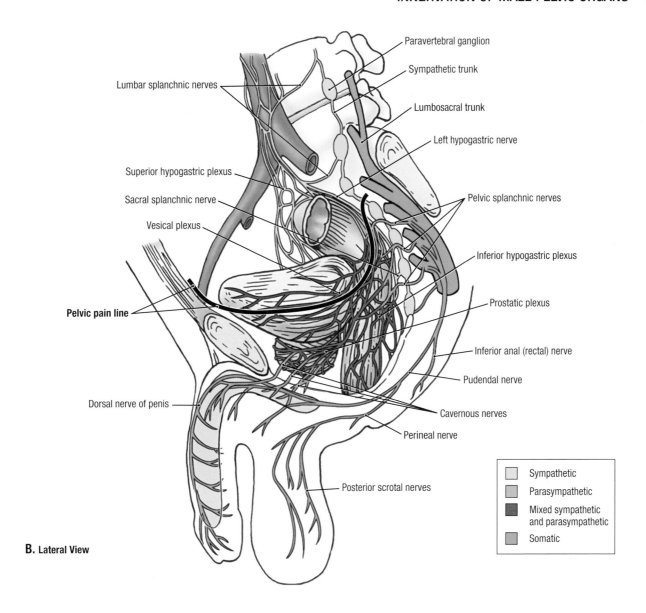

B. Lateral View

- Paravertebral ganglion
- Sympathetic trunk
- Lumbosacral trunk
- Left hypogastric nerve
- Pelvic splanchnic nerves
- Inferior hypogastric plexus
- Prostatic plexus
- Inferior anal (rectal) nerve
- Pudendal nerve
- Cavernous nerves
- Perineal nerve
- Posterior scrotal nerves

Lumbar splanchnic nerves
Superior hypogastric plexus
Sacral splanchnic nerve
Vesical plexus
Pelvic pain line
Dorsal nerve of penis

Legend:
- Sympathetic
- Parasympathetic
- Mixed sympathetic and parasympathetic
- Somatic

3.32   INNERVATION OF MALE PELVIS AND PERINEUM *(CONTINUED)*

A. Overview. **B.** Innervation of prostate and external genitalia.

- The primary function of the sacral sympathetic trunks is to provide post-synaptic fibers to the sacral plexus for sympathetic innervation of the lower limb.
- The peri-arterial plexuses of the ovarian, superior rectal, and internal iliac arteries are minor routes by which sympathetic fibers enter the pelvis. Their primary function is vasomotion of the arteries they accompany.
- The hypogastric plexuses (superior and inferior) are networks of sympathetic and visceral afferent nerve fibers.
- The superior hypogastric plexus carries fibers conveyed to and from the aortic (intermesenteric) plexus by the L3 and L4 splanchnic nerves. The superior hypogastric plexus divides into right and left hypogastric nerves that merge with the parasympathetic pelvic splanchnic nerves to form the inferior hypogastric plexuses.

- The fibers of the inferior hypogastric plexuses continue to the pelvic viscera upon which they form pelvic plexuses, e.g., prostatic nerve plexus.
- The pelvic splanchnic nerves convey presynaptic parasympathetic fibers from the S2–S4 spinal cord segments, which make up the sacral outflow of the parasympathetic system.
- Visceral afferents conveying unconscious reflex sensation follow the course of the parasympathetic fibers retrogradely to the spinal sensory ganglia of S2–S4, as do those transmitting pain sensations from the viscera inferior to the pelvic pain line (structures that do not contact the peritoneum plus the distal sigmoid colon and rectum). Visceral afferent fibers conducting pain from structures superior to the pelvic pain line (structures in contact with the peritoneum, except for the distal sigmoid colon and rectum) follow the sympathetic fibers retrogradely to inferior thoracic and superior lumbar spinal ganglia.

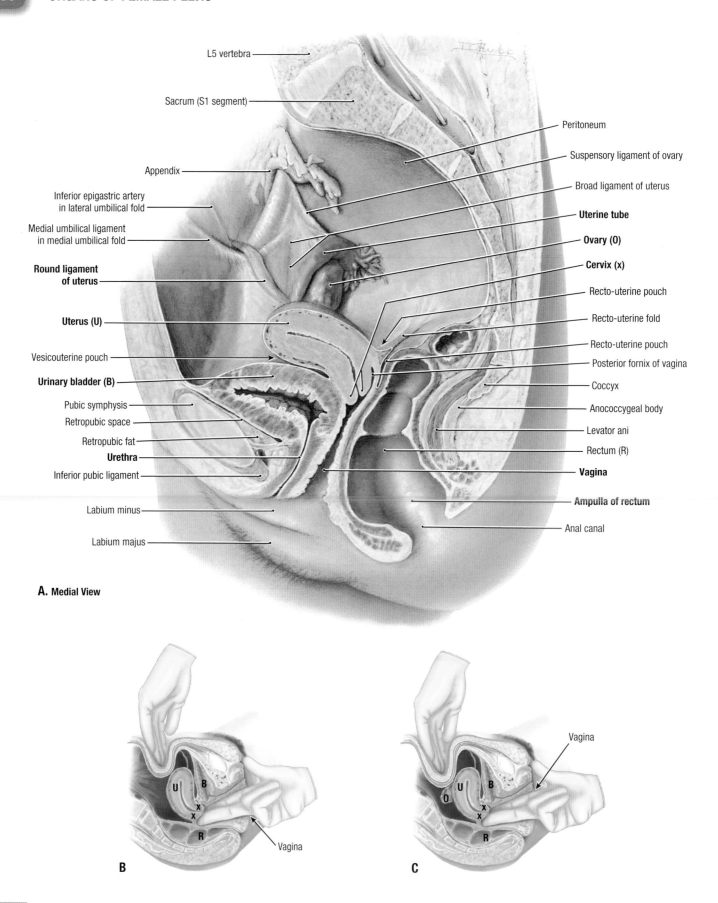

L5 vertebra

Sacrum (S1 segment)

Appendix

Inferior epigastric artery
in lateral umbilical fold

Medial umbilical ligament
in medial umbilical fold

**Round ligament
of uterus**

Uterus (U)

Vesicouterine pouch

Urinary bladder (B)

Pubic symphysis

Retropubic space

Retropubic fat

Urethra

Inferior pubic ligament

Labium minus

Labium majus

Peritoneum

Suspensory ligament of ovary

Broad ligament of uterus

Uterine tube

Ovary (O)

Cervix (x)

Recto-uterine pouch

Recto-uterine fold

Recto-uterine pouch

Posterior fornix of vagina

Coccyx

Anococcygeal body

Levator ani

Rectum (R)

Vagina

Ampulla of rectum

Anal canal

A. Medial View

B

Vagina

C

Vagina

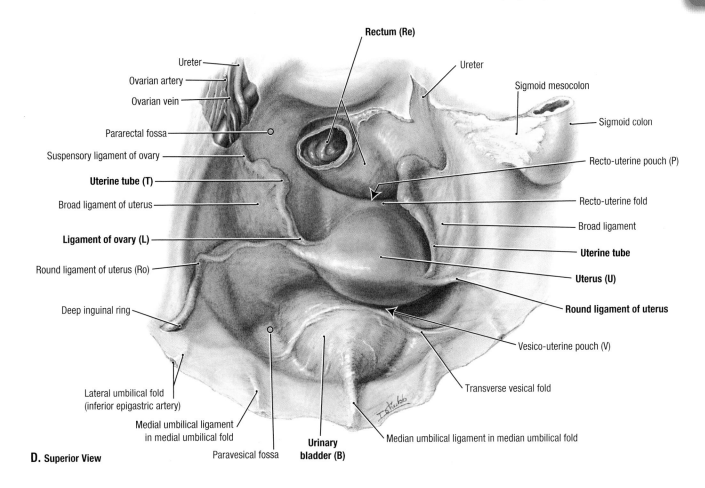

Rectum (Re)

Ureter

Ovarian artery

Ovarian vein

Pararectal fossa

Suspensory ligament of ovary

Uterine tube (T)

Broad ligament of uterus

Ligament of ovary (L)

Round ligament of uterus (Ro)

Deep inguinal ring

Lateral umbilical fold
(inferior epigastric artery)

Medial umbilical ligament
in medial umbilical fold

D. Superior View

Paravesical fossa

**Urinary
bladder (B)**

Median umbilical ligament in median umbilical fold

Transverse vesical fold

Vesico-uterine pouch (V)

Round ligament of uterus

Uterus (U)

Uterine tube

Broad ligament

Recto-uterine fold

Recto-uterine pouch (P)

Sigmoid colon

Sigmoid mesocolon

Ureter

Ovary
(not seen in A
as it lies on the
posterior aspect
of the broad ligament)

E. Laparoscopic View of Normal Female Pelvis

| 3.33 | **FEMALE PELVIC ORGANS IN SITU** *(CONTINUED)* |

A. Median section. The adult uterus is typically *anteverted* (tipped antereosuperiorly relative to the axis of the vagina) and *anteflexed* (flexed or bent anteriorly relative to the cervix, creating the *angle of flexion*) so that its mass lies over the bladder. The cervix, opening on the anterior wall of the vagina, has a short, round, anterior lip and a long, thin, posterior lip. **B. Bimanual palpation of uterus. C. Bimanual palpation of uterine adnexa** (e.g., ovaries). **D.** True pelvis with peritoneum intact, viewed from above. The uterus is usually asymmetrically placed. The round ligament of the female takes the same subperitoneal course as the ductus deferens of the male.

E. Laparoscopy involves inserting a laparoscope into the peritoneal cavity through a small incision below the umbilicus. Insufflation of inert gas creates a pneumoperitoneum to provide space to visualize the pelvic organs. Additional openings (ports) can be made to introduce other instruments for manipulation or to enable therapeutic procedures (e.g., ligation of the uterine tubes).

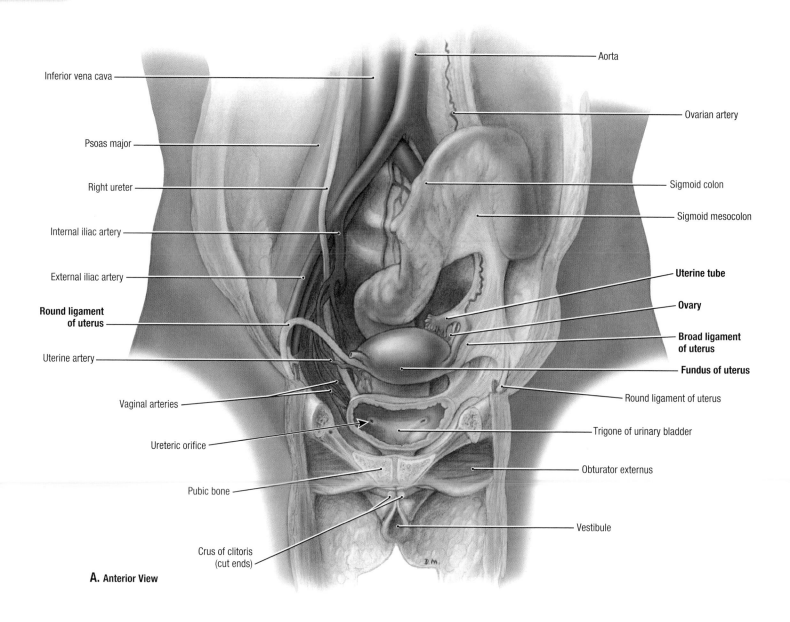

Inferior vena cava

Psoas major

Right ureter

Internal iliac artery

External iliac artery

Round ligament of uterus

Uterine artery

Vaginal arteries

Ureteric orifice

Pubic bone

Crus of clitoris (cut ends)

Aorta

Ovarian artery

Sigmoid colon

Sigmoid mesocolon

Uterine tube

Ovary

Broad ligament of uterus

Fundus of uterus

Round ligament of uterus

Trigone of urinary bladder

Obturator externus

Vestibule

A. Anterior View

3.34   FEMALE GENITAL ORGANS

A. Dissection. Part of the pubic bones, the anterior aspect of the bladder, and—on the specimen's right side—the uterine tube, ovary, broad ligament, and peritoneum covering the lateral wall of the pelvis have been removed. **B. Lifetime changes in uterine size and proportion** (body to cervical ratio, e.g., 2:1). All these stages represent normal anatomy for the particular age and reproductive status of the woman.

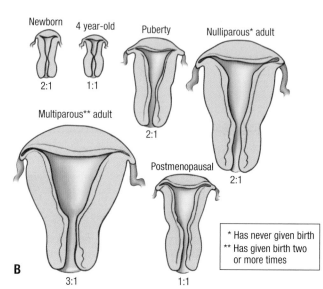

Newborn   4 year-old   Puberty   Nulliparous* adult

2:1   1:1   2:1

Multiparous** adult

Postmenopausal

2:1

3:1   1:1

B

* Has never given birth
** Has given birth two or more times

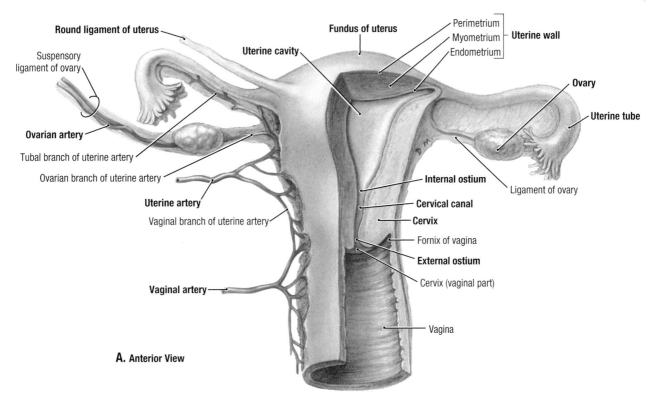

Round ligament of uterus

Suspensory ligament of ovary

Ovarian artery

Tubal branch of uterine artery

Ovarian branch of uterine artery

Uterine artery

Vaginal branch of uterine artery

Vaginal artery

Fundus of uterus

Uterine cavity

Perimetrium
Myometrium — Uterine wall
Endometrium

Ovary

Uterine tube

Internal ostium

Ligament of ovary

Cervical canal

Cervix

Fornix of vagina

External ostium

Cervix (vaginal part)

Vagina

A. Anterior View

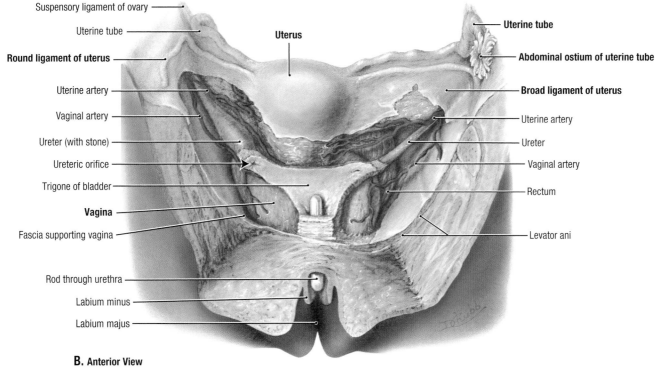

Suspensory ligament of ovary

Uterine tube

Round ligament of uterus

Uterine artery

Vaginal artery

Ureter (with stone)

Ureteric orifice

Trigone of bladder

Vagina

Fascia supporting vagina

Rod through urethra

Labium minus

Labium majus

Uterus

Uterine tube

Abdominal ostium of uterine tube

Broad ligament of uterus

Uterine artery

Ureter

Vaginal artery

Rectum

Levator ani

B. Anterior View

3.35 UTERUS AND ITS ADNEXA

A. Blood supply. On the specimen's left side, part of the uterine wall with the round ligament and the vaginal wall have been cut away to expose the cervix, uterine cavity, and thick muscular wall of the uterus, the myometrium. On the specimen's right side, the ovarian artery (from the aorta) and uterine artery (from the internal iliac) supply the ovary, uterine tube, and uterus and anastomose in the broad ligament along the lateral aspect of the uterus. The uterine artery sends a uterine branch to supply the uterine body and fundus and a vaginal branch to supply the cervix and vagina. **B.** Uterus and broad ligament. The pubic bones and bladder, trigone excepted, are removed, as a continued dissection from Figure 3.34.

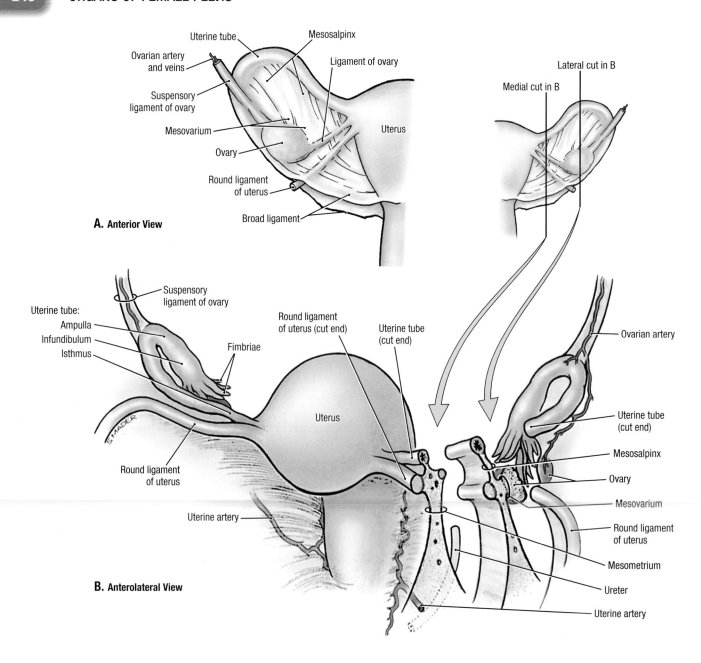

A. Anterior View

B. Anterolateral View

3.36 UTERUS AND BROAD LIGAMENT

A. and B. Two paramedian sections show "mesenteries" with the prefix meso-. "Salpinx" is the Greek word for trumpet or tube, "metro" for uterus. The mesentery of the uterus and uterine tube is called the broad ligament. The major part of the broad ligament, the *mesometrium*, is attached to the uterus. The ovary is attached to the broad ligament by a mesentery of its own, called the *mesovarium*; to the uterus by the ligament of the ovary; and near the pelvic brim, by the suspensory ligament of the ovary containing the ovarian vessels. The part of the broad ligament superior to the level of the mesovarium is called the *mesosalpinx*. **C. Hysterectomy** (excision of the uterus) is performed through the lower anterior abdominal wall or through the vagina. Because the uterine artery crosses superior to the ureter near the lateral fornix of the vagina, the ureter is in danger of being inadvertently clamped or severed when the uterine artery is tied off during a hysterectomy.

C. Medial View

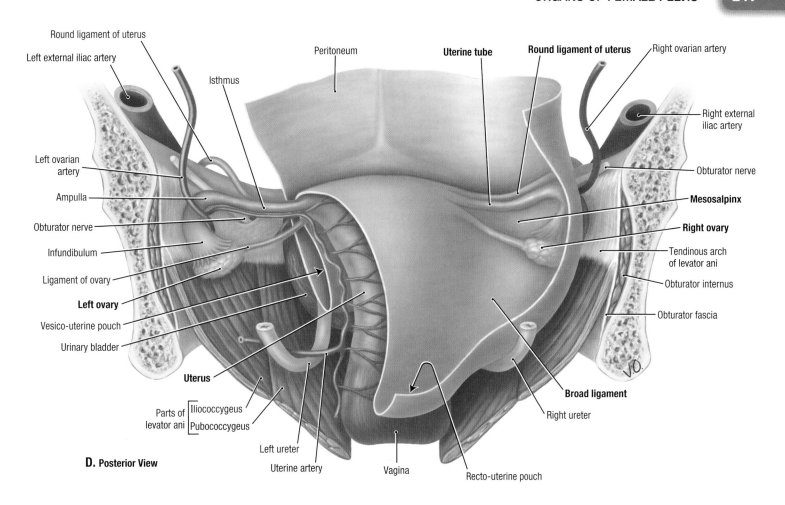

Round ligament of uterus

Left external iliac artery

Isthmus

Peritoneum

Uterine tube

Round ligament of uterus

Right ovarian artery

Right external iliac artery

Left ovarian artery

Ampulla

Obturator nerve

Infundibulum

Ligament of ovary

Left ovary

Vesico-uterine pouch

Urinary bladder

Obturator nerve

Mesosalpinx

Right ovary

Tendinous arch of levator ani

Obturator internus

Obturator fascia

Uterus

Parts of levator ani { Iliococcygeus / Pubococcygeus }

Left ureter

Uterine artery

Vagina

Recto-uterine pouch

Broad ligament

Right ureter

D. Posterior View

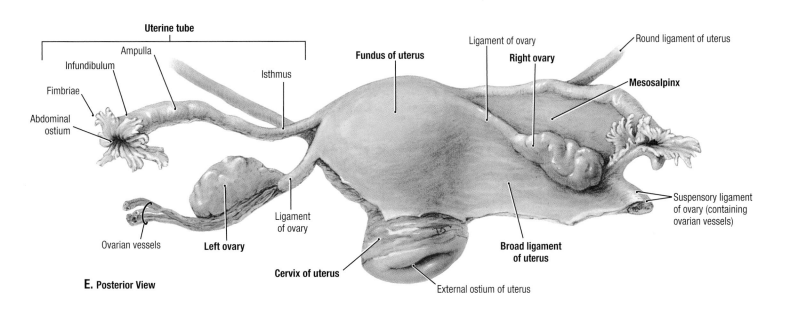

Uterine tube

Ampulla

Infundibulum

Fimbriae

Abdominal ostium

Isthmus

Fundus of uterus

Ligament of ovary

Right ovary

Round ligament of uterus

Mesosalpinx

Ovarian vessels

Left ovary

Ligament of ovary

Cervix of uterus

External ostium of uterus

Broad ligament of uterus

Suspensory ligament of ovary (containing ovarian vessels)

E. Posterior View

3.36   **UTERUS AND BROAD LIGAMENT** *(CONTINUED)*

D. Uterus in situ. **E.** Uterus and adnexa, removed from cadaver.

Small intestine

Falciform ligament

Fundus of uterus

Placenta

Chorionic lamina with blood vessels

Umbilicus (maternal)

Umbilical cord (with umbilical arteries and vein)

Peritoneum

Perimetrium ⎤
            ⎥ of uterus
Myometrium ⎦

Linea alba

Median umbilical ligament

Cervix of uterus

Vesico-uterine pouch

Pubic symphysis

Urinary bladder

Vagina

Urethra

Amniotic cavity (filled with amniotic fluid)

Recto-uterine pouch

of cervical canal ⎡ Internal os
           ⎢ Mucus plug
           ⎣ External os

Coccyx

Rectal ampulla

Perineal body

A

3.37 **PREGNANT UTERUS**

A. Median section; fetus is intact.

B. Anteroposterior View

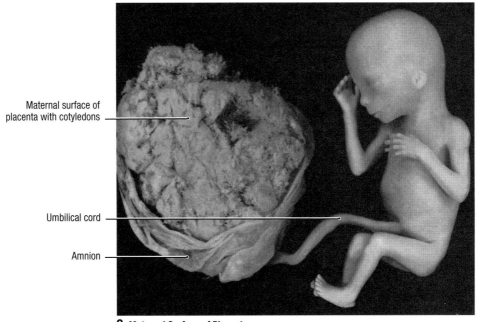

Maternal surface of
placenta with cotyledons

Umbilical cord

Amnion

C. Maternal Surface of Placenta

| 3.37 | **PREGNANT UTERUS** *(CONTINUED)* |

B. Radiograph of fetus. **C.** Photograph of an 18-week-old fetus connected to the placenta by the umbilical cord.

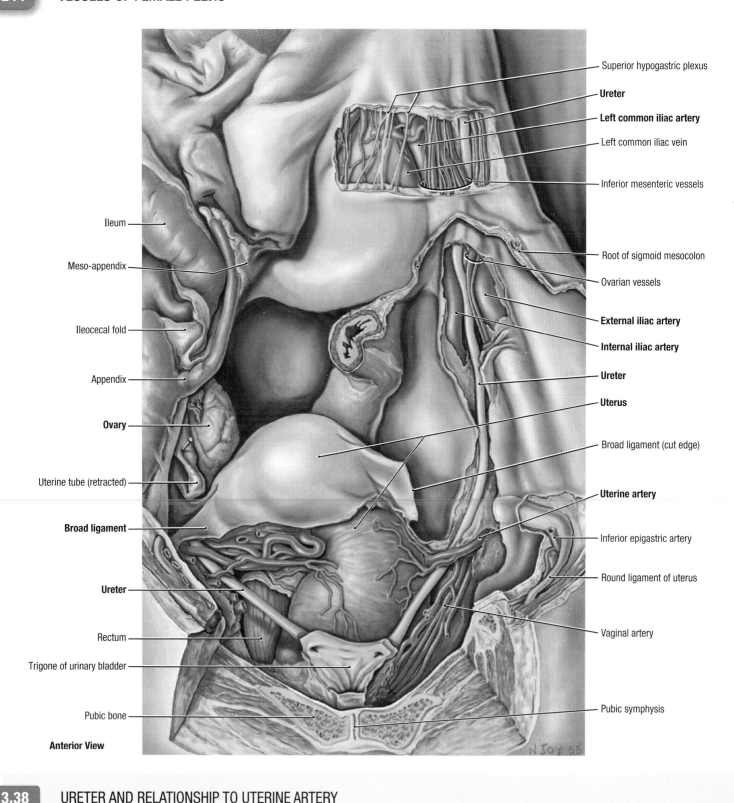

Superior hypogastric plexus

Ureter

Left common iliac artery

Left common iliac vein

Inferior mesenteric vessels

Ileum

Meso-appendix

Root of sigmoid mesocolon

Ovarian vessels

Ileocecal fold

External iliac artery

Internal iliac artery

Appendix

Ureter

Ovary

Uterus

Broad ligament (cut edge)

Uterine tube (retracted)

Uterine artery

Broad ligament

Inferior epigastric artery

Round ligament of uterus

Ureter

Rectum

Vaginal artery

Trigone of urinary bladder

Pubic bone

Pubic symphysis

Anterior View

N JOY 55

| **3.38** | URETER AND RELATIONSHIP TO UTERINE ARTERY |

- Most of the pubic symphysis and most of the bladder (except the trigone) have been removed as in Figure 3.34B.
- The left ureter is crossed by the ovarian vessels and nerves; the apex of the inverted V-shaped root of the sigmoid mesocolon is situated anterior to the left ureter.
- The left ureter crosses the external iliac artery at the bifurcation of the common iliac artery and then descends anterior to the internal iliac artery;

its course is subperitoneal from where it enters the pelvis to where it passes deep to the broad ligament and is crossed by the uterine artery. **Injury of the ureter** may occur in this region when the uterine artery is ligated and cut during hysterectomy.

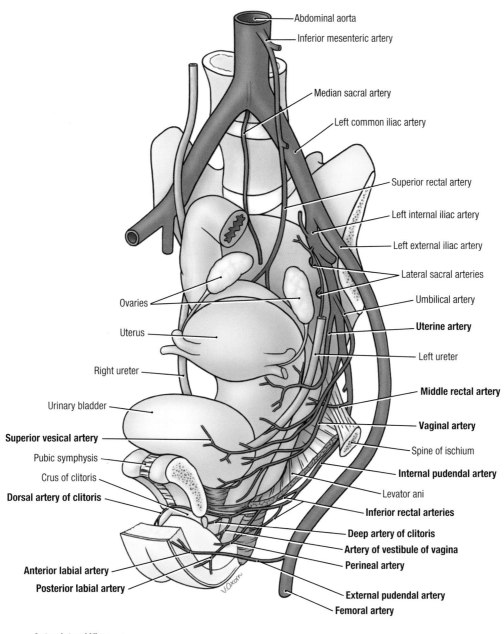

Abdominal aorta

Inferior mesenteric artery

Median sacral artery

Left common iliac artery

Superior rectal artery

Left internal iliac artery

Left external iliac artery

Lateral sacral arteries

Umbilical artery

Uterine artery

Left ureter

Middle rectal artery

Vaginal artery

Spine of ischium

Internal pudendal artery

Levator ani

Inferior rectal arteries

Deep artery of clitoris

Artery of vestibule of vagina

Perineal artery

External pudendal artery

Femoral artery

Ovaries

Uterus

Right ureter

Urinary bladder

Superior vesical artery

Pubic symphysis

Crus of clitoris

Dorsal artery of clitoris

Anterior labial artery

Posterior labial artery

Anterolateral View

3.39   ARTERIAL SUPPLY OF FEMALE PELVIS AND PERINEUM

- The blood supply of the uterus is mainly from the *uterine arteries*, with potential collateral supply from the ovarian arteries.
- The arteries supplying the superior part of the vagina derive from the *uterine arteries*; the arteries supplying the middle and inferior parts of the vagina derive from the *vaginal* and *internal pudendal arteries*.
- The superior vesical arteries supply the anterosuperior parts of the bladder; the vaginal arteries supply the postero-inferior parts of the bladder.

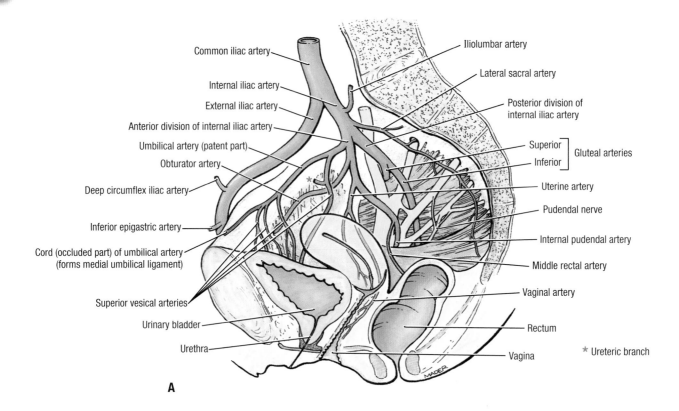

Common iliac artery

Internal iliac artery

External iliac artery

Anterior division of internal iliac artery

Umbilical artery (patent part)

Obturator artery

Deep circumflex iliac artery

Inferior epigastric artery

Cord (occluded part) of umbilical artery
(forms medial umbilical ligament)

Superior vesical arteries

Urinary bladder

Urethra

Iliolumbar artery

Lateral sacral artery

Posterior division of
internal iliac artery

Superior ⎤
          ⎥ Gluteal arteries
Inferior ⎦

Uterine artery

Pudendal nerve

Internal pudendal artery

Middle rectal artery

Vaginal artery

Rectum

Vagina

* Ureteric branch

A

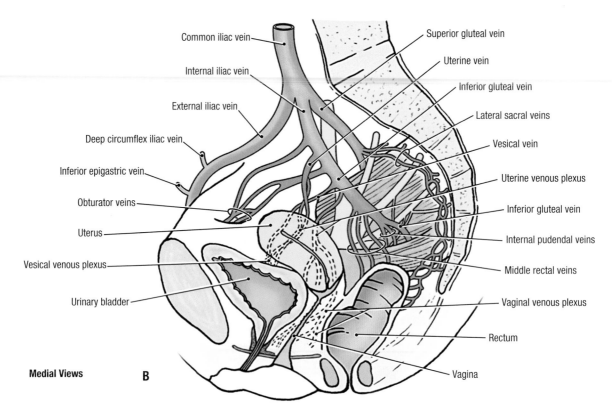

Common iliac vein

Internal iliac vein

External iliac vein

Deep circumflex iliac vein

Inferior epigastric vein

Obturator veins

Uterus

Vesical venous plexus

Urinary bladder

Superior gluteal vein

Uterine vein

Inferior gluteal vein

Lateral sacral veins

Vesical vein

Uterine venous plexus

Inferior gluteal vein

Internal pudendal veins

Middle rectal veins

Vaginal venous plexus

Rectum

Vagina

Medial Views   **B**

| 3.40 | ARTERIES AND VEINS OF FEMALE PELVIS |

A. Arteries in situ. **B.** Pelvic veins and venous plexuses. **C.** Arteries isolated from **A**.

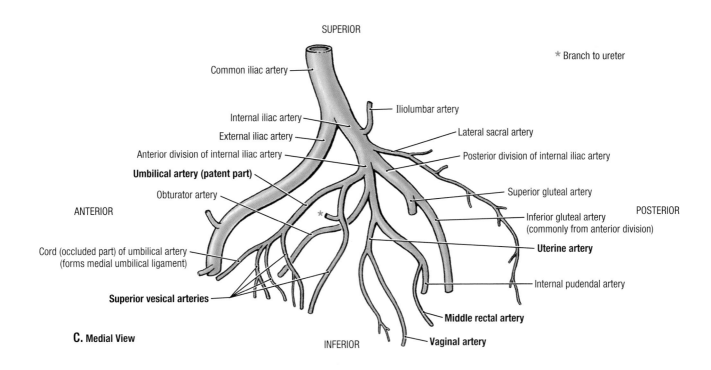

SUPERIOR

Common iliac artery

* Branch to ureter

Iliolumbar artery

Internal iliac artery

External iliac artery

Lateral sacral artery

Anterior division of internal iliac artery

Posterior division of internal iliac artery

Umbilical artery (patent part)

Superior gluteal artery

Obturator artery

ANTERIOR

POSTERIOR

Inferior gluteal artery
(commonly from anterior division)

Uterine artery

Cord (occluded part) of umbilical artery
(forms medial umbilical ligament)

Internal pudendal artery

Superior vesical arteries

Middle rectal artery

C. Medial View

INFERIOR **Vaginal artery**

3.40   ARTERIES AND VEINS OF FEMALE PELVIS *(CONTINUED)*

TABLE 3.7 *ARTERIES OF FEMALE PELVIS*

Artery	Origin	Course	Distribution
Internal iliac	Common iliac artery	Passes over pelvic brim and descends into pelvic cavity	Main blood supply to pelvic organs, gluteal muscles, and perineum
Anterior division of internal iliac artery	Internal iliac artery	Passes anteriorly along lateral wall of pelvis, dividing into visceral, obturator, and internal iliac arteries	Pelvic viscera and muscles of superior medial thigh and perineum
Umbilical	Anterior division of internal iliac artery	Short pelvic course, gives off superior vesical arteries	Superior aspect of urinary bladder
Superior vesical artery	Patent proximal part of umbilical artery	Usually multiple, pass to superior aspect of urinary bladder	Superior aspect of urinary bladder
Obturator		Runs antero-inferiorly on lateral pelvic wall	Pelvic muscles, nutrient artery to ilium, head of femur, and muscles of medial compartment of thigh
Uterine		Runs anteromedially in base of broad ligament/superior cardinal ligament; gives rise to vaginal branch, then crosses ureter superiorly to reach lateral aspect of uterine cervix	Uterus, ligaments of uterus, medial parts of uterine tube and ovary, and superior vagina
Vaginal	Anterior division of internal iliac artery	Divides into vaginal and inferior vesical branches	Vaginal branch: lower vagina, vestibular bulb, and adjacent rectum; inferior vesical branch: fundus of urinary bladder
Middle rectal		Descends in pelvis to inferior part of rectum	Inferior part of rectum
Internal pudendal		Exits pelvis via greater sciatic foramen and enters perineum (ischio-anal fossa) via lesser sciatic foramen	Main artery to perineum including muscles of anal canal and perineum, skin and urogenital triangle and erectile bodies
Posterior division of internal iliac artery	Internal iliac artery	Passes posteriorly and gives rise to parietal branches	Pelvic wall and gluteal region
Iliolumbar	Posterior division of internal iliac artery	Ascends anterior to sacro-iliac joint and posterior to common iliac vessels and psoas major	Iliacus, psoas major, quadratus lumborum muscles, and cauda equina in vertebral canal
Lateral sacral (superior and inferior)		Run on anteromedial aspect of piriformis	Piriformis muscle, structures in sacral canal, and erector spinae muscles
Ovarian	Abdominal aorta	Crosses pelvic brim and descends in suspensory ligament to ovary	Abdominal and/or pelvic ureter, ovary, and ampullary end of uterine tube

Lumbar (caval/aortic)
Inferior mesenteric
Common iliac
Internal iliac
External iliac
Superficial inguinal
Deep inguinal
Sacral
→ Direction of flow

A. Inferior mesenteric artery
Abdominal aorta
Left ovarian artery
Left common iliac artery
Left internal iliac artery
Left external iliac artery
Left ureter
Left femoral artery
Urinary bladder
Urethra

Anterior Views

B. Uterine tube and ovary
Uterus
Vagina

C. Clitoris
Vaginal orifice
Labium minus

3.41   LYMPHATIC DRAINAGE OF FEMALE PELVIS AND PERINEUM

A. Pelvic urinary system. **B.** Internal genital organs. **C.** Vulva. **D.** Zones of pelvis and perineum initially draining into specific groups of lymph nodes.

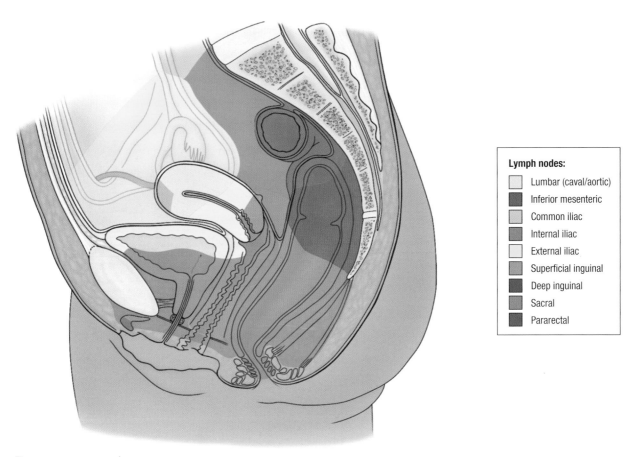

Lymph nodes:

☐ Lumbar (caval/aortic)

■ Inferior mesenteric

☐ Common iliac

■ Internal iliac

☐ External iliac

■ Superficial inguinal

■ Deep inguinal

■ Sacral

■ Pararectal

D

3.41   *LYMPHATIC DRAINAGE OF FEMALE PELVIS AND PERINEUM (CONTINUED)*

TABLE 3.8 LYMPHATIC DRAINAGE OF STRUCTURES OF FEMALE PELVIS AND PERINEUM

Lymph Node Group	Structures Typically Draining to Lymph Node Group
Lumbar	Gonads and associated structures (along ovarian vessels), ovary, uterine tube (except isthmus and intra-uterine parts), fundus of uterus, common iliac nodes
Inferior mesenteric	Superiormost rectum, sigmoid colon, descending colon, pararectal nodes
Common iliac	External and internal iliac lymph nodes
Internal iliac	Inferior pelvic structures, deep perineal structures, sacral nodes, base of bladder, inferior pelvic ureter, anal canal (above pectinate line), inferior rectum, middle and upper vagina, cervix, body of uterus, sacral nodes
External iliac	Anterosuperior pelvic structures, deep inguinal nodes, superior bladder, superior pelvic ureter, upper vagina, cervix, lower body of uterus
Superficial inguinal	Lower limb, superficial drainage of inferolateral quadrant of trunk, including anterior abdominal wall inferior to umbilicus, gluteal region, superolateral uterus (near attachment of round ligament), skin of perineum including vulva, ostium of vagina (inferior to hymen), prepuce of clitoris, peri-anal skin, anal canal inferior to pectinate line
Deep inguinal	Glans of clitoris, superficial inguinal nodes
Sacral	Postero-inferior pelvic structures, inferior rectum, inferior vagina
Pararectal	Superior rectum

3.42 INNERVATION OF FEMALE PELVIC VISCERA

- Pelvic splanchnic nerves (S2–S4) supply parasympathetic motor fibers to the uterus and vagina (and vasodilator fibers to the erectile tissue of the clitoris and bulb of the vestibule; not shown).
- Presynaptic sympathetic fibers pass through the lumbar splanchnic nerves to synapse in prevertebral ganglia; the postsynaptic fibers travel through the superior and inferior hypogastric plexuses to reach the pelvic viscera.
- Visceral afferent fibers conducting pain from intraperitoneal viscera travel with the sympathetic fibers to the T12–L2 spinal ganglia. Visceral afferent fibers conducting pain from subperitoneal viscera travel with parasympathetic fibers to the S2–S4 spinal ganglia.
- Somatic sensation from the opening of the vagina also passes to the S2–S4 spinal ganglia via the pudendal nerve.
- Muscular contractions of the uterus are hormonally induced.

Innervation:
- · · · · Presynaptic sympathetic
- ——— Postsynaptic sympathetic
- · · · · Presynaptic parasympathetic
- ——— Postsynaptic parasympathetic
- ——— Visceral afferent running with sympathetic and parasympathetic fibers
- ——— Somatic sensory
- ——— Somatic motor

Spinal cord

Spinal ganglion

T12
L1
L2
L3
L4
L5
S1
S2
S3
S4
S5

Upper lumbar sympathetic trunk

Lumbar splanchnic nerves

Spinal ganglia

Pelvic splanchnic nerves

Pelvic plexus

Sacral plexus

Prevertebal (sympathetic) ganglia

Para-aortic plexus

Peri-arterial plexus of ovarian artery

Superior hypogastric plexus

Inferior hypogastric plexuses

Uterine plexus

Pudendal nerve

Ovarian plexus

Pelvic intra-peritoneal viscera

Pelvic plexus

Lower limit of peritoneum (pelvic pain line)

Uterovaginal plexus

Cervix

Pelvic sub-peritoneal viscera

Pelvic plexus

Vagina

Pudendal nerve

Perineum

Enteric (parasympathetic) ganglion

Anterior View

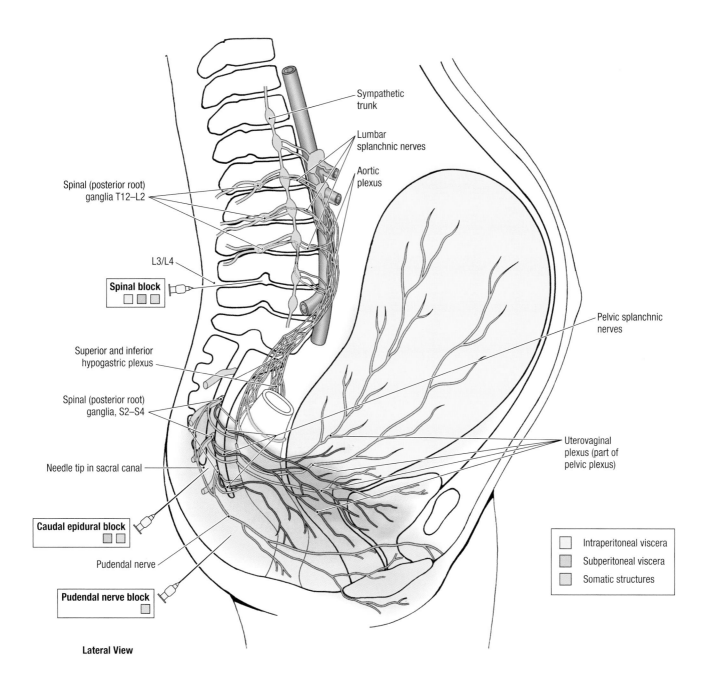

Sympathetic trunk

Lumbar splanchnic nerves

Aortic plexus

Spinal (posterior root) ganglia T12–L2

L3/L4

Spinal block

Superior and inferior hypogastric plexus

Spinal (posterior root) ganglia, S2–S4

Needle tip in sacral canal

Caudal epidural block

Pudendal nerve

Pudendal nerve block

Lateral View

Pelvic splanchnic nerves

Uterovaginal plexus (part of pelvic plexus)

- [ ] Intraperitoneal viscera
- [ ] Subperitoneal viscera
- [ ] Somatic structures

3.43 INNERVATION OF PELVIC VISCERA DURING PREGNANCY; NERVE BLOCKS

- A **spinal block**, in which the anesthetic agent is introduced with a needle into the spinal subarachnoid space at the L3–L4 vertebral level produces complete anesthesia inferior to approximately the waist level. The perineum, pelvic floor, and birth canal are anesthetized, and motor and sensory functions of the entire lower limbs, as well as sensation of uterine contractions, are temporarily eliminated.
- With the **caudal epidural block**, the anesthetic agent is administered using an in-dwelling catheter in the sacral canal. The entire birth canal, pelvic floor, and most of the perineum are anesthetized, but the lower limbs are not usually affected. The mother is aware of her uterine contractions.
- A **pudendal nerve block** is a peripheral nerve block that provides local anesthesia over the S2–S4 dermatomes (most of the perineum) and the inferior quarter of the vagina. It does not block pain from the superior birth canal (uterine cervix and superior vagina), so the mother is able to feel uterine contractions.

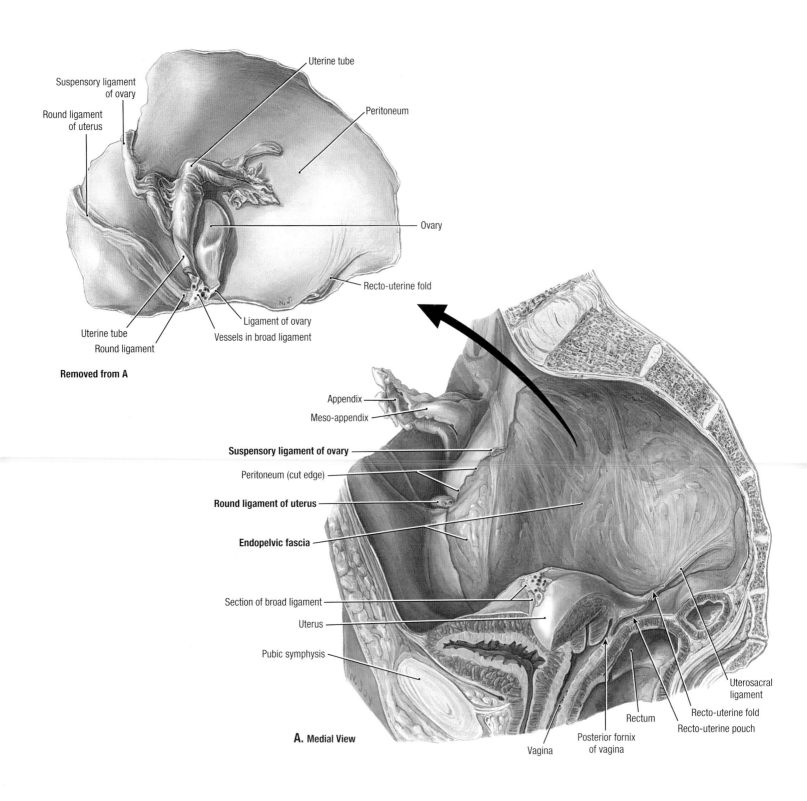

Suspensory ligament of ovary

Round ligament of uterus

Uterine tube

Peritoneum

Ovary

Recto-uterine fold

Uterine tube

Round ligament

Ligament of ovary

Vessels in broad ligament

Removed from A

Appendix

Meso-appendix

Suspensory ligament of ovary

Peritoneum (cut edge)

Round ligament of uterus

Endopelvic fascia

Section of broad ligament

Uterus

Pubic symphysis

Uterosacral ligament

Recto-uterine fold

Recto-uterine pouch

Rectum

Posterior fornix of vagina

Vagina

A. Medial View

3.44   SERIAL DISSECTION OF AUTONOMIC NERVES OF FEMALE PELVIS

A. Broad ligament and peritoneum of the lateral wall of the pelvic cavity have been removed to expose the endopelvic fascia.

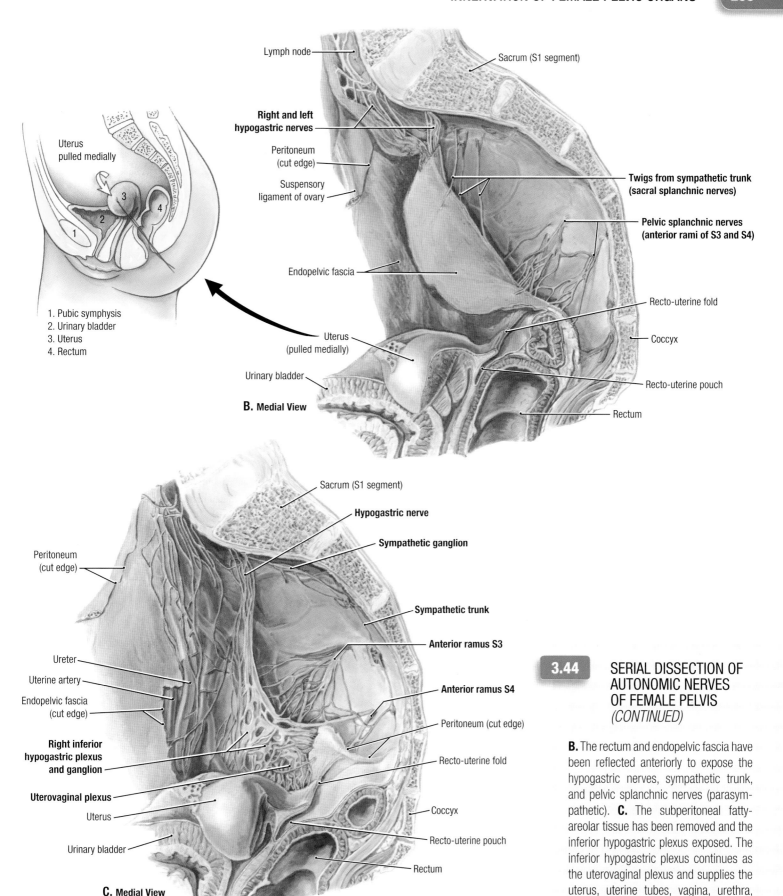

Uterus
pulled medially

1. Pubic symphysis
2. Urinary bladder
3. Uterus
4. Rectum

Lymph node

Sacrum (S1 segment)

**Right and left
hypogastric nerves**

Peritoneum
(cut edge)

**Twigs from sympathetic trunk
(sacral splanchnic nerves)**

Suspensory
ligament of ovary

**Pelvic splanchnic nerves
(anterior rami of S3 and S4)**

Endopelvic fascia

Recto-uterine fold

Coccyx

Uterus
(pulled medially)

Recto-uterine pouch

Urinary bladder

Rectum

B. Medial View

Sacrum (S1 segment)

Hypogastric nerve

Sympathetic ganglion

Peritoneum
(cut edge)

Sympathetic trunk

Anterior ramus S3

Ureter

Uterine artery

Anterior ramus S4

Endopelvic fascia
(cut edge)

Peritoneum (cut edge)

**Right inferior
hypogastric plexus
and ganglion**

Recto-uterine fold

Uterovaginal plexus

Uterus

Coccyx

Urinary bladder

Recto-uterine pouch

Rectum

C. Medial View

3.44

**SERIAL DISSECTION OF
AUTONOMIC NERVES
OF FEMALE PELVIS**
(CONTINUED)

B. The rectum and endopelvic fascia have
been reflected anteriorly to expose the
hypogastric nerves, sympathetic trunk,
and pelvic splanchnic nerves (parasympathetic). **C.** The subperitoneal fatty-
areolar tissue has been removed and the
inferior hypogastric plexus exposed. The
inferior hypogastric plexus continues as
the uterovaginal plexus and supplies the
uterus, uterine tubes, vagina, urethra,
greater vestibular glands, erectile tissue
of the clitoris, and bulb of the vestibule.

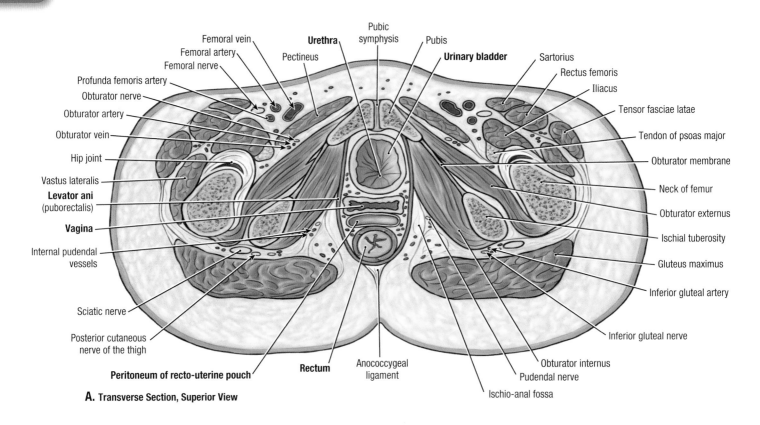

Femoral vein
Femoral artery
Femoral nerve
Pectineus
Pubic symphysis
Urethra
Pubis
Urinary bladder
Sartorius
Rectus femoris
Iliacus
Tensor fasciae latae
Tendon of psoas major
Obturator membrane
Neck of femur
Obturator externus
Ischial tuberosity
Gluteus maximus
Inferior gluteal artery

Profunda femoris artery
Obturator nerve
Obturator artery
Obturator vein
Hip joint
Vastus lateralis
Levator ani (puborectalis)
Vagina
Internal pudendal vessels
Sciatic nerve
Posterior cutaneous nerve of the thigh
Peritoneum of recto-uterine pouch
Rectum
Anococcygeal ligament
Ischio-anal fossa
Pudendal nerve
Obturator internus
Inferior gluteal nerve

A. Transverse Section, Superior View

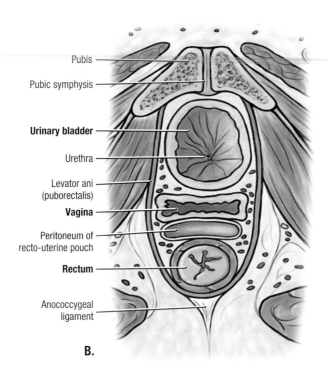

Pubis
Pubic symphysis
Urinary bladder
Urethra
Levator ani (puborectalis)
Vagina
Peritoneum of recto-uterine pouch
Rectum
Anococcygeal ligament

B.

3.45   TRANSVERSE SECTION THROUGH FEMALE PELVIS

A. Transverse section through the ischial tuberosities. **B.** Enlargement of central part of section including the bladder, vagina, rectum, and recto-uterine pouch.

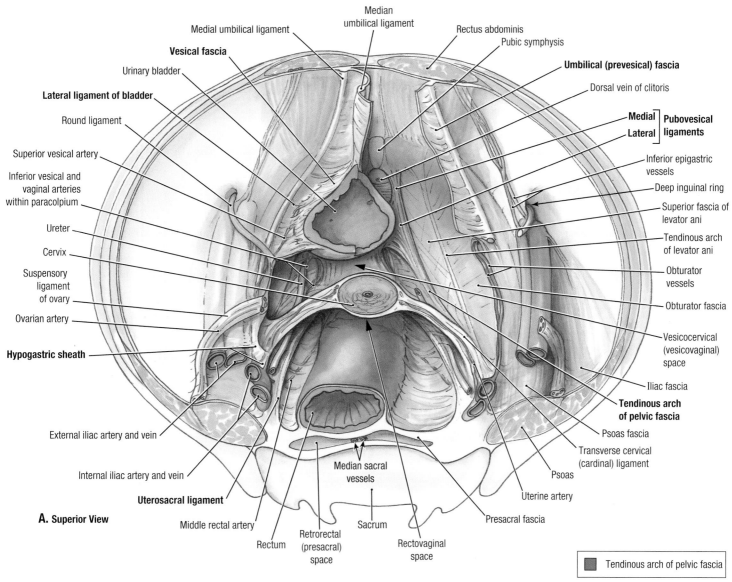

Median umbilical ligament

Medial umbilical ligament

Vesical fascia

Urinary bladder

Lateral ligament of bladder

Round ligament

Superior vesical artery

Inferior vesical and vaginal arteries within paracolpium

Ureter

Cervix

Suspensory ligament of ovary

Ovarian artery

Hypogastric sheath

External iliac artery and vein

Internal iliac artery and vein

Uterosacral ligament

Middle rectal artery

Rectum

Retrorectal (presacral) space

Sacrum

Median sacral vessels

Rectovaginal space

Rectus abdominis

Pubic symphysis

Umbilical (prevesical) fascia

Dorsal vein of clitoris

Medial ⎤ **Pubovesical**
Lateral ⎦ **ligaments**

Inferior epigastric vessels

Deep inguinal ring

Superior fascia of levator ani

Tendinous arch of levator ani

Obturator vessels

Obturator fascia

Vesicocervical (vesicovaginal) space

Iliac fascia

Tendinous arch of pelvic fascia

Psoas fascia

Transverse cervical (cardinal) ligament

Psoas

Uterine artery

Presacral fascia

A. Superior View

3.46 PELVIC FASCIA AND SUPPORTING MECHANISM OF CERVIX AND UPPER VAGINA

A. Greater and lesser pelvis demonstrating pelvic viscera and endopelvic fascia. **B.** Schematic illustration of fascial ligaments and areolar spaces at level of tendinous arch of pelvic fascia.

- Note the parietal pelvic fascia covering the obturator internus and levator ani muscles and the visceral pelvic fascia surrounding the pelvic organs. These membranous fasciae are continuous where the organs penetrate the pelvic floor, forming a tendinous arch of pelvic fascia bilaterally.
- The endopelvic fascia lies between, and is continuous with, both visceral and parietal layers of pelvic fascia. The loose, areolar portions of the endopelvic fascia have been removed; the fibrous, condensed portions remain. Note the condensation of this fascia into the hypogastric sheath, containing the vessels to the pelvic viscera, the ureters, and (in the male) the ductus deferens.
- Observe the ligamentous extensions of the hypogastric sheath: the lateral ligament of the urinary bladder, the transverse cervical ligament at the base of the broad ligament, and a less prominent lamina posteriorly containing the middle rectal vessels.

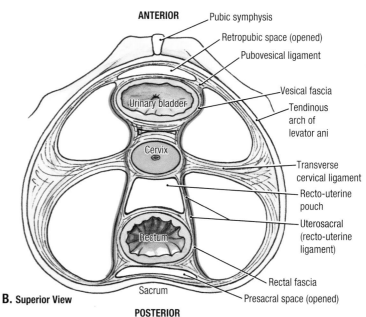

▬ Tendinous arch of pelvic fascia

ANTERIOR

Pubic symphysis

Retropubic space (opened)

Pubovesical ligament

Urinary bladder

Vesical fascia

Tendinous arch of levator ani

Cervix

Transverse cervical ligament

Recto-uterine pouch

Uterosacral (recto-uterine ligament)

Rectum

Rectal fascia

Sacrum

Presacral space (opened)

B. Superior View

POSTERIOR

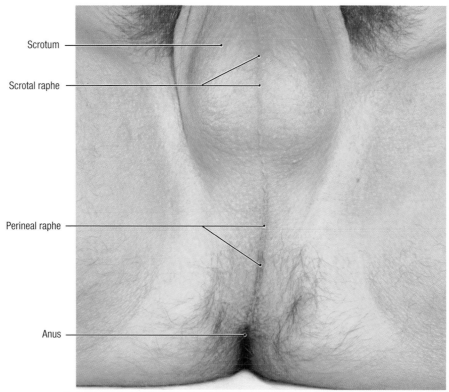

Scrotum

Scrotal raphe

Perineal raphe

Anus

A. Inferior View

Pubic hairs covering pubic region

Root of penis

Body of penis

Corona of glans

Glans penis

Scrotum

Perineal raphe

Anus

B. Inferior View

3.47   SURFACE ANATOMY OF MALE PERINEUM

A. Scrotum and anal region. **B.** Penis, scrotum, and anal region.

Mons pubis

Anterior commissure
of labia majora

Prepuce of clitoris

Labium majus

Labium minus

A. **Anterior View**

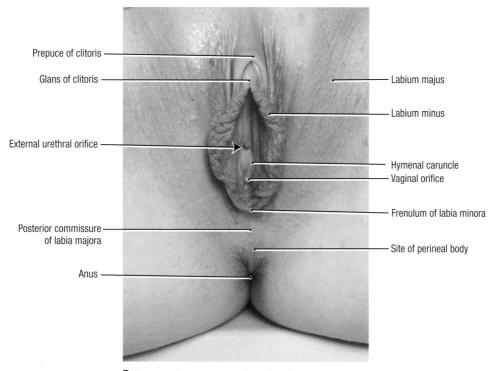

Prepuce of clitoris

Glans of clitoris

Labium majus

Labium minus

External urethral orifice

Hymenal caruncle
Vaginal orifice

Frenulum of labia minora

Posterior commissure
of labia majora

Site of perineal body

Anus

B. **Antero-inferior View (Lithotomy Position)**

3.48   **SURFACE ANATOMY OF THE FEMALE PERINEUM**

A. External genitalia (pudendum; vulva), standing position. **B.** Vestibule of vagina and the external urethral and vaginal orifices opening into it (recumbent position).

A. Inferior View

Urethra
Urogenital hiatus
Vagina
Rectum
Pubococcygeus (1)
Iliococcygeus (2)
Coccygeus (3)

(1 + 2 Levator ani)
(1 + 2 + 3 Pelvic diaphragm)

Male   Female

External urethral sphincter
Compressor urethrae
Bulbo-urethral gland within deep transverse perineal
Urethrovaginal sphincter
Deep transverse perineal
Smooth muscle

B. Inferior View

Dorsal nerve and vessels of penis
Dorsal nerve and vessels of clitoris
Deep perineal vessels covered with perineal membrane

C. Inferior View

| 3.49 | MALE AND FEMALE PERINEAL COMPARTMENTS |

A.–F. Sequential demonstration of structures of the perineal compartments, from deep to superficial. **A.–C.** Deep perineal compartment (superior to perineal membrane). **A.** Pelvic diaphragm. **B.** Muscles of deep perineal compartment. **C.** Deep perineal vessels and nerves, covered by perineal membrane on right side.

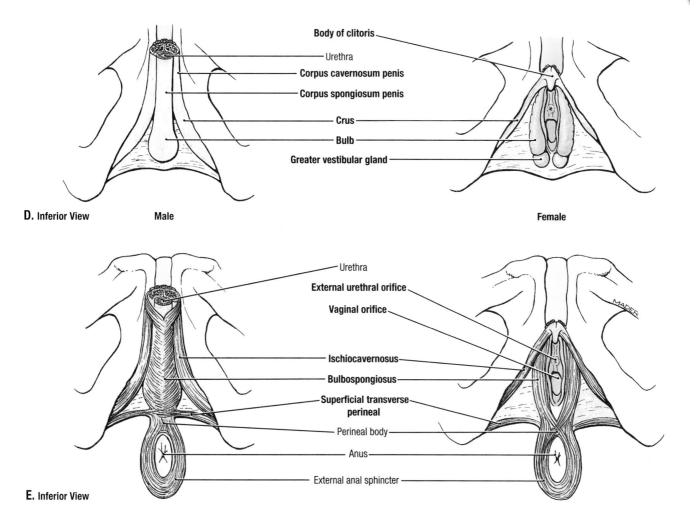

Body of clitoris

Urethra

Corpus cavernosum penis

Corpus spongiosum penis

Crus

Bulb

Greater vestibular gland

D. Inferior View   **Male**   **Female**

Urethra

External urethral orifice

Vaginal orifice

Ischiocavernosus

Bulbospongiosus

**Superficial transverse
perineal**

Perineal body

Anus

External anal sphincter

E. Inferior View

- - Urogenital
triangle

- - Anal triangle

F. Inferior View

3.49   MALE AND FEMALE PERINEAL COMPARTMENTS *(CONTINUED)*

D.–F. Superficial perineal compartment (inferior to perineal membrane). **D.** Erectile bodies. **E.** Muscles of superficial perineal compartment. **F.** Superficial muscles imposed on surface anatomy of perineum.

TABLE 3.9 MUSCLES OF PERINEUM

Muscle	Origin	Course and Insertion	Innervation	Main Action
External anal sphincter	Skin and fascia surrounding anus; coccyx via anococcygeal ligament	Passes around lateral aspects of anal canal; insertion into perineal body	Inferior anal (rectal) nerve, a branch of pudendal nerve (S2–S4)	Constricts anal canal during peristalsis, resisting defecation; supports and fixes perineal body and pelvic floor
Bulbospongiosus	*Male:* median raphe on ventral surface of bulb of penis; perineal body	*Male:* surrounds lateral aspects of bulb of penis and most proximal part of body of penis, inserting into perineal membrane, dorsal aspect of corpora spongiosum and cavernosa, and fascia of bulb of penis		*Male:* supports and fixes perineal body/pelvic floor; compresses bulb of penis to expel last drops of urine/semen; assists erection by compressing outflow via deep perineal vein and by pushing blood from bulb into body of penis
	Female: perineal body	*Female:* passes on each side of lower vagina, enclosing bulb and greater vestibular gland; inserts onto pubic arch and fascia of corpora cavernosa of clitoris	Muscular (deep) branch of perineal nerve, a branch of the pudendal nerve (S2–S4)	*Female:* supports and fixes perineal body/pelvic floor; "sphincter" of vagina; assists in erection of clitoris (and perhaps bulb of vestibule); compresses greater vestibular gland
Ischiocavernosus	Internal surface of ischiopubic ramus and ischial tuberosity	Embraces crus of penis or clitoris, inserting onto the inferior and medial aspects of the crus and to the perineal membrane medial to the crus		Maintains erection of penis or clitoris by compressing outflow veins and pushing blood from the root of penis or clitoris into the body of penis or clitoris
Superficial transverse perineal	Internal surface of ischiopubic ramus and ischial tuberosity	Passes along inferior aspect of posterior border of perineal membrane to perineal body		Supports and fixes perineal body (pelvic floor) to support abdominopelvic viscera and resist increased intra-abdominal pressure
Deep transverse perineal (male only)		Passes along superior aspect of posterior border of perineal membrane to perineal body, and external anal sphincter	Muscular (deep) branch of perineal nerve	
Smooth muscle (female only)	Ischiopubic rami	Passes to lateral wall of urethra and vagina	Autonomic nerves	Quantity of smooth muscle increases with age; function uncertain
External urethral sphincter		Surrounds urethra superior to perineal membrane; in males, also ascends anterior aspect of prostate		Compresses urethra to maintain urinary continence
Compressor urethrae (females only)	Internal surface of ischiopubic ramus	Continuous with external urethral sphincter	Dorsal nerve of penis or clitoris, terminal branch of pudendal nerve (S2–S4)	Compresses urethra; with pelvic diaphragm; assists in elongation of urethra
Urethrovaginal sphincter (females only)	Anterior side of urethra	Continuous with compressor urethrae; extends posteriorly on lateral wall of urethra and vagina to interdigitate with fibers from opposite side of perineal body		Compresses urethra and vagina

Oelrich TM. The urethral sphincter muscle in the male. *Am J Anat* 1980;158:229–246.
Oelrich TM. The striated urogenital sphincter muscle in the female. *Anat Rec* 1983;205:223–232.
Mirilas P, Skandalakis JE. Urogenital diaphragm: an erroneous concept casting its shadow over the sphincter urethrae and deep perineal space. *J Am Coll Surg* 2004;198:279–290.
DeLancey JO. Correlative study of paraurethral anatomy. *Obstet Gynecol* 1986;68:91–97.

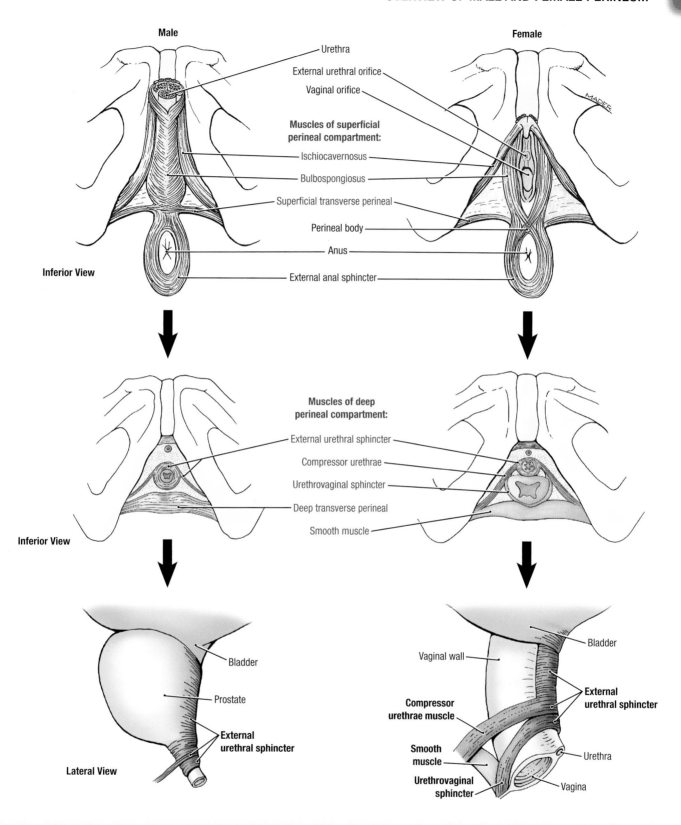

Male

Urethra

Female

External urethral orifice

Vaginal orifice

Muscles of superficial perineal compartment:

Ischiocavernosus

Bulbospongiosus

Superficial transverse perineal

Perineal body

Anus

External anal sphincter

Inferior View

Muscles of deep perineal compartment:

External urethral sphincter

Compressor urethrae

Urethrovaginal sphincter

Deep transverse perineal

Smooth muscle

Inferior View

Bladder

Prostate

External urethral sphincter

Lateral View

Bladder

Vaginal wall

External urethral sphincter

Compressor urethrae muscle

Smooth muscle

Urethra

Urethrovaginal sphincter

Vagina

| **3.50** | **MUSCLES OF PERINEUM** |

A potential subcutaneous perineal space (pouch) lies between the membranous layer of the subcutaneous tissue of the perineum and the perineal fascia (investing fascia of the superficial perineal muscles). The superficial perineal compartment (pouch) is an enclosed compartment bounded inferiorly by the perineal fascia and superiorly by the perineal membrane. The deep compartment is bounded inferiorly by the perineal membrane and continues superiorly to the (inferior investing fascia of the) pelvic diaphragm (Oelich, 1980, 1983; DeLancy 1986; Mirilus, 2004).

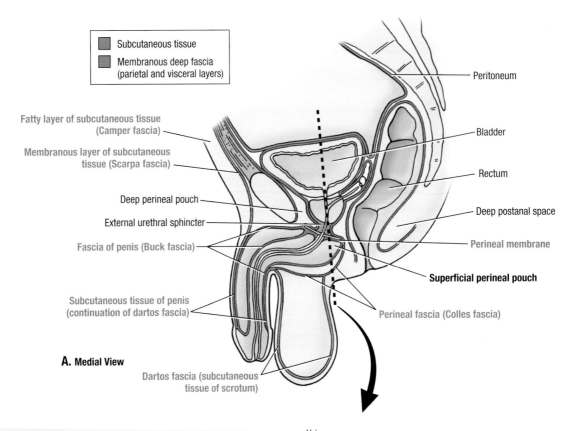

A. Medial View

Subcutaneous tissue
Membranous deep fascia
(parietal and visceral layers)

Fatty layer of subcutaneous tissue
(Camper fascia)
Membranous layer of subcutaneous
tissue (Scarpa fascia)
Deep perineal pouch
External urethral sphincter
Fascia of penis (Buck fascia)
Subcutaneous tissue of penis
(continuation of dartos fascia)
Dartos fascia (subcutaneous
tissue of scrotum)

Peritoneum
Bladder
Rectum
Deep postanal space
Perineal membrane
Superficial perineal pouch
Perineal fascia (Colles fascia)

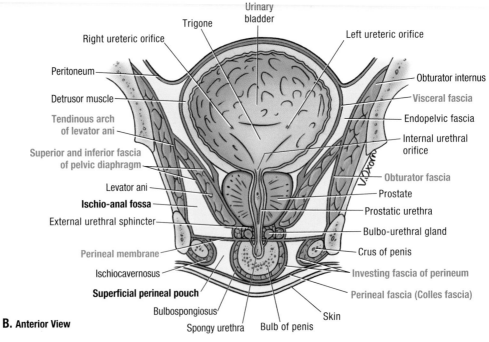

B. Anterior View

Urinary bladder
Trigone
Right ureteric orifice
Peritoneum
Detrusor muscle
Tendinous arch
of levator ani
Superior and inferior fascia
of pelvic diaphragm
Levator ani
Ischio-anal fossa
External urethral sphincter
Perineal membrane
Ischiocavernosus
Superficial perineal pouch
Bulbospongiosus
Spongy urethra

Left ureteric orifice
Obturator internus
Visceral fascia
Endopelvic fascia
Internal urethral
orifice
Obturator fascia
Prostate
Prostatic urethra
Bulbo-urethral gland
Crus of penis
Investing fascia of perineum
Perineal fascia (Colles fascia)
Skin
Bulb of penis

3.51   PERINEAL FASCIA AND PERINEAL COMPARTMENTS

A. Fascia of male perineum, median section. **B.** Compartments of male perineum, coronal section.

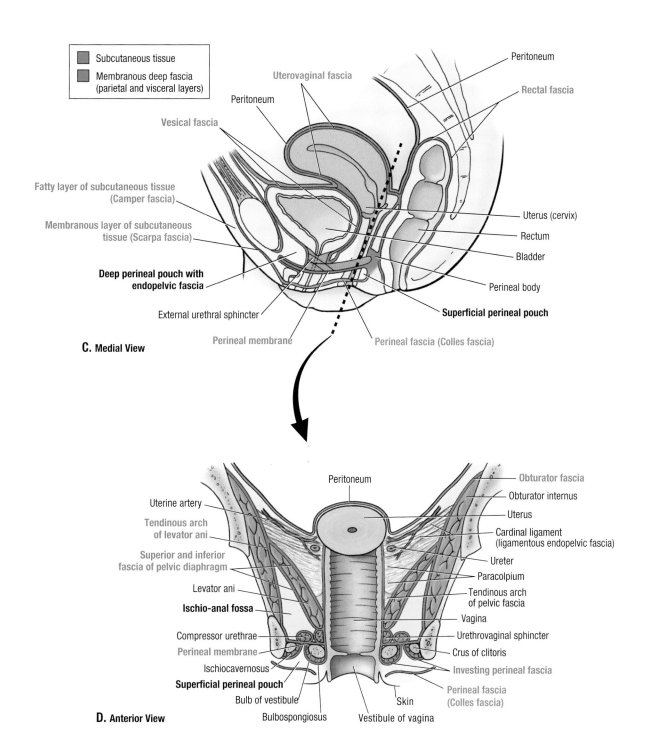

Subcutaneous tissue

Membranous deep fascia
(parietal and visceral layers)

Uterovaginal fascia

Peritoneum

Vesical fascia

Fatty layer of subcutaneous tissue
(Camper fascia)

Membranous layer of subcutaneous
tissue (Scarpa fascia)

**Deep perineal pouch with
endopelvic fascia**

External urethral sphincter

Perineal membrane

C. Medial View

Peritoneum

Rectal fascia

Uterus (cervix)

Rectum

Bladder

Perineal body

Superficial perineal pouch

Perineal fascia (Colles fascia)

Uterine artery

Tendinous arch
of levator ani

Superior and inferior
fascia of pelvic diaphragm

Levator ani

Ischio-anal fossa

Compressor urethrae

Perineal membrane

Ischiocavernosus

Superficial perineal pouch

Bulb of vestibule

D. Anterior View

Bulbospongiosus

Peritoneum

Obturator fascia

Obturator internus

Uterus

Cardinal ligament
(ligamentous endopelvic fascia)

Ureter

Paracolpium

Tendinous arch
of pelvic fascia

Vagina

Urethrovaginal sphincter

Crus of clitoris

Investing perineal fascia

Perineal fascia
(Colles fascia)

Skin

Vestibule of vagina

3.51   PERINEAL FASCIA AND PERINEAL COMPARTMENTS *(CONTINUED)*

C. Fascia of female perineum, median section. **D.** Compartments of female perineum, coronal section.
Tendinous arch of levator ani = thickening of obturator fascia providing origin for levator ani; tendinous arch of
pelvic fascia = thickening where somatic and parietal membranous pelvic fascias merge.

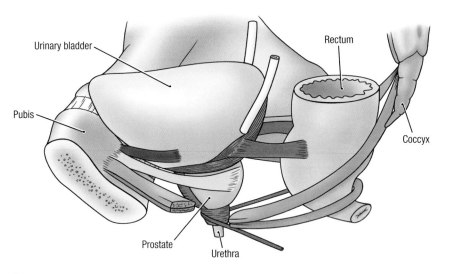

Urinary bladder

Rectum

Pubis

Coccyx

Prostate

Urethra

MALE:

Puboprostaticus

Pubococcygeus

Puborectalis

Muscle of uvula

Rectovesicalis

Muscles compressing urethra:

Internal urethral sphincter

Pubovesicalis

External urethral sphincter

A. Left Lateral View, Male

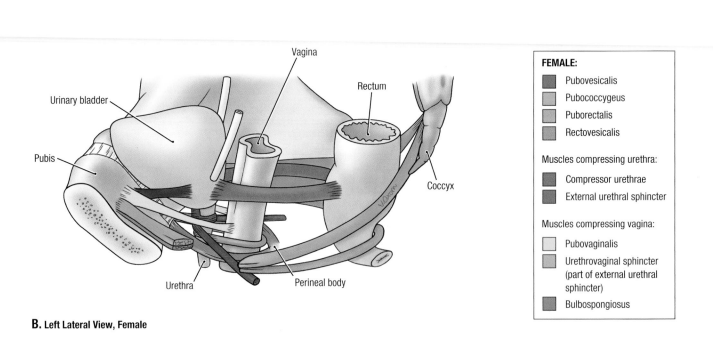

Vagina

Rectum

Urinary bladder

Pubis

Coccyx

Urethra

Perineal body

FEMALE:

Pubovesicalis

Pubococcygeus

Puborectalis

Rectovesicalis

Muscles compressing urethra:

Compressor urethrae

External urethral sphincter

Muscles compressing vagina:

Pubovaginalis

Urethrovaginal sphincter
(part of external urethral
sphincter)

Bulbospongiosus

B. Left Lateral View, Female

3.52 SUPPORTING AND COMPRESSOR/SPHINCTERIC MUSCLES OF PELVIS

A. Male. **B.** Female.

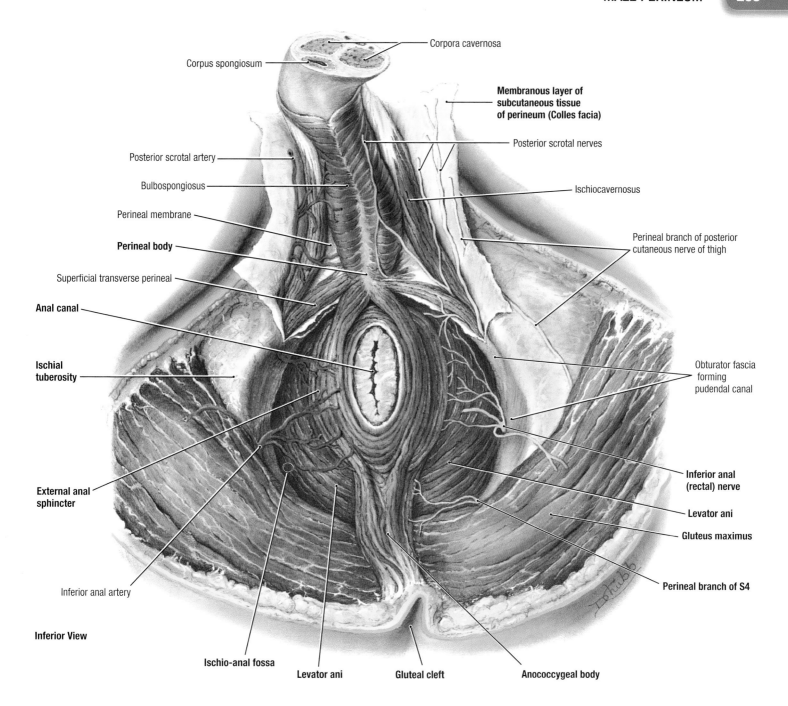

Corpora cavernosa

Corpus spongiosum

**Membranous layer of
subcutaneous tissue
of perineum (Colles facia)**

Posterior scrotal nerves

Posterior scrotal artery

Ischiocavernosus

Bulbospongiosus

Perineal membrane

Perineal body

Perineal branch of posterior
cutaneous nerve of thigh

Superficial transverse perineal

Anal canal

**Ischial
tuberosity**

Obturator fascia
forming
pudendal canal

**External anal
sphincter**

**Inferior anal
(rectal) nerve**

Levator ani

Gluteus maximus

Inferior anal artery

Perineal branch of S4

Inferior View

Ischio-anal fossa   Levator ani   Gluteal cleft   Anococcygeal body

---

3.53   **DISSECTION OF MALE PERINEUM I**

Superficial dissection.

- The membranous layer of subcutaneous tissue of the perineum was incised and reflected, opening the subcutaneous perineal compartment (pouch) in which the cutaneous nerves course.
- The perineal membrane is exposed between the three paired muscles of the superficial compartment; although not evident here, the muscles are individually ensheathed with investing fascia.
- The anal canal is surrounded by the external anal sphincter. The superficial fibers of the sphincter anchor the anal canal anteriorly to the perineal body and posteriorly, via the anococcygeal body (ligament), to the coccyx and skin of the gluteal cleft.

- Ischio-anal (ischiorectal) fossae, from which fat bodies have been removed, lie on each side of the external anal sphincter. The fossae are also bound medially and superiorly by the levator ani, laterally by the ischial tuberosities and obturator internus fascia, and posteriorly by the gluteus maximus overlying the sacrotuberous ligaments. An anterior recess of each ischio-anal fossa extends superior to the perineal membrane.
- In the lateral wall of the fossa, the inferior anal (rectal) nerve emerges from the pudendal canal and, with the perineal branch of S4, supplies the voluntary external anal sphincter and perianal skin; most cutaneous twigs have been removed.

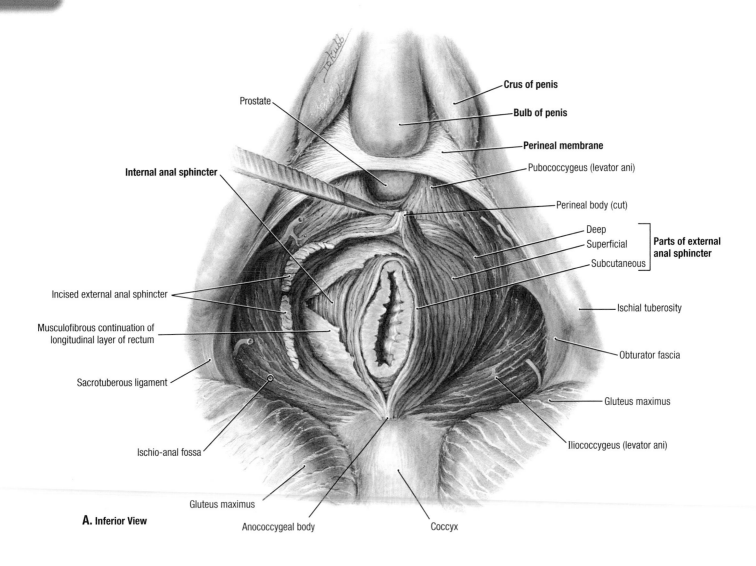

Prostate

Internal anal sphincter

Incised external anal sphincter

Musculofibrous continuation of
longitudinal layer of rectum

Sacrotuberous ligament

Ischio-anal fossa

Gluteus maximus

A. Inferior View

Anococcygeal body

Crus of penis

Bulb of penis

Perineal membrane

Pubococcygeus (levator ani)

Perineal body (cut)

Deep
Superficial
Subcutaneous

**Parts of external
anal sphincter**

Ischial tuberosity

Obturator fascia

Gluteus maximus

Iliococcygeus (levator ani)

Coccyx

3.54 DISSECTION OF THE MALE PERINEUM II

A. The superficial perineal muscles have been removed, revealing the
roots of the erectile bodies (crura and bulb) of the penis, attached to the
ischiopubic rami and perineal membrane. On the left side, the superficial and deep parts of the external anal sphincter were incised and
reflected; the underlying musculofibrous continuation of the outer longitudinal layer of the muscular layer of the rectum is cut to reveal thickening of the inner circular layer that comprises the internal anal sphincter.
B. Rupture of the spongy urethra in the bulb of the penis results in
extravasation (abnormal passage) **of urine** into the subcutaneous
perineal compartment. The attachments of the membranous layer
of subcutaneous tissue determine the direction and restrictions of
flow of the extravasated urine. Urine and blood may pass deep to the
continuations of the membranous layer in the scrotum, penis, and
inferior abdominal wall. The urine cannot pass laterally and inferiorly
into the thighs because the membranous layer fuses with the fascia
lata (deep fascia of the thigh), nor posteriorly into the anal triangle
due to continuity with the perineal membrane and perineal body.

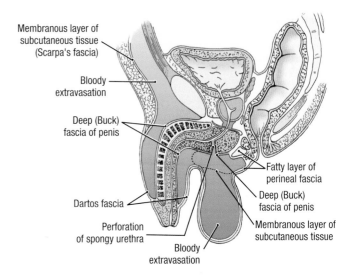

Membranous layer of
subcutaneous tissue
(Scarpa's fascia)

Bloody
extravasation

Deep (Buck)
fascia of penis

Dartos fascia

Perforation
of spongy urethra

Bloody
extravasation

Fatty layer of
perineal fascia

Deep (Buck)
fascia of penis

Membranous layer of
subcutaneous tissue

B. Medial view (from left)

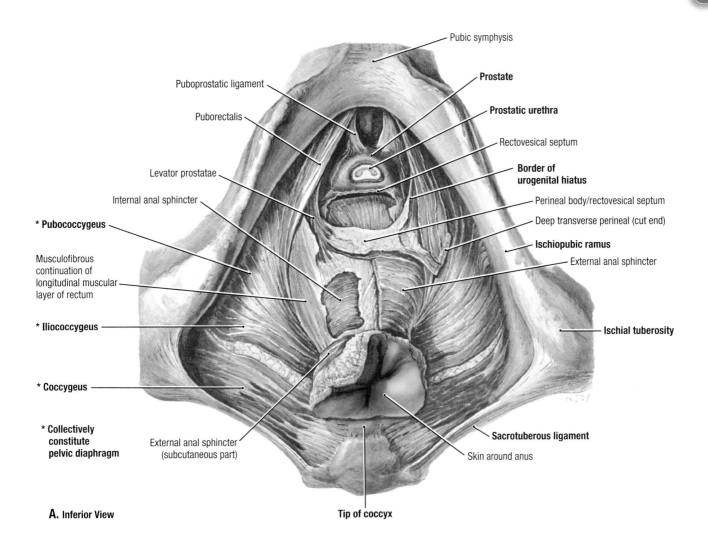

Pubic symphysis

Puboprostatic ligament

Prostate

Puborectalis

Prostatic urethra

Rectovesical septum

Levator prostatae

**Border of
urogenital hiatus**

Internal anal sphincter

Perineal body/rectovesical septum

* Pubococcygeus

Deep transverse perineal (cut end)

Ischiopubic ramus

Musculofibrous
continuation of
longitudinal muscular
layer of rectum

External anal sphincter

* Iliococcygeus

Ischial tuberosity

* Coccygeus

*** Collectively
constitute
pelvic diaphragm**

External anal sphincter
(subcutaneous part)

Sacrotuberous ligament

Skin around anus

A. Inferior View

Tip of coccyx

3.55   DISSECTION OF THE MALE PERINEUM III

A. The perineal membrane and structures superficial to it have been removed. The prostatic urethra, base of the prostate, and rectum are visible through the urogenital hiatus of the pelvic diaphragm. The osseofibrous boundaries are demonstrated. **B. Rupture of the intermediate part of the urethra** results in extravasation of urine and blood into the deep perineal compartment. The fluid may pass superiorly through the urogenital hiatus and distribute extraperitoneally around the prostate and bladder.

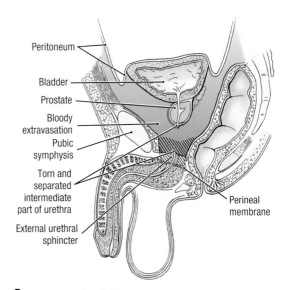

Peritoneum

Bladder

Prostate

Bloody
extravasation

Pubic
symphysis

Torn and
separated
intermediate
part of urethra

External urethral
sphincter

Perineal
membrane

B. Medial View (from left)

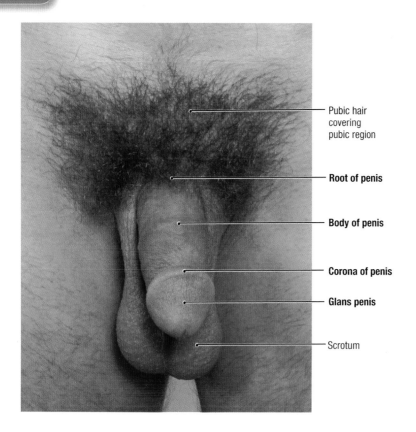

Pubic hair covering pubic region

Root of penis

Body of penis

Corona of penis

Glans penis

Scrotum

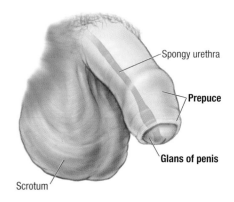

Spongy urethra

Prepuce

Glans of penis

Scrotum

B. Right Anterolateral View

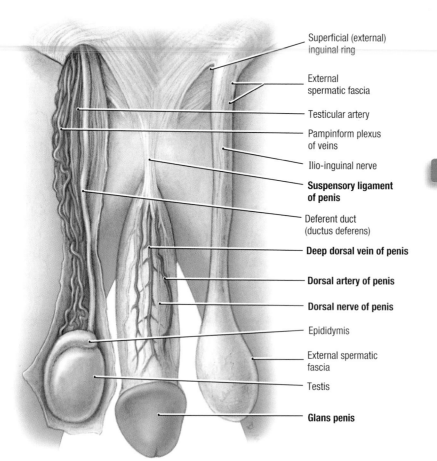

Superficial (external) inguinal ring

External spermatic fascia

Testicular artery

Pampiniform plexus of veins

Ilio-inguinal nerve

Suspensory ligament of penis

Deferent duct (ductus deferens)

Deep dorsal vein of penis

Dorsal artery of penis

Dorsal nerve of penis

Epididymis

External spermatic fascia

Testis

Glans penis

C. Anterior View

3.56

GLANS, PREPUCE, AND NEUROVASCULAR BUNDLE OF PENIS

A. Surface anatomy, penis circumcised. **B.** Uncircumcised penis. **C.** Vessels and nerves of penis and contents of spermatic cord.

In **C:**

- The superficial and deep fasciae covering the penis are removed to expose the midline deep dorsal vein and the bilateral dorsal arteries and nerves of the penis. The triangular suspensory ligament of the penis attaches to the region of the pubic symphysis and blends with the deep fascia of the penis.
- On the specimen's left, the spermatic cord passes through the external inguinal ring and picks up a covering of external spermatic fascia from the margins of the superficial inguinal ring.
- On the specimen's right, the coverings of the spermatic cord and testis are incised and reflected, and the contents of the cord are separated.

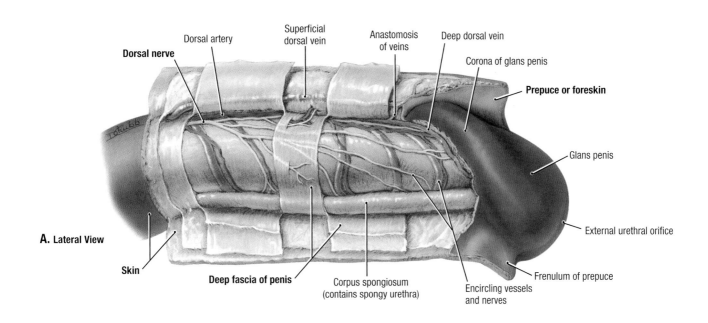

A. Lateral View

Dorsal nerve

Dorsal artery

Superficial dorsal vein

Anastomosis of veins

Deep dorsal vein

Corona of glans penis

Prepuce or foreskin

Glans penis

External urethral orifice

Frenulum of prepuce

Encircling vessels and nerves

Corpus spongiosum (contains spongy urethra)

Deep fascia of penis

Skin

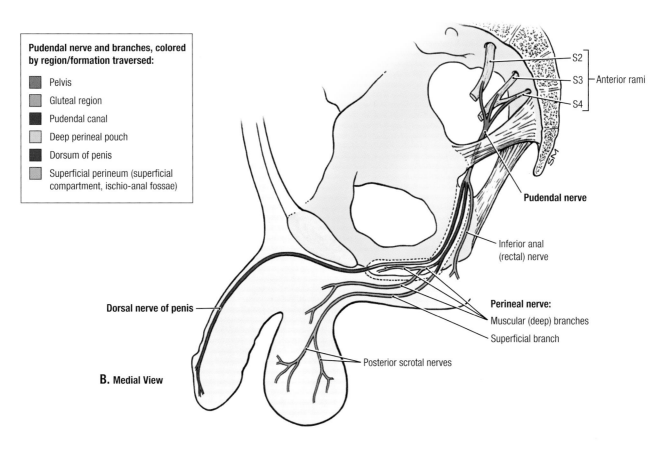

Pudendal nerve and branches, colored by region/formation traversed:

- Pelvis
- Gluteal region
- Pudendal canal
- Deep perineal pouch
- Dorsum of penis
- Superficial perineum (superficial compartment, ischio-anal fossae)

S2

S3　Anterior rami

S4

Pudendal nerve

Inferior anal (rectal) nerve

Perineal nerve:

Muscular (deep) branches

Superficial branch

Posterior scrotal nerves

Dorsal nerve of penis

B. Medial View

3.57　　**LAYERS AND NERVES OF PENIS**

A. Dissection. The skin, subcutaneous tissue, and deep fascia of the penis and prepuce are reflected separately. **B.** Distribution of pudendal nerve, right hemipelvis. Five regions transversed by the nerve are demonstrated.

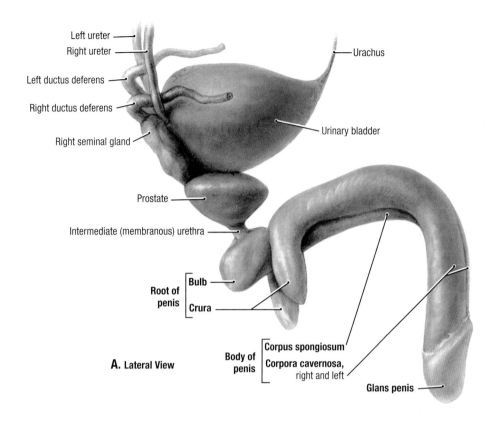

Left ureter

Right ureter

Left ductus deferens

Right ductus deferens

Right seminal gland

Urachus

Urinary bladder

Prostate

Intermediate (membranous) urethra

Root of penis
- Bulb
- Crura

Body of penis
- Corpus spongiosum
- Corpora cavernosa, right and left

Glans penis

A. Lateral View

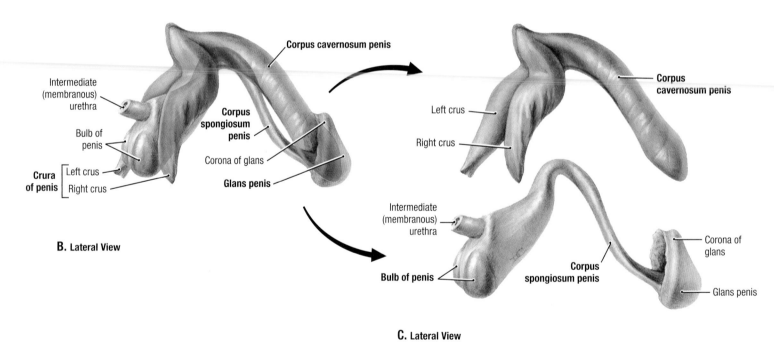

Corpus cavernosum penis

Intermediate (membranous) urethra

Bulb of penis

Crura of penis
- Left crus
- Right crus

Corpus spongiosum penis

Corona of glans

Glans penis

B. Lateral View

Corpus cavernosum penis

Left crus

Right crus

Intermediate (membranous) urethra

Bulb of penis

Corpus spongiosum penis

Corona of glans

Glans penis

C. Lateral View

3.58   MALE UROGENITAL SYSTEM, ERECTILE BODIES

A. Pelvic components of genital and urinary tracts and erectile bodies of perineum. **B.** Dissection of male erectile bodies (corpora cavernosa and corpus spongiosum). **C.** Corpus spongiosum and corpora cavernosa, separated. The corpora cavernosa are bent where the penis is suspended by the suspensory ligament of the penis from the pubic symphysis. The corpus spongiosum extends posteriorly as the bulb of the penis and terminates anteriorly as the glans.

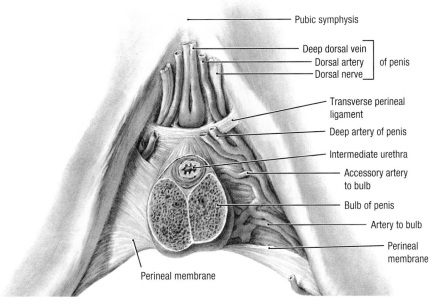

- Pubic symphysis
- Deep dorsal vein ┐
- Dorsal artery | of penis
- Dorsal nerve ┘
- Transverse perineal ligament
- Deep artery of penis
- Intermediate urethra
- Accessory artery to bulb
- Bulb of penis
- Artery to bulb
- Perineal membrane
- Perineal membrane

A. Anterior/Inferior View

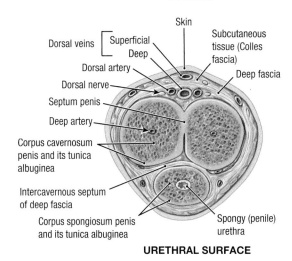

DORSUM

- Skin
- Dorsal veins ┐ Superficial
- │ Deep
- Subcutaneous tissue (Colles fascia)
- Dorsal artery
- Deep fascia
- Dorsal nerve
- Septum penis
- Deep artery
- Corpus cavernosum penis and its tunica albuginea
- Intercavernous septum of deep fascia
- Corpus spongiosum penis and its tunica albuginea
- Spongy (penile) urethra

URETHRAL SURFACE

C. Transverse Section

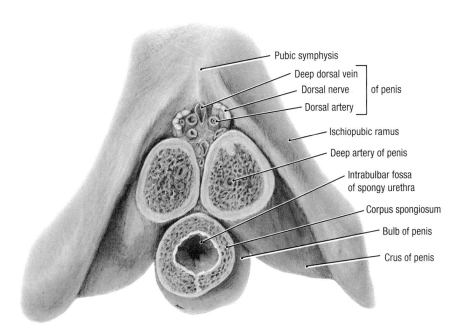

- Pubic symphysis
- Deep dorsal vein ┐
- Dorsal nerve | of penis
- Dorsal artery ┘
- Ischiopubic ramus
- Deep artery of penis
- Intrabulbar fossa of spongy urethra
- Corpus spongiosum
- Bulb of penis
- Crus of penis

B. Anterior View

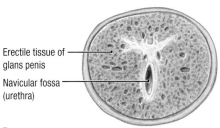

- Erectile tissue of glans penis
- Navicular fossa (urethra)

D. Transverse Section

- Corona of glans penis
- Septum penis
- Corpus cavernosum penis
- Spongy (penile)urethra
- Corpus spongiosum penis

E. Transverse Section

3.59 CROSS SECTIONS OF PENIS

A. Transverse section through bulb of penis with crura removed. The bulb is cut posterior to the entry of the intermediate urethra. On the left side, the perineal membrane is partially removed, opening the deep perineal compartment. **B.** The crura and bulb of penis have been sectioned obliquely. The spongy urethra is dilated within the bulb of the penis. **C.** Transverse section through body of penis. **D.** Transverse section through the proximal part of the glans penis. **E.** Transverse section through the distal part of the glans penis.

Lateral View

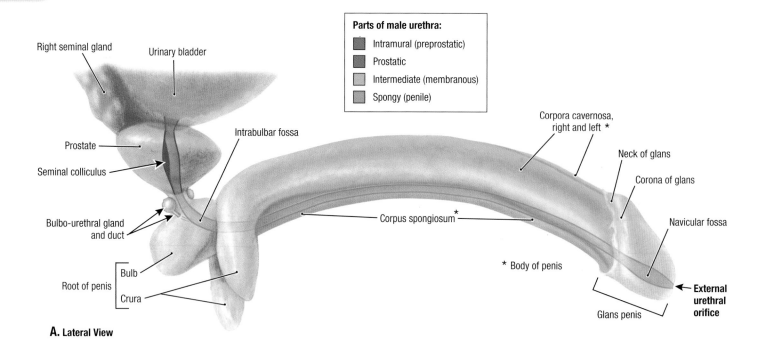

Parts of male urethra:
- Intramural (preprostatic)
- Prostatic
- Intermediate (membranous)
- Spongy (penile)

Right seminal gland

Urinary bladder

Prostate

Seminal colliculus

Bulbo-urethral gland and duct

Root of penis
- Bulb
- Crura

Intrabulbar fossa

Corpora cavernosa, right and left *

Neck of glans

Corona of glans

Corpus spongiosum *

Navicular fossa

* Body of penis

Glans penis

External urethral orifice

A. Lateral View

Dorsal vein of penis

Corpora cavernosa penis

Adductors

Femoral artery and vein

Bulb of penis

Intrabulbar fossa of spongy urethra

Sciatic nerve

Ischio-anal fossa

Gluteus maximus

Spermatic cord

Obturator externus

Superficial perineal muscles

Levator ani (puborectalis)

Anal canal

Ischial tuberosity

External urethral orifice

Glans penis

Frenulum of prepuce

Navicular fossa

Urethral lacuna

Orifices of urethral glands

Corpus spongiosum penis

Spongy (penile) urethra

Skin

B. Transverse Section, Inferior View

C. Urethal Aspect of Distal Penis

3.60 URETHRA

A. Urethra and related structures. **B.** Transverse section of body passing through the bulb of the penis. **C.** Spongy urethra, interior. A longitudinal incision was made on the urethral surface of the penis and carried through the floor of the urethra, allowing a view of the dorsal surface of the interior of the urethra.

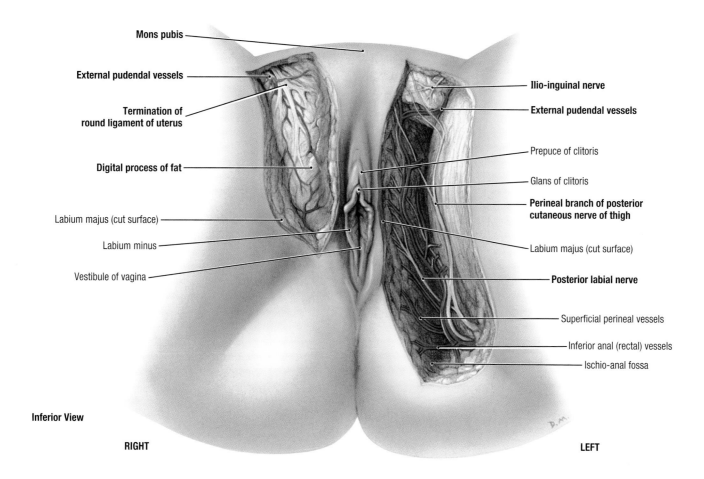

Mons pubis

External pudendal vessels

Termination of
round ligament of uterus

Digital process of fat

Labium majus (cut surface)

Labium minus

Vestibule of vagina

Ilio-inguinal nerve

External pudendal vessels

Prepuce of clitoris

Glans of clitoris

Perineal branch of posterior
cutaneous nerve of thigh

Labium majus (cut surface)

Posterior labial nerve

Superficial perineal vessels

Inferior anal (rectal) vessels

Ischio-anal fossa

Inferior View

RIGHT

LEFT

3.61 **FEMALE PERINEUM I**

Superficial dissection.
On the right side of the specimen:
- A long digital process of fat lies deep to the fatty subcutaneous tissue and descends into the labium majus.
- The round ligament of the uterus ends as a branching band of fascia that spreads out superficial to the fatty digital process.

On the left side of the specimen:
- Most of the fatty digital process is removed.
- The mons pubis is the rounded fatty prominence anterior to the pubic symphysis and bodies of the pubic bones.
- The posterior labial vessels and nerves (S2, S3) are joined by the perineal branch of the posterior cutaneous nerve of thigh (S1, S2, S3) and run anterior to the mons pubis. At the mons pubis, the vessels anastomose with the external pudendal vessels, and the nerves overlap in supply with the ilio-inguinal nerve (L1).

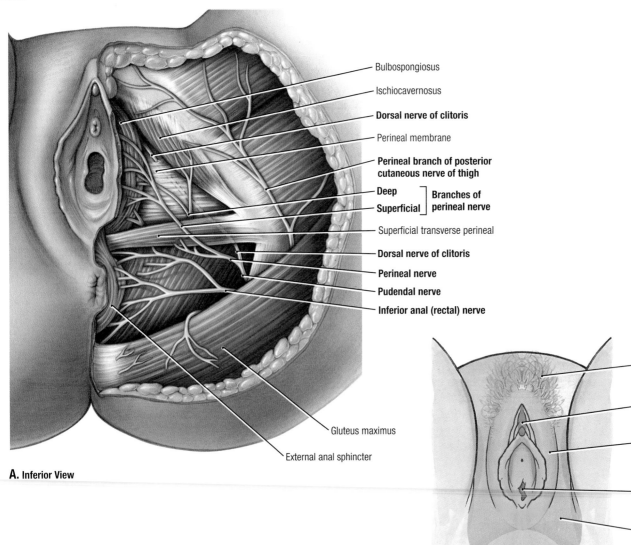

Bulbospongiosus

Ischiocavernosus

Dorsal nerve of clitoris

Perineal membrane

Perineal branch of posterior cutaneous nerve of thigh

Deep ⎤ Branches of
Superficial ⎦ perineal nerve

Superficial transverse perineal

Dorsal nerve of clitoris

Perineal nerve

Pudendal nerve

Inferior anal (rectal) nerve

Gluteus maximus

External anal sphincter

A. Inferior View

Anterior labial nerve

Dorsal nerve of clitoris

Posterior labial nerves

Deep perineal nerve

Perineal branch of posterior cutaneous nerve of thigh

Inferior rectal (anal) nerve

Inferior clunial nerves

B. Inferior View

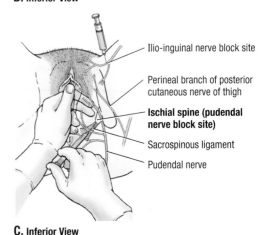

Ilio-inguinal nerve block site

Perineal branch of posterior cutaneous nerve of thigh

Ischial spine (pudendal nerve block site)

Sacrospinous ligament

Pudendal nerve

C. Inferior View

3.62   INNERVATION OF THE FEMALE PERINEUM

A. and B. The anterior aspect of the perineum is supplied by anterior labial nerves, derived from the ilio-inguinal nerve and genital branch of the genitofemoral nerve. The pudendal nerve is the main nerve of the perineum. Posterior labial nerves, derived from the superficial perineal nerve, supply most of the vulva. The deep perineal nerve supplies the orifice of the vagina and superficial perineal muscles; and the dorsal nerve of the clitoris supplies deep perineal muscles and sensations to the clitoris. The inferior anal (rectal) nerve, also from the pudendal nerve, innervates the external anal sphincter and the perianal skin. The lateral perineum is supplied by the perineal branch of the posterior cutaneous nerve of the thigh. **C.** To relieve the pain experienced during childbirth, **pudendal nerve block anesthesia** may be performed by injecting a local anesthetic agent into the tissue surrounding the pudendal nerve, near the ischial spine. A pudendal nerve block does not abolish sensations from the anterior and lateral parts of the perineum. Therefore, **an anesthetic block of the ilio-inguinal and/or perineal branch of the posterior cutaneous nerve of the thigh** may also need to be performed.

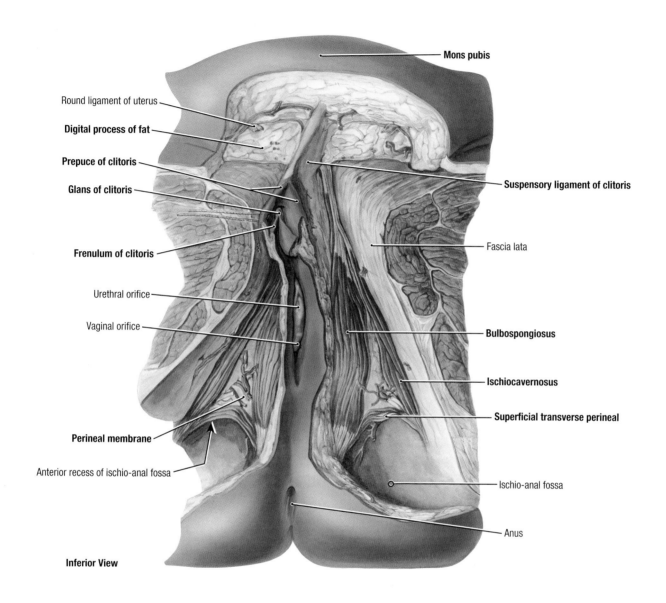

Mons pubis

Round ligament of uterus

Digital process of fat

Prepuce of clitoris

Glans of clitoris

Frenulum of clitoris

Urethral orifice

Vaginal orifice

Perineal membrane

Anterior recess of ischio-anal fossa

Inferior View

Suspensory ligament of clitoris

Fascia lata

Bulbospongiosus

Ischiocavernosus

Superficial transverse perineal

Ischio-anal fossa

Anus

3.63 **FEMALE PERINEUM II**

- Note the thickness of the subcutaneous fatty tissue of the mons pubis and the encapsulated digital process of fat deep to this. The suspensory ligament of the clitoris descends from the linea alba.

- Anteriorly, each labium minus forms two laminae or folds: the lateral laminae of the labia pass on each side of the glans clitoris and unite, forming a hood that partially or completely covers the glans, the prepuce (foreskin) of the clitoris. The medial laminae of the labia merge posterior to the glans, forming the frenulum of the clitoris.

- There are three muscles on each side: bulbospongiosus, ischiocavernosus, and superficial transverse perineal; the perineal membrane is visible between them.

- The bulbospongiosus muscle overlies the bulb of the vestibule and the great vestibular gland. In the male, the muscles of the two sides are united by a median raphe; in the female, the orifice of the vagina separates the right from the left.

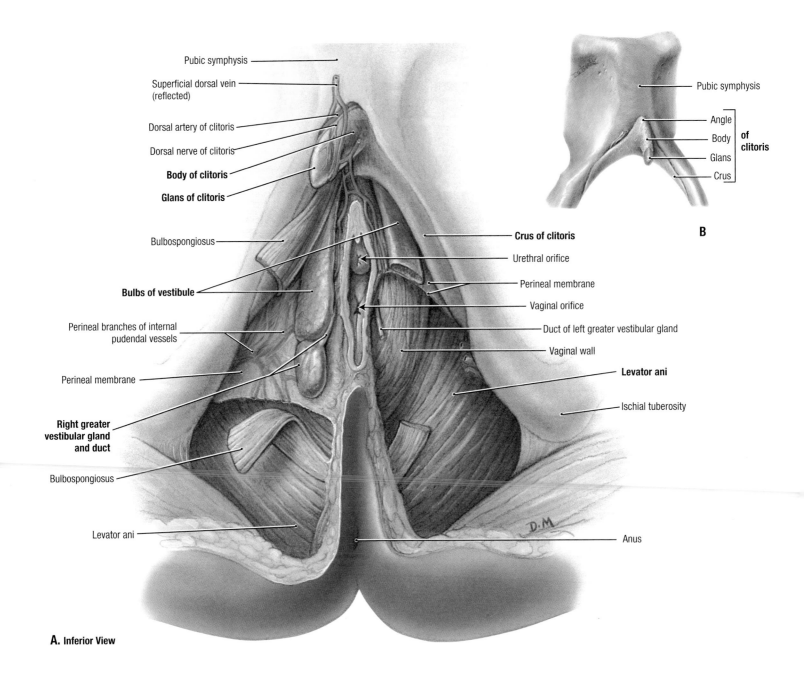

Pubic symphysis

Superficial dorsal vein (reflected)

Dorsal artery of clitoris

Dorsal nerve of clitoris

Body of clitoris

Glans of clitoris

Bulbospongiosus

Bulbs of vestibule

Perineal branches of internal pudendal vessels

Perineal membrane

Right greater vestibular gland and duct

Bulbospongiosus

Levator ani

Pubic symphysis

Angle
Body
Glans
Crus
of clitoris

B

Crus of clitoris

Urethral orifice

Perineal membrane

Vaginal orifice

Duct of left greater vestibular gland

Vaginal wall

Levator ani

Ischial tuberosity

Anus

D.M

A. Inferior View

3.64   **FEMALE PERINEUM III**

A. Deeper dissection. **B.** Clitoris.
In **A:**

- The bulbospongiosus muscle is reflected on the right side and mostly removed on the left side; the posterior portion of the bulb of the vestibule and the greater vestibular gland have been removed on the left side.
- The glans and body of the clitoris is displaced to the right so that the distribution of the dorsal vessels and nerve of the clitoris can be seen.
- Homologues of the bulb of the penis, the bulbs of the vestibule exist as two masses of elongated erectile tissue that lie along the sides of the vaginal orifice; veins connect the bulbs of the vestibule to the glans of the clitoris.

- On the specimen's right side, the greater vestibular gland is situated at the posterior end of the bulb; both structures are covered by bulbospongiosus muscle.
- On the specimen's left side, the bulb, gland, and perineal membrane are cut away, thereby revealing the external aspect of the vaginal wall.

In **B:**

- The body of the clitoris, composed of two crura (corpora cavernosa), is capped by the glans.

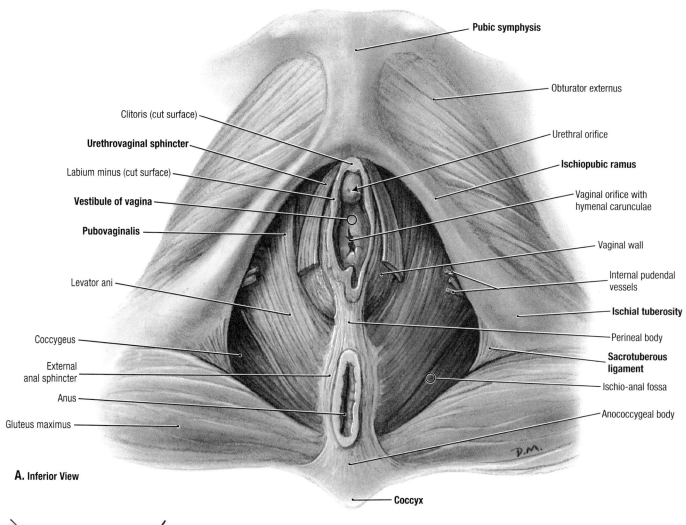

Pubic symphysis

Clitoris (cut surface)

Urethrovaginal sphincter

Labium minus (cut surface)

Vestibule of vagina

Pubovaginalis

Levator ani

Coccygeus

External anal sphincter

Anus

Gluteus maximus

Obturator externus

Urethral orifice

Ischiopubic ramus

Vaginal orifice with hymenal carunculae

Vaginal wall

Internal pudendal vessels

Ischial tuberosity

Perineal body

Sacrotuberous ligament

Ischio-anal fossa

Anococcygeal body

A. Inferior View

Coccyx

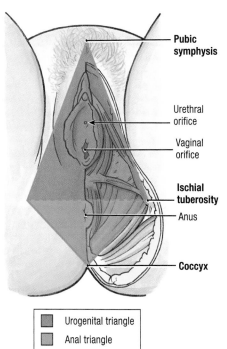

Pubic symphysis

Urethral orifice

Vaginal orifice

Ischial tuberosity

Anus

Coccyx

☐ Urogenital triangle
☐ Anal triangle

B. Inferior View

3.65   **FEMALE PERINEUM IV**

A. Deep perineal compartment. The perineal membrane and smooth muscle corresponding in position to the deep transverse perineal muscle in the male have been removed.

- The most anterior and medial part of the levator ani muscle, the pubovaginalis, passes posterior to the vaginal orifice.
- The urethrovaginal sphincter, part of the external urethral sphincter of the female, rests on the urethra and straddles the vagina.
- The labia minora (cut short here) bound the vestibule of the vagina.

A. and B. The osseoligamentous boundaries of the diamond-shaped perineum are the pubic symphysis, ischiopubic rami, ischial tuberosities, sacrotuberous ligaments, and coccyx. For descriptive purposes, a transverse line connecting the ischial tuberosities subdivides the diamond into urogenital and anal triangles.

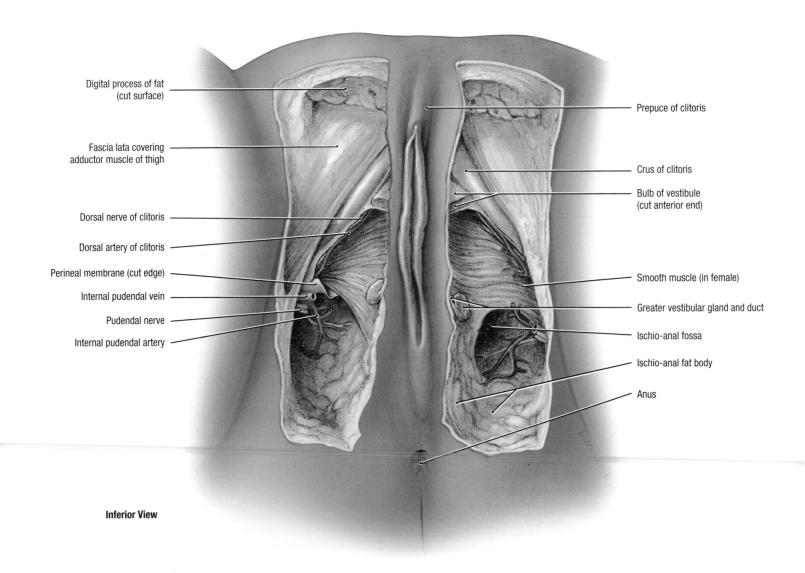

Digital process of fat
(cut surface)

Fascia lata covering
adductor muscle of thigh

Dorsal nerve of clitoris

Dorsal artery of clitoris

Perineal membrane (cut edge)

Internal pudendal vein

Pudendal nerve

Internal pudendal artery

Prepuce of clitoris

Crus of clitoris

Bulb of vestibule
(cut anterior end)

Smooth muscle (in female)

Greater vestibular gland and duct

Ischio-anal fossa

Ischio-anal fat body

Anus

Inferior View

3.66   FEMALE PERINEUM V

This is a different dissection than the previous series, with the vulva undissected centrally but the perineum dissected deeply on each side. Although most of the perineal membrane and bulbs of the vestibule have been removed, the greater vestibular glands (structures of the superficial perineal compartment) have been left in place. The development and extent of the smooth muscle layer corresponding in position to the voluntary deep transverse perineal muscles of the male are highly variable, being relatively extensive in this case, blending centrally with voluntary fibers of the external urethral sphincter and the perineal body.

The greater vestibular glands are usually not palpable, but are so when infected. Occlusion of the vestibular gland duct can predispose the individual to **infection of the vestibular gland.** The gland is the site or origin of most **vulvar adenocarcinomas** (cancers). **Bartholinitis**, inflammation of the greater vestibular (Bartholin) glands, may result from a number of pathogenic organisms. Infected glands may enlarge to a diameter of 4 to 5 cm and impinge on the wall of the rectum. Occlusion of the vestibular gland duct without infection can result in the accumulation of mucin (**Bartholin cyst**).

A. Transverse Section

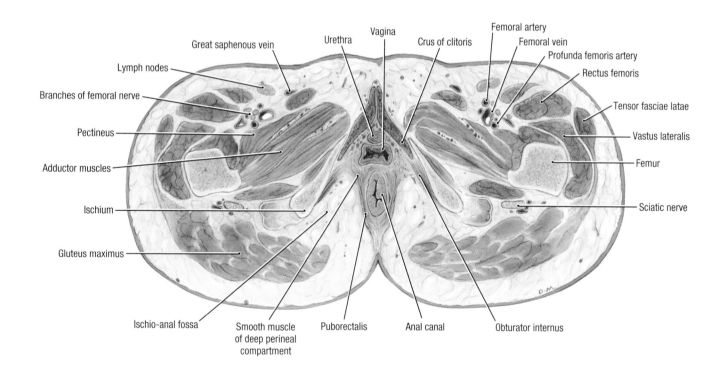

B. Transverse Section

3.67 **FEMALE PERINEUM V**

A. Section through vagina and urethra at base of urinary bladder. **B.** Section through vagina, urethra, and crura of clitoris.

A

B

C

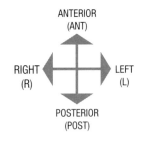

ANTERIOR (ANT)

RIGHT (R) — LEFT (L)

POSTERIOR (POST)

A	**Anus**	**LA**	**Levator ani**
Ad	Adductor muscles	Max	Gluteus maximus
Bi	Biceps femoris tendon	Med	Gluteus medius
Bu	**Bulb of penis**	Min	Gluteus minimus
Cav	**Corpus cavernosum penis**	OE	Obturator externus
CC	Coccygeus	OI	Obturator internus
Cox	Coccyx	OV	Obturator vessels and nerve
Cr	**Crus of penis**		
DD	Ductus deferens	**P**	**Prostate**
DVP	Dorsal vein of penis	**PB**	**Perineal body**
EA	External iliac artery	Pec	Pectineus
EAS	External anal sphincter	PF	Profunda femoris artery
EV	External iliac vein	Pir	Piriformis
F	Femur	**PR**	**Puborectalis**
FA	Femoral artery	PS	Psoas
FN	Femoral nerve	PV	Pudendal vessels and nerves
FV	Femoral vein	QF	Quadratus femoris
GC	Gluteal cleft	**R**	**Rectum**
GSV	Great saphenous vein	RA	Rectus abdominis
GT	Greater trochanter	RF	Rectus femoris
GV	Superior gluteal vein	**RP**	**Root of penis**
HdF	Head of femur	Sar	Sartorius
I	Body of ischium	Sc	Spermatic cord
IA	Internal iliac artery	SC	Sigmoid colon
IAF	**Ischio-anal fossa (pararectal fat)**	**SG**	**Seminal gland**
		SM	Sigmoidal vessels in mesentery of sigmoid colon
IC	**Ischiocavernosus**		
IE	Inferior epigastric vessels	Sn	Sciatic nerve
IL	Iliacus	SP	Superior ramus of pubis
IP	Iliopsoas	SR	Sacrum
IPR	Ischiopubic ramus	Sy	Pubic symphysis
IR	Inferior pubic ramus	**U**	**Urethra**
IS	Ischial spine	**UB**	**Urinary bladder**
IT	Ischial tuberosity	VI	Vastus intermedius
IV	Internal iliac vein		

(Organs/structures of male pelvis and perineum are in boldface)

3.68 TRANSVERSE (AXIAL) MRIs AND SECTIONAL SPECIMEN OF MALE PELVIS AND PERINEUM, INFERIOR VIEWS

A.–D. MRIs. **E.** Anatomical section.

3.68 TRANSVERSE (AXIAL) MRIs AND SECTIONAL SPECIMEN OF MALE PELVIS AND PERINEUM, INFERIOR VIEWS (*CONTINUED*)

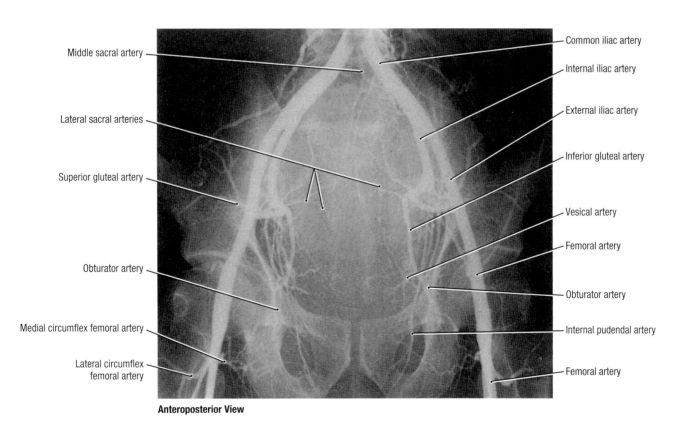

Middle sacral artery

Lateral sacral arteries

Superior gluteal artery

Obturator artery

Medial circumflex femoral artery

Lateral circumflex femoral artery

Common iliac artery

Internal iliac artery

External iliac artery

Inferior gluteal artery

Vesical artery

Femoral artery

Obturator artery

Internal pudendal artery

Femoral artery

Anteroposterior View

3.69 PELVIC ANGIOGRAPHY

A

SUPERIOR

RIGHT — LEFT

INFERIOR

B

C

A	**Anus**	LS	Lumbosacral trunk
Ad	Adductors	OE	Obturator externus
CA	Common iliac artery	**OI**	**Obturator internus**
Cav	**Corpus cavernosum penis**	**P**	**Prostate**
Cs	**Corpus spongiosum penis**	Pec	Pectineus
CV	Common iliac vein	PS	Psoas
DC	Descending colon	Pu	Pubic bone
EA	External iliac artery	**PV**	**Pelvic vessels and nerves**
EV	External iliac vein	**R**	**Rectum**
FA	Femoral artery	**Sac**	**Sacrum**
FV	Femoral vein	SC	Sigmoid colon
HdF	Head of femur	**SG**	**Seminal gland**
IL	Iliacus	**Sy**	**Pubic symphysis**
In	Small intestine	**U**	**Urethra**
IR	**Inferior rectal nerve and vessels**	**UB**	**Urinary bladder**
LA	**Levator ani**		

3.70   CORONAL MRIs OF MALE PELVIS AND PERINEUM, ANTERIOR VIEWS

MALE

Median Section, Male

FEMALE

Median Section, Female

Median MRI Scan, Male

Median MRI Scan, Female

Male:

A	Anus
B	Bulb of penis
Co	Coccyx
Cav	Corpus cavernosum penis
Cs	Corpus spongiosum penis
P	Prostate
PP	Prostatic venous plexus
R	Rectum
RA	Rectus abdominis
RF	Retropubic fat
RVP	Rectovesical pouch
S	Sacrum
SG	Seminal gland
SN	Sacral nerves
Sy	Pubic symphysis
UB	Urinary bladder

SUPERIOR

ANTERIOR — POSTERIOR

INFERIOR

Female:

B	Body of uterus
C	Cervix of uterus
Co	Coccyx
E	Endometrium
EF	Endopelvic fascia
F	Fundus of uterus
M	Myometrium
R	Rectum
RA	Rectus abdominis
S	Sacrum
Sy	Pubic symphysis
UB	Urinary bladder
V	Vagina
VU	Vesico-uterine pouch

3.71   MEDIAN MRIs OF MALE AND FEMALE PELVIS AND PERINEUM

A

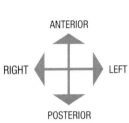

ANTERIOR

RIGHT — LEFT

POSTERIOR

B

C

A	**Anus**	**M**	**Myometrium**
AC	Acetabulum	Max	Gluteus maximus
Ad	Adductor muscles	OE	Obturator externus
AS	Anterior superior iliac spine	**OI**	**Obturator internus**
BC	Body of clitoris	**Ov**	**Ovary**
CC	Crus of clitoris	ONV	Obturator nerve and vessels
EA	External iliac artery	Pd	Pudendal nerve and vessels
EF	Endopelvic fascia	Pec	Pectineus
EV	External iliac vein	PIR	Piriformis
FA	Femoral artery	**Pm**	**Perineal membrane**
FN	Femoral nerve	**Pu**	**Pubic bone**
FV	Femoral vein	QF	Quadratus femoris
GC	Gluteal cleft	**R**	**Rectum**
HdF	Head of femur	RA	Rectus abdominis
I	Ilium	**RF**	**Recto-uterine fold**
IAF	**Ischio-anal fossa**	**RL**	**Round ligament**
IE	Inferior epigastric vessels	**S**	**Sacrum**
In	Intestine	SP	Superior ramus of pubis
IP	Iliopsoas	Sy	Pubic symphysis
IPR	Ischiopubic ramus	**U**	**Uterus**
IT	Ischial tuberosity	**UB**	**Urinary bladder**
LA	**Levator ani**	**Ur**	**Urethra**
Lin	Linea alba	**V**	**Vagina**
LM	**Labia majus**	**Ve**	**Vestibule**

3.72   TRANSVERSE (AXIAL) MRIs AND SECTIONAL SPECIMENS OF FEMALE PELVIS AND PERINEUM, INFERIOR VIEWS

A.–C. MRIs.

D

E

ANTERIOR

RIGHT · LEFT

POSTERIOR

F

G

3.72 TRANSVERSE (AXIAL) MRIs AND SECTIONAL SPECIMENS OF FEMALE PELVIS
AND PERINEUM, INFERIOR VIEWS (CONTINUED)

D. and F. MRIs. **E. and G.** Anatomical sections.

A

B

SUPERIOR

RIGHT ← → LEFT

INFERIOR

BL	**Broad ligament**	OE	Obturator externus
E	**Endometrium**	**OI**	**Obturator internus**
F	**Ovarian follicle**	P	Pectineus
FU	**Fundus of uterus**	**PM**	**Perineal membrane**
HdF	Head of femur	**S**	**Sigmoid colon**
I	Ilium	**Sc**	**Sacrum**
IA	Internal iliac artery	SI	Sacro-iliac joint
IV	Internal iliac vein	**U**	**Urethra**
IS	**Internal urethral sphincter**	**UB**	**Urinary bladder**
LS	Lumbosacral trunk	**Ut**	**Uterus**
M	**Myometrium**	**V**	**Vagina**
O	**Ovary**		

3.73 CORONAL MRIs OF FEMALE PELVIS AND PERINEUM, ANTERIOR VIEWS

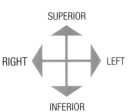

Urinary bladder (distended) (1)

Vagina (2)

Cervix (3)

Intestine (4)

Fundus of uterus (5)

Endometrium (6)

Myometrium (7)

V.Oxorn

A. Longitudinal Section

ANTERIOR

INFERIOR ← → SUPERIOR

POSTERIOR

Longitudinal US Section

3.74 ULTRASOUND SCANS OF FEMALE PELVIS

A. Median (transabdominal) ultrasound scan and orientation drawing (numbers in parentheses correspond to labels on the ultrasound scan).

B. Transverse (Axial) Scan

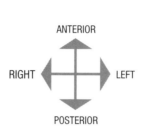

ANTERIOR

RIGHT | LEFT

POSTERIOR

C. Transverse (Axial) Scan

Urinary bladder (distended) (*1*)

Broad ligament (*6*)

Right ovary (*2*)

Left ovary (*7*)

Broad ligament (*3*)

Ovarian follicle (*8*)

Uterus (*4*)

Endometrium and endometrial canal (*9*)

Intestine (*5*)

Myometrium (*10*)

V.Oxorn

B and C

D

D. Sagittal Scan

3.74 **ULTRASOUND SCANS OF FEMALE PELVIS** *(CONTINUED)*

B. and C. Transabdominal axial (transverse) scan through uterus and ovaries. **Transabdominal US scanning** requires a fully distended urinary bladder to displace the bowel loops from the pelvis and to provide an acoustical window through which to observe pelvic anatomy.

D. Transvaginal sagittal scan of left ovary (numbers in parentheses correspond to labels on the ultrasound scans). **Transvaginal and transrectal ultrasonography** enables the placing of the probe closer to the structures of interest, allowing increased resolution.

A. Coronal Section

B. Hysterosalpingogram of Normal Uterus, Anteroposterior View

KEY for B:		
UC Uterine cavity	P Pararectal fossae	VS Vaginal speculum
▲▲ Uterine tubes	C Catheter in cervical canal	

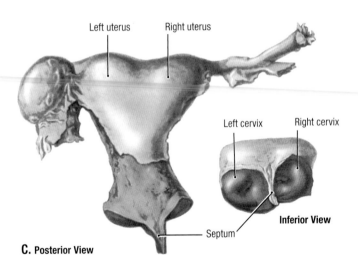

C. Posterior View

Inferior View

D. Hysterosalpingogram of Bicornate Uterus, Anteroposterior View

KEY for D:		
1 and 2 Uterine cavities	F Uterine tubes	
E Cervical canal	I Isthmus of uterine tubes	

3.75   RADIOGRAPH OF UTERUS AND UTERINE TUBES (HYSTEROSALPINGOGRAM)

A. Coronal section of uterus. **B.** During *hysterosalpingography*, radiopaque material is injected into the uterus through external os of the uterus. If normal, contrast medium travels through the triangular uterine cavity (UC) and uterine tubes (*arrowheads*) and passes into the pararectal fossae *(P)* of the peritoneal cavity. The female genital tract is in direct communication with the peritoneal cavity and is, therefore, a potential pathway for the spread of an infection from the vagina and uterus. **C.** Illustration of duplicated uterus. **D.** Hysterosalpingogram of a bicornate ("two-horned") uterus.

Back

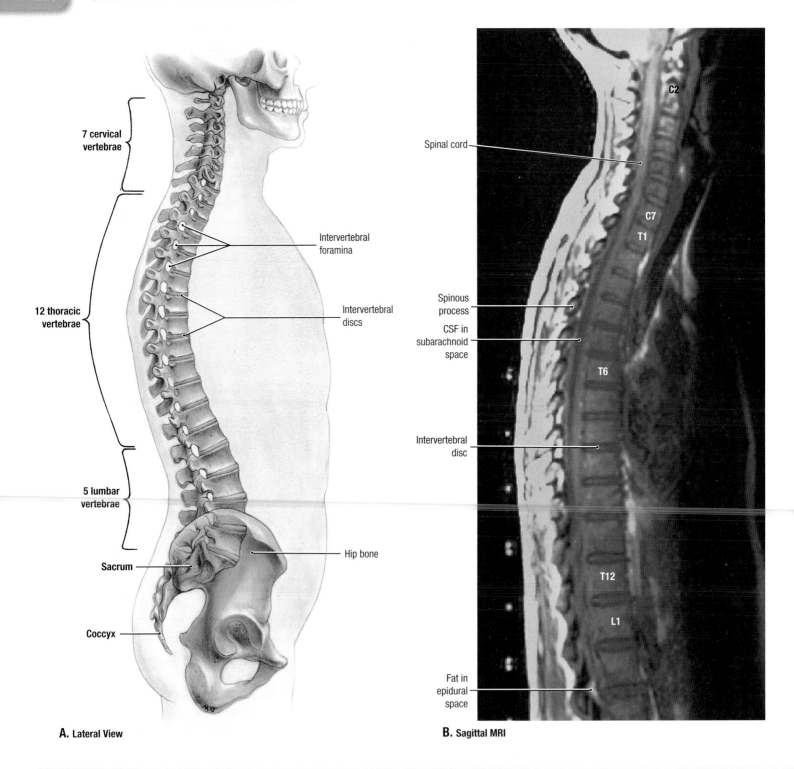

A. Lateral View

B. Sagittal MRI

4.1 **OVERVIEW OF VERTEBRAL COLUMN**

A. Vertebral column showing articulation with skull and hip bone. **B.** Sagittal MRI, lateral view.

- The vertebral column usually consists of 24 separate (presacral) vertebrae, 5 fused vertebrae in the sacrum, and variably 4 fused or separate coccygeal vertebrae. Of the 24 separate vertebrae, 12 support ribs (thoracic), 7 are in the neck (cervical), and 5 are in the lumbar region (lumbar).
- Vertebrae contributing to the posterior walls of the thoracic and pelvic cavities are concave anteriorly; elsewhere (in the cervical and lumbar regions) they are convex anteriorly.

- The spinal nerves exit the vertebral (spinal) canal via the intervertebral (IV) foramina. There are 8 cervical, 12 thoracic, 5 lumbar, 5 sacral, and 1 to 2 coccygeal spinal nerves.
- Note the size and shape of the vertebral bodies, the direction of the spinous processes, cerebrospinal fluid (CSF) in the subarachnoid space, and the spinal cord in the vertebral canal (in **B**).

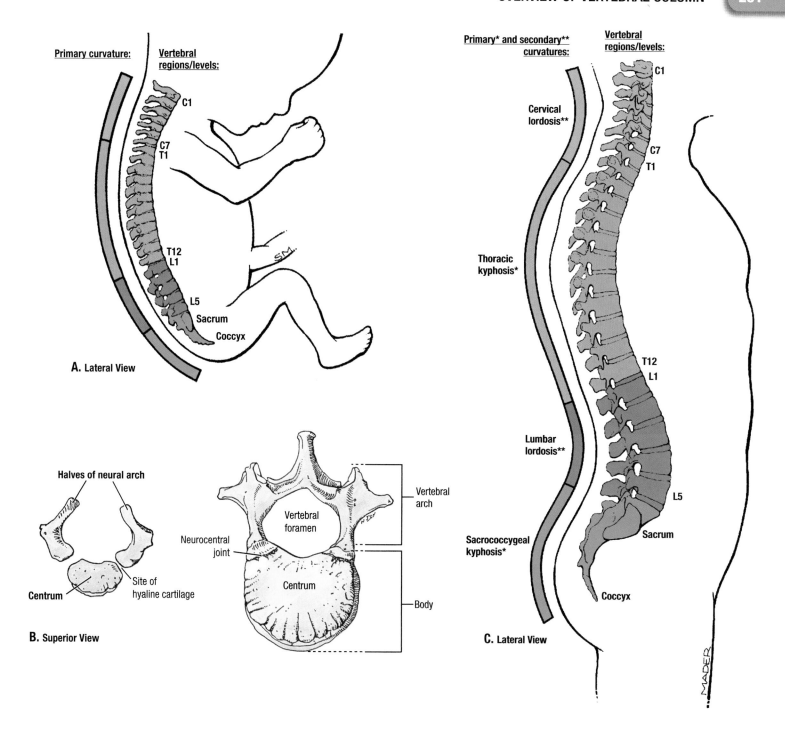

A. Lateral View

B. Superior View

Halves of neural arch

Centrum

Site of hyaline cartilage

Neurocentral joint

Vertebral foramen

Centrum

Vertebral arch

Body

Primary curvature:

Vertebral regions/levels:

C1

C7
T1

T12
L1

L5

Sacrum

Coccyx

Primary* and secondary** curvatures:

Vertebral regions/levels:

Cervical lordosis**

Thoracic kyphosis*

Lumbar lordosis**

Sacrococcygeal kyphosis*

C1

C7
T1

T12
L1

L5

Sacrum

Coccyx

C. Lateral View

4.2   CURVATURES OF VERTEBRAL COLUMN

A. Fetus. Note the C-shaped curvature of the fetal spine, which is concave anteriorly over its entire length. **B.** Development of the vertebrae. At birth, a vertebra consists of three bony parts (two halves of the neural arch and the centrum) united by hyaline cartilage. At age 2, the halves of each neural arch begin to fuse, proceeding from the lumbar to the cervical region; at approximately age 7, the arches begin to fuse to the centrum, proceeding from the cervical to lumbar regions. **C.** Adult. The four curvatures of the adult vertebral column include the cervical lordosis, which is convex anteriorly and lies between vertebrae C1 and T2; the thoracic kyphosis, which is concave anteriorly, between vertebrae T2 and T12; the lumbar lordosis, convex anteriorly and lying between T12 and the lumbosacral joint; and the sacrococcygeal kyphosis, concave anteriorly and spanning from the lumbosacral joint to the tip of the coccyx. The anteriorly concave thoracic kyphosis and sacrococcygeal kyphosis are primary curves, and the anteriorly convex cervical lordosis and lumbar lordosis are secondary curves that develop after birth. The cervical lordosis develops when the child begins to hold the head up, and the lumbar kyphosis develops when the child begins to walk.

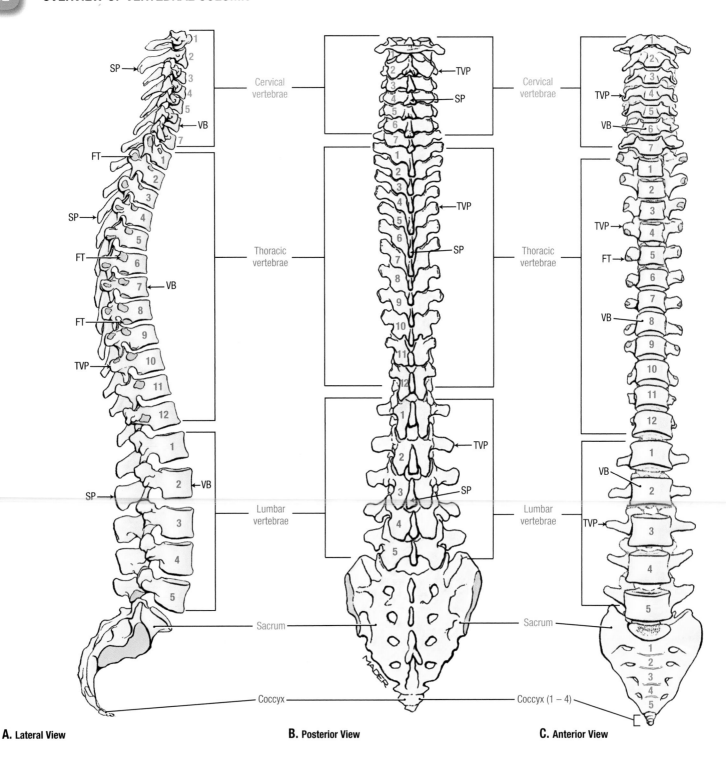

A. Lateral View

B. Posterior View

C. Anterior View

| 4.3 | THREE VIEWS OF VERTEBRAL COLUMN |

- The vertebral bodies (*VB*) vary in size and shape.
- Transverse processes (*TVP*) in the cervical region are directed laterally, inferiorly, and anteriorly. In the thoracic region, the vertebrae have facets for articulation with the ribs (*FT*); the TVPs are directed laterally, posteriorly, and superiorly; and are stout. In the lumbar region, the TVPs point laterally and are long and slender.

- Generally, spinous processes (*SP*) are bifid in Caucasians in the cervical region, long and spinelike in the thoracic region, and stout and oblong in the lumbar region. The cervical and thoracic SPs often overlap the adjacent, inferior vertebrae.

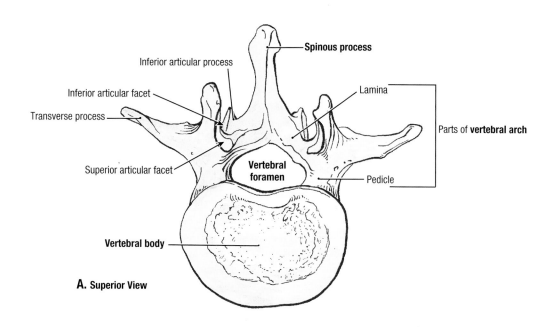

Inferior articular process

Spinous process

Inferior articular facet

Lamina

Transverse process

Parts of **vertebral arch**

Superior articular facet

Vertebral foramen

Pedicle

Vertebral body

A. **Superior View**

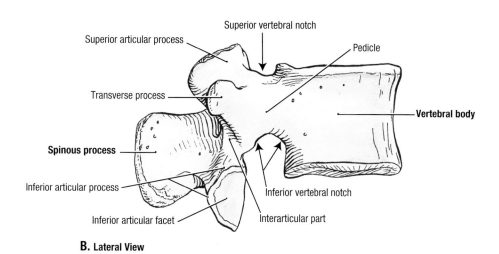

Superior articular process

Superior vertebral notch

Pedicle

Transverse process

Vertebral body

Spinous process

Inferior articular process

Inferior vertebral notch

Inferior articular facet

Interarticular part

B. **Lateral View**

4.4   TYPICAL VERTEBRA

A typical vertebra (e.g., the 2nd lumbar vertebra) consists of the following parts:

- A vertebral body, situated anteriorly, functions to support weight.
- The vertebral arch consists of two columnar pedicles, one on each side, which arise from the body, and two flat plates called laminae that unite posteriorly in the midline. The vertebral foramen is enclosed by the vertebral body and arch. Collectively, the vertebral foramina constitute the vertebral canal, in which the spinal cord lies. The function of a vertebral arch is to protect the spinal cord.

- Three processes, two transverse and one spinous, provide attachment for muscles and are the levers that help move the vertebrae.
- Four articular processes, two superior and two inferior, each have an articular facet. The articular processes project superiorly and inferiorly from the vertebral arch and come into apposition with the articular facet of the corresponding processes of the vertebrae above and below. The direction of the articular facets determines the nature of the movement between adjacent vertebrae.

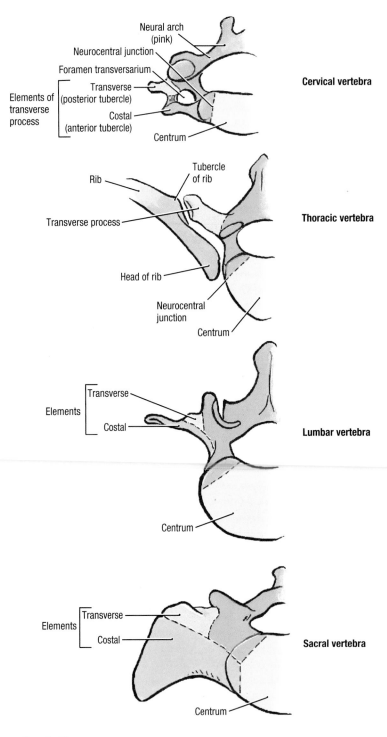

Superior Views

4.5   HOMOLOGOUS PARTS OF VERTEBRAE

A rib is a free costal element in the thoracic region; in the cervical and lumbar regions, it is represented by the anterior part of a transverse process, and in the sacrum, by the anterior part of the lateral mass. The heads of the ribs (thoracic region) articulate with the sides of the vertebral bodies posterior to the neurocentral junction and the tubercles of the ribs articulate with the transverse processes of the vertebrae.

Cervical vertebrae

Uncus of body (uncinate process)

Superior articular facet

Foramen transversarium

Uncus of body (uncinate process)

Zygapophysial (facet) joint

Inferior articular facet

Thoracic vertebrae

Superior articular facet

Facet for tubercle of rib

Superior articular facet

Zygapophysial (facet) joint

Facets for head of rib

Inferior articular facet

→ flexion
← extension
↓ lateral flexion to right
↑ lateral flexion to left
↻ rotation to left
↻ rotation to right

Lumbar vertebrae

Transverse process

Superior articular facet

Zygapophysial (facet) joint

Inferior articular facet

Superior Views - arrows indicate direction of movement of superior adjacent vertebra (not shown) relative to the inferior vertebra (shown here)

Lateral Views - arrows indicate direction of movement of the superior and inferior vertebra relative to each other

4.6   VERTEBRAL FEATURES AND MOVEMENTS

Direction of movement is indicated by *arrows*.

- In the thoracic and lumbar regions, the articular processes/facets lie posterior to the vertebral bodies and in the cervical region posterolateral to the bodies. Superior articular facets in the cervical region face mainly superiorly, in the thoracic region, mainly posteriorly, and in the lumbar region, mainly medially. The change in direction is gradual from cervical to thoracic but abrupt from thoracic to lumbar.

- Although movements between adjacent vertebrae are relatively small, especially in the thoracic region, the summation of all the small movements produces a considerable range of movement of the vertebral column as a whole.

- Movements of the vertebral column are freer (have greater range of motion) in the cervical and lumbar regions than in the thoracic region. Lateral bending is freest in the cervical and lumbar regions; flexion of the vertebral column is greatest in the cervical region; extension is most marked in the lumbar region, but the interlocking articular processes prevent rotation.

- The thoracic region is most stable because of the external support gained from the articulations of the ribs and costal cartilages with the sternum. The direction of the articular facets permits rotation, but flexion, extension, and lateral bending are severely restricted.

A. Lateral View

B. Lateral View

C. Lateral View

D. Lateral View

E. Anterior View

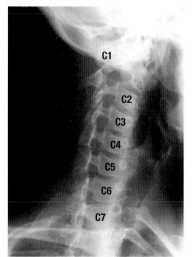

F. Oblique View

4.7   SURFACE ANATOMY WITH RADIOGRAPHIC CORRELATION OF SELECTED MOVEMENTS OF THE CERVICAL SPINE

A. Extension of the neck. **B.** Radiograph of the extended cervical spine. **C.** Flexion of the neck. **D.** Radiograph of the flexed cervical spine. **E.** Head turned (rotated) to left. **F.** Radiograph of cervical spine rotated to left.

A. Lateral View

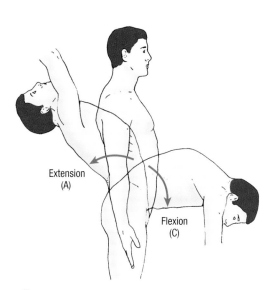

Extension
(A)

Flexion
(C)

B. Lateral View

L1
L2
L3
L4
L5

C. Lateral View

Lateral flexion
(E)

D. Anterior View

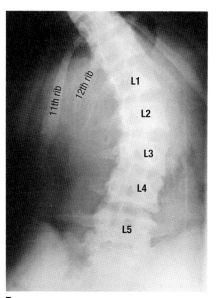

11th rib
12th rib

L1
L2
L3
L4
L5

E. Anteroposterior View

4.8 SURFACE ANATOMY WITH RADIOGRAPHIC CORRELATION OF SELECTED MOVEMENTS OF THE LUMBAR SPINE

A. Radiograph of the extended lumbar spine. **B.** Flexion and extension of the trunk. **C.** Radiograph of the flexed lumbar spine. **D.** Lateral flexion (side flexion) of the trunk. **E.** Radiograph of the lumbar spine during lateral bending.

The range of movement of the vertebral column is limited by the thickness, elasticity, and compressibility of the IV discs; shape and orientation of the zygapophysial joints; tension of the joint capsules of the zygapophysial joints; resistance of the ligaments and back muscles; connection to thoracic (rib) cage and bulk of surrounding tissue.

Posterior tubercle
Posterior arch
Superior articular facet
Foramen transversarium
Transverse process
Anterior arch
Anterior tubercle
Atlas (C1)

Inferior articular process
Transverse process
Superior articular facet
Dens (odontoid process)
Axis (C2)

Transverse process:
Posterior tubercle
Groove for spinal nerve
Anterior tubercle
C3

Foramen transversarium
C4

Spinous process
Uncus of body (uncinate process)
Body
C5

Articular process
Inferior
Superior
C6

C7

Superior Views

TABLE 4.1 TYPICAL CERVICAL VERTEBRAE (C3–C7)a

Part	Distinctive Characteristics
Body	Small and wider from side to side than anteroposteriorly; superior surface is concave with an uncus of body (uncinate process bilaterally); inferior surface is convex
Vertebral foramen	Large and triangular
Transverse processes	Foramina transversaria small or absent in vertebra C7; vertebral arteries and accompanying venous and sympathetic plexuses pass through foramina, except C7 foramina, which transmits only small accessory vertebral veins; anterior and posterior tubercles separated by groove for spinal nerve
Articular processes	Superior articular facets directed superoposteriorly; inferior articular facets directed infero-anteriorly; obliquely placed facets are most nearly horizontal in this region
Spinous process	Short (C3–C5) and bifid, only in Caucasians (C3–C5); process of C6 is long but that of C7 is longer; C7 is called "vertebra prominens"

aC1 and C2 vertebrae are atypical.

4.9   CERVICAL VERTEBRAE

The bodies of the cervical vertebrae can be dislocated in neck injuries with less force than is required to fracture them. Because of the large vertebral canal in the cervical region, slight dislocation can occur without damaging the spinal cord. When a cervical vertebra is severely dislocated, it injures the spinal cord. If the dislocation does not result in "facet jumping" with locking of the displaced articular processes, the cervical vertebrae may self-reduce ("slip back into place") so that a radiograph may not indicate that the cord has been injured. MRI may reveal the resulting soft tissue damage.

Aging of the IV disc combined with the changing shape of the vertebrae results in an increase in compressive forces at the periphery of the vertebral bodies, where the disc attaches. In response **osteophytes** (bony spurs) commonly develop around the margins of the vertebral body, especially along the outer attachment of the IV disc. Similarly, as altered mechanics place greater stresses on the zygapophysial joints, osteophytes develop along the attachments of the joint capsules, especially those of the superior articular process.

Atlas (C1) — Anterior arch / Anterior tubercle — C1

C2

Uncovertebral joint

Dens — **Axis (C2)**
Body

Uncovertebral joint

C3

Transverse process — Anterior tubercle / Posterior tubercle / Groove for spinal nerve

C4

Uncus of body (uncinate process)

C5

C6

C7

A. Anterior View

Posterior arch

Posterior tubercle

Anterior tubercle of **atlas (C1)**

Axis (C2)

Zygapophysial joint

Column of articular processes

Anterior tubercle

Groove for spinal nerve

Lamina

Posterior tubercle

Spinous processes

C7

B. Lateral View

External occipital protuberance

Posterior atlanto-occipital membrane

C1

Posterior arch of atlas

Nuchal ligament

Interspinous ligament

Supraspinous ligament

Ligamentum flavum

Spinous process of C7 vertebra

C7

Anterior longitudinal ligament

C. Lateral View

4.10   CERVICAL SPINE

A. and B. Articulated cervical vertebrae. **C.** Ligaments.

A. Anteroposterior View

Uncinate process of body of C5

Uncovertebral joint

Pedicle

1st rib

Transverse process of T2

Clavicle

Spinous process of T2

C3

C7

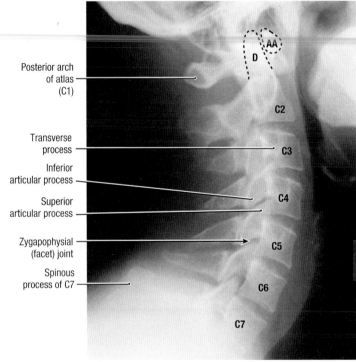

B. Lateral View

Posterior arch of atlas (C1)

Transverse process

Inferior articular process

Superior articular process

Zygapophysial (facet) joint

Spinous process of C7

AA

D

C2

C3

C4

C5

C6

C7

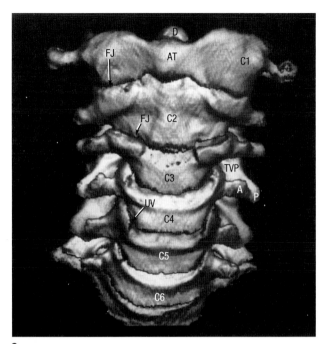

C. Anterior View

D

FJ   AT   C1

FJ   C2

TVP

C3   A   P

UV   C4

C5

C6

A	Anterior tubercle of transverse process	PA	Posterior arch of C1
AA	Anterior arch of C1	PT	Posterior tubercle of C1
AT	Anterior tubercle of C1	SF	Superior articular facet of C1
C1–C7	Vertebrae	SP	Spinous process
D	Dens (odontoid) process of C2	T	Foramen transversarium
FJ	Zygapophysial (facet) joint	TVP	Transverse process
La	Lamina	UV	Uncovertebral joint
P	Posterior tubercle of transverse process	VC	Vertebral canal

D. Posterior View

AT

AA   AA

D

T   C1   T

SF

VC

PA   PA

PT

C2   C3

La   La

FJ   C4

SP

4.11   IMAGING OF THE CERVICAL SPINE

A. and B. Radiographs. The arrowheads demarcate the margins of the *(black)* column of air in the trachea.
C. and D. Three-dimensional (3D) reconstructed computed tomographic (CT) images.

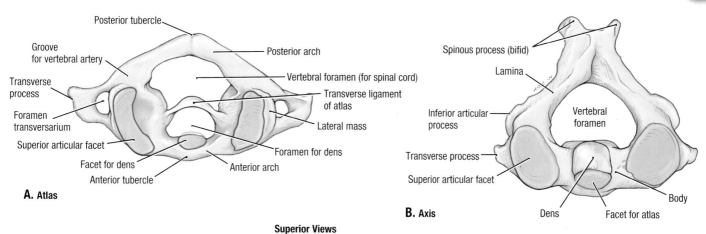

A. Atlas

Posterior tubercle
Posterior arch
Groove for vertebral artery
Vertebral foramen (for spinal cord)
Transverse process
Transverse ligament of atlas
Foramen transversarium
Lateral mass
Superior articular facet
Foramen for dens
Facet for dens
Anterior arch
Anterior tubercle

B. Axis

Spinous process (bifid)
Lamina
Inferior articular process
Vertebral foramen
Transverse process
Superior articular facet
Body
Dens
Facet for atlas

Superior Views

C. Anteroposterior View

Atlanto-occipital joints
Median atlanto-axial joint
Lateral atlanto-axial joints

A	Lateral mass of atlas
D	Dens of axis
C2	Axis

D

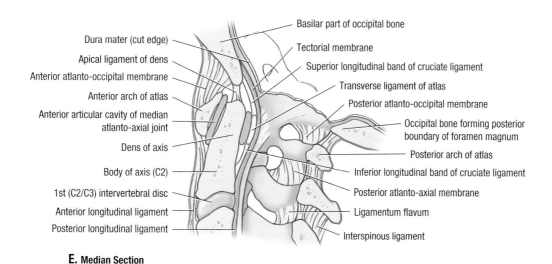

Dura mater (cut edge)
Basilar part of occipital bone
Apical ligament of dens
Tectorial membrane
Anterior atlanto-occipital membrane
Superior longitudinal band of cruciate ligament
Anterior arch of atlas
Transverse ligament of atlas
Anterior articular cavity of median atlanto-axial joint
Posterior atlanto-occipital membrane
Dens of axis
Occipital bone forming posterior boundary of foramen magnum
Body of axis (C2)
Posterior arch of atlas
1st (C2/C3) intervertebral disc
Inferior longitudinal band of cruciate ligament
Anterior longitudinal ligament
Posterior atlanto-axial membrane
Posterior longitudinal ligament
Ligamentum flavum
Interspinous ligament

E. Median Section

4.12 ATLAS AND AXIS AND THE ATLANTO-AXIAL JOINT

A. Atlas. **B.** Axis. **C.** Radiograph taken through the open mouth. **D.** Articulated atlas and axis. **E.** Median section with ligaments.

Occipital bone

Anterior atlanto-occipital membrane

Joint capsule of atlanto-occipital joint

Atlas

Joint capsule of lateral atlanto-axial joint

Anterior atlanto-axial membrane

Axis

A. Anterior View

Anterior longitudinal ligament

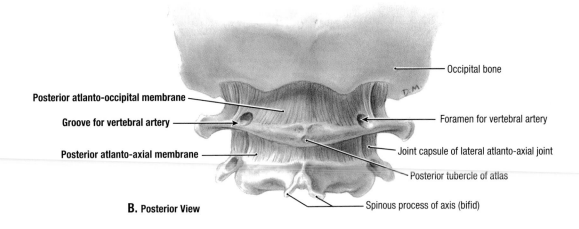

Occipital bone

Posterior atlanto-occipital membrane

Groove for vertebral artery

Foramen for vertebral artery

Posterior atlanto-axial membrane

Joint capsule of lateral atlanto-axial joint

Posterior tubercle of atlas

B. Posterior View

Spinous process of axis (bifid)

Basilar artery

Foramen magnum (dashed line)

Vertebral artery traversing foramina transversaria

Atlas

Tectorial membrane

Posterior arch of atlas

Axis

C. Posterior View

4.13 **CRANIOVERTEBRAL JOINTS AND VERTEBRAL ARTERY**

A. Anterior atlanto-axial and atlanto-occipital membranes. The anterior longitudinal ligament ascends to blend with, and form a central thickening in, the anterior atlanto-axial and atlanto-occipital membranes. **B.** Posterior atlanto-axial and atlanto-occipital membranes. Inferior to the axis (C2 vertebra), ligamenta flava occur in this position. **C.** Tectorial membrane and vertebral artery. The tectorial membrane is a superior continuation of the posterior longitudinal ligament superior to the body of the axis. After coursing through the foramina transversaria of vertebrae C6–C1, the vertebral arteries turn medially, grooving the superior aspect of the posterior arch of the atlas and piercing the posterior atlanto-occipital membrane (**B**). The right and left vertebral arteries traverse the foramen magnum and merge intracranially, forming the basilar artery.

Dorsum sellae

Oculomotor nerve (CN III)

Trochlear nerve (CN IV)

Trigeminal nerve (CN V)

Abducent nerve (CN VI)

Facial nerve (CN VII)

Intermediate nerve (CN VII)

Vestibulocochlear nerve (CN VIII)

Glossopharyngeal nerve (CN IX)

Vagus nerve (CN X)

Spinal accessory nerve (CN XI)

Tectorial membrane

Hypoglossal nerve (CN XII)

Cruciform ligament

Superior band

Transverse ligament of atlas (transverse band)

Inferior band

Alar ligament

Spinal nerve C1

Vertebral artery

Accessory atlanto-axial ligament

Post ramus of spinal nerve C1

Posterior arch of atlas (cut)

Tectorial membrane
(reflected)

A. Posterior View

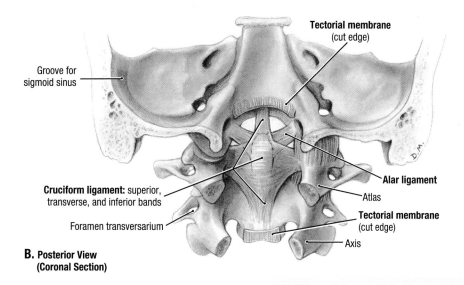

Tectorial membrane
(cut edge)

Groove for
sigmoid sinus

Alar ligament

Cruciform ligament: superior,
transverse, and inferior bands

Atlas

Tectorial membrane
(cut edge)

Foramen transversarium

Axis

B. Posterior View
(Coronal Section)

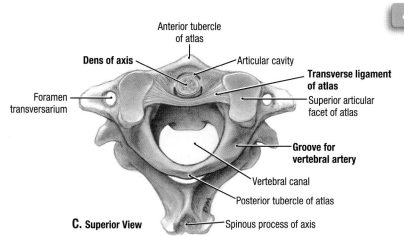

Anterior tubercle
of atlas

Dens of axis

Articular cavity

**Transverse ligament
of atlas**

Foramen
transversarium

Superior articular
facet of atlas

**Groove for
vertebral artery**

Vertebral canal

Posterior tubercle of atlas

C. Superior View

Spinous process of axis

4.14   LIGAMENTS OF ATLANTO-OCCIPITAL AND
ATLANTO-AXIAL JOINTS

A. Cranial nerves and dura mater of posterior cranial fossa with dura mater
and tentorial membrane incised and removed to reveal the medial atlanto-
axial joint. **B.** The alar ligaments serve as check ligaments for the rotary
movements of the atlanto-axial joints. **B. and C.** The transverse ligament of
the atlas, the transverse band of the cruciform ligament, provides the posterior wall of a socket that receives the dens of the axis, forming a pivot joint.

Fracture of atlas. The atlas is a bony ring, with two wedge-
shaped lateral masses, connected by relatively thin anterior and
posterior arches and the transverse ligament of the atlas (see Figs.
4.12A & C). Vertical forces (e.g., striking the head on bottom of pool)
may force the lateral masses apart fracturing one or both of the anterior or posterior arches. If the force is sufficient, rupture of the transverse ligament of the atlas will also occur.

B. Median Section

TABLE 4.2 THORACIC VERTEBRAE

Part	Distinctive Characteristics
Body	Heart shaped; has one or two costal facets for articulation with head of rib
Vertebral foramen	Circular and smaller than those of cervical and lumbar vertebrae
Transverse processes	Long and extend posterolaterally; length diminishes from T1 to T12; T1–T10 have transverse costal facets for articulation with a tubercle of ribs 1–10 (ribs 11 and 12 have no tubercle and do not articulate with a transverse process)
Articular processes	Superior articular facets directed posteriorly and slightly laterally; inferior articular facets directed anteriorly and slightly medially
Spinous process	Long and slopes postero-inferiorly; tip extends to level of vertebral body below

4.15   THORACIC VERTEBRAE

A. Features. **B.** MRI scan of thoracic spine, median section.

Transverse process

Spinous process

Lamina

Vertebral foramen

Pedicle

Vertebral body

T1 **T2** **T3** **T4**

Superior four thoracic vertebrae (T1-T4)

T5 **T6** **T7** **T8**

Middle four thoracic vertebrae (T5-T8)

T9 **T10** **T11** **T12**

C. Superior Views

Inferior four thoracic vertebrae (T9-T12)

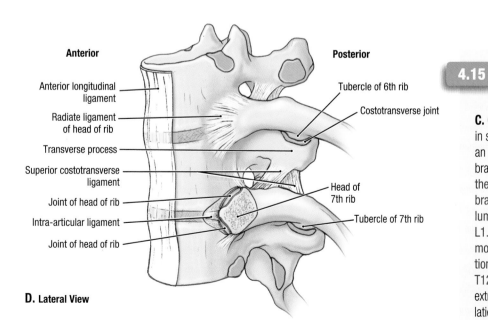

Anterior

Posterior

Anterior longitudinal ligament

Radiate ligament of head of rib

Transverse process

Superior costotransverse ligament

Joint of head of rib

Intra-articular ligament

Joint of head of rib

Tubercle of 6th rib

Costotransverse joint

Head of 7th rib

Tubercle of 7th rib

D. Lateral View

| 4.15 | **THORACIC VERTEBRAE** (*CONTINUED*) |

C. Comparative anatomy. The vertebral bodies increase in size as the vertebral column descends, each bearing an increasing amount of weight transferred by the vertebra above. **Fracture of thoracic vertebrae**. Although the characteristics of the superior aspect of vertebra T12 are distinctly thoracic, its inferior aspect has lumbar characteristics for articulation with vertebra L1. The abrupt transition allowing primarily rotational movements with vertebra T11 while disallowing rotational movements with vertebral L1 makes vertebra T12 especially susceptible to fracture. **D.** Intra- and extra-articular ligaments of the costovertebral articulations. Typically, the head of each rib articulates with the bodies of two adjacent vertebrae and the IV disc between them, and the tubercle of the rib articulates with the transverse process of the inferior vertebra.

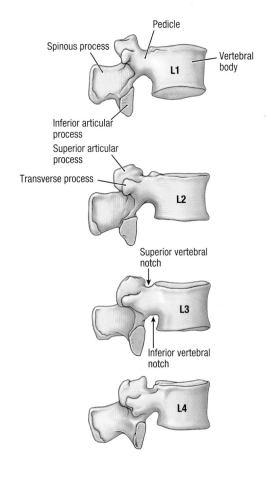

Pedicle

Spinous process

Vertebral body

L1

Inferior articular process

Superior articular process

Transverse process

L2

Superior vertebral notch

L3

Inferior vertebral notch

L4

L5

A. Lateral Views

B. Lateral View

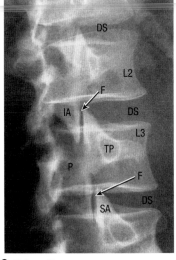

C. Oblique View

TABLE 4.3 LUMBAR VERTEBRAE

Part	Distinctive Characteristics
Body	Massive; kidney shaped when viewed superiorly
Vertebral	Triangular; larger than in thoracic vertebrae and foramen smaller than in cervical vertebrae
Transverse	Long and slender; accessory process on posterior surface of base of each transverse process
Articular processes	Superior articular facets directed posteromedially (or medially); inferior articular facets directed anterolaterally (or laterally); mammillary process on posterior surface of each superior articular process
Spinous process	Short and sturdy; thick, broad, and rectangular

4.16   LUMBAR VERTEBRAE

A, E, and F. Features. **B, C, and D.** Radiographs **G.** Laminectomy. A **laminectomy** is the surgical excision of one or more spinous processes and their supporting laminae in a particular region of the vertebral column (number 1 in **G.**). The term is also commonly used to denote the removal of most of the vertebral arch by transecting the pedicles (number 2 in **G.**). Laminectomies provide access to the vertebral canal to relieve pressure on the spinal cord or nerve roots, commonly caused by a tumor or herniated IV disc.

Key for B, C and D

F	Zygapophysial (facet) joint	P	Pedicle
DS	Intervertebral disc space	SA	Superior articular process
IA	Inferior articular process	SP	Spinous process
IV	Intervertebral foramen	T12–L5	Vertebral bodies
L	Lamina	TP	Transverse process

D. Superior View

E. Superior View

F. Posterior View

G. Superior View, Sites of Laminectomy (1 and 2)

4.16 LUMBAR VERTEBRAE (*CONTINUED*)

Superior vertebral notch

Superior articular process

Intervertebral (IV) foramen

Intervertebral (IV) disc

Joint capsule of zygapophysial (facet) joint

Ligamentum flavum

Anulus fibrosus of IV disc (dissected to show lamellae)

Inferior articular facet

A. Lateral View

Inferior vertebral notch

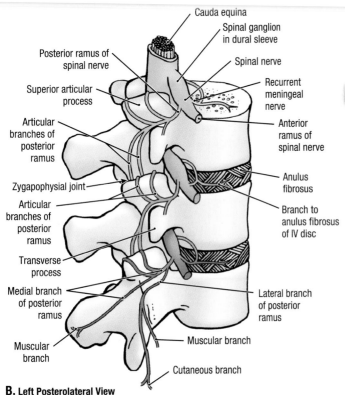

Cauda equina

Spinal ganglion in dural sleeve

Posterior ramus of spinal nerve

Spinal nerve

Superior articular process

Recurrent meningeal nerve

Articular branches of posterior ramus

Anterior ramus of spinal nerve

Zygapophysial joint

Anulus fibrosus

Articular branches of posterior ramus

Branch to anulus fibrosus of IV disc

Transverse process

Medial branch of posterior ramus

Lateral branch of posterior ramus

Muscular branch

Muscular branch

Cutaneous branch

B. Left Posterolateral View

4.17   STRUCTURE AND INNERVATION OF INTERVERTEBRAL DISCS AND ZYGAPOPHYSIAL JOINTS

A. Intervertebral discs and intervertebral foramen. Sections have been removed from the superficial layers of the anulus fibrosus of the inferior IV disc to show the change in direction of the fibers in the concentric layers of the anulus. Note that the IV discs form the inferior half of the anterior boundary of the IV foramen. **B.** Innervation of zygapophysial joints and the anulus fibrosus of IV discs.

When the **zygapophysial joints are injured** or develop osteophytes during aging (osteoarthritis), the related spinal nerves are affected. This causes pain along the distribution pattern of the dermatomes and spasm in the muscles derived from the associated myotomes (a myotome consists of all the muscles or parts of muscles receiving innervation from one spinal nerve). Denervation of lumbar zygapophysial joints is a procedure that may be used for treatment of back pain caused by disease of these joints. The nerves are sectioned near the joints or are destroyed by radiofrequency percutaneous rhizolysis (root dissolution). The denervation process is directed at the articular branches of two adjacent posterior rami of the spinal nerves because each joint receives innervation from both the nerve exiting that level and the superjacent nerve.

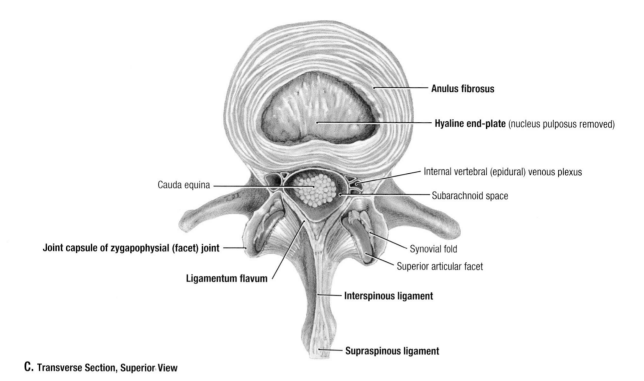

Anulus fibrosus

Hyaline end-plate (nucleus pulposus removed)

Internal vertebral (epidural) venous plexus

Cauda equina

Subarachnoid space

Joint capsule of zygapophysial (facet) joint

Synovial fold

Superior articular facet

Ligamentum flavum

Interspinous ligament

Supraspinous ligament

C. Transverse Section, Superior View

Left common iliac artery

Zygapophysial (facet) joints

L4-L5 Intervertebral IV disc

Psoas major

Superior articular process of L4 vertebra

Cauda equina in lumbar cistern

Lamina

Inferior articular process of L5 vertebra

Spinous process

D. Transverse (Axial) CT Scan

4.17   STRUCTURE AND INNERVATION OF INTERVERTEBRAL DISCS AND ZYGAPOPHYSIAL JOINTS (*CONTINUED*)

C. Transverse section. The nucleus pulposus has been removed, and the cartilaginous epiphysial plate exposed. There are fewer rings of the anulus fibrosus posteriorly, and consequently, this portion of the annulus fibrosus is thinner. The ligamentum flavum, interspinous, and supraspinous ligaments are continuous. **D.** CT image of L4/L5 IV disc.

Superior articular process

T9 vertebra

Zygapophysial (facet) joint

Pedicle (cut)

Ligamentum flavum

Lamina

Pedicle (cut)

Posterior longitudinal ligament

Nucleus pulposus

Anulus fibrosus

Body

Anterior longitudinal ligament

Intervertebral disc

A. Anterior View

4.18   INTERVERTEBRAL DISCS: LIGAMENTS AND MOVEMENTS

A. Anterior longitudinal ligament and ligamenta flava. The pedicles of vertebrae T9 to T11 were sawed through, and the posterior aspect of the bodies is shown in **B.**

B. Posterior longitudinal ligament. **C.** IV disc during loading and movement.

- The anterior and posterior longitudinal ligaments are ligaments of the vertebral bodies; the ligamenta flava are ligaments of the vertebral arches.
- The anterior longitudinal ligament consists of broad, strong, fibrous bands, thickened centrally, that are attached to the IV discs and vertebral bodies

anteriorly and are perforated by the foramina for arteries and veins passing to and from the vertebral bodies.

- The ligamenta flava, composed of elastic fibers, extend between adjacent laminae; right and left ligaments converge in the median plane. They extend laterally to the articular processes, where they blend with the joint capsule of the zygapophysial joints.

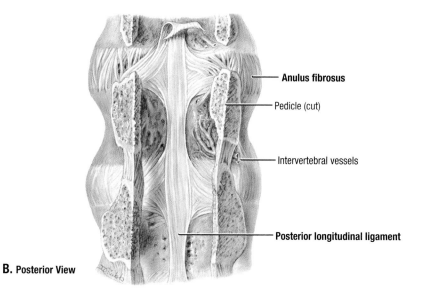

Anulus fibrosus

Pedicle (cut)

Intervertebral vessels

Posterior longitudinal ligament

B. Posterior View

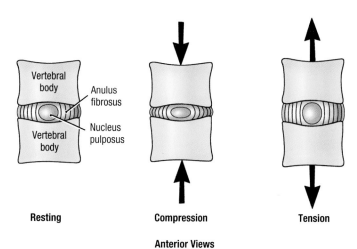

Vertebral body

Anulus fibrosus

Nucleus pulposus

Vertebral body

Resting   Compression   Tension

Anterior Views

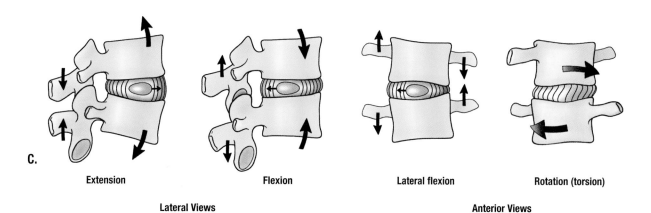

C.

Extension   Flexion   Lateral flexion   Rotation (torsion)

Lateral Views   **Anterior Views**

INTERVERTEBRAL DISCS: LIGAMENTS AND MOVEMENTS (*CONTINUED*)

- The posterior longitudinal ligament is a narrow band passing from disc to disc, spanning the posterior surfaces of the vertebral bodies (in **B**). The ligament is diamond shaped posterior to each IV disc, where it exchanges fibers with the anulus fibrosus; the ligament extends to the sacrum inferiorly and becomes the tectorial membrane cranially.

- The movement or loading of the IV disc changes its shape and the position of the nucleus pulposus. Flexion and extension movements cause compression and tension simultaneously.

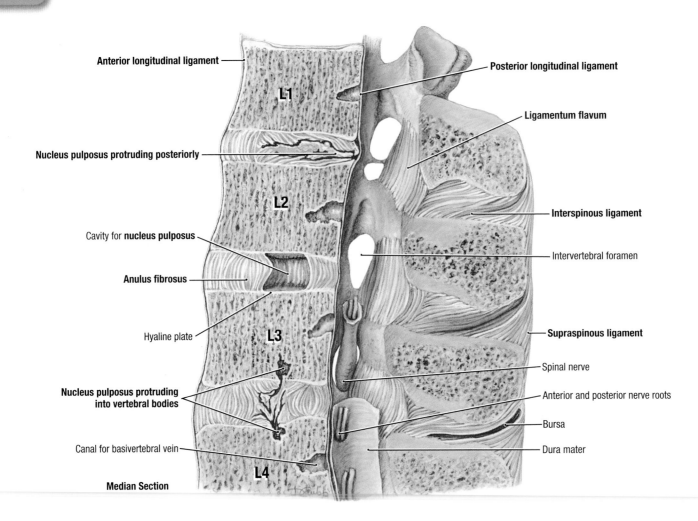

Anterior longitudinal ligament

Nucleus pulposus protruding posteriorly

L1

L2

Cavity for **nucleus pulposus**

Anulus fibrosus

Hyaline plate

L3

Nucleus pulposus protruding into vertebral bodies

Canal for basivertebral vein

L4

Median Section

Posterior longitudinal ligament

Ligamentum flavum

Interspinous ligament

Intervertebral foramen

Supraspinous ligament

Spinal nerve

Anterior and posterior nerve roots

Bursa

Dura mater

4.19   LUMBAR REGION OF VERTEBRAL COLUMN

The nucleus pulposus of the normal disc between vertebrae L2 and L3 has been removed from the enclosing anulus fibrosus.

- The ligamentum flavum extends from the superior border and adjacent part of the posterior aspect of one lamina to the inferior border and adjacent part of the anterior aspect of the lamina above and extends laterally to become continuous with the fibrous capsule of the zygapophysial joint.
- The obliquely placed interspinous ligament unites the superior and inferior borders of two adjacent spines.
- The bursa between L3 and L4 spines is presumably the result of habitual hyperextension, which brings the lumbar spines into contact.

The nucleus pulposus of the disc between L1 and L2 has herniated posteriorly through the anulus. **Herniation** or **protrusion of the gelatinous nucleus pulposus** into or through the anulus fibrosus is a well-recognized cause of low back and lower limb pain. If degeneration of the posterior longitudinal ligament and wearing of the anulus fibrosus has occurred, the nucleus pulposus may herniate into the vertebral canal and compress the spinal cord or nerve roots of spinal nerves in the cauda equina. Herniations usually occur posterolaterally, where the anulus is relatively thin and does not receive support from either the posterior or anterior longitudinal ligaments.

Median section

L1

L2

L3

L4

L5

Sacrum

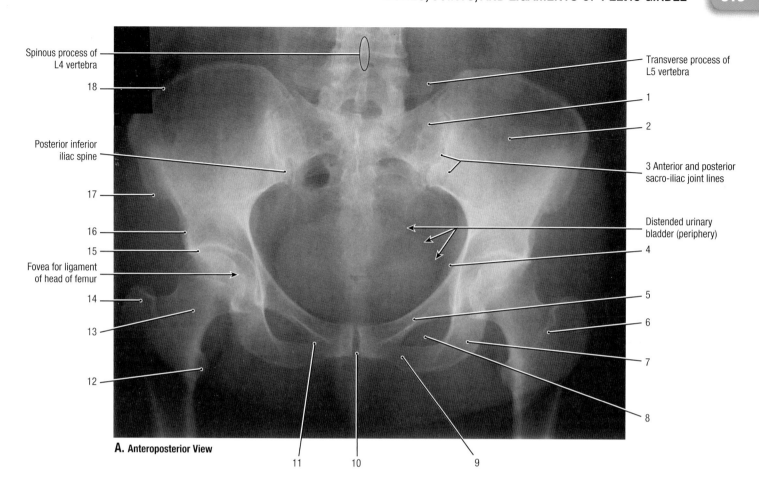

Spinous process of L4 vertebra

Posterior inferior iliac spine

Fovea for ligament of head of femur

18
17
16
15
14
13
12

11   10   9

Transverse process of L5 vertebra

1
2

3 Anterior and posterior sacro-iliac joint lines

Distended urinary bladder (periphery)

4

5
6
7
8

A. Anteroposterior View

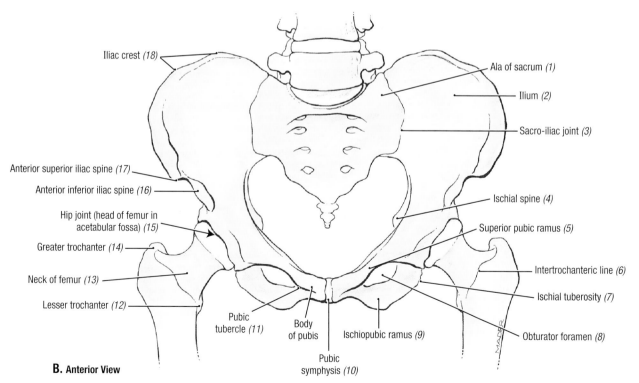

Iliac crest (18)

Anterior superior iliac spine (17)

Anterior inferior iliac spine (16)

Hip joint (head of femur in acetabular fossa) (15)

Greater trochanter (14)

Neck of femur (13)

Lesser trochanter (12)

Pubic tubercle (11)

Body of pubis

Pubic symphysis (10)

Ala of sacrum (1)

Ilium (2)

Sacro-iliac joint (3)

Ischial spine (4)

Superior pubic ramus (5)

Intertrochanteric line (6)

Ischial tuberosity (7)

Obturator foramen (8)

Ischiopubic ramus (9)

B. Anterior View

4.20   **PELVIS**

A. Radiograph of pelvis. **B.** Bony pelvis with articulated femora.

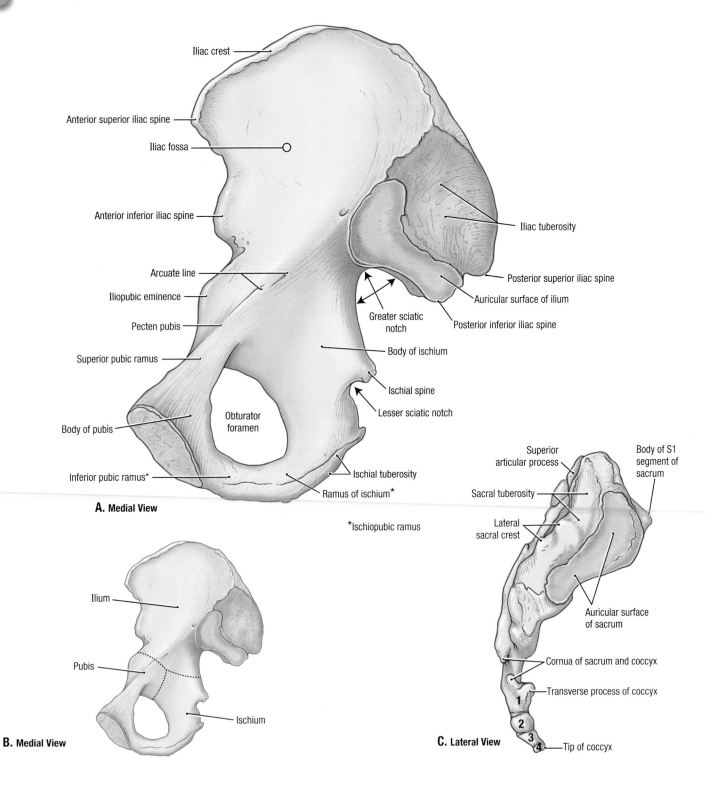

A. Medial View

Iliac crest

Anterior superior iliac spine

Iliac fossa

Anterior inferior iliac spine

Arcuate line

Iliopubic eminence

Pecten pubis

Superior pubic ramus

Body of pubis

Inferior pubic ramus*

Obturator foramen

Ramus of ischium*

Iliac tuberosity

Posterior superior iliac spine

Auricular surface of ilium

Posterior inferior iliac spine

Greater sciatic notch

Body of ischium

Ischial spine

Lesser sciatic notch

Ischial tuberosity

*Ischiopubic ramus

B. Medial View

Ilium

Pubis

Ischium

C. Lateral View

Superior articular process

Sacral tuberosity

Lateral sacral crest

Body of S1 segment of sacrum

Auricular surface of sacrum

Cornua of sacrum and coccyx

Transverse process of coccyx

1
2
3
4

Tip of coccyx

4.21   HIP BONE, SACRUM, AND COCCYX

A. Features of hip bone. **B.** Ilium, ischium, and pubis. **C.** Sacrum and coccyx. Vertebral column is fused to the sacrum.

- Each hip bone consists of three bones: ilium, ischium, and pubis.
- Anterosuperiorly, the auricular, ear-shaped surface of the sacrum articulates with the auricular surface of the ilium; the sacral and iliac tuberosities are for the attachment of the posterior sacro-iliac and interosseous sacro-iliac ligaments.

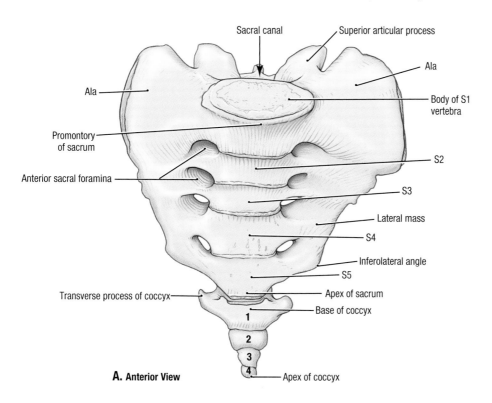

Sacral canal
Superior articular process
Ala
Ala
Promontory of sacrum
Body of S1 vertebra
Anterior sacral foramina
S2
S3
Lateral mass
S4
Inferolateral angle
S5
Transverse process of coccyx
Apex of sacrum
Base of coccyx
1
2
3
4
Apex of coccyx

A. Anterior View

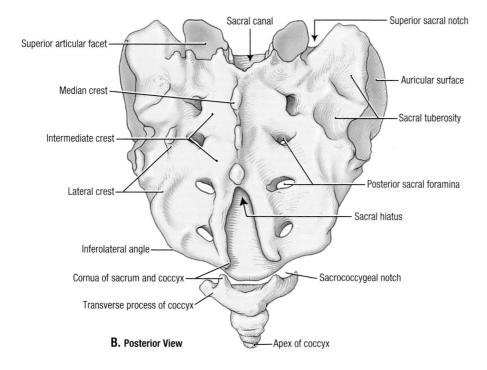

Sacral canal
Superior sacral notch
Superior articular facet
Median crest
Auricular surface
Intermediate crest
Sacral tuberosity
Lateral crest
Posterior sacral foramina
Sacral hiatus
Inferolateral angle
Cornua of sacrum and coccyx
Sacrococcygeal notch
Transverse process of coccyx
Apex of coccyx

B. Posterior View

| 4.22 | **SACRUM AND COCCYX** |

A. Pelvic (anterior) surface. **B.** Dorsal (posterior surface). **C.** Sacrum in youth.

- In **A,** the bodies of the five sacral vertebrae are demarcated in the mature sacrum by four transverse lines ending laterally in four pairs of anterior sacral foramina. The coccyx has four vertebrae (segments)—the first having a pair of transverse processes and a pair of cornua (horns).
- The costal (lateral) elements of the coccygeal vertebrae begin to fuse around puberty. The bodies begin to fuse from inferior to superior at about the 17th to 18th year, with fusion usually completed by the 23rd year.

1
2
3
4
5

C. Anterior View

Transverse process of L5 vertebra

Anterior longitudinal ligament

Iliac crest

Iliolumbar ligament

Ilium

L5/S1 intervertebral disc

Greater sciatic foramen

Anterior sacro-iliac ligament

Sacrotuberous ligament

Sacrospinous ligament

Sacrum

Coccyx

Anterior sacrococcygeal ligament

A. Anterior View

4.23   LUMBAR AND PELVIC LIGAMENTS

- The anterior sacro-iliac ligament is part of the fibrous capsule of the sacro-iliac joint anteriorly and spans between the lateral aspect of the sacrum and the ilium, anterior to the auricular surfaces.

During **pregnancy,** the pelvic joints and ligaments relax, and pelvic movements increase. The sacro-iliac interlocking mechanism is less effective because the relaxation permits greater rotation of the pelvis and contributes to the lordotic posture often assumed during pregnancy with the change in the center of gravity. Relaxation of the sacro-iliac joints and pubic symphysis permits as much as 10% to 15% increase in diameters (mostly transverse), facilitating passage of the fetus through the pelvic canal. The coccyx is also allowed to move posteriorly.

B. Posterior View

Transverse processes of L5 vertebra

Supraspinous ligament

Iliolumbar ligament

Posterior sacro-iliac ligament

Ilium

Posterior superior iliac spine

Sacrospinous ligament

Ischial spine

Greater sciatic foramen

Posterior sacrococcygeal ligaments

Lesser sciatic foramen

Sacrotuberous ligament

Ischial tuberosity

4.23   LUMBAR AND PELVIC LIGAMENTS (*CONTINUED*)

- The sacrotuberous ligaments attach the sacrum, ilium, and coccyx to the ischial tuberosity; the sacrospinous ligaments unite the sacrum and coccyx to the ischial spine. The sacrotuberous and sacrospinous ligaments convert the sciatic notches of the hip bones into greater and lesser sciatic foramina.
- The fibers of the posterior sacro-iliac ligament vary in obliquity; the superior fibers are shorter and lie between the ilium and superior part of the sacrum; the longer, obliquely oriented inferior fibers span between the posterior superior iliac spine and the inferior part of the sacrum, also blending with the sacrotuberous ligament.
- The interosseous sacro-iliac ligament lies deep to the posterior sacro-iliac ligament (see Fig. 4.24).
- The iliolumbar ligaments unite the ilia and transverse processes of L5; the lumbosacral portions of the ligaments descend to the alae of the sacrum and blend with the anterior sacro-iliac ligaments.

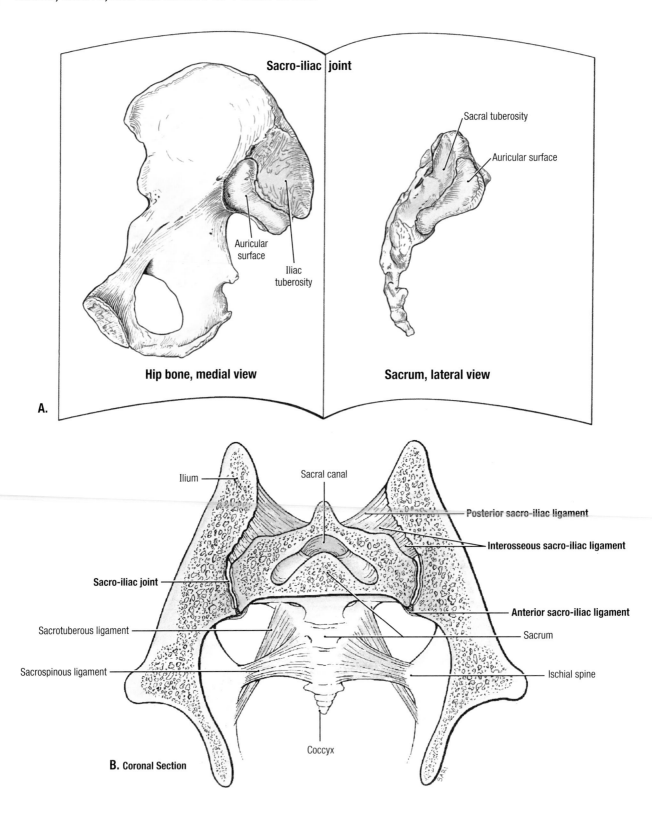

Hip bone, medial view

Sacrum, lateral view

A.

B. Coronal Section

4.24 ARTICULAR SURFACES OF SACRO-ILIAC JOINT AND LIGAMENTS

A. Articular surfaces. Note the auricular surface (articular area, *blue*) of the sacrum and hip bone and the roughened areas superior and posterior to the auricular areas (*orange*) for the attachment of the interosseous sacro-iliac ligament. **B.** Sacro-iliac ligaments. Note the sacro-iliac joints and the strong interosseous sacro-iliac ligament that lies inferior and anterior to the posterior sacro-iliac ligament. The interosseous sacro-iliac ligament consists of short fibers connecting the sacral tuberosity to the iliac tuberosity. The sacrum is suspended from the ilia by the posterior and interosseous sacro-iliac ligaments.

Interosseous
sacro-iliac
ligament

Iliacus   Psoas   Sacral   S1   Ala of   Ilium
canal   nerve   sacrum

A. Transverse (axial) CT Scan

Ala of sacrum

Posterior joint line

Anterior joint line

Sacral foramina

Lateral mass of sacrum

B. Anteroposterior View

<table>
<tr><td>**4.25**</td><td>**IMAGING OF SACRO-ILIAC JOINT**</td></tr>
</table>

A. CT scan. The sacro-iliac joint is indicated by *arrows*. Note that the articular surfaces of the ilium and sacrum have irregular shapes that result in partial interlocking of the bones. The sacro-iliac joint is oblique, with the anterior aspect of the joint situated lateral to the posterior aspect of the joint. **B.** Radiograph. Due to the oblique placement of the sacro-iliac joints, the anterior and posterior joint lines appear separately.

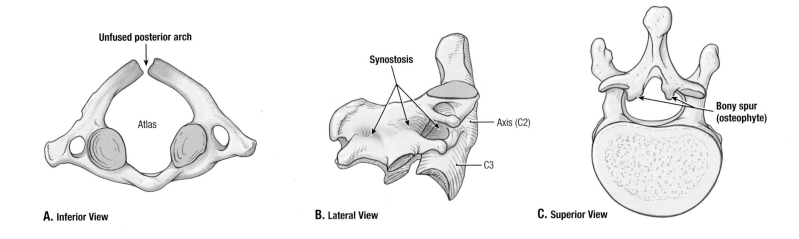

Unfused posterior arch

Atlas

A. Inferior View

Synostosis

Axis (C2)

C3

B. Lateral View

Bony spur
(osteophyte)

C. Superior View

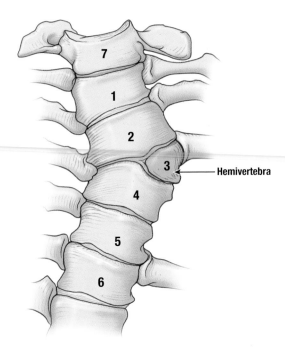

7

1

2

3 — Hemivertebra

4

5

6

D. Anterior View

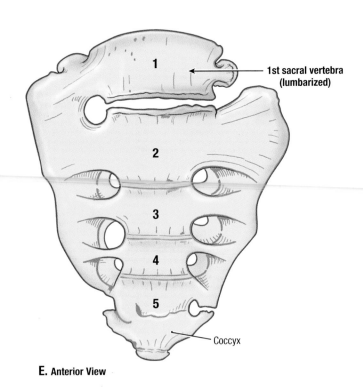

1 — 1st sacral vertebra
(lumbarized)

2

3

4

5

Coccyx

E. Anterior View

ANOMALIES OF VERTEBRAE

A. Unfused posterior arch of the atlas. The centrum fused to the right and left halves of the neural arch, but the arch did not fuse in the midline posteriorly. **B. Synostosis (fusion) of vertebrae C2 (axis) and C3. C. Bony spurs.** Sharp bony spurs may grow from the laminae inferiorly into the ligamenta flava, thereby reducing the lengths of the functional portions of these ligaments. When the vertebral column is flexed, the ligaments may be torn. **D. Hemivertebra.** The entire right half of vertebra T3

and the corresponding rib are absent. The left lamina and the spine are fused with those of T4, and the left IV foramen is reduced in size. Observe the associated scoliosis (lateral curvature of the spine). **E. Transitional lumbosacral vertebra.** Here, the 1st sacral vertebra is partly free (lumbarized). Not uncommonly, the 5th lumbar vertebra may be partly fused to the sacrum (sacralized).

A. Sagittal Section

Spinous process of L4

Defect (spondylolysis)

L5

L5

Posterior View

Anterior displacement (spondylolisthesis)

Sacrum

Sacral canal

L4

L5

S1

Defect

Sacral canal

B. Lateral View

L3

L4

L5

Pedicle

Pars interarticularis (neck)

Superior articular process

Inferior articular process

Transverse process

Broken neck at "Scotty dog" indicates spondylolysis

C. Oblique View

4.27

SPONDYLOLYSIS AND SPONDYLOLISTHESIS

A. Articulated and isolated spondylolytic L5 vertebra. The vertebra has an oblique defect (spondylolysis) through the interarticular part (pars interarticularis). The interarticular part is the region of the lamina of a lumbar vertebra between the superior and inferior articular processes. The defect may be traumatic or congenital in origin. Also, the vertebral body of L5 has slipped anteriorly (spondylolisthesis). **B and C.** Radiographs.

In **B**, the *dotted line* following the posterior vertebral margins of L5 and the sacrum shows the anterior displacement of L5 (*arrow*). In **C**, note the superimposed outline of a dog: the neck is the transverse process, the eye is the pedicle, and the ear is the superior articular process. The lucent (dark) cleft across the "neck" of the dog is the **spondylolysis**; the anterior displacement (*arrow*) is the **spondylolisthesis**.

Site of nuchal ligament

Spinal (posterior) part of deltoid

Teres major

Latissimus dorsi

External oblique

Posterior median furrow

Gluteus medius

Gluteus maximus

Posterior View

Descending (superior) part of trapezius

Transverse (middle) part of trapezius

Ascending (inferior) part of trapezius

Erector spinae

Site of posterior superior iliac spine (PSIS)

Intergluteal cleft

4.28   SURFACE ANATOMY OF BACK

- The arms are abducted, so the scapulae have rotated superiorly on the thoracic wall.
- The latissimus dorsi and teres major muscles form the posterior axillary fold.
- The trapezius muscle has three parts: descending, transverse, and ascending.

- Note the deep median furrow that separates the longitudinal bulges formed by the contracted erector spinae group of muscles;
- Dimples (depressions) indicate the site of the posterior superior iliac spines, which usually lie at the level of the sacro-iliac joints.

Occipitalis

Occipital artery

Occipital lymph node

Descending (superior) part of trapezius

Levator scapulae

Rhomboid minor

Rhomboid major

Deltoid

Subtrapezial plexus
(spinal accessory nerve (CN XI) and
branches of C3, C4 anterior rami)

Trapezius

Latissimus dorsi

External oblique

Thoracolumbar fascia

Gluteal fascia (covering gluteus medius)

Gluteus maximus

Posterior View

Greater occipital nerve (posterior ramus of C2 spinal nerve)

3rd occipital nerve (posterior ramus of C3)

Lesser occipital nerve (anterior ramus of C2)

Cutaneous branches of posterior rami

Transverse (middle) part of trapezius

Ascending (inferior) part of trapezius

Triangle of auscultation

Cutaneous branches of posterior rami

Posterior branches of lateral cutaneous branches

Lateral cutaneous branch of iliohypogastric nerve
(anterior ramus of L1)

Cutaneous branches of posterior rami of L1 to L3
(superior clunial nerves)

4.29   SUPERFICIAL MUSCLES OF BACK

On the *left*, the trapezius muscle is reflected. Observe two layers: the trapezius and latissimus dorsi muscles,
and the levator scapulae and rhomboids minor and major. These axio-appendicular muscles help attach the
upper limb to the trunk.

Nuchal ligament

Sternocleidomastoid
Splenius
Trapezius
Levator scapulae
Posterior scalene
Serratus posterior superior
Trapezius (cut surface)

Rhomboid minor

Rhomboid major

Serratus anterior

Thoracolumbar fascia
10th rib

Serratus posterior inferior
(aponeurosis)

External oblique

Internal oblique
Aponeurosis of internal oblique

Iliac crest

Posterior View

Semispinalis capitis
Sternocleidomastoid
Splenius
Levator scapulae
Rhomboid minor

Deltoid

Rhomboid major

Teres major
Serratus anterior
8th rib
Angle of rib

Serratus posterior inferior (belly)

Latissimus dorsi
External oblique
Lumbar triangle
Gluteal fascia (covering gluteus medius)
Gluteus maximus

4.30   INTERMEDIATE MUSCLES OF BACK

The trapezius and latissimus dorsi muscles are largely cut away on both sides. On the *left,* the rhomboid muscles have been severed, allowing the vertebral border of the scapula to be raised from the thoracic wall. The serratus posterior superior and inferior form the intermediate layer of muscles, passing from the vertebral spines to the ribs; the two muscles slope in opposite directions and are muscles of respiration. The thoracolumbar fascia extends laterally to the angles of the ribs, becoming thin superiorly and passing deep to the serratus posterior superior muscle. The fascia gives attachment to the latissimus dorsi and serratus posterior inferior muscles (see Fig. 4.35).

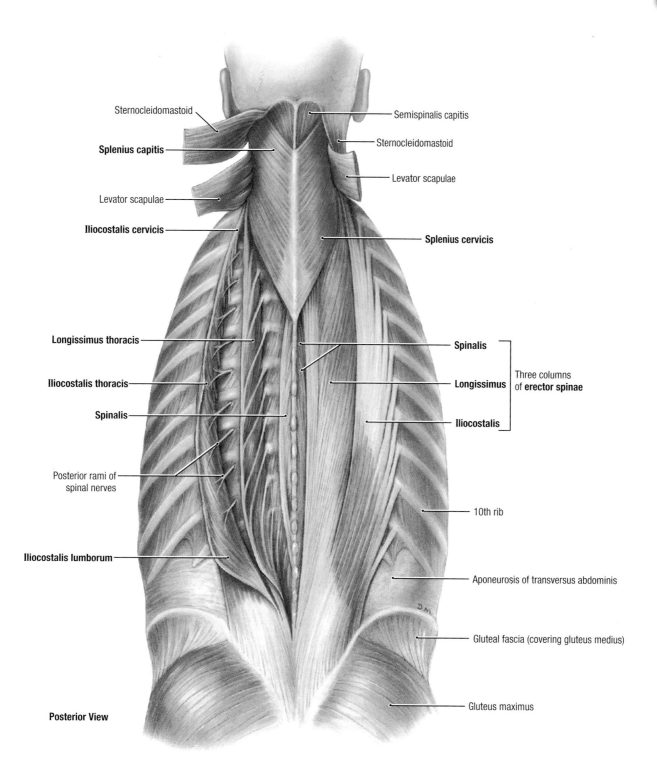

Sternocleidomastoid

Semispinalis capitis

Splenius capitis

Sternocleidomastoid

Levator scapulae

Levator scapulae

Iliocostalis cervicis

Splenius cervicis

Longissimus thoracis

Spinalis

Three columns of **erector spinae**

Iliocostalis thoracis

Longissimus

Spinalis

Iliocostalis

Posterior rami of spinal nerves

10th rib

Iliocostalis lumborum

Aponeurosis of transversus abdominis

Gluteal fascia (covering gluteus medius)

Gluteus maximus

Posterior View

| 4.31 | DEEP MUSCLES OF BACK: SPLENIUS AND ERECTOR SPINAE |

On the *right* of the body, the erector spinae muscles are in situ, lying between the spinous processes medially and the angles of the ribs laterally. The erector spinae are split into three longitudinal columns: iliocostalis laterally, longissimus in the middle, and spinalis medially. On the *left,* the longissimus muscle is pulled laterally to show the insertion into the transverse processes and ribs; not shown here are its extensions to the neck and head, longissimus cervicis and capitis.

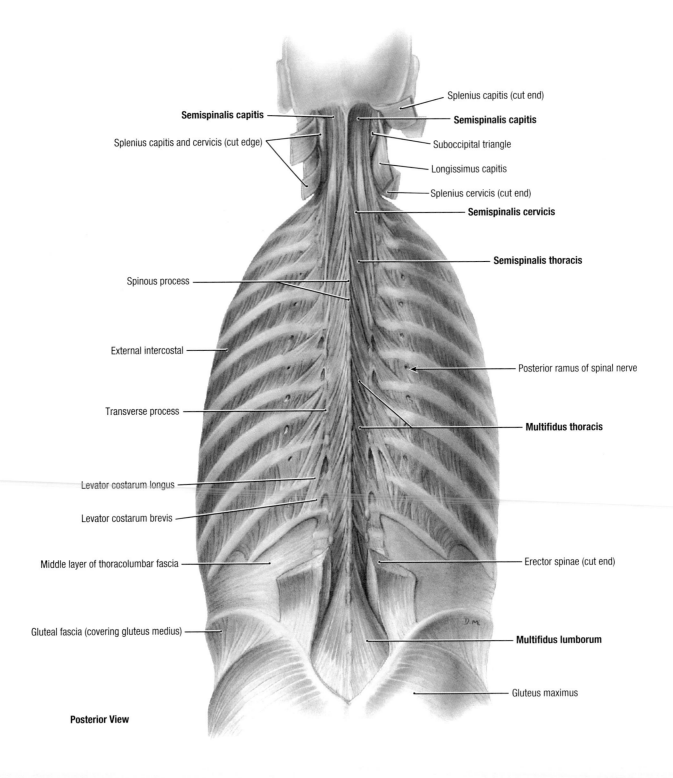

Splenius capitis (cut end)

Semispinalis capitis

Suboccipital triangle

Longissimus capitis

Splenius cervicis (cut end)

Semispinalis cervicis

Semispinalis thoracis

Posterior ramus of spinal nerve

Multifidus thoracis

Erector spinae (cut end)

Multifidus lumborum

Gluteus maximus

Semispinalis capitis

Splenius capitis and cervicis (cut edge)

Spinous process

External intercostal

Transverse process

Levator costarum longus

Levator costarum brevis

Middle layer of thoracolumbar fascia

Gluteal fascia (covering gluteus medius)

Posterior View

4.32

DEEP MUSCLES OF BACK: SEMISPINALIS AND MULTIFIDUS

- The semispinalis, multifidus, and rotatores muscles constitute the transverso spinalis group of deep muscles. In general, their bundles pass obliquely in a superomedial direction, from transverse processes to spinous processes in successively deeper layers. The bundles of semispinalis span approximately five interspaces, those of multifidus, approximately three, and those of rotatores, one or two.

- The semispinalis (thoracis, cervicis, and capitis) muscles span the lower thoracic region to the skull.
- The multifidus muscle extends from the sacrum to the spine of the axis. In the lumbosacral region it emerges from the aponeurosis of the erector spinae, and extends from the sacrum, and mammillary processes of the lumbar vertebrae, to insert into spinous processes approximately three segments higher.

Tip of transverse process

Superior costotransverse ligament

Neck of rib

Posterior ramus of spinal nerve

Tubercle of rib

Rotatores brevis

Rotatores longus

External intercostal

Superior costotransverse ligament

Levator costarum longus

Lateral costotransverse ligaments

Dura mater

Spinal cord

Posterior longitudinal ligament

Posterior costotransverse ligament

Posterior View

4.33   ## ROTATORES AND COSTOTRANSVERSE LIGAMENTS

- Of the three layers of transversospinalis, or oblique muscles of the back (semispinalis, multifidus, rotatores), the rotatores are the deepest and shortest. They pass from the root of one transverse process superomedially to the junction of the transverse process and lamina of the vertebra above. Rotatores longus span two vertebrae.
- The levatores costarum pass from the tip of one transverse process inferiorly to the rib below; some span two ribs.

- The superior costotransverse ligament splits laterally into two sheets, between which lie the levatores costarum and external intercostal muscles; the posterior ramus passes posterior to this ligament.
- The lateral costotransverse ligament is strong and joins the tubercle of the rib to the tip of the transverse process. It forms the posterior aspect of the joint capsule of the costotransverse joint.

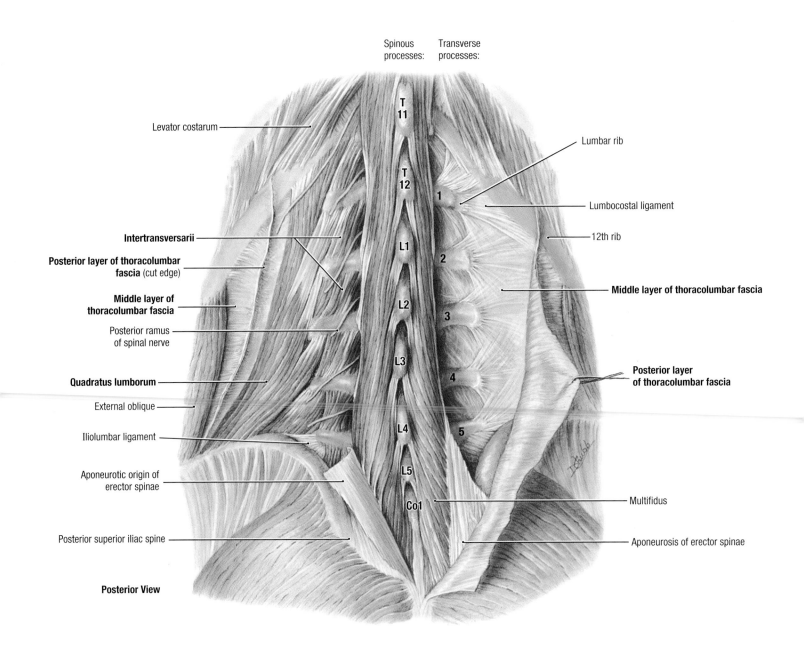

Spinous processes:

Transverse processes:

Levator costarum

T 11

Lumbar rib

T 12

1

Lumbocostal ligament

Intertransversarii

12th rib

Posterior layer of thoracolumbar fascia (cut edge)

L1

2

Middle layer of thoracolumbar fascia

Middle layer of thoracolumbar fascia

L2

3

Posterior ramus of spinal nerve

L3

4

Posterior layer of thoracolumbar fascia

Quadratus lumborum

External oblique

L4

5

Iliolumbar ligament

L5

Aponeurotic origin of erector spinae

Co1

Multifidus

Posterior superior iliac spine

Aponeurosis of erector spinae

Posterior View

4.34 **BACK: MULTIFIDUS, QUADRATUS LUMBORUM, AND THORACOLUMBAR FASCIA**

Right: After removal of erector spinae at the L1 level, the middle layer of thoracolumbar fascia extends from the tip of each lumbar transverse process in a fan-shaped manner. A short lumbar rib is present at the level of L1. *Left:* After removal of the posterior and middle layers of thoracolumbar fascia, the lateral border of the quadratus lumborum muscle is oblique, and the medial border is in continuity with the intertransversarii.

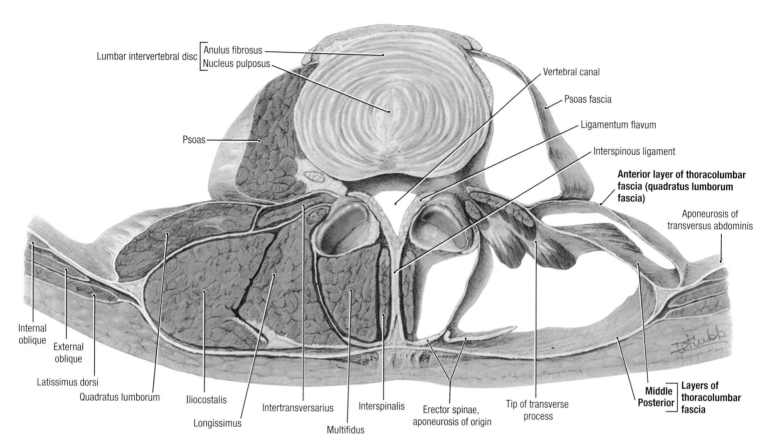

Lumbar intervertebral disc [Anulus fibrosus
Nucleus pulposus]

Psoas

Vertebral canal

Psoas fascia

Ligamentum flavum

Interspinous ligament

Anterior layer of thoracolumbar fascia (quadratus lumborum fascia)

Aponeurosis of transversus abdominis

Internal oblique

External oblique

Latissimus dorsi

Quadratus lumborum

Iliocostalis

Longissimus

Intertransversarius

Interspinalis

Multifidus

Erector spinae, aponeurosis of origin

Tip of transverse process

Middle
Posterior] Layers of thoracolumbar fascia

Transverse Section (Dissected), Superior View

4.35   TRANSVERSE SECTION OF BACK MUSCLES AND THORACOLUMBAR FASCIA

- On the *left,* the muscles are seen in their fascial sheaths or compartments; on the *right,* the muscles have been removed from their sheaths.
- The deep back muscles extend from the pelvis to the cranium and are enclosed in fascia. This fascia attaches medially to the nuchal ligament, the tips of the spinous processes, the supraspinous ligament, and the median crest of the sacrum. The lateral attachment of the fascia is to the cervical transverse processes, the angles of the ribs, and the aponeurosis of transversus abdominis. The thoracic and lumbar parts of the fascia are named thoracolumbar fascia.
- The aponeurosis of transversus abdominis and posterior aponeurosis of internal oblique muscles split into two strong sheets, the middle and

posterior layers of thoracolumbar fascia. The anterior layer of thoracolumbar fascia is the deep fascia of the quadratus lumborum (quadratus lumborum fascia). The posterior layer of the thoracolumbar fascia provides proximal attachment for the latissimus dorsi muscle and, at a higher level, the serratus posterior inferior muscle.

Back strain is a common back problem that usually results from extreme movements of the vertebral column, such as extension or rotation. Back strain refers to some stretching or microscopic tearing of muscle fibers and/or ligaments of the back. The muscles usually involved are those producing movements of the lumbar IV joints.

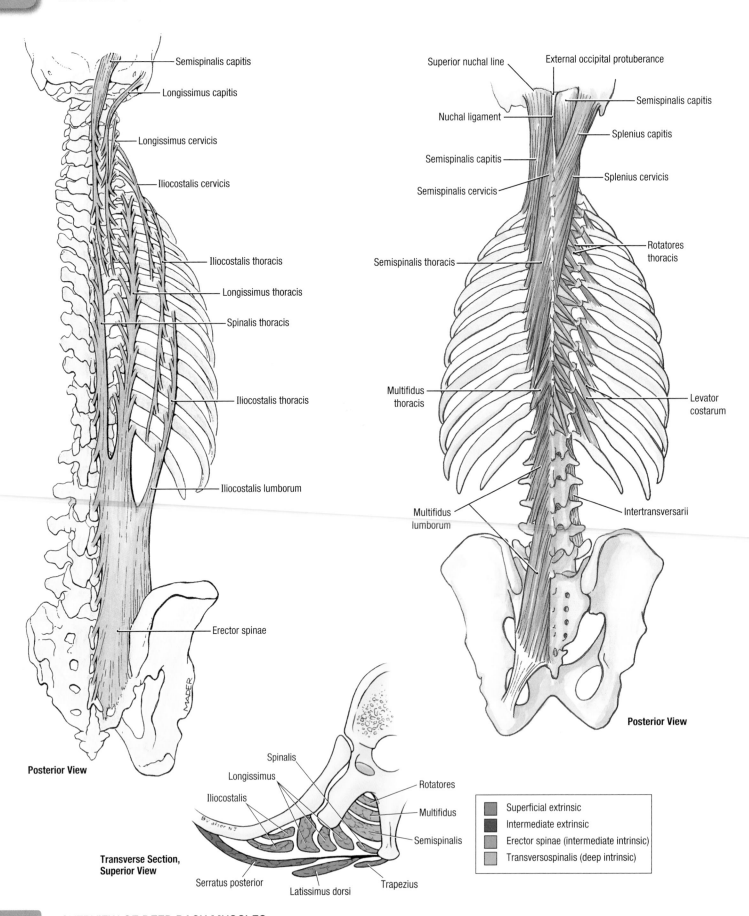

Semispinalis capitis

Longissimus capitis

Longissimus cervicis

Iliocostalis cervicis

Iliocostalis thoracis

Longissimus thoracis

Spinalis thoracis

Iliocostalis thoracis

Iliocostalis lumborum

Erector spinae

Posterior View

Superior nuchal line

External occipital protuberance

Nuchal ligament

Semispinalis capitis

Semispinalis capitis

Splenius capitis

Semispinalis cervicis

Splenius cervicis

Semispinalis thoracis

Rotatores thoracis

Multifidus thoracis

Levator costarum

Multifidus lumborum

Intertransversarii

Posterior View

Spinalis

Longissimus

Iliocostalis

Rotatores

Multifidus

Semispinalis

Transverse Section, Superior View

Serratus posterior

Latissimus dorsi

Trapezius

Superficial extrinsic

Intermediate extrinsic

Erector spinae (intermediate intrinsic)

Transversospinalis (deep intrinsic)

4.36 OVERVIEW OF DEEP BACK MUSCLES

TABLE 4.4 *INTRINSIC BACK MUSCLES*[a]

Muscles	Caudal (Inferior) Attachment	Rostral (Superior) Attachment	Nerve Supply[b]	Main Actions
Superficial layer				
Splenius	Nuchal ligament and spinous processes of C7–T6 vertebrae	*Splenius capitis:* fibers run superolaterally to mastoid process of temporal bone and lateral third of superior nuchal line of occipital bone *Splenius cervicis:* posterior tubercles of transverse processes of C1–C3/C4 vertebrae		*Acting unilaterally:* laterally flex neck and rotate head to side of active muscles; *Acting bilaterally:* extend head and neck
Intermediate layer				*Acting unilaterally:* laterally bend vertebral column to side of active muscles
Erector spinae	Arises by a broad tendon from posterior part of iliac crest, posterior surface of sacrum, sacral and inferior lumbar spinous processes, and supraspinous ligament	*Iliocostalis (lumborum, thoracis, and cervicis):* fibers run superiorly to angles of lower ribs and cervical transverse processes *Longissimus (thoracis, cervicis, and capitis):* fibers run superiorly to ribs between tubercles and angles to transverse processes in thoracic and cervical regions, and to mastoid process of temporal bone *Spinalis (thoracis, cervicis, and capitis):* fibers run superiorly to spinous processes in the upper thoracic region and to skull	Posterior rami of spinal nerves	*Acting bilaterally:* extend vertebral column and head; as back is flexed, control movement by gradually lengthening their fibers
Deep layer				
Transversospinalis	*Semispinalis:* arises from thoracic and cervical transverse processes *Multifidus:* arises from sacrum and ilium, transverse processes of T1–L5, and articular processes of C4–C7 *Rotatores:* arise from transverse processes of vertebrae; best developed in thoracic region	*Semispinalis: thoracis, cervicis, and capitis:* fibers run superomedially to occipital bone and spinous processes in thoracic and cervical regions, spanning four to six segments *Multifidus (lumborum, thoracis, and cervicis):* fibers pass superomedially to spinous processes, spanning two to four segments *Rotatores (thoracis and cervicis):* Pass superomedially and attach to junction of lamina and transverse process of vertebra of origin or into spinous process above their origin, spanning one to two segments		**Extension** *Semispinalis:* extends head and thoracic and cervical regions of vertebral column and rotates them contralaterally *Multifidus:* stabilizes vertebrae during local movement of vertebral column *Rotatores:* Stabilize vertebrae and assist with local extension and rotary movements of vertebral column; may function as organ of proprioception
Minor deep layer				
Interspinales	Superior surfaces of spinous processes of cervical and lumbar vertebrae	Inferior surfaces of spinous processes of vertebrae superior to vertebrae of origin	Posterior rami of spinal nerves	Aid in extension and rotation of vertebral column
Intertransversarii	Transverse processes of cervical and lumbar vertebrae	Transverse processes of adjacent vertebrae	Posterior and anterior rami of spinal nerves	Aid in lateral flexion of vertebral column *Acting bilaterally:* stabilize vertebral column
Levatores costarum	**Medial attachment:** Tips of transverse processes of C7 and T1–T11 vertebrae	**Lateral attachment:** Pass inferolaterally and insert on rib between its tubercle and angle	Posterior rami of C8–T11 spinal nerves	Elevate ribs, assisting inspiration Assist with lateral flexion of vertebral column

[a]See figures on opposite page.
[b]Most back muscles are innervated by posterior rami of spinal nerves, but a few are innervated by anterior rami. Intertransversarii of cervical region are supplied by anterior rami.

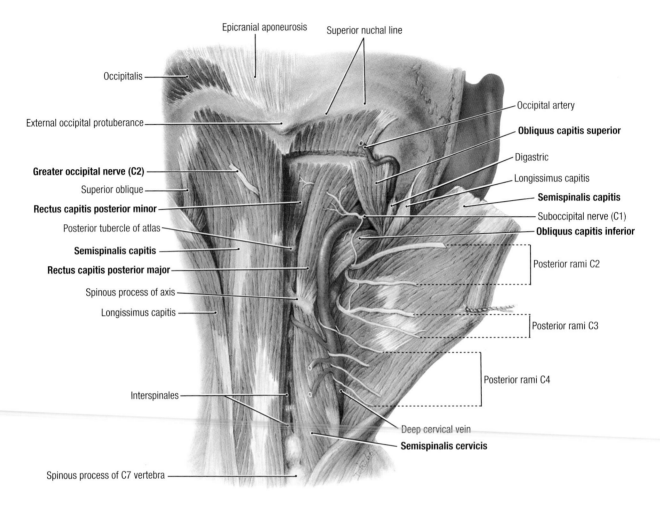

Epicranial aponeurosis

Superior nuchal line

Occipitalis

External occipital protuberance

Greater occipital nerve (C2)

Superior oblique

Rectus capitis posterior minor

Posterior tubercle of atlas

Semispinalis capitis

Rectus capitis posterior major

Spinous process of axis

Longissimus capitis

Interspinales

Spinous process of C7 vertebra

Occipital artery

Obliquus capitis superior

Digastric

Longissimus capitis

Semispinalis capitis

Suboccipital nerve (C1)

Obliquus capitis inferior

Posterior rami C2

Posterior rami C3

Posterior rami C4

Deep cervical vein

Semispinalis cervicis

Posterior View

4.37 SUBOCCIPITAL REGION I

The trapezius, sternocleidomastoid, and splenius muscles are removed. The right semispinalis capitis muscle is cut and reflected laterally.

- The semispinalis capitis, the great extensor muscle of the head and neck, forms the posterior wall of the suboccipital region. It is pierced by the greater occipital nerve (posterior ramus of C2) and has free medial and lateral borders at this level.
- The greater occipital nerve, when followed caudally, leads to the inferior border of the obliquus capitis inferior muscle, around which it turns. Following the inferior border of the obliquus capitis inferior muscle medially from the nerve leads to the spinous process of the axis; followed laterally, this leads to the transverse process of the atlas.
- Five muscles (all paired) are attached to the spinous process of the axis: obliquus capitis inferior, rectus capitis posterior major, semispinalis cervicis, multifidus, and interspinalis; the latter two are largely concealed by the semispinalis cervicis.

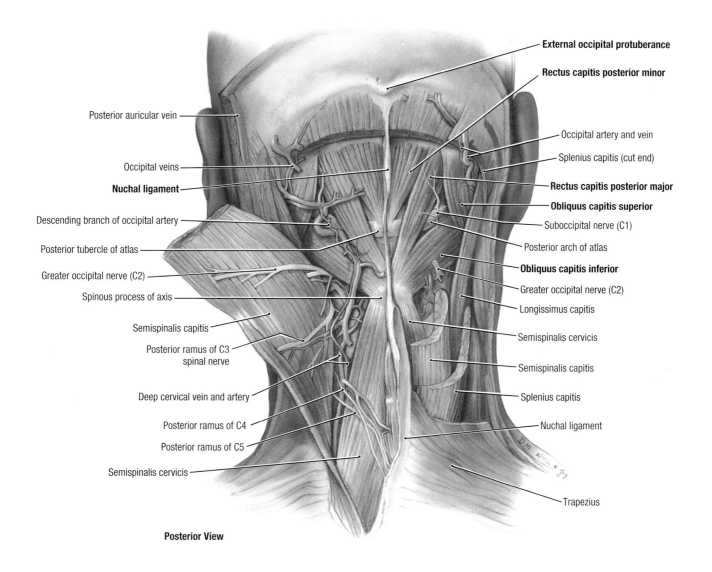

Posterior auricular vein

Occipital veins

Nuchal ligament

Descending branch of occipital artery

Posterior tubercle of atlas

Greater occipital nerve (C2)

Spinous process of axis

Semispinalis capitis

Posterior ramus of C3 spinal nerve

Deep cervical vein and artery

Posterior ramus of C4

Posterior ramus of C5

Semispinalis cervicis

Posterior View

External occipital protuberance

Rectus capitis posterior minor

Occipital artery and vein

Splenius capitis (cut end)

Rectus capitis posterior major

Obliquus capitis superior

Suboccipital nerve (C1)

Posterior arch of atlas

Obliquus capitis inferior

Greater occipital nerve (C2)

Longissimus capitis

Semispinalis cervicis

Semispinalis capitis

Splenius capitis

Nuchal ligament

Trapezius

4.38   SUBOCCIPITAL REGION II

The semispinalis capitis is reflected on the *left* and removed on the *right* side of the body; neck is flexed.

- The suboccipital region contains four pairs of structures: two straight muscles, the rectus capitis posterior major and minor; two oblique muscles, the obliquus capitis superior and obliquus capitis inferior; two nerves (posterior rami), C1 suboccipital (motor) and C2 greater occipital (sensory); and two arteries, the occipital and vertebral.
- The nuchal ligament, which represents the cervical part of the supraspinous ligament, is a median, thin, fibrous partition attached to the spinous processes of cervical vertebrae and the external occipital protuberance.
- The suboccipital triangle is bounded by three muscles: obliquus capitis superior and inferior and rectus capitis posterior major.
- The suboccipital nerve (posterior ramus of C1) supplies the three muscles bounding the suboccipital triangle and also the rectus capitis minor muscle and communicates with the greater occipital nerve.
- The occipital veins along with the suboccipital nerve (posterior ramus of C1) emerge through the suboccipital triangle to join the deep cervical vein.
- The posterior arch of the atlas forms the floor of the suboccipital triangle.

A. Posterior View

- Trapezius (cut)
- **Rectus capitis posterior minor**
- **Semispinalis capitis** (cut)
- **Rectus capitis posterior major**
- Occipital artery
- **Obliquus capitis superior**
- **Obliquus capitis inferior**
- Greater occipital nerve (C2)
- **Semispinalis capitis** (cut)
- Splenius (incised and retracted)
- Trapezius (cut)
- Superior nuchal line
- Inferior nuchal line
- Suboccipital nerve (C1)
- Posterior atlanto-occipital membrane
- Vertebral artery
- Transverse process of C1 vertebra
- Posterior arch C1
- Spinal ganglion of C2 spinal nerve
- Transverse process of C2 vertebra

B. Lateral View

- Sternocleidomastoid
- Splenius capitis
- Levator scapulae
- Trapezius
- Acromion

C. Anterior View

- Rectus capitis anterior
- Rectus capitis lateralis
- Transverse process of atlas (C1)
- Longus capitis
- Scalene muscles
- Longus colli
- C6
- T3

4.39   MUSCLES OF BASE OF SKULL

A. Suboccipital region. **B.** Lateral cervical region. **C.** Prevertebral muscles.

TABLE 4.5 MUSCLES OF ATLANTO-OCCIPITAL AND ATLANTO-AXIAL JOINTS

Movements of Atlanto-Occipital Joints

Flexion	Extension	Lateral Bending
Longus capitis Rectus capitis anterior Anterior fibers of sternocleidomastoid	Rectus capitis posterior major and minor Obliquus capitis superior Semispinalis capitis Splenius capitis Longissimus capitis Trapezius	Sternocleidomastoid Longissimus capitis Rectus capitis lateralis Splenius capitis

Rotation of Atlanto-Axial Joints[a]

Ipsilateral[b]	Contralateral
Obliquus capitis inferior Rectus capitis posterior, major and minor Longissimus capitis Splenius capitis	Sternocleidomastoid Semispinalis capitis

[a]Rotation is the specialized movement at these joints. Movement of one joint involves the other.
[b]Same side to which head is rotated.

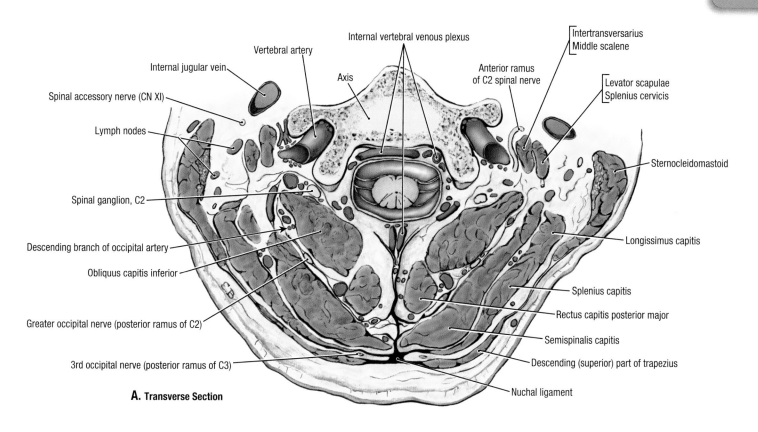

Internal vertebral venous plexus

Vertebral artery

Internal jugular vein

Axis

Spinal accessory nerve (CN XI)

Intertransversarius
Middle scalene

Anterior ramus
of C2 spinal nerve

Levator scapulae
Splenius cervicis

Lymph nodes

Sternocleidomastoid

Spinal ganglion, C2

Descending branch of occipital artery

Longissimus capitis

Obliquus capitis inferior

Splenius capitis

Greater occipital nerve (posterior ramus of C2)

Rectus capitis posterior major

Semispinalis capitis

3rd occipital nerve (posterior ramus of C3)

Descending (superior) part of trapezius

Nuchal ligament

A. Transverse Section

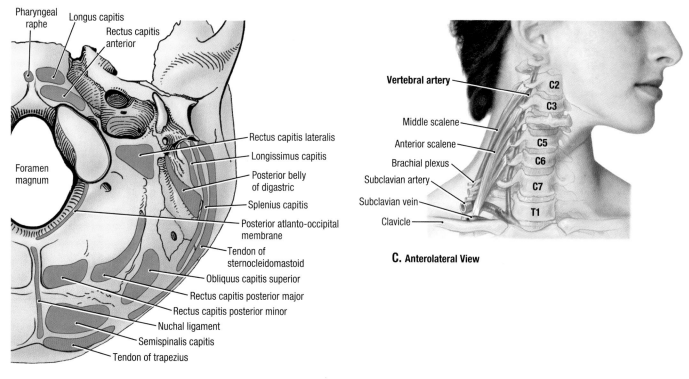

Pharyngeal raphe

Longus capitis

Rectus capitis anterior

Vertebral artery

C2

C3

Middle scalene

Anterior scalene

C5

Brachial plexus

C6

Rectus capitis lateralis

Longissimus capitis

Posterior belly of digastric

Splenius capitis

C7

Subclavian artery

Subclavian vein

T1

Clavicle

Foramen magnum

Posterior atlanto-occipital membrane

Tendon of sternocleidomastoid

Obliquus capitis superior

Rectus capitis posterior major

Rectus capitis posterior minor

Nuchal ligament

Semispinalis capitis

Tendon of trapezius

C. Anterolateral View

B. Inferior View

4.40   NUCHAL REGION

A. Transverse section at the level of the axis. **B.** Muscle attachments on the inferior aspect of the skull. **C.** Vertebral artery.

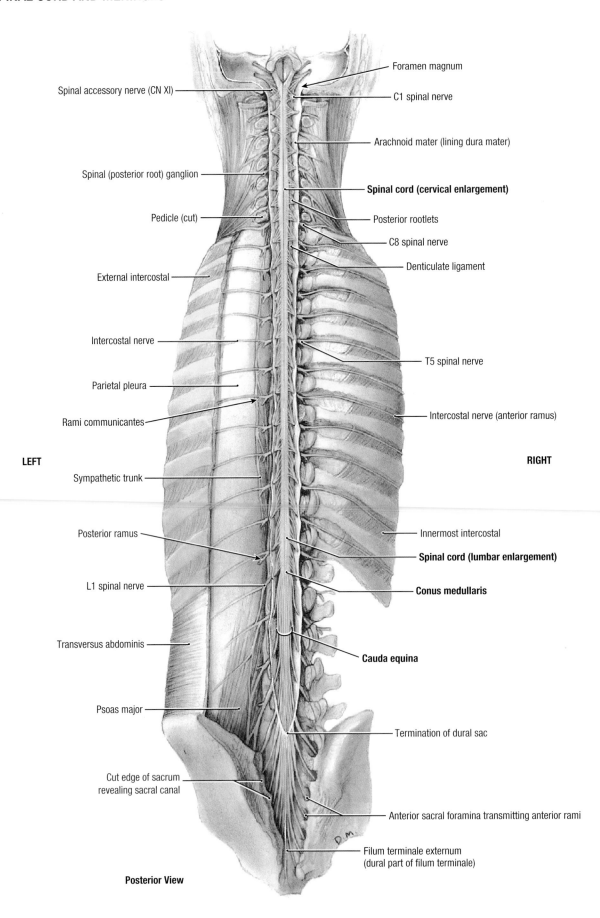

Foramen magnum

Spinal accessory nerve (CN XI)

C1 spinal nerve

Arachnoid mater (lining dura mater)

Spinal (posterior root) ganglion

Spinal cord (cervical enlargement)

Posterior rootlets

Pedicle (cut)

C8 spinal nerve

Denticulate ligament

External intercostal

Intercostal nerve

T5 spinal nerve

Parietal pleura

Rami communicantes

Intercostal nerve (anterior ramus)

LEFT

RIGHT

Sympathetic trunk

Innermost intercostal

Posterior ramus

Spinal cord (lumbar enlargement)

Conus medullaris

L1 spinal nerve

Transversus abdominis

Cauda equina

Psoas major

Termination of dural sac

Cut edge of sacrum
revealing sacral canal

Anterior sacral foramina transmitting anterior rami

Filum terminale externum
(dural part of filum terminale)

Posterior View

Posterior rootlets

Anterior rootlets

Denticulate ligament

Denticulate ligament

Anterior root

Posterior rootlets (cut)

Spinal cord

Dura mater

Arachnoid mater

A. Posterior View

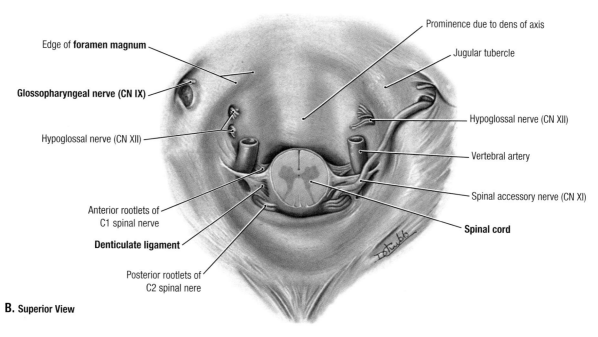

Prominence due to dens of axis

Edge of **foramen magnum**

Jugular tubercle

Glossopharyngeal nerve (CN IX)

Hypoglossal nerve (CN XII)

Hypoglossal nerve (CN XII)

Vertebral artery

Spinal accessory nerve (CN XI)

Anterior rootlets of
C1 spinal nerve

Spinal cord

Denticulate ligament

Posterior rootlets of
C2 spinal nere

B. Superior View

4.42   SPINAL CORD AND MENINGES

A. Dural sac cut open. The denticulate ligament anchors the cord to the dural sac between successive nerve roots by means of strong, toothlike processes. The anterior nerve roots (rootlets) lie anterior to the denticulate ligament, and the posterior nerve roots (rootlets) lie posterior to the ligament. **B.** Structures of vertebral canal seen through foramen magnum. The spinal cord, vertebral arteries, spinal accessory nerve (CN XI), and most superior part of the denticulate ligament pass through the foramen magnum within the meninges.

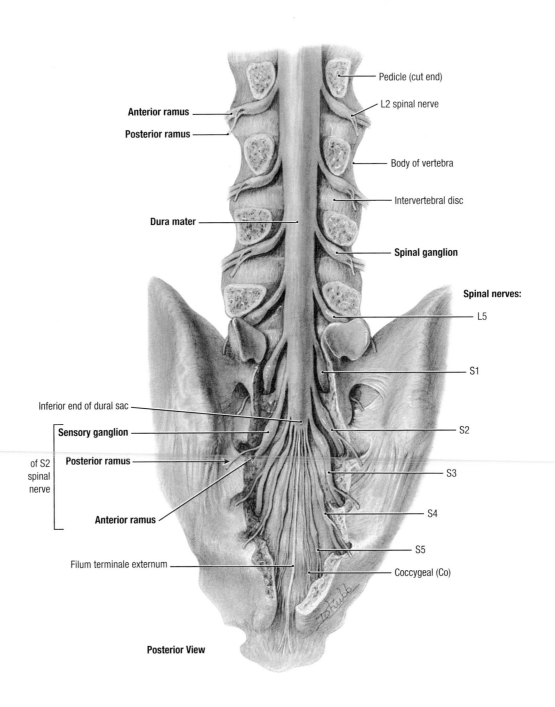

Pedicle (cut end)

L2 spinal nerve

Anterior ramus

Posterior ramus

Body of vertebra

Intervertebral disc

Dura mater

Spinal ganglion

Spinal nerves:

L5

S1

Inferior end of dural sac

S2

Sensory ganglion

of S2 spinal nerve

Posterior ramus

S3

S4

Anterior ramus

S5

Filum terminale externum

Coccygeal (Co)

Posterior View

4.43   INFERIOR END OF DURAL SAC I

The posterior parts of the lumbar vertebrae and sacrum were removed.
- The inferior limit of the dural sac is at the level of the posterior superior iliac spine (body of 2nd sacral vertebra); the dura continues as the filum terminale externum.
- The lumbar spinal ganglia are in the IV foramina, and the sacral spinal ganglia are somewhat asymmetrically placed within the sacral canal.
- The posterior rami are smaller than the anterior rami.

A. Posterior View

Labels (left image, top to bottom):
- Spinal cord
- Posterior root
- T12 spinal nerve
- Radicular branch of spinal vein
- L1 spinal nerve
- L2 spinal nerve
- Posterior root
- Anterior root
- L3 spinal nerve
- L4 spinal nerve
- L5 spinal nerve (in dural sleeve)
- Dura mater
- Arachnoid mater
- Denticulate ligament
- **Conus medullaris**
- Posterior rootlets
- **Filum terminale internum**
- **Cauda equina**
- Subarachnoid space
- Pedicle of L5 vertebra
- Superior articular process of sacrum

B. Myelogram

Labels (right image):
- Pedicle
- Body of L2 vertebra
- Contrast medium in subarachnoid space within the dural sleeve around the spinal nerve roots
- Cauda equina in cerebrospinal fluid
- Nerve rootlet in cerebrospinal fluid
- Lumbar cistern (inferior part)

| 4.44 | **INFERIOR END OF DURAL SAC II** |

A. Inferior dural sac and lumbar cistern of subarachnoid space, opened. **B.** Myelogram of the lumbar region of the vertebral column. Contrast medium was injected into the subarachnoid space. **C.** Termination of spinal cord, in situ, sagittal section.

- The conus medullaris, or conical lower end of the spinal cord, continues as a glistening thread, the filum terminale internum, which descends with the posterior and anterior nerve roots; these constitute the cauda equina.
- In the adult, the spinal cord usually ends at the level of the disc between vertebrae L1 and L2. Variations: 95% of cords end within the limits of the bodies of L1 and L2, whereas 3% end posterior to the inferior half of T12, and 2% posterior to L3.
- The subarachnoid space usually ends at the level of the disc between S1 and S2, but it can be more inferior.

To obtain a **sample of CSF from the lumbar cistern**, a lumbar puncture needle, fitted with a stylet, is inserted into the subarachnoid space. Flexion of the vertebral column facilitates insertion of the needle by stretching the ligamenta flava and spreading the laminae and spinous processes apart. The needle is inserted in the midline between the spinous processes of the L3 and L4 (or the L4 and L5) vertebrae. At these levels in adults, there is little danger of damaging the spinal cord.

Labels (C):
- Spinal cord
- **Conus medullaris**
- **Filum terminale internum**
- Subarachnoid space (lumbar cistern) containing cerebrospinal fluid and nerve roots
- Filum terminale externum
- L2
- S2

C. Sagittal Section

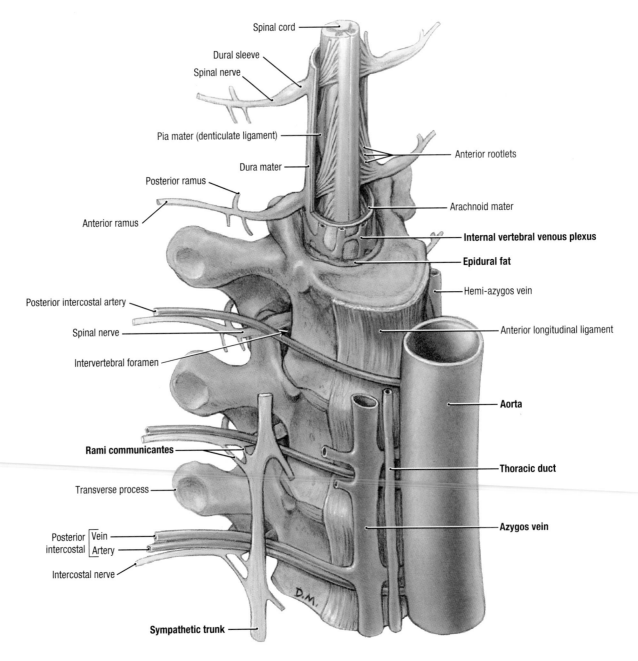

Spinal cord

Dural sleeve

Spinal nerve

Pia mater (denticulate ligament)

Anterior rootlets

Dura mater

Posterior ramus

Arachnoid mater

Anterior ramus

Internal vertebral venous plexus

Epidural fat

Posterior intercostal artery

Hemi-azygos vein

Spinal nerve

Anterior longitudinal ligament

Intervertebral foramen

Aorta

Rami communicantes

Transverse process

Thoracic duct

Posterior intercostal { Vein / Artery

Azygos vein

Intercostal nerve

Sympathetic trunk

Right Anterolateral View

4.45 SPINAL CORD AND PREVERTEBRAL STRUCTURES

The vertebrae have been removed superiorly to expose the spinal cord and meninges.
- The aorta descends to the left of the midline, with the thoracic duct and azygos vein to its right.
- Typically, the azygos vein is on the right side of the vertebral bodies, and the hemi-azygos vein is on the left.
- The thoracic sympathetic trunk and ganglia lie lateral to the thoracic vertebrae; the rami communicantes connect the sympathetic ganglia with the spinal nerve.
- A sleeve of dura mater surrounds the spinal nerves and blends with the sheath (epineurium) of the spinal nerve.
- The dura mater is separated from the walls of the vertebral canal by epidural fat and the internal vertebral venous plexus.

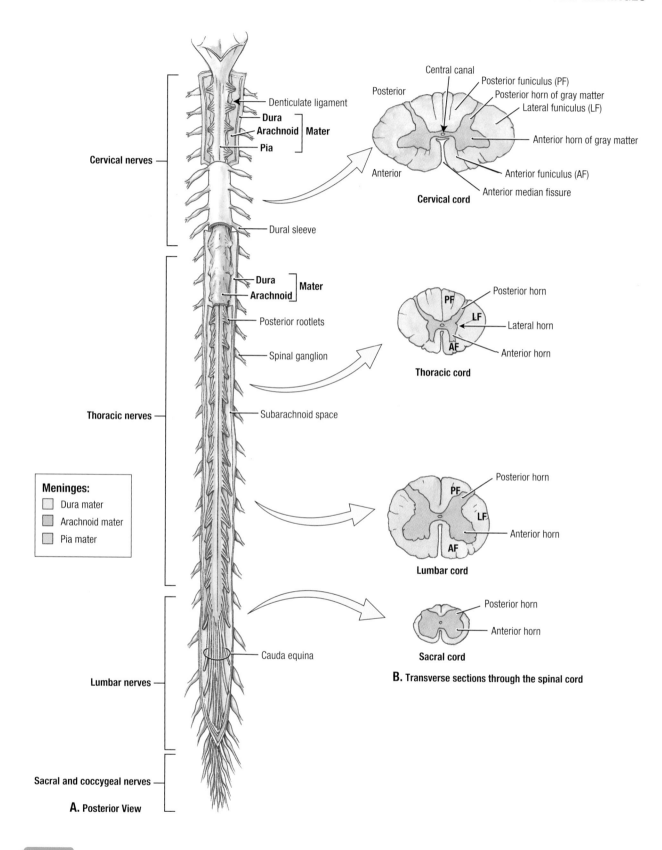

Denticulate ligament

Dura
Arachnoid } Mater
Pia

Cervical nerves

Central canal
Posterior
Posterior funiculus (PF)
Posterior horn of gray matter
Lateral funiculus (LF)

Anterior horn of gray matter

Anterior
Anterior funiculus (AF)
Anterior median fissure

Cervical cord

Dural sleeve

Dura } Mater
Arachnoid

Posterior rootlets

Spinal ganglion

Posterior horn

PF
LF — Lateral horn
AF — Anterior horn

Thoracic cord

Thoracic nerves

Subarachnoid space

Meninges:
☐ Dura mater
☐ Arachnoid mater
☐ Pia mater

Posterior horn

PF
LF
AF — Anterior horn

Lumbar cord

Posterior horn

Anterior horn

Sacral cord

Cauda equina

B. Transverse sections through the spinal cord

Lumbar nerves

Sacral and coccygeal nerves

A. Posterior View

4.46 ISOLATED SPINAL CORD AND SPINAL NERVE ROOTS WITH COVERINGS AND REGIONAL SECTIONS

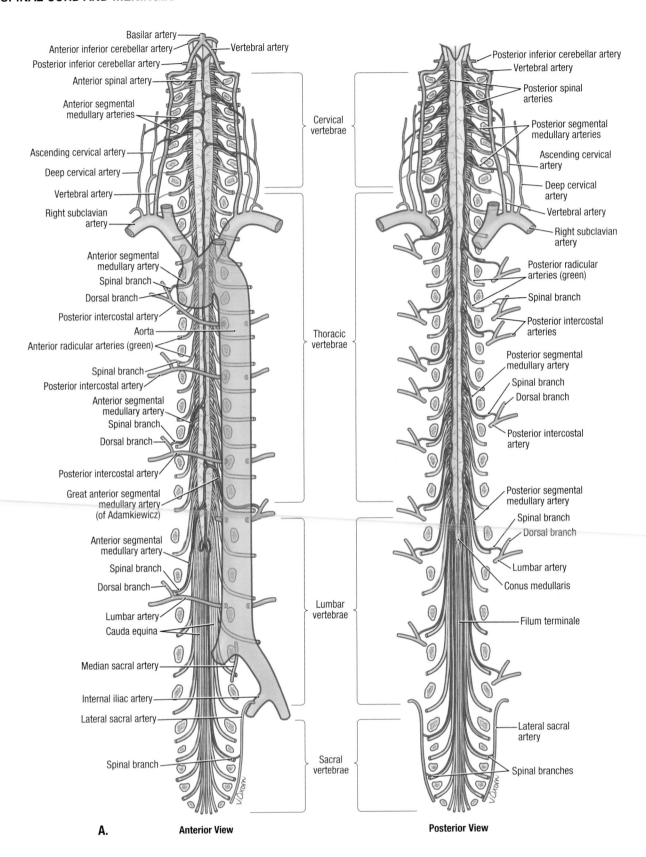

A.   **Anterior View**

                         Posterior View

4.47   BLOOD SUPPLY OF SPINAL CORD

A. Arteries of spinal cord. The segmental reinforcements of blood supply from the segmental medullary arteries are important in supplying blood to the anterior and posterior spinal arteries. Fractures, dislocations, and fracture-dislocations may interfere with the blood supply to the spinal cord from the spinal and medullary arteries.

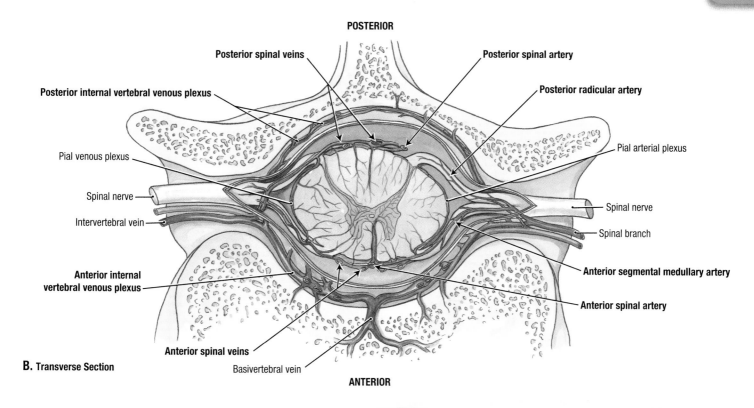

POSTERIOR

Posterior spinal veins

Posterior spinal artery

Posterior internal vertebral venous plexus

Posterior radicular artery

Pial venous plexus

Pial arterial plexus

Spinal nerve

Spinal nerve

Intervertebral vein

Spinal branch

Anterior internal vertebral venous plexus

Anterior segmental medullary artery

Anterior spinal artery

Anterior spinal veins

Basivertebral vein

B. Transverse Section

ANTERIOR

4.47   ## BLOOD SUPPLY OF SPINAL CORD (*CONTINUED*)

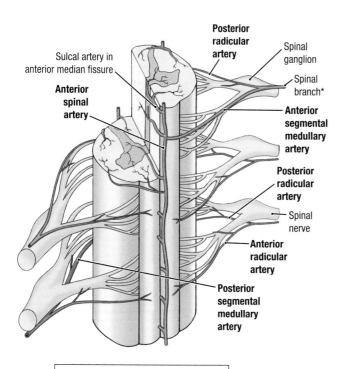

Sulcal artery in anterior median fissure

Posterior radicular artery

Spinal ganglion

Spinal branch*

Anterior spinal artery

Anterior segmental medullary artery

Posterior radicular artery

Spinal nerve

Anterior radicular artery

Posterior segmental medullary artery

* Spinal branches arise from the vertebral, intercostal, lumbar, or sacral artery, depending on level of spinal cord.

C. Anterolateral View

B. Arterial supply and venous drainage. **C.** Segmental medullary and radicular arteries. Three longitudinal arteries supply the spinal cord: an anterior spinal artery, formed by the union of branches of vertebral arteries, and paired posterior spinal arteries, each of which is a branch of either the vertebral artery or the posterior inferior cerebellar artery.

- The spinal arteries run longitudinally from the medulla oblongata of the brainstem to the conus medullaris of the spinal cord. By themselves, the anterior and posterior spinal arteries supply only the short superior part of the spinal cord. The circulation to much of the spinal cord depends on segmental medullary and radicular arteries.

- The anterior and posterior segmental medullary arteries enter the IV foramen to unite with the spinal arteries to supply blood to the spinal cord. The great anterior segmental medullary artery (Adamkiewicz artery) occurs on the left side in 65% of people. It reinforces the circulation to two thirds of the spinal cord.

- Posterior and anterior roots of the spinal nerves and their coverings are supplied by posterior and anterior radicular arteries, which run along the nerve roots. These vessels do not reach the posterior or anterior spinal arteries.

- The 3 anterior and 3 posterior spinal veins are arranged longitudinally; they communicate freely with each other and are drained by up to 12 anterior and posterior medullary and radicular veins. The veins draining the spinal cord join the internal vertebral plexus in the epidural space.

Ischemia. Deficiency of blood supply (ischemia) of the spinal cord affects its function and can lead to muscle weakness and paralysis. The spinal cord may also suffer circulatory impairment if the segmental medullary arteries, particularly the great anterior segmental medullary artery (of Adamkiewicz), are narrowed by obstructive arterial disease or aortic clamping during surgery.

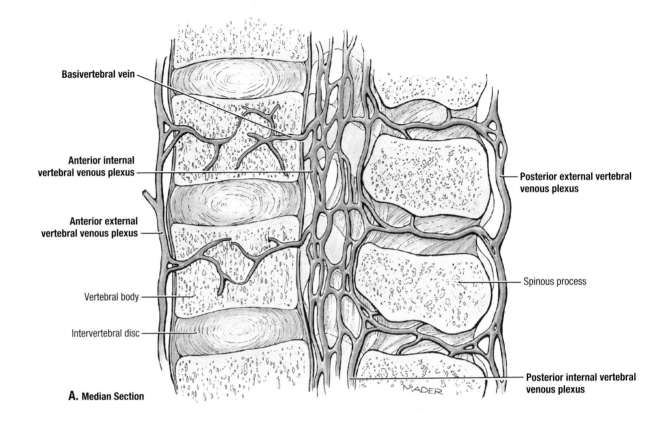

Basivertebral vein

Anterior internal
vertebral venous plexus

Anterior external
vertebral venous plexus

Vertebral body

Intervertebral disc

Posterior external vertebral
venous plexus

Spinous process

Posterior internal vertebral
venous plexus

A. Median Section

Posterior external vertebral
venous plexus

Posterior internal vertebral
venous plexus

Anterior internal vertebral
venous plexus

Intervertebral vein

Lumbar vein

Ascending lumbar
vein

Basivertebral vein

Vertebral body

Anterior external vertebral
venous plexus

B. Superior View

4.48   VERTEBRAL VENOUS PLEXUSES

A. Median section of lumbar spine. **B.** Superior view of lumbar vertebra with the vertebral body sectioned transversely.

- There are internal and external vertebral venous plexuses, communicating with each other and with both systemic veins and the portal system. **Infection and tumors can spread** from the areas drained by the systemic and portal veins to the vertebral venous system and lodge in the vertebrae, spinal cord, brain, or skull.

- The internal vertebral venous plexus, located in the vertebral canal, consists of a plexus of thin-walled, valveless veins that surround the dura mater. Cranially, the internal venous plexus communicates through the foramen magnum with the occipital and basilar sinuses; at each spinal segment, the plexus receives veins from the spinal cord and a basivertebral vein from the vertebral body. The plexus is drained by IV veins that pass through the intervertebral and sacral foramina to the vertebral, intercostal, lumbar, and lateral sacral veins.

- The anterior external vertebral venous plexus is formed by veins that course through the body of each vertebra. Veins that pass through the ligamenta flava form the posterior external vertebral venous plexus. In the cervical region, these plexuses communicate with the occipital and deep cervical veins. In the thoracic, lumbar, and pelvic regions, the azygos (or hemi-azygos), ascending lumbar, and lateral sacral veins, respectively, further link segment to segment.

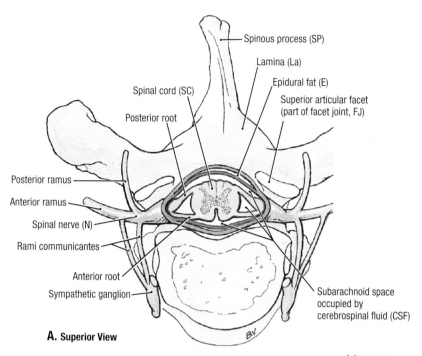

Spinous process (SP)
Lamina (La)
Epidural fat (E)
Superior articular facet
(part of facet joint, FJ)
Spinal cord (SC)
Posterior root
Posterior ramus
Anterior ramus
Spinal nerve (N)
Rami communicantes
Anterior root
Sympathetic ganglion
Subarachnoid space
occupied by
cerebrospinal fluid (CSF)

A. Superior View

B. Transverse (axial) MRI (T1 algorithm)

Interneuron
Posterior horn
of gray matter
Posterior rootlet
Posterior root
Spinal ganglion
Cell body
Spinal nerve
Posterior ramus
Posterior ramus
Anterior ramus
Anterior ramus
Anterior horn
of gray matter
Anterior root
Skin
Anterior rootlets
Spinal cord
Sympathetic ganglion
Skeletal muscle

Somatic (general) sensory
Somatic motor

C. Schematic Illustration

4.49 ## OVERVIEW OF SOMATIC NERVOUS SYSTEM

A. Spinal cord in situ in vertebral canal. **B.** Axial (transverse) MRI of lumbar spine. **C.** Components of typical spinal nerve. The somatic nervous system, or voluntary nervous system, composed of somatic parts of the CNS and PNS, provides general sensory and motor innervation to all parts of the body (G. *soma*), except the viscera in the body cavities, smooth muscle, and glands.

The somatic (general) sensory fibers transmit sensations of touch, pain, temperature, and position from sensory receptors. The somatic motor fibers permit voluntary and reflexive movement by causing contraction of skeletal muscles, such as occurs when one touches a candle flame.

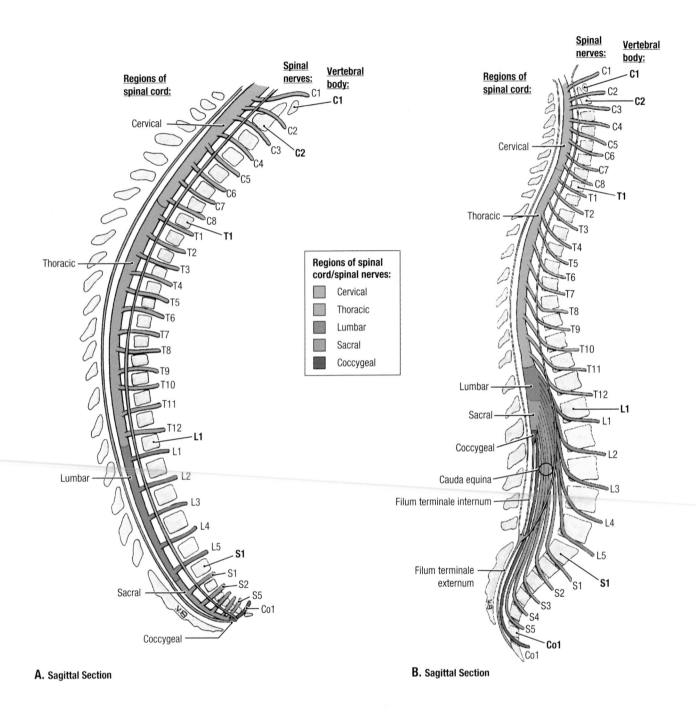

A. Sagittal Section

B. Sagittal Section

Regions of spinal cord/spinal nerves:
- Cervical
- Thoracic
- Lumbar
- Sacral
- Coccygeal

4.50 SPINAL CORD AND SPINAL NERVES

A. Spinal cord at 12 weeks gestation. **B.** Spinal cord of an adult.

- Early in development, the spinal cord and vertebral (spinal) canal are nearly equal in length. The canal grows longer, so spinal nerves have an increasingly longer course to reach the IV foramen at the correct level for their exit. The spinal cord of adults terminates between vertebral bodies L1–L2. The remaining spinal nerves, seeking their IV foramen of exit, form the cauda equina.
- All 31 pairs of spinal nerves—8 cervical (C), 12 thoracic (T), 5 lumbar (L), 5 sacral (S), and 1 coccygeal (Co)—arise from the spinal cord and exit through the IV foramina in the vertebral column.

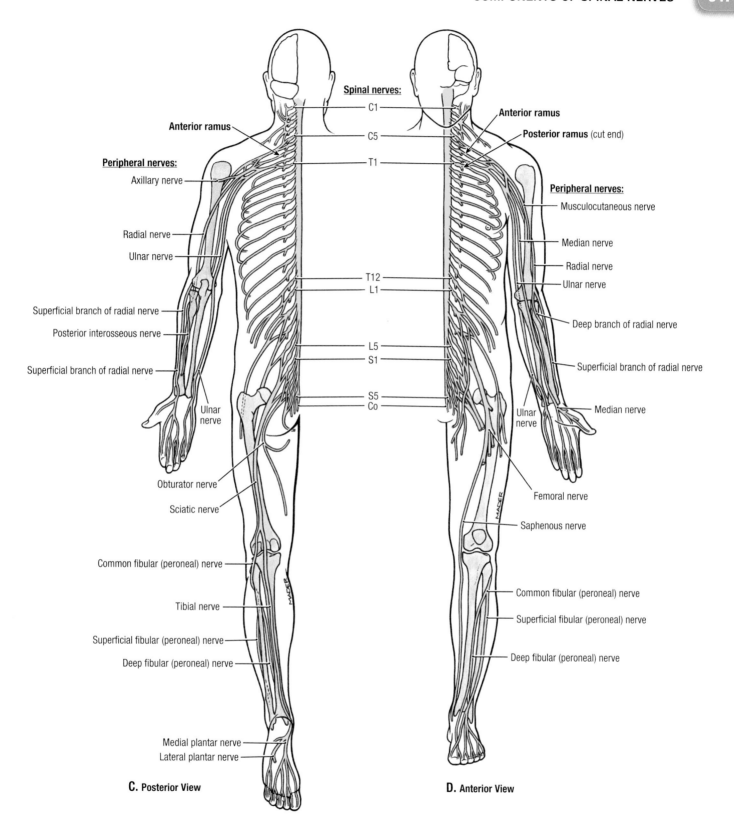

Spinal nerves:
C1
C5
T1
T12
L1
L5
S1
S5
Co

Anterior ramus

Peripheral nerves:
Axillary nerve
Radial nerve
Ulnar nerve
Superficial branch of radial nerve
Posterior interosseous nerve
Superficial branch of radial nerve
Ulnar nerve
Obturator nerve
Sciatic nerve
Common fibular (peroneal) nerve
Tibial nerve
Superficial fibular (peroneal) nerve
Deep fibular (peroneal) nerve
Medial plantar nerve
Lateral plantar nerve

C. Posterior View

Anterior ramus
Posterior ramus (cut end)

Peripheral nerves:
Musculocutaneous nerve
Median nerve
Radial nerve
Ulnar nerve
Deep branch of radial nerve
Superficial branch of radial nerve
Median nerve
Ulnar nerve
Femoral nerve
Saphenous nerve
Common fibular (peroneal) nerve
Superficial fibular (peroneal) nerve
Deep fibular (peroneal) nerve

D. Anterior View

4.50 SPINAL CORD AND SPINAL NERVES (*CONTINUED*)

C. and D. Peripheral nerves.
- The anterior rami supply nerve fibers to the anterior and lateral regions of the trunk and upper and lower limbs.

- The posterior rami supply nerve fibers to synovial joints of the vertebral column, deep muscles of the back, and overlying skin.

Anterolateral View

A.

Inferior View

Posterior View

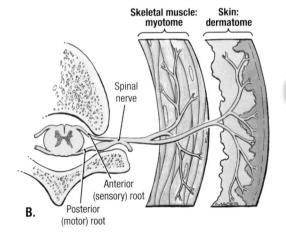

Skeletal muscle: myotome   Skin: dermatome

Spinal nerve

Anterior (sensory) root

Posterior (motor) root

B.

4.51   DERMATOMES

A.–C. Dermatome map (Foerster, 1933). The Keegan and Garrett (1948) dermatome map is not included here. The two schemes are similar in the trunk but differ in the limbs, where both are presented. **B.** Schematic illustration of a dermatome and myotome. The unilateral area of skin innervated by the general sensory fibers of a single spinal nerve is called a dermatome. From clinical studies of lesions in the posterior roots or spinal nerves, dermatome maps have been devised that indicate the typical patterns of innervation of the skin by specific spinal nerves.

Lateral rotation (shoulder)
C5

Medial rotation (shoulder)
C6, C7, C8

Finger flexion
C7, **C8**

Adduction (shoulder)
C6, C7, C8

Abduction (shoulder)
C5

Lateral rotation (hip)
L5, S1

Medial rotation (hip)
L1, L2, L3

Finger extension
C7, C8

Adduction (hip)
L1, L2, L3

Abduction (hip)
L5, S1

A. Anterior View

The movements associated with each **bolded** segment are most commonly tested to determine the neurologic level of a lesion.

Flexion (elbow)
C5, **C6**

Extension (elbow)
C6, **C7**

Extension (wrist)
C6, C7

Flexion (wrist)
C6, **C7**

B. Lateral View

Supination (forearm)
C6

Pronation (forearm)
C7, C8

C. Anterior View

Abduction
T1

Abduction
T1

Adduction
T1

**Abduction and Adduction of Digits
(Metacarpophalangeal Joints)**

D. Anterior View

Extension (shoulder)
C6, C7, C8

Flexion (shoulder)
C5

Extension (hip)
L4, L5

Flexion (hip)
L2, L3

Flexion (knee)
L5, S1

Extension (knee)
L3, L4

Dorsiflexion (ankle)
L4, L5

Plantarflexion (ankle)
S1, S2

E. Lateral View

4.52   MYOTOMES

Somatic motor (general somatic efferent) fibers transmit impulses to skeletal (voluntary) muscles. The unilateral muscle mass receiving innervation from the somatic motor fibers conveyed by a single spinal nerve is a myotome. Each skeletal muscle is innervated by the somatic motor fibers of several spinal nerves; therefore, the muscle myotome will consist of several segments. The muscle myotomes have been grouped by joint movement to facilitate clinical testing. The intrinsic muscles of the hand constitute a single myotome—T1.

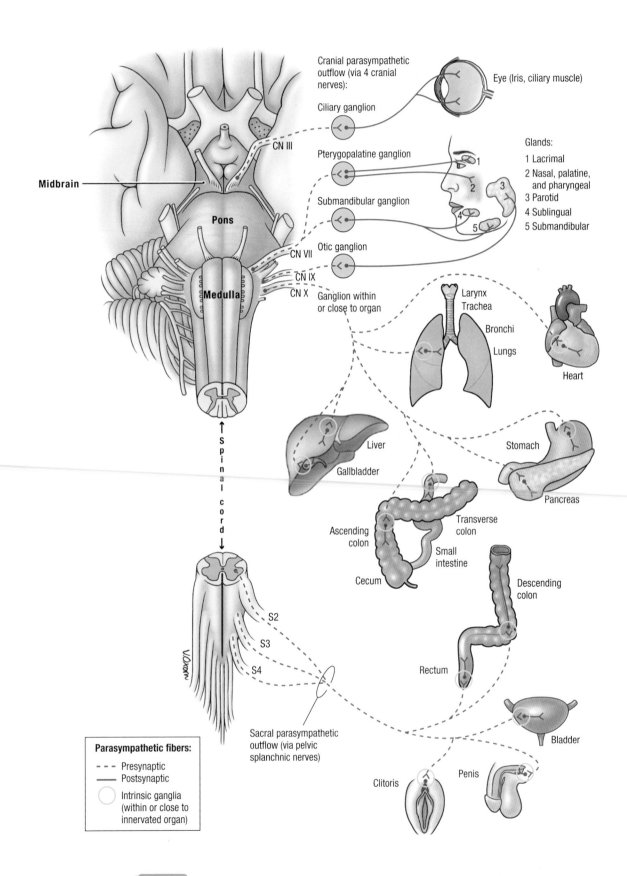

Cranial parasympathetic outflow (via 4 cranial nerves):

Ciliary ganglion

Eye (Iris, ciliary muscle)

CN III

Midbrain

Pterygopalatine ganglion

Glands:
1 Lacrimal
2 Nasal, palatine, and pharyngeal
3 Parotid
4 Sublingual
5 Submandibular

Pons

Submandibular ganglion

Otic ganglion

CN VII

CN IX

CN X

Medulla

Ganglion within or close to organ

Larynx
Trachea

Bronchi

Lungs

Heart

Spinal cord

Liver

Gallbladder

Stomach

Pancreas

Ascending colon

Transverse colon

Small intestine

Cecum

Descending colon

S2

S3

S4

Rectum

Sacral parasympathetic outflow (via pelvic splanchnic nerves)

Bladder

Parasympathetic fibers:
- - - Presynaptic
——— Postsynaptic
◯ Intrinsic ganglia (within or close to innervated organ)

Clitoris

Penis

4.53   DISTRIBUTION OF PARASYMPATHETIC NERVE FIBERS

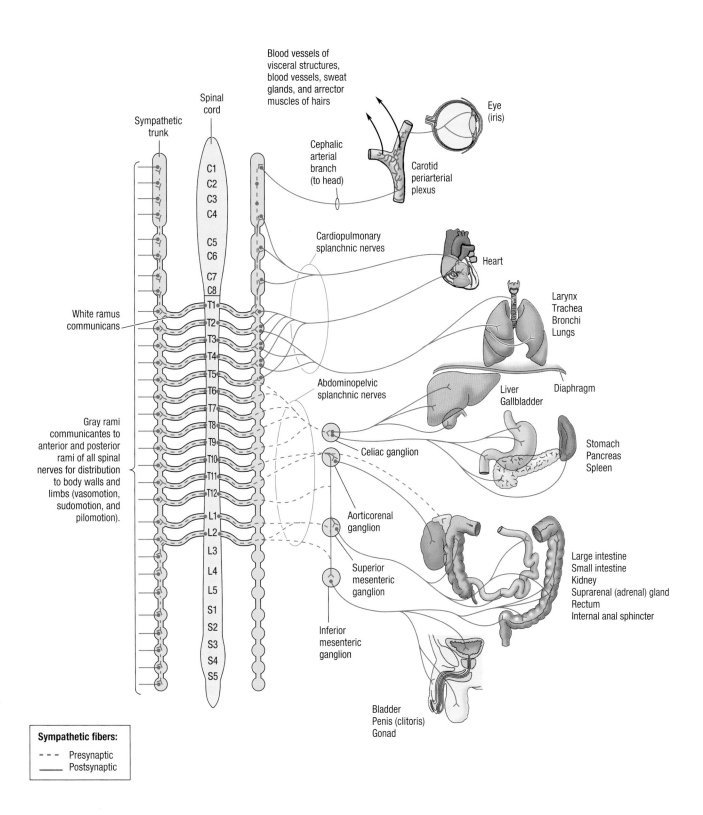

Sympathetic trunk

Spinal cord

Blood vessels of visceral structures, blood vessels, sweat glands, and arrector muscles of hairs

Cephalic arterial branch (to head)

Eye (iris)

Carotid periarterial plexus

C1
C2
C3
C4
C5
C6
C7
C8
T1
T2
T3
T4
T5
T6
T7
T8
T9
T10
T11
T12
L1
L2
L3
L4
L5
S1
S2
S3
S4
S5

White ramus communicans

Gray rami communicantes to anterior and posterior rami of all spinal nerves for distribution to body walls and limbs (vasomotion, sudomotion, and pilomotion).

Cardiopulmonary splanchnic nerves

Heart

Larynx
Trachea
Bronchi
Lungs

Diaphragm

Abdominopelvic splanchnic nerves

Liver
Gallbladder

Celiac ganglion

Stomach
Pancreas
Spleen

Aorticorenal ganglion

Superior mesenteric ganglion

Large intestine
Small intestine
Kidney
Suprarenal (adrenal) gland
Rectum
Internal anal sphincter

Inferior mesenteric ganglion

Bladder
Penis (clitoris)
Gonad

Sympathetic fibers:

- - - Presynaptic
——— Postsynaptic

4.54 DISTRIBUTION OF SYMPATHETIC NERVE FIBERS

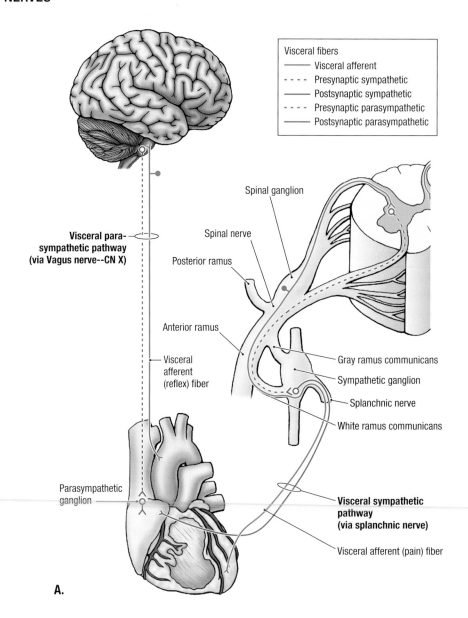

Visceral fibers
—— Visceral afferent
- - - - Presynaptic sympathetic
—— Postsynaptic sympathetic
- - - - Presynaptic parasympathetic
—— Postsynaptic parasympathetic

Spinal ganglion

Spinal nerve

Posterior ramus

Visceral para-sympathetic pathway (via Vagus nerve--CN X)

Anterior ramus

Visceral afferent (reflex) fiber

Gray ramus communicans

Sympathetic ganglion

Splanchnic nerve

White ramus communicans

Parasympathetic ganglion

Visceral sympathetic pathway (via splanchnic nerve)

Visceral afferent (pain) fiber

A.

4.55   VISCERAL AFFERENT AND VISCERAL EFFERENT (MOTOR) INNERVATION

A. Schematic illustration. Visceral afferent fibers have important relationships to the CNS, both anatomically and functionally. We are usually unaware of the sensory input of these fibers, which provides information about the condition of the body's internal environment. This information is integrated in the CNS, often triggering visceral or somatic reflexes or both. Visceral reflexes regulate blood pressure and chemistry by altering such functions as heart and respiratory rates and vascular resistance. Visceral sensation that reaches a conscious level is generally categorized as pain that is usually poorly localized and may be perceived as hunger or nausea. However, adequate stimulation may elicit true pain. Most visceral/reflex (unconscious) sensation and some pain travel in visceral afferent fibers that accompany the parasympathetic fibers retrograde. Most visceral pain impulses (from the heart and most organs of the peritoneal cavity) travel along visceral afferent fibers accompanying sympathetic fibers.

Visceral efferent (motor) innervation. The efferent nerve fibers and ganglia of the ANS are organized into two systems or divisions.

1. Sympathetic (thoracolumbar) division. In general, the effects of sympathetic stimulation are catabolic (preparing the body for "flight or fight").
2. Parasympathetic (craniosacral) division. In general, the effects of parasympathetic stimulation are anabolic (promoting normal function and conserving energy).

Conduction of impulses from the CNS to the effector organ involves a series of two neurons in both sympathetic and parasympathetic systems. The cell body of the presynaptic (preganglionic) neuron (first neuron) is located in the gray matter of the CNS. Its fiber (axon) synapses on the cell body of a postsynaptic (postganglionic) neuron, the second neuron in the series. The cell bodies of such second neurons are located in autonomic ganglia outside the CNS, and the postsynaptic fibers terminate on the effector organ (smooth muscle, modified cardiac muscle, or glands).

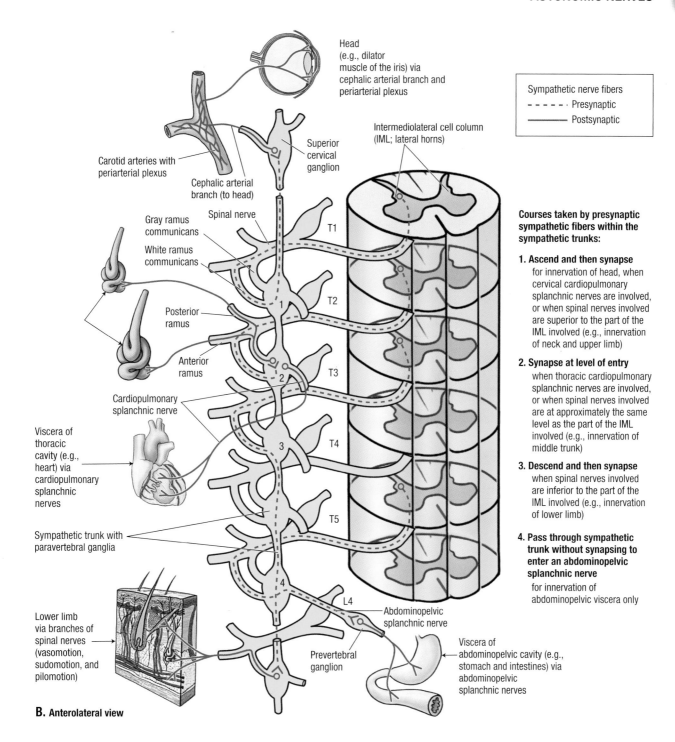

Head
(e.g., dilator
muscle of the iris) via
cephalic arterial branch and
periarterial plexus

Intermediolateral cell column
(IML; lateral horns)

Carotid arteries with
periarterial plexus

Cephalic arterial
branch (to head)

Superior
cervical
ganglion

Sympathetic nerve fibers
- - - - - Presynaptic
————— Postsynaptic

Gray ramus
communicans

White ramus
communicans

Spinal nerve

T1

Posterior
ramus

T2

Anterior
ramus

Cardiopulmonary
splanchnic nerve

T3

Viscera of
thoracic
cavity (e.g.,
heart) via
cardiopulmonary
splanchnic
nerves

T4

Sympathetic trunk with
paravertebral ganglia

T5

Lower limb
via branches of
spinal nerves
(vasomotion,
sudomotion, and
pilomotion)

L4

Abdominopelvic
splanchnic nerve

Prevertebral
ganglion

Viscera of
abdominopelvic cavity (e.g.,
stomach and intestines) via
abdominopelvic
splanchnic nerves

B. Anterolateral view

**Courses taken by presynaptic
sympathetic fibers within the
sympathetic trunks:**

1. **Ascend and then synapse**
   for innervation of head, when
   cervical cardiopulmonary
   splanchnic nerves are involved,
   or when spinal nerves involved
   are superior to the part of the
   IML involved (e.g., innervation
   of neck and upper limb)

2. **Synapse at level of entry**
   when thoracic cardiopulmonary
   splanchnic nerves are involved,
   or when spinal nerves involved
   are at approximately the same
   level as the part of the IML
   involved (e.g., innervation of
   middle trunk)

3. **Descend and then synapse**
   when spinal nerves involved
   are inferior to the part of the
   IML involved (e.g., innervation
   of lower limb)

4. **Pass through sympathetic
   trunk without synapsing to
   enter an abdominopelvic
   splanchnic nerve**
   for innervation of
   abdominopelvic viscera only

4.55   VISCERAL AFFERENT AND VISCERAL EFFERENT (MOTOR) INNERVATION (*CONTINUED*)

B. Courses taken by sympathetic motor fibers. Presynaptic fibers
all follow the same course until they reach the sympathetic trunks. In
the sympathetic trunks, they follow one of four possible courses. Fibers
involved in providing sympathetic innervation to the body wall and limbs
or viscera above the level of the diaphragm follow paths 1 to 3. They
synapse in the paravertebral ganglia of the sympathetic trunks. Fibers
involved in innervating abdominopelvic viscera follow path 4 to prevertebral ganglion via abdominopelvic splanchnic nerves. Postsynaptic fibers
usually don't ascend or descend within the sympathetic trunks, exiting at
the level of synapse.

A. Inferior View

B. Inferior View

1	Site of retropharyngeal space
2	Longus colli
3	Longus capitis
4	Parotid gland
5	Retromandibular vein
6	Stylopharyngeus
7	Styloglossus
8	Stylohyoid muscle and ligament/process
9	Internal carotid artery
10	Internal jugular vein
11	Rectus capitis lateralis
12	Posterior belly of digastric
13	Anterior arch of atlas (C1 vertebra)
14	Lateral mass of atlas (C1)
15	Posterior arch of atlas (C1)
16	Vertebral artery
17	Transverse ligament of atlas (C1)
18	Transverse process of atlas (C1)
19	Spinal cord
20	Rectus capitis posterior major
21	Obliquus capitis inferior
22	Obliquus capitis superior
23	Spinous process of atlas (C1)
24	Longissimus capitis
25	Rectus capitis posterior minor
26	Semispinalis capitis
27	Sternocleidomastoid
28	Splenius capitis
29	Trapezius
30	Fatty mass
31	Dens of axis (C2 vertebra)
32	Anterior tubercle of atlas (C1)
33	Inferior articular facet of atlas (C1)
34	Foramen magnum
35	Foramen transversarium
36	Posterior tubercle of atlas (C1)
37	Mastoid process
38	Occipital bone of skull
39	External occipital protuberance
40	Ramus of mandible

ANTERIOR

RIGHT ⟷ LEFT

POSTERIOR

C. Postero-inferior View

4.56 IMAGING OF SUPERIOR NUCHAL REGION AT LEVEL OF ATLAS

A. Transverse section of specimen. **B.** Transverse computed tomographic (CT) scan. **C.** Three-dimensional (3D) CT of the base of the skull and atlas.

A. Inferior View

B. Inferior View

1	Linea alba	6	Latissimus dorsi	11	Multifidus	16	Spinous process
2	Rectus abdominis	7	Descending aorta	12	Rotatores	17	Cauda equina
3	External oblique	8	Inferior vena cava	13	Iliocostalis	18	Psoas major
4	Internal oblique	9	Spinalis	14	4th lumbar vertebra	19	Quadratus lumborum
5	Transversus abdominis	10	Longissimus	15	Transverse process		

4.57   IMAGING OF LUMBAR SPINE AT L4

A. Transverse section of specimen. **B.** Transverse computed tomographic (CT) scan.

A. Inferior View

B. Inferior View

1	Rectus abdominis	6	Internal iliac vein	10	2nd sacral vertebra	14	Erector spinae
2	External oblique	7	Anterior rami	11	Sacro-iliac joint	15	Gluteus minimis
3	Internal oblique	8	Superior gluteal vessels	12	Sacral nerve root	16	Gluteus medius
4	Iliopsoas	9	Body of ilium	13	Multifidus	17	Gluteus maximus
5	Internal iliac artery						

4.58   IMAGING OF SACRO-ILIAC JOINT

A. Transverse section of specimen. **B.** Transverse computed tomographic (CT) scan.

A.

B.

C.

D.

AR	Anterior ramus	LL	Left lung	SG	Suprarenal gland
C1-T1	Vertebrae	M	Medulla oblongata	SI	Small intestine
Cr	Crus of diaphragm	MP	Mastoid process	SN	Spinal nerve
CSF	Cerebrospinal fluid in subarachnoid space	P	Psoas muscle	Sp	Spleen
D	Dens (odontoid) process of C2	PR	Posterior ramus	St	Sternocleidomastoid
HA	Hemi-azygos vein	RK	Right kidney	ST	Stomach
IV	Intervertebral disc	RL	Right lung	VA	Vertebral artery
L	Liver	S	Spinal cord		
LK	Left kidney	SF	Splenic flexure		

4.59 CORONAL MRI SCANS OF CERVICAL AND THORACIC SPINE

A. and **B.** Cervical spine. **C.** and **D.** Thoracic spine.

Lower Limb

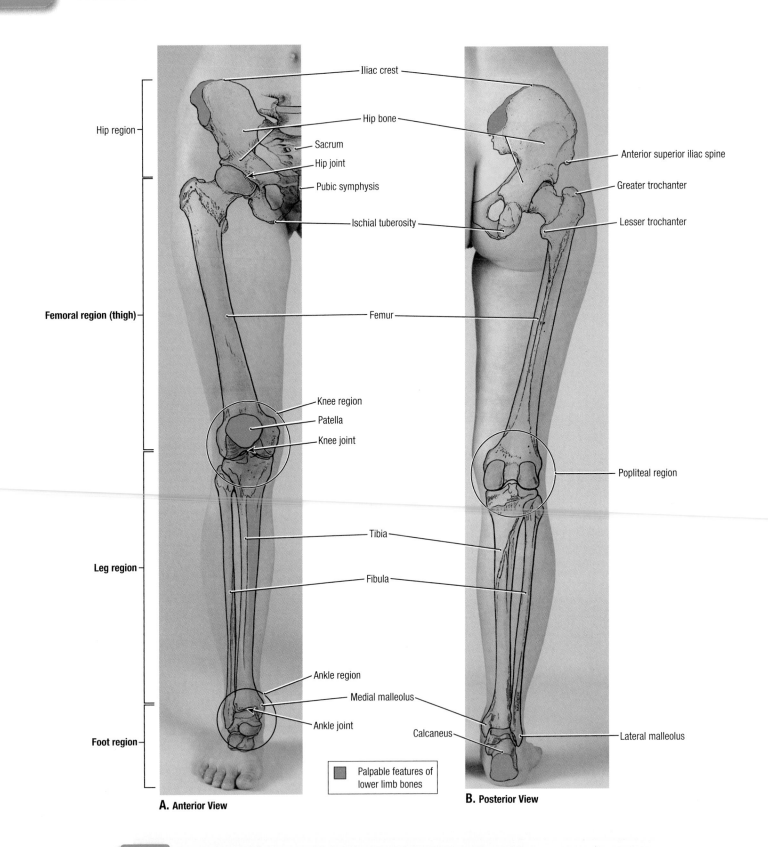

A. Anterior View

B. Posterior View

5.1   REGIONS, BONES, AND MAJOR JOINTS OF LOWER LIMB

The hip bones meet anteriorly at the pubic symphysis and articulate with the sacrum posteriorly. The femur articulates with the hip bone proximally and the tibia distally. The tibia and fibula are the bones of the leg that join the foot at the ankle.

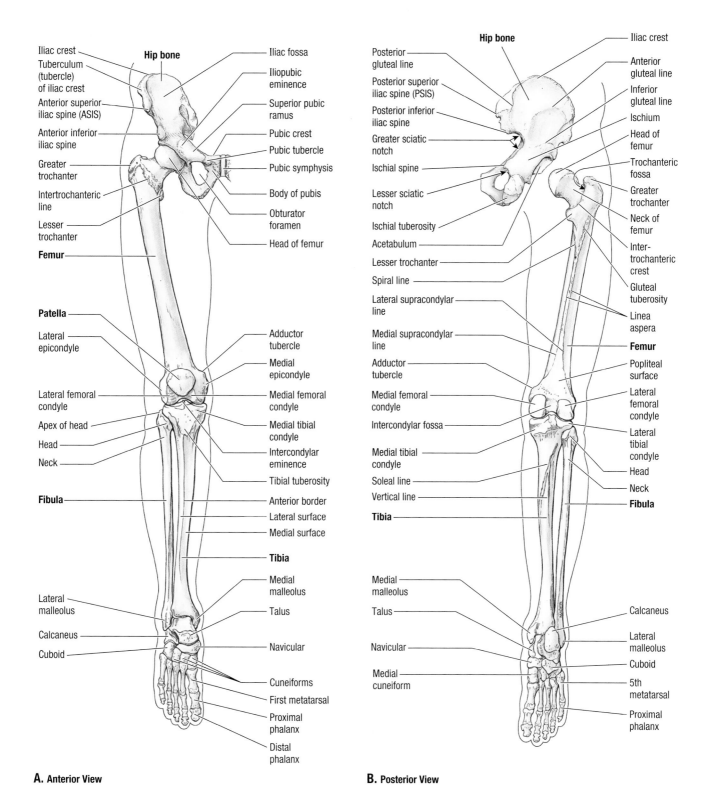

A. Anterior View

Iliac crest
Tuberculum (tubercle) of iliac crest
Anterior superior iliac spine (ASIS)
Anterior inferior iliac spine
Greater trochanter
Intertrochanteric line
Lesser trochanter
Femur

Hip bone

Iliac fossa
Iliopubic eminence
Superior pubic ramus
Pubic crest
Pubic tubercle
Pubic symphysis
Body of pubis
Obturator foramen
Head of femur

Patella
Lateral epicondyle
Lateral femoral condyle
Apex of head
Head
Neck
Fibula

Adductor tubercle
Medial epicondyle
Medial femoral condyle
Medial tibial condyle
Intercondylar eminence
Tibial tuberosity
Anterior border
Lateral surface
Medial surface
Tibia
Medial malleolus
Talus
Navicular
Cuneiforms
First metatarsal
Proximal phalanx
Distal phalanx

Lateral malleolus
Calcaneus
Cuboid

B. Posterior View

Posterior gluteal line
Posterior superior iliac spine (PSIS)
Posterior inferior iliac spine
Greater sciatic notch
Ischial spine
Lesser sciatic notch
Ischial tuberosity
Acetabulum
Lesser trochanter
Spiral line
Lateral supracondylar line
Medial supracondylar line
Adductor tubercle
Medial femoral condyle
Intercondylar fossa
Medial tibial condyle
Soleal line
Vertical line
Tibia

Hip bone

Iliac crest
Anterior gluteal line
Inferior gluteal line
Ischium
Head of femur
Trochanteric fossa
Greater trochanter
Neck of femur
Inter-trochanteric crest
Gluteal tuberosity
Linea aspera
Femur
Popliteal surface
Lateral femoral condyle
Lateral tibial condyle
Head
Neck
Fibula

Medial malleolus
Talus
Navicular
Medial cuneiform

Calcaneus
Lateral malleolus
Cuboid
5th metatarsal
Proximal phalanx

5.2   FEATURES OF BONES OF LOWER LIMB

The foot is in full plantar flexion. The hip joint is disarticulated in **B** to demonstrate the acetabulum of the hip bone and the entire head of the femur.

A. Anterior View

Pubis

Ilium (I)

Ischium (S)

Femur (F)

Tibia

Fibula

Talus

Calcaneus

Cuboid

Metatarsals

Phalanges

B. Anteroposterior View

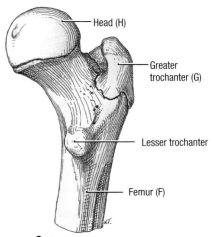

Head (H)

Greater trochanter (G)

Lesser trochanter

Femur (F)

C. Posterior View

D. Anteroposterior View

| 5.3 | POSTNATAL LOWER LIMB DEVELOPMENT |

A. Bones of lower limb at birth. The hip bone can be divided into three primary parts: ilium, ischium, and pubis. The diaphyses (bodies) of the long bones are well ossified. Some epiphyses (growth plates) and tarsal bones have begun to ossify, including the distal epiphysis of the femur and proximal epiphysis of the tibia, calcaneus, talus, and cuboid. **B. and D.** Anteroposterior radiographs of postmortem specimens of newborns show the bony (*white*) and cartilaginous *(gray)* components of the femur and hip bone. **C.** Epiphyses at proximal end of femur. The epiphysis of the head of the femur begins to ossify during the 1st year, that of the greater trochanter before the 5th year, and that of the

lesser trochanter before the 14th year. These usually fuse completely with the body (shaft) before the end of the 18th year.

Dislocated epiphysis of femoral head. In older children and adolescents (10 to 17 years of age), the epiphysis of the femoral head may slip away from the femoral neck because of weakness of the epiphyseal plate. This injury may be caused by acute trauma or repetitive microtraumas that place increased shearing stress on the epiphysis, especially with abduction and lateral rotation.

Tibia

Epiphysial plate

Synovial folds

Medial cuneiform

Epiphysis

1st metatarsal

Proximal phalanx

Distal phalanx

Talus

Calcaneus

Navicular

E. Sagittal Section

Epiphysial plate

Tibia

Synovial folds

Talus

2nd metatarsal

Calcaneus

Epiphysis

Navicular

Middle cuneiform

Epiphysis of
calcaneus

F. Sagittal Section

5.3 POSTNATAL LOWER LIMB DEVELOPMENT (*CONTINUED*)

E. Foot of child age 4. **F.** Foot of child age 10.

- In the foot of the younger child **(E),** epiphyses of long bones (tibia, metatarsals, and phalanges) ossify like short bones, with the ossification centers being enveloped in cartilage. Ossification has already extended to the surface of the larger tarsal bones.
- In the foot of the older child **(F),** ossification has spread to the dorsal and plantar surfaces of all tarsal bones in view, and cartilage persists on the articular surfaces only.
- The traction epiphysis of the calcaneus for the calcaneal tendon and plantar aponeurosis begins to ossify from the ages of 6 to 10 years.
- The first metatarsal bone is similar to a phalanx in that its epiphysis is at the base instead of the head, as in the second and other metatarsal bones.

- The tuberosity of the calcaneus and the sesamoid bones of the first and the heads of the second to fifth metatarsals (here the second) support the longitudinal arch of the foot; the medial part of the longitudinal arch is higher and more mobile than the lateral.

Fractures involving epiphysial plates. The primary ossification center for the superior end of the tibia appears shortly after birth and joins the shaft of the tibia during adolescence (usually 16 to 18 years of age). Tibial fractures in children are more serious if they involve the epiphysial plates because continued normal growth of bone may be jeopardized. Disruption of the epiphysial plate at the tibial tuberosity may cause inflammation of the tuberosity and chronic recurring pain during adolescence (Osgood-Schlatter disease), especially in young athletes.

A. Anterior View

L2
L3
L4
Psoas

Femoral nerve (L2–L4)

Iliacus

Obturator nerve (L2–L4)

Rectus femoris
Pectineus
Sartorius

Obturator externus
Posterior branch
Anterior branch

Anterior compartment of thigh

Vastus lateralis
Vastus intermedius
Vastus medialis
Articularis genu

Adductor brevis
Adductor longus
Adductor magnus
Gracilis

Medial compartment of thigh

Innervation of thigh:
- Anterior compartment
- Medial compartment
- Posterior compartment

Common fibular (peroneal) nerve (L4–S2)

Superficial fibular (peroneal) nerve (L4–S1)

Deep fibular (peroneal) nerve (L5–S2)

Tibialis anterior

Lateral compartment of leg

Fibularis (peroneus) longus
Fibularis (peroneus) brevis

Extensor hallucis longus

Extensor digitorum longus

Anterior compartment of leg

Fibularis (peroneus) tertius

Extensor digitorum brevis

Innervation of leg:
- Anterior compartment
- Lateral compartment
- Posterior compartment of leg and sole of foot

B. Posterior View

Superior gluteal nerve
Inferior gluteal nerve

Gluteal compartment

Sciatic nerve (tibial and common fibular)

Semitendinosus
Biceps femoris (long head)
Semitendinosus
Adductor magnus
Semimembranosus
Biceps femoris (short head)

Posterior compartment of thigh

Tibial nerve (L4–S3)

Common fibular (peroneal) nerve (L4–S2)

Gastrocnemius
Popliteus

Plantaris
Gastrocnemius

Posterior compartment of leg

Soleus

Flexor digitorum longus

Tibialis posterior

Posterior compartment of leg

Flexor hallucis longus

Medial plantar nerve (L4–L5)

Abductor hallucis

Flexor digitorum brevis
Flexor hallucis brevis
Lumbrical to 2nd digit

Lateral plantar nerve (S1–S2)

All other muscles in sole of foot

TABLE 5.1 MOTOR NERVES OF LOWER LIMB

Nerve	Origin	Course	Distribution
Femoral		Passes deep to midpoint of inguinal ligament, lateral to femoral vessels, dividing into muscular and cutaneous branches in femoral triangle	Anterior thigh muscles
Obturator	Lumbar plexus (L2–L4)	Traverses lesser pelvis to enter thigh via obturator foramen and then divides; its anterior branch descends between adductor longus and adductor brevis; its posterior branch descends between adductor brevis and adductor magnus	*Anterior branch:* adductor longus, adductor brevis, gracilis, and pectineus; *Posterior branch:* obturator externus and adductor magnus
Sciatic	Sacral plexus (L4–S3)	Enters gluteal region through greater sciatic foramen, usually passing inferior to piriformis, descends in posterior compartment of thigh, bifurcating at apex of popliteal fossa into tibial and common fibular (peroneal) nerves	Muscles of posterior thigh, leg and sole and dorsum of foot
Tibial	Sciatic nerve	Terminal branch of sciatic nerve arising at apex of popliteal fossa; descends through popliteal fossa with popliteal vessels, continuing in deep posterior compartment of leg with posterior tibial vessels; bifurcates into medial and lateral plantar nerves	Hamstring muscles of posterior compartment of thigh, muscles of posterior compartment of leg, and sole of foot
Common fibular (peroneal)		Terminal branch of sciatic nerve arising at apex of popliteal fossa; follows medial border of biceps femoris and its tendon to wind around neck of fibula deep to fibularis longus, where it bifurcates into superficial and deep fibular nerves	Short head of biceps femoris, muscles of anterior and lateral compartments of leg, and dorsum of foot
Superficial fibular (peroneal)	Common fibular nerve	Arises deep to fibularis longus on neck of fibula and descends in lateral compartment of the leg; pierces crural fascia in distal third of leg to become cutaneous	Muscles of lateral compartment of leg
Deep fibular (peroneal)		Arises deep to fibularis longus on neck of fibula; passes through extensor digitorum longus into anterior compartment, descending on interosseous membrane; crosses ankle joint and enters dorsum of foot	Muscles of anterior compartment of leg and dorsum of foot

Lateral cutaneous branch of subcostal nerve (T12)

Femoral branch — Genitofemoral nerve

Genital branch

Ilioinguinal nerve

Lateral cutaneous nerve of thigh, anterior branches

Cutaneous branch of obturator nerve

Anterior cutaneous branches of femoral nerve (lateral group)

Anterior cutaneous branches of femoral nerve (medial group)

Infrapatellar branch of saphenous nerve

Saphenous nerve (from femoral nerve)

Lateral sural cutaneous nerve (from common fibular nerve)

Superficial fibular (peroneal) nerve becoming dorsal digital nerves

Lateral dorsal cutaneous nerve of foot (termination of sural nerve)

Deep fibular (peroneal) nerve

A. Anterior View

Superior clunial nerves (posterior rami) L1 L2 L3

Lateral cutaneous branch of iliohypogastric nerve

Medial clunial nerves (posterior rami) S1 S2 S3

Lateral cutaneous nerve of thigh (posterior branches)

Inferior clunial nerves (branches of posterior cutaneous nerve of thigh)

Cutaneous branches of obturator nerve

Lateral cutaneous nerve of thigh (continuation of anterior branches)

Posterior cutaneous nerve of thigh

Lateral sural cutaneous nerve (from common fibular nerve)

Saphenous nerve (from femoral nerve)

Medial sural cutaneous nerve (from tibial nerve)

Communicating branch of lateral sural cutaneous nerve

Sural nerve

Medial calcaneal branches of tibial nerve

Lateral plantar nerve

Medial plantar nerve

B. Posterior View

5.5 **CUTANEOUS NERVES OF LOWER LIMB**

Cutaneous nerves in the subcutaneous tissue supply the skin of the lower limb. The cutaneous innervation of the lower limb reflects both the original segmental innervation of the skin via separate spinal nerves in its dermatomal pattern (Fig. 5.8) and the result of plexus formation of segmental peripheral nerves. In **B**, the medial sural cutaneous nerve (*sural* is Latin for calf) is joined between the popliteal fossa and posterior aspect of the ankle by a communicating branch of the lateral sural cutaneous nerve to form the sural nerve. The level of the junction is variable and is low in this specimen.

TABLE 5.2 CUTANEOUS NERVES OF LOWER LIMB

Nerve	Origin (Contributing Spinal Nerves)	Course	Distribution to Skin of Lower Limb
Subcostal (lateral cutaneous branch)	T12 anterior ramus	Descends over iliac crest	Hip region inferior to anterior part of iliac crest and anterior to greater trochanter
Iliohypogastric	Lumbar plexus (L1; occasionally T12)	Parallels iliac crest	Lateral cutaneous branch supplies superolateral quadrant of buttock
Ilio-inguinal	Lumbar plexus (L1; occasionally T12)	Passes through inguinal canal	Inguinal fold; femoral branch supplies skin over medial femoral triangle
Genitofemoral	Lumbar plexus (L1–L2)	Descends anterior surface of psoas major	Femoral branch supplies skin over lateral part of femoral triangle; genital branch supplies anterior scrotum or labia majora
Lateral cutaneous nerve of thigh	Lumbar plexus (L2–L3)	Passes deep to inguinal ligament, 2–3 cm medial to anterior superior iliac spine	Skin on anterior and lateral aspects of thigh
Anterior cutaneous branches	Lumbar plexus via femoral nerve (L2–L4)	Arise in femoral triangle; pierce fascia lata along the path of sartorius muscle	Skin of anterior and medial aspects of thigh
Cutaneous branch of obturator nerve	Lumbar plexus via obturator nerve (L2–L4)	Following its descent between adductors longus and brevis, obturator nerve pierces fascia lata to reach the skin of thigh	Skin of middle part of medial thigh
Posterior cutaneous nerve of thigh	Sacral plexus (S1–S3)	Enters gluteal region via greater sciatic foramen deep to gluteus maximus; then descends deep to fascia lata; terminal branches pierce fascia lata	Supply skin of posterior thigh and popliteal fossa
Saphenous nerve	Lumbar plexus via femoral nerve (L3–L4)	Traverses adductor canal but does not pass through adductor hiatus	Skin on medial side of leg and foot
Superficial fibular nerve	Common fibular nerve (L4–S1)	After supplying fibular muscles, perforates deep fascia of leg	Skin of anterolateral leg and dorsum of foot
Deep fibular nerve	Common fibular nerve (L5)	After supplying muscles on dorsum of foot, pierces deep fascia superior to heads of 1st and 2nd metatarsals	Skin of web between great and 2nd toes
Sural nerve	Tibial and common fibular nerves (S1–S2)	Medial sural cutaneous branch of tibial nerve and lateral sural cutaneous branch of common fibular nerve merge at varying levels on posterior leg	Skin of posterolateral leg and lateral margin of foot
Medial plantar nerve	Tibial nerve (L4–L5)	Passes between first and second layers of plantar muscles	Skin of medial side of sole, and plantar aspect, sides, and nail beds of medial 3½ toes
Lateral plantar nerve	Tibial nerve (S1–S2)	Passes between first and second layers of plantar muscles	Skin of lateral sole, and plantar aspect, sides, and nail beds of lateral 1½ toes
Calcaneal nerves	Tibial and sural nerves (S1–S2)	Branches over calcaneal tuberosity	Skin of heel
Superior clunial nerves	L1–L3 posterior rami	Course laterally/inferiorly in subcutaneous tissue	Skin overlying superior and central parts of buttock
Medial clunial nerves	S1–S3 posterior rami	From dorsal sacral foramina; enter overlying subcutaneous tissue	Skin of medial buttock and intergluteal cleft
Inferior clunial nerves	Posterior cutaneous nerve of thigh (S2-S3)	Arise deep to gluteus maximus; emerge from beneath inferior border of muscle	Skin of inferior buttock (overlying gluteal fold)

TABLE 5.3 *NERVE LESIONS*

Nerve Injury	Injury Description	Impairments	Clinical Aspects
Femoral nerve	Trauma at femoral triangle Pelvic fracture	Flexion of thigh is weakened Extension of leg is lost Sensory loss on anterior thigh and medial leg	Loss of knee jerk reflex Anesthesia on anterior thigh
Obturator nerve	Anterior hip dislocation Radical retropubic prostatectomy	Adduction of thigh is lost Sensory loss on medial thigh	
Superior gluteal nerve	Surgery Posterior hip dislocation Poliomyelitis	Gluteus medius and minimus function is lost Ability to pull contralateral pelvis up to level and abduction of thigh are lost	Gluteus medius limp or "waddling gait" Positive Trendelenburg sign Contralateral
Inferior gluteal nerve	Surgery Posterior hip dislocation	Gluteus maximus function is lost Ability to rise from a seated position, climb stairs or incline, or jump is lost	Patient will lean the body trunk backward at heel strike
Common fibular nerve	Blow to lateral aspect of leg Fracture of neck of fibula	Eversion of foot is lost Dorsiflexion of foot is lost Extension of toes is lost Sensory loss on anterolateral leg and dorsum of foot	Patient will present with foot plantar flexed ("foot drop") and inverted Patient cannot stand on heels "Foot slap"
Tibial nerve at popliteal fossa	Trauma at popliteal fossa	Inversion of foot is weakened Plantar flexion of foot is lost Sensory loss on sole of foot	Patient will present with foot dorsiflexed and everted Patient cannot stand on toes

Myotatic (Deep Tendon) Reflex	Spinal Cord Segments
Quadriceps (knee joint)	L3/L4
Calcaneal (Achilles; ankle jerk)	S1/S2

5.6   MYOTOMES AND DEEP TENDON REFLEXES

A. Myotomes. Somatic motor (general somatic efferent) fibers transmit impulses to skeletal (voluntary) muscles. The unilateral muscle mass receiving innervation from the somatic motor fibers conveyed by a single spinal nerve is a myotome. Each skeletal muscle is usually innervated by the somatic motor fibers of several spinal nerves; therefore, the muscle myotome will consist of several segments. The muscle myotomes have been grouped by joint movement to facilitate clinical testing.

B. Myotactic (deep tendon) reflexes. A myotatic (stretch) reflex is an involuntary contraction of a muscle in response to being stretched. Deep tendon reflexes (e.g., "knee jerk") are monosynaptic stretch reflexes that are elicited by briskly tapping the tendon with a reflex hammer. Each tendon reflex is mediated by specific spinal nerves. Stretch reflexes control muscle tone (e.g., in antigravity, muscles that keep the body upright against gravity).

TABLE 5.4 NERVE ROOT (ANTERIOR RAMUS) LESIONS

Compressed Nerve Root	Dermatome Affected	Muscles Affected	Movement Weakness/Deficit	Nerve and Reflex Involved
L4	L4: medial surface of leg; big toe	Quadriceps	Extension of knee	Femoral nerve ↓ Knee jerk
L5	L5: lateral surface of leg; dorsum of foot	Tibialis anterior Extensor hallucis longus Extensor digitorum longus	Dorsiflexion of ankle (patient cannot stand on heels) Extension of toes	Common fibular nerve No reflex loss
S1	S1: posterior surface of lower limb; little toe	Gastrocnemius Soleus	Plantar flexion of ankle (patient cannot stand on toes) Flexion of toes	Tibial nerve ↓ Ankle jerk

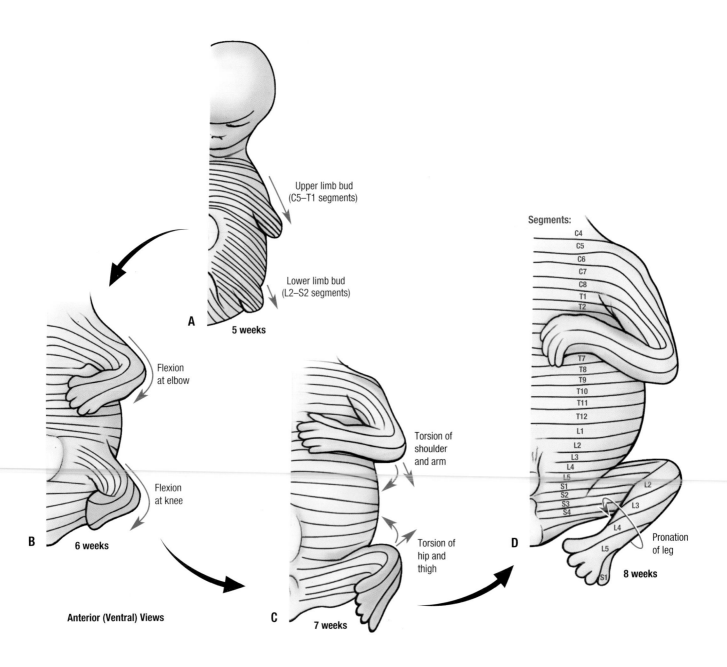

Upper limb bud
(C5–T1 segments)

Lower limb bud
(L2–S2 segments)

A **5 weeks**

Flexion
at elbow

Flexion
at knee

B **6 weeks**

Anterior (Ventral) Views

Torsion of
shoulder
and arm

Torsion of
hip and
thigh

C **7 weeks**

Segments:

C4
C5
C6
C7
C8
T1
T2

T7
T8
T9
T10
T11
T12
L1
L2
L3
L4
L5
S1
S2
S3
S4

L2
L3
L4
L5
S1

Pronation
of leg

D **8 weeks**

5.7 ROTATION OF LIMBS DURING DEVELOPMENT; EFFECT ON LOWER LIMB DERMATOME PATTERN

A. During early development, the trunk is divided into segments (metameres) that correspond to, and receive innervation from, the corresponding spinal cord segments. During the 4th week of development, the upper limb buds appear as elevations of the C5 to T1 segments of the ventrolateral body wall. Following the cranial-to-caudal pattern of development the lower limb buds appear about a week later (5th week). The lower limb buds grow laterally from broader bases formed by the L2 to S2 segments.

B. The distal ends of the limb buds flatten into paddlelike hand plates and foot plates that are elongated in the craniocaudal axis. Initially, both the thumb and the great toe are on the cranial sides of the developing hand and foot, directed superiorly, with the palms and soles directed anteriorly.

Where gaps develop between the precursors of the long bones (future elbow and knee joints), flexures occur. At first, the limbs bend anteriorly, so that the elbow and knee are directed laterally, causing the palm and sole to be directed medially (toward the trunk).

C. By the end of the 7th week, the proximal parts of the upper and lower limbs undergo a 90-degree torsion around their long axes, but in opposite directions, so that the elbow becomes directed caudally and posteriorly and the knee cranially and anteriorly.

D. In the lower limb, the torsion of the proximal limb is accompanied by a permanent pronation (twisting) of the leg, so that the foot becomes oriented with the great toe on the medial side.

A. Anterior View

B. Posterior View

C. Anterior View

D. Posterior View

5.8 ## DERMATOMES OF LOWER LIMB

The dermatomal, or segmental, pattern of distribution of sensory nerve fibers persists despite the merging of spinal nerves in plexus formation during development. Two different dermatome maps are commonly used. **A. and B.** The dermatome pattern of the lower limb according to Foerster (1933) is preferred by many because of its correlation with clinical findings. **C. and D.** The dermatome pattern of the lower limb according to Keegan and Garrett (1948) is preferred by others for its aesthetic uniformity and obvious correlation with development. Although depicted as distinct zones, adjacent dermatomes overlap considerably, except along the axial line.

A. Anterior View

Aorta
External iliac artery
Common iliac artery
Deep circumflex iliac artery
Internal iliac artery
Inferior epigastric artery
Superficial circumflex iliac artery
Profunda femoris artery (deep artery of thigh)
External pudendal artery
Lateral circumflex femoral artery
Obturator artery
Medial circumflex femoral artery
Perforating arteries
Femoral artery
Descending genicular artery
Descending branch
Popliteal artery
Superior medial genicular artery
Superior lateral genicular artery
Inferior lateral genicular artery
Inferior medial genicular artery
Geniculate anastomosis
Anterior tibial recurrent artery
Anterior tibial artery
Perforating branch of fibular (peroneal) artery
Plantar anastomosis
Lateral malleolar artery
Medial malleolar artery
Lateral tarsal artery
Dorsal artery of foot (dorsalis pedis artery)
Arcuate artery
Medial tarsal artery
Dorsal digital arteries
Deep plantar artery
1st dorsal metatarsal artery

B. Posterior View

Superior gluteal artery
Inferior gluteal artery
Cruciate anastomosis
Medial circumflex femoral artery
Lateral circumflex femoral artery
Profunda femoris artery (deep artery of thigh)
Perforating arteries
Femoral artery
Hiatus in adductor magnus
Geniculate anastomosis
Superior medial genicular artery
Superior lateral genicular artery
Popliteal artery
Inferior lateral genicular artery
Inferior medial genicular artery
Anterior tibial artery
Fibular (peroneal) artery
Posterior tibial artery
Perforating branch
Plantar anastomosis
Medial plantar artery
Lateral plantar artery
Plantar arch
Deep plantar artery
Plantar metatarsal artery
Plantar digital arteries

5.9   OVERVIEW OF ARTERIES OF LOWER LIMB

The arteries often anastomose or communicate to form networks to ensure blood supply distal to the joint throughout the range of movement (cruciate, geniculate and plantar anastomoses). If a main channel is slowly occluded, the smaller alternate channels can usually increase in size, providing a **collateral circulation** that ensures the blood supply to structures distal to the blockage.

Inferior vena cava

External iliac vein

Deep circumflex iliac vein

Common iliac vein

Internal iliac vein

Inferior epigastric vein

Medial circumflex femoral vein

Lateral circumflex femoral vein

Obturator vein

**Profunda femoris vein
(deep vein of thigh)**

Great saphenous vein

Femoral vein

Perforating veins

Descending genicular vein

Lateral superior genicular vein

Medial superior genicular vein

Lateral inferior genicular vein

Medial inferior genicular vein

Anterior tibial veins

Dorsal venous arch

A. Anterior View

Superior gluteal vein

Internal pudendal vein

Inferior gluteal vein

**Profunda femoris vein
(deep vein of thigh)**

Femoral vein

Descending genicular vein

Lateral superior genicular vein

Popliteal vein

Lateral inferior genicular vein

Medial inferior genicular vein

Circumflex fibular vein

Fibular (peroneal) vein

Posterior tibial veins

Plantar venous arch

Plantar digital veins

B. Posterior View

Accompanying veins
(L. *venae comitantes*)

Artery

Vascular
sheath

C.

5.10   DEEP VEINS OF LOWER LIMB

A. and B. Deep veins lie internal to the deep fascia. Although only the anterior and posterior tibial veins are depicted as paired structures in this schematic illustration, typically in the limbs deep veins occur as multiple, generally parallel, continually interanastomosing accompanying veins (L., venae comitantes) surrounding and sharing the name of the artery they accompany. **C.** Accompanying veins.

Superficial circumflex iliac vein

Superficial epigastric vein

Femoral vein

Superficial external pudendal vein

Great saphenous vein

Lateral cutaneous vein of thigh

Medial cutaneous vein of thigh

Great saphenous vein

Site of saphenous cutdown

Medial malleolus

A. Anteromedial View

Great saphenous vein

Small saphenous vein

Small saphenous vein

B. Posterior View

Sites where perforating veins penetrate deep fascia

Small (short) saphenous vein

Lateral malleolus

Dorsal venous arch

Common dorsal digital veins

C. Lateral View

5.11   SUPERFICIAL VEINS OF LOWER LIMB

Blood is continuously shunted from the superficial veins in the subcutaneous tissue to deep veins via the perforating veins. **Vein grafts** obtained by surgically harvesting parts of the great saphenous vein are used to bypass obstructions in blood vessels (e.g., a coronary artery). When used as a bypass, the vein is reversed so that the valves do not obstruct blood flow. Because there are so many anastomosing leg veins, removal of the great saphenous vein rarely affects circulation seriously, provided the deep veins are intact.

Saphenous cut down. The great saphenous vein can be located by making a skin incision anterior to the medial malleolus. This procedure is used to insert a cannula for prolonged administration of blood, electrolytes, drugs etc.

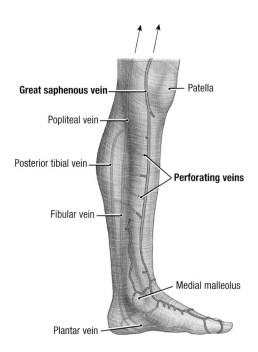

Great saphenous vein

Patella

Popliteal vein

Posterior tibial vein

Perforating veins

Fibular vein

Medial malleolus

Plantar vein

A. Medial View

B. Medial View, Varicose Veins

Great saphenous vein

Patella

Great saphenous vein

Great saphenous vein

Medial malleolus

Dorsal venous arch

C. Anteromedial View, Normal Veins

5.12   DRAINAGE AND SURFACE ANATOMY OF SUPERFICIAL VEINS OF LOWER LIMB

A. Schematic diagram of drainage of superficial veins. Blood is shunted from the superficial veins (e.g., great saphenous vein) to the deep veins (e.g., fibular and posterior tibial veins) via perforating veins that penetrate the deep fascia. Muscular compression of deep veins assists return of blood to the heart against gravity. **B. Varicose veins** form when either the deep fascia or the valves of the perforating veins are incompetent. This allows the muscular compression that normally propels blood toward the heart to push blood from the deep to the superficial veins. Consequently, superficial veins become enlarged and tortuous. **C.** Normal veins, distended following exercise.

Superficial inguinal lymph nodes (superior group)

Femoral vein

Superficial inguinal lymph nodes (inferior group)

Great saphenous vein

Superficial lymphatic vessels

Great saphenous vein

Deep inguinal lymph nodes

A. Anteromedial View

Great saphenous vein

Medial border of patella

Medial malleolus

B. Anteromedial View

Popliteal vein

Popliteal lymph nodes (superficial nodes)

Small saphenous vein

C. Posterior View

5.13 SUPERFICIAL LYMPHATIC DRAINAGE OF LOWER LIMB

The superficial lymphatic vessels converge on and accompany the saphenous veins and their tributaries in the superficial fascia. The lymphatic vessels along the great saphenous vein drain into the superficial inguinal lymph nodes; those along the small saphenous vein drain into the popliteal lymph nodes. Lymph from the superficial inguinal nodes drains to the deep inguinal and external iliac nodes. Lymph from the popliteal nodes ascends through deep lymphatic vessels accompanying the deep blood vessels to the deep inguinal nodes. In **B,** note that the great saphenous vein lies anterior to the medial malleolus and a hand's breadth posterior to the medial border of the patella. **Lymph nodes enlarge** when diseased. Abrasions and minor sepsis, caused by pathogenic micro-organisms or their toxins in the blood or other tissues, may produce slight enlargement of the superficial inguinal nodes (lymphadenopathy) in otherwise healthy people. Malignancies (e.g., of the external genitalia and uterus) and perineal abscesses also result in enlargement of these nodes.

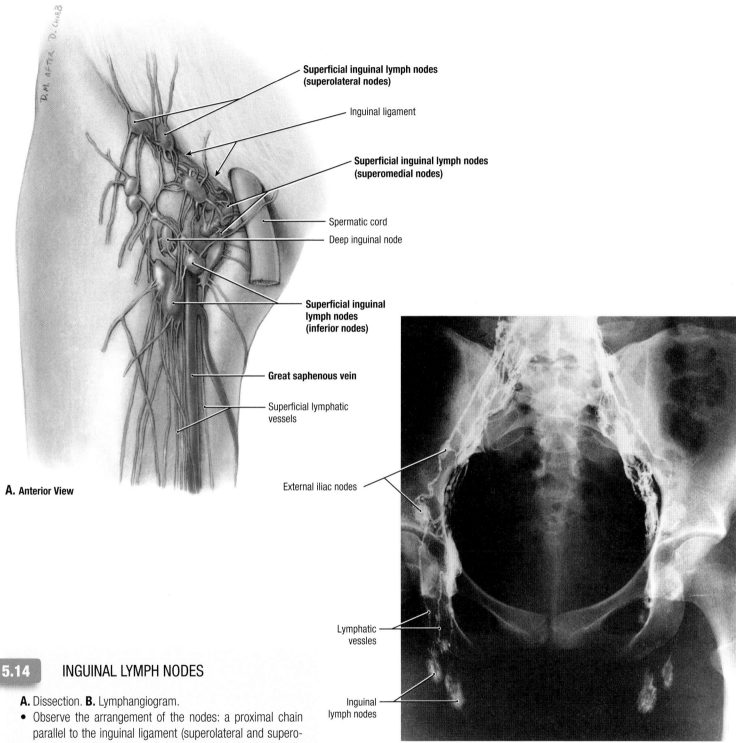

Superficial inguinal lymph nodes (superolateral nodes)

Inguinal ligament

Superficial inguinal lymph nodes (superomedial nodes)

Spermatic cord

Deep inguinal node

Superficial inguinal lymph nodes (inferior nodes)

Great saphenous vein

Superficial lymphatic vessels

A. Anterior View

External iliac nodes

Lymphatic vessels

Inguinal lymph nodes

B. Anteroposterior View

5.14 **INGUINAL LYMPH NODES**

A. Dissection. **B.** Lymphangiogram.

- Observe the arrangement of the nodes: a proximal chain parallel to the inguinal ligament (superolateral and supero-medial superficial inguinal lymph nodes) and a distal chain on the sides of the great saphenous vein (inferior superficial inguinal lymph nodes). Efferent vessels leave these nodes and pass deep to the inguinal ligament to enter the deep inguinal and external iliac nodes. Some of the lymphatic vessels traverse the femoral canal, and others ascend alongside the femoral artery and vein, some inside the femoral sheath, and some outside it.
- Note the anastomosis between the lymph vessels.

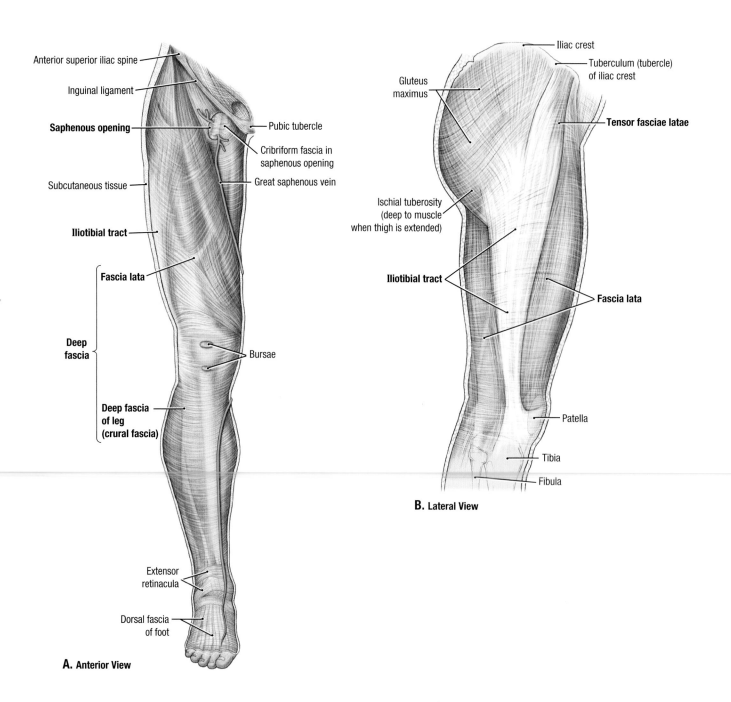

Anterior superior iliac spine

Inguinal ligament

Saphenous opening

Subcutaneous tissue

Iliotibial tract

Fascia lata

Deep fascia

Deep fascia of leg (crural fascia)

Pubic tubercle

Cribriform fascia in saphenous opening

Great saphenous vein

Bursae

Extensor retinacula

Dorsal fascia of foot

A. Anterior View

Iliac crest

Tuberculum (tubercle) of iliac crest

Gluteus maximus

Tensor fasciae latae

Ischial tuberosity (deep to muscle when thigh is extended)

Iliotibial tract

Fascia lata

Patella

Tibia

Fibula

B. Lateral View

5.15 FASCIA AND MUSCULOFASCIAL COMPARTMENTS OF LOWER LIMB

A. Anterior skin and subcutaneous tissue have been removed to reveal the deep fascia of the thigh (fascia lata) and leg (crural fascia). **B.** Lateral skin and subcutaneous tissue have been removed to reveal the fascia lata. The fascia lata is thick laterally and forms the iliotibial tract. The iliotibial tract serves as a common aponeurosis for the gluteus maximus and tensor fasciae latae muscles.

One of the most common causes of lateral knee pain in endurance athletes (e.g., runners, cyclers, hikers) is **iliotibial tract (band) syndrome (ITBS)**. Friction of the IT tract against the lateral epicondyle of the femur with flexion and extension of the knee (e.g., during running) may result in the inflammation of the IT tract over the lateral aspect of the knee or its attachment to the dorsolateral tubercle (Gerdy tubercle). ITBS may also occur in the hip region, especially in older individuals.

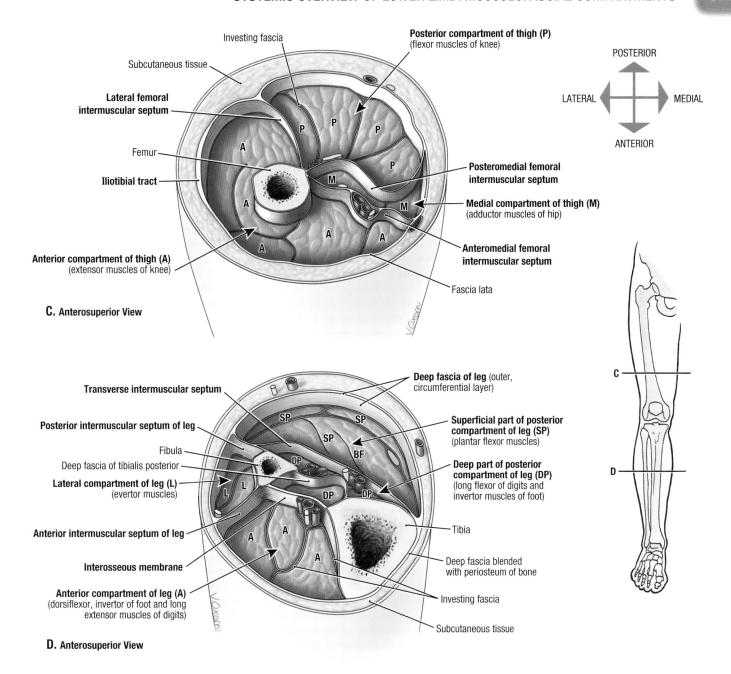

C. Anterosuperior View

D. Anterosuperior View

5.15   FASCIA AND MUSCULOFASCIAL COMPARTMENTS OF LOWER LIMB (*CONTINUED*)

C. and D. The fascial compartments of the thigh **(C)** and leg **(D)** are demonstrated in transverse section. The fascial compartments contain muscles that generally perform common functions and share common innervation, and contain the spread of infection. While both thigh and leg have anterior and posterior compartments, the thigh also includes a medial compartment and the leg a lateral compartment. Trauma to muscles and/or vessels in the compartments may produce hemorrhage, edema, and inflammation of the muscles. Because the septa, deep fascia, and bony attachments firmly bound the compartments, increased volume resulting from these processes raises intracompartmental pressure. In **compartment syndromes,** structures within or distal to the compressed area become ischemic and may become permanently injured (e.g., compression of capillary beds results in denervation and consequent paralysis of muscles). A **fasciotomy** (incision of bounding fascia or septum) may be performed to relieve the pressure in the compartment and restore circulation.

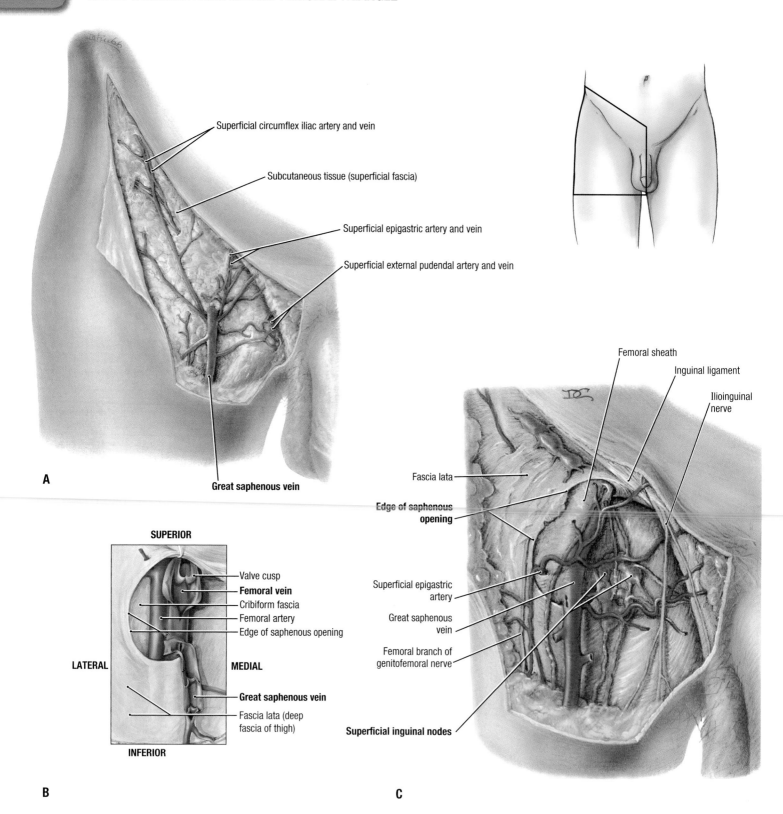

A

Superficial circumflex iliac artery and vein

Subcutaneous tissue (superficial fascia)

Superficial epigastric artery and vein

Superficial external pudendal artery and vein

Great saphenous vein

B

SUPERIOR

Valve cusp
Femoral vein
Cribiform fascia
Femoral artery
Edge of saphenous opening

LATERAL   MEDIAL

Great saphenous vein

Fascia lata (deep fascia of thigh)

INFERIOR

C

Femoral sheath

Inguinal ligament

Ilioinguinal nerve

Fascia lata

Edge of saphenous opening

Superficial epigastric artery

Great saphenous vein

Femoral branch of genitofemoral nerve

Superficial inguinal nodes

5.16   SUPERFICIAL INGUINAL VESSELS AND SAPHENOUS OPENING

A. Superficial inguinal vessels. The arteries are branches of the femoral artery, and the veins are tributaries of the great saphenous vein. **B.** Valves of the proximal part of femoral and great saphenous veins. **C.** Saphenous opening.

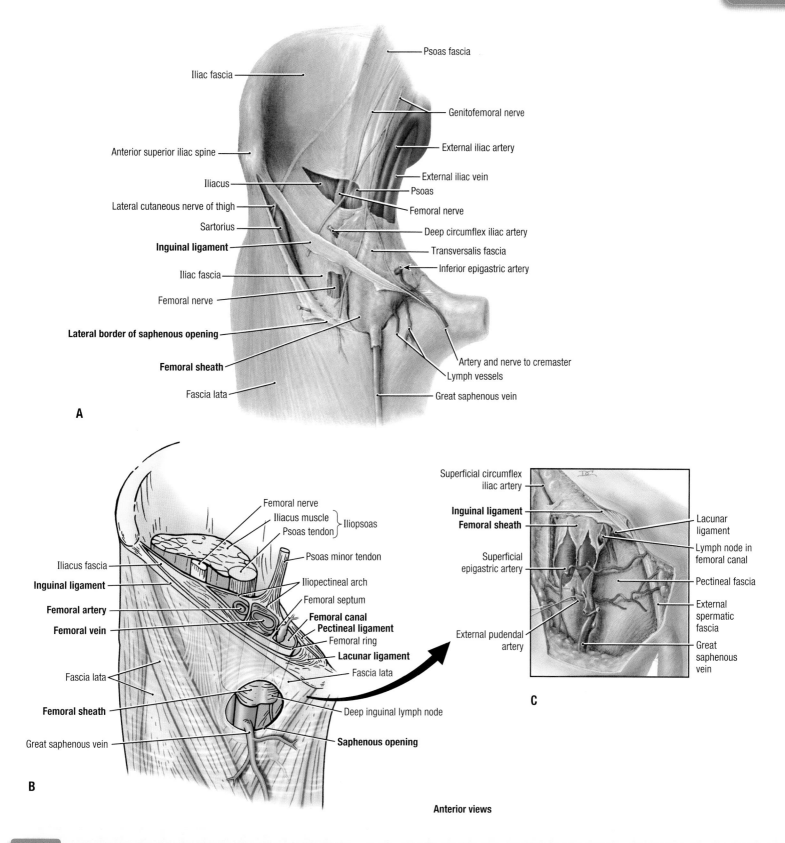

A. Dissection. **B.** Schematic illustration. The femoral sheath contains the femoral artery, vein, and lymph vessels, but the femoral nerve, lying posterior to the iliacus fascia, is outside the femoral sheath. **C.** Femoral sheath and femoral ring. The three compartments of the femoral sheath are the lateral for the femoral artery; intermediate for the femoral vein; and medial for the femoral canal. The base of the femoral canal is formed by the small (about 1 cm wide) proximal opening at its abdominal end, the femoral ring. This opening is closed by extraperitoneal fatty tissue.

5.17   FEMORAL SHEATH AND INGUINAL LIGAMENT

Anterior views

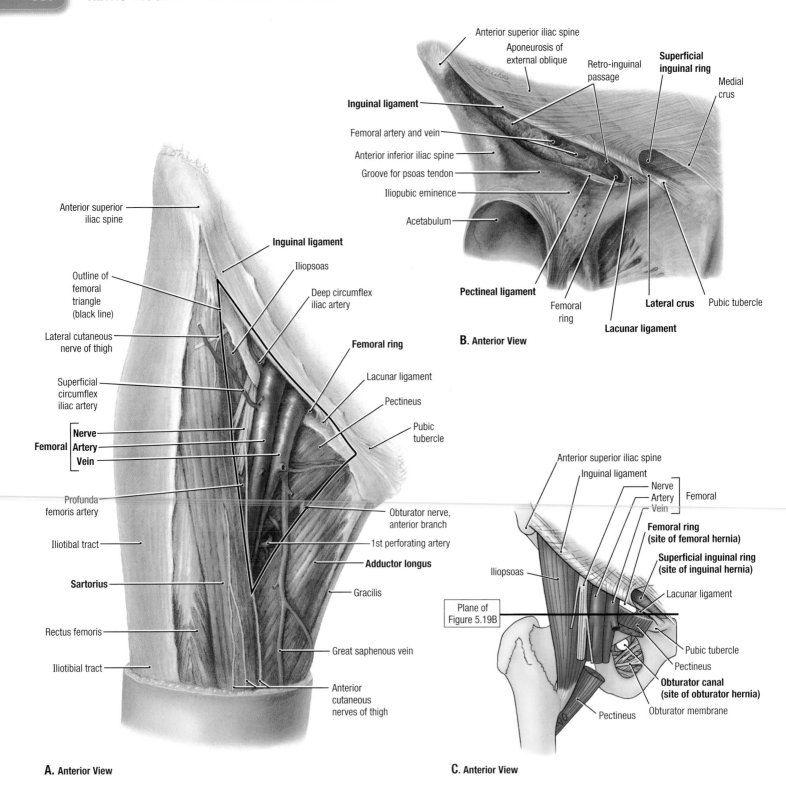

A. Anterior View

- Anterior superior iliac spine
- Outline of femoral triangle (black line)
- Lateral cutaneous nerve of thigh
- Superficial circumflex iliac artery
- **Nerve**
- **Femoral** **Artery**
- **Vein**
- Profunda femoris artery
- Iliotibal tract
- **Sartorius**
- Rectus femoris
- Iliotibial tract

- **Inguinal ligament**
- Iliopsoas
- Deep circumflex iliac artery
- **Femoral ring**
- Lacunar ligament
- Pectineus
- Pubic tubercle
- Obturator nerve, anterior branch
- 1st perforating artery
- **Adductor longus**
- Gracilis
- Great saphenous vein
- Anterior cutaneous nerves of thigh

B. Anterior View

- Anterior superior iliac spine
- Aponeurosis of external oblique
- Retro-inguinal passage
- **Superficial inguinal ring**
- Medial crus
- **Inguinal ligament**
- Femoral artery and vein
- Anterior inferior iliac spine
- Groove for psoas tendon
- Iliopubic eminence
- Acetabulum
- **Pectineal ligament**
- Femoral ring
- **Lateral crus**
- **Lacunar ligament**
- Pubic tubercle

C. Anterior View

- Anterior superior iliac spine
- Inguinal ligament
- Nerve
- Artery — Femoral
- Vein
- **Femoral ring (site of femoral hernia)**
- **Superficial inguinal ring (site of inguinal hernia)**
- Lacunar ligament
- Iliopsoas
- Plane of Figure 5.19B
- Pubic tubercle
- Pectineus
- **Obturator canal (site of obturator hernia)**
- Obturator membrane
- Pectineus

5.18 STRUCTURES PASSING TO/FROM FEMORAL TRIANGLE VIA RETRO-INGUINAL PASSAGE

A. Dissection. The boundaries of the femoral triangle are the inguinal ligament superiorly (base of triangle), the medial border of the sartorius (lateral side), and the lateral border of the adductor longus (medial side). The point at which the lateral and medial sides converge inferiorly forms the apex. The femoral triangle is bisected by the femoral vessels. **B.** Retro-inguinal passage between the inguinal ligament anteriorly and the bony pelvis posteriorly. **C.** The iliopsoas muscle, the femoral nerve, artery, and vein, and the lymphatic vessels draining the inguinal nodes pass deep to the inguinal ligament to enter the anterior thigh or return to the trunk. Three potential sites for **hernia formation** are indicated. **Pulsations of the femoral artery** can be felt distal to the inguinal ligament, midway between the anterior superior iliac spine and the pubic tubercle.

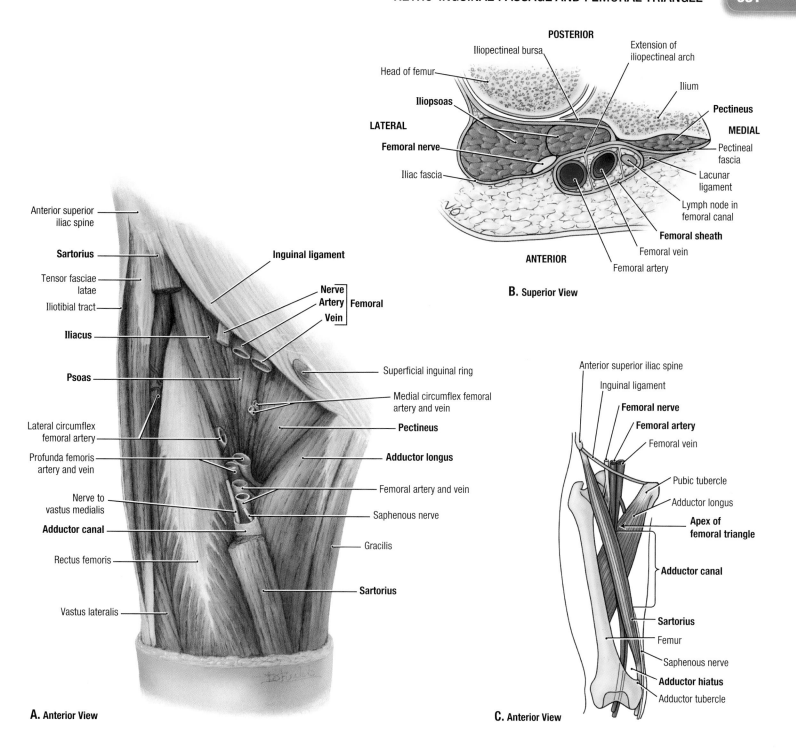

B. Superior View

A. Anterior View

C. Anterior View

5.19 **FLOOR OF FEMORAL CANAL AND RETRO-INGUINAL PASSAGE**

A. Dissection. Portions of the sartorius muscle, femoral vessels, and femoral nerve have been removed revealing the floor of the femoral triangle, formed by the iliopsoas laterally and the pectineus medially. At the apex of the triangle the femoral vessels, saphenous nerve, and the nerve to the vastus medialis pass deep to the sartorius into the adductor (subsartorial) canal. **B.** Transverse section of the femoral triangle at the level of head of femur. (Level of section is indicated in Fig. 5.18 **C.**) The iliopsoas and femoral nerve traverse the retro-inguinal passage and femoral triangle in a fascial sheath separate from the femoral vessels, which are contained within the femoral sheath. **C.** Schematic illustration of course of femoral vessels. The adductor canal extends from the apex of the femoral triangle to the adductor hiatus, by which the vessels enter and leave the popliteal fossa.

Sartorius

Rectus femoris

Vastus intermedius

Adductor longus

Vastus lateralis

Vastus medialis

Patella

Patellar ligament

A. Anterior View

B. Anteromedial View

5.20 SURFACE ANATOMY OF ANTERIOR AND MEDIAL ASPECTS OF THIGH

Patellar tendinitis (jumper's knee) is caused by continuous overloading of the knee extensor mechanism, resulting in microtears of the tendon. The most vulnerable site is where the patellar ligament (tendon) attaches to the patella. This overuse injury can result in degeneration and tearing of the tendon.

Iliacus

Anterior superior
iliac spine

Fascia lata

**Tensor
fasciae latae**

Sartorius

Rectus femoris

Iliotibial tract

Vastus lateralis

**Lateral patellar
retinaculum**

Patellar ligament

Tendon of psoas minor

Psoas major

Pubic tubercle

Pectineus

Adductor longus

Gracilis

Vastus medialis

Patella

**Medial patellar
retinaculum**

Sartorius

A

Iliacus

Tensor fasciae latae

Rectus femoris
(proximal end)

Gluteus minimus

Iliotibial tract

Vastus intermedius

Vastus lateralis

Rectus femoris
(distal end)

Patellar ligament

Psoas major

Adductor longus
(proximal end)

Adductor brevis

Pectineus
(distal end)

Adductor longus
(distal end)

Gracilis

Adductor magnus

Vastus medialis

Sartorius
(distal end)

Medial meniscus

Sartorius tendon

Gracilis tendon

Tibia

B

Anterior Views

5.21   **ANTERIOR AND MEDIAL THIGH MUSCLES, SUPERFICIAL AND DEEP
DISSECTIONS**

A. Superficial dissection. **B.** Deep dissection. The central portions of the muscle bellies of the sartorius, rectus
femoris, pectineus, and adductor longus muscles have been removed. **Weakness of the vastus medialis or
vastus lateralis,** resulting from arthritis or trauma to the knee joint, for example, can result in abnormal
patellar movement and loss of joint stability.

Iliopsoas

Anterior superior iliac spine

Tensor fasciae latae

Sartorius

Rectus femoris

Adductor longus

Vastus lateralis

Iliotibial tract

Vastus medialis

Patella

Sartorius attachment

Femoral artery, vein, and nerve

Pectineus

Gracilis

Rectus femoris

Vastus lateralis

Vastus medialis

Quadriceps tendon

Patellar ligament

Gracilis

Pectineus

Adductor brevis

Adductor longus

Vastus intermedius

Attachments cut:

Vastus lateralis

Vastus medialis

Rectus femoris

Gracilis attachment

A   B   C   D

Anterior Views

5.22   ANTERIOR AND MEDIAL THIGH MUSCLES, SCHEMATIC ILLUSTRATIONS

A.–D. Sequential views from superficial to deep.

A "hip pointer," which is a **contusion of the iliac crest,** usually occurs at its anterior part (e.g., where the sartorius attaches to the anterior superior iliac spine). This is one of the most common injuries to the hip region, usually occurring in association with collision sports. Contusions cause bleeding from ruptured capillaries and infiltration of blood into the muscles, tendons, and other soft tissues. The term hip pointer may also refer to avulsion of bony muscle attachments, for example, of the sartorius or rectus femoris from the anterior superior or inferior iliac spines or of the iliopsoas from the lesser trochanter of the femur. However, these injuries should be called **avulsion fractures.**

A person with a **paralyzed quadriceps** cannot extend the leg against resistance and usually presses on the distal end of the thigh during walking to prevent inadvertent flexion of the knee joint.

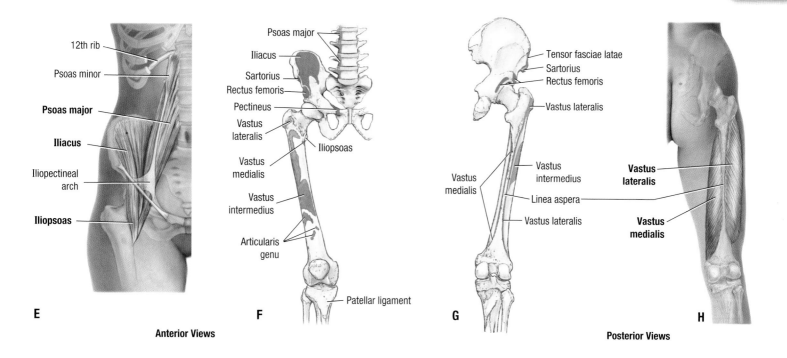

Anterior Views

Posterior Views

5.22   **ANTERIOR AND MEDIAL THIGH MUSCLES, SCHEMATIC ILLUSTRATIONS (*CONTINUED*)**

E. Iliopsoas. **F. and G.** Attachments of anterior muscles of thigh. **H.** Posterior attachment of vastus medialis and lateralis.

TABLE 5.5   MUSCLES OF ANTERIOR THIGH

Muscle	Proximal Attachment[a]	Distal Attachment[a]	Innervation[b]	Main Actions
Iliopsoas				
Psoas major	Lateral aspects of T12–L5 vertebrae and IV discs; transverse processes of all lumbar vertebrae	Lesser trochanter of femur	Anterior rami of lumbar nerves (**L1, L2,** and L3)	Flexes and stabilizes[c] hip joint
Iliacus	Iliac crest, iliac fossa, ala of sacrum and anterior sacro-iliac ligaments	Tendon of psoas major, lesser trochanter, and femur distal to it	Femoral nerve (L2 and L3)	
Tensor fasciae latae	Anterior superior iliac spine and anterior part of iliac crest	Iliotibial tract that attaches to lateral condyle of tibia	Superior gluteal (L4 and L5)	Abducts, medially rotates, and flexes hip joint; helps to keep knee extended; steadies trunk on thigh
Sartorius	Anterior superior iliac spine and superior part of notch inferior to it	Superior part of medial surface of tibia	Femoral nerve (L2 and L3)	Flexes, abducts, and laterally rotates hip joint; flexes knee joint[d]
Quadriceps femoris				
Rectus femoris	Anterior inferior iliac spine and ilium superior to acetabulum	Base of patella and by patellar ligament to tibial tuberosity; medial and lateral vasti also attach to tibia and patella via aponeuroses (medial and lateral patellar retinacula)	Femoral nerve (L2, **L3,** and **L4**)	Extends knee joint; rectus femoris also steadies hip joint and helps iliopsoas to flex hip joint
Vastus lateralis	Greater trochanter and lateral lip of linea aspera of femur			
Vastus medialis	Intertrochanteric line and medial lip of linea aspera of femur			
Vastus intermedius	Anterior and lateral surfaces of body of femur			

[a]See also Figure 5.22 for muscle attachments.
[b]Numbers indicate spinal cord segmental innervation of nerves (e.g., L1, L2, and L3 indicate that nerves supplying psoas major are derived from first three lumbar segments of the spinal cord; boldface type [**L1, L2**] indicates main segmental innervation). Damage to one or more of these spinal cord segments or to motor nerve roots arising from these segments results in paralysis of the muscles concerned.
[c]Psoas major is also a postural muscle that helps control deviation of trunk and is active during standing.
[d]Four actions of sartorius (L. *sartor,* tailor) produce the once-common cross-legged sitting position used by tailors—hence the name.

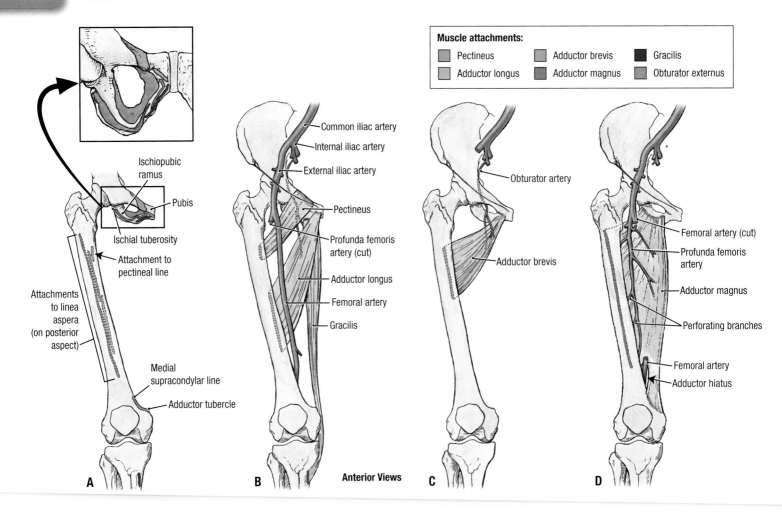

Muscle attachments:
- Pectineus
- Adductor longus
- Adductor brevis
- Adductor magnus
- Gracilis
- Obturator externus

A. Overview of attachments. **B.** Pectineus, adductor longus, and gracilis. **C.** Adductor brevis. **D.** Adductor magnus.

Anterior Views

5.23   ATTACHMENTS OF MUSCLES OF MEDIAL ASPECT OF THIGH

TABLE 5.6 MUSCLES OF MEDIAL THIGH

Muscle	Proximal Attachment	Distal Attachment[a]	Innervation[b]	Main Actions
Pectineus	Superior pubic ramus	Pectineal line of femur, just inferior to lesser trochanter	Femoral nerve (**L2** and L3) may receive a branch from obturator nerve	Adducts and flexes hip joint; assists with medial rotation of hip joint
Adductor longus	Body of pubis inferior to pubic crest	Middle third of linea aspera of femur	Obturator nerve, anterior branch (L2, **L3**, and L4)	Adducts hip joint
Adductor brevis	Body of pubis and inferior pubic ramus	Pectineal line and proximal part of linea aspera of femur	Obturator nerve (L2, **L3**, and L4)	Adducts hip joint and, to some extent, flexes it
Adductor magnus	Inferior pubic ramus, ramus of ischium (adductor part), and ischial tuberosity	Gluteal tuberosity, linea aspera, medial supracondylar line (adductor part), and adductor tubercle of femur (hamstring part)	*Adductor part:* obturator nerve (L2, **L3**, and **L4**) *Hamstring part:* tibial part of sciatic nerve (**L4**)	Adducts hip joint; its adductor part also flexes hip joint, and its hamstring part extends it
Gracilis	Body of pubis and inferior pubic ramus	Superior part of medial surface of tibia	Obturator nerve (**L2** and L3)	Adducts hip joint, flexes knee joint, and helps rotate it medially
Obturator externus	Margins of obturator foramen and obturator membrane	Trochanteric fossa of femur	Obturator nerve (L3 and **L4**)	Laterally rotates hip joint; steadies head of femur in acetabulum

Collectively, the first five muscles listed are the adductors of the thigh, but their actions are more complex (e.g., they act as flexors of the hip joint during flexion of the knee joint and are active during walking).
[a]See Figure 5.22 for muscle attachments.
[b]See Table 5.1 for explanation of segmental innervation.

External iliac artery and vein

Psoas

Obturator internus

Adductor longus

Adductor magnus

Rectus femoris

Sartorius

Vastus medialis

3 tendons merging to
form pes anserinus

A. Medial View

Sacrum

Piriformis

Sacrospinous ligament

Coccygeus

Internal pudendal artery

Gluteus maximus

Semitendinosus

Gracilis

Semimembranosus

Semitendinosus

Gastrocnemius, medial head (cut)

Soleus

Gracilis

Semitendinosus

Sartorius

Pes anserinus

B. Anterior View

Forming
pes anserinus:

Gracilis

Semitendinosus

Sartorius

C. Medial View

| 5.24 | MUSCLES OF MEDIAL ASPECT OF THIGH |

A. Dissection. **B.** Muscular tripod. The sartorius, gracilis, and semitendinosus muscles form an inverted tripod arising from three different components of the hip bone. These muscles course within three different compartments, perform three different functions, and are innervated by three different nerves yet share a common distal attachment. **C.** Distal attachment of sartorius, gracilis, and semitendinosus muscles. All three tendons become thin and aponeurotic and are collectively referred to as the pes anserinus. The gracilis is a relatively weak member of the adductor group and hence can be removed without noticeable loss of its actions on the leg. Surgeons often **transplant the gracilis**, or part of it, with its nerve and blood vessels to replace a damaged muscle in the hand, for example.

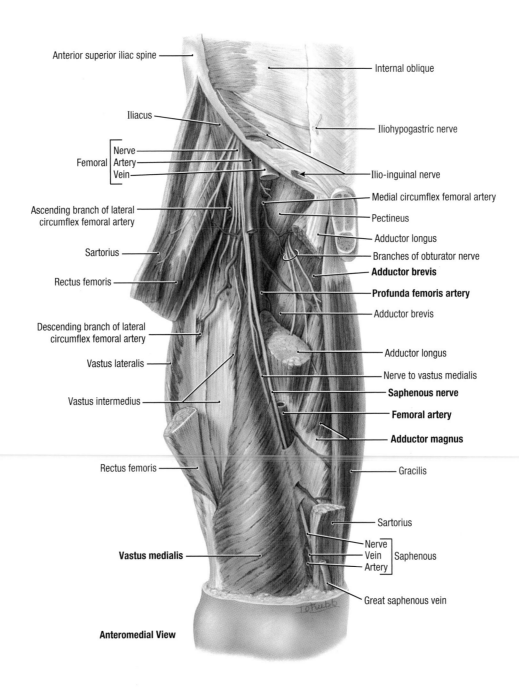

Anterior superior iliac spine

Iliacus

Femoral — Nerve / Artery / Vein

Ascending branch of lateral circumflex femoral artery

Sartorius

Rectus femoris

Descending branch of lateral circumflex femoral artery

Vastus lateralis

Vastus intermedius

Rectus femoris

Vastus medialis

Internal oblique

Iliohypogastric nerve

Ilio-inguinal nerve

Medial circumflex femoral artery

Pectineus

Adductor longus

Branches of obturator nerve

Adductor brevis

Profunda femoris artery

Adductor brevis

Adductor longus

Nerve to vastus medialis

Saphenous nerve

Femoral artery

Adductor magnus

Gracilis

Sartorius

Nerve / Vein / Artery — Saphenous

Great saphenous vein

Anteromedial View

5.25   ANTEROMEDIAL ASPECT OF THIGH

- The limb is rotated laterally.
- The femoral nerve breaks up into several nerves on entering the thigh.
- The femoral artery lies between two motor territories: that of the obturator nerve, which is medial, and that of the femoral nerve, which is lateral. No motor nerve crosses anterior to the femoral artery, but the twig to the pectineus muscle crosses posterior to the femoral artery.
- The nerve to the vastus medialis muscle and the saphenous nerve accompany the femoral artery into the adductor canal. The saphenous nerve and

artery and their anastomotic accompanying vein emerge from the canal distally between the sartorius and gracilis muscles.

- The profunda femoris artery (deep artery of thigh) is the largest branch of the femoral artery and the chief artery to the thigh. It arises from the femoral artery in the femoral triangle. In the middle third of the thigh, it is separated from the femoral artery and vein by the adductor longus. It gives off three or four perforating arteries that wrap around the posterior aspect of the femur and supply the adductor magnus, hamstring and vastus lateralis muscles.

A. Lateral View

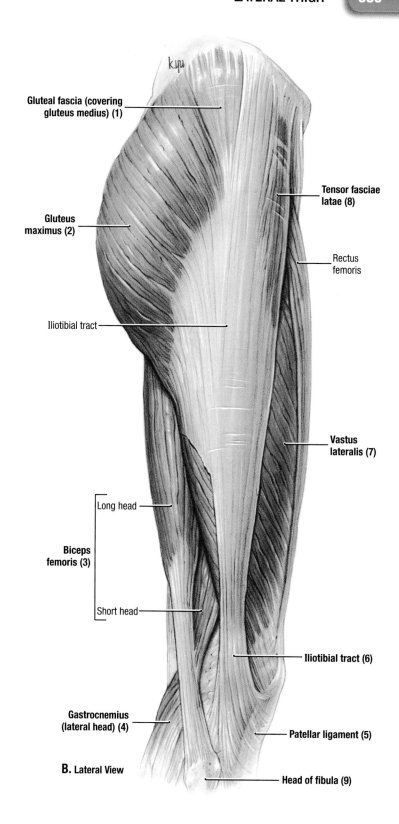

Gluteal fascia (covering gluteus medius) (1)

Gluteus maximus (2)

Iliotibial tract

Biceps femoris (3)

Long head

Short head

Gastrocnemius (lateral head) (4)

B. Lateral View

Tensor fasciae latae (8)

Rectus femoris

Vastus lateralis (7)

Iliotibial tract (6)

Patellar ligament (5)

Head of fibula (9)

5.26   **LATERAL ASPECT OF THIGH**

A. Surface anatomy (*numbers* refer to structures in **B**). **B.** Dissection showing the iliotibial tract, a thickening of the fascia lata, which serves as a tendon for the gluteus maximus and tensor fasciae latae. The iliotibial tract attaches to the anterolateral (Gerdy) tubercle of the lateral condyle of the tibia. The biceps femoris tendon attaches on the head of the fibula.

Key for B

Proximal muscular attachment

Distal muscular attachment

Ligamentous attachment

Iliac crest

Tuberculum of iliac crest

Anterior superior iliac spine

Anterior inferior iliac spine

Rim of acetabulum

Head of femur

Greater trochanter

Intertrochanteric line

Lesser trochanter

Iliac fossa

Iliopubic eminence

Superior ramus of pubis

Pubic tubercle

Pubic symphysis

Pubic crest

Pecten pubis

Body of pubis

Obturator foramen

Ramus of ischium

Inferior ramus of pubis

Ischial tuberosity

Ischiopubic ramus

Femur

Patella

Adductor tubercle

Medial epicondyle

Lateral epicondyle

Lateral femoral condyle

Medial femoral condyle

Apex of head

Medial and lateral tibial condyles

Head

Neck

Tuberosity

Fibula

Tibia

A. Anterior View

Iliacus

Sartorius

Rectus femoris

Gluteus minimus

Vastus lateralis

Iliopsoas

Vastus medialis

Pectineus

Adductor longus

Gracilis

Obturator externus

Adductor brevis

Adductor magnus

Vastus intermedius

Aricularis genu

Adductor magnus

Iliotibial tract

Biceps femoris

Patellar ligament

B. Anterior View

5.27   BONES OF THE THIGH AND PROXIMAL LEG

A. Bony features. **B.** Muscle attachment sites.

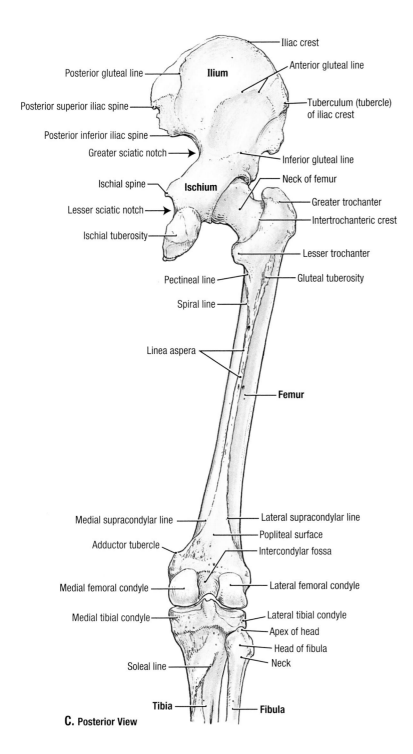

Iliac crest

Posterior gluteal line

Ilium

Anterior gluteal line

Posterior superior iliac spine

Tuberculum (tubercle) of iliac crest

Posterior inferior iliac spine

Greater sciatic notch

Inferior gluteal line

Ischial spine

Ischium

Neck of femur

Lesser sciatic notch

Greater trochanter

Intertrochanteric crest

Ischial tuberosity

Lesser trochanter

Pectineal line

Gluteal tuberosity

Spiral line

Linea aspera

Femur

Medial supracondylar line

Lateral supracondylar line

Adductor tubercle

Popliteal surface

Intercondylar fossa

Medial femoral condyle

Lateral femoral condyle

Medial tibial condyle

Lateral tibial condyle

Apex of head

Head of fibula

Neck

Soleal line

Tibia   **Fibula**

C. Posterior View

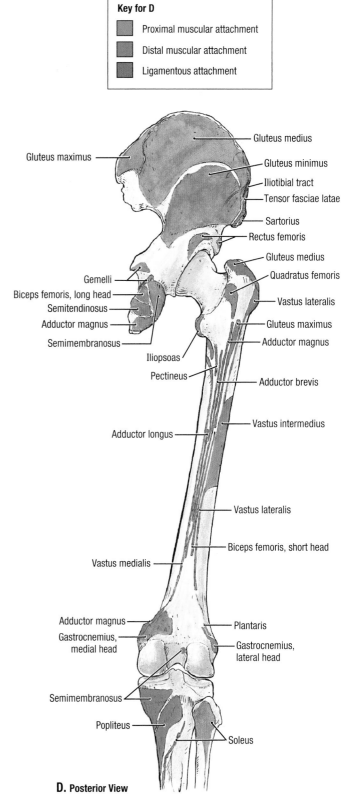

Key for D	
	Proximal muscular attachment
	Distal muscular attachment
	Ligamentous attachment

Gluteus maximus

Gluteus medius

Gluteus minimus

Iliotibial tract

Tensor fasciae latae

Sartorius

Rectus femoris

Gluteus medius

Gemelli

Quadratus femoris

Biceps femoris, long head

Semitendinosus

Vastus lateralis

Adductor magnus

Gluteus maximus

Semimembranosus

Adductor magnus

Iliopsoas

Pectineus

Adductor brevis

Adductor longus

Vastus intermedius

Vastus lateralis

Biceps femoris, short head

Vastus medialis

Adductor magnus

Plantaris

Gastrocnemius, medial head

Gastrocnemius, lateral head

Semimembranosus

Popliteus

Soleus

D. Posterior View

5.27

BONES OF THE THIGH AND PROXIMAL LEG
(CONTINUED)

C. Bony features. **D.** Muscle attachment sites.

Gluteus medius (7)

Gluteus maximus (6)

Iliotibial tract (5)

Adductor magnus

Semitendinosus

Long head of
biceps femoris

Semimembranosus (1)

Short head
of biceps femoris

Sciatic nerve

Gracilis

Biceps femoris (4)

Tibial nerve

Common fibular
(peroneal) nerve

Tibial nerve

Plantaris

**Common
fibular nerve**

Gastrocnemius,
medial head (2)

Gastrocnemius,
lateral head (3)

A. Posterior View

B. Posterior View

5.28   MUSCLES OF THE GLUTEAL REGION AND POSTERIOR THIGH I

A. Surface anatomy (*numbers* refer to structures in **B**). **B.** Superficial dissection of muscles of gluteal region
and posterior thigh (hamstring muscles consisting of semimembranosus, semitendinosus, and biceps femoris). **Hamstring strains** (pulled and/or torn hamstrings) are common in running, jumping, and quick-start sports. The muscular exertion required to excel in these sports may tear part of the proximal attachments of the hamstrings from the ischial tuberosity.

Gluteus medius

Piriformis

Superior gemellus

Obturator internus

Inferior gemellus

Quadratus femoris

Adductor magnus

Sciatic nerve

Hamstrings

Biceps femoris

Semitendinosus

Semimembranosus

Oblique popliteal ligament

Gastrocnemius, medial head

C. Posterior View

Iliotibial tract

**Greater trochanter
(location of
trochanteric bursa)**

Gluteus maximus

Iliotibial tract

Bellies of gastrocnemius
(cut)

Plantaris

Popliteus

Soleus

Gastrocnemius, lateral head

Gluteus minimus

Tensor fasciae latae

Gluteus medius (cut)

Piriformis

Superior gemellus

Obturator internus

Inferior gemellus

**Ischial tuberosity
(location of ischial bursa)**

Hamstring muscles (cut)

**Quadratus
femoris**

Gluteus maximus

**Adductor
magnus**

Adductor
part

Hamstring
part

Iliotibial tract

Popliteal vein

Popliteal artery

Vastus medialis

Adductor tubercle

Semimembranosus

Oblique popliteal ligament

**Biceps femoris,
short head**

Biceps femoris
long head (cut)

Plantaris

Popliteus

Soleus

D. Posterior View

5.28   MUSCLES OF GLUTEAL REGION AND POSTERIOR THIGH (*CONTINUED*) II AND III

C. Muscles of gluteal region and posterior thigh with gluteus maximus reflected. **D.** Adductor magnus muscle. The adductor magnus has two parts: one belongs to the adductor group, innervated by the obturator nerve and the other to the hamstring group, innervated by the tibial portion of the sciatic nerve. The trochanteric bursa separates the superior fibers of the gluteus maximus from the greater trochanter of the femur and the ischial bursa separates the inferior part of the gluteus maximus from the ischial tuberosity. Diffuse deep pain in the lateral thigh region (e.g., during stair climbing) may be caused by **trochanteric bursitis.** It is characterized by point tenderness over the greater trochanter, with pain radiating along the iliotibial tract. **Ischial bursitis** results from excessive friction between the ischial bursae and ischial tuberosities (e.g., as from cycling).

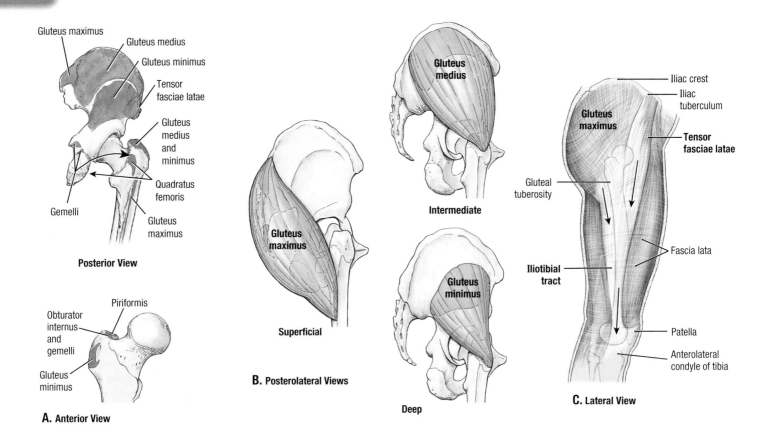

5.29 MUSCLES OF GLUTEAL REGION

A. Attachments. **B.** Relationship of gluteal muscles. **C.** Gluteus maximus and tensor fasciae latae.

TABLE 5.7 MUSCLES OF GLUTEAL REGION

Muscle	Proximal Attachment[a] (*Red*)	Distal Attachment[a] (*Blue*)	Innervation[b]	Main Actions
Gluteus maximus	Ilium posterior to posterior gluteal line, dorsal surface of sacrum and coccyx, sacrotuberous ligament	Iliotibial tract that inserts into lateral condyle of tibia; some fibers to gluteal tuberosity	Inferior gluteal nerve (L5, **S1, S2**)	Extends hip joint and assists in lateral rotation; steadies thigh and assists in raising trunk from flexed position
Gluteus medius	External surface of ilium between anterior and posterior gluteal lines; gluteal fascia	Lateral surface of greater trochanter of femur	Superior gluteal nerve (**L5**, S1)	Abducts and medially rotates hip joint[c]; keeps pelvis level when opposite leg is off ground and advances pelvis during swing phase of gait; TFL also contributes to stability of extended knee
Gluteus minimus	External surface of ilium between anterior and inferior gluteal lines	Anterior surface of greater trochanter of femur		
Tensor fasciae latae (TFL)	Anterior superior iliac spine and iliac crest	Iliotibial tract that attaches to lateral condyle (Gerdy tubercle) of tibia		
Piriformis	Anterior surface of sacrum and sacrotuberous ligament	Superior border of greater trochanter of femur	Anterior rami of S1 and S2	Laterally rotate extended hip joint and abduct flexed hip joint; steady femoral head in acetabulum
Obturator internus	Pelvic surface of obturator membrane and surrounding bones	Medial surface of greater trochanter of femur by common tendons	Nerve to obturator internus (L5, S1)	
Superior gemellus	Ischial spine			
Inferior gemellus	Ischial tuberosity			
Quadratus femoris	Lateral border of ischial tuberosity	Quadrate tubercle on intertrochanteric crest of femur	Nerve to quadratus femoris (L5, S1)	Laterally rotates hip joint,[d] steadies femoral head in acetabulum

[a]See Figure 5.22 for muscle attachments.
[b]See Table 5.1 for explanation of segmental innervation.
[c]Gluteus medius and minimus: anterior fibers medially rotate hip joint and posterior fibers laterally rotate hip joint.
[d]There are six lateral rotators of the hip joint: piriformis, obturator internus, gemelli (superior and inferior), quadratus femoris, and obturator externus. These muscles also stabilize the hip joint.

Posterior Views

5.30   MUSCLES OF POSTERIOR THIGH

A. Attachments. **B.** Superficial layer. **C.** Intermediate layer. **D.** Deep layer.

TABLE 5.8 MUSCLES OF POSTERIOR THIGH (HAMSTRING)

Muscle[a]	Proximal Attachment[a] (*Red*)	Distal Attachment[a] (*Blue*)	Innervation[b]	Main Actions
Semitendinosus	Ischial tuberosity	Medial surface of superior part of tibia	Tibial division of sciatic nerve (L5, S1, and S2)	Extend hip joint; flex knee joint and rotate it medially; when hip and knee joints are flexed, can extend trunk
Semimembranosus		Posterior part of medial condyle of tibia; reflected attachment forms oblique popliteal ligament to lateral femoral condyle		
Biceps femoris	*Long head:* ischial tuberosity; *Short head:* linea aspera and lateral supracondylar line of femur	Lateral side of head of fibula; tendon is split at this site by fibular collateral ligament of knee	*Long head:* tibial division of sciatic nerve (L5, S1, and S2); *Short head:* common fibular (peroneal) division of sciatic nerve (L5, S1, and S2)	Flexes knee joint and rotates it laterally; extends hip joint (e.g., when initiating a walking gait)

[a]See Figure 5.22 for muscle attachments.
[b]See Table 5.1 for explanation of segmental innervation.

Gluteus maximus

Superior gluteal artery

Piriformis

Gluteus medius

Inferior gluteal artery and nerve

Superior gemellus

Internal pudendal artery

Obturator internus

Pudendal nerve

Inferior gemellus

Nerve to obturator internus

Sacrotuberous ligament

Branch of medial circumflex femoral artery

Trochanteric bursa

Quadratus femoris

Posterior cutaneous nerve of thigh

Gluteofemoral bursa

Sciatic nerve

Branch of medial circumflex femoral artery

Adductor magnus

Biceps femoris, long head

1st perforating artery

Semitendinosus

Semimembranosus

Nerve to
Semimembranosus
Semitendinosus
Adductor magnus

2nd perforating artery

A. Posterior View

Biceps femoris, short head

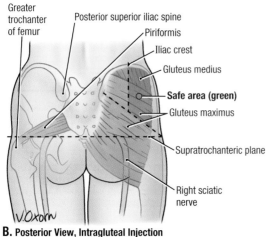

Greater
trochanter
of femur

Posterior superior iliac spine

Piriformis

Iliac crest

Gluteus medius

Safe area (green)

Gluteus maximus

Supratrochanteric plane

Right sciatic
nerve

V.Oxorn

B. Posterior View, Intragluteal Injection

5.31

MUSCLES OF GLUTEAL REGION AND POSTERIOR THIGH IV

A. Dissection. The gluteus maximus muscle is split superiorly and inferiorly, and the middle part is excised; two cubes remain to identify its nerve. The gluteus maximus is the only muscle to cover the greater trochanter; it is apo-neurotic and has underlying bursae where it glides on the trochanter (trochan-teric bursa) and the aponeurosis of the vastus lateralis muscle (gluteofemoral bursa). **B. Intragluteal injection.** Injections can be made safely only into the superolateral part of the buttock to avoid injury to the sciatic and glu-teal nerves. This site has a rich vascular network from the superior gluteal vessels that lie between the gluteus medius and minimus muscles.

Posterior superior iliac spine

Gluteus minimus

Piriformis

Superior gluteal artery and nerve

Gluteus medius

Sacrotuberous ligament

Superior gemellus

Pudendal nerve

Obturator internus tendon

Internal pudendal artery

Inferior gemellus

Nerve to obturator internus

Greater trochanter

Tip of coccyx

Obturator externus tendon

Medial circumflex femoral artery

Sciatic nerve

Quadratus femoris

Inferior gluteal nerve and artery

Posterior cutaneous
nerve of thigh

Gluteus maximus

Biceps femoris, long head

Semitendinosus

Posterior cutaneous nerve
of thigh

Semimembranosus

1st perforating artery

Iliotibial tract

Adductor magnus

Intermuscular septum

Gracilis

Biceps femoris, short head

Sciatic nerve

2nd perforating artery

Semimembranosus

Semitendinosus

Biceps femoris, long head

A. Posterior View

Abductors
(Gluteus medius, minimus, and
tensor fasciae latae)

Iliotibial
tract

B   C

Posterior Views

5.32   MUSCLES OF GLUTEAL REGION AND POSTERIOR THIGH V

A. The proximal three quarters of the gluteus maximus muscle is reflected, and parts of the gluteus medius and the three hamstring muscles are excised. The superior gluteal vessels and nerves emerge superior to the piriformis muscle; all other vessels and nerves emerge inferior to it. **B.** When the weight is borne by one limb, the muscles on the supported side fix the pelvis so that it does not sag to the unsupported side, keeping the pelvis level. **C.** When the right **abductors are paralyzed,** owing to a lesion of the right superior gluteal nerve, fixation by these muscles is lost and the pelvis tilts to the unsupported left side (positive Trendelenburg sign).

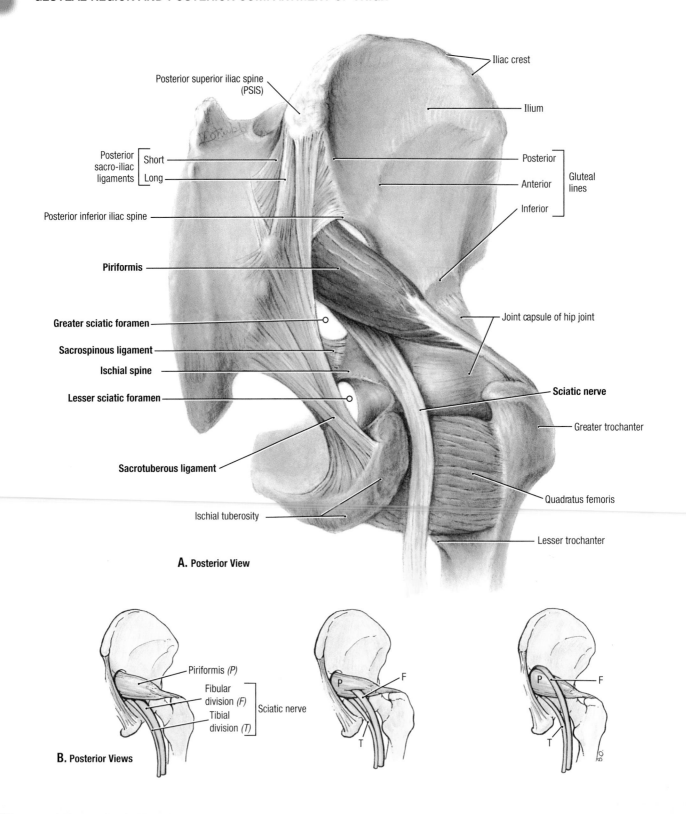

Iliac crest

Posterior superior iliac spine (PSIS)

Ilium

Posterior sacro-iliac ligaments — Short / Long

Posterior

Anterior

Inferior

Gluteal lines

Posterior inferior iliac spine

Piriformis

Greater sciatic foramen

Sacrospinous ligament

Ischial spine

Lesser sciatic foramen

Joint capsule of hip joint

Sciatic nerve

Greater trochanter

Sacrotuberous ligament

Quadratus femoris

Ischial tuberosity

Lesser trochanter

A. Posterior View

Piriformis *(P)*

Fibular division *(F)*

Tibial division *(T)*

Sciatic nerve

P F

P F

T

T

B. Posterior Views

| 5.33 | LATERAL ROTATORS OF HIP, SCIATIC NERVE, AND LIGAMENTS OF GLUTEAL REGION |

A. Piriformis and quadratus femoris. In the anatomical position the tip of the coccyx lies superior to the level of the ischial tuberosity and inferior to that of the ischial spine. The lateral border of the sciatic nerve lies midway between the lateral surface of the greater trochanter and the medial surface of the ischial tuberosity.

B. Relationship of sciatic nerve to piriformis muscle. Of 640 limbs studied in Dr. Grant's laboratory, in 87%, the tibial and fibular (peroneal) divisions passed inferior to the piriformis (*left*); in 12.2%, the fibular (peroneal) division passed through the piriformis (*center*); and in 0.5% the fibular (peroneal) division passed superior to the piriformis (*right*).

Iliac crest

Posterior superior iliac spine (PSIS)

Ilium

Posterior inferior iliac spine (PIIS)

Greater sciatic foramen

Sacrospinous ligament

Ischium

Capsule of hip joint

Piriformis

Superior gemellus*

Greater trochanter

Inferior gemellus*

Obturator externus

Obturator internus*

* Triceps coxae

Sacrotuberous ligament

Ischial tuberosity

Lesser trochanter

C. Posterior View

Obturator internus and gemelli

Obturator externus

Piriformis

D. Posteromedial View

5.33   **LATERAL ROTATORS OF HIP, SCIATIC NERVE, AND LIGAMENTS OF GLUTEAL REGION (*CONTINUED*)**

C. Obturator internus, obturator externus, and superior and inferior gemelli.
- The obturator internus is located partly in the pelvis, where it covers most of the lateral wall of the lesser pelvis. It leaves the pelvis through the lesser sciatic foramen, makes a right-angle turn, becomes tendinous, and receives the distal attachments of the gemelli before attaching to the medial surface of the greater trochanter (trochanteric fossa).
- The obturator externus extends from the external surface of the obturator membrane and surrounding bone of the pelvis to the posterior aspect of the greater trochanter, passing directly under the acetabulum and neck of the femur.

- **Sciatic nerve block.** Sensation conveyed by the sciatic nerve can be blocked by injecting an anesthetic agent a few centimeters inferior to the midpoint of the line joining the PSIS and the superior border of the greater trochanter. Paresthesia radiates to the foot because of anesthesia of the plantar nerves, which are terminal branches of the tibial nerve derived from the sciatic nerve.
- **Common fibular nerve compression at piriformis.** In the approximately 12% of people in whom the common fibular division of the sciatic nerve passes through the piriformis, this muscle may compress the nerve.

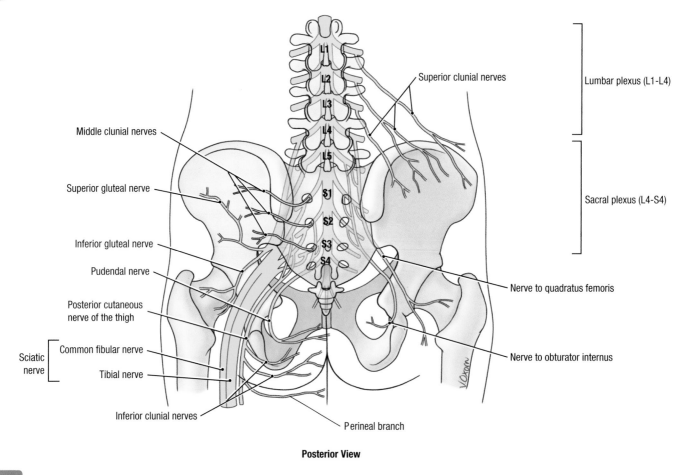

Posterior View

5.34 NERVES OF GLUTEAL REGION

TABLE 5.9 NERVES OF GLUTEAL REGION

Nerve	Origin	Course	Distribution in Gluteal Region
Clunial (superior, middle, and inferior)	*Superior:* posterior rami of L1–L3 nerves *Middle:* posterior rami of S1–S3 nerves *Inferior:* posterior cutaneous nerve of thigh	*Superior nerves* cross iliac crest; *middle nerves* exit through posterior sacral foramina and enter gluteal region; *inferior nerves* curve around inferior border of gluteus maximus	Gluteal region as far laterally as greater trochanter
Sciatic	Sacral plexus (L4–S3)	Exits pelvis via greater sciatic foramen inferior to piriformis to enter gluteal region	No muscles in gluteal region
Posterior cutaneous nerve of thigh	Sacral plexus (S1–S3)	Exits pelvis via greater sciatic foramen inferior to piriformis, emerges from inferior border of gluteus maximus coursing deep to fascia lata	Skin of buttock via inferior cluneal branches, skin over posterior thigh and popliteal fossa; skin of lateral perineum and upper medial thigh via perineal branch
Superior gluteal	Anterior rami of L4–S1 nerves	Exits pelvis via greater sciatic foramen superior to piriformis; courses between gluteus medius and minimus	Gluteus medius, gluteus minimus, and TFL
Inferior gluteal	Anterior rami of L5–S2 nerves	Exits pelvis via greater sciatic foramen inferior to piriformis, dividing into multiple branches	Gluteus maximus
Nerve to quadratus femoris	Anterior rami of L4–S1 nerves	Exits pelvis via greater sciatic foramen deep to sciatic nerve	Posterior hip joint, inferior gemellus, and quadratus femoris
Pudendal	Anterior rami of S2–S4 nerves	Exits pelvis via greater sciatic foramen inferior to piriformis; descends posterior to sacrospinous ligament; enters perineum (pudendal canal) through lesser sciatic foramen	No structures in gluteal region (supplies most of perineum)
Nerve to obturator internus	Anterior rami of L5–S2 nerves	Exits pelvis via greater sciatic foramen inferior to piriformis; descends posterior to ischial spine; enters lesser sciatic foramen and passes to obturator internus	Superior gemellus and obturator internus

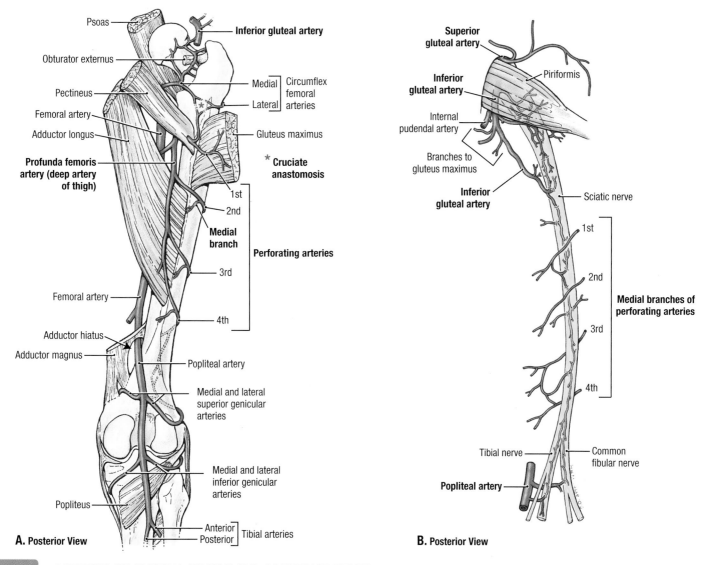

A. Posterior View

B. Posterior View

5.35   ARTERIES OF GLUTEAL REGION AND POSTERIOR THIGH

TABLE 5.10 ARTERIES OF GLUTEAL REGION AND POSTERIOR THIGH

Artery	Origin	Course	Distribution
Superior gluteal		Enters gluteal region through greater sciatic foramen superior to piriformis; divides into superficial and deep branches; anastomoses with inferior gluteal and medial circumflex femoral arteries	*Superficial branch:* superior gluteus maximus *Deep branch:* runs between gluteus medius and minimus, supplying both and tensor fasciae latae
Inferior gluteal		Enters gluteal region through greater sciatic foramen inferior to piriformis; descends on medial side of sciatic nerve; anastomoses with superior gluteal artery and participates in cruciate anastomosis of thigh	Inferior gluteus maximus, obturator internus, quadratus femoris, and superior parts of hamstring muscles
Internal pudendal	Internal iliac	Enters gluteal region through greater sciatic foramen; descends posterior to ischial spine; exits gluteal region via lesser sciatic foramen to perineum	No structures in gluteal region (supplies external genitalia and muscles in perineal region)
Perforating arteries		Perforate aponeurotic portion of adductor magnus attachment and medial intermuscular septum to enter and supply muscular branches to posterior compartment; then pierce lateral intermuscular septum to enter posterolateral aspect of anterior compartment	Hamstring muscles in posterior compartment; posterior portion of vastus lateralis in anterior compartment; femur (via femoral nutrient arteries); reinforce arterial supply of sciatic nerve
Lateral circumflex femoral	Profunda femoris (may arise from femoral)	Passes laterally deep to sartorius and rectus femoris; enter gluteal region	Anterior part of gluteal region
Medial circumflex femoral		Passes medially and posteriorly between pectineus and iliopsoas; enters gluteal region	Supplies most blood to head and neck of femur; hip region

Anterior superior iliac spine

Anterior inferior iliac spine

Acetabular labrum

Head of femur

Pectineus

Pectineal fascia

Rectus femoris

Pectineal ligament

Pubic tubercle

Iliofemoral ligament

Anterior branch

Posterior branch

Obturator nerve

Greater trochanter

Obturator externus

Intertrochanteric line

Lesser trochanter

A. Anterior View

Piriformis

Fovea (pit) for ligament of head of femur

Obturator internus and gemelli

Gluteus minimus

Vastus lateralis

Iliofemoral ligament

Iliopsoas

Key for B

Proximal muscular attachment

Distal muscular attachment

Ligamentous attachment

B. Anterior View

5.36   HIP JOINT

A. Iliofemoral ligament. **B.** Muscle attachments of anterior aspect of the proximal femur. In **A:**

- The head of the femur is exposed just medial to the iliofemoral ligament and faces superiorly, medially, and anteriorly. At the site of the subtendinous bursa of psoas, the capsule is weak or (as in this specimen) partially deficient, but it is guarded by the psoas tendon.

- The iliofemoral ligament, shaped like an inverted "Y." Superiorly it is attached deep to the rectus femoris muscle; the ligament becomes tight on medial rotation of the femur.

- The pectineus muscle is thin, and its fascia blends with the pectineal ligament.

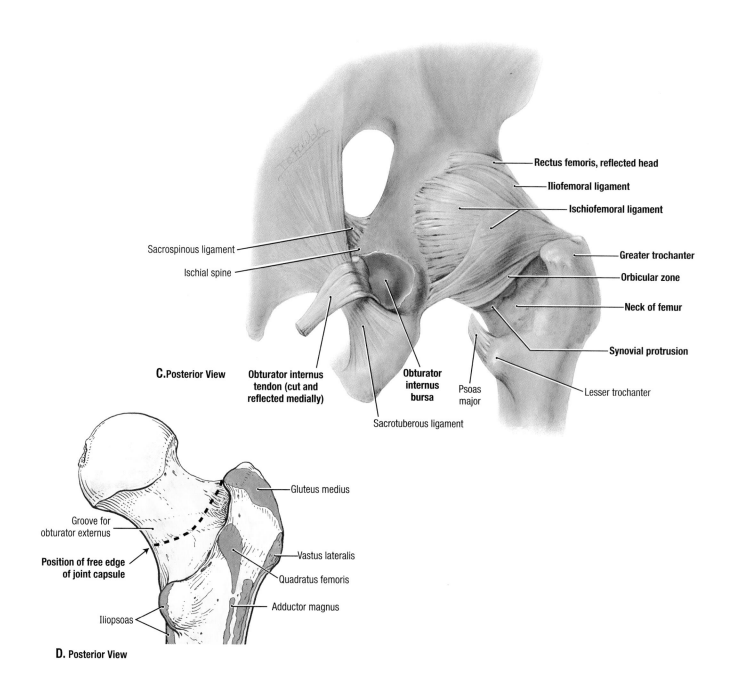

C. Posterior View

Rectus femoris, reflected head
Iliofemoral ligament
Ischiofemoral ligament
Greater trochanter
Orbicular zone
Neck of femur
Synovial protrusion
Lesser trochanter
Psoas major
Obturator internus bursa
Obturator internus tendon (cut and reflected medially)
Sacrotuberous ligament
Ischial spine
Sacrospinous ligament

D. Posterior View

Gluteus medius
Vastus lateralis
Quadratus femoris
Adductor magnus
Iliopsoas
Position of free edge of joint capsule
Groove for obturator externus

5.36   **HIP JOINT** (*CONTINUED*)

C. Ischiofemoral ligament. **D.** Muscle attachments onto the posterior aspect of proximal femur. In **C:**

- The fibers of the capsule spiral to become taut during extension and medial rotation of the femur.

- The synovial membrane protrudes inferior to the fibrous capsule and forms a bursa for the tendon of the obturator externus muscle. Note the large subtendinous bursa of the obturator internus at the lesser sciatic notch, where the tendon turns 90 degrees to attach to the greater trochanter.

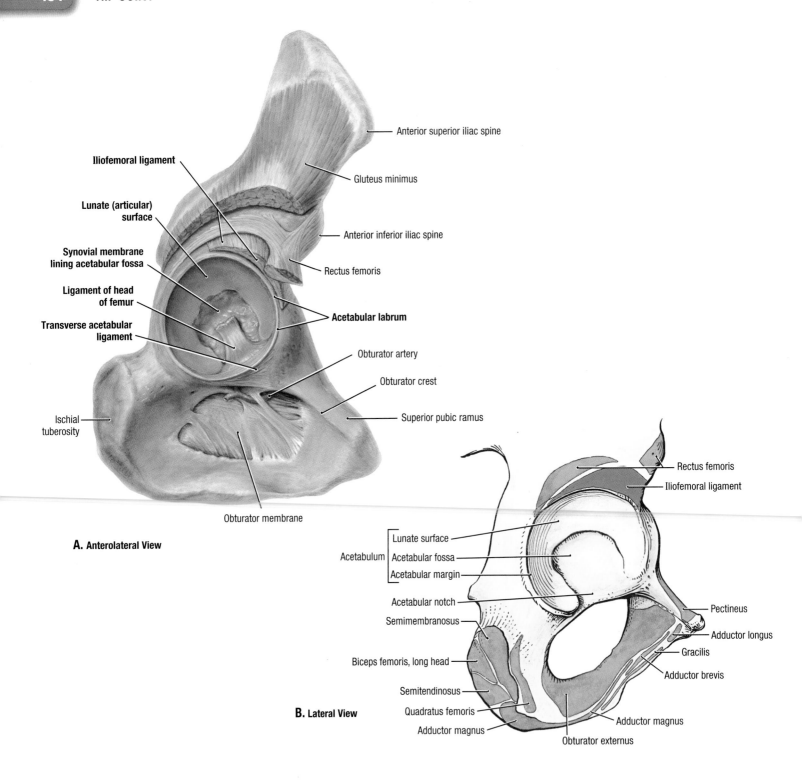

A. Anterolateral View

B. Lateral View

5.37   ACETABULAR REGION

A. Dissection of acetabulum. **B.** Muscle attachments of acetabular region.
In **A:**
- The transverse acetabular ligament bridges the acetabular notch.
- The acetabular labrum is attached to the acetabular rim and transverse acetabular ligament and forms a complete ring around the head of the femur.

- The ligament of the head of the femur lies between the head of the femur and the acetabulum. These fibers are attached superiorly to the pit (fovea) on the head of the femur and inferiorly to the transverse acetabular ligament and the margins of the acetabular notch. The artery of the ligament of the head of the femur passes through the acetabular notch and into the ligament of the head of the femur.

Anterior gluteal line

Iliac crest

Posterior gluteal line

Anterior superior iliac spine

Posterior superior iliac spine

Inferior gluteal line

Anterior inferior iliac spine

Posterior inferior iliac spine

Greater sciatic notch

Lunate surface

Acetabular fossa

Acetabulum

Ischial spine

Acetabular notch

Lesser sciatic notch

Body of ischium

Pubic tubercle

Obturator foramen

SART

Ischial tuberosity

Inferior pubic ramus*

Ramus of ischium*

A. Lateral View

*Ischiopubic ramus

Ilium

Site of triradiate cartilage

Pubis

Ischium

B. Lateral View

5.38   HIP BONE

A. Features of the lateral aspect. In the anatomical position, the anterior superior iliac spine and pubic tubercle are in the same coronal plane, and the ischial spine and superior end of the pubic symphysis are in the same horizontal plane; the internal aspect of the body of the pubis faces superiorly, and the acetabulum faces inferolaterally. **B.** Hip bone in youth. The three parts of the hip bone (ilium, ischium, and pubis) meet in the acetabulum at the triradiate synchondrosis. One or more primary centers of ossification appear in the triradiate cartilage at approximately the 12th year. Secondary centers of ossification appear along the length of the iliac crest, at the anterior inferior iliac spine, the ischial tuberosity, and the pubic symphysis at about puberty; fusion is usually complete by age 23.

A. Anteroposterior View

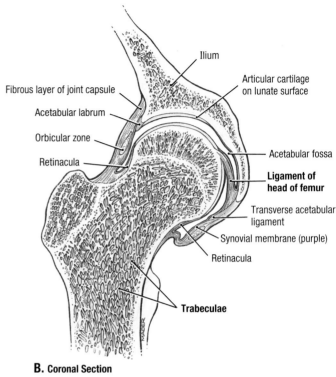

Ilium

Articular cartilage on lunate surface

Fibrous layer of joint capsule

Acetabular labrum

Orbicular zone

Retinacula

Acetabular fossa

Ligament of head of femur

Transverse acetabular ligament

Synovial membrane (purple)

Retinacula

Trabeculae

B. Coronal Section

C. Hip Prosthesis

5.39   RADIOGRAPH AND CORONAL SECTION OF HIP JOINT

A. Radiograph. On the femur, note the greater (*G*) and lesser (*L*) trochanters, the intertrochanteric crest (*I*), and the pit or fovea (*F*) for the ligament of the head. On the pelvis, note the roof (*A*) and posterior rim (*P*) of the acetabulum and the "teardrop" appearance (*T*) caused by the superimposition of structures at the inferior margin of the acetabulum. **B.** Coronal section. Observe the bony trabeculae projecting into the head of the femur. The ligament of the head of the femur becomes taut during adduction of the hip joint, such as when crossing the legs. **C. Hip replacement.** The hip joint is subject to severe traumatic injury and degenerative disease. **Osteoarthritis of the hip joint**, characterized by pain, edema, limitation of motion, and erosion of articular cartilage, is a common cause of disability. During hip replacement, a metal prosthesis anchored to the femur by bone cement replaces the femoral head and neck. A plastic socket is cemented to the hip bone to replace the acetabulum. See Figure 5.41 clinical blue text.

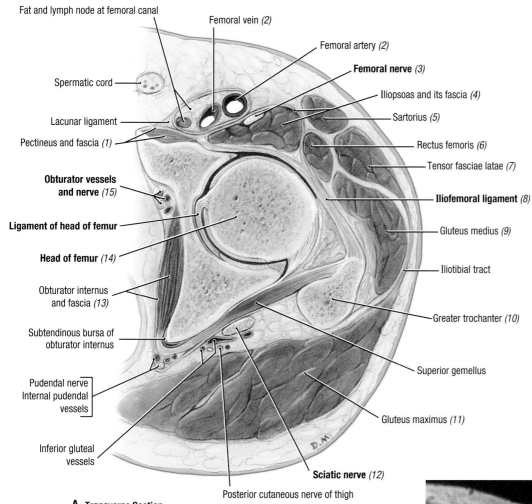

Fat and lymph node at femoral canal

Femoral vein (2)

Femoral artery (2)

Femoral nerve (3)

Iliopsoas and its fascia (4)

Spermatic cord

Sartorius (5)

Lacunar ligament

Rectus femoris (6)

Pectineus and fascia (1)

Tensor fasciae latae (7)

Obturator vessels and nerve (15)

Iliofemoral ligament (8)

Ligament of head of femur

Gluteus medius (9)

Head of femur (14)

Iliotibial tract

Obturator internus and fascia (13)

Greater trochanter (10)

Subtendinous bursa of obturator internus

Superior gemellus

Pudendal nerve
Internal pudendal vessels

Gluteus maximus (11)

Inferior gluteal vessels

Sciatic nerve (12)

Posterior cutaneous nerve of thigh

A. Transverse Section, Inferior View

5.40 TRANSVERSE SECTION THROUGH THIGH AT LEVEL OF HIP JOINT

A. Transverse section. **B.** MRI (*numbers* refer to structures in **A**). In **A**:
- The fibrous capsule of the joint is thick where it forms the iliofemoral ligament and thin posterior to the subtendinous bursa of psoas and tendon.
- The femoral sheath, enclosing the femoral artery, vein, lymph node, lymph vessels, and fat, is free, except posteriorly where, between the psoas and pectineus muscles, it is attached to the capsule of the hip joint.
- The femoral vein is located at the interval between the psoas and pectineus muscles. The femoral nerve lies between the iliacus muscle and fascia.

B. Transverse MRI

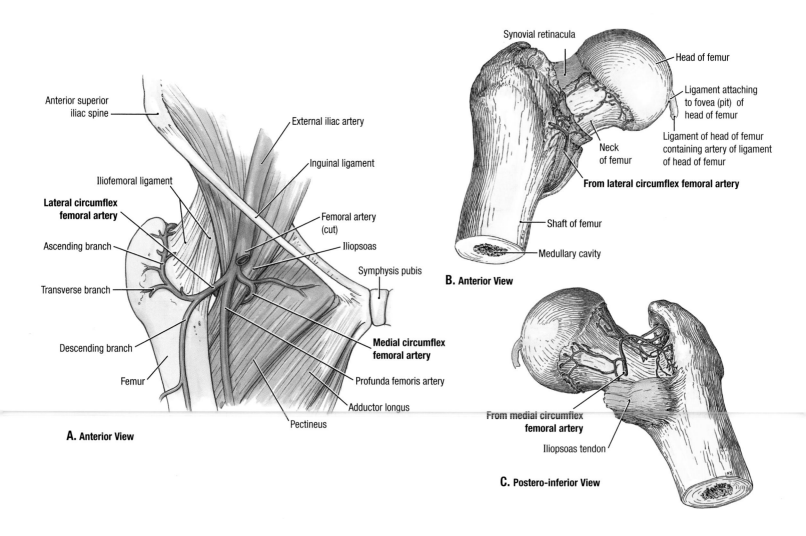

Anterior superior iliac spine

Iliofemoral ligament

Lateral circumflex femoral artery

Ascending branch

Transverse branch

Descending branch

Femur

External iliac artery

Inguinal ligament

Femoral artery (cut)

Iliopsoas

Symphysis pubis

Medial circumflex femoral artery

Profunda femoris artery

Adductor longus

Pectineus

A. Anterior View

Synovial retinacula

Head of femur

Ligament attaching to fovea (pit) of head of femur

Neck of femur

Ligament of head of femur containing artery of ligament of head of femur

From lateral circumflex femoral artery

Shaft of femur

Medullary cavity

B. Anterior View

From medial circumflex femoral artery

Iliopsoas tendon

C. Postero-inferior View

5.41 BLOOD SUPPLY TO HEAD OF FEMUR

A. Medial and lateral circumflex femoral arteries in femoral triangle. **B.** Branches of lateral circumflex femoral artery. **C.** Branches of medial circumflex femoral artery.

- Branches of the medial and lateral circumflex femoral arteries ascend on the posterosuperior and postero-inferior parts of the neck of the femur. The vessels ascend in synovial retinacula—reflections of synovial membrane along the neck of the femur. The retinacula (in **B** and **C**) have been mostly removed; thus, the vessels can be clearly visualized.
- The branches of the medial and lateral circumflex femoral arteries perforate the bone just distal to the head of the femur, where they anastomose with branches from the artery of the ligament of the head of the femur and with medullary branches located within the shaft of the femur.
- The ligament of the head of the femur usually contains the artery of the ligament of the head of the femur, a branch of the obturator artery. The

artery enters the head of the femur only when the center of the ossification has extended to the pit (fovea) for the ligament of the head (12th to 14th year). When present, this anastomosis persists even in advanced age; however, in 20% of persons, it is never established.

Fractures of the femoral neck often disrupt the blood supply to the head of the femur. The medial circumflex femoral artery supplies most of the blood to the head and neck of the femur and is often torn when the femoral neck is fractured. In some cases, the blood supplied by the artery of the ligament of the head may be the only blood received by the proximal fragment of the femoral head, which may be inadequate. If the blood vessels are ruptured, the fragment of bone may receive no blood and undergo aseptic avascular necrosis.

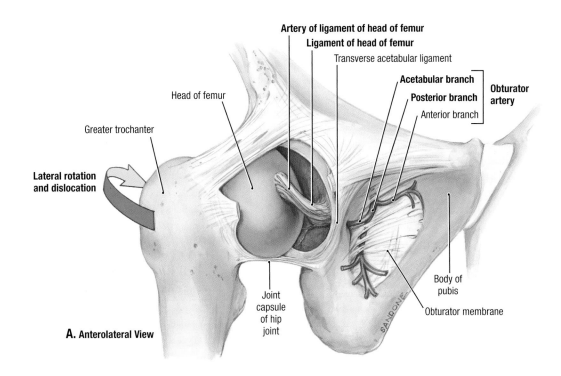

Artery of ligament of head of femur
Ligament of head of femur
Transverse acetabular ligament
Acetabular branch
Posterior branch
Anterior branch
Obturator artery

Head of femur

Greater trochanter

Lateral rotation and dislocation

Body of pubis

Obturator membrane

Joint capsule of hip joint

A. Anterolateral View

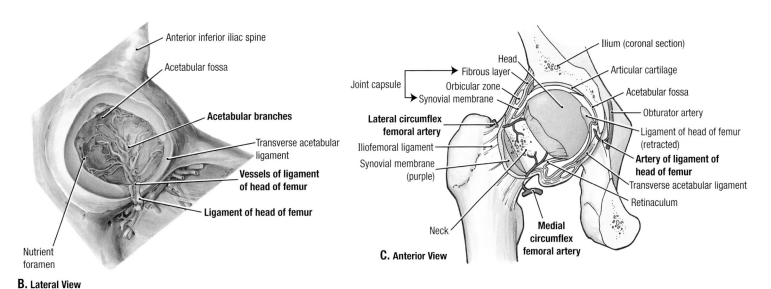

Anterior inferior iliac spine

Acetabular fossa

Acetabular branches

Transverse acetabular ligament

Vessels of ligament of head of femur

Ligament of head of femur

Nutrient foramen

B. Lateral View

Ilium (coronal section)
Head
Fibrous layer
Joint capsule
Orbicular zone
Synovial membrane
Articular cartilage
Acetabular fossa
Obturator artery
Ligament of head of femur (retracted)
Artery of ligament of head of femur
Transverse acetabular ligament
Retinaculum

Lateral circumflex femoral artery
Iliofemoral ligament
Synovial membrane (purple)

Neck

Medial circumflex femoral artery

C. Anterior View

5.42 BLOOD VESSELS OF ACETABULAR FOSSA AND LIGAMENT OF HEAD OF FEMUR

A. Obturator artery. The hip joint has been dislocated to reveal the ligament of the head of the femur. The obturator artery divides into anterior and posterior branches, and the acetabular branch arises from the posterior branch. The artery of the ligament of the head of the femur is a branch of the acetabular artery and can be seen traveling in the ligament to the head of the femur. **B.** Acetabular artery and vein. The acetabular branches (artery and vein) pass through the acetabular foramen and enter the acetabular fossa, where they diverge in the fatty areolar tissue. The branches radiate to the margin of the fossa, where they enter nutrient foramina. **C.** Blood supply of the head and neck of the femur. A section of bone has been removed from the femoral neck.

A. Posterior View

B. Posterior View

Semimembranosus (1)

Branch communicating with inferior gluteal vein

Sartorius

Gracilis

Semitendinosus (2)

MEDIAL

Small saphenous vein

Medial sural cutaneous nerve

Gastrocnemius, medial head (3)

Biceps femoris (6)

Tibial nerve

Popliteal vein

Popliteal artery

LATERAL

Common fibular (peroneal) nerve

Lateral sural cutaneous nerve

Communicating fibular (peroneal) nerve

Gastrocnemius, lateral head (5)

Soleus (4)

5.43 POPLITEAL FOSSA

A. Surface anatomy (*numbers* refer to structures in **B**). **B.** Superficial dissection.

- The two heads of the gastrocnemius muscle are embraced on the medial side by the semimembranosus muscle, which is overlaid by the semitendinosus muscle, and on the lateral side by the biceps femoris muscle.
- The small saphenous vein runs between the two heads of the gastrocnemius muscle. Deep to this vein is the medial sural cutaneous nerve, which, followed proximally, leads to the tibial nerve. The tibial nerve is superficial to the popliteal vein, which, in turn, is superficial to the popliteal artery.

Because the popliteal artery is deep in the popliteal fossa, it may be difficult to feel the **popliteal pulse.** Palpation of this pulse is commonly performed by placing the person in the prone position with the knee flexed to relax the popliteal fascia and hamstrings. The pulsations are best felt in the inferior part of the fossa. Weakening or loss of the popliteal pulse is a sign of femoral artery obstruction.

Gracilis

Semitendinosus

Semimembranosus

Medial sural cutaneous nerve

Tibial nerve

Nerve to gastrocnemius,
medial head

MEDIAL

Popliteus

Plantaris tendon

Soleus

Gastrocnemius, medial head

Posterior View

Biceps femoris

Sural communicating branch

Common fibular (peroneal) nerve

Sural nerve

Nerve to | Gastrocnemius, lateral head
          | Soleus

Plantaris

LATERAL

Nerve to popliteus

Gastrocnemius, lateral head

5.44   NERVES OF POPLITEAL FOSSA

The two heads of the gastrocnemius muscle are separated. A cutaneous branch of the tibial nerve joins a cutaneous branch of the common fibular (peroneal) nerve to form the sural nerve. In this specimen, the junction is high; usually it is 5 to 8 cm proximal to the ankle.

All motor branches in this region emerge from the tibial nerve, one branch from its medial side and the others from its lateral side; hence, it is safer to dissect on the medial side.

Gracilis

Semitendinosus

Semimembranosus

Popliteal vein

Tibial nerve

MEDIAL

Popliteal artery

Superior medial genicular artery

Semitendinosus

Semimembranosus

Semimembranosus bursa

Gastrocnemius, medial head

Inferior medial genicular artery

Popliteus fascia

Soleus

Plantaris

Gastrocnemius

Biceps femoris, long head

Biceps femoris, short head

Lateral intermuscular septum

Common fibular (peroneal) nerve

Femur

Biceps femoris

Superior lateral genicular artery

LATERAL

Gastrocnemius, lateral head

Plantaris

Inferior lateral genicular artery

Popliteus

Nerve to popliteus

Posterior View

5.45   DEEP DISSECTION OF POPLITEAL FOSSA

The common fibular (peroneal) nerve follows the posterior border of the biceps femoris muscle and, in this specimen, gives off two cutaneous branches. The popliteal artery lies on the floor of the popliteal fossa. The floor is formed by the femur, capsule of the knee joint, and popliteus muscle and fascia. The popliteal artery gives off genicular branches that also lie on the floor of the fossa. A **popliteal aneurysm** (abnormal dilation of all or part of the popliteal artery) usually causes edema (swelling) and pain in the popliteal fossa. If the femoral artery has to be ligated, blood can bypass the occlusion through the genicular anastomosis and reach the popliteal artery distal to the ligation.

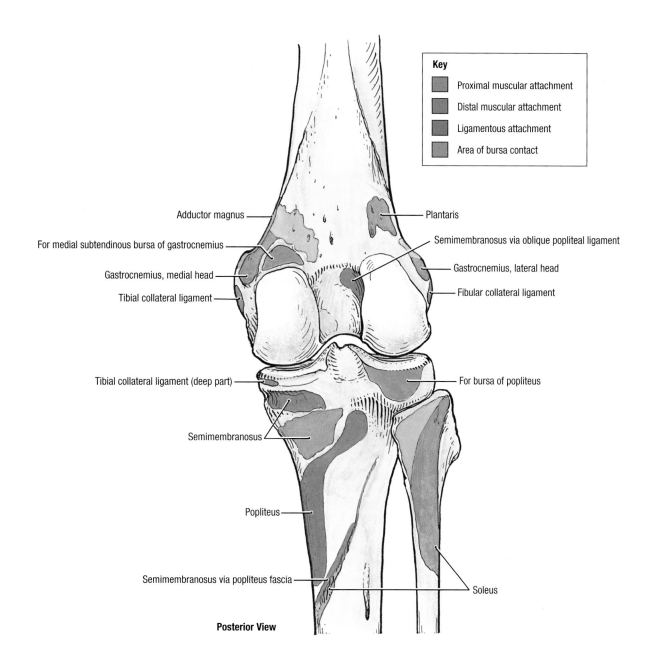

Key
- Proximal muscular attachment
- Distal muscular attachment
- Ligamentous attachment
- Area of bursa contact

Adductor magnus

For medial subtendinous bursa of gastrocnemius

Gastrocnemius, medial head

Tibial collateral ligament

Tibial collateral ligament (deep part)

Semimembranosus

Popliteus

Semimembranosus via popliteus fascia

Plantaris

Semimembranosus via oblique popliteal ligament

Gastrocnemius, lateral head

Fibular collateral ligament

For bursa of popliteus

Soleus

Posterior View

5.46 ATTACHMENT OF MUSCLES OF POPLITEAL REGION

Lighter tones are secondary attachments.

Rectus femoris *(1)*

Sartorius

Vastus lateralis *(9)*

Vastus medialis *(2)*

Iliotibial tract *(10)*

Patella *(7)*

Sartorius tendon

Biceps femoris *(6)*

Lateral patellar retinaculum

Patellar ligament *(3)*

Medial patellar retinaculum

Head of fibula *(5)*

Tibial tuberosity (4)

A. Anterior View

5.47   ANTERIOR ASPECT OF KNEE

A. Distal thigh and knee regions. Note that the tendons of the four parts of the quadriceps unite to form the quadriceps tendon, a broad band that attaches to the patella. The patellar ligament, a continuation of the quadriceps tendon, attaches the patella to the tibial tuberosity. The lateral and medial patellar retinacula, formed largely by continuation of the iliotibial tract, and investing fascia of the vasti muscles, maintains alignment of the patella and patellar ligament. The retinacula also form the anterolateral and anteromedial portions of the fibrous layer of the joint capsule of the knee.

B. Anterior Views

C. Anterior Views

Anterior superior iliac spine

↓ Line of gravity

Normal Q-angle

Normal alignment

↓ Q-angle

Genu varum

↑ Q-angle

Genu valgum

5.47   **ANTERIOR ASPECT OF KNEE** (*CONTINUED*)

B. Surface anatomy (numbers refer to structures in **A**). The femur is placed diagonally within the thigh, whereas the tibia is almost vertical within the leg, creating an angle at the knee between the long axes of the bones. The angle between the two bones, referred to clinically as the **Q-angle,** is assessed by drawing a line from the anterior superior iliac spine to the middle of the patella and extrapolating a second (vertical) line passing through the middle of the patella and tibial tuberosity. The Q-angle is typically greater in adult females, owing to their wider pelves. **C. Genu valgum and genu varum.**

A medial angulation of the leg in relation to the thigh, in which the femur is abnormally vertical and the Q-angle is small, is a deformity called genu varum (bowleg) that causes unequal weight bearing resulting in arthrosis (destruction of knee cartilages), and an overstressed fibular collateral ligament. A lateral angulation of the leg (large Q-angle, >17 degrees) in relation to the thigh is called genu valgum (knock-knee). This results in excess stress and degeneration of the lateral structures of the knee joint.

Subcutaneous prepatellar bursa

Patella

Synovial fold

Joint capsule consisting
of patellar retinaculum

Iliotibial tract (cut)

Synovial membrane

Articular cartilage

Infrapatellar synovial fold

Alar fold

Infrapatellar fat pad

Synovial fold

Articular cartilage

Patella

Subcutaneous prepatellar bursa (opened)

Tibial collateral ligament (cut)

Medial femoral condyle

Medial meniscus

Articular cartilage of medial tibial plateau

Fibrous layer of joint capsule

A. Anterior View

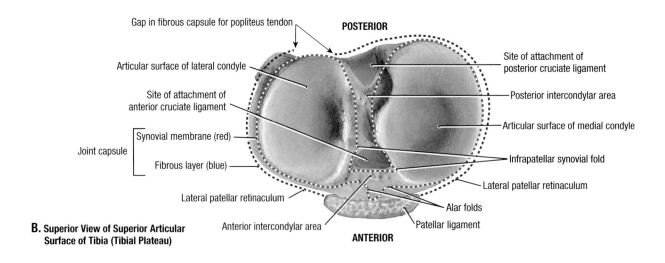

Gap in fibrous capsule for popliteus tendon

POSTERIOR

Articular surface of lateral condyle

Site of attachment of
anterior cruciate ligament

Joint capsule

Synovial membrane (red)

Fibrous layer (blue)

Lateral patellar retinaculum

Anterior intercondylar area

Site of attachment of
posterior cruciate ligament

Posterior intercondylar area

Articular surface of medial condyle

Infrapatellar synovial fold

Lateral patellar retinaculum

Alar folds

Patellar ligament

**B. Superior View of Superior Articular
Surface of Tibia (Tibial Plateau)**

ANTERIOR

5.48   FIBROUS LAYER AND SYNOVIAL MEMBRANE OF JOINT CAPSULE

A. Dissection. **B.** Attachment of the layers of the joint capsule to the tibia. The fibrous layer (*blue dotted line*) and synovial membrane (*red dotted line*) are adjacent on each side, but they part company centrally to accommodate intercondylar and infrapatellar structures that are intracapsular (inside the fibrous layer) but extra-articular (excluded from the articular cavity by synovial membrane).

A. Anterior View

Patellar surface
Groove for lateral meniscus
Popliteus tendon
Lateral meniscus
Coronary ligament (cut edge)
Fibular collateral ligament
Biceps femoris, extension to deep fascia of leg
Patellar ligament
Inferior facets (1)
Middle facets (2)
Superior facets (3)

Groove for medial meniscus
Notch for anterior cruciate ligament
Posterior cruciate ligament
Anterior cruciate ligament
Medial meniscus
Coronary ligament (cut edge)
Tibial collateral ligament
Sartorius
Apex of patella
Nonarticular area
Medial vertical facet (4)
Base of patella
Quadriceps tendon

B. Inferior View

Patellar surface
Groove for medial meniscus
Groove for lateral meniscus
13 mm
Lateral condyle
Medial condyle
Anterior cruciate ligament

C. Superior View

Posterior cruciate ligament
Fibula
Anterior cruciate ligament
Medial meniscus
Transverse ligament of knee
Lateral meniscus

D. Posterior View

INFERIOR
LATERAL
Inferior facet
MEDIAL
Medial vertical facet
Middle facet
Superior facet
SUPERIOR

5.49   ARTICULAR SURFACES AND LIGAMENTS OF KNEE JOINT

A. Flexed knee joint with patella reflected. There are indentations on the sides of the femoral condyles at the junction of the patellar and tibial articular areas. The lateral tibial articular area is shorter than the medial one. The notch at the anterolateral part of the intercondylar notch is for the anterior cruciate ligament on full extension. **B.** Distal femur. **C.** Tibial plateaus. **D.** Articular surfaces of patella. The three paired facets (superior, middle, and inferior) on the posterior surface of the patella articulate with the patellar surface of the femur successively during (1) extension, (2) slight flexion, (3) flexion, and the most medial vertical facet on the patella (4) articulates during full flexion with the crescentic facet on the medial margin of the intercondylar notch of the femur. When the **patellar dislocation** occurs, it nearly always dislocates laterally. The tendency toward lateral dislocation is normally counterbalanced by the medial, more horizontal pull of the powerful vastus medialis. In addition, the more anterior projection of the lateral femoral condyle and deeper slope for the large lateral patellar facet provides a mechanical deterrent to lateral dislocation. An imbalance of the lateral pull and the mechanisms resisting it result in abnormal tracking of the patella within the patellar groove and chronic patellar pain, even if actual dislocation does not occur.

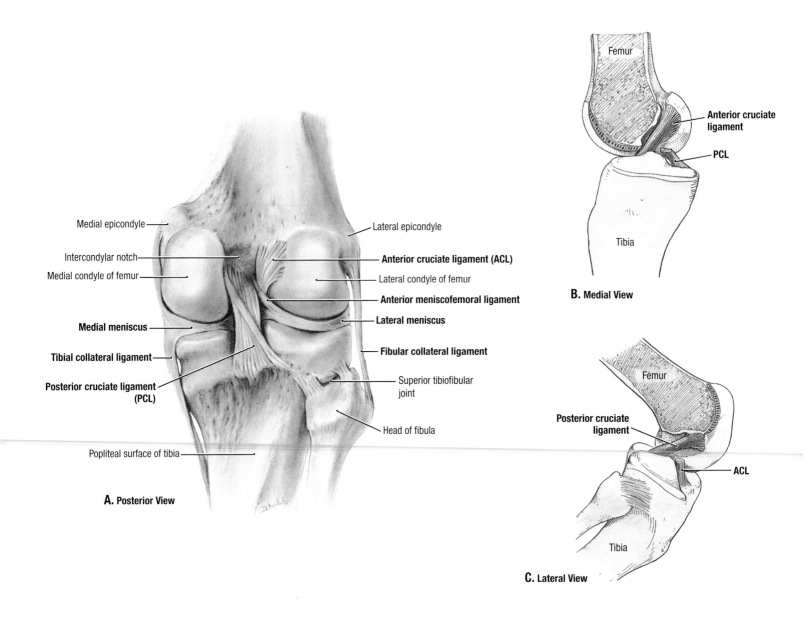

A. Posterior View

B. Medial View

C. Later al View

5.50   LIGAMENTS OF KNEE JOINT

A. Posterior aspect of joint. The bandlike tibial (medial) collateral ligament is attached to the medial meniscus, and the cordlike fibular (lateral) collateral ligament is separated from the lateral meniscus by the width of the popliteus tendon (removed). The posterior cruciate ligament is joined by a cord from the lateral meniscus called the anterior meniscofemoral ligament. The posterior meniscofemoral ligament attaches to the medial condyle of the femur just posterior to the attachment of the posterior cruciate ligament. **B.** Anterior cruciate ligament (ACL). **C.** Posterior cruciate ligament (PCL). In each illustration, half the femur is sagittally sectioned and removed with the proximal part of the corresponding cruciate ligament. Note that the posterior cruciate ligament prevents the femur from sliding anteriorly on the tibia, particularly when the

knee is flexed. The anterior cruciate ligament prevents the femur from sliding posteriorly on the tibia, preventing hyperextension of the knee, and limits medial rotation of the femur when the foot is on the ground (i.e., when the leg is fixed). **Injury to the knee joint** is frequently caused by a blow to the lateral side of the extended knee or excessive lateral twisting of the flexed knee, which disrupts the tibial collateral ligament and concomitantly tears and/or detaches the medial meniscus from the joint capsule. This injury is common in athletes who twist their flexed knees while running (e.g., in football and soccer). The anterior cruciate ligament, which serves as a pivot for rotary movements of the knee, is taut during flexion and may also tear subsequent to the rupture of the tibial collateral ligament.

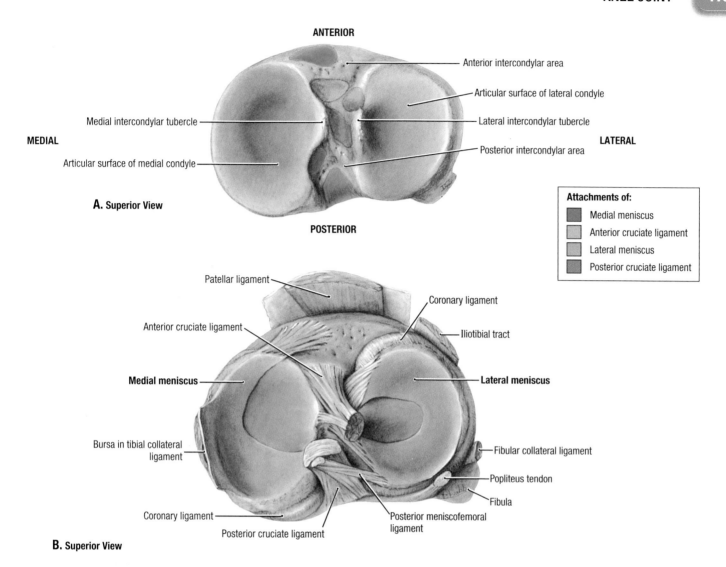

ANTERIOR

Anterior intercondylar area

Articular surface of lateral condyle

Medial intercondylar tubercle

Lateral intercondylar tubercle

MEDIAL

LATERAL

Posterior intercondylar area

Articular surface of medial condyle

A. Superior View

POSTERIOR

Attachments of:
- Medial meniscus
- Anterior cruciate ligament
- Lateral meniscus
- Posterior cruciate ligament

Patellar ligament

Coronary ligament

Anterior cruciate ligament

Iliotibial tract

Medial meniscus

Lateral meniscus

Bursa in tibial collateral ligament

Fibular collateral ligament

Popliteus tendon

Fibula

Coronary ligament

Posterior meniscofemoral ligament

Posterior cruciate ligament

B. Superior View

5.51 CRUCIATE LIGAMENTS AND MENISCI

A. Attachments sites on tibia. **B.** Menisci in situ.

- The lateral tibial condyle is flatter, shorter from anterior to posterior, and more circular. The medial condyle is concave, longer from anterior to posterior, and more oval.
- The menisci conform to the shapes of the surfaces on which they rest. Because the horns of the lateral meniscus are attached close together and its coronary ligament is slack, this meniscus can slide anteriorly and posteriorly on the (flat) condyle; because the horns of the medial meniscus are attached further apart, its movements on the (concave) condyle are restricted.

Arthroscopy is an endoscopic examination that allows visualization of the interior of the knee joint cavity with minimal disruption of tissue. The arthroscope and one (or more) additional canula(e) are inserted through tiny incisions, known as portals. The second canula is for passage of specialized tools (e.g., manipulative probes or forceps) or equipment for trimming, shaping, or removing damaged tissue. This technique allows removal of torn menisci, loose bodies in the joint such as bone chips, and debridement (the excision of devitalized articular cartilaginous material in advanced cases of arthritis). Ligament repair or replacement may also be performed using an arthroscope.

Normal lateral meniscus

Trimming torn lateral meniscus

C. Femoral condyle (F), Tibial plateau (T), Lateral meniscus (LM)

Vastus medialis

Adductor magnus

Medial superior genicular artery

Gastrocnemius

Semimembranosus

Tibial collateral ligament

Coronary ligament (part of ligament removed)

Medial meniscus

Medial inferior genicular artery

Gracilis

Semitendinosus } **Pes anserinus**

Sartorius

Popliteus fascia

A. Medial View

Adductor magnus

Gastrocnemius

Tibial collateral ligament

Tibial collateral ligament

Semimembranosus

Patellar ligament

Pes anserinus { Sartorius

Gracilis

Semitendinosus

Tibial collateral ligament

B. Medial View

5.52 MEDIAL ASPECT OF KNEE

A. Dissection. The bandlike part of the tibial collateral ligament attaches to the medial epicondyle of the femur, bridges superficial to the insertion of the semimembranosus muscle, and crosses the medial inferior genicular artery. Distally, the ligament is crossed by the three tendons forming the pes anserinus (sartorius, gracilis, and semitendinosus). **B.** Bones, showing muscle and ligament attachment sites.

Lateral intermuscular septum

Vastus lateralis

Lateral superior genicular artery

Iliotibial tract

Gastrocnemius, lateral head

Fibular collateral ligament

Popliteus tendon

Lateral meniscus

Lateral inferior genicular artery

Common fibular (peroneal) nerve

Biceps femoris tendon

A. Lateral View

Gastrocnemius

Fibular collateral ligament

Popliteus

Biceps femoris

Fibular collateral ligament

Iliotibial tract [attaches to anterolateral (Gerdy) tubercle]

Patellar ligament

B. Lateral View

5.53   LATERAL ASPECT OF KNEE

A. Dissection. **B.** Bones, showing muscle and ligament attachments. Three structures arise from the lateral epicondyle and are uncovered by reflecting the biceps muscle: the gastrocnemius muscle is posterosuperior; the popliteus muscle is antero-inferior; and the fibular collateral ligament is in between, crossing superficial to the popliteus muscle. The lateral inferior genicular artery courses along the lateral meniscus.

A. Medial View

B. Lateral View

5.54   ARTICULARIS GENU AND BURSAE OF KNEE REGION

A. Articularis genu (articular muscle of the knee). This muscle lies deep to the vastus intermedius muscle and consists of fibers arising from the anterior surface of the femur proximally and attaching into the synovial membrane distally. The articularis genu pulls the synovial membrane of the suprapatellar bursa (*dotted line*) superiorly during extension of the knee so that it will not be caught between the patella and femur within the knee joint. **B.** Lateral aspect of knee. Latex was injected into the articular cavity and fixed with acetic acid. The distended synovial membrane was exposed and cleaned. The gastrocnemius muscle was reflected proximally, and the biceps femoris muscle and the iliotibial tract were reflected distally. The extent of the synovial capsule: superiorly, it rises superior to the patella, where it rests on a layer of fat that allows it to glide freely with movements of the joint; this superior

part is called the suprapatellar bursa; posteriorly, it rises as high as the origin of the gastrocnemius muscle; laterally, it curves inferior to the lateral femoral epicondyle, where the popliteus tendon and fibular collateral ligament are attached; and inferiorly, it bulges inferior to the lateral meniscus, overlapping the tibia (the coronary ligament is removed to show this). **Prepatellar bursitis** (housemaid's knee) is usually a friction bursitis caused by friction between the skin and the patella. The suprapatellar bursa communicates with the articular cavity of the knee joint; consequently, abrasions or penetrating wounds superior to the patella may result in **suprapatellar bursitis** caused by bacteria entering the bursa from the torn skin. The infection may spread to the knee joint. **C.** Posterior aspect of knee.

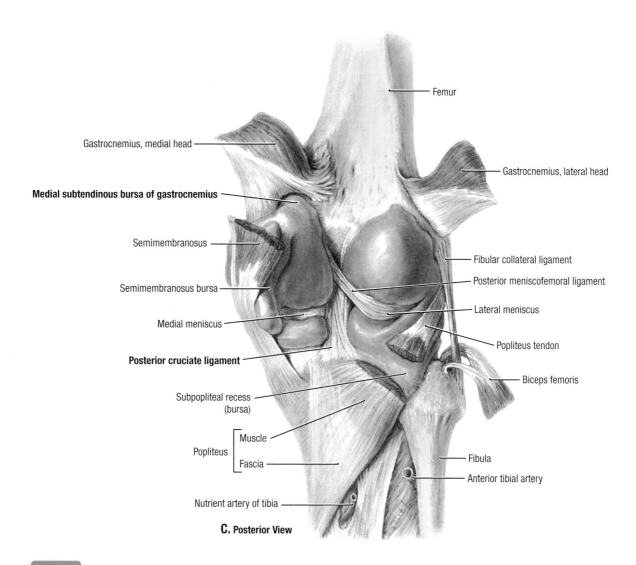

Femur

Gastrocnemius, medial head

Medial subtendinous bursa of gastrocnemius

Semimembranosus

Semimembranosus bursa

Medial meniscus

Posterior cruciate ligament

Subpopliteal recess (bursa)

Popliteus — Muscle

Popliteus — Fascia

Nutrient artery of tibia

Gastrocnemius, lateral head

Fibular collateral ligament

Posterior meniscofemoral ligament

Lateral meniscus

Popliteus tendon

Biceps femoris

Fibula

Anterior tibial artery

C. Posterior View

5.54   ARTICULARIS GENU AND BURSAE OF KNEE REGION (*CONTINUED*), DISTENDED KNEE JOINT

TABLE 5.11 BURSAE AROUND KNEE

Bursa	Location	Structural Features or Functions
Suprapatellar	Located between femur and tendon of quadriceps femoris	Held in position by articular muscle of knee; communicates freely with synovial cavity of knee joint
Popliteus	Located between tendon of popliteus and lateral condyle of tibia	Opens into synovial cavity of knee joint, inferior to lateral meniscus
Anserine	Separates tendons of sartorius, gracilis, and semitendinosus from tibia and tibial collateral ligament	Area where tendons of these muscles attach to tibia (pes anserinus) resembles the foot of a goose (L. *pes*, foot; L. *anser,* goose)
Medial subtendinous bursa of gastrocnemius	Lies deep to proximal attachment of tendon of medial head of gastrocnemius	Extension of synovial cavity of knee joint
Semimembranosus	Located between medial head of gastrocnemius and semimembranosus tendon	Related to the distal attachment of semimembranosus
Subcutaneous prepatellar	Lies between skin and anterior surface of patella	Allows free movement of skin over patella during movements of leg
Subcutaneous infrapatellar	Located between skin and tibial tuberosity	Helps knee to withstand pressure when kneeling
Deep infrapatellar	Lies between patellar ligament and anterior surface of tibia	Separated from knee joint by infrapatellar fat pad

Descending branch of lateral circumflex femoral artery

Popliteal artery

Superior lateral genicular artery

Inferior lateral genicular artery

Anterior tibial recurrent artery

Anterior tibial artery

Femoral artery

Descending genicular artery

Saphenous branch

Superior medial genicular artery

Middle genicular artery

Inferior medial genicular artery

Posterior tibial artery

A. Anterior View

Adductor magnus

Superior medial genicular artery

Semimembranosus

Inferior medial genicular artery

Posterior tibial artery

Popliteal artery

Superior lateral genicular artery

Branches of middle genicular artery

Inferior lateral genicular artery

Popliteus

Anterior tibial artery

Soleus

Nancy Joy

B. Posterior View

5.55   ANASTOMOSES AROUND KNEE

A. Genicular anastomosis on the anterior aspect of the knee. **B.** Popliteal artery in popliteal fossa.

- The popliteal artery runs from the adductor hiatus (in the adductor magnus muscle) proximally to the inferior border of the popliteus muscle distally, where it bifurcates into the anterior and posterior tibial arteries.
- The three anterior relations of the popliteal artery include the femur (fat intervening), the joint capsule of the knee; and the popliteus muscle.
- Five genicular branches of the popliteal artery supply the capsule and ligaments of the knee joint. The genicular arteries are the superior lateral, superior medial, middle, inferior lateral, and inferior medial genicular arteries.

Adductor magnus

Vastus medialis

Descending genicular artery
(from femoral artery)

**Superior medial
genicular artery**

Tibial collateral ligament

Synovial membrane

Medial meniscus

Coronary ligament

Patellar ligament

**Inferior medial
genicular artery**

Tibial collateral ligament
superficial part

C. Anteromedial View

Synovial membrane

**Superior lateral
genicular artery**

Biceps femoris

Patella

Fibular collateral
ligament

**Inferior lateral
genicular artery**

Lateral meniscus

Coronary ligament

**Anterior tibial
recurrent artery**

D. Anterolateral View

5.55 ANASTOMOSES AROUND KNEE (*CONTINUED*)

C. Medial aspect of the knee showing superior and inferior medial genicular arteries. **D.** Lateral aspect of the knee showing superior and inferior lateral genicular arteries.

The genicular arteries participate in the formation of the periarticular genicular anastomosis, a network of vessels surrounding the knee that provides collateral circulation capable of maintaining blood supply to the leg during full knee flexion, which may kink the popliteal artery. Other contributors to this important anastomosis are the descending genicular artery, a branch of the femoral artery, superomedially; descending branch of the lateral circumflex femoral artery, superolaterally; and anterior tibial recurrent artery, a branch of the anterior tibial artery, inferolaterally.

A. Anteroposterior View

B. Skyline View (Knee in Flexion)

C. Transverse MRI

5.56 IMAGING OF THE KNEE AND PATELLOFEMORAL ARTICULATION

A. Anteroposterior radiograph of knee. **B.** Radiograph of patella (knee joint flexed). *FE,* femur; *FP,* fat pad; *P,* patella; *PJ,* patellofemoral joint. **C.** Transverse MRI showing the patellofemoral joint.

Pain deep to the patella often results from excessive running; hence, this type of pain is often called "runner's knee." The pain results from repetitive microtrauma caused by abnormal tracking of the patella relative to the patellar surface of the femur, a condition known as the **patellofemoral syndrome**. This syndrome may also result from a direct blow to the patella and from osteoarthritis of the patellofemoral compartment (degenerative wear and tear of articular cartilages). In some cases, strengthening of the vastus medialis corrects patellofemoral dysfunction. This muscle tends to prevent lateral dislocation of the patella resulting from the Q-angle because the vastus medialis attaches to and pulls on the medial border of the patella. Hence, weakness of the vastus medialis predisposes the individual to patellofemoral dysfunction and patellar dislocation.

Femur

Posterior cruciate ligament *(7)*

Anterior cruciate ligament *(6)*

Lateral meniscus *(1)*

Tibial collateral ligament *(5)*

Fibular collateral ligament *(2)*

Medial meniscus *(4)*

Proximal tibiofibular joint

Tibia

Head of fibula *(3)*

Anserine bursa

A. Coronal Section

Lateral View

B. Coronal MRI

C. Coronal MRI

5.57   CORONAL SECTION AND MRIs OF KNEE

A. Section through intercondylar notch of femur, tibia, and fibula. **B.** MRI through intercondylar notch of femur and tibia. **C.** MRI through femoral condyles tibia and fibula. *Numbers* in MRIs refer to structures in **A.** *VM*, vastus medialis; *EL*, epiphyseal line; *IT*, iliotibial tract; *FC*, femoral condyle; *BF*, biceps femoris; *ST*, semitendinosus; *LG*, lateral head of gastrocnemius; *MG*, medial head of gastrocnemius; *PV*, popliteal vein; *PA*, popliteal artery; *F*, fat in popliteal fossa; *MF*, meniscofemoral ligament.

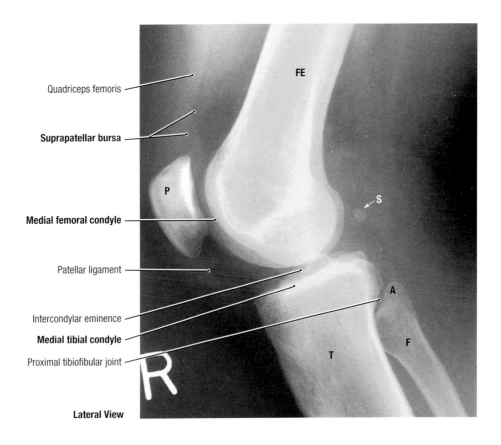

Quadriceps femoris

Suprapatellar bursa

Medial femoral condyle

Patellar ligament

Intercondylar eminence

Medial tibial condyle

Proximal tibiofibular joint

Lateral View

5.58   RADIOGRAPH OF KNEE

Lateral radiograph of flexed knee. *FE*, femur; *T*, tibia; *F*, fibula; *A*, apex of fibula; *S*, fabella; *P*, patella. The fabella is an inconsistent sesamoid bone in the lateral head of gastrocnemius muscle.

A. Sagittal MRI

5.59   SAGITTAL SECTION AND MRIs OF KNEE

A. MRI through medial aspect of intercondylar notch of femur showing cruciate ligaments. **B.** Illustration of section through lateral aspect of intercondylar notch of femur. **C.** MRI through medial femoral and tibial condyles. *Numbers* in MRIs refer to structures in **A.** *SM*, semimembranosus; *ST*, semitendinosus; *MG*, medial head of gastrocnemius; *VM*, vastus medialis; *PF*, prefemoral fat; *SF*, suprapatellar fat; *AM*, anterior horn of medial meniscus; *PM*, posterior horn of medial meniscus; *PV*, popliteal vessels.

Biceps femoris

Quadriceps tendon (1)

Suprapatellar bursa (3)

Patella (2)

Subcutaneous prepatellar bursa

Cavity of knee joint

Infrapatellar fat pad (4)

Patellar ligament (5)

Deep infrapatellar bursa

Tibial tuberosity (6)

Subcutaneous infrapatellar bursa

Fat in popliteal fossa (11)

Femur(F)

Fibrous layer of capsule of knee joint (10)

Synovial membrane

Posterior cruciate ligament (9)

Anterior cruciate ligament (8)

Tibia (T)

Lateral head of gastrocnemius

Popliteus (7)

B. Sagittal Section

Anterior View

C. Sagittal MRI

VM

SM

F

ST

10 — AM

PM — 10

T

MG

SAGITTAL SECTION AND MRIs OF KNEE (*CONTINUED*)

A. Anterior View

B. Anterior View

5.60 ANTERIOR LEG—SUPERFICIAL MUSCLES

A. Surface anatomy (*numbers* refer to structures labeled in **B**). **B.** Dissection. The muscles of the anterior compartment are ankle dorsiflexors/toe extensors. They are active in walking as they concentrically contract to raise the forefoot to clear the ground during the swing phase of the gait cycle and eccentrically contract to lower the forefoot to the ground after the heel strike of the stance phase.

Shin splints, edema, and pain in the area of the distal third of the tibia, result from repetitive microtrauma of the anterior compartment muscles, especially the tibialis anterior. This produces a mild form of **anterior compartment syndrome**. The pain commonly occurs during traumatic injury or athletic overexertion of the muscles. Edema and muscle-tendon inflammation causes swelling that reduces blood flow to the muscles. The swollen ischemic muscles are painful and tender to pressure.

Key for A
- Proximal muscular attachment
- Distal muscular attachment
- Ligamentous attachment

A. Attachments. **B.** Features of bones.

5.61 FEATURES OF BONES AND MUSCLE ATTACHMENTS: ANTERIOR LEG AND DORSUM OF FOOT

TABLE 5.12 MUSCLES OF ANTERIOR COMPARTMENT OF LEG

Muscle	Proximal Attachment	Distal Attachment	Innervation[a]	Main Actions
Tibialis anterior	Lateral condyle and superior half of lateral surface of tibia	Medial and inferior surfaces of medial cuneiform and base of first metatarsal	Deep fibular (peroneal) nerve (L4–L5)	Dorsiflexes ankle joint and inverts foot
Extensor hallucis longus	Middle part of anterior surface of fibula and interosseous membrane	Dorsal aspect of base of distal phalanx of great toe (hallux)		Extends great toe and dorsiflexes ankle joint
Extensor digitorum longus	Lateral condyle of tibia and superior three fourths of anterior surface of interosseous membrane	Middle and distal phalanges of lateral four digits	Deep fibular (peroneal) nerve (L5–S1)	Extends lateral four digits and dorsiflexes ankle joint
Fibularis (peroneus)	Inferior third of anterior surface of fibula and interosseus membrane	Dorsum of base of fifth metatarsal		Dorsiflexes ankle joint and aids tertius in eversion of foot

[a]See Table 5.1 for explanation of segmental innervation.

A. Anterior View

B. Anterolateral View

5.62 ANTERIOR LEG—DEEP MUSCLES, NERVES, AND VESSELS

TABLE 5.13 COMMON, SUPERFICIAL, AND DEEP FIBULAR (PERONEAL) NERVES

Nerve	Origin	Course	Distribution/Structure(S) Supplied
Common fibular	Sciatic nerve	Forms as sciatic nerve bifurcates at the apex of popliteal fossa and follows medial border of biceps femoris; winds around neck of fibula, dividing into superficial and deep fibular nerves	Skin on lateral part of posterior aspect of leg via the lateral sural cutaneous nerve; lateral aspect of knee joint via its articular branch
Superficial fibular	Common fibular nerve	Arises deep to fibularis longus and descends in lateral compartment of leg; pierces crural fascia at distal third of leg to become cutaneous	Fibularis longus and brevis and skin on distal third of anterolateral surface of leg and dorsum of foot
Deep fibular	Common fibular nerve	Arises deep to fibularis longus; passes through extensor digitorum longus, descends on interosseous membrane, and continues on dorsum of foot	Anterior muscles of leg, dorsum of foot, and skin of first interdigital cleft; dorsal aspect of joints crossed via articular branches

C. Anterolateral View

Iliotibial tract

Head of fibula

Common fibular (peroneal) nerve

Fibularis (peroneus) longus

Superficial fibular (peroneal) nerve

Fibularis (peroneus) brevis

Patellar ligament

Anterior tibial recurrent nerve and artery

Tuberosity of tibia

Anterior border of tibia

Lateral surface of tibia

Interosseous membrane

Anterior (extensor) surface of fibula

Deep fibular (peroneal) nerve

Anterior tibial artery

Perforating branch of fibular (peroneal) artery

Fibularis (peroneus) longus

Anterior lateral malleolar artery

Inferior fibular (peroneal) retinaculum

Extensor digitorum brevis

Fibularis (peroneus) brevis

Perforating branches of metatarsal arteries

Dorsal metatarsal arteries

Dorsal digital arteries

Superior extensor retinaculum

Lateral branch of deep fibular nerve to joints and extensor digitorum brevis

Anterior medial malleolar artery

Medial branch of deep fibular nerve to joints and 1st and 2nd digits

Lateral tarsal artery

Dorsalis pedis artery (dorsal artery of foot)

Arcuate artery

D. Lateral View

Common fibular (peroneal) nerve

Fibularis (peroneus) longus

Superficial fibular (peroneal) nerve

Apex of head

Biceps femoris

Fibular collateral ligament

Head of fibula

Neck of fibula

Deep fibular (peroneal) nerve

Superficial fibular (peroneal) nerve

E. Anterior View

Lateral condyle

Tibiofibular joint and anterior ligament of fibular head

Head of fibula

Anterior tibial artery

Interosseous membrane

Perforating branch of fibular artery

Tibiofibular syndesmosis and anterior tibiofibular ligament

Inferior transverse ligament (part of posterior tibio-fibular ligament)

Lateral malleolus

Tuberosity of tibia

5.62   ANTERIOR LEG—DEEP MUSCLES, NERVES, AND VESSELS (*CONTINUED*)

A. Overview of motor innervation. **B.** Deep dissection of the anterior compartment of the leg. The muscles are separated to display the anterior tibial artery and deep fibular nerve. **C.** Neurovascular structures. **D.** Relations of common fibular nerve and branches to the proximal fibula. **E.** Interosseous membrane.

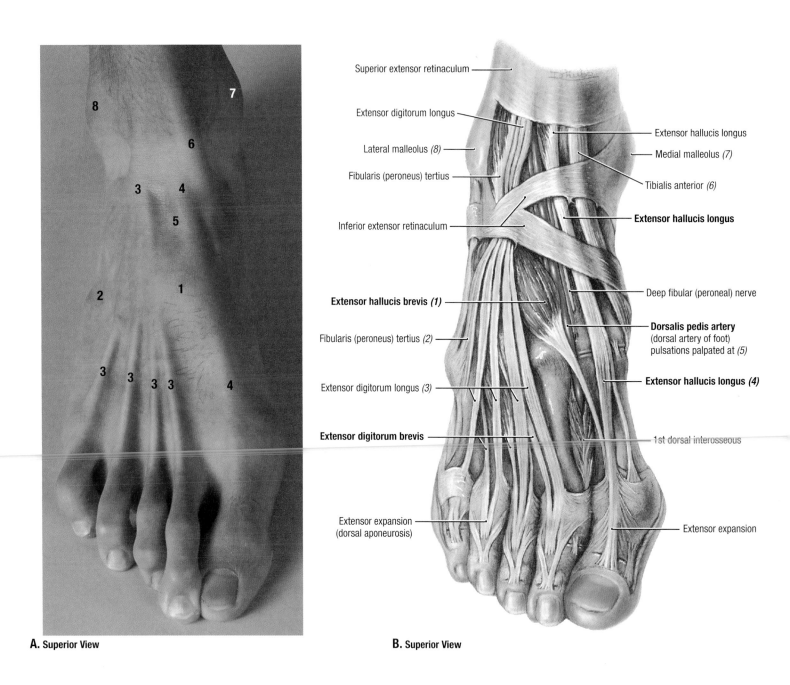

A. Superior View

B. Superior View

5.63 DORSUM OF FOOT

A. Surface anatomy (*numbers* refer to structures labeled in **B**). **B.** Dissection. The dorsal vein of foot and deep fibular nerve are cut.

At the ankle, the dorsalis pedis artery (dorsal artery of foot) and deep fibular nerve lie midway between the malleoli. On the dorsum of the foot, the dorsal artery of foot is crossed by the extensor hallucis brevis muscle and disappears between the two heads of the first dorsal interosseous muscle.

Clinically, knowing the location of the belly of the extensor digitorum brevis is important for distinguishing this muscle from abnormal edema. Contusion and tearing of the muscle fibers and associated blood vessels

result in a **hematoma in extensor digitorum brevis**, producing edema anteromedial to the lateral malleolus. Most people who have not seen this inflamed muscle assume they have a severely sprained ankle.

The **dorsalis pedis pulse** may be palpated with the feet slightly dorsiflexed. The pulse is usually easy to palpate because the dorsal arteries of the foot are subcutaneous and pass along a line from the extensor retinaculum to a point just lateral to the extensor hallucis longus tendon. A diminished or absent dorsalis pedis pulse usually suggests vascular insufficiency resulting from arterial disease.

A. Superior View

B. Superior View

| 5.64 | ATTACHMENTS OF MUSCLES AND ARTERIES OF DORSUM OF FOOT |

A. Attachments. **B.** Arterial supply.

TABLE 5.14 ARTERIAL SUPPLY TO DORSUM OF FOOT

Artery	Origin	Course	Distribution
Dorsalis pedis (dorsal artery of foot)	Continuation of anterior tibial artery distal to talocrural joint	Descends anteromedially to 1st interosseous space and divides into deep plantar and arcuate arteries	Dorsal surface of foot
Lateral tarsal artery	From dorsalis pedis artery (dorsal artery of foot)	Runs an arched course laterally beneath extensor digitorum brevis to anastomose with branches of arcuate artery	
Arcuate artery		Runs laterally from 1st interosseous space across bases of lateral four metatarsals, deep to extensor tendons	
Deep plantar artery		Passes to sole of foot and joins plantar arch	Sole of foot
Metatarsal arteries 1st	From deep plantar artery	Run between metatarsals to clefts of toes where each vessel divides into two dorsal digital arteries.	Dorsal surface of foot
2nd to 4th	From arcuate artery	Perforating arteries connect to plantar arch and plantar metatarsal arteries.	
Dorsal digital arteries	From metatarsal arteries	Pass to sides of adjoining digits	Digits

Iliotibial tract

Biceps femoris tendon

Common fibular (peroneal) nerve

Gastrocnemius lateral head

Fibularis (peroneus) longus

Soleus

Tibialis anterior

Superficial fibular (peroneal) nerve

Fibularis (peroneus) longus

Calcaneal tendon

Fibularis (peroneus) longus

Fibularis (peroneus) brevis

Fibularis (peroneus) tertius

Patellar retinaculum

Patella

Fibular collateral ligament

Deep (crural) fascia of leg

Extensor digitorum longus

Extensor hallucis longus

Fibularis (peroneus) tertius

Extensor digitorum brevis

Extensor hallucis brevis

Extensor digitorum longus

A. Anterolateral View

B. Anterolateral View

5.65 MUSCLES OF LATERAL LEG AND FOOT

A. Surface anatomy. **B.** Dissection.

- The two fibular (peroneal) muscles both attach to two thirds of the fibula, the fibularis (peroneus) longus muscle to the proximal two thirds, and the fibularis (peroneus) brevis muscle to the distal two thirds. Where they overlap, the fibularis brevis muscle lies anteriorly.
- The fibularis (peroneus) longus muscle enters the foot by hooking around the cuboid and traveling medially to the base of the first metatarsal and medial cuneiform.

- **Common fibular (peroneal) nerve lesion.** The nerve lies in contact with the neck of the fibula deep to the fibularis longus muscle, where it is vulnerable to injury (**B,** *red circle*). This injury may have serious implications because the nerve supplies the extensor and everter muscle groups, with loss of function resulting in foot-drop (inability to dorsiflex the ankle) and difficulty in everting the foot.

C. Lateral View

D. Lateral View

E. Lateral View

5.65 MUSCLES OF LATERAL LEG AND FOOT (*CONTINUED*)

C. Fibularis (peroneus) longus. **D.** Fibularis (peroneus) brevis. **E.** Attachments sites on fibula.

TABLE 5.15 *MUSCLES OF LATERAL COMPARTMENT OF LEG*

Muscle	Proximal Attachment	Distal Attachment	Innervation[a]	Main Actions
Fibularis (peroneus) longus	Head and superior two thirds of lateral surface of fibula	Base of first metatarsal and medial cuneiform	Superficial fibular (peroneal) nerve (L5, S1, and S2)	Evert foot and weakly plantar flex ankle joint
Fibularis (peroneus) brevis	Inferior two thirds of lateral surface of fibula	Dorsal surface of tuberosity on lateral side of base of fifth metatarsal		

[a]See Table 5.1 for explanation of segmental innervation

A. Lateral View

Small saphenous vein

Sural nerve

Calcaneal tendon (1)

Anterior inferior tibiofibular ligament

Anterior talofibular ligament*

Talus

Inferior extensor retinaculum

*Components of lateral
ligament of ankle*

Lateral malleolus (6)

Extensor digitorum longus (2)

Extensor digitorum brevis (3)

Fibularis (peroneus) tertius

**Superior fibular (peroneal)
retinaculum**

*Calcaneofibular ligament

Calcaneus

Subtalar joint

Abductor digiti minimi

Tuberosity of 5th metatarsal

**Inferior fibular
(peroneal) retinaculum**

Fibularis (peroneus) brevis (4)

Calcaneocuboid joint

B. Lateral View

Fibularis (peroneus) longus (5)

5.66 SYNOVIAL SHEATHS AND TENDONS AT ANKLE

A. Surface anatomy (*numbers* refer to structures labeled in **B**). **B.** Tendons at the lateral aspect of the ankle.

Fibularis (peroneus) longus

Fibularis (peroneus) brevis

Tendon of ⎡ Fibularis longus
          ⎣ Fibularis brevis

D. Anterolateral View

Tibialis anterior

Inferior extensor retinaculum

Extensor digitorum longus and fibularis (peroneus) tertius

Dorsalis pedis artery

Extensor hallucis longus

Deep fibular nerve

Extensor hallucis brevis

Extensor digitorum brevis

Fibularis (peroneus) tertius

Fibularis (peroneus) brevis

Fibularis (peroneus) longus

C. Anterolateral View

of talus
Body   Neck   Head
Navicular
Middle ⎤ Cuneiforms
Lateral ⎦

Metatarsals

Lateral tubercle

Phalanges

Cuboid

Groove for fibularis (peroneus) longus

Base

Tuberosity of 5th metatarsal

Tubercle

Head

E. Lateral View   Calcaneus   **Fibular (peroneal) trochlea**

5.66   **SYNOVIAL SHEATHS AND TENDONS AT ANKLE (*CONTINUED*)**

C. Synovial sheaths of tendons on the anterolateral aspect of the ankle. The tendons of the fibularis (peroneus) longus and fibularis (peroneus) brevis muscles are enclosed in a common synovial sheath posterior to the lateral malleolus. This sheath splits into two, one for each tendon, posterior to the fibular (peroneal) trochlea. **D.** Schematic illustration of fibularis longus and brevis. **E.** Lateral aspect of bones of foot.

A   **B**   **C**   **D**

5.67   MUSCLES OF POSTERIOR LEG

A. and B. Muscles of superficial compartment. **C. and D.** Muscles of deep compartment.

TABLE 5.16 MUSCLES OF POSTERIOR COMPARTMENT OF LEG

Muscle	Proximal Attachment	Distal Attachment	Innervation[a]	Main Actions
Superficial muscles				
Gastrocnemius	*Lateral head:* lateral aspect of lateral condyle of femur			Plantar flexes ankle joint when knee joint is extended; raises heel during walking, and flexes knee joint
	Medial head: popliteal surface of femur, superior to medial condyle	Posterior surface of calcaneus via calcaneal tendon (tendocalcaneus)	Tibial nerve (S1 and S2)	
Soleus	Posterior aspect of head of fibula, superior fourth of posterior surface of fibula, soleal line and medial border of tibia			Plantar flexes ankle joint (independent of knee position) and steadies leg on foot
Plantaris	Inferior end of lateral supracondylar line of femur and oblique popliteal ligament			Weakly assists gastrocnemius in plantar flexing ankle joint and flexing knee joint
Deep muscles				
Popliteus	Lateral surface of lateral condyle of femur and lateral meniscus	Posterior surface of tibia, superior to soleal line		Unlocks fully extended knee joint (laterally rotates femur 5 degrees on planted tibia); weakly flexes knee joint
Flexor hallucis longus	Inferior two thirds of posterior surface of fibula and inferior part of interosseous membrane	Base of distal phalanx of great toe (hallux)	Tibial nerve (**L4**, L5, and S1)	Flexes great toe at all joints and plantar flexes ankle joint; supports medial longitudinal arch of foot
Flexor digitorum longus	Medial part of posterior surface of tibia inferior to soleal line, and by a broad tendon to fibula	Bases of distal phalanges of lateral four digits	Tibial nerve (**S2** and S3)	Flexes lateral four digits and plantar flexes ankle joint; supports longitudinal arches of foot
Tibialis posterior	Interosseous membrane, posterior surface of tibia inferior to soleal line and posterior surface of fibula	Tuberosity of navicular, cuneiform, and cuboid and bases of metatarsals 2–4	Tibial nerve (L4 and L5)	Plantar flexes ankle joint and inverts foot

[a]See Table 5.1 for explanation of segmental innervation.

Gastrocnemius, medial head

Plantaris

Gastrocnemius, lateral head

Semimembranosus

Popliteus

Soleus

Tibialis posterior

Flexor digitorum longus

Flexor hallucis longus

Fibularis (peroneus) brevis

For bursa of calcaneal tendon

Calcaneal tendon

A. Posterior View

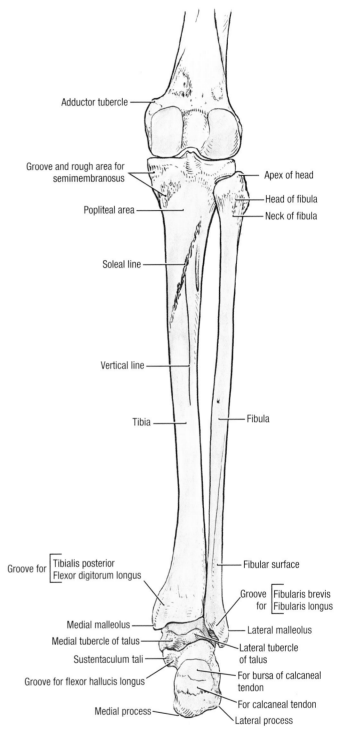

Adductor tubercle

Groove and rough area for semimembranosus

Apex of head

Head of fibula

Neck of fibula

Popliteal area

Soleal line

Vertical line

Tibia

Fibula

Groove for Tibialis posterior / Flexor digitorum longus

Fibular surface

Groove for Fibularis brevis / Fibularis longus

Medial malleolus

Lateral malleolus

Medial tubercle of talus

Lateral tubercle of talus

Sustentaculum tali

For bursa of calcaneal tendon

Groove for flexor hallucis longus

For calcaneal tendon

Medial process

Lateral process

B. Posterior View

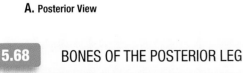

5.68 BONES OF THE POSTERIOR LEG

A. Muscle attachments. **B.** Features of bones.

Tibial fractures. The tibial shaft is narrowest at the junction of its middle and inferior thirds, which is the most frequent site of fracture. Unfortunately, this area of the bone also has the poorest blood supply.

Fibular fractures. These commonly occur 2 to 6 cm proximal to the distal end of the lateral malleolus and are often associated with fracture/

dislocations of the ankle joint, which are combined with tibial fractures. When a person slips and the foot is forced into an excessively inverted position, the ankle ligaments tear, forcibly tilting the talus against the lateral malleolus and shearing it off.

A. Posterior View

B. Posterior View

Semitendinosus

Semimembranosus *(1)*

Gracilis

Sartorius

Gastrocnemius, medial head *(2)*

Flexor digitorum longus

Tibialis posterior

Flexor retinaculum

Biceps femoris *(8)*

Tibial nerve

Common fibular (peroneal) nerve

Medial sural cutaneous nerve

Gastrocnemius, lateral head *(7)*

Soleus *(6)*

Fibularis (peroneus) longus *(4)*

Fibularis (peroneus) brevis *(5)*

Calcaneal tendon *(3)*

Superior fibular (peroneal) retinaculum

5.69 POSTERIOR LEG, SUPERFICIAL MUSCLES OF POSTERIOR COMPARTMENT

A. Surface anatomy (*numbers* refer to structures labeled in **B**). **B.** Dissection. **Gastrocnemius strain** (tennis leg) is a painful calf injury resulting from partial tearing of the medial belly of the muscle at or near its musculotendinous junction. It is caused by overstretching the muscle during simultaneous full extension of the knee joint and dorsiflexion of the ankle joint.

Semitendinosus

Semimembranosus

Gastrocnemius medial head

Medial inferior genicular vessels

Gastrocnemius

Flexor digitorum longus

Tibialis posterior

Biceps femoris

Popliteal vein

Tibial nerve

Gastrocnemius, lateral head

Common fibular (peroneal) nerve

Soleus

Fibularis (peroneus) longus

Fibularis (peroneus) brevis

Flexor hallucis longus

Calcaneal tendon

C. Posterior View

Gastrocnemius, medial head

Gastrocnemius, lateral head

Semimembranosus

Popliteus

Soleus

Tibialis posterior

Flexor digitorum longus

Flexor hallucis longus

Fibularis (peroneus) brevis

For bursa of calcaneal tendon

Calcaneal tendon

D. Posterior View

5.69   **POSTERIOR LEG, SUPERFICIAL MUSCLES OF POSTERIOR COMPARTMENT** (*CONTINUED*)

C. Dissection revealing soleus. **D.** Bones of leg showing muscle attachments. Inflammation of the calcaneal tendon due to microscopic tears of collagen fibers in the tendon, particularly just superior to its attachment to the calcaneus, results in **calcaneal tendinitis**, which causes pain during walking. **Calcaneal tendon rupture** is probably the most severe acute muscular problem of the leg. Following complete rupture of the tendon, passive dorsiflexion is excessive, and the person cannot plantar flex against resistance.

A. Posterior View

B. Posterior View

Semimembranosus

Tibial nerve

Popliteus

Common fibular (peroneal) nerve

Popliteus fascia

Soleus

Fibula

Tibialis posterior

Fibular (peroneal) artery

Extensor digitorum longus

Posterior tibial artery

Tibial nerve

Flexor hallucis longus

Deep (crural) fascia of leg

Transverse intermuscular septum

Flexor retinaculum

Tibialis posterior

Flexor digitorum longus

Calcaneal tendon

Soleus

Tibialis posterior

Flexor digitorum longus

Flexor hallucis longus

Medial malleolus

Grooves for tendon of flexor hallucis longus

For bursa of calcaneal tendon

Calcaneal tendon

5.70 POSTERIOR LEG, DEEP MUSCLES OF POSTERIOR COMPARTMENT

A. Superficial dissection. The calcaneal (Achilles) tendon is cut, the gastrocnemius muscle is removed, and only a horseshoe-shaped proximal part of the soleus muscle remains in place. **B.** Bones of leg showing muscle attachments. **Calcaneal bursitis** results from inflammation of the bursa of the calcaneal tendon located between the calcaneal tendon and the superior part of the posterior surface of the calcaneus. Calcaneal bursitis causes pain posterior to the heel and occurs commonly during long-distance running, basketball, and tennis. It is caused by excessive friction on the bursa as the calcaneal tendon continuously slides over it.

Semimembranosus

Tibial collateral ligament

Pes anserinus:

Sartorius

Gracilis

Semitendinosus

Popliteus fascia

Soleus

Tibial nerve

Flexor digitorum longus

Tibialis posterior

Posterior tibial artery and veins

Flexor retinaculum

Popliteal artery

Popliteal vein

Biceps femoris

Common fibular (peroneal) nerve

Popliteus and nerve

Soleus

Anterior tibial artery and vein

Posterior intermuscular septum

Tibialis posterior and nerve

Fibular (peroneal) artery

Flexor hallucis longus

Transverse intermuscular septum

Calcaneal tendon

C. Posterior View

Calcaneal tendon

Flexor hallucis longus

Flexor digitorum longus

Calcaneus

Tibialis posterior

Flexor digitorum longus

Quadratus plantae

Flexor hallucis longus

D. Anteromedial View

Tibialis posterior

Flexor hallucis longus

Flexor digitorum longus

E. Plantar View

5.70   **POSTERIOR LEG, DEEP MUSCLES OF POSTERIOR COMPARTMENT (*CONTINUED*)**

C. Deeper dissection. The flexor hallucis longus and flexor digitorum longus are pulled apart, and the posterior tibial artery is partly excised. The tibialis posterior lies deep to the two long digital flexors. **D.** Crossing of muscles (tendons) of the deep compartment superoposterior to the medial malleolus and into the sole of the foot. **E.** Bones of foot showing muscle attachments.

Saphenous nerve

Great (long) saphenous vein *(1)*

Deep fascia of leg

Transverse intermuscular septum

Flexor hallucis longus

Posterior tibial artery

Tibial nerve

Flexor digitorum longus

Tibialis posterior *(2)*

Flexor retinaculum:

Superficial part

Deep part

Calcaneal tendon *(3)*

Abductor hallucis and nerve

Medial plantar artery and nerve

Lateral plantar nerve and artery *(4)*

Medial calcaneal branches

A. Medial View

Flexor digitorum longus

Medial malleolus

Medial (deltoid) ligament

Flexor hallucis longus

Tibialis posterior

Calcaneal tendon

Bursa of calcaneal tendon

Quadratus plantae

Osseofibrous tunnel

Sustentaculum tali

Medial tubercle of talus

Attachment of abductor hallucis

B. Medial View

C. Medial View

5.71   MEDIAL ANKLE REGION

A. Dissection. The calcaneal tendon and posterior part of the abductor hallucis were excised. **B.** Schematic illustration of the tendons passing posterior to medial malleolus. **C.** Surface anatomy (*numbers* refer to structures labeled in **A**).

- The posterior tibial artery and the tibial nerve lie between the flexor digitorum longus and flexor hallucis longus muscles and divide into medial and lateral plantar branches.

- The tibialis posterior and flexor digitorum longus tendons occupy separate osseofibrous tunnels posterior to the medial malleolus.

- The **posterior tibial pulse** can usually be palpated between the posterior surface of the medial malleolus and the medial border of the calcaneal tendon.

Soleus

Calcaneal tendon

Flexor hallucis longus

Flexor digitorum longus

Tibialis posterior

Medial malleolus

Tibialis anterior

Calcaneus

Fibularis (peroneus) longus

Fibularis (peroneus) brevis

Quadratus plantae

Flexor digitorum longus

Slip from flexor hallucis longus

Flexor hallucis longus

Lumbricals

Flexor digitorum longus

A. Posteromedial View

Flexor hallucis longus

Flexor digitorum longus

Tibialis posterior

Tibialis anterior

Medial malleolus

Medial (deltoid)
ligament of ankle

Calcaneal
tendon

Quadratus plantae

Tibialis posterior

Flexor digitorum longus

Flexor hallucis longus

1st metatarsal

Flexor hallucis brevis

Medial sesamoid bone

B. Medial View

5.72   MEDIAL ANKLE AND FOOT

A. Tendons of deep compartment of the leg traced to their distal attachments in the sole of the foot. **B.** Foot raised as in walking and sesamoid bones of the great toe. The sesamoid bones of the great toe are located on each side of a bony ridge on the 1st metatarsal.

- The sesamoid bones are a "footstool" for the first metatarsal, giving it increased height.
- By inserting into the flexor digitorum longus muscle, the quadratus plantae muscle modifies the oblique pull of the flexor tendons.
- The flexor hallucis longus muscle uses three pulleys: a groove on the posterior aspect of the distal end of the tibia, a groove on the posterior aspect of the talus, and a groove inferior to the sustentaculum tali.
- The flexor digitorum longus muscle crosses superficial to the tibialis posterior, superoposterior to the medial malleolus.

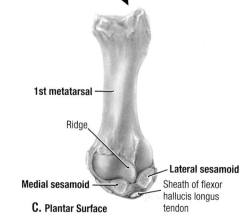

1st metatarsal

Ridge

Medial sesamoid

Lateral sesamoid

Sheath of flexor
hallucis longus
tendon

C. Plantar Surface

Femoral artery

Medial superior
genicular artery

Popliteal artery

Medial inferior
genicular artery

Posterior tibial
artery

Anterior tibial
artery

Fibular (peroneal)
artery

Posterior tibial
artery

Lateral plantar
artery

Medial plantar
artery

Dorsalis pedis
artery

Plantar
arch

A. **Medial View**

Anterior tibial artery

**Perforating branch
of fibular (peroneal) artery**

Dorsalis pedis artery
(dorsal artery of foot)

Calcaneal branch

B. **Lateral View**

Popliteal
artery

Anterior tibial
artery

**Fibular (peroneal)
artery**

Flexor hallucis
longus

Communicating
branch

Posterior tibial artery

C. **Posterior View**

Popliteal artery

Popliteus

**Anterior tibial
artery**

**Posterior tibial
artery**

D. **Posterior View**

5.73 POPLITEAL ARTERIOGRAM AND ARTERIAL ANOMALIES

A. Popliteal arteriogram. The femoral artery becomes the popliteal artery at the adductor
hiatus. The anterior tibial artery continues as the dorsalis pedis (dorsal artery of the foot).
The posterior tibial artery terminates as the medial and lateral plantar arteries; its major
branch is the fibular artery. **B. Anomalous dorsalis pedis artery**. The perforating
branch of the fibular artery rarely continues as the dorsalis pedis artery, but when
it does, the anterior tibial artery ends proximal to the ankle or is a slender vessel.
C. Absence of posterior tibial artery. Compensatory enlargement of the fibular
artery was found to occur in approximately 5% of limbs. **D. High division of popliteal artery**. Along with the anterior tibial artery descending anterior to the popliteus
muscle; this anomaly was found to occur in approximately 2% of limbs.

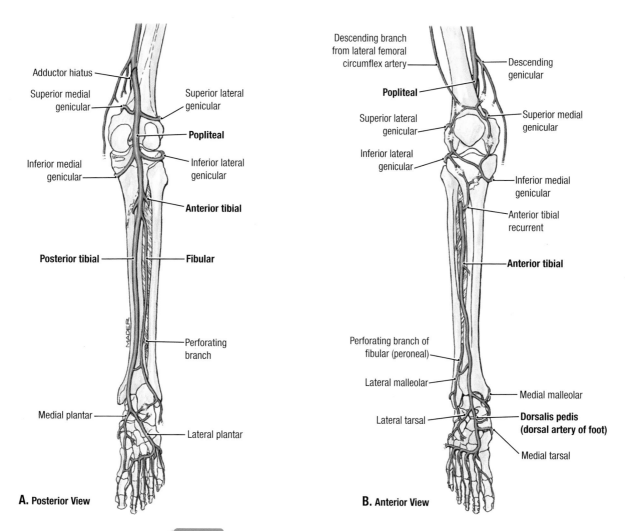

A. Posterior View

B. Anterior View

5.74   ARTERIAL SUPPLY OF LEG AND FOOT

TABLE 5.17 ARTERIAL SUPPLY OF LEG AND FOOT

Artery	Origin	Course	Distribution in Leg
Popliteal	Continuation of femoral artery at adductor hiatus	Passes through popliteal fossa to leg; divides into anterior and posterior tibial arteries at lower border of popliteus	Lateral and medial aspects of knee via genicular arteries
Anterior tibial	From popliteal	Passes between tibia and fibula into anterior compartment through gap superior to interosseous membrane; descends between tibialis anterior and extensor digitorum longus muscles	Anterior compartment
Dorsalis pedis (dorsal artery of foot)	Continuation of anterior tibial artery distal to talocrural joint	Descends to first interosseous space; pierces first dorsal interosseous muscle as deep plantar artery; joins deep plantar arch	Muscles on dorsum of foot
Posterior tibial	From popliteal	Passes through posterior compartment; divides into medial and lateral plantar arteries posterior to medial malleolus	Posterior and lateral compartments, nutrient artery passes to tibia
Fibular (peroneal)		Descends in posterior compartment adjacent to posterior intermuscular septum	Posterior compartment: perforating branches supply lateral compartment
Medial plantar	From posterior tibial	In foot between abductor hallucis and flexor digitorum brevis muscles	Supplies mainly muscles of great toe and skin on medial side of sole of foot
Lateral plantar		Runs anterolaterally deep to abductor hallucis and flexor digitorum brevis, and then arches medially to form deep plantar arch	Supplies lateral aspect of sole of foot

B. Transverse Section

- Articular cavity
- Tibia
- **Anterior ligament of head of fibula**
- **Posterior ligament of head of fibula**
- Synovial membrane
- Fibula

Articular facet for tibia

Articular facet for fibula

- Head of fibula
- **Posterior ligament of fibular head**
- Opening for anterior tibial vessels
- **Interosseous membrane**
- Tibia
- Fibula
- Opening for perforating branch of fibular artery
- **Posterior tibiofibular ligament**
- Inferior transverse ligament

A. Posterior View

- Anterior border
- Nutrient foramen
- Extensor surface for { Extensor digitorum longus / Fibularis (peroneus) tertius / Extensor hallucis longus }
- Extensor surface for tibialis anterior
- **Interosseous border**
- Surface for tibialis posterior
- Surface for tibialis posterior
- Medial crest
- Tibia
- **Interosseous border**
- Anterior border

Key for D
- ▨ Proximal muscular attachment
- ▨ Ligamentous attachment

- Surface for flexor hallucis longus
- **For interosseous tibiofibular ligament**
- Articular facets for { Tibia / Talus }
- Malleolar fossa for posterior talofibular ligament
- Fibular notch for interosseous tibiofibular ligament
- Articular facets for fibula
- Talus
- Calcaneus

Tibia
- Anterior tibiofibular ligament
- **Interosseous ligament**
- Posterior tibiofibular ligament
- Fibula

C. Transverse Section

D. Fibula, Medial View   **Lateral View**

5.75   TIBIOFIBULAR JOINT AND TIBIOFIBULAR SYNDESMOSIS

A. Overview. **B.** Tibiofibular joint. **C.** Tibiofibular syndesmosis. **D.** Tibia and fibula, disarticulated.

- The superior tibiofibular joint (proximal tibiofibular joint) is a plane type of synovial joint between the flat facet on the fibular head and a similar facet located posterolaterally on the lateral tibial condyle. The tense joint capsule surrounds the joint and attaches to the margins of the articular surfaces of the fibula and tibia.

- The tibiofibular syndesmosis is a fibrous joint. This articulation is essential for stability of the ankle joint because it keeps the lateral malleolus firmly against the lateral surface of the talus. The strong interosseous tibiofibular ligament is continuous superiorly with the interosseous membrane and forms the principal connection between the distal ends of the tibia and fibula.

A. Plantar View

Flexor digitorum longus

Flexor hallucis longus

Fibrous digital sheaths

Superficial transverse metatarsal ligament

Plantar digital nerves and arteries

Plantar aponeurosis

Plantar fascia

Plantar fascia

Cutaneous branches of lateral plantar vessels and nerves

Cutaneous branches of medial plantar nerve and artery

Medial calcaneal branches of tibial nerve and calcaneal branches of posterior tibial artery

Fat pad

B. Plantar View

Sesamoid bones of 1st metatarsal

Heads of 2nd to 5th metatarsals

Tuberosity of calcaneus

C. Plantar View

5.76   **SOLE OF FOOT, SUPERFICIAL**

A. Surface anatomy. **B.** Dissection. Plantar aponeurosis and fascia, with neurovascular structures. **C.** Weight-bearing areas.

- The weight of the body is transmitted to the talus from the tibia and fibula. It is then transmitted to the tuberosity of the calcaneus, the heads of the second to fifth metatarsals, and the sesamoid bones of the first digit.

Plantar fasciitis, strain and inflammation of the plantar aponeurosis, may result from running and high-impact aerobics, especially when inappropriate footwear is worn. It causes pain on the plantar surface of the heel and on the medial aspect of the foot. Point tenderness is located at the proximal attachment of the plantar aponeurosis to the medial tubercle of the calcaneus and on the medial surface of this bone. The pain increases with passive extension of the great toe and may be further exacerbated by dorsiflexion of the ankle and/or weight bearing.

Plantar Views

5.77   FIRST LAYER OF MUSCLES OF SOLE OF FOOT

A. Bones. **B.** Overview. **C.** Dissection. Muscles and neurovascular structures.

TABLE 5.18 MUSCLES IN SOLE OF FOOT—FIRST LAYER

Muscle	Proximal Attachment	Distal Attachment	Innervation	Actions[a]
Abductor hallucis	Medial process of tuberosity of calcaneus, flexor retinaculum, and plantar aponeurosis	Medial side of base of proximal phalanx of first digit	Medial plantar nerve (S2–S3)	Abducts and flexes first digit
Flexor digitorum brevis	Medial process of tuberosity of calcaneus, plantar aponeurosis, and intermuscular septa	Both sides of middle phalanges of lateral four digits		Flexes lateral four digits
Abductor digiti minimi	Medial and lateral processes of tuberosity of calcaneus, plantar aponeurosis, and intermuscular septa	Lateral side of base of proximal phalanx of fifth digit	Lateral plantar nerve (S2–S3)	Abducts and flexes fifth digit

[a]Although individual actions are described, the primary function of the intrinsic muscles of the foot is to act collectively to resist forces that stress (attempt to flatten) the arches of the foot.

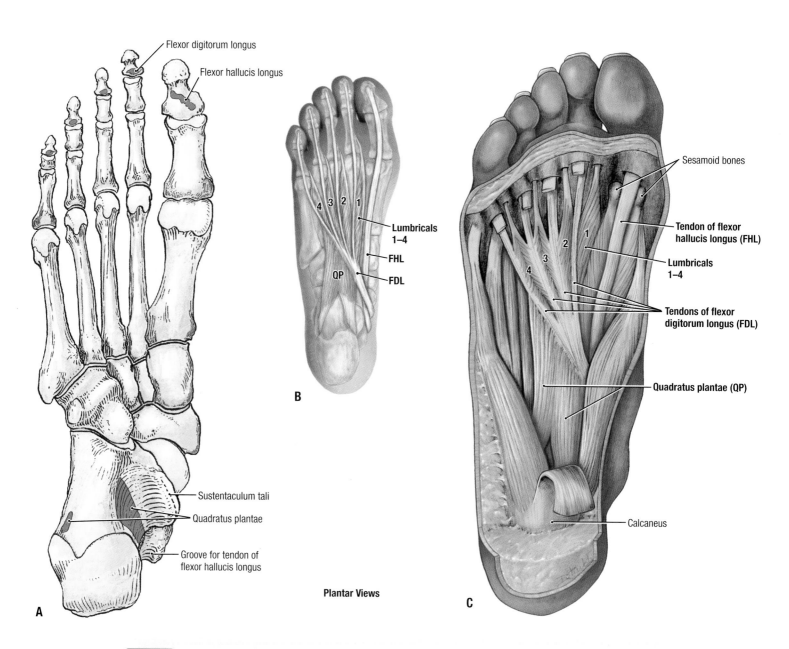

Flexor digitorum longus

Flexor hallucis longus

Lumbricals 1–4

FHL

QP

FDL

Sustentaculum tali

Quadratus plantae

Groove for tendon of flexor hallucis longus

A

B

Plantar Views

Sesamoid bones

Tendon of flexor hallucis longus (FHL)

Lumbricals 1–4

Tendons of flexor digitorum longus (FDL)

Quadratus plantae (QP)

Calcaneus

C

5.78   SECOND LAYER OF MUSCLES OF SOLE OF FOOT

A. Bony attachments. **B.** Overview. **C.** Dissection.

TABLE 5.19 MUSCLES IN SOLE OF FOOT—SECOND LAYER

Muscle	Proximal Attachment	Distal Attachment	Innervation	Actions[a]
Quadratus plantae	Medial surface and lateral margin of plantar surface of calcaneus	Posterolateral margin of tendon of flexor digitorum longus	Lateral plantar nerve (S2–S3)	Assists flexor digitorum longus in flexing lateral four digits
Lumbricals	Tendons of flexor digitorum longus	Medial aspect of extensor expansion over lateral four digits	*Medial one:* medial plantar nerve (S2–S3); *Lateral three:* lateral plantar nerve (S2–S3)	Flex proximal phalanges and extend middle and distal phalanges of lateral four digits

[a]Although individual actions are described, the primary function of the intrinsic muscles of the foot is to act collectively to resist forces that stress (attempt to flatten) the arches of the foot.

Plantar digital arteries

Plantar metatarsal arteries

Deep plantar arch

Deep plantar artery (1st perforating artery)

Perforating arteries (to dorsal metatarsal arteries)

Deep branch

Superficial branch

Medial plantar artery

Lateral plantar artery

Posterior tibial artery

Calcaneal branch

AHT
AHO
FDM
FHB

Adductor hallucis, transverse head (AHT)

Flexor digiti minimi (FDM)

Deep branch of lateral plantar artery and nerve

Lateral plantar nerve

Lateral plantar artery

Fibrous digital sheath

Plantar ligament (plate)

Deep transverse metatarsal ligament

Adductor hallucis, oblique head (AHO)

Lateral head ⎱ **Flexor hallucis brevis**
Medial head ⎰ **(FHB)**

Flexor hallucis longus tendon

Medial plantar nerve

A   B   C

Plantar Views

5.79   THIRD LAYER OF MUSCLES AND ARTERIAL SUPPLY OF SOLE OF FOOT

A. Arterial supply. **B.** Overview. **C.** Dissection. Muscles and neurovascular structures.

TABLE 5.20 MUSCLES IN SOLE OF FOOT—THIRD LAYER

Muscle	Proximal Attachment	Distal Attachment	Innervation	Actions[a]
Flexor hallucis brevis	Plantar surfaces of cuboid and lateral cuneiforms	Both sides of base of proximal phalanx of first digit	Medial plantar nerve (S2–S3)	Flexes proximal phalanx of first digit
Adductor hallucis	*Oblique head:* bases of metatarsals 2–4; *Transverse head:* plantar ligaments of metatarsophalangeal joints	Tendons of both heads attach to lateral side of base of proximal phalanx of first digit	Deep branch of lateral plantar nerve (S2–S3)	Adducts first digit; assists in maintaining transverse arch of foot
Flexor digiti minimi	Base of fifth metatarsal	Base of proximal phalanx of fifth digit	Superficial branch of lateral plantar nerve (S2–S3)	Flexes proximal phalanx of fifth digit, thereby assisting with its flexion

[a]Although individual actions are described, the primary function of the intrinsic muscles of the foot is to act collectively to resist forces that stress (attempt to flatten) the arches of the foot.

A. Adductor Flexor brevis / Abductor Flexor brevis — Hallucis

Flexor digiti minimi
2nd dorsal interosseous (D2)
1st plantar interosseous (P1)
1st dorsal interosseous (D1)
Adductor hallucis
Fibularis (peroneus) longus
Tibialis anterior

3rd dorsal interosseous (D3)
4th dorsal interosseous (D4)
2nd plantar interosseous (P2)
3rd plantar interosseous (P3)

Flexor digiti minimi
Groove for tendon of fibularis longus
Tibialis posterior

B. Plantar interossei:
3rd
2nd
1st
Dorsal interossei:
Second
First
Fibularis longus
Tibialis posterior

C. Flexor digitorum longus
Flexor digitorum brevis
Flexor hallucis longus
Heads of metatarsals
Sesamoid bones
Plantar ligament (plate)
Medial head / Lateral head / Tendon of origin — Flexor hallucis brevis
Fibularis longus tendon
Flexor digiti minimi brevis
Fibularis (peroneus) longus tendon
Tibialis posterior
Plantar calcaneonavicular (spring) ligament
Long plantar ligament
Abductor hallucis
Abductor digiti minimi
Tuberosity of calcaneus

D3 D2
D4 P2 P1 D1
P3

Plantar Views

5.80 FOURTH LAYER OF MUSCLES OF SOLE OF FOOT

A. Bony attachments of muscles of third and fourth layers. **B.** Overview. **C.** Dissection. Muscles and ligaments.

TABLE 5.21 MUSCLES IN SOLE OF FOOT—FOURTH LAYER

Muscle	Proximal Attachment	Distal Attachment	Innervation	Actions[a]
Plantar interossei (three muscles; P1–P3)	Plantar aspect of medial sides of shafts of metatarsals 3–5	Medial sides of bases of proximal phalanges of third to fifth digits	Lateral plantar nerve (S2–S3)	Adduct digits 3–5 and flex metatarsophalangeal joints
Dorsal interossei (four muscles; D1–D4)	Adjacent sides of shafts of metatarsals 1–5	First: medial side of proximal phalanx of second digit. Second to fourth: lateral sides of second to fourth digits		Abduct digits 2–4 and flex metatarsophalangeal joints

[a]Although individual actions are described, the primary function of the intrinsic muscles of the foot is to act collectively to resist forces that stress (attempt to flatten) the arches of the foot.

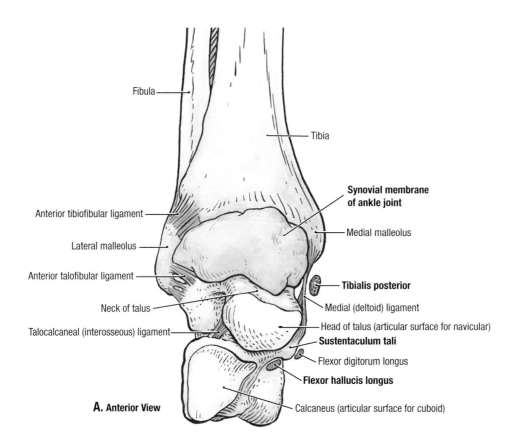

Fibula

Tibia

Anterior tibiofibular ligament

Synovial membrane of ankle joint

Lateral malleolus

Medial malleolus

Anterior talofibular ligament

Tibialis posterior

Neck of talus

Medial (deltoid) ligament

Talocalcaneal (interosseous) ligament

Head of talus (articular surface for navicular)

Sustentaculum tali

Flexor digitorum longus

Flexor hallucis longus

A. Anterior View

Calcaneus (articular surface for cuboid)

B. Anteroposterior View

5.81   JOINT CAVITY OF ANKLE JOINT

A. Ankle joint with joint cavity distended with injected latex. **B.** Radiograph of joints of ankle region. *L,* lateral malleolus; *M,* medial malleolus; *T,* talus; *TF,* tibiofibular syndesmosis.

- The anterior articular surfaces of the calcaneus and head of the talus are each convex from side to side; thus the foot can be inverted and everted at the transverse tarsal joint.
- Note the relations of the tendons to the sustentaculum tali: the flexor hallucis longus inferior to it, flexor digitorum longus along its medial aspect, and tibialis posterior superior to it and in contact with the medial (deltoid) ligament.

Fibularis (peroneus) brevis

Anterior (extensor) surface

Interosseous membrane

Subcutaneous area

Anterior tibiofibular ligament

Lateral malleolus

Anterior talofibular ligament

Talocalcaneal (interosseous) ligament

Bifurcate ligament
(calcaneocuboid ligament)

Cuboid bone

Lateral cuneiform bone

Dorsal intermetatarsal ligaments

Tibialis anterior

Medial malleolus

Medial (deltoid) ligament

Dorsal talonavicular ligament

Navicular bone

Dorsal cuneonavicular ligaments

Medial cuneiform bone

Dorsal tarsometatarsal ligaments

1st metatarsal bone

Anterosuperior View

5.82   ANKLE JOINT AND LIGAMENTS OF DORSUM OF FOOT

Dissection. The ankle joint is plantar flexed, and its anterior capsular fibers are removed.

- All muscles attached to the fibula except the biceps femoris pull inferiorly on the bone during contraction. The oblique fibers of the interosseous membrane and ligaments uniting the fibula to the tibia resist this inferior pull but allow the fibula to be forced superiorly during full dorsiflexion of the ankle.
- The bifurcate ligament, a Y-shaped ligament consisting of calcaneocuboid and calcaneonavicular ligaments, and the talonavicular ligament are the primary dorsal ligaments of the transverse tarsal joint.

A **Pott fracture-dislocation of the ankle** occurs when the foot is forcibly everted. This action pulls on the extremely strong medial (deltoid) ligament, often avulsing the medial malleolus and compressing the lateral malleolus against the talus, shearing off the malleolus or, more often, fracturing the fibula superior to the tibiofibular syndesmosis.

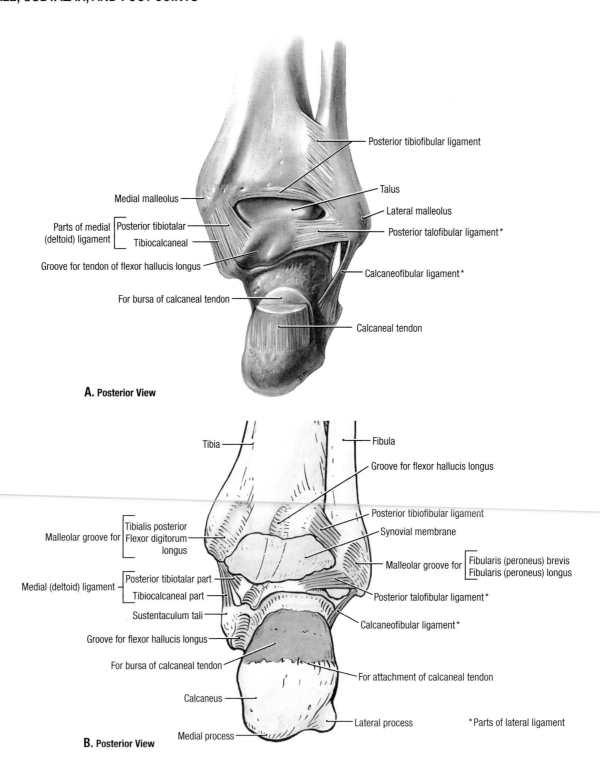

Posterior tibiofibular ligament

Talus

Medial malleolus

Lateral malleolus

Parts of medial (deltoid) ligament { **Posterior tibiotalar**
Tibiocalcaneal }

Posterior talofibular ligament*

Groove for tendon of flexor hallucis longus

Calcaneofibular ligament*

For bursa of calcaneal tendon

Calcaneal tendon

A. Posterior View

Tibia

Fibula

Groove for flexor hallucis longus

Malleolar groove for { **Tibialis posterior**
Flexor digitorum longus }

Posterior tibiofibular ligament

Synovial membrane

Malleolar groove for { **Fibularis (peroneus) brevis**
Fibularis (peroneus) longus }

Medial (deltoid) ligament { **Posterior tibiotalar part**
Tibiocalcaneal part }

Posterior talofibular ligament*

Sustentaculum tali

Calcaneofibular ligament*

Groove for flexor hallucis longus

For bursa of calcaneal tendon

For attachment of calcaneal tendon

Calcaneus

Lateral process

*Parts of lateral ligament

Medial process

B. Posterior View

| 5.83 | POSTERIOR ASPECT OF ANKLE JOINT |

A. Dissection. **B.** Ankle joint with joint cavity distended with latex. Observe the grooves for the flexor hallucis longus muscle, which crosses the middle of the ankle joint posteriorly, the two tendons posterior to the medial malleolus, and the two tendons posterior to the lateral malleolus.

- The posterior aspect of the ankle joint is strengthened by the transversely oriented posterior tibiofibular and posterior talofibular ligaments.

- The calcaneofibular ligament stabilizes the joint laterally, and the posterior tibiotalar and tibiocalcanean parts of the medial (deltoid) ligament stabilize it medially.

- The groove for the flexor hallucis tendon is between the medial and lateral tubercles of the talus and continues inferior to the sustentaculum tali.

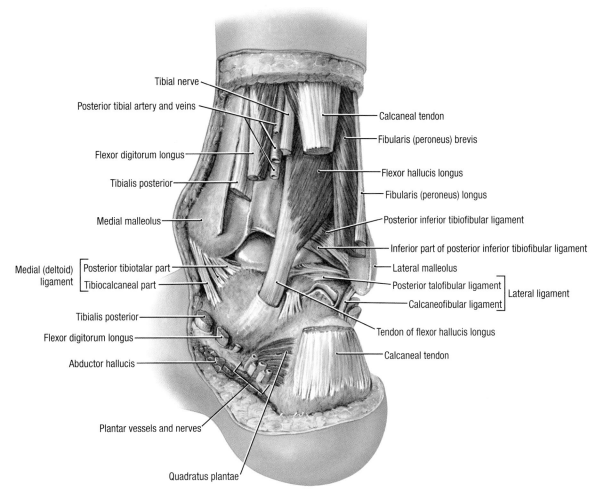

Tibial nerve

Posterior tibial artery and veins

Flexor digitorum longus

Tibialis posterior

Medial malleolus

Medial (deltoid) ligament — Posterior tibiotalar part

Tibiocalcaneal part

Tibialis posterior

Flexor digitorum longus

Abductor hallucis

Plantar vessels and nerves

Quadratus plantae

Calcaneal tendon

Fibularis (peroneus) brevis

Flexor hallucis longus

Fibularis (peroneus) longus

Posterior inferior tibiofibular ligament

Inferior part of posterior inferior tibiofibular ligament

Lateral malleolus

Posterior talofibular ligament — Lateral ligament

Calcaneofibular ligament

Tendon of flexor hallucis longus

Calcaneal tendon

Posteromedial View

5.84   POSTEROMEDIAL ANKLE

- The flexor hallucis longus muscle is midway between the medial and lateral malleoli; the tendons of the flexor digitorum and tibialis posterior are medial to it, and the tendons of the fibularis longus and brevis are lateral to it.
- The strongest parts of the ligaments of the ankle are those that prevent anterior displacement of the leg bones, namely, the posterior part of the medial ligament (posterior tibiotalar), the posterior talofibular, and calcaneofibular and tibiocalcaneal parts.

Tarsal tunnel syndrome, the entrapment and compression of the tibial nerve, occurs when there is edema and tightness in the ankle involving the synovial sheaths of the tendons of muscles in the posterior compartment of the leg. The area involved is from the medial malleolus to the calcaneus. The heel pain results from compression of the tibial nerve by the flexor retinaculum.

Medial (deltoid) ligament of ankle joint

Medial malleolus

Groove for tibialis posterior

Neck of talus

Dorsal talonavicular ligament

Tibionavicular part of medial ligament

Navicular

1st cuneiform bone

Posterior tibiotalar part

Calcaneal tendon

Medial tubercle of talus

Groove for flexor hallucis longus

Bursa of calcaneal tendon

Calcaneus

Plantar calcaneonavicular ligament

Sustentaculum tali

Tibiocalcaneal part

Tibialis posterior

A. Medial View

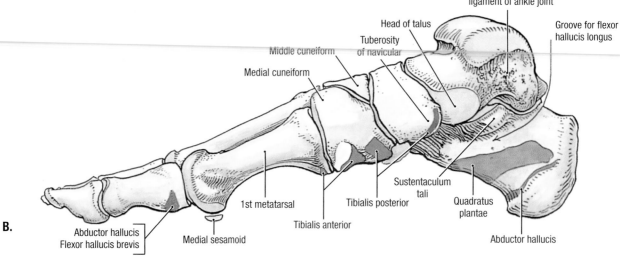

For medial (deltoid) ligament of ankle joint

Head of talus

Tuberosity of navicular

Middle cuneiform

Medial cuneiform

Groove for flexor hallucis longus

1st metatarsal

Tibialis posterior

Sustentaculum tali

Quadratus plantae

Tibialis anterior

Abductor hallucis

Abductor hallucis Flexor hallucis brevis

Medial sesamoid

B.

5.85   MEDIAL LIGAMENTS OF ANKLE REGION

A. Dissection. **B.** Bones. The joint capsule of the ankle joint is reinforced medially by the large, strong medial (deltoid) ligament that attaches proximally to the medial malleolus and fans out from it to attach distally to the talus, calcaneus, and navicular via four adjacent and continuous parts: the tibionavicular part, the tibiocalcaneal part, and the anterior and posterior tibiotalar parts. The medial ligament stabilizes the ankle joint during eversion of the foot and prevents subluxation (partial dislocation) of the ankle joint.

A   **Medial Views**

A	Calcaneal (Achilles) tendon
Ca	Calcaneus
Cb	Cuboid
Cu	Cuneiforms
F	Fat
L	Lateral malleolus
MT	Metatarsal
N	Navicular
S	Sustentaculum tali
Su	Superimposed tibia and fibula
T	Talus
TS	Tarsal sinus

B

5.86   RADIOGRAPHS OF ANKLE AND FOOT

A. Superolateral View

Tibialis anterior
Calcaneal tendon
Tibia
Fibula
Synovial fold
Anterior tibiofibular ligament
Talonavicular ligament
Lateral malleolus
Cervical ligament
Calcaneonavicular ligament
Calcaneocuboid ligament — Bifurcate ligament
Head of talus
*Anterior talofibular ligament
Bursa of calcaneal tendon
Middle cuneiform
*Calcaneofibular ligament
Lateral cuneiform
Lateral talocalcaneal ligament
Calcaneus
Talocalcaneal interosseous ligament (in tarsal sinus)
Fibularis (peroneus) longus
Fibularis (peroneus) brevis
Dorsal calcaneocuboid ligament
Cuboid

B. Lateral View

M
L
T
Ca
TS
Ca
N
Cb

C. Lateral View (Abbreviations refer to structures identified in **B.**)

Tibia
Medial malleolus (M)
Anterior tibiofibular ligament
Talus (T)
Anterior talofibular ligament*
Talonavicular ligament
Navicular (N)
Lateral malleolus
Calcaneonavicular
Calcaneocuboid ligaments — Bifurcate ligament
Cuboid (Cb)
*Calcaneofibular ligament
*Parts of lateral liagment of ankle
Calcaneus (Ca)
Lateral talocalcaneal ligament
Talocalcaneal interosseous ligament (in tarsal sinus, TS)
Cervical ligament
Dorsal calcaneocuboid ligament

5.87   LATERAL LIGAMENTS OF ANKLE REGION

A. Dissection with foot inverted by underlying wedge. **B.** Lateral radiograph. **C.** Dissection. (Abbreviations refer to structures identified in **B.**)

The ankle joint is reinforced laterally by the lateral ligament of the ankle, which consists of three separate ligaments: (1) anterior talofibular ligament, a flat, weak band; (2) calcaneofibular ligament, a round cord directed postero-inferiorly; and (3) posterior talofibular ligament, a strong, medially directed horizontal ligament (see Fig. 5.83).

Ankle sprains (partial or fully torn ligaments) are common injuries. Ankle sprains nearly always result from forceful inversion of the weight-bearing plantar flexed foot. The anterior talofibular ligament is most commonly injured, resulting in instability of the ankle. The calcaneofibular is also often torn.

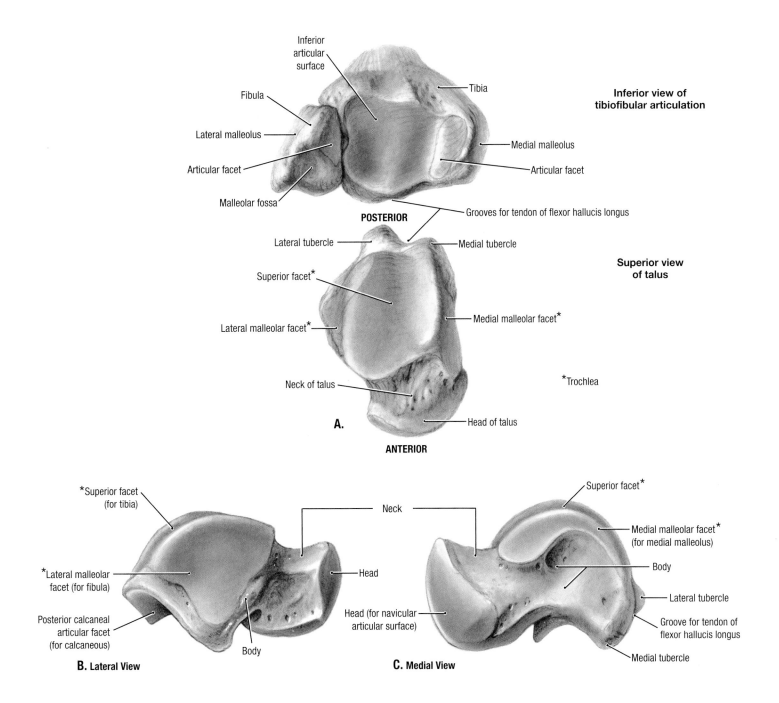

Inferior articular surface

Fibula

Lateral malleolus

Articular facet

Malleolar fossa

Tibia

Inferior view of tibiofibular articulation

Medial malleolus

Articular facet

Grooves for tendon of flexor hallucis longus

POSTERIOR

Lateral tubercle

Superior facet*

Lateral malleolar facet*

Medial tubercle

Superior view of talus

Medial malleolar facet*

Neck of talus

*Trochlea

Head of talus

A.

ANTERIOR

*Superior facet (for tibia)

*Lateral malleolar facet (for fibula)

Posterior calcaneal articular facet (for calcaneous)

Neck

Head

Head (for navicular articular surface)

Body

B. Lateral View

Superior facet*

Medial malleolar facet* (for medial malleolus)

Body

Lateral tubercle

Groove for tendon of flexor hallucis longus

Medial tubercle

C. Medial View

5.88

ARTICULAR SURFACES OF ANKLE JOINT

A. Superior aspect of talus separated from distal ends of tibia and fibula. The superior articular surface of the talus is broader anteriorly than posteriorly; hence the medial and lateral malleoli, which grasp the sides of the talus, tend to be forced apart in dorsiflexion. The fully dorsiflexed position is stable compared with the fully plantar flexed position. In plantar flexion, when the tibia and fibula articulate with the narrower posterior part of the superior articular surface of the talus, some side-to-side movement of the joint is allowed, accounting for the instability of the joint in this position. **B.** Lateral aspect of talus. The lateral, triangular articular area is for articulation with the lateral malleolus. **C.** Medial aspect of talus. The comma-shaped articular area is for articulation with the medial malleolus.

Fractures of the talar neck may occur during severe forceful dorsiflexion of the ankle, for example, from a motor vehicle accident. In some cases the body of the talus dislocates posteriorly.

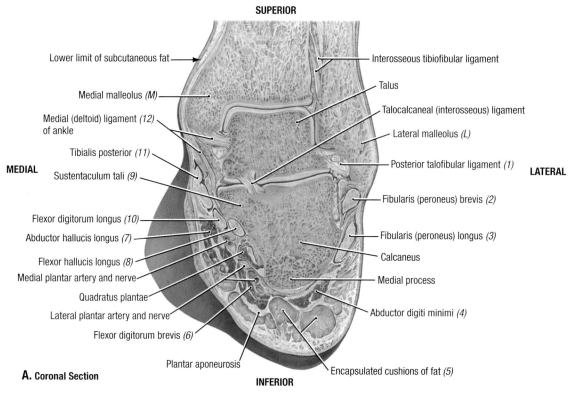

SUPERIOR

Lower limit of subcutaneous fat → Interosseous tibiofibular ligament

Medial malleolus *(M)* Talus

Medial (deltoid) ligament *(12)* of ankle Talocalcaneal (interosseous) ligament

Tibialis posterior *(11)* Lateral malleolus *(L)*

Sustentaculum tali *(9)* Posterior talofibular ligament *(1)*

MEDIAL LATERAL

Flexor digitorum longus *(10)* Fibularis (peroneus) brevis *(2)*

Abductor hallucis longus *(7)* Fibularis (peroneus) longus *(3)*

Flexor hallucis longus *(8)* Calcaneus

Medial plantar artery and nerve Medial process

Quadratus plantae Abductor digiti minimi *(4)*

Lateral plantar artery and nerve

Flexor digitorum brevis *(6)*

Plantar aponeurosis Encapsulated cushions of fat *(5)*

A. Coronal Section INFERIOR

B. Coronal MRI

5.89   CORONAL SECTION AND MRI THROUGH ANKLE

A. Coronal section. **B.** Coronal MRI (*numbers* in **B** refer to structures labeled in **A**).

- The tibia rests on the talus, and the talus rests on the calcaneus; between the calcaneus and the skin are several encapsulated cushions of fat.
- The lateral malleolus descends farther inferiorly than the medial malleolus.
- The talocalcaneal (interosseous) ligament between the talus and calcaneus separates the subtalar, or posterior talocalcaneal joint from the talocalcaneonavicular joint.

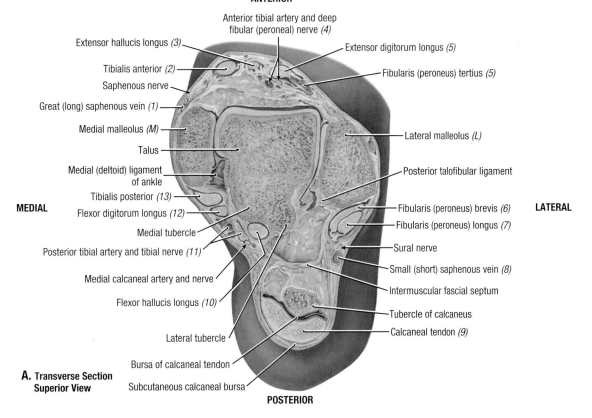

ANTERIOR

Anterior tibial artery and deep
fibular (peroneal) nerve *(4)*

Extensor hallucis longus *(3)*

Extensor digitorum longus *(5)*

Tibialis anterior *(2)*

Fibularis (peroneus) tertius *(5)*

Saphenous nerve

Great (long) saphenous vein *(1)*

Medial malleolus *(M)*

Lateral malleolus *(L)*

Talus

Medial (deltoid) ligament
of ankle

Posterior talofibular ligament

Tibialis posterior *(13)*

MEDIAL

Flexor digitorum longus *(12)*

Fibularis (peroneus) brevis *(6)*

LATERAL

Medial tubercle

Fibularis (peroneus) longus *(7)*

Posterior tibial artery and tibial nerve *(11)*

Sural nerve

Medial calcaneal artery and nerve

Small (short) saphenous vein *(8)*

Flexor hallucis longus *(10)*

Intermuscular fascial septum

Lateral tubercle

Tubercle of calcaneus

Bursa of calcaneal tendon

Calcaneal tendon *(9)*

A. Transverse Section
Superior View

Subcutaneous calcaneal bursa

POSTERIOR

B. Transverse MRI

5.90   **TRANSVERSE SECTION AND MRI THROUGH ANKLE**

A. Transverse section. **B.** Transverse MRI (*numbers* in **B** refer to structures labeled in **A**).

- The body of the talus is wedge shaped and positioned between the malleoli, which are bound to it by the medial (deltoid) and posterior talofibular ligaments.
- The flexor hallucis longus muscle lies within its osseofibrous sheath between the medial and lateral tubercles of the talus.
- There is a small, inconstant subcutaneous bursa superficial to the calcaneal tendon and a large, constant bursa of calcaneal tendon deep to it.

Medial cuneiform bone

Lateral cuneiform bone

Cuboid bone

Navicular

Bifurcate ligament (calcaneocuboid ligament)

Tuberosity

Anterior talar articular surface

Plantar calcaneonavicular (spring) ligament

Cervical ligament

Medial (deltoid) ligament

Groove for tibialis posterior

Sustentaculum tali

Talocalcaneal interosseous ligament

Middle talar articular surface

Posterior talocalcaneal ligament

Groove for flexor hallucis longus

Calcaneofibular ligament

Posterior talar articular surface

Joint capsule of ankle joint (cut)

Calcaneus

A. Superior View

Calcaneal tendon (cut edge)

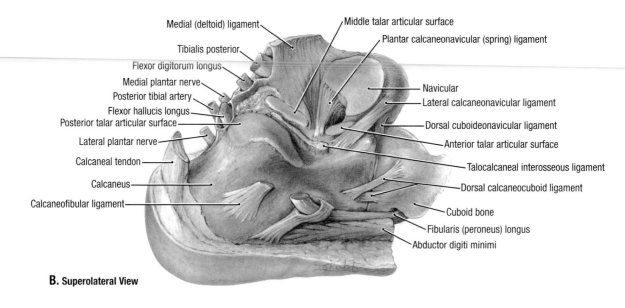

Medial (deltoid) ligament

Middle talar articular surface

Plantar calcaneonavicular (spring) ligament

Tibialis posterior

Flexor digitorum longus

Medial plantar nerve

Posterior tibial artery

Flexor hallucis longus

Navicular

Lateral calcaneonavicular ligament

Posterior talar articular surface

Dorsal cuboideonavicular ligament

Lateral plantar nerve

Anterior talar articular surface

Calcaneal tendon

Talocalcaneal interosseous ligament

Calcaneus

Dorsal calcaneocuboid ligament

Calcaneofibular ligament

Cuboid bone

Fibularis (peroneus) longus

Abductor digiti minimi

B. Superolateral View

5.91 JOINTS OF INVERSION AND EVERSION

The joints of inversion and eversion are the subtalar (posterior talocalcaneal) joint, talocalcaneonavicular joint, and transverse tarsal (combined calcaneocuboid and talonavicular) joint. **A.** Posterior and middle parts of foot with talus removed. **B.** Posterior part of foot with talus removed. The convex posterior talar facet is separated from the concave middle, and anterior facets by the talocalcaneal (interosseous) ligament within the tarsal sinus.

Calcaneal fractures. A hard fall onto the heel, for example, from a ladder, may fracture the calcaneous into several pieces, resulting in a comminuted fracture. A calcaneal fracture is usually disabling because it disrupts the subtalar (talocalcaneal) joint.

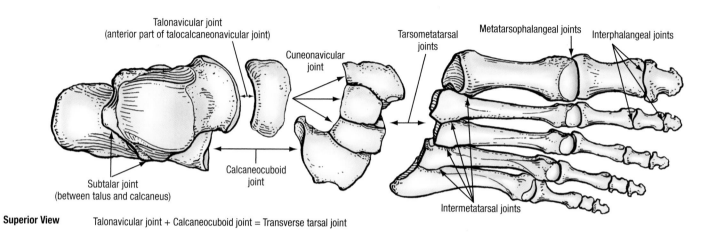

Talonavicular joint
(anterior part of talocalcaneonavicular joint)

Cuneonavicular joint

Tarsometatarsal joints

Metatarsophalangeal joints

Interphalangeal joints

Subtalar joint
(between talus and calcaneus)

Calcaneocuboid joint

Intermetatarsal joints

Superior View   Talonavicular joint + Calcaneocuboid joint = Transverse tarsal joint

5.92   JOINTS OF FOOT

TABLE 5.22 JOINTS OF FOOT

Joint	Type	Articular Surface	Joint Capsule	Ligaments	Movements
Subtalart	Synovial (plane) joint	Inferior surface of body of talus articulates with superior surface of calcaneus	Attached to margins of articular surfaces	Medial, lateral, and posterior talocalcaneal ligaments support capsule; talocalcaneal (interosseous) ligament binds bones together	Inversion and eversion of foot
Talocalcaneo-navicular	Synovial joint; talonavicular part is a pivot joint	Head of talus articulates with calcaneus and navicular bones	Incompletely encloses joint	Plantar calcaneonavicular ("spring") ligament supports head of talus	Gliding and rotary movements
Calcaneocuboid	Synovial (plane) joint	Anterior end of calcaneus articulates with posterior surface of cuboid	Encloses joint	Dorsal calcaneocuboid ligament, plantar calcaneocuboid ligament, and long plantar ligament support joint capsule	Inversion and eversion of foot
Cuneonavicular	Synovial (plane) joint	Anterior navicular articulates with posterior surface of cuneiforms	Common joint capsule	Dorsal and plantar ligaments	Limited gliding movement
Tarsometatarsal	Synovial (plane) joint	Anterior tarsal bones articulate with bases of metatarsal bones	Encloses joint	Dorsal, plantar, and interosseous ligaments	Gliding or sliding
Intermetatarsal	Synovial (plane) joint	Bases of metatarsal bones articulate with each other	Encloses each joint	Dorsal, plantar, and interosseous ligaments bind bones together	Little individual movement
Metatarsophalangeal	Synovial (condyloid) joint	Heads of metatarsal bones articulate with bases of proximal phalanges	Encloses each joint	Collateral ligaments support capsule on each side; plantar ligament supports plantar part of capsule	Flexion, extension, and some abduction, adduction and circumduction
Interphalangeal	Synovial (hinge) joint	Head of proximal or middle phalanx articulates with base of phalanx distal to it	Encloses each joint	Collateral and plantar ligaments support joints	Flexion and extension

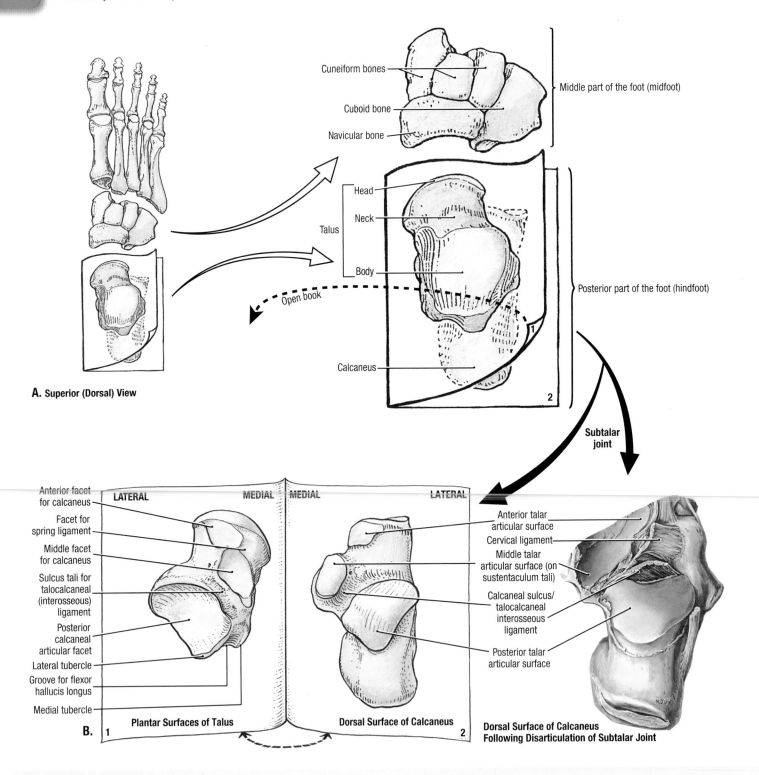

A. Superior (Dorsal) View

Cuneiform bones

Cuboid bone

Navicular bone

Middle part of the foot (midfoot)

Head

Neck

Talus

Body

Calcaneus

Posterior part of the foot (hindfoot)

Open book

Subtalar joint

Anterior facet for calcaneus

Facet for spring ligament

Middle facet for calcaneus

Sulcus tali for talocalcaneal (interosseous) ligament

Posterior calcaneal articular facet

Lateral tubercle

Groove for flexor hallucis longus

Medial tubercle

LATERAL   MEDIAL   MEDIAL   LATERAL

Plantar Surfaces of Talus   **Dorsal Surface of Calcaneus**

Anterior talar articular surface

Cervical ligament

Middle talar articular surface (on sustentaculum tali)

Calcaneal sulcus/ talocalcaneal interosseous ligament

Posterior talar articular surface

Dorsal Surface of Calcaneus Following Disarticulation of Subtalar Joint

B.

5.93   TALOCALCANEAL JOINT

A. Bones of foot, with "closed book" inserted in joint plane of subtalar joint.
B. "Open book" view of the bony surfaces of talocalcaneal joints. The plantar surface of the talus and dorsal surface of the calcaneus are displayed as pages in a book.

• The joints of inversion and eversion are the subtalar (posterior talocalcaneal) joint, talocalcaneonavicular joint, and transverse tarsal (combined calcaneocuboid and talonavicular) joint.

• The talus participates in the ankle joint, of the posterior and anterior talocalcaneal joints, and of the talonavicular joint.

• The posterior and anterior talocalcaneal joints are separated from each other by the sulcus tali and calcaneal sulcus, which, when the talus and calcaneus are in articulation, become the tarsal sinus.

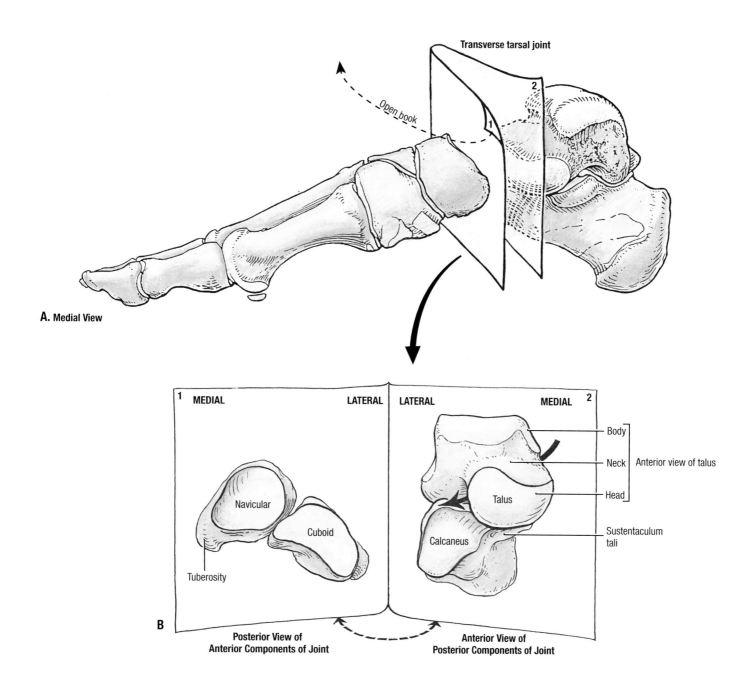

5.94   TRANSVERSE TARSAL JOINT

A. Bones of foot, with "closed book" inserted in joint plane of transverse tarsal joint. **B.** Articular surfaces of transverse tarsal joint. This compound joint includes the talonavicular and calcaneocuboid articulations. The posterior surfaces of the navicular and cuboid bones and the anterior surfaces of the talus and calcaneus are displayed as pages in an "open book". The *black arrow* traverses the tarsal sinus, in which the talocalcaneal (interosseous) ligament is located.

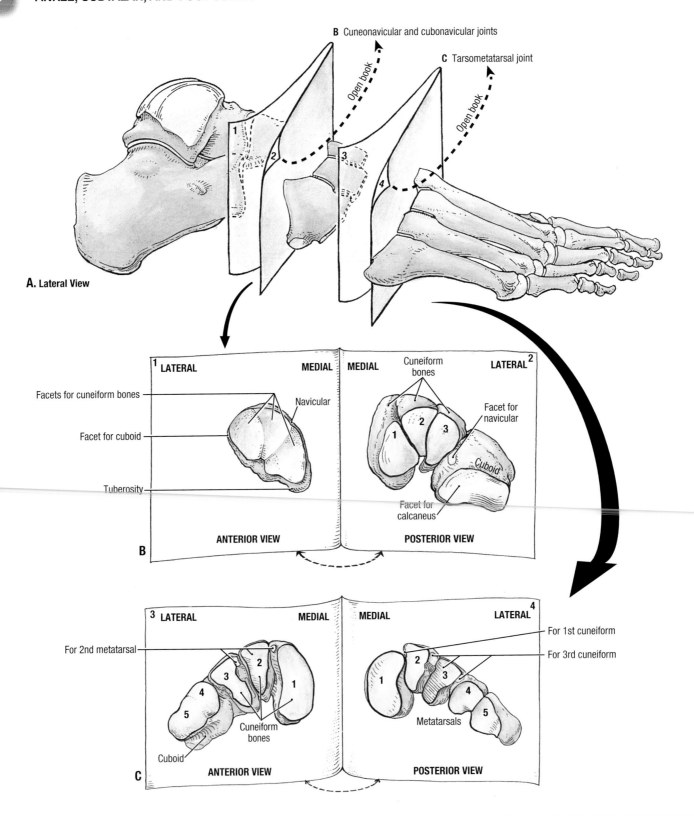

B Cuneonavicular and cubonavicular joints

C Tarsometatarsal joint

Open book

Open book

A. Lateral View

B

1 LATERAL   MEDIAL   MEDIAL   LATERAL 2

Facets for cuneiform bones

Navicular

Facet for cuboid

Cuneiform bones

Facet for navicular

Cuboid

Tuberosity

Facet for calcaneus

ANTERIOR VIEW   POSTERIOR VIEW

C

3 LATERAL   MEDIAL   MEDIAL   LATERAL 4

For 2nd metatarsal

For 1st cuneiform

For 3rd cuneiform

Cuneiform bones

Metatarsals

Cuboid

ANTERIOR VIEW   POSTERIOR VIEW

5.95   CUNEONAVICULAR, CUBONAVICULAR, AND TARSOMETATARSAL JOINTS

A. Bones of foot, with "closed book" inserted in indicated joint planes. **B.** "Open book" view of the bony surfaces of the cuneonavicular and cubonavicular joints. **C.** "Open book" view of the bony surfaces of the tarsometatarsal joints.

Metatarsal fractures (dancer's fracture) usually occur when the dancer loses balance, putting full body weight on the metatarsal. **Fatigue fractures of the metatarsals,** usually transverse, may result from prolonged walking with repeated stress on the metatarsals.

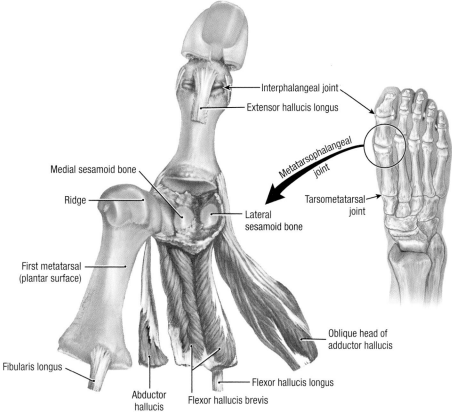

Interphalangeal joint

Extensor hallucis longus

Metatarsophalangeal joint

Tarsometatarsal joint

Medial sesamoid bone

Ridge

Lateral sesamoid bone

First metatarsal (plantar surface)

Oblique head of adductor hallucis

Fibularis longus

Flexor hallucis longus

Abductor hallucis

Flexor hallucis brevis

A. Superior View of Phalanges and Nail, Right Great Toe, Medial View of First Metetarsal

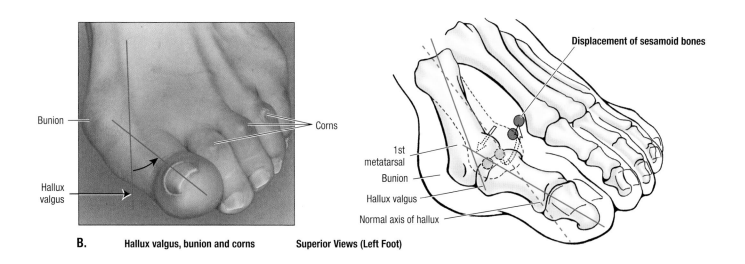

Bunion

Corns

Hallux valgus

Displacement of sesamoid bones

1st metatarsal

Bunion

Hallux valgus

Normal axis of hallux

B.   **Hallux valgus, bunion and corns**   **Superior Views (Left Foot)**

5.96   METATARSOPHALANGEAL JOINT OF GREAT TOE

A. First metatarsal and sesamoid bones of the right great toe. The sesamoid bones of the great toe (hallux) are bound together and located on each side of a bony ridge on the first metatarsal. **B. Hallux valgus** is a foot deformity caused by pressure from footwear and degenerative joint disease. It is characterized by lateral deviation of the base of the first metatarsal and base of the proximal phalanx of the great toe (L. *hallux*). In some people, the deviation is so great that the 1st toe overlaps the 2nd toe. These individuals are unable to move their 1st digit away from their 2nd digit because the sesamoid bones under the head of the 1st metatarsal are displaced and lie in the space between the heads of the 1st and 2nd metatarsals. In addition, a subcutaneous bursa may form owing to pressure and friction against the shoe. When tender and inflamed, the bursa is called a **bunion.**

Metatarsal bone

Plantar intermetatarsal ligaments

Plantar tarsometatarsal ligaments

Plantar tarsometatarsal ligaments

Medial cuneiform bone

Cuboid bone

Tibialis anterior

Tendon of fibularis (peroneus) longus

Navicular bone

Plantar calcaneocuboid
(short plantar) ligament

Plantar calcaneonavicular (spring) ligament

Long plantar ligament

Sustentaculum tali

Medial malleolus

Tibialis posterior

Groove for tendon of flexor hallucis longus

Calcaneus

A. Plantar View

5.97   LIGAMENTS OF SOLE OF FOOT

A. Dissection of superficial ligaments. **B.** Bones lying deep to ligaments of **A**.
In **A**:

- The head of the talus is exposed between the sustentaculum tali of the calcaneus and the navicular.
- Note the insertions of three long tendons: fibularis (peroneus) longus, tibialis anterior, and tibialis posterior.
- The tendon of the fibularis (peroneus) longus muscle crosses the sole of the foot in the groove anterior to the ridge of the cuboid, is bridged by some fibers of the long plantar ligament, and inserts into the base of the first metatarsal.
- Observe the slips of the tibialis posterior tendon extending to the bones anterior to the transverse tarsal joint.

Groove ⎤
Tuberosity ⎦ of cuboid

Medial cuneiform

Cuboid

Navicular

Tuberosity

Head of talus

Sustentaculum tali

Groove for tendon of
flexor hallucis longus

Medial tubercle

Tuberosity of calcaneus

B. Plantar View

Fifth metatarsal

First metatarsal

Plantar tarsometatarsal ligaments

Plantar intermetatarsal ligaments

1st cuneiform bone

Plantar cuneocuboid ligament

Plantar cuneonavicular ligaments

Plantar cubonavicular ligament

Navicular bone

Plantar calcaneocuboid
(short plantar) ligament

Plantar calcaneonavicular
(spring) ligament

Anterior tubercle of calcaneus

Sustentaculum tali

Medial (deltoid) ligament

Calcaneus

C. Plantar View

Cuboid

Medial cuneiform

Plantar calcaneocuboid
(short plantar) ligament

Plantar calcaneonavicular
(spring) ligament

Medial (deltoid) ligament

Calcaneus

D. Plantar View

| 5.97 | LIGAMENTS OF SOLE OF FOOT (*CONTINUED*) |

C. Dissection of the deep ligaments. **D.** Support for head of talus. The head of the talus is supported by the plantar calcaneonavicular ligament (spring ligament) and the tendon of the tibialis posterior.

- The plantar calcaneocuboid (short plantar) and plantar calcaneonavicular (spring) ligaments are the primary plantar ligaments of the transverse tarsal joint.
- The ligaments of the anterior foot diverge laterally and posteriorly from each side of the long axis of the third metatarsal and third cuneiform; hence a posterior thrust received by the first metatarsal, as when rising on the big toe while in walking, is transmitted directly to the navicular and talus by the first cuneiform and indirectly by the second metatarsal, second cuneiform, third metatarsal, and third cuneiform.
- A posterior thrust received by the fourth and fifth metatarsals is transmitted directly to the cuboid and calcaneus.

A. Superior View

Calcaneus

Body ⎤
Neck ⎥ Talus
Head ⎦

Navicular

Cuboid

Lateral (3rd) cuneiform
Middle (2nd) cuneiform
Medial (1st) cuneiform

Metatarsals (1-5)

Proximal phalanx

Middle phalanx

Distal phalanx

Medial longitudinal arch
Lateral longitudinal arch

B. Normal Arch

Medial Views

C. Fallen Arch

D. Medial View

Tibialis anterior
Tibialis posterior
Flexor hallucis longus
Fibularis longus
Intrinsic plantar muscles

Dynamic support

Passive support (Four (1-4) layers)

(1) Plantar aponeurosis

Short plantar ligament (3)

Long plantar ligament (2)

Plantar calcaneonavicular (spring) ligament (4)

5.98   ARCHES OF FOOT

A. Medial and lateral longitudinal arches. **B.** Normal arch. **C.** Fallen arch. **D.** Supports of the longitudinal arches.

Pes planus (flatfeet). Acquired flatfeet ("fallen arches") are likely to be secondary to dysfunction of the tibialis posterior due to trauma, degeneration with age, or denervation. In the absence of normal passive or dynamic support, the plantar calcaneonavicular ligament fails to support

the head of the talus. Consequently, the head of the talus displaces inferomedially. As a result flattening of the medial longitudinal arch occurs **(C)** along with lateral deviation of the forefoot. Flatfeet are common in older people, particularly if they undertake much unaccustomed standing or gain weight rapidly, adding stress on the muscles and increasing strain on the ligaments supporting the arches.

Patella

A. Posterior View

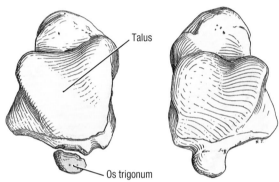

Talus

Os trigonum

B. Superior Views

Femur

Fabella

Fibula

Tibia

C. Lateral View

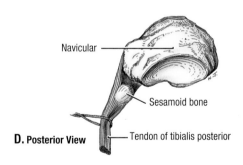

Navicular

Sesamoid bone

Tendon of tibialis posterior

D. Posterior View

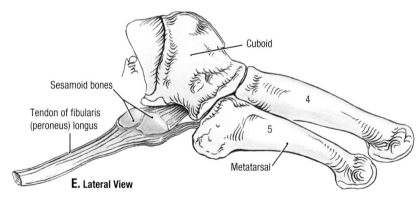

Cuboid

Sesamoid bones

Tendon of fibularis (peroneus) longus

4

5

Metatarsal

E. Lateral View

5.99 BONY ANOMALIES

A. Bipartite patella. Occasionally, the superolateral angle of the patella ossifies independently and remains discrete. **B. Os trigonum.** The lateral (posterior) tubercle of the talus has a separate center of ossification that appears from the ages of 7 to 13 years; when this fails to fuse with the body of the talus, as in the left bone of this pair, it is called an os trigonum. It was found in Dr. Grant's lab in 7.7% of 558 adult feet; 22 were paired, and 21 were unpaired. **C. Fabella.** A sesamoid bone in the lateral head of the gastrocnemius muscle was present in 21.6% of 116 limbs. **D. Sesamoid bone in the tendon of tibialis posterior.** A sesamoid bone was found in 23% of 348 adults. **E. Sesamoid bone in the tendon of fibularis (peroneus) longus.** A sesamoid bone was found in 26% of 92 specimens. In this specimen, it is bipartite, and the fibularis (peroneus) longus muscle has an additional attachment to the 5th metatarsal bone.

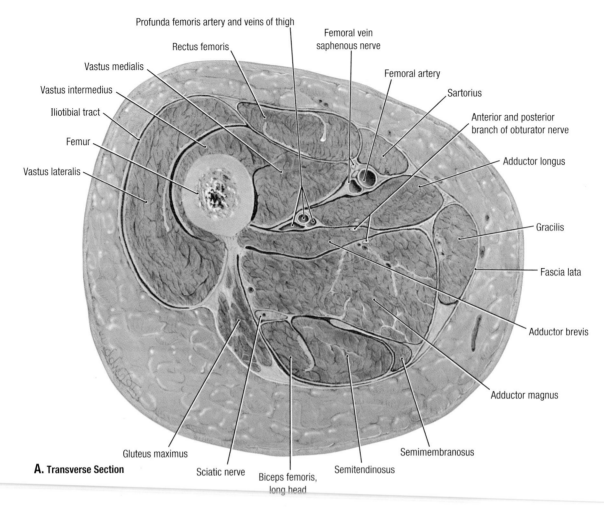

Profunda femoris artery and veins of thigh
Rectus femoris
Vastus medialis
Vastus intermedius
Iliotibial tract
Femur
Vastus lateralis

Femoral vein
saphenous nerve
Femoral artery
Sartorius
Anterior and posterior
branch of obturator nerve
Adductor longus

Gracilis
Fascia lata
Adductor brevis
Adductor magnus
Semimembranosus

Gluteus maximus
Sciatic nerve
Biceps femoris,
long head
Semitendinosus

A. Transverse Section

B. Transverse MRI

A and B

Level of Section

5.100   TRANSVERSE SECTIONS AND MRIs OF THIGH

A. Anatomical section of proximal thigh. **B.** Transverse MRI of proximal thigh.

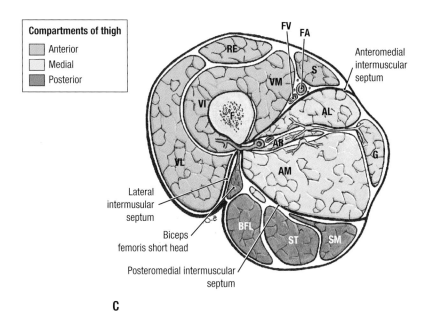

Compartments of thigh
- Anterior
- Medial
- Posterior

C

Transverse MRI

D. Transverse MRI

Level of Section

E. Coronal MRI

Key

AB	Adductor brevis
AL	Adductor longus
AM	Adductor magnus
AS	Anteromedial intermuscular septum
BF	Biceps femoris
BFL	Long head of biceps femoris
BFS	Short head of biceps femoris
F	Femur
FA	Femoral artery
FL	Fascia lata
FV	Femoral vein
G	Gracilis
GM	Gluteus maximus
GSV	Great saphenous vein

H	Head of femur
IT	Iliotibial tract
LS	Lateral intermuscular septum
OE	Obturator externus
PS	Posterior intermuscular septum
RF	Rectus femoris
S	Sartorius
SM	Semimembranosus
SN	Sciatic nerve
ST	Semitendinosus
TFL	Tensor fasciae latae
UB	Urinary bladder
VI	Vastus intermedius
VL	Vastus lateralis
VM	Vastus medialis

5.100

TRANSVERSE SECTIONS AND MRIs OF THIGH (*CONTINUED*)

C. Diagrammlatic anatomical section and transverse (axial) MRI of midthigh. **D.** Transverse (axial) MRI of distal thigh. **E.** Coronal MRI.

The thigh has three compartments, each with its own nerve supply and primary function: anterior group extends the knee and is supplied by the femoral nerve; medial group adducts the hip and is supplied by the obturator nerve; posterior group flexes the knee and is supplied by the sciatic nerve.

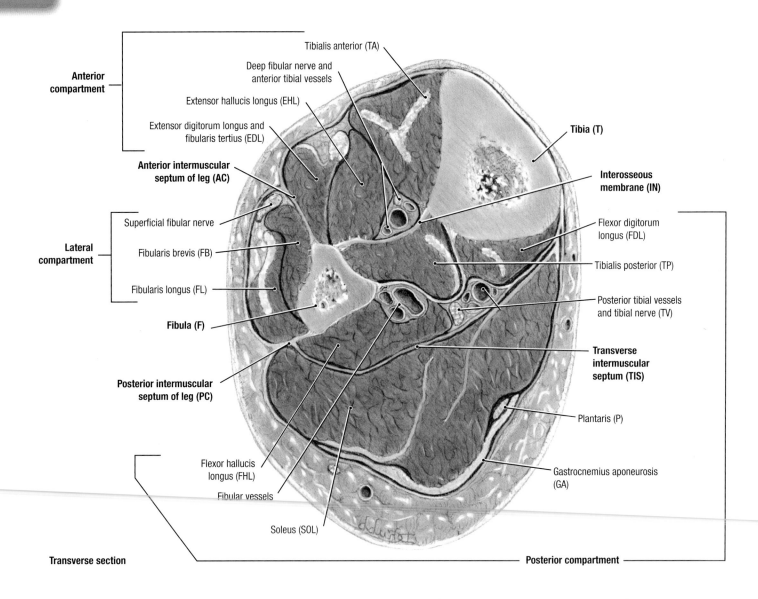

Anterior compartment

Tibialis anterior (TA)

Deep fibular nerve and anterior tibial vessels

Extensor hallucis longus (EHL)

Extensor digitorum longus and fibularis tertius (EDL)

Anterior intermuscular septum of leg (AC)

Superficial fibular nerve

Lateral compartment

Fibularis brevis (FB)

Fibularis longus (FL)

Fibula (F)

Posterior intermuscular septum of leg (PC)

Flexor hallucis longus (FHL)

Fibular vessels

Soleus (SOL)

Transverse section

Tibia (T)

Interosseous membrane (IN)

Flexor digitorum longus (FDL)

Tibialis posterior (TP)

Posterior tibial vessels and tibial nerve (TV)

Transverse intermuscular septum (TIS)

Plantaris (P)

Gastrocnemius aponeurosis (GA)

Posterior compartment

5.101 TRANSVERSE SECTION OF LEG

Boundaries of anterior, lateral, and posterior compartments of leg. Anterior compartment: tibia, interosseous membrane, fibula, anterior intermuscular septum, and crural fascia. Lateral compartment: fibula, anterior and posterior intermuscular septa, and the crural fascia. Posterior compartment: tibia, interosseous membrane, fibula, posterior intermuscular septum, and crural fascia. The posterior compartment is subdivided by the transverse intermuscular septum into superficial and deep subcompartments.

Compartmental infections in the leg. Because the septa and deep fascia forming the boundaries of the leg compartments are strong, the increased volume consequent to infection with suppuration (formation of pus) increases intracompartmental pressure. Inflammation within the anterior and posterior compartments spreads chiefly in a distal direction; however a purulent infection in the lateral compartment can ascend proximally into the popliteal fossa, presumably along the course of the fibular nerve. **Fasciotomy** may be necessary to relieve compartmental pressure and debride (remove by scraping) pockets of infection.

Level of Section

A. Transverse MRI

D. Coronal MRI

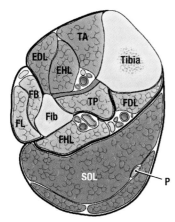

B. Transverse Section and MRI

Key for B

Anterior compartment	
Lateral compartment	
Posterior compartment	

C. Transverse MRI

Key	
AC	Anterior intermuscular septum
AV	Anterior tibial vessels and deep fibular nerve
EDL	Extensor digitorum longus
EHL	Extensor hallucis longus
F	Fibula
FB	Fibularis brevis
FDL	Flexor digitorum longus
FHL	Flexor hallucis longus
FL	Fibularis longus
GA	Gastrocnemius aponeurosis
G	Gracilis
GM	Gluteus maximus
GSV	Great saphenous vein
HF	Head of fibula
IN	Interosseous membrane
LG	Lateral head of gastrocnemius
MG	Medial head of gastrocnemius
MM	Medial malleolus
P	Popliteus
PC	Posterior intermuscular septum
SOL	Soleus
SSV	Small saphenous vein
T	Tibia
TA	Tibialis anterior
Ta	Talus
TC	Calcaneal tendon
TP	Tibialis posterior
TV	Tibial nerve and posterior tibial vessels

5.102 MRIs OF LEG

A., B. and C. Transverse (axial) MRIs. **D.** Coronal MRI.

Transverse Sections

Compact bone

Spongy bone

Spongy bone

Compact bone

Medullary (marrow) cavity

Femur

A. Anterior View

Transverse Sections

T

F

Compact bone

T

Spongy bone

F

T

Fibula (F)   Tibia (T)

F

T

F

T

B. Anterior View

N Joy

5.103   TRANSVERSE SECTIONS THROUGH FEMUR, TIBIA AND FIBULA

A. Femur. **B.** Tibia and fibula. Note the differences in thickness of the compact and spongy bone and in the width of the medullary (marrow) cavity. Compact and spongy bones are distinguished by the relative amount of solid matter and by the number and size of the spaces they contain. All bones have a superficial thin layer of compact bone around a central mass of spongy bone, except where the latter is replaced by the medullary (marrow) cavity. Within the medullary cavity of adult bones and between the spicules (trabeculae) of spongy bone, yellow (fatty) or red (blood cell and platelet forming) bone marrow or both are found.

Upper Limb

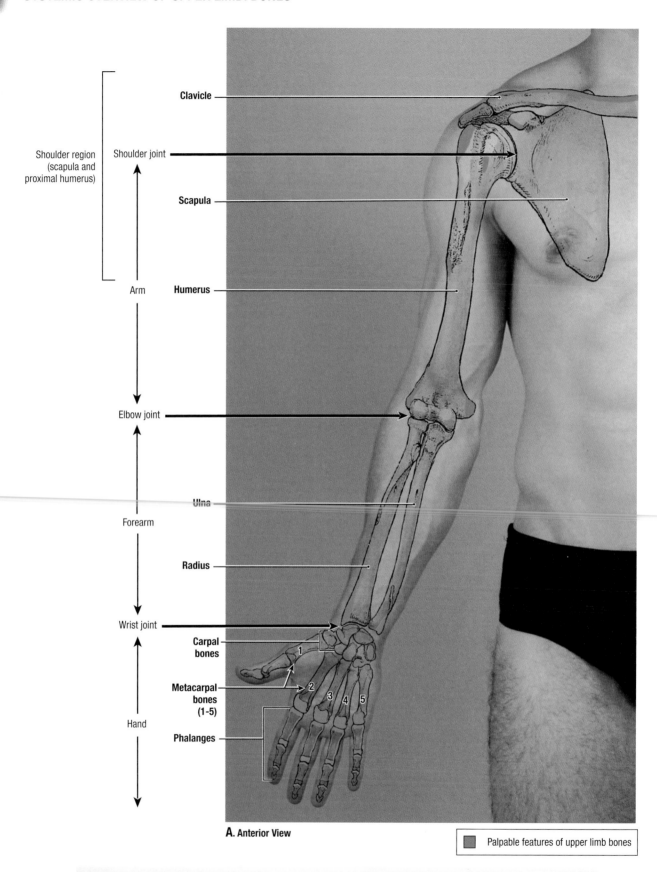

Shoulder region
(scapula and
proximal humerus)

Arm

Forearm

Hand

Clavicle

Shoulder joint

Scapula

Humerus

Elbow joint

Ulna

Radius

Wrist joint

Carpal
bones

Metacarpal
bones
(1–5)

Phalanges

A. Anterior View

Palpable features of upper limb bones

6.1   REGIONS, BONES, AND MAJOR JOINTS OF UPPER LIMB

The joints divide the upper limb into four main regions: the shoulder, arm, forearm, and hand.

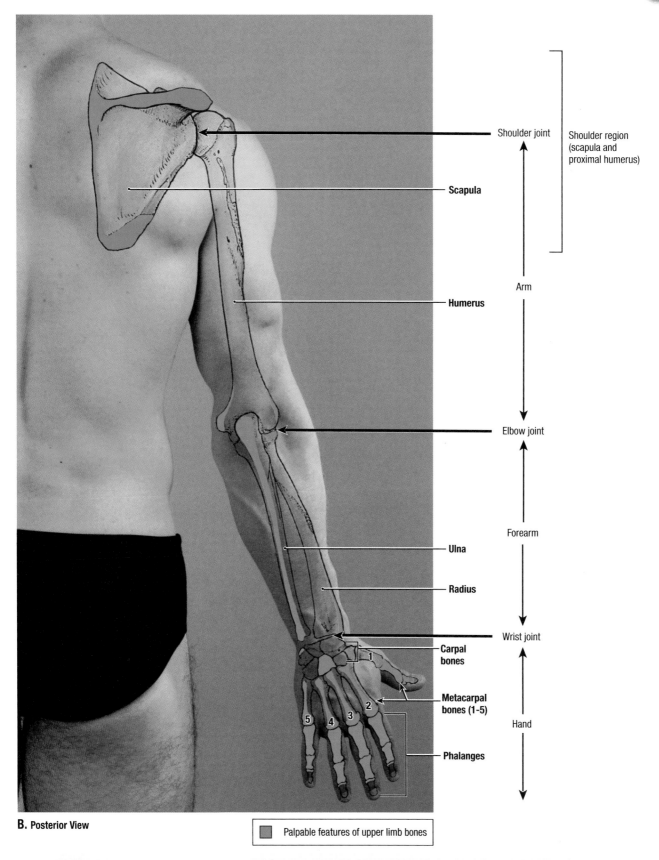

Shoulder joint

Shoulder region (scapula and proximal humerus)

Scapula

Arm

Humerus

Elbow joint

Forearm

Ulna

Radius

Wrist joint

Carpal bones

Metacarpal bones (1-5)

Hand

Phalanges

B. Posterior View

Palpable features of upper limb bones

6.1 REGIONS, BONES, AND MAJOR JOINTS OF UPPER LIMB *(CONTINUED)*

The pectoral (shoulder) girdle is an incomplete ring of bones formed by the right and left scapulae and clavicles and is joined medially to the manubrium of the sternum.

Clavicle

B. Clavicle, Superior View

LATERAL   MEDIAL

Scapula

Shaft (body) of humerus

Radius   Ulna

A. Anterior View

Metacarpals

Phalanges

C. Proximal Humerus, Anterior View

Coracoid process

Acromion

Medial border

Inferior angle

D. Scapula, Anterior View

Capitulum   Medial epicondyle

Trochlea

E. Distal Humerus, Anterior View

F. Proximal Radius, Anterior View

G. Proximal Ulna, Medial View

H. Distal Radius, Anterior View

I. Distal Ulna, Anterior View

6.2   OSSIFICATION AND SITES OF EPIPHYSES OF BONES OF UPPER LIMB

A. Upper limb bones at birth. Only the diaphyses of the long bones and scapula are ossified. The epiphyses, carpal bones, coracoid process, medial border of the scapula, and acromion are still cartilaginous. **B.–I.** Sites of epiphyses (*darker orange regions*).

- The ends of the long bones are ossified by the formation of one or more secondary centers of ossification; these epiphyses develop from birth to approximately 20 years of age in the clavicle, humerus, radius, ulna, metacarpals, and phalanges.

Epiphyses. Without knowledge of bone growth and the appearance of bones in radiographic and other diagnostic images at various ages, a displaced epiphysial plate could be mistaken for a fracture, and separation of an epiphysis could be interpreted as a displaced piece of fractured bone. Knowledge of the patient's age and the location of epiphyses can prevent these errors.

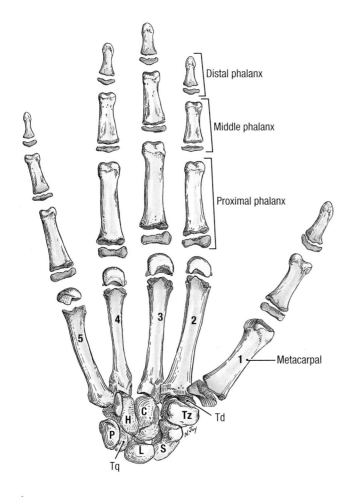

J. Anterior View (Right Hand)

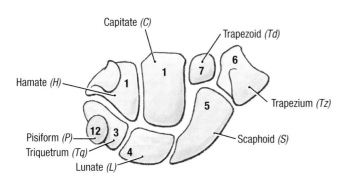

Numbers: approximate age of ossification of carpal bones in years

K. Anterior View

L. Antero-posterior View, Right Hand

Epiphyses in radiographs appear as radiolucent lines

6.2   **OSSIFICATION AND SITES OF EPIPHYSES OF BONES OF UPPER LIMB** *(CONTINUED)*

J. Sequence of ossification of carpal bones. **K.** Ossification of bones of hand. Note the phalanges have a single proximal epiphysis and metacarpals 2, 3, 4, and 5 have single distal epiphyses. The 1st metacarpal behaves as a phalanx by having proximal epiphysis. Short-lived epiphyses may appear at the other ends of metacarpals 1 and/or 2. There are individual and gender differences in sequence and timing of ossification. **L.** Radiographs of stages of ossification of wrist and hand. *Top*, a 2½-year-old child; the lunate is ossifying, and the distal radial epiphysis *(R)* is present (*C*, capitate; *H*, hamate; *Tq*, triquetrum; *L*, lunate). *Bottom*, an 11-year-old child. All carpal bones are ossified (*S*, scaphoid; *Td*, trapezoid; *Tz*, trapezium; *arrowhead*, pisiform), and the distal epiphysis of the ulna *(U)* has ossified.

A. Superior Surface

Acromial end
Clavicle
Shaft
Sternal facet (articular surface)
Deltoid tubercle

B. Inferior Surface

Acromial facet (articular surface)
Deltoid tubercle
Clavicle
Impression for costoclavicular ligament
Subclavian groove
Trapezoid line*
Conoid tubercle*
Sternal end
*Tuberosity for coracoclavicular ligament (conoid and trapezoid parts)

C. Anterior View

Humerus
Radial fossa
Coronoid fossa
Lateral epicondyle
Medial epicondyle
Capitulum
Trochlea

Trochlear notch
Radial notch
Olecranon
Head
Neck
Coronoid process
Tuberosity
Tuberosity of ulna
Supinator fossa
Anterior oblique line
Ulna
Radius

D. Anterior View

Acromial end of clavicle
Lesser tubercle
Coracoid process
Acromion of scapula
Superior border
Greater tubercle
Superior angle
Crest of lesser tubercle
Clavicle
Sternal end
Crest of greater tubercle
Suprascapular notch
Intertubercular sulcus (bicipital groove)
Scapula
Surgical neck
Medial (vertebral) border
Body of scapula
Subscapular fossa
Inferior angle
Deltoid tuberosity
Lateral border
Shaft of humerus
Humerus
Lateral supra-epicondylar ridge
Medial supra-epicondylar ridge
Radial fossa
Coronoid fossa
Lateral epicondyle
Medial epicondyle
Capitulum
Trochlea
Head of radius
Neck of radius
Coronoid process
Tuberosity of radius
Tuberosity of ulna
Anterior oblique line
Ulna
Shaft of radius
Shaft of ulna
Radius
Styloid process of radius
Head of ulna articulating with ulnar notch of radius
Styloid process of ulna
Carpal bones
Proximal phalanx
Metacarpal bones
Distal phalanx
Proximal
Middle
Distal
Phalanges

6.3 FEATURES OF BONES OF UPPER LIMB

A. and B. Clavicle. **C.** Anterior aspect of disarticulated distal end of humerus and proximal end of radius and ulna. **D.** Anterior aspect of articulated upper limb.

E. Posterior View:
- Superior border
- Spine of scapula
- Superior angle
- Supraspinous fossa
- Head of scapula
- Neck of scapula
- Infraspinous fossa
- Medial (vertebral) border
- **Scapula**
- Lateral border
- Inferior angle
- Acromioclavicular joint
- Acromion
- Acromial angle
- Greater tubercle
- Head of humerus
- Surgical neck of humerus
- Anatomical neck of humerus
- Deltoid tuberosity
- Radial groove
- Shaft of humerus
- **Humerus**
- Medial supra-epicondylar ridge
- Lateral supra-epicondylar ridge
- Lateral epicondyle
- Medial epicondyle
- Head of radius
- Olecranon articulating with olecranon fossa of humerus
- Posterior oblique line
- Posterior border
- **Ulna**
- **Radius**
- Head of ulna
- Dorsal radial tubercle
- Styloid process
- Styloid process of radius
- **Carpal bones**
- **Metacarpal bones**
- 1, 2, 3, 4, 5
- Proximal phalanx
- Distal phalanx
- **Phalanges**: Proximal, Middle, Distal

E. Posterior View

F. Lateral View:
- Acromion
- Supraspinous fossa
- Supraglenoid tubercle
- Coracoid process
- Spine
- Glenoid cavity
- Infraglenoid tubercle
- Infraspinous fossa
- Lateral border
- Inferior angle

F. Lateral View

G. Posterior View:
- **Humerus**
- Olecranon fossa
- Medial epicondyle
- Lateral epicondyle
- Groove for ulnar nerve
- Trochlea
- Olecranon
- Head
- Neck
- Supinator crest
- Tuberosity
- Posterior border
- Posterior oblique line
- **Ulna**
- **Radius**

G. Posterior View

6.3 FEATURES OF BONES OF UPPER LIMB *(CONTINUED)*

E. Posterior aspect of articulated upper limb bones. **F.** Lateral aspect of scapula. **G.** Posterior aspect of disarticulated distal end of humerus and proximal ends of radius and ulna.

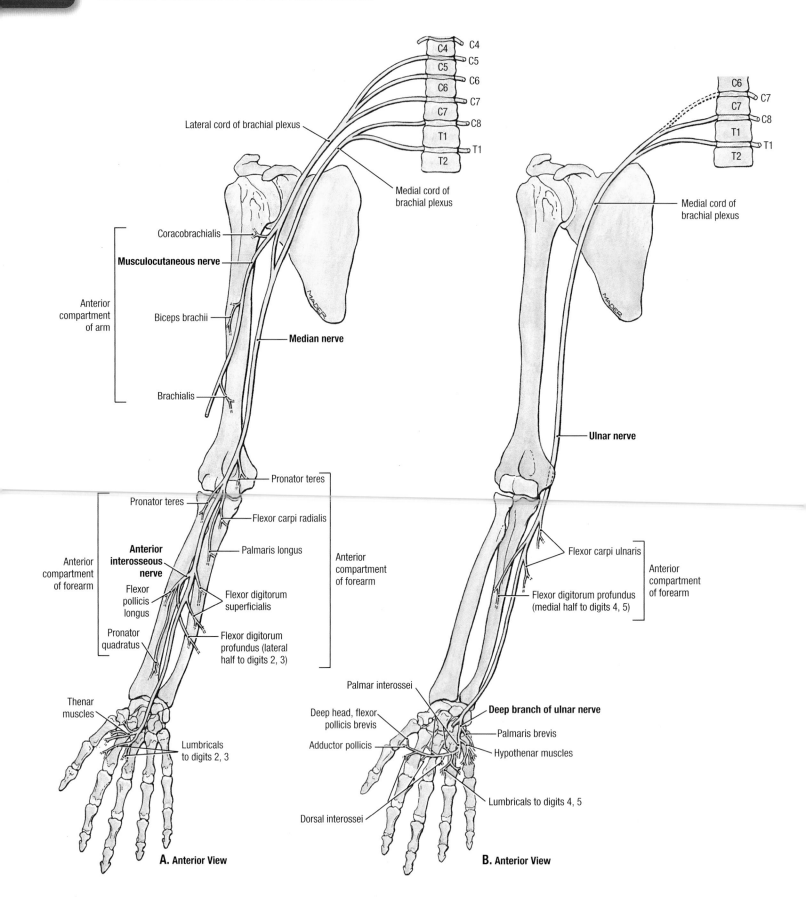

C4
C5
C6
C7
C8
T1
T2

C4
C5
C6
C7
C8
T1

Lateral cord of brachial plexus

Medial cord of brachial plexus

Coracobrachialis

Musculocutaneous nerve

Anterior compartment of arm

Biceps brachii

Median nerve

Brachialis

Pronator teres

Pronator teres

Flexor carpi radialis

Anterior interosseous nerve

Palmaris longus

Anterior compartment of forearm

Flexor pollicis longus

Flexor digitorum superficialis

Pronator quadratus

Flexor digitorum profundus (lateral half to digits 2, 3)

Thenar muscles

Lumbricals to digits 2, 3

A. Anterior View

C6
C7
C8
T1
T2

Medial cord of brachial plexus

Ulnar nerve

Flexor carpi ulnaris

Flexor digitorum profundus (medial half to digits 4, 5)

Anterior compartment of forearm

Palmar interossei

Deep head, flexor pollicis brevis

Deep branch of ulnar nerve

Adductor pollicis

Palmaris brevis

Hypothenar muscles

Lumbricals to digits 4, 5

Dorsal interossei

B. Anterior View

6.4 OVERVIEW OF MOTOR INNERVATION OF UPPER LIMB

C. Posterior View

6.4   OVERVIEW OF MOTOR INNERVATION OF UPPER LIMB *(CONTINUED)*

A. Musculocutaneous and median nerves. The musculocutaneous nerve innervates all the muscles of the anterior compartment of the arm. The median nerve innervates muscles of the anterior compartment of the forearm (with $1\frac{1}{2}$ exceptions that are innervated by the ulnar nerve), the lumbricals to digits 2 and 3, and the intrinsic muscles of the thumb (thenar muscles) with $1\frac{1}{2}$ exceptions that are innervated by the ulnar nerve. **B.** Ulnar nerve. The ulnar nerve innervates the flexor carpi ulnaris and ulnar half of the flexor digitorum profundus in the forearm, the hypothenar and interosseus muscles of the hand, the lumbricals to digits 3 and 4, and $1\frac{1}{2}$ thenar muscles (adductor pollicis and the deep head of the flexor pollicis brevis). **C.** Radial nerve. The radial nerve innervates all muscles of the posterior compartments of the arm and forearm.

Supraclavicular nerves (C3, C4)

Superior lateral cutaneous nerve of arm **(from axillary nerve)**

Intercostobrachial nerve

Medial cutaneous nerve of arm **(from medial cord of brachial plexus)**

Inferior lateral cutaneous nerve of arm **(from radial nerve)**

Posterior cutaneous nerve of forearm **(from radial nerve)**

Lateral cutaneous nerve of forearm **(from musculocutaneous nerve)**

Posterior cutaneous nerve of forearm **(from radial nerve)**

Lateral cutaneous nerve of forearm **(from musculo-cutaneous nerve)**

Posterior branch

Anterior branch

Radial nerve, superficial branch

Median nerve

Medial cutaneous nerve of forearm

Posterior branch

Medial cutaneous nerve of forearm **(from medial cord of brachial plexus)**

Anterior branch

Dorsal (cutaneous) branch of ulnar nerve

Ulnar nerve

Median nerve

Superficial branch of radial nerve

Palmar (cutaneous) branches of

Ulnar nerve, superficial branch

A. Anterior View

Supraclavicular nerves (C3, C4)

Superior lateral cutaneous nerve of arm **(from axillary nerve)**

Intercostobrachial nerve **(from 2nd/3rd intercostal nerve)**

Posterior cutaneous nerve of arm **(from radial nerve)**

Medial cutaneous nerve, of forearm, posterior branches

Inferior lateral cutaneous nerve of arm

Posterior cutaneous nerve of forearm

Posterior cutaneous nerve of forearm

From radial nerve

Lateral cutaneous nerve of forearm, posterior branch

Dorsal (cutaneous) branch of ulnar nerve

Dorsal digital branches

Radial nerve, superficial branch

Communicating branches

Median nerve, palmar digital branches

B. Posterior View

6.5   CUTANEOUS NERVES OF UPPER LIMB

TABLE 6.1 CUTANEOUS NERVES OF UPPER LIMB[a]

Nerve	Spinal Nerve components	Source	Course/Distribution
Supraclavicular nerves	C3–C4	Cervical plexus	Pass anterior to clavicle, immediately deep to platysma, and supply the skin over the clavicle and superolateral aspect of the pectoralis major muscle
Superior lateral cutaneous nerve of arm	C5–C6	Axillary nerve (posterior cord of brachial plexus)	Emerges from posterior margin of deltoid to supply skin over lower part of this muscle and the lateral side of the midarm
Inferior lateral cutaneous nerve of arm		Radial nerve (posterior cord of brachial plexus)	Arises with the posterior cutaneous nerve of forearm; pierces lateral head of triceps brachii to supply skin over the inferolateral aspect of the arm
Posterior cutaneous nerve of arm			Arises in axilla and supplies skin on posterior surface of the arm to olecranon
Posterior cutaneous nerve of forearm	C5–C8		Arises with the inferior lateral cutaneous nerve of the arm; pierces lateral head of triceps brachii to supply skin over the posterior aspect of the arm
Superficial branch of radial nerve			Arises in cubital fossa; supplies lateral (radial) half of the dorsal aspect of hand and thumb, and proximal portion of the dorsal aspects of digits 2 and 3, and the lateral (radial) half of dorsal aspect of digit 4
Lateral cutaneous nerve of forearm	C6–C7	Musculocutaneous nerve (lateral cord of brachial plexus)	Arises between biceps brachii and brachialis muscle as continuation of musculocutaneous nerve distal to branch to brachialis; emerges in cubital fossa lateral to biceps tendon and median cubital vein; supplies skin along radial (lateral) border of forearm to base of thenar eminence
Median nerve	C6–C7 (via lateral root); C8–T1 (via medial root)	Lateral and medial cords of brachial plexus	Courses with brachial artery in arm and deep to flexor digitorum superficialis in forearm; distal to origin of palmar cutaneous branch, traverses carpal tunnel to supply skin of palmar aspect of radial $3\frac{1}{2}$ digits and adjacent palm, plus distal dorsal aspects of same, including nail beds
Ulnar nerve	(C7), C8–T1		Courses with brachial, superior ulnar collateral, and ulnar arteries; supplies skin of palmar and dorsal aspects of medial (ulnar) $1\frac{1}{2}$ digits and palm and dorsum of hand proximal to those digits
Medial cutaneous nerve of forearm	C8–T1	Medial cord of brachial plexus	Pierces deep fascia with basilic vein in midarm; divides into anterior and posterior branches supplying skin over anterior and medial surfaces of forearm to wrist
Medial cutaneous nerve of arm	C8–T2		Smallest and most medial branch of brachial plexus; communicates with intercostobrachial nerve, then descends medial to brachial artery and basilic vein to innervate skin of distal medial arm
Intercostobrachial nerve	T2	Lateral cutaneous branch of 2nd intercostal nerve	Arises distal to angle of 2nd rib; supplies skin of axilla and proximal medial arm

[a]See Table 6.16 on Lesions of nerves of upper limb at end of chapter.

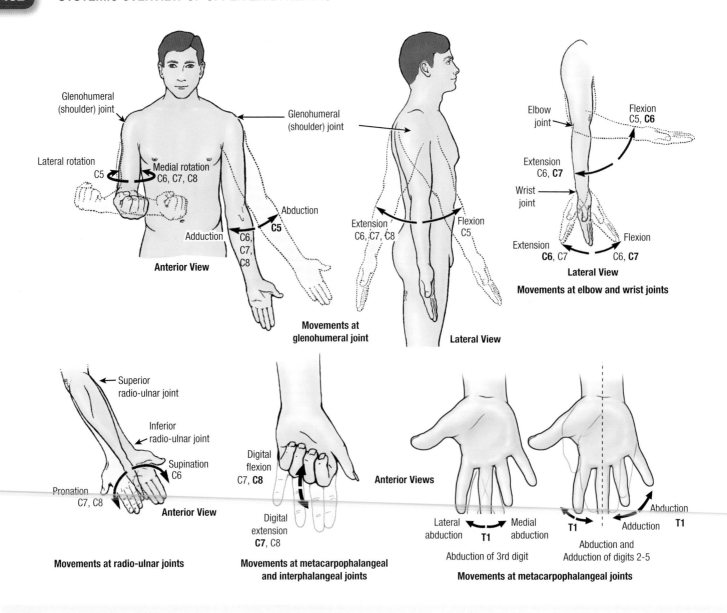

Glenohumeral (shoulder) joint

Glenohumeral (shoulder) joint

Lateral rotation C5

Medial rotation C6, C7, C8

Abduction C5

Adduction C6, C7, C8

Anterior View

Movements at glenohumeral joint

Extension C6, C7, C8

Flexion C5

Lateral View

Elbow joint

Flexion C5, **C6**

Extension C6, **C7**

Wrist joint

Extension **C6**, C7

Flexion C6, **C7**

Lateral View

Movements at elbow and wrist joints

Superior radio-ulnar joint

Inferior radio-ulnar joint

Supination C6

Pronation C7, C8

Anterior View

Movements at radio-ulnar joints

Digital flexion C7, **C8**

Digital extension **C7**, C8

Movements at metacarpophalangeal and interphalangeal joints

Anterior Views

Lateral abduction

Medial abduction

T1

Abduction of 3rd digit

T1

Adduction

T1

Abduction

Abduction and Adduction of digits 2-5

Movements at metacarpophalangeal joints

MYOTOMES AND MYOTATIC (DEEP TENDON STRETCH) REFLEXES

Myotomes. Somatic motor (general somatic efferent) fibers transmit impulses to skeletal (voluntary) muscles. The unilateral muscle mass receiving information from the somatic motor fibers conveyed by a single spinal nerve is a myotome. The movements associated with each bolded segment in Table 6.2 are most commonly tested to determine the neurologic level of a lesion.

Myotatic reflexes. A myotatic reflex (deep tendon or stretch reflex) is an involuntary contraction of a muscle in response to sudden stretching. Myotatic reflexes are elicited by briskly tapping the tendon with a reflex hammer. Each tendon reflex is mediated by specific spinal nerves. Stretch reflexes control muscle tone.

TABLE 6.2 *CLINICAL MANIFESTATIONS OF NERVE ROOT COMPRESSION: UPPER LIMB (UL)*

Herniated Disc Between	Compressed Nerve Roots	Dermatomes Affected	Muscles Affected	Movement Weakness	Nerve and Myotatic Reflex Involved
C4 and C5	**C5**	C5 Shoulder Lateral surface UL	Deltoid	Abduction of shoulder	Axillary nerve ↓ Biceps jerk
C5 and C6	**C6**	C6 Thumb	Biceps Brachialis Brachioradialis	Flexion of elbow Supination/pronation of forearm	Musculocutaneous nerve ↓ Biceps jerk ↓ Brachioradialis jerk
C6 and C7	**C7**	C7 Posterior surface UL Middle and index fingers	Triceps Wrist extensors	Extension of elbow Extension of wrist	Radial nerve ↓ Triceps reflex

TABLE 6.3 *DERMATOMES OF UPPER LIMB*

Spinal Segment/Nerve(s)	Description of Dermatome(s)
C3, C4	Region at base of neck extending laterally over shoulder
C5	Lateral aspect of arm (i.e., superior aspect of abducted arm)
C6	Lateral forearm and thumb
C7	Middle and ring fingers (or middle 3 fingers) and center of posterior aspect of forearm
C8	Little finger, medial side of hand and forearm (i.e., inferior aspect of abducted arm)
T1	Medial aspect of forearm and inferior arm
T2	Medial aspect of superior arm and skin of axilla[a]

[a]Not indicated on the Keegan and Garrett dermatome map. However, pain experienced during a heart attack, considered to be mediated by T1 and T2, is commonly described as "radiating down the medial side of the left arm").

A. Anterior View

B. Posterior View

C. Anterior View

D. Posterior View

6.7 DERMATOMES OF UPPER LIMB

The dermatomal or segmental pattern of distribution of sensory nerve fibers persists despite the merging of spinal nerves in plexus formation during development. Two different dermatome maps are commonly used. **A.** and **B.** The dermatome pattern of the upper limb according to Foerster (1933) is preferred by many because of its correlation with clinical findings. In the Foerster schema, dermatomes C6–T1 are displaced from the trunk to limbs. **C.** and **D.** The dermatome pattern of the upper limb according to Keegan and Garrett (1948) is preferred by others for its correlation with development. Although depicted as distinct zones, adjacent dermatomes overlap considerably except along the axial line.

Superficial cervical artery
Dorsal scapular artery
Suprascapular artery
Axillary artery
(begins lateral to
border of 1st rib)
Thoraco-acromial artery
Posterior
Circumflex humeral artery
Anterior
Deltoid (ascending) branch
Brachial artery
(begins at inferior
border of teres major)
Profunda brachii
artery (deep artery
of arm)
Collateral arteries { Middle / Radial }
Radial recurrent artery
Common interosseous artery
Radial artery
Ulnar artery
Anterior interosseous artery
Deep palmar arch
Superficial palmar arch

Cervicodorsal trunk*
Thyrocervical trunk
Vertebral artery
Right subclavian artery
Right and left common carotid arteries
Left subclavian artery
Brachiocephalic trunk
Arch of aorta
1st rib
Subscapular artery
Internal thoracic artery
Lateral thoracic artery
Superior ulnar collateral artery
Inferior ulnar collateral artery
Anterior / Posterior } Ulnar recurrent arteries

A. Anterior View

6.8 ARTERIES AND ARTERIAL ANASTOMOSES OF UPPER LIMB

A. The arteries often anastomose or communicate to form networks to ensure blood supply distal to the joint throughout the range of movement. **Arterial occlusion.** If a main channel is occluded, the smaller alternate channels can usually increase in size, providing a collateral circulation that ensures the blood supply to structures distal to the blockage. However, collateral pathways require time to develop; they are usually insufficient to compensate for sudden occlusions.

*See Weiglein AH, Moriggl B, Schalk C, Künzel KH, Müller U. Arteries in the posterior cervical triangle in man. *Clin Anat* 2005 Nov;18(8):553-557.

B. Posterior View

- Dorsal scapular artery
- Levator scapulae
- Rhomboid minor
- Anastomoses with intercostal arteries
- Suprascapular artery
- Axillary artery
- Subscapular artery
- Circumflex scapular artery
- Thoracodorsal artery
- Brachial artery
- Teres major

C. Anterior View

- Teres major
- Deltoid branch
- **Brachial artery**
- Profunda brachii artery (deep artery of arm)
- Superior ulnar collateral artery
- Inferior ulnar collateral artery
- Collateral arteries { Middle / Radial }
- Radial recurrent artery
- **Ulnar artery**
- **Radial artery**
- Anterior
- Posterior } Ulnar recurrent arteries
- Recurrent
- Common
- Anterior
- Posterior } Interosseous arteries

D — **Anterior View (Palmar Aspect)**

- Radial artery
- Ulnar artery
- Superficial palmar branch
- Radial artery
- Princeps pollicis
- Radialis indicis
- Anterior interosseous artery
- **Palmar carpal arch**
- **Deep palmar arch**
- Palmar metacarpal arteries
- **Superficial palmar arch**
- Common palmar digital arteries
- Proper palmar digital artery gives rise to a dorsal branch

Lateral View (isolated third digit)

- Radius
- Posterior interosseous artery
- Anterior interosseous artery
- Dorsal carpal branch of ulnar artery
- **Dorsal carpal arch**
- Perforating branches
- Dorsal metacarpal arteries
- Dorsal digital arteries
- Dorsal branches of proper palmar digital arteries

Posterior View (Dorsum of Hand)

- Radial artery
- Dorsal carpal branch
- Dorsalis pollicis
- Dorsalis indicis

6.8 ARTERIES AND ARTERIAL ANASTOMOSES OF UPPER LIMB *(CONTINUED)*

B. Scapular anastomoses. **C.** Anastomoses of the elbow. **D.** Anastomoses of the hand. Joints receive blood from articular arteries that arise from vessels around joints.

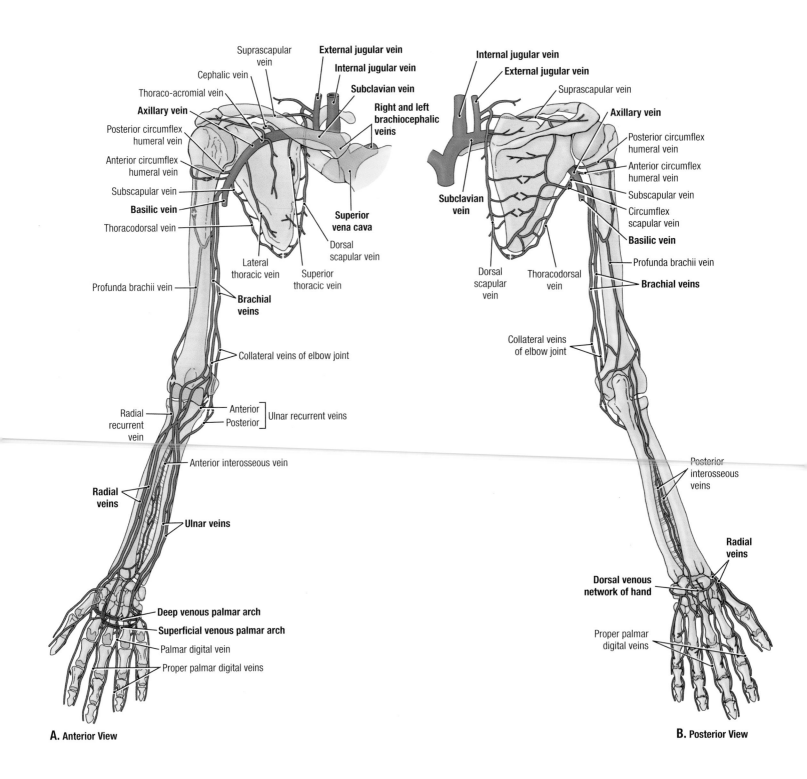

Suprascapular vein

Cephalic vein

Thoraco-acromial vein

Axillary vein

Posterior circumflex humeral vein

Anterior circumflex humeral vein

Subscapular vein

Basilic vein

Thoracodorsal vein

Profunda brachii vein

External jugular vein

Internal jugular vein

Subclavian vein

Right and left brachiocephalic veins

Superior vena cava

Dorsal scapular vein

Lateral thoracic vein

Superior thoracic vein

Brachial veins

Collateral veins of elbow joint

Radial recurrent vein

Anterior
Posterior } Ulnar recurrent veins

Anterior interosseous vein

Radial veins

Ulnar veins

Deep venous palmar arch

Superficial venous palmar arch

Palmar digital vein

Proper palmar digital veins

A. Anterior View

Internal jugular vein

External jugular vein

Suprascapular vein

Axillary vein

Posterior circumflex humeral vein

Anterior circumflex humeral vein

Subscapular vein

Circumflex scapular vein

Basilic vein

Profunda brachii vein

Brachial veins

Subclavian vein

Dorsal scapular vein

Thoracodorsal vein

Collateral veins of elbow joint

Posterior interosseous veins

Radial veins

Dorsal venous network of hand

Proper palmar digital veins

B. Posterior View

6.9   OVERVIEW OF DEEP VEINS OF UPPER LIMB

Deep veins lie internal to the deep fascia and occur as paired, continually interanastomosing "accompanying veins" (L., *venae comitantes*) surrounding and sharing the name of the artery they accompany.

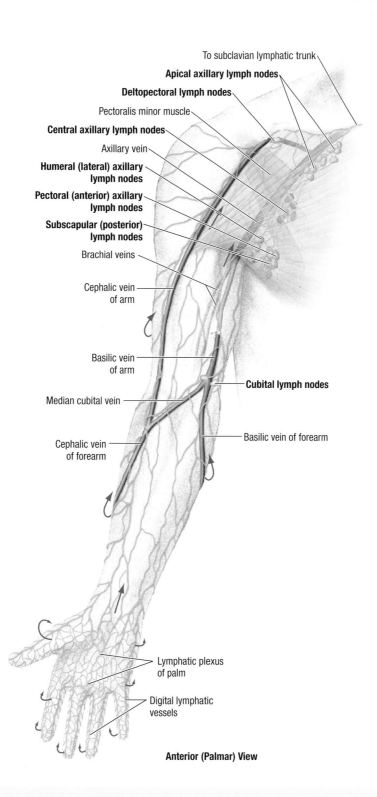

To subclavian lymphatic trunk

Apical axillary lymph nodes

Deltopectoral lymph nodes

Pectoralis minor muscle

Central axillary lymph nodes

Axillary vein

Humeral (lateral) axillary lymph nodes

Pectoral (anterior) axillary lymph nodes

Subscapular (posterior) lymph nodes

Brachial veins

Cephalic vein of arm

Basilic vein of arm

Cubital lymph nodes

Median cubital vein

Basilic vein of forearm

Cephalic vein of forearm

Lymphatic plexus of palm

Digital lymphatic vessels

Anterior (Palmar) View

6.10   SUPERFICIAL VENOUS AND LYMPHATIC DRAINAGE OF UPPER LIMB

Superficial lymphatic vessels arise from lymphatic plexuses in the digits, palm, and dorsum of the hand and ascend with the superficial veins of the upper limb. The superficial lymphatic vessels ascend through the forearm and arm, converging toward the cephalic and especially to the basilic vein to reach the axillary lymph nodes. Some lymph passes through the cubital nodes at the elbow and the deltopectoral (infraclavicular) nodes at the shoulder. Deep lymphatic vessels accompany the neurovascular bundles of the upper limb and end primarily in the humeral (lateral) and central axillary lymph nodes.

Deltoid

Pectoralis major

Clavipectoral (deltopectoral) triangle

Cephalic vein

Basilic vein

Median cubital vein

Median vein of forearm

Cephalic vein of forearm

Basilic vein of forearm

Perforating veins

A. Anterior View

Dorsal digital veins

Dorsal digital venous arches

Superficial dorsal veins

Dorsal venous network of hand

Basilic vein

Cephalic vein

B. Posterior View

Palmar digital veins

Transverse anastomoses

Basilic vein

Cephalic vein

C. Anterior View

6.11   SUPERFICIAL VENOUS DRAINAGE OF UPPER LIMB

A. Forearm, arm, and pectoral region. **B.** Dorsal surface of hand. **C.** Palmar surface of hand. The *arrows* indicate where perforating veins penetrate the deep fascia. Blood is continuously shunted from these superficial veins in the subcutaneous tissue to deep veins via the perforating veins.

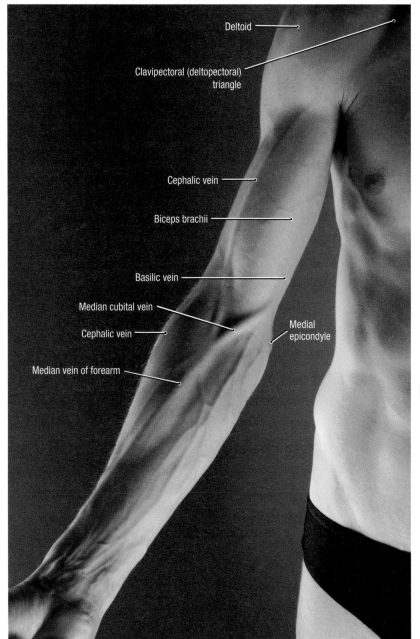

Deltoid

Clavipectoral (deltopectoral)
triangle

Cephalic vein

Biceps brachii

Basilic vein

Median cubital vein

Cephalic vein

Median vein of forearm

Medial
epicondyle

D. Anterior View

Superficial
dorsal veins

Cephalic
vein

Dorsal venous
network of hand

E. Posterior View

6.11   SUPERFICIAL VENOUS DRAINAGE OF UPPER LIMB *(CONTINUED)*

D. Surface anatomy of veins of forearm and arm. **E.** Surface anatomy of veins of the dorsal surface of hand.

Because of the prominence and accessibility of the superficial veins, they are commonly used for **venipuncture** (puncture of a vein to draw blood or inject a solution). By applying a tourniquet to the arm, the venous return is occluded, and the veins distend and usually are visible and/or palpable. Once a vein is punctured, the tourniquet is removed so that when the needle is removed the vein will not bleed extensively. The median cubital vein is commonly used for venipuncture. The veins forming the dorsal venous network of the hand and the cephalic and basilic veins arising from it are commonly used for long-term introduction of fluids **(intravenous feeding)**. The cubital veins are also a site for the **introduction of cardiac catheters** to secure blood samples from the great vessels and chambers of the heart.

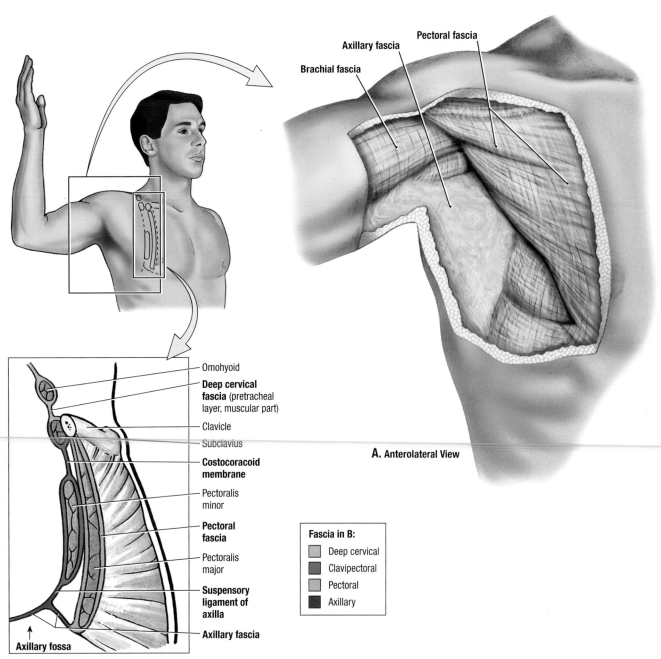

A. Anterolateral View

B. Sagittal Section

Fascia in B:
- Deep cervical
- Clavipectoral
- Pectoral
- Axillary

6.12   DEEP FASCIA OF UPPER LIMB—AXILLARY AND CLAVIPECTORAL FASCIA

A. Axillary fascia. The axillary fascia forms the floor of the axillary fossa and is continuous with the pectoral fascia covering the pectoralis major muscle and the brachial fascia of the arm. **B.** Clavipectoral fascia. The clavipectoral fascia extends from the axillary fascia to enclose the pectoralis minor and subclavius muscles and then attaches to the clavicle. The part of the clavipectoral fascia superior to the pectoralis minor is the costocoracoid membrane, and the part of the clavipectoral fascia inferior to the pectoralis minor is the suspensory ligament of the axilla. The suspensory ligament of the axilla, an extension of the axillary fascia, supports the axillary fascia and pulls the axillary fascia and the skin inferior to it superiorly when the arm is abducted, forming the axillary fossa or "armpit."

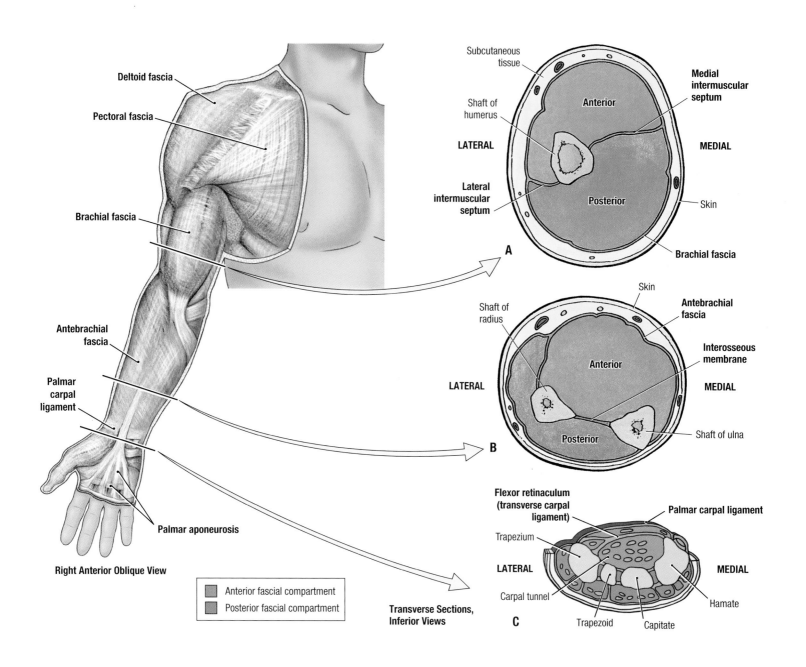

Right Anterior Oblique View

Anterior fascial compartment
Posterior fascial compartment

Transverse Sections, Inferior Views

6.13   DEEP FASCIA OF UPPER LIMB, BRACHIAL AND ANTEBRACHIAL FASCIA

A. Brachial fascia. The brachial fascia is the deep fascia of the arm and is continuous superiorly with the pectoral and axillary layers of fascia. Medial and lateral intermuscular septa extend from the deep aspect of the brachial fascia to the humerus, dividing the arm into anterior and posterior musculofascial compartments. **B.** Antebrachial fascia. The antebrachial fascia surrounds the forearm and is continuous with the brachial fascia and deep fascia of the hand. The interosseous membrane separates the forearm into anterior and posterior musculofascial compartments. Distally the fascia thickens to form the palmar carpal ligament, which is continuous with the flexor retinaculum and dorsally with the extensor expansion. The deep fascia of the hand is continuous with the antebrachial fascia, and on the palmar surface of the hand it thickens to form the palmar aponeurosis. **C.** Flexor retinaculum (transverse carpal ligament). The flexor retinaculum extends between the medial and lateral carpal bones to form the carpal tunnel.

Supraclavicular nerves (C3 and C4)

Platysma (reflected superiorly)

Clavicle

Deltoid

Clavipectoral (deltopectoral) triangle

Cephalic vein

Cephalic vein in deltopectoral groove

Clavicular head of pectoralis major

Intercostobrachial nerve (T2)

Sternocostal head of pectoralis major

Posterior branch of lateral pectoral cutaneous branch of intercostal nerve

Lateral mammary branch of lateral pectoral cutaneous branches of intercostal nerve

Serratus anterior

Abdominal part of pectoralis major

Platysma

Pectoral fascia covering pectoralis major

Subcutaneous tissue

Lateral mammary branches of lateral pectoral cutaneous branches of intercostal nerves

Medial mammary branches of anterior pectoral cutaneous branches of intercostal nerves

Anterior View

6.14   SUPERFICIAL DISSECTION, MALE PECTORAL REGION

- The platysma muscle, which usually descends to the 2nd or 3rd rib, is cut short on the right side and, together with the supraclavicular nerves, is reflected on the left side.
- The exposed intermuscular bony strip of the clavicle is subcutaneous and subplatysmal.
- The cephalic vein passes deeply to join the axillary vein in the clavipectoral (deltopectoral) triangle.
- The cutaneous innervation of the pectoral region by the supraclavicular nerves (C3 and C4) and upper thoracic nerves (T2–T6); the brachial plexus (C5–T1) does not supply cutaneous branches to the pectoral region.

Anterior axillary fold

Deltoid

Deltopectoral groove

Clavipectoral (deltopectoral) triangle

Clavicle

Suprasternal (jugular) notch

Clavicle

Posterior axillary fold

Axillary fossa

Serratus anterior

Abdominal part of pectoralis major

Sternocostal head of pectoralis major

Clavicular head of pectoralis major

6.15 SURFACE ANATOMY, MALE PECTORAL REGION

The clavipectoral (deltopectoral) triangle is the depressed area just inferior to the lateral part of the clavicle, bounded by the clavicle superiorly, the deltoid laterally, and the clavicular head of pectoralis major medially. The clavipectoral triangle and the intermuscular deltopectoral groove extending from its inferior apex demarcate an "internervous plane" (plane not crossed by motor nerves) for an **anterior or deltopectoral surgical incision** to approach to the axilla, shoulder joint, or proximal humerus.

When the arm is abducted and then adducted against resistance, the two heads of the pectoralis major are visible and palpable. As this muscle extends from the thoracic wall to the arm, it forms the anterior axillary fold. Digitations of the serratus anterior appear inferolateral to the pectoralis major. The coracoid process of the scapula is covered by the anterior part of deltoid; however, the tip of the process can be felt on deep palpation in the clavipectoral triangle. The deltoid forms the contour of the shoulder.

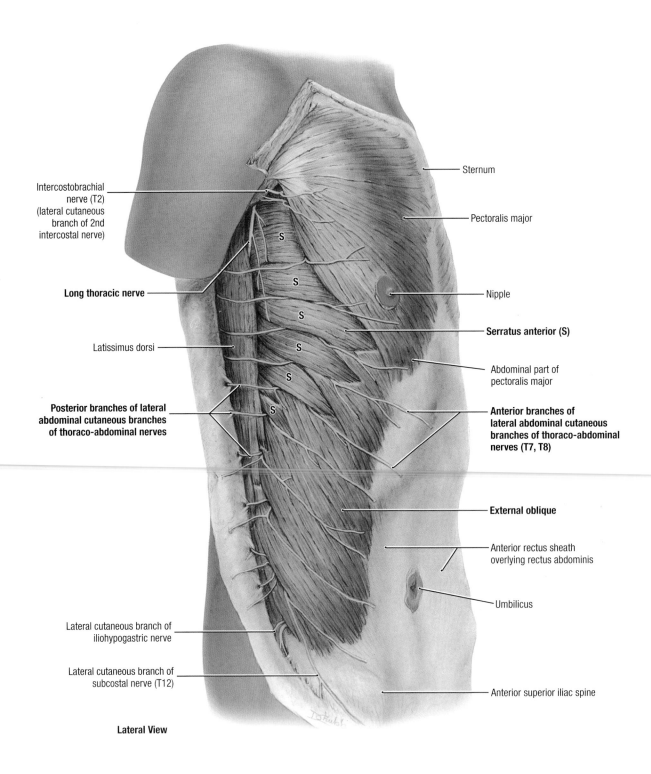

Intercostobrachial nerve (T2) (lateral cutaneous branch of 2nd intercostal nerve)

Long thoracic nerve

Latissimus dorsi

Posterior branches of lateral abdominal cutaneous branches of thoraco-abdominal nerves

Lateral cutaneous branch of iliohypogastric nerve

Lateral cutaneous branch of subcostal nerve (T12)

Sternum

Pectoralis major

Nipple

Serratus anterior (S)

Abdominal part of pectoralis major

Anterior branches of lateral abdominal cutaneous branches of thoraco-abdominal nerves (T7, T8)

External oblique

Anterior rectus sheath overlying rectus abdominis

Umbilicus

Anterior superior iliac spine

Lateral View

6.16   SUPERFICIAL DISSECTION OF TRUNK

- The slips of the serratus anterior interdigitate with the external oblique.
- The long thoracic nerve (nerve to serratus anterior) lies on the lateral (superficial) aspect of the serratus anterior; this nerve is vulnerable to damage from **stab wounds** and during surgery (e.g., radical mastectomy).
- The anterior and posterior branches of the lateral thoracic and abdominal cutaneous branches of intercostal and thoraco-abdominal nerves are dissected.

Axillary fossa

Posterior axillary fold

Anterior axillary fold

Latissimus dorsi

Serratus anterior

External oblique

Anterolateral View

Clavicular head of pectoralis major

Sternocostal head of pectoralis major

Body of sternum

Nipple

Abdominal part of pectoralis major

External oblique

Site of anterior rectus sheath overlaying rectus abdominis

Umbilicus

Linea semilunaris

Anterior superior iliac spine

6.17 | **SURFACE ANATOMY OF ANTEROLATERAL ASPECT OF TRUNK**

When the arm is abducted and then adducted against resistance, the sternocostal part of the pectoralis major can be seen and palpated. If the anterior axillary fold bounding the axilla is grasped between the fingers and thumb, the inferior border of the sternocostal head of the pectoralis major can be felt. Several digitations of the serratus anterior are visible inferior to the anterior axillary fold. The posterior axillary fold is composed of skin and muscular tissue (latissimus dorsi and teres major) bounding the axilla posteriorly.

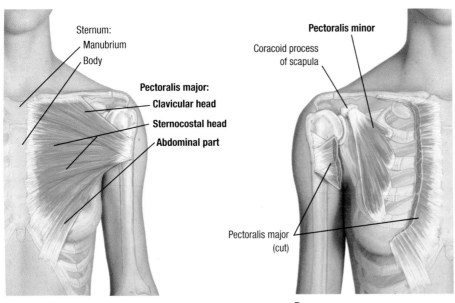

A. Anterior View

B. Anterior View

C. Anterior View

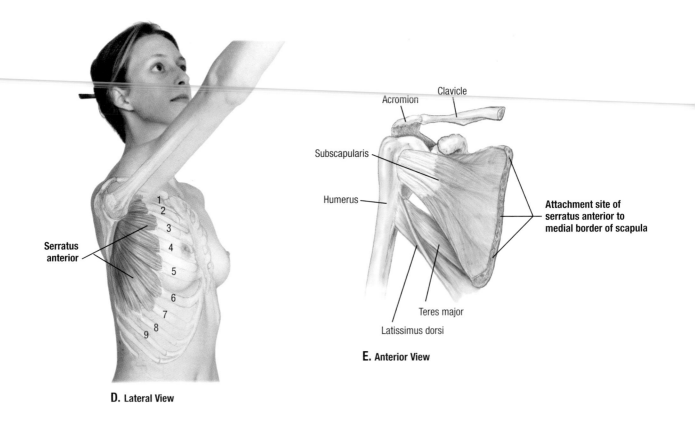

D. Lateral View

E. Anterior View

6.18   PECTORALIS MAJOR AND MINOR AND SERRATUS ANTERIOR

A. Pectoralis major. **B.** Pectoralis minor. **C.** Subclavius. **D. and E.** Serratus anterior and its scapular attachment.

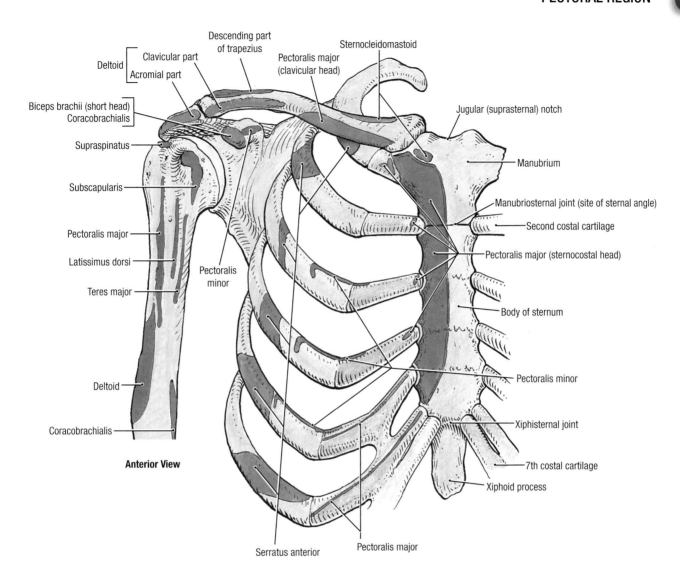

Descending part of trapezius

Clavicular part

Deltoid

Acromial part

Biceps brachii (short head)
Coracobrachialis

Supraspinatus

Subscapularis

Pectoralis major

Latissimus dorsi

Teres major

Pectoralis minor

Deltoid

Coracobrachialis

Anterior View

Serratus anterior

Pectoralis major (clavicular head)

Sternocleidomastoid

Jugular (suprasternal) notch

Manubrium

Manubriosternal joint (site of sternal angle)

Second costal cartilage

Pectoralis major (sternocostal head)

Body of sternum

Pectoralis minor

Xiphisternal joint

7th costal cartilage

Xiphoid process

Pectoralis major

6.19   ANTERIOR ATTACHMENTS OF ANTERIOR AND POSTERIOR AXIO-APPENDICULAR AND SCAPULOHUMERAL MUSCLES

TABLE 6.4 ANTERIOR AXIO-APPENDICULAR MUSCLES

Muscle	Proximal Attachment (*red*)	Distal Attachment (*blue*)	Innervation[a]	Main Actions
Pectoralis major	*Clavicular head:* anterior surface of medial half of clavicle *Sternocostal head:* anterior surface of sternum, superior six costal cartilages *Abdominal part:* aponeurosis of external oblique muscle	Crest of greater tubercle of intertubercular sulcus (lateral lip of bicipital groove)	Lateral and medial pectoral nerves; clavicular head (C5 and **C6**), sternocostal head (**C7, C8**, and T1)	Adducts and medially rotates humerus at shoulder joint; draws scapula anteriorly and inferiorly Acting alone: clavicular head flexes shoulder joint, and sternocostal head extends it from the flexed position
Pectoralis minor	3rd to 5th ribs near their costal cartilages	Medial border and superior surface of coracoid process of scapula	Medial pectoral nerve (C8 and T1)	Stabilizes scapula by drawing it inferiorly and anteriorly against thoracic wall
Subclavius	Junction of 1st rib and its costal cartilage	Inferior surface of middle third of clavicle	Nerve to subclavius (**C5** and C6)	Anchors and depresses clavicle at sternoclavicular joint
Serratus anterior	External surfaces of lateral parts of 1st to 8th–9th ribs	Anterior surface of medial border of scapula (see Fig. 6.18E.)	Long thoracic nerve (C5, **C6**, and **C7**)	Protracts scapula and holds it against thoracic wall; rotates scapula

[a]Numbers indicate spinal cord segmental innervation (e.g., C5 and C6 indicate that nerves supplying the clavicular head of pectoralis major are derived from 5th and 6th cervical segments of spinal cord). Boldface numbers indicate the main segmental innervation. Damage to these segments or to motor nerve roots arising from them results in paralysis of the muscles concerned.

Pectoralis minor

Deltoid branch of
thoraco-acromial artery

Acromial branches
of thoraco-acromial vein
and artery

Thoraco-acromial artery

Lateral pectoral nerve

Deltoid

Clavicular branch of
thoraco-acromial artery

Clavipectoral fascia
(costocoracoid membrane)

Cephalic vein

Medial pectoral
nerve

Clavicular head of
pectoralis major

Posterior tendon

Pectoral branches of
thoraco-acromial artery

Anterior tendon

Sternocostal head of
pectoralis major

Latissimus dorsi

Anterior View

6.20   ANTERIOR WALL OF AXILLA AND CLAVIPECTORAL FASCIA

A. Anterior wall of axilla. The clavicular head of the pectoralis major is excised, except for two cubes of muscle
that remain to identify the branches of the lateral pectoral nerve.
- The clavipectoral fascia superior to the pectoralis minor (costocoracoid membrane) is pierced by the
cephalic vein, the lateral pectoral nerve, and the thoraco-acromial vessels.
- The pectoralis minor and clavipectoral fascia are pierced by the medial pectoral nerve.
- Observe the insertion of the pectoralis major from deep to superficial: inferior part of the sternocostal head,
superior part of the sternocostal head (posterior tendon), and clavicular head (anterior tendon)

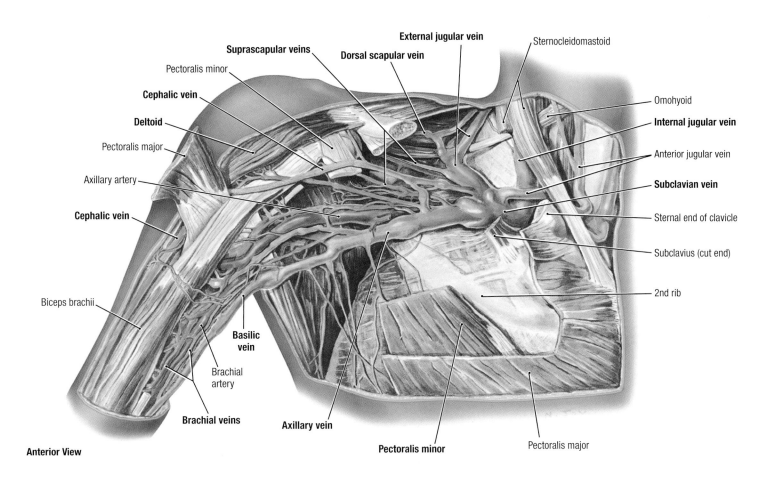

Anterior View

6.21 VEINS OF AXILLA

- The basilic vein joins the brachial veins to become the axillary vein near the inferior border of teres major, the axillary vein becomes the subclavian vein at the lateral border of the 1st rib, and the subclavian joins the internal jugular to become the brachiocephalic vein posterior to the sternal end of the clavicle.
- Numerous valves, enlargements in the vein, are shown.
- The cephalic vein in this specimen bifurcates to end in the axillary and external jugular veins.

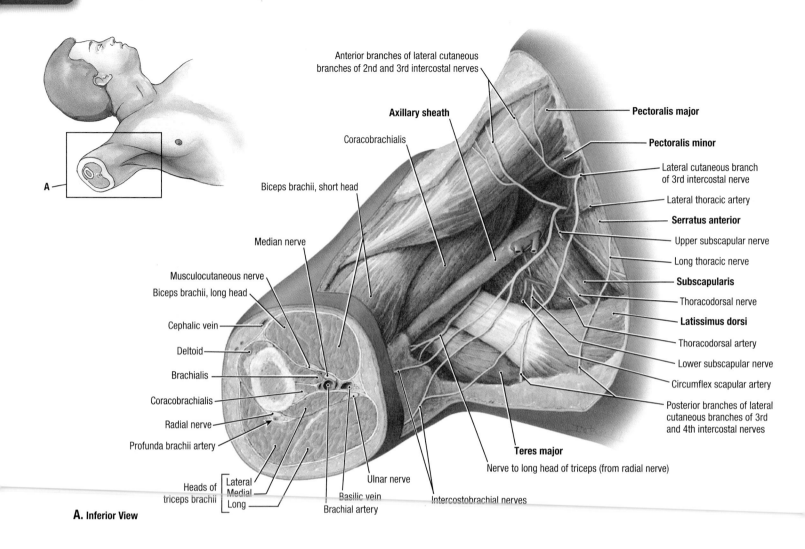

Anterior branches of lateral cutaneous branches of 2nd and 3rd intercostal nerves

Axillary sheath

Coracobrachialis

Biceps brachii, short head

Median nerve

Musculocutaneous nerve

Biceps brachii, long head

Cephalic vein

Deltoid

Brachialis

Coracobrachialis

Radial nerve

Profunda brachii artery

Heads of triceps brachii { Lateral / Medial / Long }

Ulnar nerve

Basilic vein

Brachial artery

Intercostobrachial nerves

Pectoralis major

Pectoralis minor

Lateral cutaneous branch of 3rd intercostal nerve

Lateral thoracic artery

Serratus anterior

Upper subscapular nerve

Long thoracic nerve

Subscapularis

Thoracodorsal nerve

Latissimus dorsi

Thoracodorsal artery

Lower subscapular nerve

Circumflex scapular artery

Posterior branches of lateral cutaneous branches of 3rd and 4th intercostal nerves

Teres major

Nerve to long head of triceps (from radial nerve)

A. Inferior View

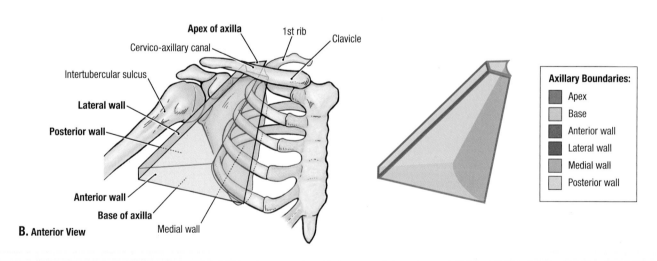

Apex of axilla   1st rib   Clavicle

Cervico-axillary canal

Intertubercular sulcus

Lateral wall

Posterior wall

Anterior wall

Base of axilla

Medial wall

B. Anterior View

Axillary Boundaries:
- Apex
- Base
- Anterior wall
- Lateral wall
- Medial wall
- Posterior wall

6.22   WALLS AND CONTENTS OF THE AXILLA

A. Dissection. **B.** Location and walls of axilla, schematic diagram.
- The walls of the axilla are anterior (formed by the pectoralis major, pectoralis minor, and subclavius muscles), posterior (formed by subscapularis, latissimus dorsi, and teres major muscles), medial (formed by the serratus anterior muscle), and lateral (formed by the intertubercular sulcus [bicipital groove] of the humerus [concealed by the biceps and coracobrachialis muscles]).
- The axillary sheath surrounds the nerves and vessels (neurovascular bundle) of the upper limb.

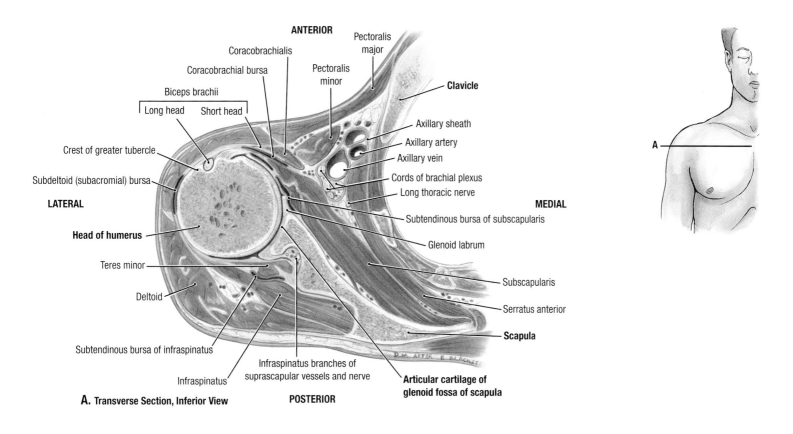

A. Transverse Section, Inferior View

B. Transverse Section, Inferior View

C. Transverse Section, Inferior View

6.23   TRANSVERSE SECTIONS THROUGH SHOULDER JOINT AND AXILLA

A. Anatomical section. **B.** Walls of axilla, schematic illustration. **C.** Walls and contents of axilla, schematic illustration.

- The intertubercular sulcus (bicipital groove) containing the tendon of the long head of the biceps brachii muscle is directed anteriorly; the short head of the biceps muscle and the coracobrachialis and pectoralis minor muscles are sectioned just inferior to their attachments to the coracoid process.
- The small glenoid cavity is deepened by the glenoid labrum.

- Bursae include the subdeltoid (subacromial) bursa, between the deltoid and greater tubercle; the subtendinous bursa of subscapularis, between the subscapularis tendon and scapula; and coracobrachial bursa, between the coracobrachialis and subscapularis.
- The axillary sheath encloses the axillary artery and vein and the three cords of the brachial plexus to form a neurovascular bundle, surrounded by axillary fat.

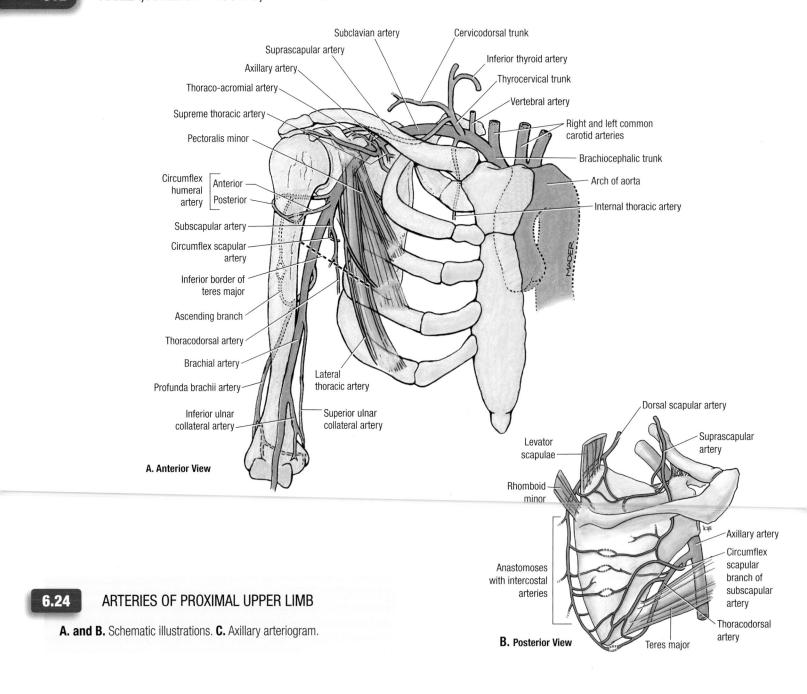

Subclavian artery
Suprascapular artery
Axillary artery
Thoraco-acromial artery
Supreme thoracic artery
Pectoralis minor
Circumflex humeral artery — Anterior / Posterior
Subscapular artery
Circumflex scapular artery
Inferior border of teres major
Ascending branch
Thoracodorsal artery
Brachial artery
Profunda brachii artery
Inferior ulnar collateral artery
Superior ulnar collateral artery
Lateral thoracic artery

Cervicodorsal trunk
Inferior thyroid artery
Thyrocervical trunk
Vertebral artery
Right and left common carotid arteries
Brachiocephalic trunk
Arch of aorta
Internal thoracic artery

A. Anterior View

Dorsal scapular artery
Suprascapular artery
Levator scapulae
Rhomboid minor
Anastomoses with intercostal arteries
Axillary artery
Circumflex scapular branch of subscapular artery
Thoracodorsal artery
Teres major

B. Posterior View

6.24 ARTERIES OF PROXIMAL UPPER LIMB

A. and B. Schematic illustrations. **C.** Axillary arteriogram.

TABLE 6.5 *ARTERIES OF PROXIMAL UPPER LIMB (SHOULDER REGION AND ARM)*

Artery	Origin	Course
Internal thoracic	Subclavian artery	Descends, inclining anteromedially, posterior to sternal end of clavicle and first costal cartilage; enters thorax to descend in parasternal plane; gives rise to perforating branches, anterior intercostal, musculophrenic, and superior epigastric arteries
Thyrocervical trunk		Ascends as a short, wide trunk, often giving rise to the suprascapular artery and/or cervicodorsal trunk and terminating by bifurcating into the ascending cervical and inferior thyroid arteries
Suprascapular	Cervicodorsal trunk from thyrocervical trunk (or as direct branch of subclavian artery[a])	Passes inferolaterally over anterior scalene muscle and phrenic nerve, subclavian artery and brachial plexus running laterally posterior and parallel to clavicle; next passes over transverse scapular ligament to supraspinous fossa, then lateral to scapular spine (deep to acromion) to infraspinous fossa

[a]See Weiglein AH, Moriggl B, Schalk C, et al. Arteries in the posterior cervical triangle. *Clinical Anatomy* 2005;18:533–537.

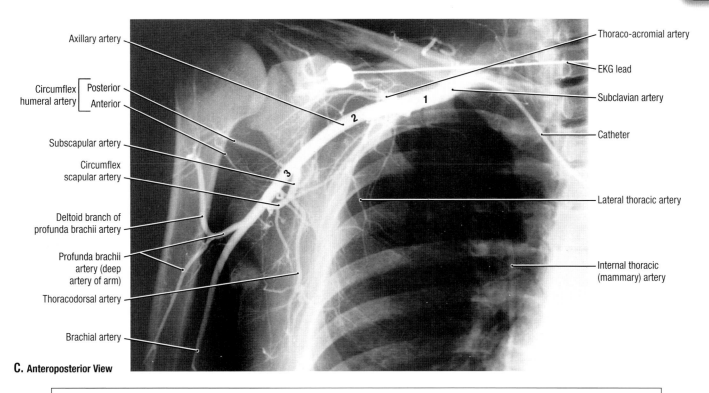

Axillary artery

Circumflex humeral artery — Posterior / Anterior

Subscapular artery

Circumflex scapular artery

Deltoid branch of profunda brachii artery

Profunda brachii artery (deep artery of arm)

Thoracodorsal artery

Brachial artery

Thoraco-acromial artery

EKG lead

Subclavian artery

Catheter

Lateral thoracic artery

Internal thoracic (mammary) artery

C. Anteroposterior View

1: First part of the axillary artery is located between the lateral border of the 1st rib and the medial border of pectoralis minor.

2: Second part of the axillary artery lies posterior to pectoralis minor.

3: Third part of the axillary artery extends from the lateral border of pectoralis minor to the inferior border of teres major, where it becomes the brachial artery.

TABLE 6.5 ARTERIES OF PROXIMAL UPPER LIMB (SHOULDER REGION AND ARM) (CONTINUED)

Artery	Origin		Course
Supreme thoracic	1st part (as only branch)		Runs anteromedially along superior border of pectoralis minor; then passes between it and pectoralis major to thoracic wall; helps supply 1st and 2nd intercostal spaces and superior part of serratus anterior
Thoraco-acromial	2nd part (medial branch)	Axillary artery	Curls around superomedial border of pectoralis minor, pierces costocoracoid membrane (clavipectoral fascia), and divides into four branches: pectoral, deltoid, acromial, and clavicular
Lateral thoracic	2nd part (lateral branch)		Descends along axillary border of pectoralis minor; follows it onto thoracic wall, supplying lateral aspect of breast
Circumflex humeral (anterior and posterior)	3rd part (sometimes via a common trunk)		Encircle surgical neck of humerus, anastomosing with each other laterally; larger posterior branch traverses quadrangular space
Subscapular	3rd part (largest branch)		Descends from level of inferior border of subscapularis along lateral border of scapula, dividing within 2–3 cm into terminal branches, the circumflex scapular and thoracodorsal arteries
Circumflex scapular	Subscapular artery		Curves around lateral border of scapula to enter infraspinous fossa, anastomosing with subscapular artery
Thoracodorsal	Near its origin		Continuation of subscapular artery; accompanies thoracodorsal nerve to enter latissimus dorsi
Profunda brachii (deep brachial) artery	Near middle of arm	Brachial artery	Accompanies radial nerve through radial groove of humerus, supplying posterior compartment of arm and participating in peri-articular arterial anastomosis around elbow joint
Superior ulnar collateral	Inferior to teres major		Accompanies ulnar nerve to posterior aspect of elbow; anastomoses with posterior ulnar recurrent artery
Inferior ulnar collateral	Superior to medial epicondyle of humerus		Passes anterior to medial epicondyle of humerus to anastomose with anterior ulnar collateral artery around elbow joint

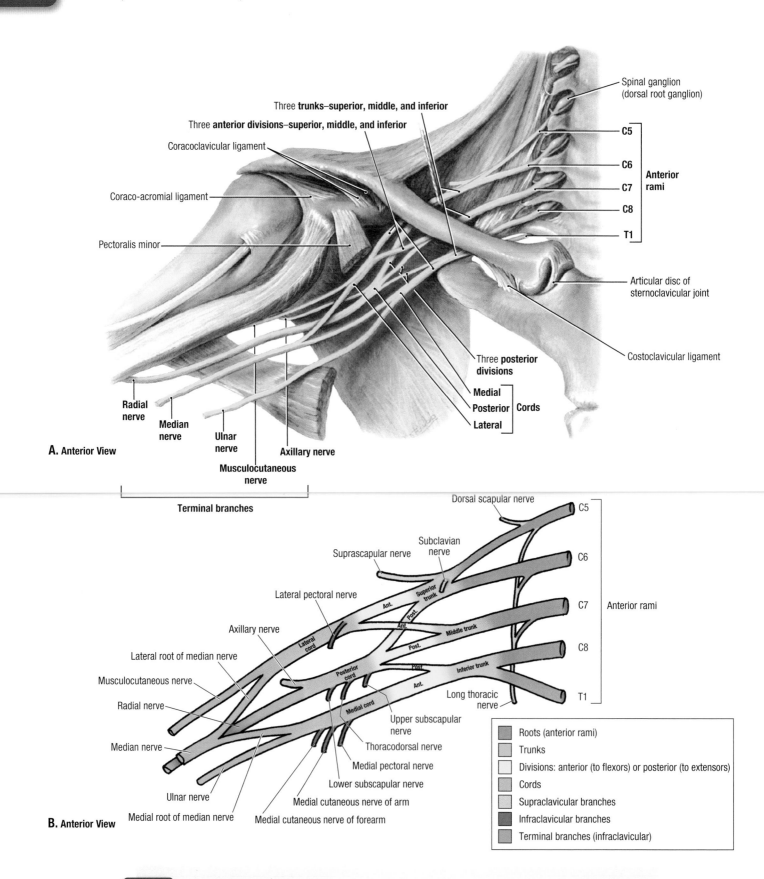

Three **trunks–superior, middle, and inferior**

Three **anterior divisions–superior, middle, and inferior**

Coracoclavicular ligament

Coraco-acromial ligament

Pectoralis minor

Spinal ganglion (dorsal root ganglion)

C5

C6 — Anterior rami

C7

C8

T1

Articular disc of sternoclavicular joint

Costoclavicular ligament

Three **posterior divisions**

Medial

Posterior — Cords

Lateral

Radial nerve

Median nerve

Ulnar nerve

Axillary nerve

Musculocutaneous nerve

A. Anterior View

Terminal branches

Dorsal scapular nerve

C5

Subclavian nerve

Suprascapular nerve

C6

Lateral pectoral nerve

Superior trunk

Ant.

Post.

C7 — Anterior rami

Axillary nerve

Ant.

Lateral cord

Middle trunk

Lateral root of median nerve

Post.

C8

Musculocutaneous nerve

Posterior cord

Post.

Inferior trunk

Radial nerve

Medial cord

Ant.

Long thoracic nerve

T1

Median nerve

Upper subscapular nerve

Thoracodorsal nerve

Ulnar nerve

Medial pectoral nerve

Medial root of median nerve

Lower subscapular nerve

Medial cutaneous nerve of arm

Medial cutaneous nerve of forearm

B. Anterior View

	Roots (anterior rami)
	Trunks
	Divisions: anterior (to flexors) or posterior (to extensors)
	Cords
	Supraclavicular branches
	Infraclavicular branches
	Terminal branches (infraclavicular)

6.25 BRACHIAL PLEXUS

A. Dissection. **B.** Schematic illustration.

TABLE 6.6 BRACHIAL PLEXUS

Nerve	Origin	Course	Distribution/Structure(s) Supplied
Supraclavicular Branches			
Dorsal scapular	Anterior ramus of C5 with a frequent contribution from C4	Pierces scalenus medius, descends on deep surface of rhomboids	Rhomboids and occasionally supplies levator scapulae
Long thoracic	Anterior rami of C5–C7	Descends posterior to C8 and T1 rami and passes distally on external surface of serratus anterior	Serratus anterior
Subclavian	Superior trunk receiving fibers from C5 and C6 and often C4	Descends posterior to clavicle and anterior to brachial plexus and subclavian artery	Subclavius and sternoclavicular joint
Suprascapular	Superior trunk receiving fibers from C5 and C6 and often C4	Passes laterally across posterior triangle of neck, through suprascapular notch deep to superior transverse scapular ligament	Supraspinatus, infraspinatus, and glenohumeral (shoulder) joint
Infraclavicular branches			
Lateral pectoral	Lateral cord receiving fibers from C5–C7	Pierces clavipectoral fascia to reach deep surface of pectoral muscles	Primarily pectoralis major but sends a loop to medial pectoral nerve that innervates pectoralis minor
Musculocutaneous	Lateral cord receiving fibers from C5–C7	Pierces coracobrachialis and descends between biceps brachii and brachialis	Coracobrachialis, biceps brachii, and brachialis; continues as lateral cutaneous nerve of forearm
Median	Lateral root of median nerve is a terminal branch of lateral cord (C6, C7); medial root of median nerve is a terminal branch of medial cord (C8, T1)	Lateral and medial roots merge to form median nerve lateral to axillary artery; crosses anterior to brachial artery to lie medial to artery in cubital fossa	Flexor muscles in forearm (except flexor carpi ulnaris, ulnar half of flexor digitorum profundus), 3½ thenar and lateral 2 lumbrical muscles in hand, and skin of palm and 3½ digits lateral to a line bisecting 4th digit and the dorsum of the distal halves of these digits
Medial pectoral	Medial cord receiving fibers from C8, T1	Passes between axillary artery and vein and enters deep surface of pectoralis minor	Pectoralis minor and part of pectoralis major
Medial cutaneous nerve of arm	Medial cord receiving fibers from C8, T1	Runs along the medial side of axillary vein and communicates with intercostobrachial nerve	Skin on medial side of arm
Medial cutaneous nerve of forearm	Medial cord receiving fibers from C8, T1	Runs between axillary artery and vein	Skin over medial side of forearm
Ulnar	Terminal branch of medial cord receiving fibers from C8, T1 and often C7	Passes down medial aspect of arm and runs posterior to medial epicondyle to enter forearm	Innervates 1½ flexor muscles in forearm (see Median nerve), 1½ thenar, 2 medial lumbricals, and all interossei muscles in hand, and skin of hand medial to a line bisecting 4th digit (ring finger) anteriorly and posteriorly
Upper subscapular	Branch of posterior cord receiving fibers from C5	Passes posteriorly and enters subscapularis	Superior portion of subscapularis
Thoracodorsal	Branch of posterior cord receiving fibers from C6 to C8	Arises between upper and lower subscapular nerves and runs inferolaterally to latissimus dorsi	Latissimus dorsi
Lower subscapular	Branch of posterior cord receiving fibers from C6	Passes inferolaterally, deep to subscapular artery and vein, to subscapularis and teres major	Inferior portion of subscapularis and teres major
Axillary	Terminal branch of posterior cord receiving fibers from C5 and C6	Passes to posterior aspect of arm through quadrangular space[a] with posterior circumflex humeral artery and then winds around surgical neck of humerus; gives rise to lateral cutaneous nerve of arm	Teres minor and deltoid, glenohumeral (shoulder) joint, and skin of superolateral arm
Radial	Terminal branch of posterior cord receiving fibers from C5 to T1	Descends posterior to axillary artery; enters radial groove to pass between long and medial heads of triceps brachii	Triceps brachii, anconeus, brachioradialis, and extensor muscles of forearm; supplies skin on posterior aspect of arm and forearm and dorsum of hand lateral to axial line of digit 4

[a]Quadrangular space is bounded superiorly by subscapularis and teres minor, inferiorly by teres major, medially by long head of triceps brachii, and laterally by humerus.

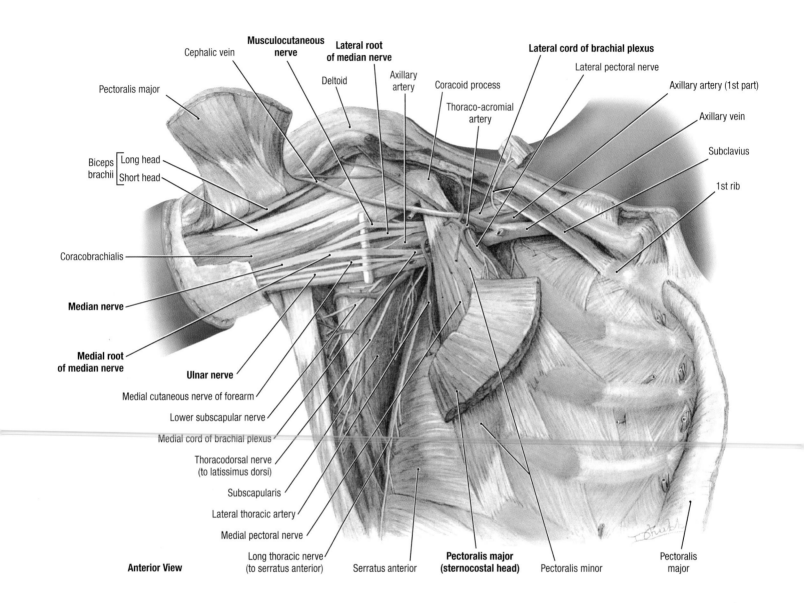

STRUCTURES OF AXILLA: DEEP DISSECTION I

- The pectoralis major muscle is reflected, and the clavipectoral fascia is removed; the cube of muscle superior to the clavicle is cut from the clavicular head of the pectoralis major muscle.
- The subclavius and pectoralis minor are the two deep muscles of the anterior wall.
- The 2nd part axillary artery passes posterior to the pectoralis minor muscle, a fingerbreadth from the tip of the coracoid process; the axillary vein lies anterior and then medial to the axillary artery.
- The median nerve, followed proximally, leads by its lateral root to the lateral cord and musculocutaneous nerve and by its medial root to the medial cord and ulnar nerve. These four nerves and the medial cutaneous nerve of the forearm are derived from the anterior divisions of the brachial plexus and are raised on a stick. The lateral root of the median nerve may occur as several strands.
- The musculocutaneous nerve enters the flexor compartment of the arm by piercing the coracobrachialis muscle.

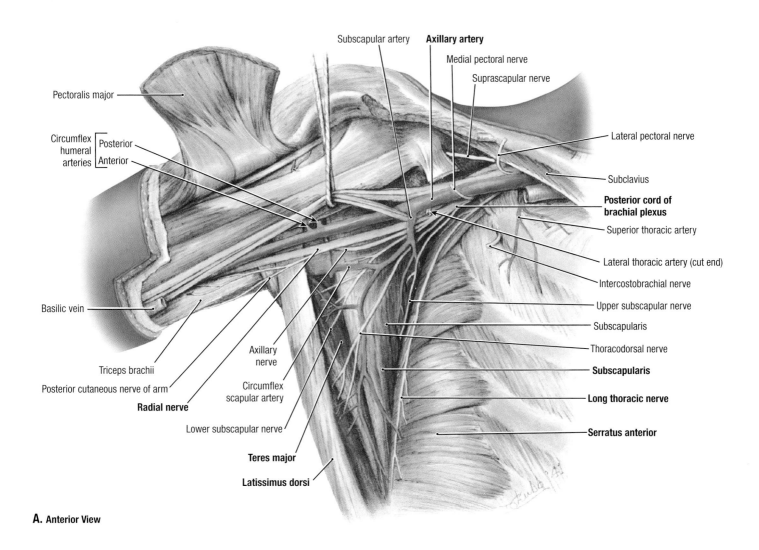

Subscapular artery

Axillary artery

Medial pectoral nerve

Suprascapular nerve

Pectoralis major

Circumflex humeral arteries — Posterior / Anterior

Lateral pectoral nerve

Subclavius

Posterior cord of brachial plexus

Superior thoracic artery

Lateral thoracic artery (cut end)

Intercostobrachial nerve

Upper subscapular nerve

Subscapularis

Thoracodorsal nerve

Subscapularis

Long thoracic nerve

Serratus anterior

Basilic vein

Axillary nerve

Triceps brachii

Circumflex scapular artery

Posterior cutaneous nerve of arm

Radial nerve

Lower subscapular nerve

Teres major

Teres major

Latissimus dorsi

A. Anterior View

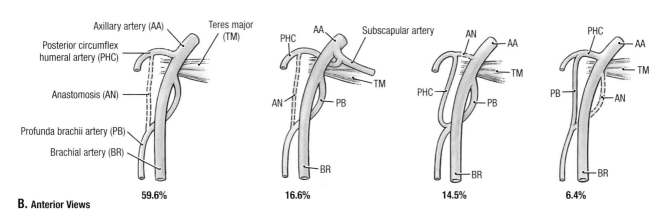

Axillary artery (AA)   Teres major (TM)

Posterior circumflex humeral artery (PHC)

Anastomosis (AN)

Profunda brachii artery (PB)

Brachial artery (BR)

PHC   AA   Subscapular artery

AN   PB

BR

59.6%   16.6%

AN   AA

PHC   TM

PB

BR

PHC   AA

TM

PB   AN

BR

14.5%   6.4%

B. Anterior Views

6.27   **POSTERIOR AND MEDIAL WALLS OF AXILLA: DEEP DISSECTION II**

A. Dissection. The pectoralis minor muscle is excised, the lateral and medial cords of the brachial plexus are retracted, and the axillary vein is removed. **B.** Variations of the posterior circumflex humeral artery and profunda brachii artery. Percentages are based on 235 specimens dissected in Dr. Grant's laboratory.

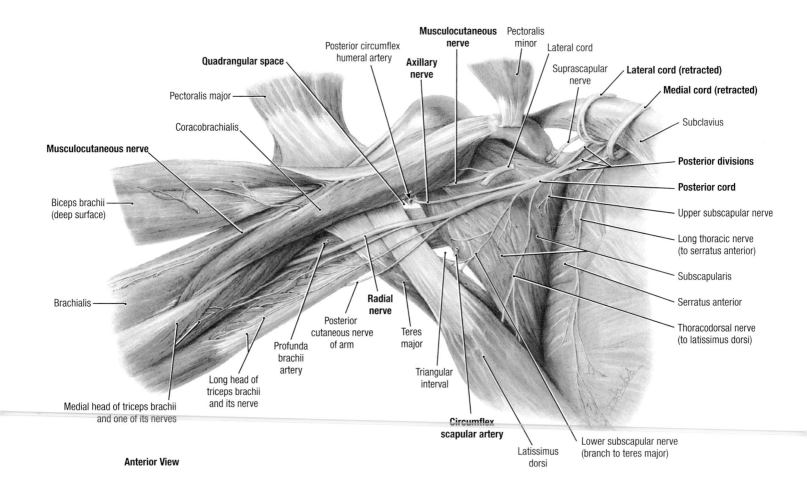

Anterior View

6.28 POSTERIOR WALL OF AXILLA, MUSCULOCUTANEOUS NERVE, AND POSTERIOR CORD: DEEP DISSECTION III

- The pectoralis major and minor muscles are reflected laterally, the lateral and medial cords of the brachial plexus are reflected superiorly, and the arteries, veins, and median and ulnar nerves are removed.
- Coracobrachialis arises with the short head of the biceps brachii muscle from the tip of the coracoid process and attaches halfway down the medial aspect of the humerus.
- The musculocutaneous nerve pierces the coracobrachialis muscle and supplies it, the biceps, and the brachialis before becoming the lateral cutaneous nerve of the forearm.
- The posterior cord of the plexus is formed by the union of the three posterior divisions; it supplies the three muscles of the posterior wall of the axilla and then bifurcates into the radial and axillary nerves.
- In the axilla, the radial nerve gives off the nerve to the long head of the triceps brachii muscle and a cutaneous branch; in this specimen, it also gives off a branch to the medial head of the triceps. It then enters the radial groove of the humerus with the profunda brachii (deep brachial) artery.
- The axillary nerve passes through the quadrangular space along with the posterior circumflex humeral artery. The borders of the quadrangular space are superiorly, the lateral border of the scapula; inferiorly, the teres major; laterally, the humerus (surgical neck); and medially, the long head of triceps brachii. The circumflex scapular artery traverses the triangular interval.

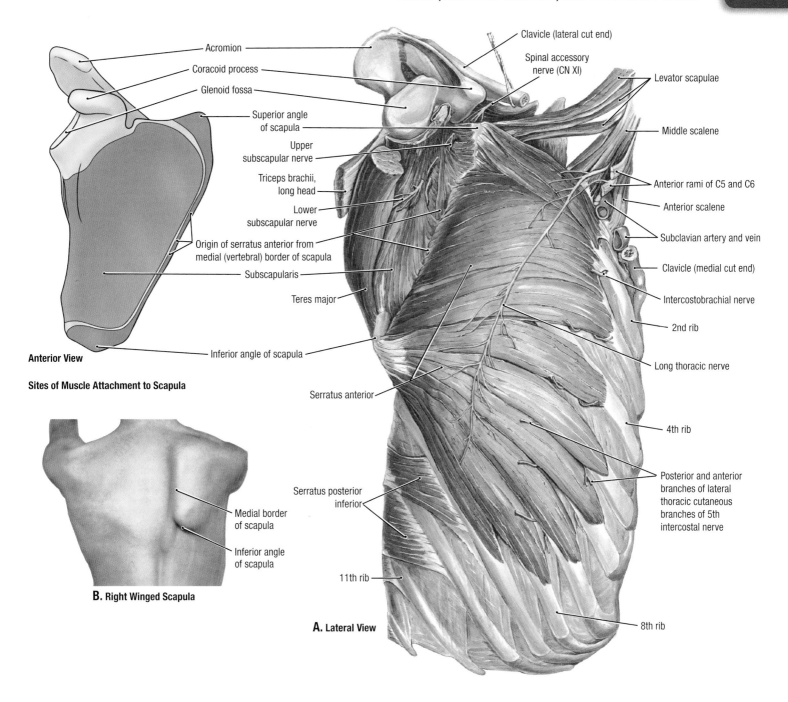

Acromion

Coracoid process

Glenoid fossa

Clavicle (lateral cut end)

Spinal accessory nerve (CN XI)

Levator scapulae

Middle scalene

Superior angle of scapula

Upper subscapular nerve

Triceps brachii, long head

Lower subscapular nerve

Origin of serratus anterior from medial (vertebral) border of scapula

Subscapularis

Teres major

Inferior angle of scapula

Anterior rami of C5 and C6

Anterior scalene

Subclavian artery and vein

Clavicle (medial cut end)

Intercostobrachial nerve

2nd rib

Long thoracic nerve

4th rib

Posterior and anterior branches of lateral thoracic cutaneous branches of 5th intercostal nerve

Serratus anterior

Serratus posterior inferior

11th rib

8th rib

Anterior View

Sites of Muscle Attachment to Scapula

Medial border of scapula

Inferior angle of scapula

B. Right Winged Scapula

A. Lateral View

6.29   SERRATUS ANTERIOR AND SUBSCAPULARIS

A. The serratus anterior muscle, which forms the medial wall of the axilla, has a fleshy belly extending from the superior 8 or 9 ribs in the midclavicular line *(right)* to the medial border of the scapula *(left)*.

- The fibers of the serratus anterior muscle from the 1st rib and the tendinous arch between the 1st and 2nd ribs (see Table 6.4) converge on the superior angle of the scapula; those from the 2nd and 3rd ribs diverge to spread thinly along the medial border; and the remainder (from the 4th to 9th ribs), which form the bulk of the muscle, converge on the inferior angle via a tendinous insertion.

- The long thoracic nerve to serratus anterior arises from spinal nerves C5, C6, and C7 and courses externally along most of the muscle's length.

Winged scapula **(B).** When the serratus anterior is paralyzed because of injury to the long thoracic nerve, the medial border of the scapula moves laterally and posteriorly, away from the thoracic wall. When the arm is abducted, the medial border and the inferior angle of the scapula pull away from the posterior thoracic wall, a deformation known as a winged scapula. In addition, the arm cannot be abducted above the horizontal position because the serratus anterior is unable to rotate the glenoid cavity superiorly.

- The trunks of the brachial plexus and the subclavian artery emerge between the anterior and middle scalene muscles; the subclavian vein is separated from the artery by the anterior scalene muscle.

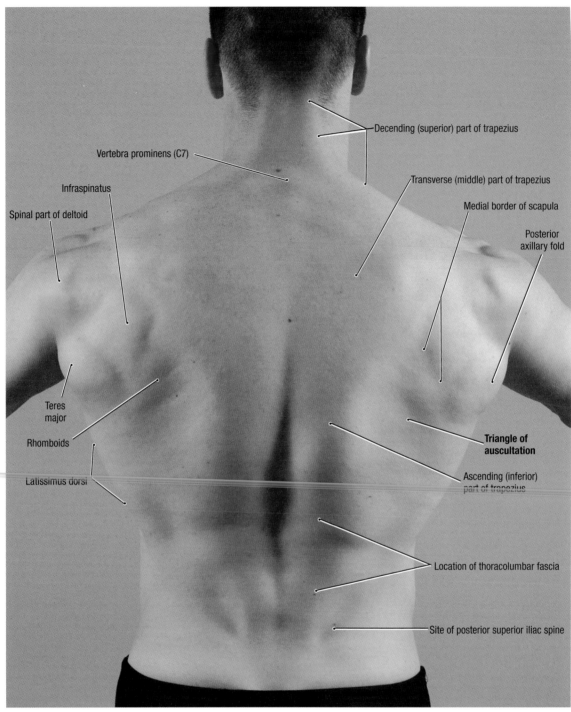

Decending (superior) part of trapezius

Vertebra prominens (C7)

Transverse (middle) part of trapezius

Infraspinatus

Medial border of scapula

Spinal part of deltoid

Posterior axillary fold

Teres major

Rhomboids

Triangle of auscultation

Latissimus dorsi

Ascending (inferior) part of trapezius

Location of thoracolumbar fascia

Site of posterior superior iliac spine

Posterior View

6.30 ## SURFACE ANATOMY OF SUPERFICIAL BACK

The superior border of the latissimus dorsi and a part of the rhomboid major are overlapped by the trapezius. The area formed by the superior border of latissimus dorsi, the medial border of the scapula, and the inferolateral border of the trapezius is called the **triangle of auscultation**. This gap in the thick back musculature is a good place to examine posterior segments of the lungs with a stethoscope. When the scapulae are drawn anteriorly by folding the arms across the thorax and the trunk is flexed, the auscultatory triangle enlarges. The teres major forms a raised oval area on the inferolateral third of the posterior aspect of the scapula when the arm is adducted against resistance. The posterior axillary fold is formed by the teres major and the tendon of the latissimus dorsi.

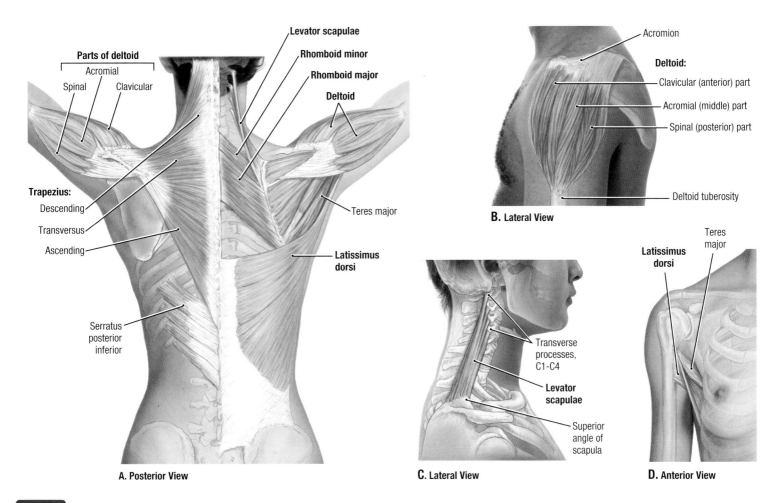

6.31 SUPERFICIAL BACK AND DELTOID MUSCLES

TABLE 6.7 SUPERFICIAL BACK (POSTERIOR AXIO-APPENDICULAR) AND DELTOID MUSCLES

Muscle	Proximal Attachment	Distal Attachment	Innervation	Main Actions
Trapezius	Medial third of superior nuchal line; external occipital protuberance, nuchal ligament, and spinous processes of C7–T12 vertebrae	Lateral third of clavicle, acromion, and spine of scapula	Spinal accessory nerve (CN XI—motor) and cervical nerves (C3–C4—sensory)	Elevates, retracts, and rotates scapula; *descending part* elevates, *transverse part* retracts, and *ascending part* depresses scapula; descending and ascending part act together in superior rotation of scapula
Latissimus dorsi	Spinous processes of inferior six thoracic vertebrae, thoracolumbar fascia, iliac crest, and inferior three or four ribs	Intertubercular sulcus (bicipital groove) of humerus	Thoracodorsal nerve (**C6, C7**, C8)	Extends, adducts, and medially rotates shoulder joint; elevates body toward arms during climbing
Levator scapulae	Posterior tubercles of transverse processes of C1–C4 vertebrae	Superior part of medial border of scapula	Dorsal scapular (C5) and cervical (C3–C4) nerves	Elevates scapula and tilts its glenoid cavity inferiorly by rotating scapula
Rhomboid minor and major	*Minor:* Inferior part of nuchal ligament and spinous processes of C7 and T1 vertebrae *Major:* spinous processes of T2–T5 vertebrae	Medial border of scapula from level of spine to inferior angle	Dorsal scapular nerve (C4–**C5**)	Retract scapula and rotate it to depress glenoid cavity; fix scapula to thoracic wall
Deltoid	Lateral third of clavicle *(clavicular part)*, acromion *(acromial part)*, and spine *(spinal part)* of scapula	Deltoid tuberosity of humerus	Axillary nerve (**C5**–C6)	*Clavicular (anterior) part:* flexes and medially rotates shoulder joint; *acromial (middle) part:* abducts shoulder joint; *spinal (posterior) part:* extends and laterally rotates shoulder joint

Occipitalis

Occipital artery

Occipital lymph node

Greater occipital nerve (posterior ramus of C2 spinal nerve)

3rd occipital nerve (posterior ramus of C3)

Descending (superior) part of trapezius

Lesser occipital nerve (anterior ramus of C2)

Levator scapulae

Rhomboid minor

Rhomboid major

Cutaneous branches of posterior rami

Deltoid

Transverse (middle) part of trapezius

Ascending (inferior) part of trapezius

Triangle of auscultation

Subtrapezial plexus (spinal accessory nerve (CN XI) and branches of C3, C4 anterior rami)

Cutaneous branches of posterior rami

Trapezius

Latissimus dorsi

Posterior branches of lateral cutaneous branches of thoraco-abdominal nerves (anterior rami)

Thoracolumbar fascia

External oblique

Lateral cutaneous branch of iliohypogastric nerve (anterior ramus of L1)

Lumbar triangle

Cutaneous branches of posterior rami of L1 to L3 (superior clunial nerves)

Gluteal fascia (covering gluteus medius)

Gluteus maximus

Posterior View

6.32 CUTANEOUS NERVES OF SUPERFICIAL BACK AND POSTERIOR AXIO-APPENDICULAR MUSCLES

The trapezius muscle is cut and reflected on the left side. A superficial or first muscle layer consists of the trapezius and latissimus dorsi muscles, and a second layer of the levator scapulae and rhomboids. Cutaneous branches of posterior rami penetrate but do not supply the superficial muscles.

TABLE 6.8 MOVEMENTS OF SCAPULA

Boldface indicates prime movers. In the *middle* and *right columns* the *dotted outlines* represent the starting position for each movement.

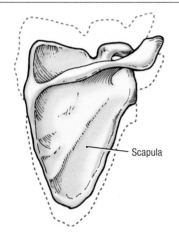

Posterior View
Elevation (red)
Depression (green)

Posterior View

Elevation:
Trapezius, descending part (1)
Levator scapulae (2)
Rhomboids (3)

Anterior View   **Posterior View**

Depression:
Trapezius, ascending part (1)
Serratus anterior, inferior part (2)
Pectoralis minor (3)

Also: Gravity, Latissimus dorsi,
Inferior part of sternocostal
head of pectoralis major

Protraction (red)
Retraction (green)

Anterior View

Protraction:
Serratus anterior (1)
Pectoralis minor (2)
Also: Pectoralis major

Posterior View

Retraction:
Trapezius, transverse part (1)
Rhomboids (2)
Latissimus dorsi (3)

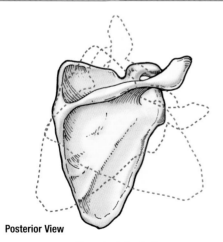

Posterior View

Upward rotation (red)
Downward rotation (green)

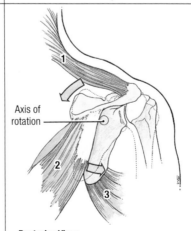

Posterior View

Upward rotation
Trapezius, descending part (1)
Trapezius, ascending part (2)
Serratus anterior, inferior part (3)

Anterior View   **Posterior View**

Downward rotation
Levator scapulae (1)
Rhomboids (2)
Latissimus dorsi (3)
Pectoralis minor (4)

Also: Gravity, Inferior part of sternocostal
head of pectoralis major

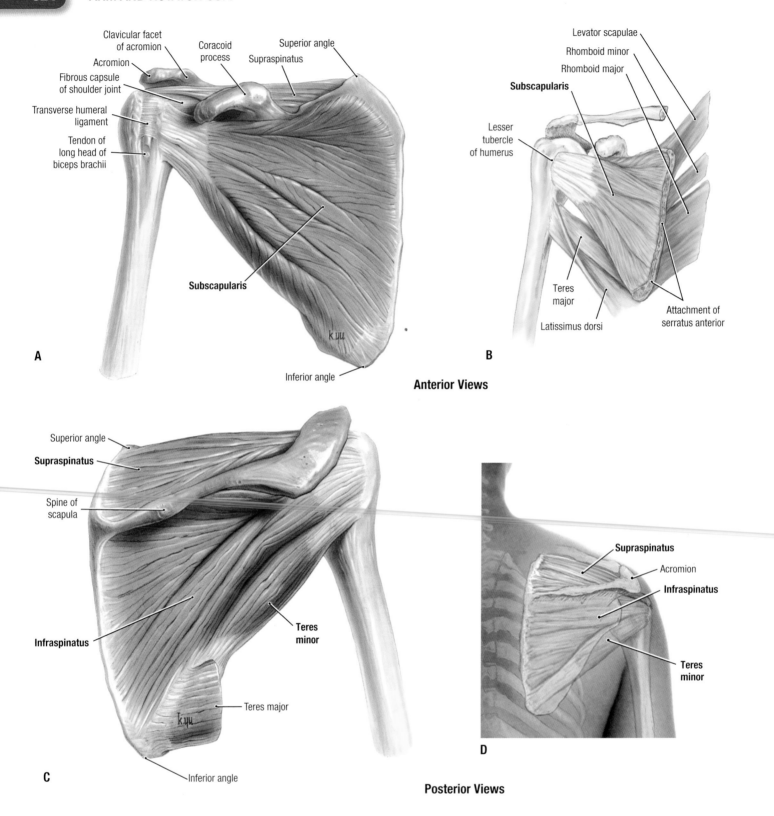

Anterior Views

Posterior Views

6.33 ROTATOR CUFF

A. and B. Subscapularis. **C. and D.** Supraspinatus, infraspinatus, and teres minor.

Four of the scapulohumeral muscles—supraspinatus, infraspinatus, teres minor, and subscapularis—are called rotator cuff muscles because they form a musculotendinous rotator cuff around the glenohumeral joint. All except the supraspinatus are rotators of the humerus.

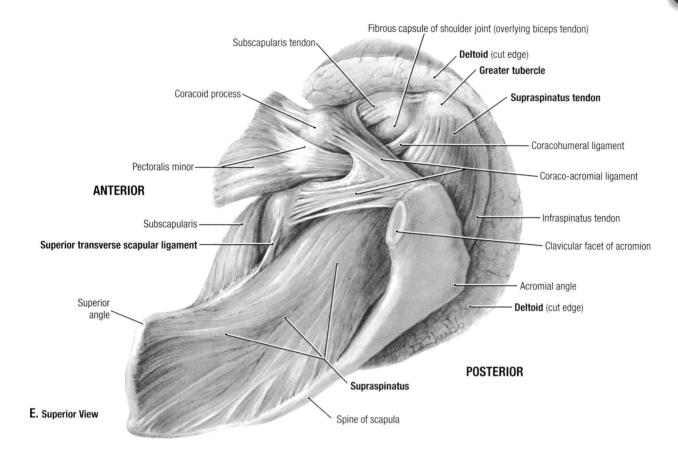

Fibrous capsule of shoulder joint (overlying biceps tendon)

Subscapularis tendon

Deltoid (cut edge)

Greater tubercle

Coracoid process

Supraspinatus tendon

Coracohumeral ligament

Pectoralis minor

Coraco-acromial ligament

ANTERIOR

Subscapularis

Infraspinatus tendon

Superior transverse scapular ligament

Clavicular facet of acromion

Superior angle

Acromial angle

Deltoid (cut edge)

POSTERIOR

Supraspinatus

E. Superior View

Spine of scapula

6.33   ROTATOR CUFF *(CONTINUED)*

E. Supraspinatus.

The supraspinatus, also part of the rotator cuff, initiates and assists the deltoid in abducting the shoulder joint. The tendons of the rotator cuff muscles blend with and reinforce the joint capsule of the glenohumeral joint, protecting the joint and giving it stability.

Injury or disease may damage the rotator cuff, producing instability of the glenohumeral joint. **Rupture or tear of the supraspinatus tendon** is the most common injury of the rotator cuff. **Degenerative tendinitis of the rotator cuff** is common, especially in older people.

TABLE 6.9 SCAPULOHUMERAL MUSCLES

Muscle	Proximal Attachment	Distal Attachment	Innervation	Main Actions
Supraspinatus (S)	Supraspinous fossa of scapula	Superior facet on greater tubercle of humerus	Suprascapular nerve (C4, **C5**, and C6)	Initiates abduction at shoulder joint and acts with rotator cuff muscles[a]
Infraspinatus (I)	Infraspinous fossa of scapula	Middle facet on greater tubercle of humerus	Suprascapular nerve (**C5** and C6)	Laterally rotates shoulder joint; helps to hold humeral head in glenoid cavity of scapula
Teres minor (T)	Superior part of lateral border of scapula	Inferior facet on greater tubercle of humerus	Axillary nerve (**C5** and C6)	
Subscapularis(S)	Subscapular fossa	Lesser tubercle of humerus	Upper and lower subscapular nerves (C5, **C6**, and C7)	Medially rotates shoulder joint and adducts it; helps to hold humeral head in glenoid cavity
Teres major[b]	Posterior surface of inferior angle of scapula	Crest of lesser tubercle (medial lip of bicipital groove) of humerus	Lower subscapular nerve (**C6** and C7)	Adducts and medially rotates shoulder joint

[a]Collectively, the supraspinatus, infraspinatus, teres minor, and subscapularis muscles are referred to as the rotator cuff muscles or "SITS" muscles. They function together during all movements of the shoulder joint to hold the head of the humerus in the glenoid cavity of scapula.
[b]Not a rotator cuff muscle.

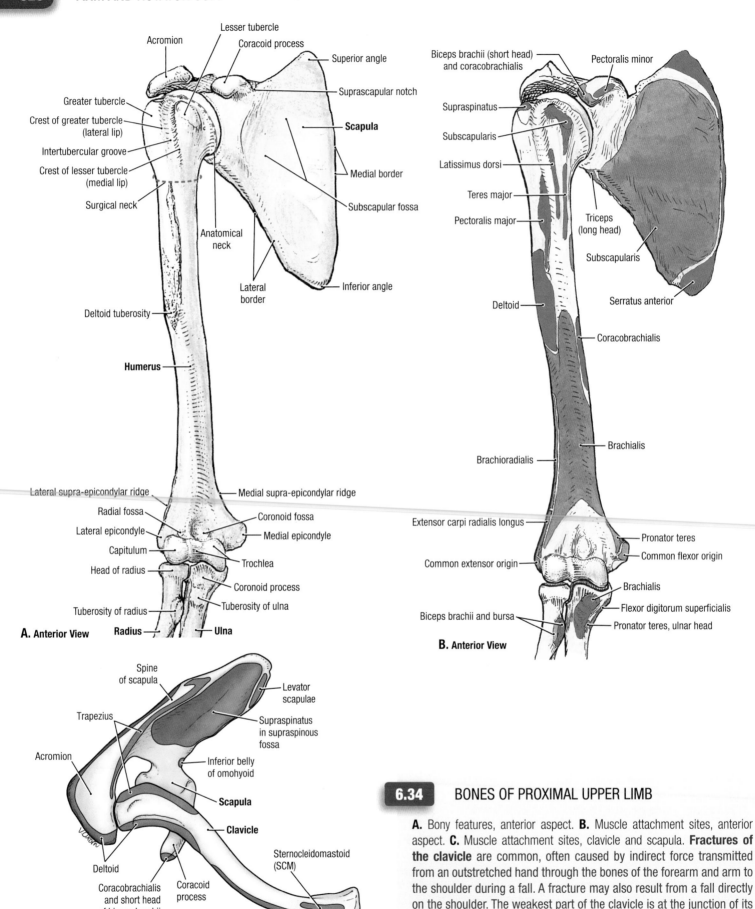

A. Anterior View

Lesser tubercle
Acromion
Coracoid process
Superior angle
Suprascapular notch
Greater tubercle
Crest of greater tubercle (lateral lip)
Intertubercular groove
Crest of lesser tubercle (medial lip)
Surgical neck
Anatomical neck
Scapula
Medial border
Subscapular fossa
Deltoid tuberosity
Humerus
Lateral border
Inferior angle
Lateral supra-epicondylar ridge
Medial supra-epicondylar ridge
Radial fossa
Coronoid fossa
Lateral epicondyle
Medial epicondyle
Capitulum
Head of radius
Trochlea
Tuberosity of radius
Coronoid process
Tuberosity of ulna
Radius
Ulna

B. Anterior View

Biceps brachii (short head) and coracobrachialis
Pectoralis minor
Supraspinatus
Subscapularis
Latissimus dorsi
Teres major
Pectoralis major
Triceps (long head)
Subscapularis
Deltoid
Serratus anterior
Coracobrachialis
Brachialis
Brachioradialis
Extensor carpi radialis longus
Pronator teres
Common flexor origin
Common extensor origin
Brachialis
Flexor digitorum superficialis
Biceps brachii and bursa
Pronator teres, ulnar head

C. Superior View

Spine of scapula
Levator scapulae
Trapezius
Supraspinatus in supraspinous fossa
Acromion
Inferior belly of omohyoid
Scapula
Clavicle
Deltoid
Sternocleidomastoid (SCM)
Coracobrachialis and short head of biceps brachii
Coracoid process
Pectoralis major

6.34   BONES OF PROXIMAL UPPER LIMB

A. Bony features, anterior aspect. **B.** Muscle attachment sites, anterior aspect. **C.** Muscle attachment sites, clavicle and scapula. **Fractures of the clavicle** are common, often caused by indirect force transmitted from an outstretched hand through the bones of the forearm and arm to the shoulder during a fall. A fracture may also result from a fall directly on the shoulder. The weakest part of the clavicle is at the junction of its middle and lateral thirds.

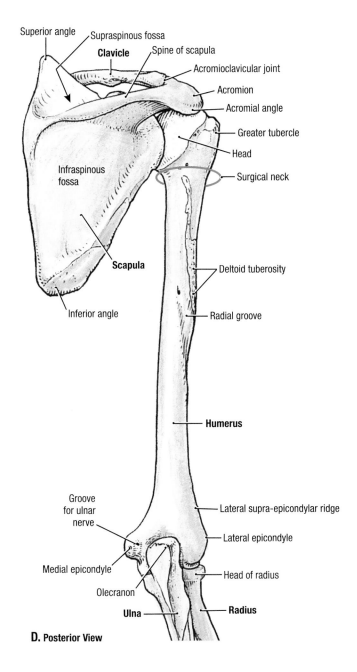

Superior angle
Suprasinous fossa
Clavicle
Spine of scapula
Acromioclavicular joint
Acromion
Acromial angle
Greater tubercle
Head
Surgical neck
Infraspinous fossa
Deltoid tuberosity
Scapula
Radial groove
Inferior angle
Humerus
Groove for ulnar nerve
Lateral supra-epicondylar ridge
Lateral epicondyle
Medial epicondyle
Head of radius
Olecranon
Ulna   **Radius**

D. Posterior View

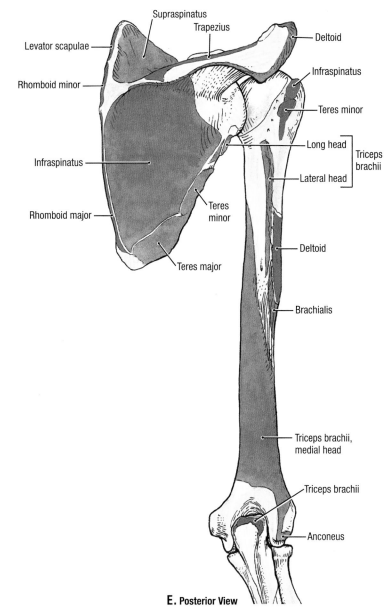

Levator scapulae
Supraspinatus
Trapezius
Deltoid
Rhomboid minor
Infraspinatus
Teres minor
Infraspinatus
Long head
Lateral head
} Triceps brachii
Rhomboid major
Teres minor
Deltoid
Teres major
Brachialis
Triceps brachii, medial head
Triceps brachii
Anconeus

E. Posterior View

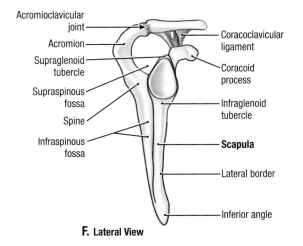

Acromioclavicular joint
Acromion
Supraglenoid tubercle
Supraspinous fossa
Spine
Infraspinous fossa
Coracoclavicular ligament
Coracoid process
Infraglenoid tubercle
Scapula
Lateral border
Inferior angle

F. Lateral View

6.34   BONES OF PROXIMAL UPPER LIMB *(CONTINUED)*

D. Bony features, posterior aspect. **E.** Muscle attachment sites, posterior aspect. **Fractures of the surgical neck of the humerus** are especially common in elderly people with **osteoporosis** (degeneration of bone). Even a low energy fall on the hand, with the force being transmitted up the forearm bones of the extended limb, may result in a fracture. **Transverse fractures of the shaft of humerus** frequently result from a direct blow to the arm. Fracture of the distal part of the humerus, near the supra-epicondylar ridges, is a **supra-epicondylar (supracondylar) fracture.**

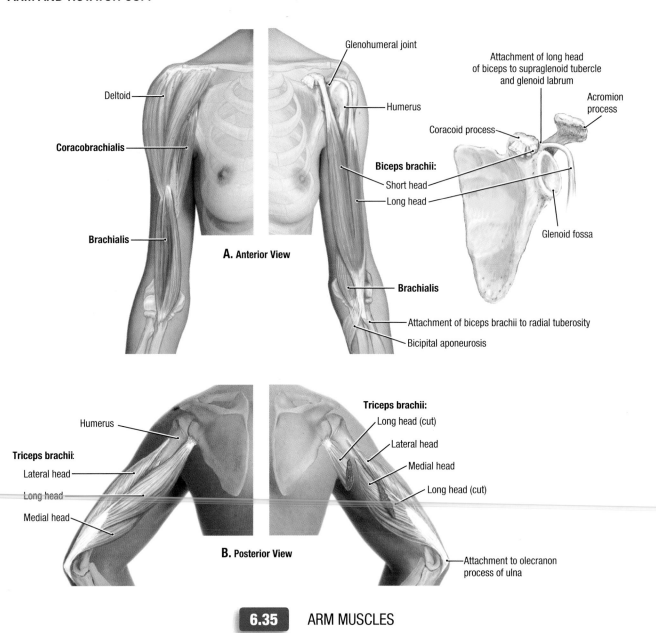

A. Anterior View

B. Posterior View

6.35 ARM MUSCLES

TABLE 6.10 ARM MUSCLES

Muscle	Proximal Attachment	Distal Attachment	Innervation	Main Actions
Biceps brachii	*Short head:* tip of coracoid process of scapula *Long head:* supraglenoid tubercle of scapula and glenoid labrum	Tuberosity of radius and fascia of forearm through bicipital aponeurosis	Musculocutaneous nerve (C5, **C6**, C7)	Supinates forearm and, when forearm is supine, flexes elbow joint; short head flexes shoulder joint; long head helps to stabilize should joint during abduction.
Brachialis	Distal half of anterior surface of humerus	Coronoid process and tuberosity of ulna	Musculocutaneous nerve (C5–C7) and radial (C5–C7)	Flexes elbow joint in all positions
Coracobrachialis	Tip of coracoid process of scapula	Middle third of medial surface of humerus	Musculocutaneous nerve (C5, **C6**, C7)	Assists with flexion and adduction of shoulder joint
Triceps brachii	*Long head:* infraglenoid tubercle of scapula *Lateral head:* posterior surface of humerus, superior to radial groove *Medial head:* posterior surface of humerus, inferior to radial groove	Proximal end of olecranon of ulna and fascia of forearm	Radial nerve (C6, **C7, C8**)	Extends the elbow joint; long head steadies head of humerus when shoulder joint is abducted
Anconeus	Lateral epicondyle of humerus	Lateral surface of olecranon and superior part of posterior surface of ulna	Radial nerve (C7–T1)	Assists triceps in extending elbow joint; stabilizes elbow joint; abducts ulna during pronation

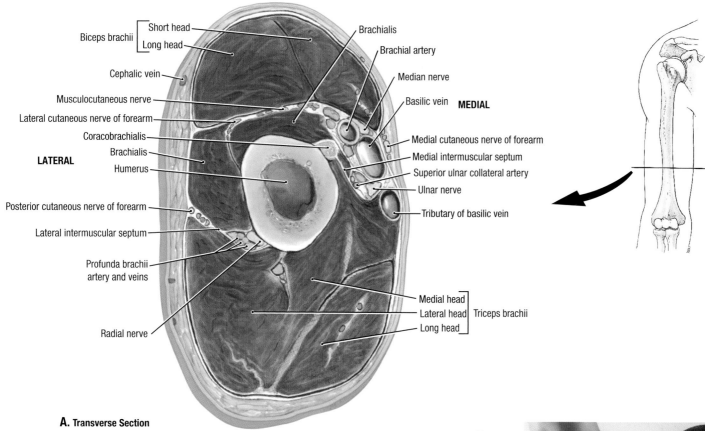

ANTERIOR (flexor compartment)

Biceps brachii — Short head
Long head

Brachialis

Brachial artery

Median nerve

Cephalic vein

Musculocutaneous nerve

Lateral cutaneous nerve of forearm

Basilic vein **MEDIAL**

Coracobrachialis

Medial cutaneous nerve of forearm

LATERAL Brachialis

Medial intermuscular septum

Humerus

Superior ulnar collateral artery

Ulnar nerve

Posterior cutaneous nerve of forearm

Tributary of basilic vein

Lateral intermuscular septum

Profunda brachii artery and veins

Medial head
Lateral head } Triceps brachii
Long head

Radial nerve

A. Transverse Section

POSTERIOR (extensor compartment)

6.36 ANTERIOR AND POSTERIOR COMPARTMENTS OF ARM

A. Anatomical section. **B.** Surface anatomy.

- Three muscles, the biceps, brachialis, and coracobrachialis, lie in the anterior compartment of the arm; the triceps brachii lies in the posterior compartment.
- The medial and lateral intermuscular septum separates these two muscle groups.
- The radial nerve and profunda brachii artery and veins serving the posterior compartment lie in contact with the radial groove of the humerus.
- The musculocutaneous nerve serving the anterior compartment lies in the plane between the biceps and the brachialis muscles.
- The median nerve crosses to the medial side of the brachial artery.
- The ulnar nerve passes posteriorly onto the medial side of the triceps muscle.
- The basilic vein (appearing here as two vessels) has pierced the deep fascia.

Olecranon

Medial epicondyle of humerus

Biceps brachii

Medial bicipital groove

Triceps brachii { Lateral head
Long head

Deltoid { Clavicular (anterior) part
Spinal (posterior) part

Axillary fossa

Teres major

Latissimus dorsi

B. Anterolateral View

Coracoid process of scapula

Fibrous capsule of shoulder joint

Supraspinatus

Greater tubercle of humerus

Tendon of pectoralis minor

Deltoid

Short head of biceps brachii

Subscapularis

Long head of biceps brachii

Coracobrachialis

Pectoralis major

Teres major

Medial border

of scapula

Inferior angle

Latissimus dorsi

Biceps brachii

Long head

of triceps brachii

Medial head

Brachialis

Brachioradialis

Bicipital aponeurosis

Tendon of biceps brachii

Pronator teres

Extensor muscles of forearm

Flexor muscles of forearm

A. Anterior View

6.37 MUSCLES OF ANTERIOR ASPECT OF ARM I

- The biceps brachii has two heads: a long head and a short head.
- When the elbow joint is flexed approximately 90° the biceps is a flexor from the supinated position of the forearm but a very powerful supinator from the pronated position.

- A triangular membranous band, the bicipital aponeurosis, runs from the biceps tendon across the cubital fossa and merges with the antebrachial (deep) fascia covering the flexor muscles on the medial side of the forearm.

Coraco-acromial ligament

Supraspinatus

Fibrous capsule of shoulder joint

Short head of biceps brachii

Transverse humeral ligament

Tendon of subscapularis

Tendon of long head of biceps brachii

Pectoralis major

Deltoid

Humerus

Lateral head of triceps brachii

Brachialis

Lateral epicondyle of humerus

Capitulum of humerus

Radius

Coracoid process
Supraspinatus

Superior angle of scapula

Pectoralis minor

Subscapularis (cut edges)

Subscapular fossa

Coracobrachialis

Teres major

Inferior angle of scapula

Latissimus dorsi

Long head

of triceps brachii

Medial head

Medial epicondyle of humerus

Tendon of biceps brachii

Ulna

B. Anterior View

6.37 MUSCLES OF ANTERIOR ASPECT OF ARM II

- The brachialis, a flattened fusiform muscle, lies posterior (deep) to the biceps and produces the greatest amount of flexion force.
- The coracobrachialis, an elongated muscle in the superomedial part of the arm, is pierced by the musculocutaneous nerve. It helps flex and adduct the arm.

- **Rupture of the tendon of the long head of the biceps** usually results from wear and tear of an inflamed tendon **(biceps tendinitis)**. Normally, the tendon is torn from its attachment to the supraglenoid tubercle of the scapula. The detached muscle belly forms a ball near the center of the distal part of the anterior aspect of the arm.

Parts of deltoid
- Clavicular (1a) (anterior)
- Acromial (1b) (middle)
- Spinal (1c) (posterior)

Triceps brachii
- Long head
- Lateral head (9)

Biceps brachii (2)

Lateral bicpital groove (★)

Brachialis (3)

Triceps tendon (8) overlying medial head

Brachioradialis (4)

Lateral epicondyle (7)

Olecranon (6)

Extensor carpi radialis longus (5)

Fascia covering anconeus and common extensor tendon

A. Lateral View

B. Lateral View

6.38   LATERAL ASPECT OF ARM

A. Dissection (*numbers* in parentheses refer to structures in **B**). **B.** Surface anatomy.

Atrophy of the deltoid occurs when the axillary nerve (C5 and C6) is severely damaged (e.g., as might occur when the surgical neck of the humerus is fractured). As the deltoid atrophies, the rounded contour of the shoulder disappears. This gives the shoulder a flattened appearance and produces a slight hollow inferior to the acromion. A loss of sensation may occur over the lateral side of the proximal part of the arm, the area supplied by the superior lateral cutaneous nerve of the arm. To test the deltoid (or the function of the axillary nerve) the shoulder joint is abducted against resistance, starting from approximately 15°. Supraspinatus initiates abduction at the shoulder joint.

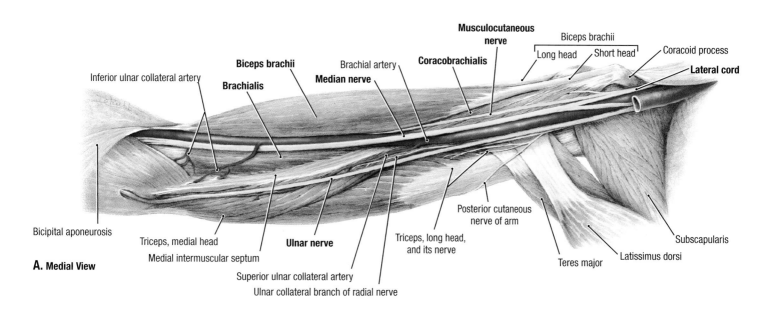

Inferior ulnar collateral artery
Biceps brachii
Brachialis
Median nerve
Brachial artery
Coracobrachialis
Musculocutaneous nerve
Biceps brachii
Long head   Short head
Coracoid process
Lateral cord
Bicipital aponeurosis
Triceps, medial head
Medial intermuscular septum
Ulnar nerve
Superior ulnar collateral artery
Ulnar collateral branch of radial nerve
Posterior cutaneous nerve of arm
Triceps, long head, and its nerve
Teres major
Latissimus dorsi
Subscapularis

A. Medial View

Cubital fossa
Brachialis
Biceps brachii
Deltopectoral groove
Deltoid
Anterior axillary fold
Basilic vein
Medial head of triceps brachii
Medial bicipital groove
Long head of triceps brachii
Posterior axillary fold
Axillary fossa

B. Medial View

6.39   **MEDIAL ASPECT OF ARM**

A. Dissection. **B.** Surface anatomy.

- The axillary artery passes just inferior to the tip of the coracoid process and courses posterior to the coracobrachialis. At the inferior border of the teres major, the axillary artery changes names to become the brachial artery and continues distally on the anterior aspect of the brachialis.
- Although collateral pathways confer some protection against gradual temporary and partial occlusion, sudden complete **occlusion or laceration of the brachial artery** creates a surgical emergency because paralysis of muscles results from ischemia within a few hours.

- The median nerve lies adjacent to the axillary and brachial arteries and then crosses the artery from lateral to medial.
- Proximally, the ulnar nerve is adjacent to the medial side of the artery, passes posterior to the medial intermuscular septum, and descends on the medial head of triceps to pass posterior to the medial epicondyle; here, the ulnar nerve is palpable.
- The superior ulnar collateral artery and ulnar collateral branch of the radial nerve (to medial head of the triceps) accompany the ulnar nerve in the arm.

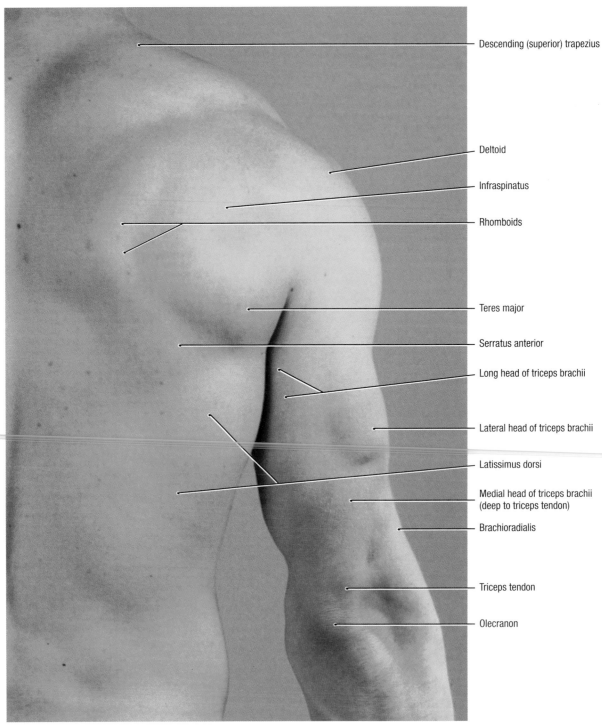

Descending (superior) trapezius

Deltoid

Infraspinatus

Rhomboids

Teres major

Serratus anterior

Long head of triceps brachii

Lateral head of triceps brachii

Latissimus dorsi

Medial head of triceps brachii
(deep to triceps tendon)

Brachioradialis

Triceps tendon

Olecranon

Posterior View

6.40 SURFACE ANATOMY OF SCAPULAR REGION AND POSTERIOR ASPECT OF ARM

The three heads of the triceps form a bulge on the posterior aspect of the arm and are identifiable in a lean individual when the elbow joint is extended from the flexed position against resistance.

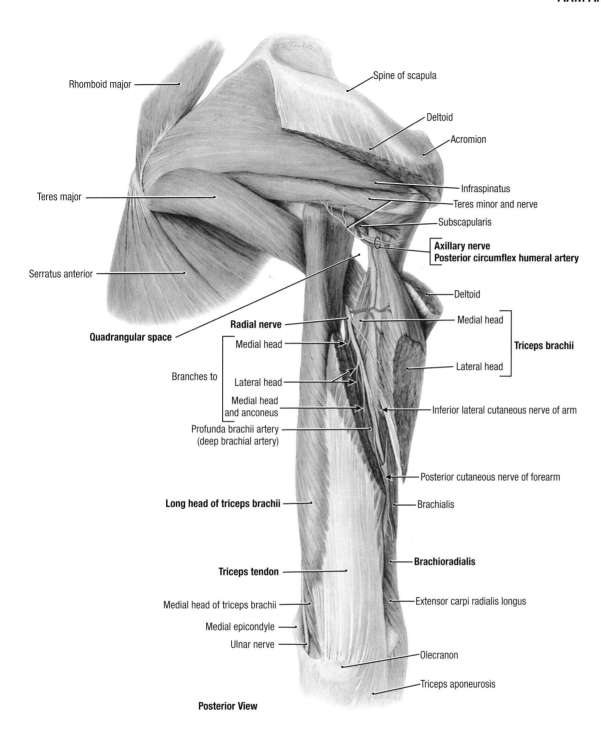

Rhomboid major

Spine of scapula

Deltoid

Acromion

Teres major

Infraspinatus

Teres minor and nerve

Subscapularis

Axillary nerve
Posterior circumflex humeral artery

Serratus anterior

Deltoid

Quadrangular space

Radial nerve

Medial head

Triceps brachii

Branches to

Medial head

Lateral head

Lateral head

Medial head
and anconeus

Inferior lateral cutaneous nerve of arm

Profunda brachii artery
(deep brachial artery)

Posterior cutaneous nerve of forearm

Long head of triceps brachii

Brachialis

Brachioradialis

Triceps tendon

Extensor carpi radialis longus

Medial head of triceps brachii

Medial epicondyle

Ulnar nerve

Olecranon

Triceps aponeurosis

Posterior View

6.41　TRICEPS BRACHII AND RELATED NERVES

- The lateral head is reflected laterally, and the medial head is attached to the deep surface of the triceps tendon, which attaches to the olecranon.
- The radial nerve and deep brachial artery pass between the proximal attachments of the long and medial heads of the triceps brachii in the middle third of the arm, directly contacting the radial groove of the humerus.
- **Midarm fracture.** The middle third of the arm is a common site for fractures of the humerus, often with associated **radial nerve trauma.** When the radial nerve is injured in the radial groove, the triceps brachii muscle typically is only weakened because only the medial head is

affected. However, the muscles in the posterior compartment of the forearm, supplied by more distal branches of the radial nerve, are paralyzed. The characteristic clinical sign of radial nerve injury is **wrist drop** (inability to extend the wrist joint and fingers at the metacarpophalangeal joints).
- The axillary nerve passes through the quadrangular space along with the posterior humeral circumflex artery.
- The ulnar nerve follows the medial border of the triceps then passes posterior to the medial epicondyle.

Suprascapular artery

Suprascapular nerve

Supraspinatus

Infraspinatus

Infraspinatus

Teres major

Triangular space

Circumflex scapular artery

Quadrangular space

Long head of
triceps brachii

Fibrous capsule of glenohumeral
(shoulder) joint

Deltoid

Teres minor

Axillary nerve

**Posterior circumflex
humeral artery**

Superior lateral cutaneous nerve of arm

Radial nerve

Profunda brachii artery (deep artery of arm)

Triangular interval

Lateral head of triceps brachii

Tendon overlying medial
head of triceps brachii

Posterior View

6.42   DORSAL SCAPULAR AND SUBDELTOID REGIONS

- The infraspinatus muscle, aided by the teres minor and spinal (posterior) fibers of the deltoid muscle, rotates the shoulder joint laterally.
- The long head of the triceps muscle passes between the teres minor (a lateral rotator) and teres major (a medial rotator).
- The long head of the triceps muscle separates the quadrangular space from the triangular interval.
- Regarding the distribution of the suprascapular and axillary nerves, each comes from C5 and C6; each supplies two muscles—the suprascapular nerve innervates the supraspinatus and infraspinatus, and the axillary nerve innervates the teres minor and deltoid muscles. Both nerves supply the shoulder joint, but only the axillary nerve has a cutaneous branch.
- **Axillary nerve injury** may occur when the glenohumeral (shoulder) joint dislocates because of its close relation to the inferior part of the joint capsule of this joint. The subglenoid displacement of the head of the humerus into the quadrangular space may damage the axillary nerve. Axillary nerve injury is indicated by paralysis of the deltoid and sensory loss over the lateral side of the proximal part of the arm.

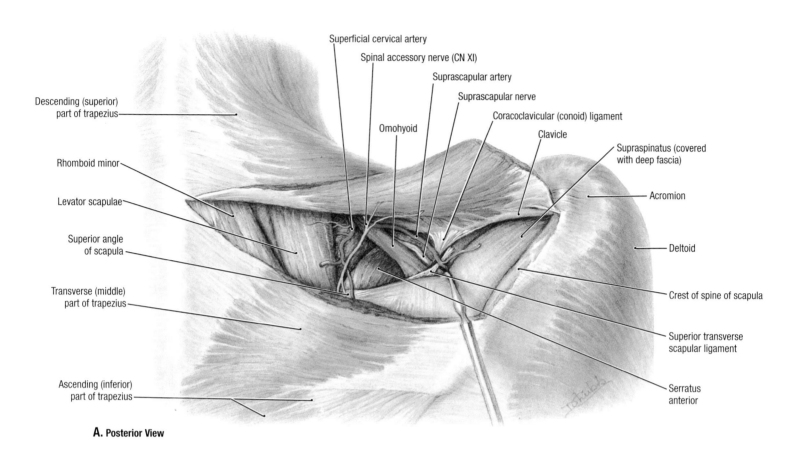

Superficial cervical artery

Spinal accessory nerve (CN XI)

Suprascapular artery

Suprascapular nerve

Coracoclavicular (conoid) ligament

Clavicle

Descending (superior) part of trapezius

Omohyoid

Supraspinatus (covered with deep fascia)

Rhomboid minor

Acromion

Levator scapulae

Deltoid

Superior angle of scapula

Crest of spine of scapula

Transverse (middle) part of trapezius

Superior transverse scapular ligament

Ascending (inferior) part of trapezius

Serratus anterior

A. Posterior View

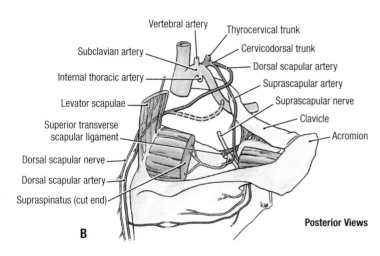

Vertebral artery

Thyrocervical trunk

Cervicodorsal trunk

Subclavian artery

Internal thoracic artery

Dorsal scapular artery

Suprascapular artery

Levator scapulae

Suprascapular nerve

Superior transverse scapular ligament

Clavicle

Dorsal scapular nerve

Acromion

Dorsal scapular artery

Supraspinatus (cut end)

Posterior Views

B

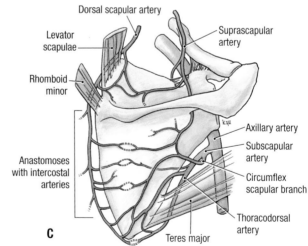

Dorsal scapular artery

Levator scapulae

Suprascapular artery

Rhomboid minor

Axillary artery

Subscapular artery

Anastomoses with intercostal arteries

Circumflex scapular branch

Thoracodorsal artery

Teres major

C

6.43   SUPRASCAPULAR REGION

A. Dissection. At the level of the superior angle of the scapula, the transverse part of the trapezius muscle is reflected. **B.** Suprascapular and dorsal scapular arteries. **C.** Scapular anastomosis.

    Several arteries join to form anastomoses on the anterior and posterior surfaces of the scapula. The importance of the collateral circulation made possible by these anastomoses becomes apparent when **ligation of a lacerated subclavian or axillary artery** is necessary or there is occlusion of these vessels. The direction of blood flow in the subscapular artery is then reversed, enabling blood to reach the third part of the axillary artery. In contrast to a sudden occlusion, slow occlusion of an artery often enables sufficient lateral circulation to develop, preventing **ischemia** (deficiency of blood).

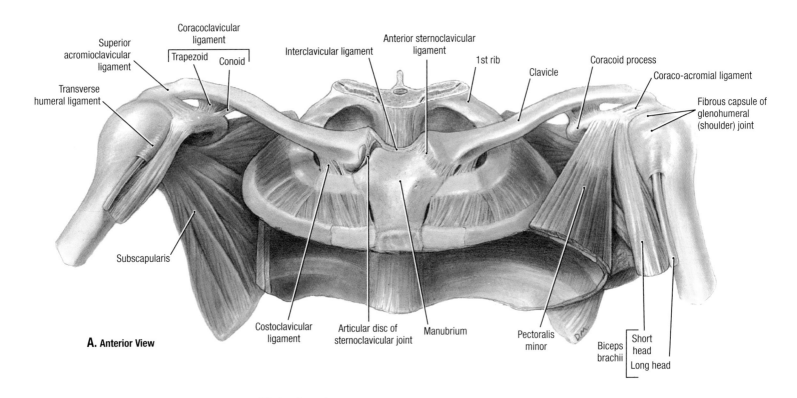

Coracoclavicular ligament

Superior acromioclavicular ligament

Trapezoid   Conoid

Interclavicular ligament

Anterior sternoclavicular ligament

1st rib

Clavicle

Coracoid process

Coraco-acromial ligament

Transverse humeral ligament

Fibrous capsule of glenohumeral (shoulder) joint

Subscapularis

Costoclavicular ligament

Articular disc of sternoclavicular joint

Manubrium

Pectoralis minor

Biceps brachii   Short head   Long head

A. Anterior View

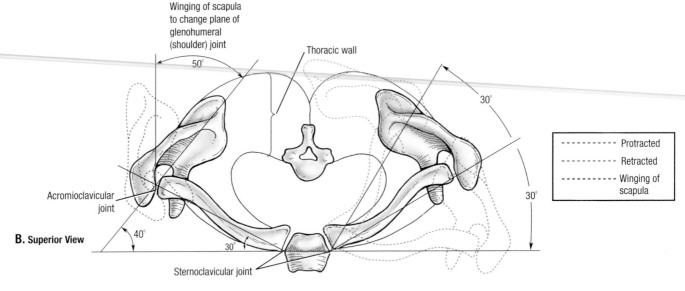

Winging of scapula to change plane of glenohumeral (shoulder) joint

50°

Thoracic wall

30°

Protracted

Retracted

Winging of scapula

Acromioclavicular joint

40°

30°

30°

B. Superior View

Sternoclavicular joint

6.44 PECTORAL GIRDLE

A. Dissection. **B.** Clavicular movements at the sternoclavicular and acromio-clavicular joints during rotation, protraction, and retraction of the scapula on the thoracic wall *(left side)* and winging of the scapula *(right side)*.

- The shoulder region includes the sternoclavicular, acromioclavicular, and shoulder (glenohumeral) joints; the mobility of the clavicle is essential to the movement of the upper limb.
- The sternoclavicular joint is the only joint connecting the upper limb (appendicular skeleton) to the trunk (axial skeleton). The articular disc of

the sternoclavicular joint divides the joint cavity into two parts and attaches superiorly to the clavicle and inferiorly to the first costal cartilage; the disc resists superior and medial displacement of the clavicle.

Paralysis of serratus anterior. In **B,** note that when the serratus anterior is paralyzed because of injury to the long thoracic nerve, the medial border of the scapula moves laterally and posteriorly away from the thoracic wall, giving the scapula the appearance of a wing **(winged scapula).** See Clinical Comment for Figure 6.29.

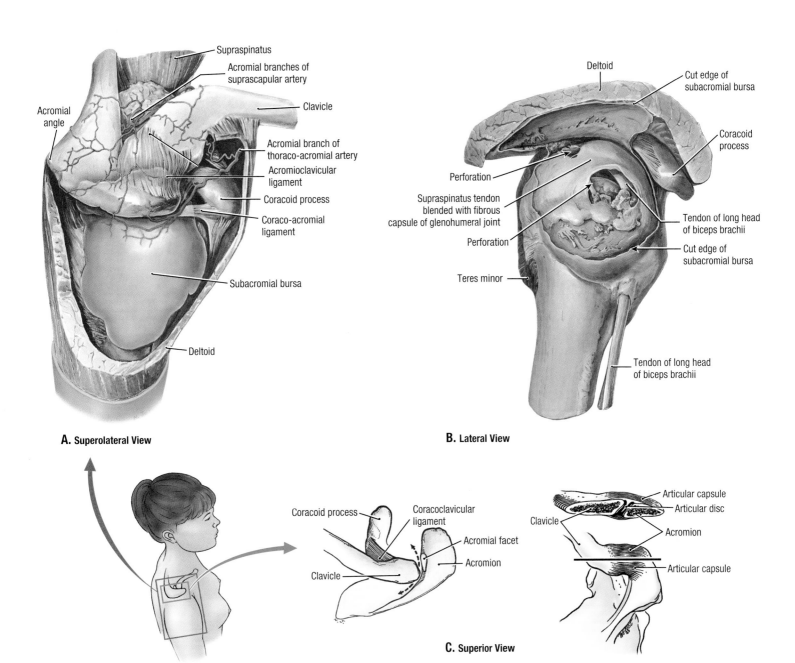

A. Superolateral View

- Supraspinatus
- Acromial branches of suprascapular artery
- Clavicle
- Acromial angle
- Acromial branch of thoraco-acromial artery
- Acromioclavicular ligament
- Coracoid process
- Coraco-acromial ligament
- Subacromial bursa
- Deltoid

B. Lateral View

- Deltoid
- Cut edge of subacromial bursa
- Coracoid process
- Perforation
- Supraspinatus tendon blended with fibrous capsule of glenohumeral joint
- Perforation
- Teres minor
- Tendon of long head of biceps brachii
- Cut edge of subacromial bursa
- Tendon of long head of biceps brachii

C. Superior View

- Coracoid process
- Coracoclavicular ligament
- Acromial facet
- Acromion
- Clavicle
- Articular capsule
- Articular disc
- Acromion
- Clavicle
- Articular capsule

6.45 SUBACROMIAL BURSA AND ACROMIOCLAVICULAR JOINT

A. Subacromial bursa. The bursa has been injected with purple latex. **B.** Acromioclavicular joint. **C. Attrition of supraspinatus tendon.** As a result of wearing away of the supraspinatus tendon and underlying capsule, the subacromial bursa and shoulder joint come into communication. The intracapsular part of the tendon of the long head of biceps muscle becomes frayed, leaving it adherent to the intertubercular groove. Of 95 dissecting room subjects in Dr. Grant's lab, none of the 18 younger than 50 years of age had a perforation, but 4 of the 19 who were 50 to 60 years and 23 of the 57 older than 60 years had perforations. The perforation was bilateral in 11 subjects and unilateral in 14.

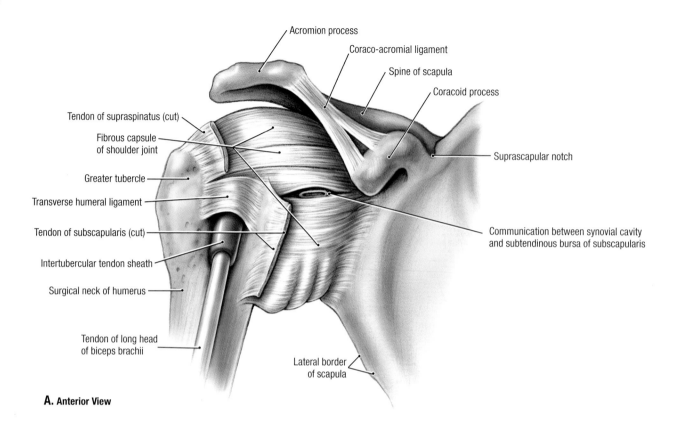

Acromion process

Coraco-acromial ligament

Spine of scapula

Coracoid process

Tendon of supraspinatus (cut)

Fibrous capsule of shoulder joint

Greater tubercle

Transverse humeral ligament

Tendon of subscapularis (cut)

Intertubercular tendon sheath

Surgical neck of humerus

Tendon of long head of biceps brachii

Suprascapular notch

Communication between synovial cavity and subtendinous bursa of subscapularis

Lateral border of scapula

A. Anterior View

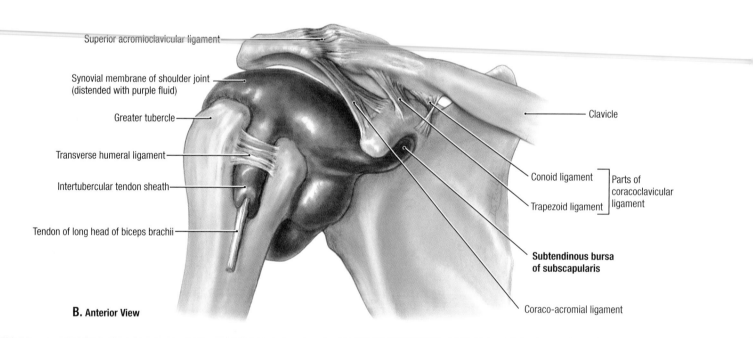

Superior acromioclavicular ligament

Synovial membrane of shoulder joint (distended with purple fluid)

Greater tubercle

Transverse humeral ligament

Intertubercular tendon sheath

Tendon of long head of biceps brachii

Clavicle

Conoid ligament | Parts of coracoclavicular ligament
Trapezoid ligament |

Subtendinous bursa of subscapularis

Coraco-acromial ligament

B. Anterior View

6.46 LIGAMENTS AND ARTICULAR CAPSULE OF GLENOHUMERAL (SHOULDER) JOINT

A. Fibrous capsule.
- The loose fibrous capsule is attached to the margin of the glenoid cavity and to the anatomical neck of the humerus.
- The strong coracoclavicular ligament provides stability to the acromioclavicular joint and prevents the scapula from being driven medially and the acromion from being driven inferior to the clavicle.

- The coraco-acromial ligament prevents superior displacement of the head of the humerus.

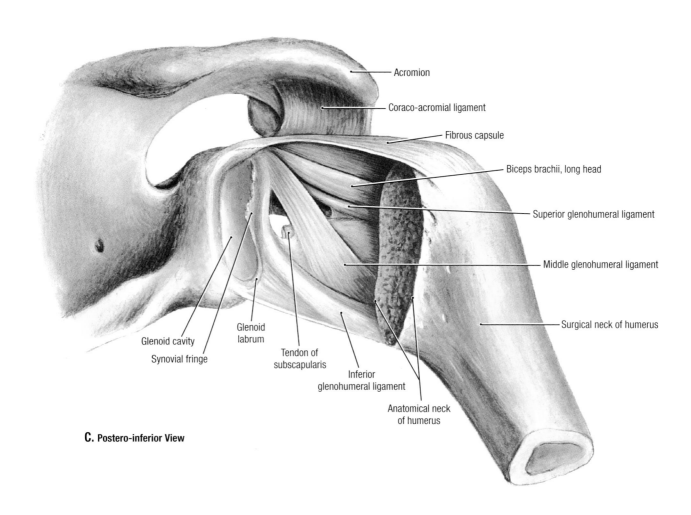

Acromion

Coraco-acromial ligament

Fibrous capsule

Biceps brachii, long head

Superior glenohumeral ligament

Middle glenohumeral ligament

Surgical neck of humerus

Glenoid cavity

Synovial fringe

Glenoid labrum

Tendon of subscapularis

Inferior glenohumeral ligament

Anatomical neck of humerus

C. Postero-inferior View

6.46   LIGAMENTS AND ARTICULAR CAPSULE OF GLENOHUMERAL (SHOULDER) JOINT *(CONTINUED)*

B. Synovial membrane of joint capsule. The synovial membrane lines the fibrous capsule and has two prolongations: (1) where it forms a synovial sheath for the tendon of the long head of the biceps muscle in its osseofibrous tunnel and (2) inferior to the coracoid process, where it forms a bursa between the subscapularis tendon and margin of the glenoid cavity—the subtendinous bursa of the subscapularis. **C.** Glenohumeral ligaments viewed from the interior of the shoulder joint.

- The joint is exposed from the posterior aspect by cutting away the thinner postero-inferior part of the capsule and sawing off the head of the humerus.
- The glenohumeral ligaments are visible from within the joint but are not easily seen externally.
- The glenohumeral ligaments and tendon of the long head of biceps brachii muscle converge on the supraglenoid tubercle.

- The slender superior glenohumeral ligament lies parallel to the tendon of the long head of biceps brachii. The middle ligament is free medially because the subtendinous bursa of subscapularis communicates with the joint cavity, usually there is only a single site of communication. In this individual there are openings on both sides of the ligament.

Because of its freedom of movement and instability, the glenohumeral joint is commonly dislocated by direct or indirect injury. Most **dislocations of the humeral head** occur in the downward (inferior) direction but are described clinically as anterior or (more rarely) posterior dislocations, indicating whether the humeral head has descended anterior or posterior to the infraglenoid tubercle and the long head of triceps. Anterior dislocation of the glenohumeral joint occurs most often in young adults, particularly athletes. It is usually caused by excessive extension and lateral rotation of the humerus.

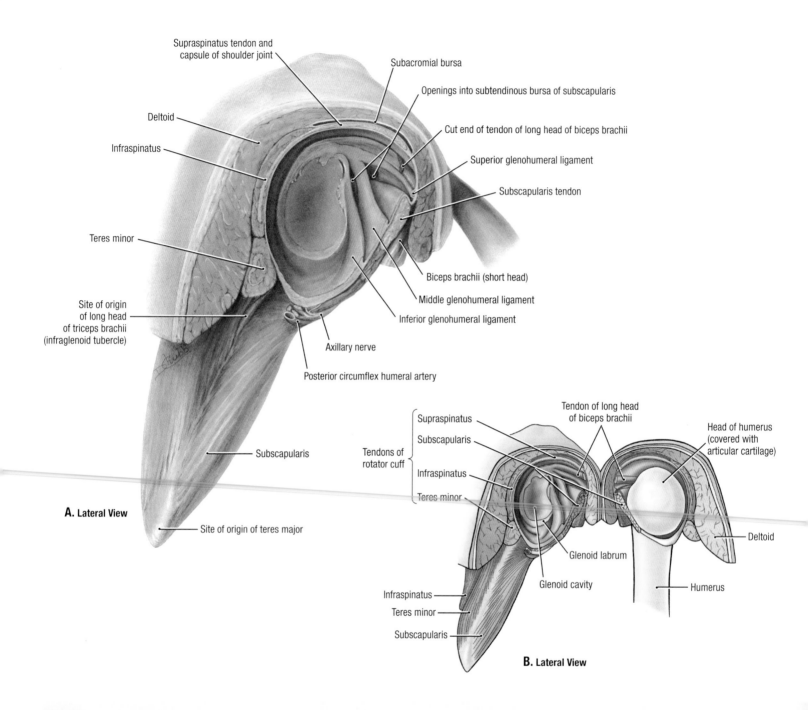

A. Lateral View

- Supraspinatus tendon and capsule of shoulder joint
- Subacromial bursa
- Openings into subtendinous bursa of subscapularis
- Deltoid
- Cut end of tendon of long head of biceps brachii
- Infraspinatus
- Superior glenohumeral ligament
- Subscapularis tendon
- Teres minor
- Biceps brachii (short head)
- Middle glenohumeral ligament
- Site of origin of long head of triceps brachii (infraglenoid tubercle)
- Inferior glenohumeral ligament
- Axillary nerve
- Posterior circumflex humeral artery
- Subscapularis
- Site of origin of teres major

B. Lateral View

- Tendon of long head of biceps brachii
- Supraspinatus
- Head of humerus (covered with articular cartilage)
- Subscapularis
- Tendons of rotator cuff
- Infraspinatus
- Teres minor
- Deltoid
- Glenoid labrum
- Infraspinatus
- Glenoid cavity
- Humerus
- Teres minor
- Subscapularis

6.47 INTERIOR OF GLENOHUMERAL (SHOULDER) JOINT AND RELATIONSHIP OF ROTATOR CUFF

A. Dissection. **B.** Schematic illustration.

- The fibrous capsule of the joint is thickened anteriorly by the three glenohumeral ligaments.
- The subacromial bursa is between the acromion and deltoid superiorly and the tendon of supraspinatus inferiorly.
- The four short rotator cuff muscles (supraspinatus, infraspinatus, teres minor, and subscapularis) cross the joint and blend with the capsule.
- The axillary nerve and posterior circumflex humeral artery are in contact with the capsule inferiorly and may be injured when the glenohumeral joint dislocates.

- Inflammation and calcification of the subacromial bursa result in pain, tenderness, and limitation of movement of the glenohumeral joint. This condition is also known as **calcific scapulohumeral bursitis.** Deposition of calcium in the supraspinatus tendon may irritate the overlying subacromial bursa, producing an inflammatory reaction, **subacromial bursitis.**

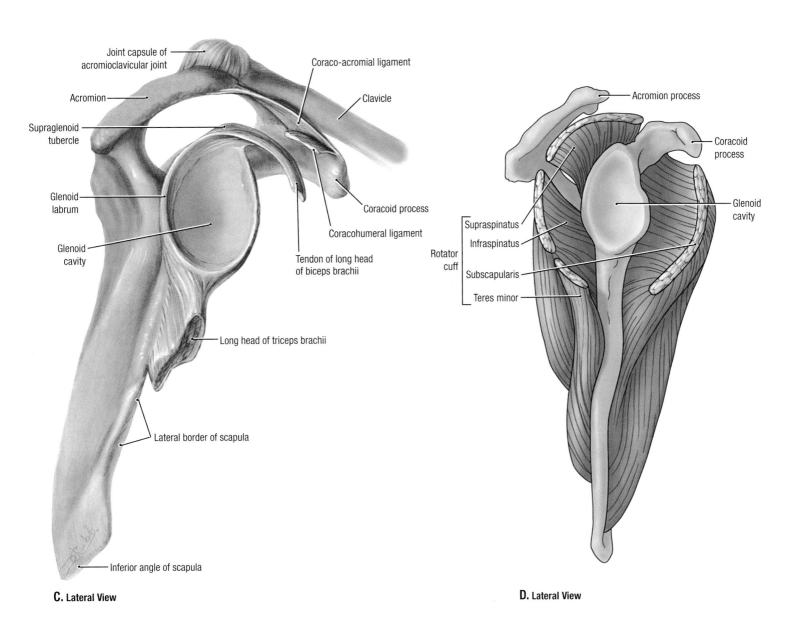

C. Lateral View

D. Lateral View

6.47 INTERIOR OF GLENOHUMERAL (SHOULDER) JOINT AND RELATIONSHIP OF ROTATOR CUFF *(CONTINUED)*

C. Dissection. **D.** Schematic illustration of the rotator cuff muscles and their relationship to the glenoid cavity.

- The coraco-acromial arch (coracoid process, coraco-acromial ligament, and acromion) prevents superior displacement of the head of the humerus.
- The long head of the triceps brachii muscle arises just inferior to the glenoid cavity; the long head of biceps just superior to it.
- The main function of the musculotendinous rotator cuff is to hold the large head of the humerus in the smaller and shallow glenoid cavity of the

scapula, both during the relaxed state (by tonic contraction) and during active abduction.

Tearing of the fibrocartilaginous glenoid labrum commonly occurs in the athletes who throw (e.g., a baseball) and in those who have shoulder instability and subluxation (partial dislocation) of the glenohumeral joint. The tear often results from sudden contraction of the biceps or forceful subluxation of the humeral head over the glenoid labrum. Usually a tear occurs in the anterosuperior part of the labrum.

Acromion

Site of acromioclavicular joint

Spine of scapula

Clavicle

Superior border of scapula

Tubercle of 1st rib

Coracoid process

Greater tubercle

Shoulder joint

Deltoid muscle

Head of humerus

Surgical neck of humerus

Infraglenoid tubercle

Axillary fat

Lateral border of scapula

Vertebral border of scapula

Rim of glenoid fossa

A. Anteroposterior View

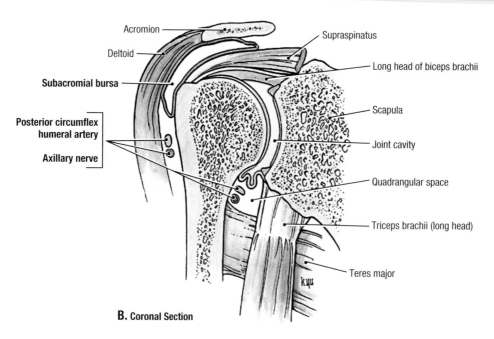

Acromion

Deltoid

Subacromial bursa

Posterior circumflex humeral artery

Axillary nerve

Supraspinatus

Long head of biceps brachii

Scapula

Joint cavity

Quadrangular space

Triceps brachii (long head)

Teres major

B. Coronal Section

6.48   IMAGING OF GLENOHUMERAL (SHOULDER) JOINT

A. Radiograph. **B.** Sectioned joint to show location of subacromial bursa and joint cavity.

C. Coronal MRI

E. Transverse MRI

D. Transverse Scan

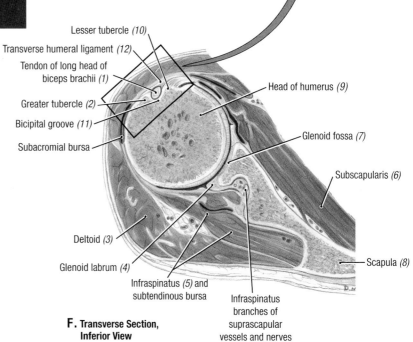

Lesser tubercle (10)
Transverse humeral ligament (12)
Tendon of long head of biceps brachii (1)
Greater tubercle (2)
Bicipital groove (11)
Subacromial bursa
Head of humerus (9)
Glenoid fossa (7)
Subscapularis (6)
Deltoid (3)
Glenoid labrum (4)
Infraspinatus (5) and subtendinous bursa
Infraspinatus branches of suprascapular vessels and nerves
Scapula (8)

F. Transverse Section, Inferior View

6.48 IMAGING OF GLENOHUMERAL (SHOULDER) JOINT *(CONTINUED)*

C. Coronal MRI. *A,* acromion; *C,* clavicle; *D,* deltoid; *GF,* glenoid cavity; *GT,* crest of greater tubercle; *H,* head of humerus; *LB,* long head of biceps brachii; *QS,* quadrangular space; *S,* scapula; *SB,* subscapularis; *SP,* supraspinatus; *SV,* suprascapular vessels and nerve; *TM,* teres minor; *TR,* trapezius. **D.** Transverse ultrasound scan of area indicated in **F. E.** Transverse MRI. **F.** Transverse section (*numbers* in **F** refer to structures labeled in **D** and **E**).

SUPERIOR

LATERAL — MEDIAL

INFERIOR

Biceps brachii

Medial epicondyle

A. Anterior View

Brachial fascia

Medial cutaneous nerve of forearm

Cephalic vein (1)

Basilic vein (3)

Cubital lymph node

Lateral cutaneous nerve of forearm

Median cubital vein (4)

Antebrachial fascia

Basilic vein of forearm (3)

Perforating vein

Bicipital aponeurosis

Median vein of forearm (2)

Cephalic vein of forearm (1)

B. Anterior View

6.49   CUBITAL FOSSA: SURFACE ANATOMY AND SUPERFICIAL DISSECTION

A. Surface anatomy. **B.** Cutaneous nerves and superficial veins (*numbers* in parentheses refer to structures in **A**).

- The cubital fossa is a triangular space (compartment) inferior to the elbow crease, roofed by deep fascia.
- In the forearm, the superficial veins (cephalic, median, basilic, and their connecting veins) make a variable, M-shaped pattern.
- The cephalic and basilic veins occupy the bicipital grooves, one on each side of the biceps brachii. In the lateral bicipital groove, the lateral

cutaneous nerve of the forearm appears just superior to the elbow crease; in the medial bicipital groove, the medial cutaneous nerve of the forearm becomes cutaneous at approximately the midpoint of the arm.

- The cubital fossa is the common site for **sampling and transfusion of blood and intravenous injections** because of the prominence and accessibility of veins. Usually, the median cubital vein or basilic vein is selected.

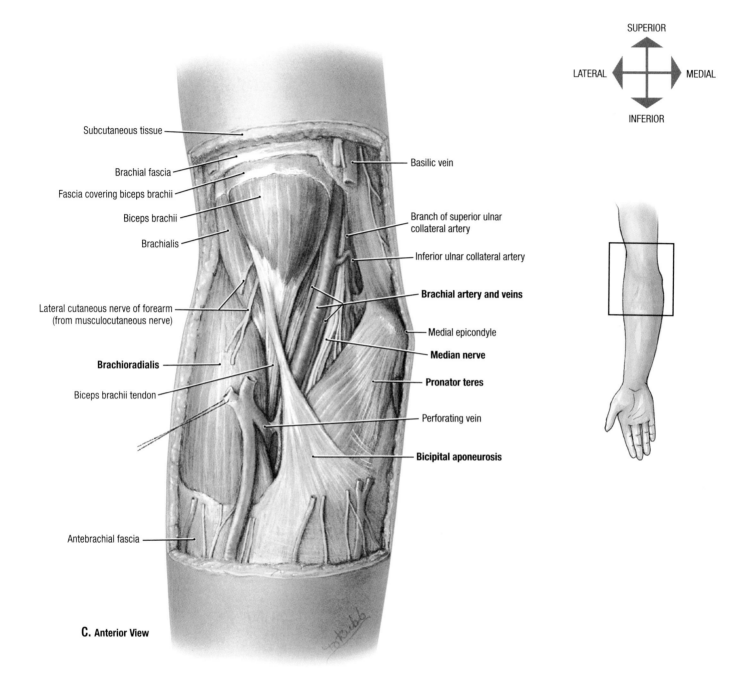

SUPERIOR

LATERAL ← → MEDIAL

INFERIOR

Subcutaneous tissue

Brachial fascia

Fascia covering biceps brachii

Biceps brachii

Brachialis

Lateral cutaneous nerve of forearm
(from musculocutaneous nerve)

Brachioradialis

Biceps brachii tendon

Antebrachial fascia

Basilic vein

Branch of superior ulnar
collateral artery

Inferior ulnar collateral artery

Brachial artery and veins

Medial epicondyle

Median nerve

Pronator teres

Perforating vein

Bicipital aponeurosis

C. Anterior View

6.49   **CUBITAL FOSSA: DEEP DISSECTION I**

C. Boundaries and contents of the cubital fossa.
- The cubital fossa is bound laterally by the brachioradialis and medially by the pronator teres and superiorly by a line joining the medial and lateral epicondyles.
- The three chief contents of the cubital fossa are the biceps brachii tendon, brachial artery, and median nerve.
- The biceps brachii tendon, on approaching its insertion, rotates through 90°, and the bicipital aponeurosis extends medially from the proximal part of the tendon.

- A fracture of the distal part of the humerus, near the supra-epicondylar ridges, is called a **supra-epicondylar (supracondylar) fracture.** The distal bone fragment may be displaced anteriorly or posteriorly. Any of the nerves or branches of the brachial vessels related to the humerus may be injured by a displaced bone fragment.

SUPERIOR

LATERAL ←→ MEDIAL

INFERIOR

Musculocutaneous nerve

Brachialis

Radial nerve

Brachioradialis

Extensor carpi radialis longus

Deep branch of radial nerve

Radial recurrent artery

Extensor carpi radialis brevis

Superficial branch of radial nerve

Radial artery

Biceps brachii

Medial intermuscular septum

Inferior ulnar collateral artery

Ulnar nerve

Brachial artery

Median nerve

Biceps brachii tendon

Superficial head of pronator teres

Ulnar artery

Deep head of pronator teres

Supinator

Flexor carpi radialis

D. Anterior View

6.49   CUBITAL FOSSA: DEEP DISSECTION II

D. Floor of the cubital fossa.

- Part of the biceps brachii muscle is excised, and the cubital fossa is opened widely, exposing the brachialis and supinator muscles in the floor of the fossa.
- The deep branch of the radial nerve pierces the supinator.
- The brachial artery lies between the biceps tendon and median nerve and divides into two branches, the ulnar and radial arteries.

- The median nerve supplies the flexor muscles. With the exception of the twig to the deep head of pronator teres, its motor branches arise from its medial side.
- The radial nerve supplies the extensor muscles. With the exception of the twig to brachioradialis, its motor branches arise from its lateral side. In this specimen, the radial nerve has been displaced laterally, so here its lateral branches appear to run medially.

A. Anterior View

- Biceps brachii
- Ulnar nerve
- Superior ulnar collateral artery
- Brachial artery
- **Supracondylar process**
- Median nerve
- Pronator teres
- **Supracondylar process**

B. Anterior View

- Tendon of long head of biceps brachii attached to intertubercular groove
- Humerus
- Long head
- Short head
- Biceps brachii
- **3rd head of biceps brachii**
- Brachialis

C. Anterior View

- Hypertrophic margin of head of humerus
- **Superior coracobrachialis**
- Musculocutaneous nerve
- Short head of biceps brachii
- Coracobrachialis
- **Attrition of long head of biceps brachii tendon**

D. Anterior View

- Cephalic vein
- Basilic vein
- Brachial artery
- Antebrachial fascia
- Radial artery
- **Superficial ulnar artery**

E. Anteromedial View

- Teres major
- **Brachial artery**
- Biceps brachii
- **Ulnar artery**
- Communicating branch from musculocutaneous nerve
- Median nerve
- **Radial artery**

F. Anterior Views

- Median nerve
- **Brachial artery**
- 5%
- 82%
- 13%

6.50   ANOMALIES

A. Supracondylar process of humerus. A fibrous band, from which the pronator teres muscle arises, joins this supra-epicondylar process to the medial epicondyle. The median nerve, often accompanied by the brachial artery, passes through the foramen formed by this band. This may be a cause of nerve entrapment. **B. Third head of biceps brachii.** In this case, there is also attrition of the biceps tendon. **C.** Attrition of the tendon of the long head of biceps brachii and presence of a coracobrachialis.

D. Superficial ulnar artery. E. Anomalous division of brachial artery. In this case, the median nerve passes between the radial and ulnar arteries, which arise high in the arm. **F. Relationship of median nerve and brachial artery.** The variable relationship of these two structures can be explained developmentally. In a study of 307 limbs in Dr. Grant's lab, portions of both primitive brachial arteries persisted in 5%, the posterior in 82%, and the anterior in 13%.

SUPERIOR

MEDIAL ← → LATERAL

INFERIOR

A. Posterior View

Triceps tendon *(2)*

Brachioradialis *(3)*

Extensor carpi
radialis longus *(4)*

Lateral epicondyle *(5)*

Common extensor
tendon

Fascia covering anconeus

Anconeus *(6)*

Medial epicondyle

Ulnar nerve

**Posterior ulnar
recurrent artery**

Tendinous arch of
cubital tunnel

Olecranon *(1)*

Aponeurosis of flexor
carpi ulnaris blended
with antebrachial fascia

B. Posterior View

6.51   **POSTERIOR ASPECT OF ELBOW I**

A. Surface anatomy. **B.** Superficial dissection (*numbers* in parentheses refer
to structures in **A**).

- The triceps brachii is attached distally to the superior surface of the olecranon and, through the deep fascia covering the anconeus, into the lateral
border of olecranon.

- The posterior surfaces of the medial epicondyle, lateral epicondyle, and
olecranon are subcutaneous and palpable.

- The ulnar nerve, also palpable, runs subfascially posterior to the medial
epicondyle; distal to this point, it disappears deep to the two heads of the
flexor carpi ulnaris.

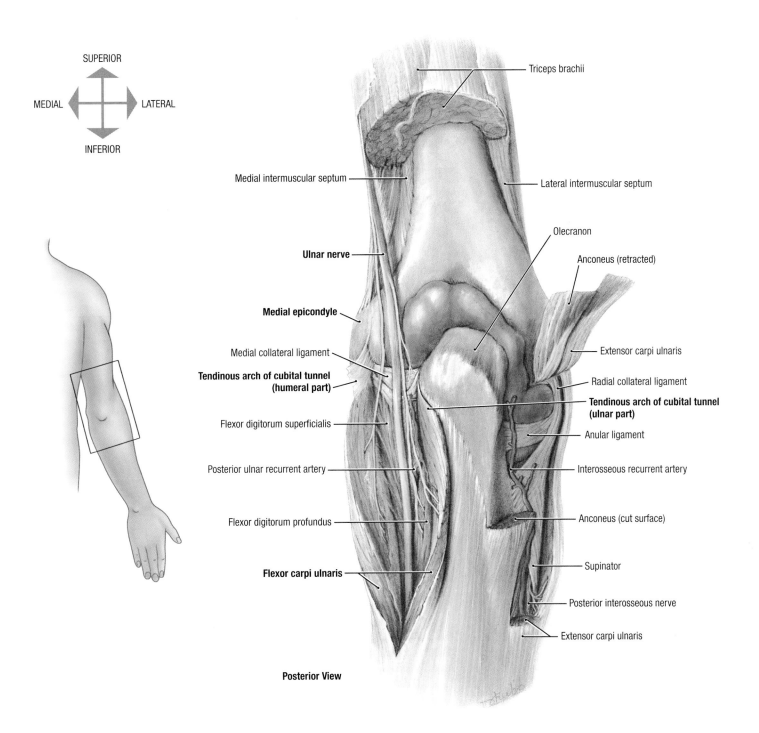

SUPERIOR

MEDIAL — LATERAL

INFERIOR

Triceps brachii

Medial intermuscular septum

Lateral intermuscular septum

Olecranon

Ulnar nerve

Anconeus (retracted)

Medial epicondyle

Medial collateral ligament

Extensor carpi ulnaris

Tendinous arch of cubital tunnel (humeral part)

Radial collateral ligament

Tendinous arch of cubital tunnel (ulnar part)

Flexor digitorum superficialis

Anular ligament

Posterior ulnar recurrent artery

Interosseous recurrent artery

Flexor digitorum profundus

Anconeus (cut surface)

Supinator

Flexor carpi ulnaris

Posterior interosseous nerve

Extensor carpi ulnaris

Posterior View

| **6.52** | **POSTERIOR ASPECT OF ELBOW II** |

Deep dissection. The distal portion of the triceps brachii muscle was removed.

• The ulnar nerve descends subfascially within the posterior compartment of the arm, passing posterior to the medial epicondyle in the groove for the ulnar nerve. Next it passes posterior to the ulnar collateral ligament of the elbow joint and then between the flexor carpi ulnaris and flexor digitorum profundus muscles.

Ulnar nerve injury occurs most commonly where the nerve passes posterior to the medial epicondyle of the humerus. The injury results when the medial part of the elbow hits a hard surface, fracturing the medial epicondyle. The ulnar nerve may be compressed in the cubital tunnel, resulting in **cubital tunnel syndrome.** The cubital tunnel is formed by the tendinous arch joining the humeral and ulnar heads of attachment of the flexor carpi ulnaris muscle. Ulnar nerve injury can result in extensive motor and sensory loss to the hand.

A. Anterior View

Lateral supra-epicondylar ridge — Medial supra-epicondylar ridge

Radial fossa — Coronoid fossa

Lateral epicondyle (common extensor orgin) — Medial epicondyle (common flexor orgin)

Capitulum — Trochlea

Trochlear notch — Olecranon

Radial notch

Head — Tubercle on coronoid process

Neck — Tuberosity of ulna

Tuberosity for { Subtendinous bursa — Biceps brachii } — Supinator fossa

Anterior oblique line

B. Posterior View

Lateral supra-epicondylar ridge

Olecranon fossa

Medial epicondyle { Flexor attachment — Groove for ulnar nerve } — Extensor attachment — Anconeus } Lateral epicondyle

Trochlea

Cutaneous triangular surface for olecranon bursa

Head

Neck

Supinator crest — Tuberosity

Posterior border

Posterior oblique line

C. Anteroposterior View

Lateral supra-epicondylar ridge — Medial supra-epicondylar ridge

Olecranon fossa

Lateral epicondyle — **Medial epicondyle**

Capitulum — Olecranon

Trochlea

Of radius { Head — Neck — Tuberosity } — Coronoid process of ulna — Proximal radio-ulnar joint — **Ulna**

D. Sagittal Section Lateral View

Triceps brachii — Brachialis

Subtendinous olecranon bursa — Fibrous capsule

Trochlea of humerus — Fat pad

Subcutaneous olecranon bursa — Synovial membrane — Coronoid process of ulna

k.yu

6.53   BONES AND IMAGING OF ELBOW REGION

A. Anterior bony features. **B.** Posterior bony features. **C.** Radiograph of elbow joint. **D.** Section of humero-ulnar joint.

The subcutaneous olecranon bursa is exposed to injury during falls on the elbow and to infection from abrasions of the skin covering the olecranon. Repeated excessive pressure and friction produces a friction **subcutaneous olecranon bursitis** (e.g., "student's elbow").

Subtendinous olecranon bursitis results from excessive friction between the triceps tendon and the olecranon. For example, it may occur due to repeated flexion-extension of the forearm during certain assembly-line jobs. The pain is severe during flexion of the forearm because of pressure exerted on the inflamed subtendinous olecranon bursa by the triceps tendon.

Proximal
radio-ulnar
joint (PR)

Anular
ligament
of radius

Radius (R)

Ulna (U)

Distal
radio-ulnar
joint (DR)

Proximal
radio-ulnar
joint (PR)

Ulna (U)

Radius (R)

Distal
radio-ulnar
joint (DR)

A. Anterior View, Supination

B. Anterior View, Pronation

6.54   SUPINATION AND PRONATION AT SUPERIOR, MIDDLE, AND INFERIOR
RADIO-ULNAR JOINTS

A. Radiograph of forearm in supination. **B.** Radiograph of forearm in pronation. The radius crosses the ulna
when the forearm is pronated. The superior and inferior radio-ulnar joints are synovial joints; the middle radio-
ulnar joint is a syndesmosis (fibrous joint) in which the interosseous ligament connects the forearm bones.

Medial epicondyle
Coronoid process
Radial tuberosity
Trochlea
Trochlear notch
Olecranon

A. Medial View

Triceps brachii
Brachioradialis
Fibrous capsule
Trochlea of humerus
Olecranon
Trochlear notch of ulna
Head
of radius — Neck
Tuberosity
Ulna

B. Sagittal MRI

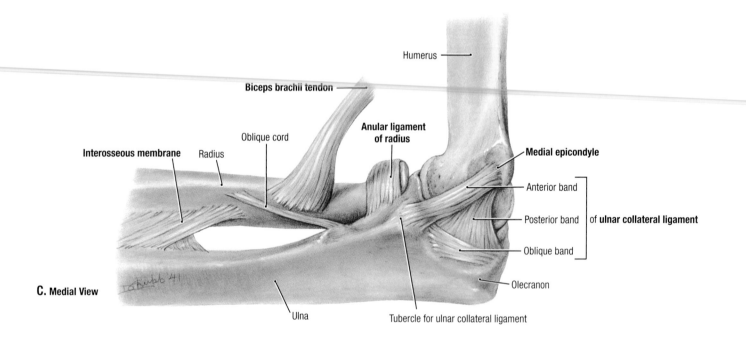

Humerus

Biceps brachii tendon

Oblique cord

Anular ligament of radius

Interosseous membrane   Radius

Medial epicondyle

Anterior band
Posterior band — of **ulnar collateral ligament**
Oblique band

Olecranon

C. Medial View

Ulna   Tubercle for ulnar collateral ligament

6.55   MEDIAL ASPECT OF BONES AND LIGAMENTS OF ELBOW REGION

A. Bony features. **B.** MRI of elbow joint. **C.** Ligaments. The anterior band of the ulnar (medial) collateral ligament is a strong, round cord that is taut when the elbow joint is extended. The posterior band is a weak fan that is taut in flexion of the joint.

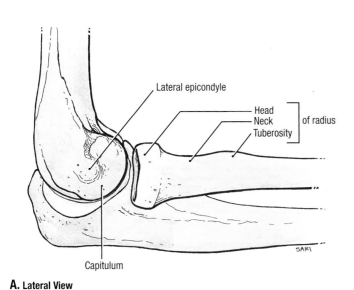

Lateral epicondyle

Head
Neck   } of radius
Tuberosity

Capitulum

A. Lateral View

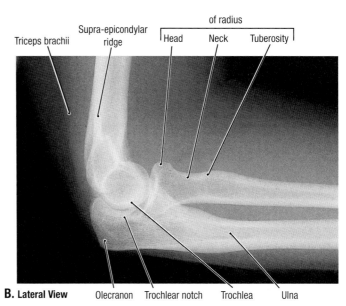

of radius

Triceps brachii   Supra-epicondylar   Head   Neck   Tuberosity
ridge

Olecranon   Trochlear notch   Trochlea   Ulna

B. Lateral View

Humerus

Lateral
supra-epidondylar
ridge

Capitulum

Head of radius

Tuberosity of radius

Neck of radius

Lateral epicondyle

Trochlear notch

Olecranon

Radial collateral ligament   **Anular ligament of radius**   Ulna   **Interosseous membrane**

C. Lateral View

6.56   LATERAL ASPECT OF BONES AND LIGAMENTS OF ELBOW REGION

A. Bony features. **B.** Lateral radiograph. **C.** Ligaments. The fan-shaped radial (lateral) collateral ligament is primarily attached to the anular ligament of the radius; superficial fibers of the lateral ligament blend with the fibrous capsule and continue onto the radius.

Humerus

Lateral epicondyle

Synovial membrane of elbow joint

Anular ligament of radius

Sacciform recess

Radius

Ulna

A. Anterior View

POSTERIOR

Nonarticular area overlaid with synovial pad of fat

Radial notch of ulna

Radial collateral ligament

Synovial fold

Anular ligament of radius

Olecranon

Synovial fat pad

Oblique part of ulnar collateral ligament

Coronoid process (articular surface)

ANTERIOR

B. Superior View

6.57 SYNOVIAL CAPSULE OF ELBOW JOINT AND ANULAR LIGAMENT

A. Synovial capsule of elbow and proximal radio-ulnar joints. The cavity of the elbow was injected with purple fluid (wax). The fibrous capsule was removed, and the synovial membrane remains. **B.** Anular ligament.

- The anular ligament secures the head of the radius to the radial notch of the ulna and with it forms a tapering columnar socket (i.e., wide superiorly, narrow inferiorly).
- The anular ligament is bound to the humerus by the radial collateral ligament of the elbow.

A common childhood injury is **subluxation and dislocation of the head of the radius** after traction on a pronated forearm (e.g., when lifting a child onto a bus). The sudden pulling of the upper limb tears or stretches the distal attachment of the less tapering anular ligament of a child. The radial head then moves distally, partially out of the anular ligament. The proximal part of the torn ligament may become trapped between the head of the radius and the capitulum of the humerus. The source of pain is the pinched anular ligament.

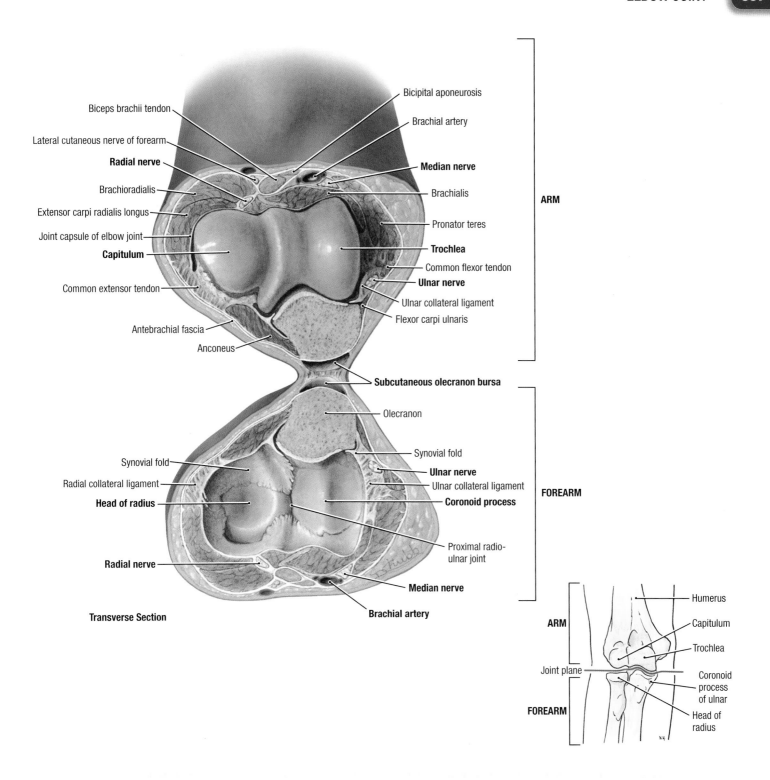

Labels (clockwise from top):
- Bicipital aponeurosis
- Brachial artery
- Biceps brachii tendon
- Lateral cutaneous nerve of forearm
- **Radial nerve**
- **Median nerve**
- Brachioradialis
- Brachialis
- Extensor carpi radialis longus
- Pronator teres
- Joint capsule of elbow joint
- **Trochlea**
- **Capitulum**
- Common flexor tendon
- **Ulnar nerve**
- Common extensor tendon
- Ulnar collateral ligament
- Flexor carpi ulnaris
- Antebrachial fascia
- Anconeus
- **Subcutaneous olecranon bursa**
- Olecranon
- Synovial fold
- Synovial fold
- **Ulnar nerve**
- Radial collateral ligament
- Ulnar collateral ligament
- **Head of radius**
- **Coronoid process**
- Proximal radio-ulnar joint
- **Radial nerve**
- **Median nerve**
- **Brachial artery**

Transverse Section

ARM / FOREARM

Inferior diagram labels:
- Humerus
- Capitulum
- Trochlea
- Joint plane
- Coronoid process of ulnar
- Head of radius
- ARM
- FOREARM

6.58   ARTICULAR SURFACES OF ELBOW JOINT

The tissue surrounding the condyles of the humerus has been sectioned in a transverse plane, followed by disarticulation of the elbow joint, revealing the articular surfaces. Compare the forearm (inferior) component with Figure 6.57B.

- Synovial folds containing fat overlie the periphery of the head of the radius and the nonarticular indentations on the trochlear notch of the ulna.
- The radial nerve is in contact with the joint capsule, the ulnar nerve is in contact with the ulnar collateral ligament, and the median nerve is separated from the joint capsule by the brachialis muscle.

TABLE 6.11 ARTERIES OF FOREARM

Radial artery

Origin:
In cubital fossa, as smaller terminal branch of brachial artery

Course/Distribution:
Runs distally under brachioradialis, lateral to flexor carpi radialis, defining boundary between the flexor and extensor compartments and supplying the radial aspect of both. Gives rise to a superficial palmar branch near the radiocarpal joint; it then transverses the anatomical snuff box to pass between the heads of the 1st dorsal interosseous muscle joining the deep branch of the ulnar artery to form the deep palmar arch

Ulnar artery

Origin: In cubital fossa, as larger terminal branch of brachial artery

Course/Distribution: Passes distally between 2nd and 3rd layers of forearm flexor muscles, supplying ulnar aspect of flexor compartment; passes superficial to flexor retinaculum at wrist, continuing as the superficial palmar arch (with superficial branch of radial) after its deep palmar branch joins the deep palmar arch

Radial recurrent artery

Origin: In cubital fossa, as 1st (lateral) branch of radial artery

Course/Distribution: Courses proximally, superficial to supinator, passing between brachioradialis and brachialis to anastomose with radial collateral artery

Anterior and posterior ulnar recurrent arteries

Origin: In and immediately distal to cubital fossa, as 1st and 2nd medial branches of ulnar artery

Course/Distribution:
Course proximally to anastomose with the inferior and superior ulnar collateral arteries, respectively, forming collateral pathways anterior and posterior to the medial epicondyle of the humerus

Common interosseous artery

Origin: Immediately distal to the cubital fossa, as 1st lateral branch of ulnar artery

Course/Distribution: Terminates almost immediately, dividing into anterior and posterior interosseous arteries

Anterior and posterior interosseous arteries

Origin: Distal to radial tubercle, as terminal branches of common interosseous

Course/Distribution: Pass to opposite sides of interosseous membrane; anterior artery runs on interosseous membrane; posterior artery runs between superficial and deep layers of extensor muscles as primary artery of compartment

Interosseous recurrent artery

Origin: Initial part of posterior interosseous artery

Course/Distribution:
Courses proximally between lateral epicondyle and olecranon, deep to anconeus, to anastomose with middle collateral artery

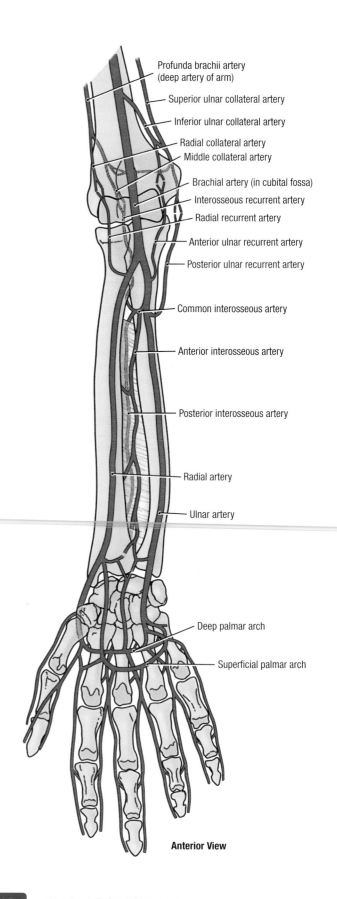

Profunda brachii artery (deep artery of arm)
Superior ulnar collateral artery
Inferior ulnar collateral artery
Radial collateral artery
Middle collateral artery
Brachial artery (in cubital fossa)
Interosseous recurrent artery
Radial recurrent artery
Anterior ulnar recurrent artery
Posterior ulnar recurrent artery
Common interosseous artery
Anterior interosseous artery
Posterior interosseous artery
Radial artery
Ulnar artery
Deep palmar arch
Superficial palmar arch

Anterior View

6.59 ARTERIES OF FOREARM

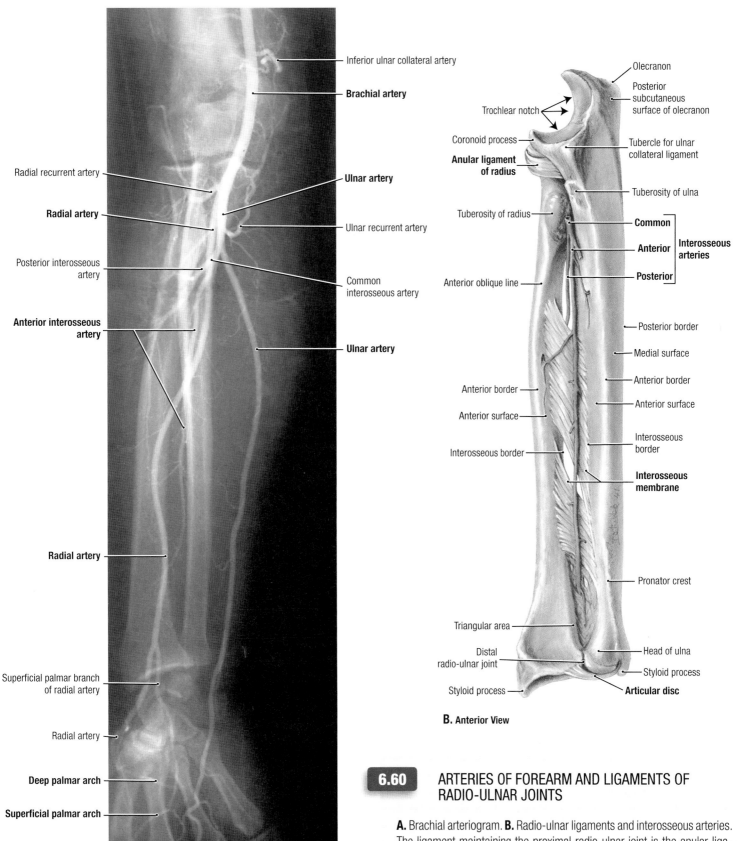

Inferior ulnar collateral artery

Brachial artery

Radial recurrent artery

Radial artery

Ulnar artery

Ulnar recurrent artery

Posterior interosseous artery

Common interosseous artery

Anterior interosseous artery

Ulnar artery

Radial artery

Superficial palmar branch of radial artery

Radial artery

Deep palmar arch

Superficial palmar arch

A. Anteroposterior View

Olecranon

Posterior subcutaneous surface of olecranon

Trochlear notch

Coronoid process

Tubercle for ulnar collateral ligament

Anular ligament of radius

Tuberosity of ulna

Tuberosity of radius

Common

Anterior — **Interosseous arteries**

Anterior oblique line

Posterior

Posterior border

Medial surface

Anterior border

Anterior border

Anterior surface

Anterior surface

Interosseous border

Interosseous border

Interosseous membrane

Pronator crest

Triangular area

Head of ulna

Distal radio-ulnar joint

Styloid process

Styloid process

Articular disc

B. Anterior View

6.60 ARTERIES OF FOREARM AND LIGAMENTS OF RADIO-ULNAR JOINTS

A. Brachial arteriogram. **B.** Radio-ulnar ligaments and interosseous arteries. The ligament maintaining the proximal radio-ulnar joint is the anular ligament, that for the distal joint is the articular disc, and that for the middle joint is the interosseous membrane. The interosseous membrane is attached to the interosseous borders of the radius and ulna, but it also spreads onto their surfaces.

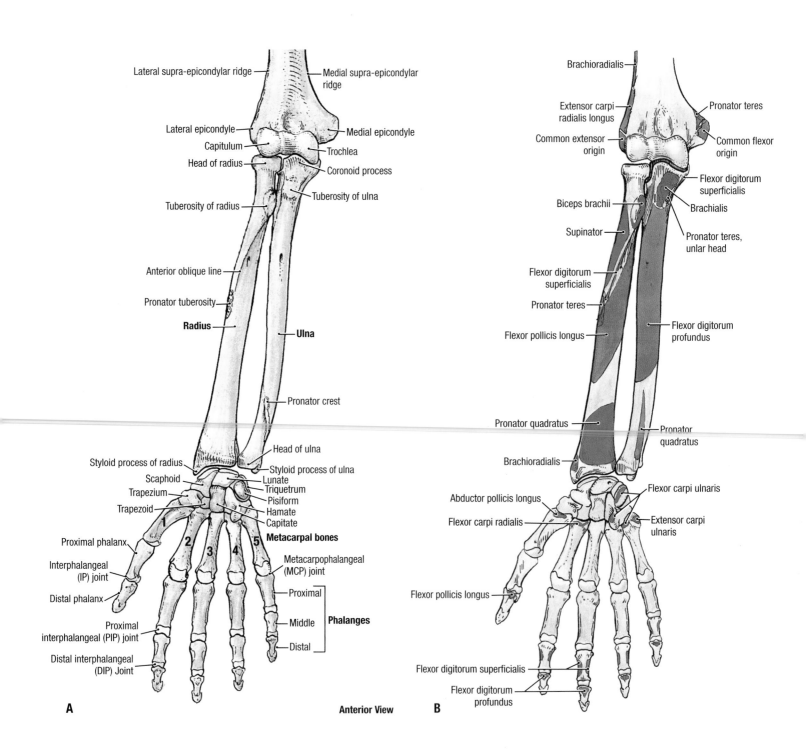

A. Bony features. **B.** Sites of muscle attachments.

6.61 BONES OF FOREARM AND HAND AND ATTACHMENTS OF FOREARM MUSCLES

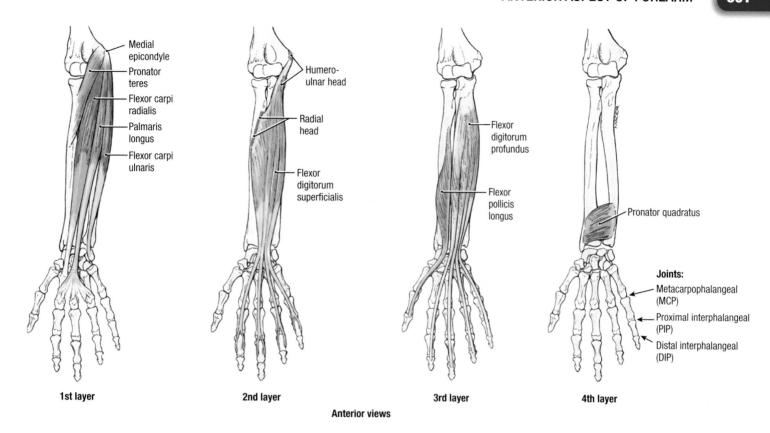

1st layer — Medial epicondyle, Pronator teres, Flexor carpi radialis, Palmaris longus, Flexor carpi ulnaris

2nd layer — Humero-ulnar head, Radial head, Flexor digitorum superficialis

3rd layer — Flexor digitorum profundus, Flexor pollicis longus

4th layer — Pronator quadratus, Joints: Metacarpophalangeal (MCP), Proximal interphalangeal (PIP), Distal interphalangeal (DIP)

Anterior views

6.62 MUSCLES OF ANTERIOR ASPECT OF FOREARM

TABLE 6.12 MUSCLES OF ANTERIOR ASPECT OF FOREARM

Muscle	Proximal Attachment	Distal Attachment	Innervation	Main Actions
Pronator teres	Medial epicondyle of humerus and coronoid process of ulna	Middle of lateral surface of radius (pronator tuberosity)	Median nerve (C6–**C7**)	Pronates forearm and flexes elbow joint
Flexor carpi radialis	Medial epicondyle of humerus	Base of 2nd and 3rd metacarpals		Flexes and abducts wrist joint
Palmaris longus		Distal half of flexor retinaculum and palmar aponeurosis	Median nerve (C7–**C8**)	Flexes wrist joint and tightens palmar aponeurosis
Flexor carpi ulnaris	*Humeral head:* medial epicondyle of humerus; *Ulnar head:* olecranon and posterior border of ulna	Pisiform, hook of hamate, and 5th metacarpal	Ulnar nerve (C7–**C8**)	Flexes and adducts wrist joint
Flexor digitorum superficialis	*Humero-ulnar head:* medial epicondyle of humerus, ulnar collateral ligament, and coronoid process of ulna *Radial head:* superior half of anterior border of radius	Bodies of middle phalanges of medial four digits	Median nerve (C7, **C8**, and T1)	Flexes PIPs of medial four digits; acting more strongly, it flexes MCPs and wrist joint
Flexor digitorum profundus	Proximal three quarters of medial and anterior surfaces of ulna and interosseous membrane	Bases of distal phalanges of medial four digits	*Medial part:* ulnar nerve (**C8**–T1) *Lateral part:* median nerve (**C8**–T1)	Flexes DIPs of medial four digits; assists with flexion of wrist joint
Flexor pollicis longus	Anterior surface of radius and adjacent interosseous membrane	Base of distal phalanx of thumb	Anterior interosseous nerve from median (**C8**–T1)	Flexes IP joints of 1st digit (thumb) and assists flexion of wrist joint
Pronator quadratus	Distal fourth of anterior surface of ulna	Distal fourth of anterior surface of radius		Pronates forearm; deep fibers bind radius and ulna together

Brachioradialis

Common flexor origin

Pronator teres

Palmaris longus

Flexor carpi radialis

Flexor carpi ulnaris

Flexor retinaculum

Palmar aponeurosis

A. Anterior View

6.63 SUPERFICIAL MUSCLES OF FOREARM AND PALMAR APONEUROSIS

- At the elbow, the brachial artery lies between the biceps tendon and median nerve. It then bifurcates into the radial and ulnar arteries.
- At the wrist, the radial artery is lateral to the flexor carpi radialis tendon, and the ulnar artery is lateral to flexor carpi ulnaris tendon.
- In the forearm, the radial artery lies between the flexor and extensor compartments. The muscles lateral to the artery are supplied by the radial nerve, and those medial to it by the median and ulnar nerves; thus, no motor nerve crosses the radial artery.
- The brachioradialis muscle slightly overlaps the radial artery, which is otherwise superficial.
- The four superficial muscles all attach proximally to the medial epicondyle of the humerus (common flexor origin).
- The palmaris longus muscle, in this specimen, has an anomalous distal belly; this muscle usually has a small belly at the common flexor origin and a long tendon that is continued into the palm as the palmar aponeurosis. The palmaris longus is absent unilaterally or bilaterally in approximately 14% of limbs.

Biceps brachii

Brachialis

Musculocutaneous nerve

Bicipital aponeurosis (reflected)

Median nerve

Brachialis

Brachial artery

Medial epicondyle of humerus (common flexor origin)

Pronator teres

Radial artery

Brachioradialis

Flexor carpi radialis

Palmaris longus

Flexor carpi ulnaris

Radial artery

Superficial branch of radial nerve

Flexor digitorum superficialis

Flexor pollicis longus

Flexor carpi radialis

Palmaris longus

Median nerve

Flexor carpi ulnaris

Ulnar artery

Ulnar nerve

Palmaris brevis

Palmar aponeurosis

Palmar digital arteries and nerves

Superficial transverse metacarpal ligament

Abductor pollicis longus

Superficial palmar branch of radial artery

B. Anterior View

A. Anterior View

Median nerve

Supinator

Pronator teres

Flexor digitorum superficialis

Flexor pollicis longus

Pronator quadratus

B. Anterior View

Biceps brachii

Median nerve

Brachial artery

Brachioradialis

Radial nerve — Superficial branch / Deep branch

Radial recurrent artery

Ulnar artery

Supinator

Pronator teres

Radial artery

Flexor digitorum superficialis, radial head

Flexor pollicis longus

Pronator quadratus

Palmar carpal branch of radial artery

Superficial palmar branch of radial artery

Flexor carpi radialis (reflected)

Ulnar nerve

Triceps brachii

Pronator teres

Flexor carpi radialis   } Reflected

Brachialis

Flexor digitorum superficialis, humero-ulnar head

Flexor carpi ulnaris
Flexor digitorum profundus   } Nerve to

Flexor carpi ulnaris

Flexor digitorum profundus

Ulnar nerve

Ulnar artery

Flexor digitorum superficialis

Pronator quadratus

Dorsal (cutaneous) branch of ulnar nerve

Dorsal carpal branch of ulnar artery

Flexor digitorum superficialis

Flexor digitorum profundus

Persisting median artery

Median nerve

Palmaris longus (reflected)

6.64   FLEXOR DIGITORUM SUPERFICIALIS AND RELATED STRUCTURES

- The flexor digitorum superficialis muscle is attached proximally to the humerus, ulna, and radius.
- The ulnar artery passes obliquely posterior to the flexor digitorum superficialis; at the medial border of the muscle, the ulnar artery joins the ulnar nerve.
- The ulnar nerve lies between the flexor digitorum profundus and flexor carpi ulnaris.
- The median nerve descends vertically posterior to the flexor digitorum superficialis and appears distally at its lateral border.
- The median artery of this specimen is a variation resulting from persistence of an embryologic vessel that usually disappears.

Median nerve

Flexor digitorum
profundus

Flexor pollicis longus

Pronator quadratus

A. Anterior View

Musculocutaneous nerve

Brachialis

Brachioradialis

Medial epicondyle
of humerus

Brachial artery

Median nerve

Radial nerve — Superficial branch

Deep branch

Flexor digitorum
superficialis (humero-
ulnar head)

Biceps brachii tendon

Extensor carpi radialis longus

Anterior
interosseous nerve

Extensor carpi radialis brevis

Posterior ulnar
recurrent artery

Supinator

Anterior
interosseous artery

Pronator teres (cut)

Flexor carpi ulnaris

Ulnar artery

Ulnar nerve

Flexor digitorum
superficialis
(radial head, cut)

3rd, 4th,
5th digits | Flexor
digitorum
profundus
muscle
Flexor pollicis longus — 2nd digit | belly for

Radial artery

Dorsal (cutaneous)
branch of ulnar nerve

Dorsal carpal branch
of ulnar artery

Pronator quadratus

Pisiform

Palmar radiocarpal ligament

Median nerve

Flexor retinaculum
(transverse carpal ligament)

Deep branch of ulnar
nerve and artery

Opponens pollicis

Flexor pollicis brevis

Opponens digiti minimi

Abductor pollicis
brevis

Abductor digiti minimi

4th lumbrical

1st lumbrical

2nd lumbrical

3rd lumbrical

B. Anterior View

6.65 DEEP FLEXORS OF DIGITS AND RELATED STRUCTURES

- The ulnar nerve enters the forearm posterior to the medial epicondyle, then descends between the flexor digitorum profundus and flexor carpi ulnaris and is joined by the ulnar artery. At the wrist the ulnar nerve and artery pass anterior to the flexor retinaculum and lateral to the pisiform to enter the palm.
- At the elbow, the ulnar nerve supplies the flexor carpi ulnaris and the medial half of the flexor digitorum profundus muscles; proximal to the wrist, it gives off the dorsal (cutaneous) branch.
- The four lumbricals arise from the flexor digitorum profundus tendons.

Layer of fat

Radial nerve

Brachialis

Deep branch

Radial nerve Superficial branch

Supinator

Anterior oblique line of radius

Ulna

Radius

Pronator quadratus

A. Anterior View

Ulnar nerve

Medial epicondyle of humerus

Ulnar nerve

Tendon of **biceps brachii**

Subtendinous bursa of biceps

Anterior interosseous nerve

Common interosseous artery

Anterior interosseous nerve

Anterior interosseous artery

Flexor digitorum profundus

Pronator teres
(distal attachment)

Flexor carpi ulnaris

Flexor pollicis longus

Tendon of brachioradialis

Pronator quadratus

2nd digit
3rd digit
4th digit
5th digit

Tendons of flexor digitorum profundus

Radial artery

Abductor pollicis longus

Flexor retinaculum
(transverse carpal ligament)

Opponens pollicis

B. Anterior View

Median nerve

Pisiform bone

Ulnar nerve and artery

Abductor digiti minimi

Opponens digiti minimi

N JoY

6.66 DEEP FLEXORS OF DIGITS AND SUPINATOR

- The five tendons of the deep digital flexors (flexor pollicis longus and flexor digitorum profundus) lie side by side as they enter the carpal tunnel.
- The deep branch of the radial nerve pierces and innervates the supinator muscle.
- The anterior interosseous nerve and artery pass deeply between the flexor pollicis longus and flexor digitorum profundus muscles to lie on the interosseous membrane.

A

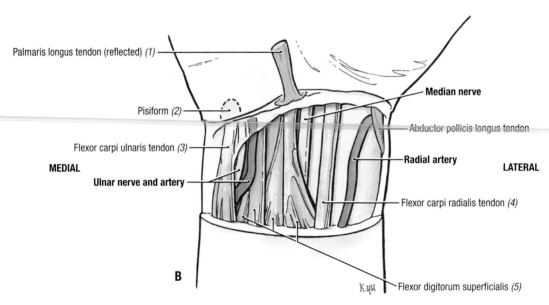

Palmaris longus tendon (reflected) *(1)*

Median nerve

Pisiform *(2)*

Abductor pollicis longus tendon

Flexor carpi ulnaris tendon *(3)*

Radial artery

MEDIAL

LATERAL

Ulnar nerve and artery

Flexor carpi radialis tendon *(4)*

B

К.ЧИ

Flexor digitorum superficialis *(5)*

Anterior Views of Right Hand and Wrist

6.67   STRUCTURES OF ANTERIOR ASPECT OF WRIST

A. Surface anatomy. **B.** Schematic illustration. **C.** Dissection.

- The distal skin incision follows the transverse skin crease at the wrist. The incision crosses the pisiform, to which the flexor carpi ulnaris muscle attaches, and the tubercle of the scaphoid, to which the tendon of flexor carpi radialis muscle is a guide.
- The palmaris longus tendon bisects the transverse skin crease; deep to the lateral margin of the tendon is the median nerve.
- The radial artery passes deep to the tendon of the abductor pollicis longus muscle.
- The flexor digitorum superficialis tendons to the 3rd and 4th digits become anterior to those of the 2nd and 5th digits.
- The recurrent branch of the median nerve to the thenar muscles lies within a circle whose center is 2.5 to 4 cm distal to the tubercle of the scaphoid.

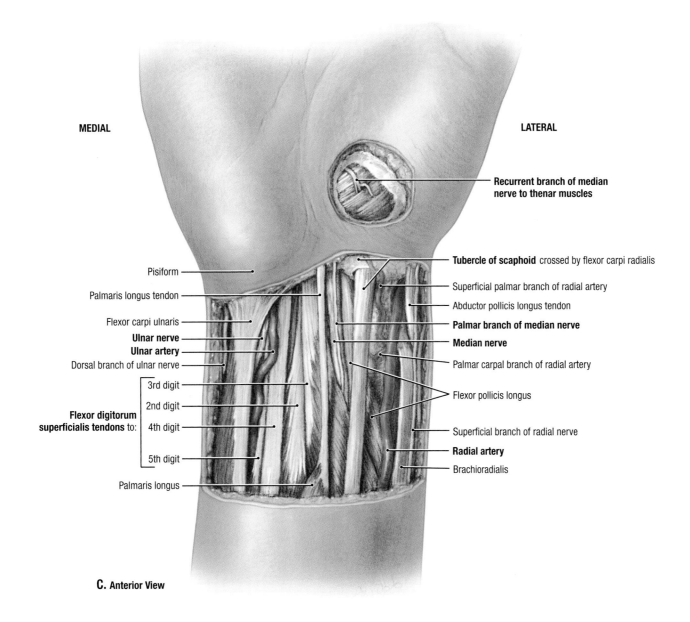

MEDIAL

LATERAL

Recurrent branch of median nerve to thenar muscles

Pisiform

Tubercle of scaphoid crossed by flexor carpi radialis

Palmaris longus tendon

Superficial palmar branch of radial artery

Flexor carpi ulnaris

Abductor pollicis longus tendon

Ulnar nerve

Palmar branch of median nerve

Ulnar artery

Median nerve

Dorsal branch of ulnar nerve

Palmar carpal branch of radial artery

3rd digit

2nd digit

Flexor pollicis longus

Flexor digitorum superficialis tendons to:

4th digit

5th digit

Superficial branch of radial nerve

Radial artery

Palmaris longus

Brachioradialis

C. Anterior View

6.67   STRUCTURES OF ANTERIOR ASPECT OF WRIST (CONTINUED)

Lesions of the median nerve usually occur in two places: the forearm and wrist. The most common site is where the nerve passes though the carpal tunnel. Lacerations of the wrist often cause median nerve injury because this nerve is relatively close to the surface. This results in paralysis of the thenar muscles and the first two lumbricals. Hence opposition of the thumb is not possible and fine control movements of the 2nd and 3rd digits are impaired. Sensation is also lost over the thumb and adjacent two and a half digits.

Median nerve injury resulting from a perforating wound in the elbow region results in loss of flexion of the proximal and distal interphalangeal joints of the 2nd and 3rd digits. The ability to flex the metacarpophalangeal joints of these digits is also affected because digital branches of the median nerve supply the 1st and 2nd lumbricals. The palmar cutaneous branch of the median nerve does not traverse the carpal tunnel. It supplies the skin of the central palm, which remains sensitive in carpal tunnel syndrome.

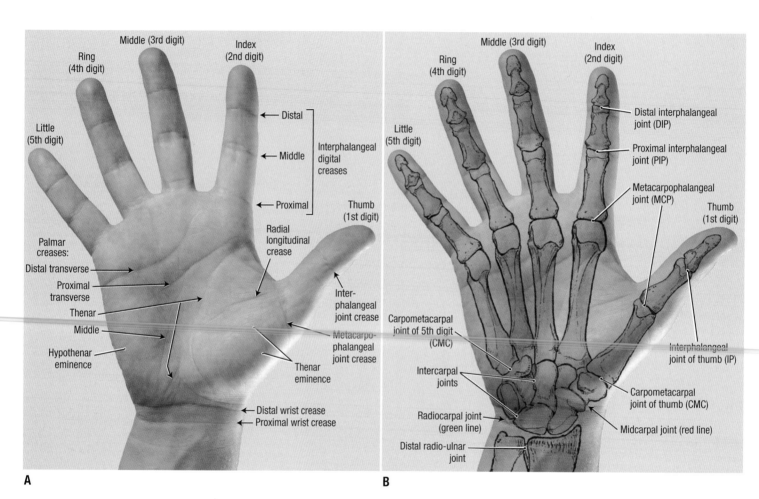

A

Anterior Views

B

6.68 SURFACE ANATOMY OF SKELETON OF HAND AND WRIST

A. Skin creases of wrist and hand. **B.** Surface projection of joints of wrist and hand. Note relationship of bones and joints to features of the hand.

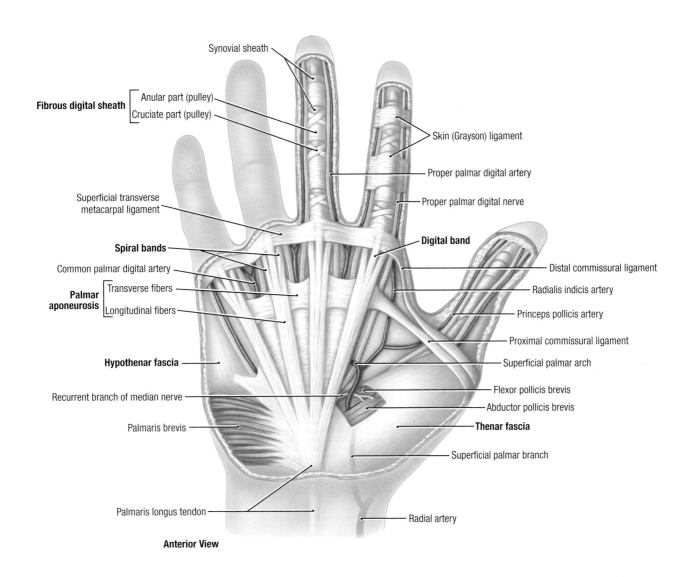

Synovial sheath

Fibrous digital sheath
- Anular part (pulley)
- Cruciate part (pulley)

Skin (Grayson) ligament

Proper palmar digital artery

Proper palmar digital nerve

Superficial transverse metacarpal ligament

Digital band

Spiral bands

Distal commissural ligament

Common palmar digital artery

Radialis indicis artery

Palmar aponeurosis
- Transverse fibers
- Longitudinal fibers

Princeps pollicis artery

Proximal commissural ligament

Hypothenar fascia

Superficial palmar arch

Recurrent branch of median nerve

Flexor pollicis brevis

Abductor pollicis brevis

Palmaris brevis

Thenar fascia

Superficial palmar branch

Palmaris longus tendon

Radial artery

Anterior View

6.69   PALMAR (DEEP) FASCIA: PALMAR APONEUROSIS, THENAR AND HYPOTHENAR FASCIA

A. Anterior view.
- The palmar fascia is thin over the thenar and hypothenar eminences, but thick centrally, where it forms the palmar aponeurosis, and in the digits, where it forms the fibrous digital sheaths.
- At the distal end (base) of the palmar aponeurosis, four bundles of digital and spiral bands continue to the bases and fibrous digital sheaths of digits 2 to 5.

B. Dupuytren contracture is a disease of the palmar fascia resulting in progressive shortening, thickening, and fibrosis of the palmar fascia and palmar aponeurosis. The fibrous degeneration of the longitudinal digital bands of the aponeurosis on the medial side of the hand pulls the 4th and

5th fingers into partial flexion at the metacarpophalangeal and proximal interphalangeal joints. The contracture is frequently bilateral. Treatment of Dupuytren contracture usually involves surgical excision of all fibrotic parts of the palmar fascia to free the fingers.

B. Dupuytren contracture

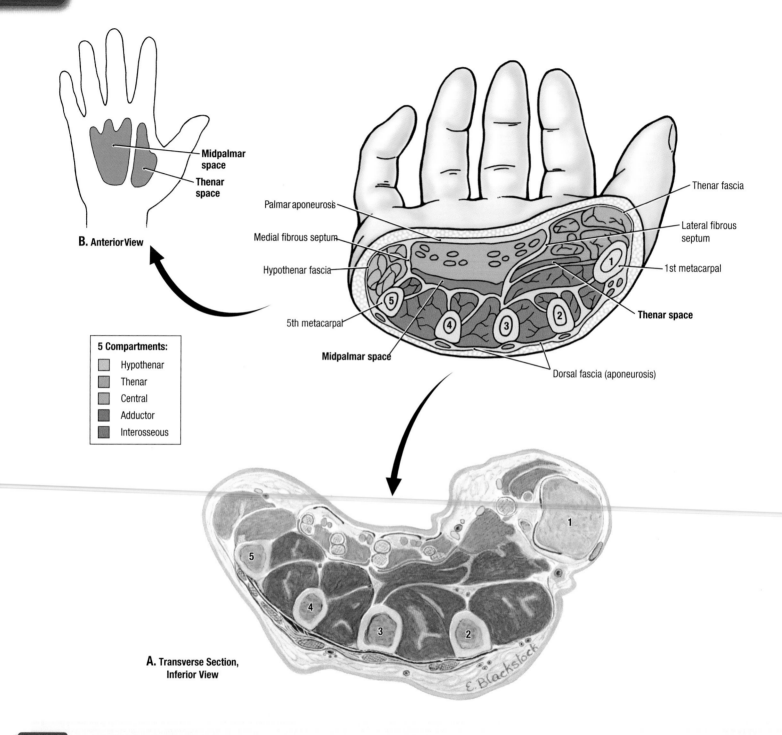

B. Anterior View

Palmar aponeurosis

Medial fibrous septum

Hypothenar fascia

5th metacarpal

Midpalmar space

Midpalmar space

Thenar space

Thenar fascia

Lateral fibrous septum

1st metacarpal

Thenar space

Dorsal fascia (aponeurosis)

5 Compartments:
- Hypothenar
- Thenar
- Central
- Adductor
- Interosseous

E. Blackslock

A. Transverse Section, Inferior View

| 6.70 | SYNOVIAL CAPSULE OF ELBOW JOINT AND ANULAR LIGAMENT |

A. Transverse section through the middle of the palm showing the fascial compartments for the musculotendinous structures of the hand. **B.** Potential fascial spaces of palm.

- The potential midpalmar space lies posterior to the central compartment, is bounded medially by the hypothenar compartment, and is related distally to the synovial sheath of the 3rd, 4th, and 5th digits.
- The potential thenar space lies posterior to the thenar compartment and is related distally to the synovial sheath of the index finger.
- The potential midpalmar and thenar spaces are separated by a septum that passes from the palmar aponeurosis to the third metacarpal.

Because the palmar fascia is thick and strong, **swellings resulting from hand infections** usually appear on the dorsum of the hand where the fascia is thinner. The potential fascial spaces of the palm are important because they may become infected. The fascial spaces determine the extent and direction of the spread of pus formed in the infected areas. Depending on the site of infection, pus will accumulate in the thenar, hypothenar, or adductor compartments. Antibiotic therapy has made infections that spread beyond one of these fascial compartments rare, but an untreated infection can spread proximally through the carpal tunnel into the forearm anterior to the pronator quadratus and its fascia.

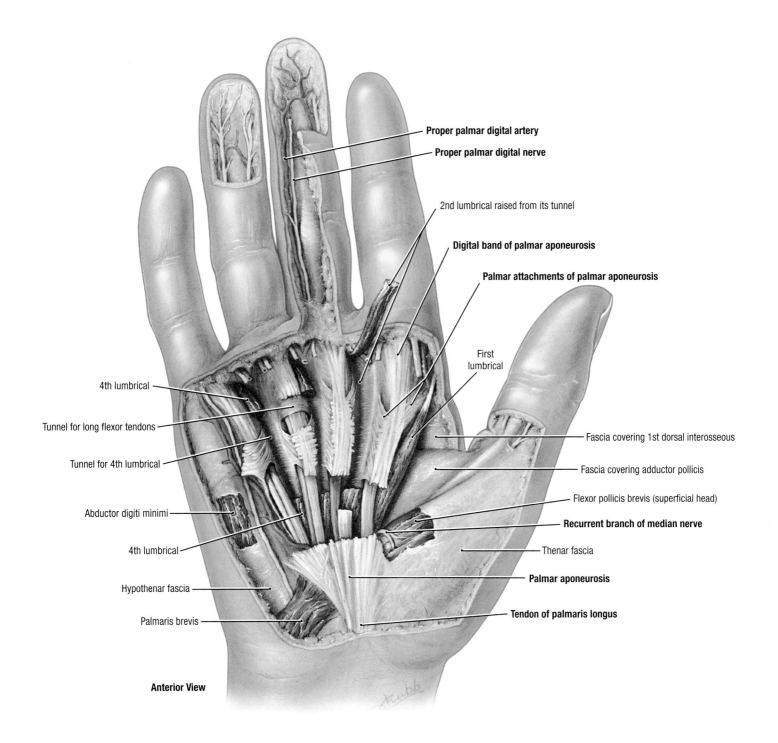

Proper palmar digital artery

Proper palmar digital nerve

2nd lumbrical raised from its tunnel

Digital band of palmar aponeurosis

Palmar attachments of palmar aponeurosis

First lumbrical

4th lumbrical

Tunnel for long flexor tendons

Tunnel for 4th lumbrical

Abductor digiti minimi

4th lumbrical

Hypothenar fascia

Palmaris brevis

Fascia covering 1st dorsal interosseous

Fascia covering adductor pollicis

Flexor pollicis brevis (superficial head)

Recurrent branch of median nerve

Thenar fascia

Palmar aponeurosis

Tendon of palmaris longus

Anterior View

6.71 PALMAR APONEUROSIS

- From the palmar aponeurosis, four longitudinal digital bands enter the fingers; the other fibers form extensive fibro-areolar septa that pass posteriorly to the palmar ligaments (see Fig. 6.78) and, more proximally, to the fascia covering the interossei. Thus, two sets of tunnels exist in the distal half of the palm: (1) tunnels for long flexor tendons and (2) tunnels for lumbricals, digital vessels, and digital nerves.
- In the dissected middle finger, note the absence of fat deep to the skin creases of the fingers.

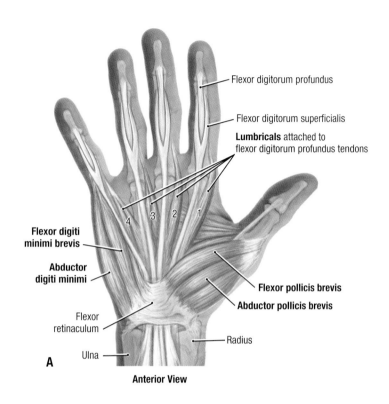

Flexor digitorum profundus

Flexor digitorum superficialis

Lumbricals attached to
flexor digitorum profundus tendons

4 3 2 1

**Flexor digiti
minimi brevis**

**Abductor
digiti minimi**

Flexor
retinaculum

Ulna

Flexor pollicis brevis

Abductor pollicis brevis

Radius

A

Anterior View

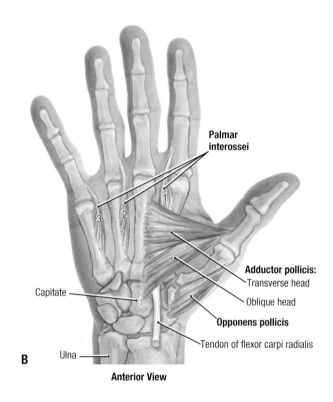

**Palmar
interossei**

3 2 1

Capitate

Adductor pollicis:
Transverse head

Oblique head

Opponens pollicis

Tendon of flexor carpi radialis

Ulna

B

Anterior View

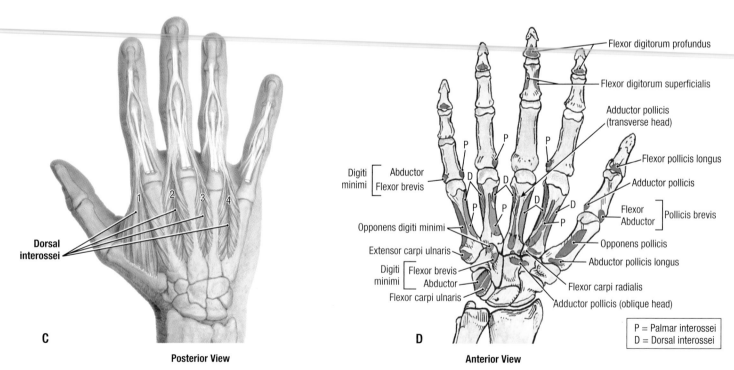

1 2 3 4

**Dorsal
interossei**

C

Posterior View

Flexor digitorum profundus

Flexor digitorum superficialis

Adductor pollicis
(transverse head)

Flexor pollicis longus

Adductor pollicis

Flexor | Pollicis brevis
Abductor |

Opponens pollicis

Abductor pollicis longus

Flexor carpi radialis

Adductor pollicis (oblique head)

Digiti | Abductor
minimi | Flexor brevis

P P P

D D

P P D D

P

Opponens digiti minimi

Extensor carpi ulnaris

Digiti | Flexor brevis
minimi | Abductor

Flexor carpi ulnaris

| P = Palmar interossei |
| D = Dorsal interossei |

D

Anterior View

6.72 MUSCULAR LAYERS OF PALM

A. Lumbricals. **B.** Adductor pollicis. **C.** Dorsal (*D*) and palmar (*P*) interossei. **D.** Bony attachments.

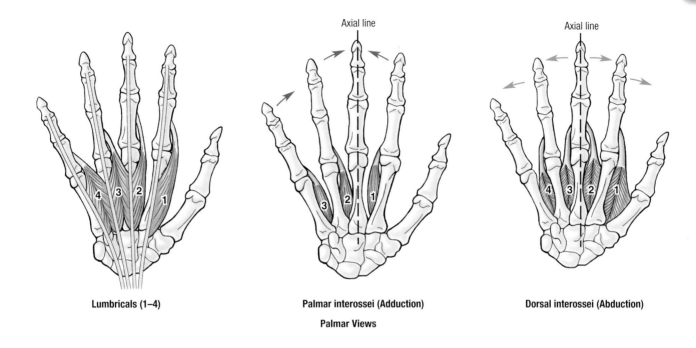

Lumbricals (1–4)   Palmar interossei (Adduction)   Dorsal interossei (Abduction)

Palmar Views

6.73   LUMBRICALS AND INTEROSSEI

TABLE 6.13 MUSCLES OF HAND

Muscle	Proximal Attachment	Distal Attachment	Innervation	Main Actions
Abductor pollicis brevis	Flexor retinaculum and tubercles of scaphoid and trapezium	Lateral side of base of proximal phalanx of thumb	Recurrent branch of median nerve (**C8** and T1)	Abducts thumb and helps oppose it
Flexor pollicis brevis	Flexor retinaculum (transverse carpal ligament) and tubercle of trapezium			Flexes thumb
Opponens pollicis		Lateral side of first metacarpal		Opposes thumb toward center of palm and rotates it medially
Adductor pollicis	*Oblique head:* bases of second and third metacarpals, capitate, and adjacent carpal bones *Transverse head:* anterior surface of shaft of third metacarpal	Medial side of base of proximal phalanx of thumb	Deep branch of ulnar nerve (C8 and **T1**)	Adducts thumb toward lateral border of palm
Abductor digiti minimi	Pisiform	Medial side of base of proximal phalanx of digit 5	Deep branch of ulnar nerve (C8 and T1)	Abducts digit 5, assists in flexion of its PIP joint
Flexor digiti minimi brevis	Hook of hamate and flexor retinaculum (transverse carpal ligament)	Medial border of fifth metacarpal		Flexes PIP joint of digit 5
Opponens digiti minimi				Draws fifth metacarpal anteriorly and rotates it, bringing digit 5 into opposition with thumb
Lumbricals 1 and 2	Lateral two tendons of flexor digitorum profundus	Lateral sides of extensor expansions of digits 2–5	Median nerve (C8 and **T1**)	Flex MCP joints and extend IP joints of digits 2–5
Lumbricals 3 and 4	Medial three tendons of flexor digitorum profundus			
Dorsal interossei 1–4	Adjacent sides of two metacarpals	Extensor expansions and bases of proximal phalanges of digits 2–4	Deep branch of ulnar nerve (C8 and **T1**)	Abduct 2–4 MCP joints; act with lumbricals to flex MCP and extend IP joints
Palmar interossei 1–3	Palmar surfaces of second, fourth, and fifth metacarpals	Extensor expansions of digits and bases of proximal phalanges of digits 2, 4, and 5		Adduct 2, 4, and 5 MCP joints; act with lumbricals to flex MCP and extend IP joints

Proper palmar digital nerve

Arterial network

Proper palmar digital artery

Proper palmar digital nerve

Proper digital nerve

Fibrous digital sheath

Flexor digitorum superficialis

Superficial palmar arch

Abductor digiti minimi

Apex of palmar aponeurosis

Palmaris brevis

Ulnar nerve

Ulnar artery

Pisiform

Dorsal carpal branch of ulnar artery

Dorsal cutaneous branch of ulnar nerve

Flexor carpi ulnaris

1st lumbrical

Radialis indicis artery

1st dorsal interosseous

Common palmar digital nerve

Adductor pollicis

Flexor pollicis brevis superficial head

Recurrent branch of median nerve

Abductor pollicis brevis

Abductor pollicis longus

Palmaris longus

Superficial palmar branch of radial artery

Radial artery

Palmaris longus tendon

A. Anterior View

6.74 SUPERFICIAL DISSECTION OF PALM, ULNAR, AND MEDIAN NERVES

A. Superficial palmar arch and digital nerves and vessels.

- The skin, superficial fascia, palmar aponeurosis, and thenar and hypothenar fasciae have been removed.
- The superficial palmar arch is formed by the ulnar artery and completed by the superficial palmar branch of the radial artery.
- The four lumbricals lie posterior to the digital vessels and nerves. The lumbricals arise from the lateral sides of the flexor digitorum profundus tendons and are inserted into the lateral sides of the dorsal expansions of the corresponding digits. The medial two lumbricals are bipennate and also arise from the medial sides of adjacent flexor digitorum profundus tendons.

- In the digits, a proper palmar digital artery and nerve lie on each side of the fibrous digital sheath.
- Note the canal (Guyon) through which the ulnar vessels and nerve pass medial to the pisiform.

Laceration of palmar (arterial) arches. Bleeding is usually profuse when the palmar (arterial) arches are lacerated. It may not be sufficient to ligate (tie off) only one forearm artery when the arches are lacerated, because these vessels usually have numerous communications in the forearm and hand and thus bleed from both ends.

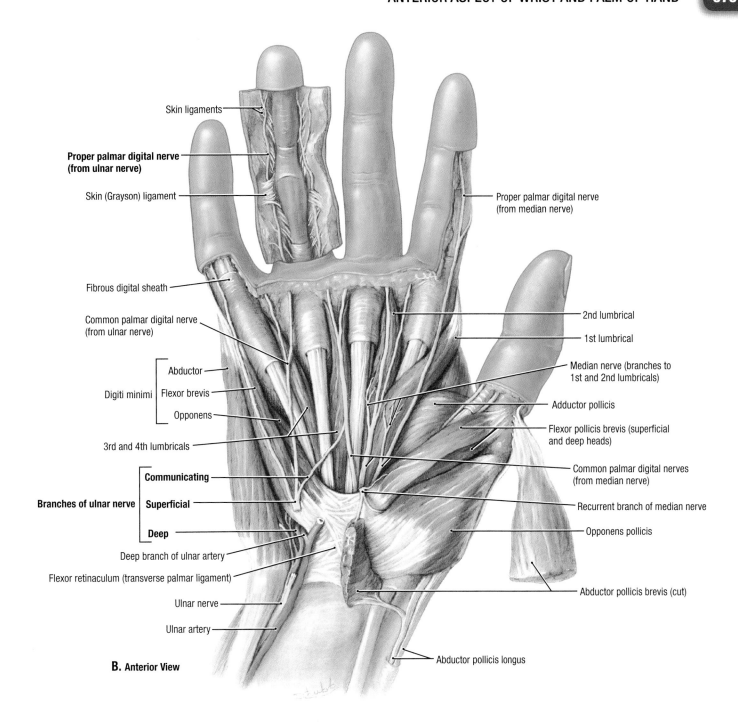

Skin ligaments

Proper palmar digital nerve (from ulnar nerve)

Skin (Grayson) ligament

Fibrous digital sheath

Common palmar digital nerve (from ulnar nerve)

Digiti minimi { Abductor / Flexor brevis / Opponens

3rd and 4th lumbricals

Branches of ulnar nerve { **Communicating** / **Superficial** / **Deep**

Deep branch of ulnar artery

Flexor retinaculum (transverse palmar ligament)

Ulnar nerve

Ulnar artery

B. Anterior View

Proper palmar digital nerve (from median nerve)

2nd lumbrical

1st lumbrical

Median nerve (branches to 1st and 2nd lumbricals)

Adductor pollicis

Flexor pollicis brevis (superficial and deep heads)

Common palmar digital nerves (from median nerve)

Recurrent branch of median nerve

Opponens pollicis

Abductor pollicis brevis (cut)

Abductor pollicis longus

6.74   SUPERFICIAL DISSECTION OF PALM, ULNAR, AND MEDIAN NERVES *(CONTINUED)*

B. Ulnar and median nerves.

Carpal tunnel syndrome results from any lesion that significantly reduces the size of the carpal tunnel or, more commonly, increases the size of some of the structures (or their coverings) that pass though it (e.g., inflammation of the synovial sheaths). The median nerve is the most sensitive structure in the carpal tunnel. The median nerve has two terminal sensory branches that supply the skin of the hand; hence paresthesia (tingling), hypothesia (diminished sensation), or anesthesia (absence of tactile sensation) may occur in the lateral three and a half digits. Recall, however, that the palmar cutaneous branch of the median nerve arises proximal to and does not pass through the carpal tunnel; thus sensation in the central palm remains unaffected. This nerve also has one terminal motor branch, the recurrent branch, which innervates the three thenar muscles. Wasting of the thenar eminence and progressive loss of coordination and strength in the thumb may occur. To relieve the compression and resulting symptoms, partial or complete surgical division of the flexor retinaculum, a procedure called **carpal tunnel release,** may be necessary. The incision for carpal tunnel release is made toward the medial side of the wrist and flexor retinaculum to avoid possible injury to the recurrent branch of the median nerve.

Synovial sheath

3

2

4

5

C

Mesotendon (forms vincula)

Osseofibrous tunnel (synovial cavity)

Tendon

Synovial sheath of digit of hand (2-5)

Synovial covering of tendon

Synovial lining of tunnel

Middle phalanx

Fibrous digital sheath

Nerve ⎫
Artery ⎬ Proper palmar digital
Vein ⎭

Synovial sheath

Tendon

B. Lateral View

Tendinous sheath of flexor pollicis longus

Flexor retinaculum (transverse carpal ligament)

Palmaris longus

Flexor digitorum superficialis and profundus in common flexor sheath

Tendinous sheath of abductor pollicis longus and extensor pollicis brevis

Flexor carpi radialis

Tendinous sheath of flexor pollicis longus

Flexor carpi ulnaris

Flexor carpi radialis

A. Anterior View

Palmar

Flexor digitorum superficialis tendon

Fibrous digital sheath

Synovial sheath

Flexor digitorum profundus tendon

Nerve ⎫
Artery ⎬ Proper palmar digital
Vein ⎭

Skin (Grayson) ligament

Extensor (dorsal) expansion

Proximal phalanx

Dorsal

C. Transverse Section (level of section indicated in A)

6.75 SYNOVIAL SHEATHS OF PALM OF HAND

A. Tendinous (synovial) sheaths of long flexor tendons of the digits. **B.** Osseofibrous tunnel and tendinous (synovial) sheath. **C.** Transverse section through the proximal phalanx.

Injuries such as puncture of a finger by a rusty nail can cause **infection of the digital synovial sheaths.** When inflammation of the tendon and synovial sheath **(tenosynovitis)** occurs, the digit swells and movement becomes painful. Because the tendons of the 2nd to 4th digits nearly always have separate synovial sheaths, the infection usually is confined to the infected digits. If the infection is untreated, however, the proximal ends of these sheaths may rupture, allowing the infection to spread to the midpalmar space. Because the synovial sheath of the little finger is usually continuous with the common flexor sheath, tenosynovitis in this finger may spread to the common flexor sheath and thus through the palm and carpal tunnel to the anterior forearm. Likewise, tenosynovitis in the thumb may spread through the continuous tendinous sheath of flexor pollicis longus.

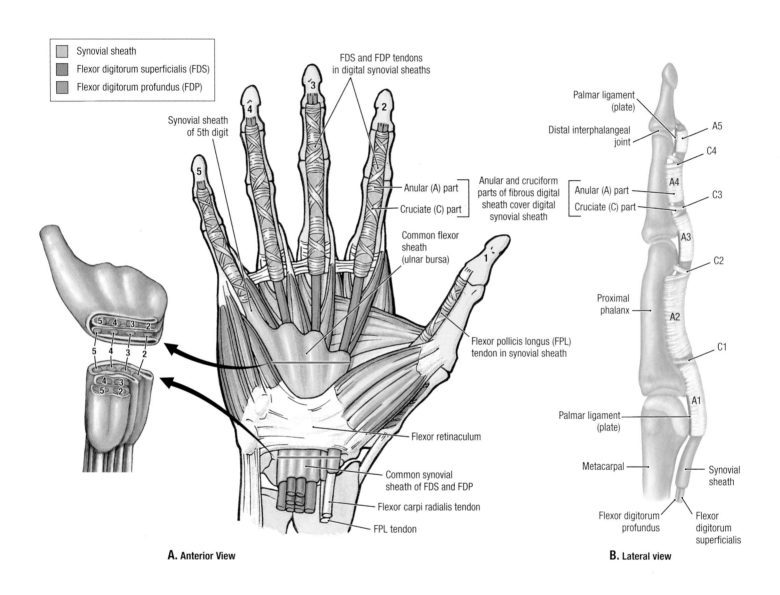

Synovial sheath

Flexor digitorum superficialis (FDS)

Flexor digitorum profundus (FDP)

FDS and FDP tendons in digital synovial sheaths

Synovial sheath of 5th digit

Anular (A) part

Cruciate (C) part

Anular and cruciate parts of fibrous digital sheath cover digital synovial sheath

Common flexor sheath (ulnar bursa)

Flexor pollicis longus (FPL) tendon in synovial sheath

Flexor retinaculum

Common synovial sheath of FDS and FDP

Flexor carpi radialis tendon

FPL tendon

A. Anterior View

Palmar ligament (plate)

Distal interphalangeal joint

A5

C4

Anular (A) part

A4

C3

Cruciate (C) part

A3

C2

Proximal phalanx

A2

C1

Palmar ligament (plate)

A1

Metacarpal

Synovial sheath

Flexor digitorum profundus

Flexor digitorum superficialis

B. Lateral view

6.76 FIBROUS DIGITAL SHEATHS

A. Fibrous digital and synovial sheaths. **B.** Anular and cruciate parts (pulleys) of the fibrous digital sheath.

Fibrous digital sheaths are the strong ligamentous tunnels containing the flexor tendons and their synovial sheaths. The sheaths extend from the heads of the metacarpals to the bases of the distal phalanges. These sheaths prevent the tendons from pulling away from the digits (bowstringing). The fibrous digital sheaths combine with the bones to form osseofibrous tunnels through which the tendons pass to reach the digits. The anular and cruciform (cruciate) parts, often referred to clinically as "pulleys," are thickened reinforcements of the fibrous digital sheaths.

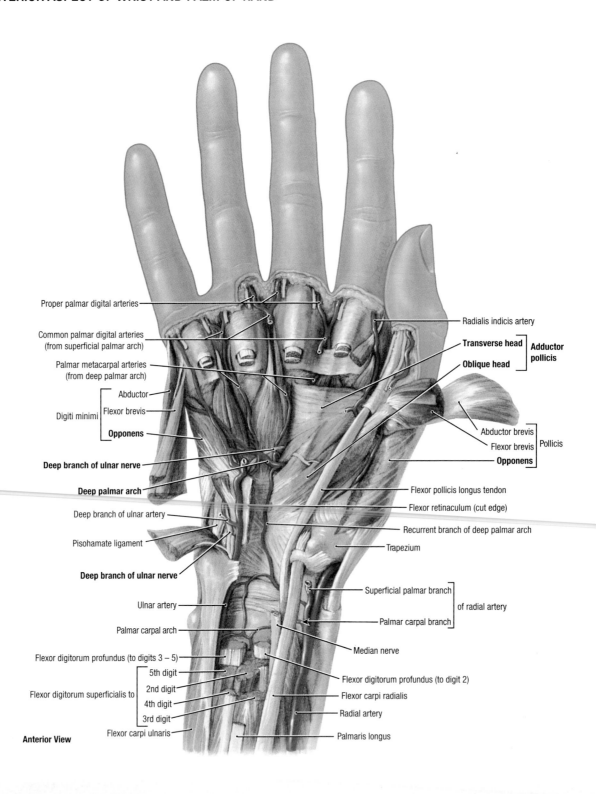

Proper palmar digital arteries

Common palmar digital arteries
(from superficial palmar arch)

Palmar metacarpal arteries
(from deep palmar arch)

Abductor

Flexor brevis

Digiti minimi

Opponens

Deep branch of ulnar nerve

Deep palmar arch

Deep branch of ulnar artery

Pisohamate ligament

Deep branch of ulnar nerve

Ulnar artery

Palmar carpal arch

Flexor digitorum profundus (to digits 3 – 5)

5th digit

2nd digit

Flexor digitorum superficialis to

4th digit

3rd digit

Flexor carpi ulnaris

Anterior View

Radialis indicis artery

Transverse head ⎤ **Adductor**
Oblique head ⎦ **pollicis**

Abductor brevis ⎤
Flexor brevis ⎥ Pollicis
Opponens ⎦

Flexor pollicis longus tendon

Flexor retinaculum (cut edge)

Recurrent branch of deep palmar arch

Trapezium

Superficial palmar branch ⎤
 ⎥ of radial artery
Palmar carpal branch ⎦

Median nerve

Flexor digitorum profundus (to digit 2)

Flexor carpi radialis

Radial artery

Palmaris longus

6.77 DEEP DISSECTION OF PALM

- The deep branch of the ulnar artery joins the radial artery to form the deep palmar arch.
- The pisohamate ligament is often considered a continuation of the tendon of flexor carpi ulnaris; thus making the pisiform a sesamoid bone.

Compression of the ulnar nerve may occur at the wrist where it passes between the pisiform and the hook of hamate. The depression between these bones is converted by the pisohamate ligament into an osseofibrous ulnar canal. **Ulnar canal syndrome** is manifest by hypoesthesia in the medial one and one half digits and weakness of the intrinsic hand muscles. Clawing of the 4th and 5th digits may occur, but in contrast to proximal nerve injury, their ability to flex is unaffected and there is no radial deviation of the wrist joint.

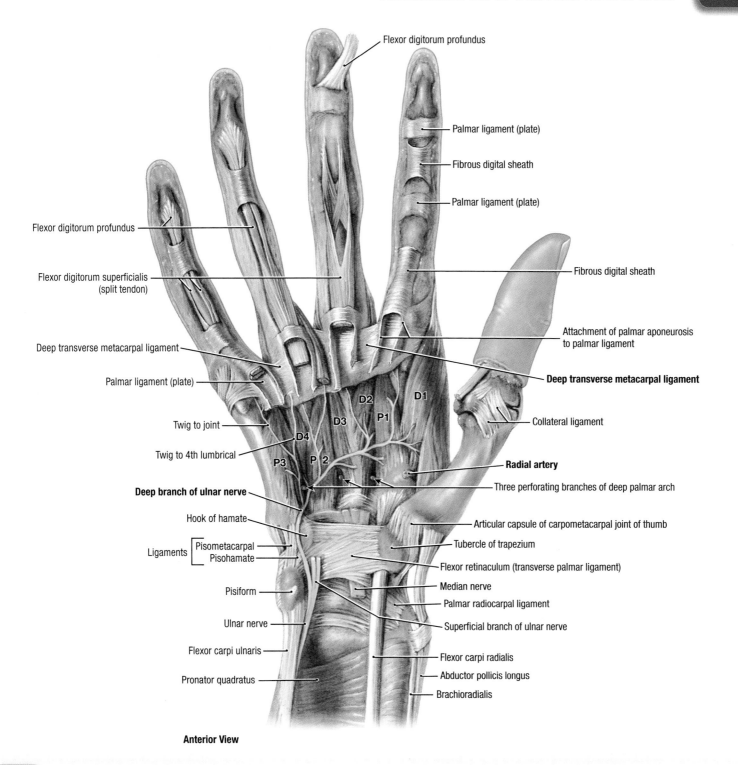

Flexor digitorum profundus

Palmar ligament (plate)

Fibrous digital sheath

Palmar ligament (plate)

Flexor digitorum profundus

Flexor digitorum superficialis (split tendon)

Fibrous digital sheath

Deep transverse metacarpal ligament

Attachment of palmar aponeurosis to palmar ligament

Palmar ligament (plate)

Deep transverse metacarpal ligament

D2

D1

Twig to joint

D3

P1

Collateral ligament

D4

Twig to 4th lumbrical

P3

P 2

Radial artery

Deep branch of ulnar nerve

Three perforating branches of deep palmar arch

Hook of hamate

Articular capsule of carpometacarpal joint of thumb

Ligaments {
Pisometacarpal
Pisohamate
}

Tubercle of trapezium

Flexor retinaculum (transverse palmar ligament)

Pisiform

Median nerve

Palmar radiocarpal ligament

Ulnar nerve

Superficial branch of ulnar nerve

Flexor carpi ulnaris

Flexor carpi radialis

Pronator quadratus

Abductor pollicis longus

Brachioradialis

Anterior View

6.78 **DEEP DISSECTION OF PALM AND DIGITS WITH DEEP BRANCH OF ULNAR NERVE**

- Three unipennate palmar (P1–P3) and four bipennate dorsal (D1–D4) interosseous muscles are illustrated; the palmar interossei adduct the fingers, and the dorsal interossei abduct the fingers in relation to the axial line, an imaginary line drawn through the long axis of the 3rd digit (see Table 6.13).
- The deep transverse metacarpal ligaments unite the palmar ligaments; the lumbricals pass anterior to the deep transverse metacarpal ligament, and the interossei pass posterior to the ligament.

- Note the ulnar (Guyon) canal through which the ulnar vessels and nerve pass medial to the pisiform.
- The pisohamate and pisometacarpal ligaments form the distal attachment of flexor carpi ulnaris.

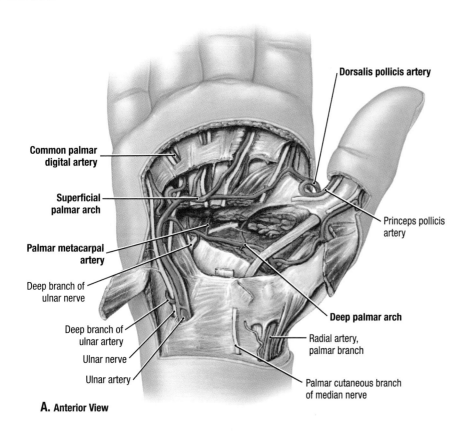

A. Anterior View

- Dorsalis pollicis artery
- Common palmar digital artery
- Superficial palmar arch
- Palmar metacarpal artery
- Deep branch of ulnar nerve
- Deep branch of ulnar artery
- Ulnar nerve
- Ulnar artery
- Princeps pollicis artery
- Deep palmar arch
- Radial artery, palmar branch
- Palmar cutaneous branch of median nerve

B. Lateral View

- Body of nail
- Distal phalanx
- Lunule
- Dorsal branch of proper palmar digital artery
- Skin ligaments
- Middle phalanx
- Proper palmar digital nerve
- Lateral band of extensor expansion
- Proper palmar digital artery
- Dorsal digital artery
- Subcutaneous tissue
- Dorsal digital branch of radial nerve
- Extensor (dorsal) expansion
- Common palmar digital nerve
- Common palmar digital artery
- Dorsal metacarpal artery
- Metacarpal

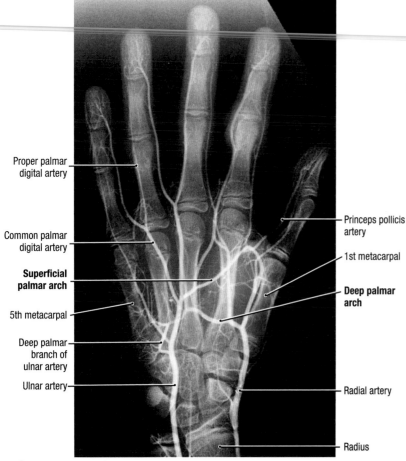

C. Anteroposterior View

- Proper palmar digital artery
- Common palmar digital artery
- Superficial palmar arch
- 5th metacarpal
- Deep palmar branch of ulnar artery
- Ulnar artery
- Princeps pollicis artery
- 1st metacarpal
- Deep palmar arch
- Radial artery
- Radius

6.79 ARTERIAL SUPPLY OF HAND

A. Dissection of palmar arterial arches. **B.** Digital vessels and nerves. **C.** Arteriogram of the hand.

- The superficial palmar arch is usually completed by the superficial palmar branch of the radial artery, but in this specimen the dorsalis pollicis artery completes the arch.

The **superficial and deep palmar (arterial) arches** are not palpable, but their surface markings are visible. The superficial palmar arch occurs at the level of the distal border of the fully extended thumb. The deep palmar arch lies approximately 1 cm proximal to the superficial palmar arch. The location of these arches should be borne in mind in wounds of the palm and when palmar incisions are made.

Intermittent bilateral attacks of **ischemia of the digits,** marked by cyanosis and often accompanied by paresthesia and pain, are characteristically brought on by cold and emotional stimuli. The condition may result from an anatomical abnormality or an underlying disease. When the cause of the condition is idiopathic (unknown) or primary, it is called **Raynaud syndrome** (disease). Since arteries receive innervation from postsynaptic fibers from the sympathetic ganglia, it may be necessary to perform a cervicodorsal presynaptic sympathectomy to dilate the digital arteries.

Radialis indicis

Princeps pollicis

Dorsalis pollicis

Dorsal carpal branch

Superficial palmar branch

Radial artery

Proper palmar digital artery gives rise to a dorsal branch

Common palmar digital arteries

Superficial palmar arch

Palmar metacarpal arteries

Deep palmar arch

Palmar carpal arch

Ulnar artery

Anterior interosseous artery

Anterior View (Palmar Aspect)

Dorsal branches of proper palmar digital arteries

Dorsal digital arteries

Dorsal metacarpal arteries

Perforating branches

Dorsal carpal arch

Dorsal carpal branch of ulnar artery

Anterior interosseous artery

Posterior interosseous artery

Radius

Lateral View (Isolated third digit)

Dorsalis indicis

Dorsalis pollicis

Princeps pollicis

Dorsal carpal arch

Radial artery

Posterior View (Dorsum of Hand)

6.80   ARTERIES OF HAND

TABLE 6.14 ARTERIES OF HAND

Artery	Origin	Course
Superficial palmar arch	Direct continuation of ulnar artery; arch is completed on lateral side by superficial branch of radial artery or another of its branches	Curves laterally deep to palmar aponeurosis and superficial to long flexor tendons; curve of arch lies across palm at level of distal border of extended thumb
Deep palmar arch	Direct continuation of radial artery; arch is completed on medial side by deep branch of ulnar artery	Curves medially, deep to long flexor tendons and is in contact with bases of metacarpals
Common palmar digital	Superficial palmar arch	Pass directly on lumbricals to webbings of digits
Proper palmar digital	Common palmar digital arteries	Run along sides of digits 2–5
Princeps pollicis	Radial artery as it turns into palm	Descends on palmar aspect of first metacarpal and divides at the base of proximal phalanx into two branches that run along sides of thumb
Radialis indicis	Radial artery, but may arise from princeps pollicis artery	Passes along lateral side of index finger to its distal end
Dorsal carpal arch	Radial and ulnar arteries	Arches within fascia on dorsum of hand

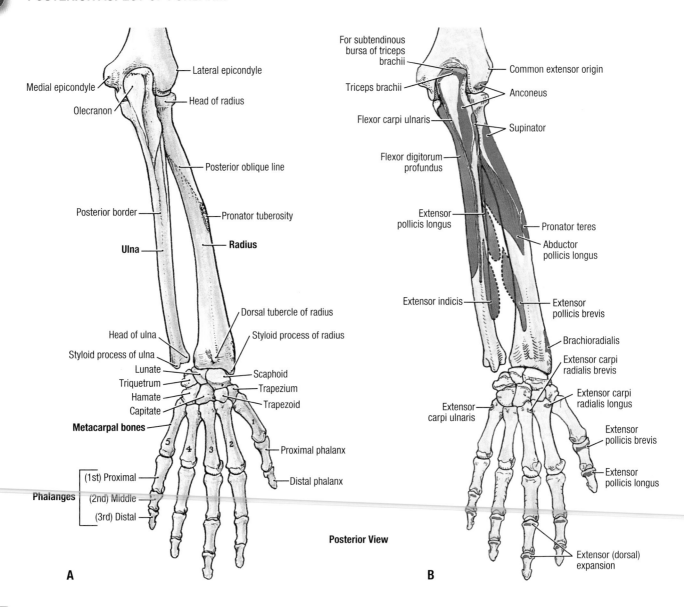

A

Medial epicondyle
Olecranon
Lateral epicondyle
Head of radius
Posterior oblique line
Posterior border
Pronator tuberosity
Ulna
Radius
Dorsal tubercle of radius
Head of ulna
Styloid process of radius
Styloid process of ulna
Lunate
Scaphoid
Triquetrum
Trapezium
Hamate
Trapezoid
Capitate
Metacarpal bones
Proximal phalanx
Distal phalanx
(1st) Proximal
(2nd) Middle
(3rd) Distal
Phalanges

B

For subtendinous bursa of triceps brachii
Triceps brachii
Common extensor origin
Anconeus
Flexor carpi ulnaris
Supinator
Flexor digitorum profundus
Extensor pollicis longus
Pronator teres
Abductor pollicis longus
Extensor indicis
Extensor pollicis brevis
Brachioradialis
Extensor carpi radialis brevis
Extensor carpi ulnaris
Extensor carpi radialis longus
Extensor pollicis brevis
Extensor pollicis longus
Extensor (dorsal) expansion

Posterior View

6.81   BONES AND MUSCLE ATTACHMENTS ON POSTERIOR ASPECT OF FOREARM AND HAND

Abduction **Adduction** **Extension** **Flexion** **Opposition** **Reposition**

6.82   MOVEMENTS OF THUMB

The thumb is rotated 90° compared to the other digits. Abduction and adduction at the MCP joint occur in a sagittal plane; flexion and extension at the MCP and IP joints occur in frontal planes, opposite to these movements at other joints.

A

Extensor
retinaculum

B

Posterior Views

6.83 MUSCLES ON POSTERIOR ASPECT OF FOREARM

A. Superficial. **B.** Deep

TABLE 6.15 MUSCLES OF POSTERIOR SURFACE OF FOREARM

Muscle	Proximal Attachment	Distal Attachment	Innervation	Main Actions
Brachioradialis (1)	Proximal two thirds of lateral supra-epicondylar ridge of humerus	Lateral surface of distal end of radius	Radial nerve (C5, **C6**, and C7)	Flexes elbow joint
Extensor carpi radialis longus (2)	Lateral supra-epicondylar ridge of humerus	Base of second metacarpal bone	Radial nerve (C6 and C7)	Extend and abduct wrist joint
Extensor carpi radialis brevis (3)		Base of third metacarpal bone	Deep branch of radial nerve (**C7** and C8)	
Extensor digitorum (4)	Lateral epicondyle of humerus	Extensor expansions of medial four digits	Posterior interosseous nerve (C7 and C8), a branch of the radial nerve	Extends medial four metacarpophalangeal joints; extends wrist joint
Extensor digiti minimi (5)		Extensor expansion of fifth digit		Extends metacarpophalangeal and interphalangeal joints of 5th digit
Extensor carpi ulnaris (6)	Lateral epicondyle of humerus and posterior border of ulna	Base of fifth metacarpal bone		Extends and adducts wrist joint
Anconeus (7)	Lateral epicondyle of humerus	Lateral surface of olecranon and superior part of posterior surface of ulna	Radial nerve (C7, C8, and T1)	Assists triceps brachii in extending elbow joint; stabilizes elbow joint; abducts ulna during pronation
Supinator (8)	Lateral epicondyle of humerus, radial collateral and anular ligaments, supinator fossa, and crest of ulna	Lateral, posterior, and anterior surfaces of proximal third of radius	Deep branch of radial nerve (C5 and **C6**)	Supinates forearm
Abductor pollicis longus (9)	Posterior surface of ulna, radius, and interosseous membrane	Base of first metacarpal bone	Posterior interosseous nerve (C7 and **C8**)	Abducts and extends carpometacarpal joint of thumb
Extensor pollicis brevis (10)	Posterior surface of radius and interosseous membrane	Base of proximal phalanx of thumb		Extends metacarpophalangeal joint of thumb
Extensor pollicis longus (11)	Posterior surface of middle third of ulna and interosseous membrane	Base of distal phalanx of thumb		Extends metacarpophalangeal and interphalangeal joints of thumb
Extensor indicis (12)	Posterior surface of ulna and interosseous membrane	Extensor expansion of second digit		Extends MCP and IP joints of 2nd digit and helps to extend wrist joint

Anconeus and its nerve

Lateral muscles:

Brachioradialis

Extensor carpi radialis longus

Extensor carpi radialis brevis

Extensor digitorum

Extensor carpi ulnaris

Extensor digiti minimi

Extensor indicis

Extensor retinaculum

Dorsal carpal branch of ulnar artery

Extensor carpi radialis brevis

Dorsal carpal arch

Perforating arteries

Dorsal metacarpal arteries

Dorsal digital arteries

A. Posterior View

Outcropping muscles of thumb:

Abductor pollicis longus

Extensor pollicis brevis

Extensor pollicis longus

Extensor pollicis longus

Radial artery in the anatomical snuff box

Dorsal carpal branch of radial artery

Extensor carpi radialis longus

Dorsalis pollicis arteries

Dorsalis indicis artery

1st dorsal interosseous

2nd dorsal interosseous

Brachioradialis

Extensor digitorum

Extensor digiti minimi

B

C

Posterior View

Anterior interosseous artery (posterior part)

Dorsal carpal branch of ulnar artery

Dorsal carpal arch

Dorsal metacarpal arteries

Dorsal digital arteries

Radial artery in snuff box

Dorsal carpal branch of radial artery

Dorsalis indicis artery

Extensor carpi radialis longus

Extensor carpi radialis brevis

Extensor carpi ulnaris

D. Posterior View

6.84 SUPERFICIAL MUSCLES OF EXTENSOR ASPECT OF FOREARM

A. Dissection. The digital extensor tendons have been reflected without disturbing the arteries because they lie on the skeletal plane. **B.** and **C.** Schematic illustrations of superficial extensor muscles. **D.** Arteries on dorsum of hand.

Anconeus

Supinator

Posterior interosseous recurrent artery

Branches of posterior interosseous nerve

Extensor digitorum

Extensor digiti minimi

Extensor carpi ulnaris

Extensor indicis

Extensor retinaculum

Extensor carpi radialis [Brevis / Longus]

Extensor pollicis longus

Dorsalis indicis artery

1st dorsal interosseous

Radialis indicis artery

1st dorsal interosseous

Deep branch of radial nerve

Brachioradialis

Extensor carpi radialis longus

Extensor carpi radialis brevis

Posterior interosseous nerve

Posterior interosseous artery

Pronator teres

Abductor pollicis longus

Extensor pollicis brevis

Extensor pollicis longus

Radial artery (in "snuff box")

Extensor pollicis brevis

Dorsalis pollicis arteries

Adductor pollicis

A. Posterolateral View

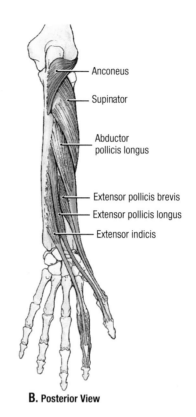

Anconeus

Supinator

Abductor pollicis longus

Extensor pollicis brevis

Extensor pollicis longus

Extensor indicis

B. Posterior View

6.85   DEEP STRUCTURES ON EXTENSOR ASPECT OF FOREARM

A. Dissection. **B.** Schematic illustration of deep extensor muscles.

- Three "outcropping" muscles of the thumb (abductor pollicis longus, extensor pollicis brevis, and extensor pollicis longus) emerge between the extensor carpi radialis brevis and the extensor digitorum.
- The laterally retracted brachioradialis and extensor carpi radialis longus and brevis muscles and supinator muscle are innervated by the deep branch of the radial nerve; the other extensor muscles are supplied by the posterior interosseous nerve, which is a continuation of the deep branch of the radial nerve that pierced the supinator.

Severance of the deep branch of the radial nerve results in an inability to extend the thumb and the metacarpophalangeal joints of the other digits. Loss of sensation does not occur because the deep branch is entirely muscular and articular in distribution.

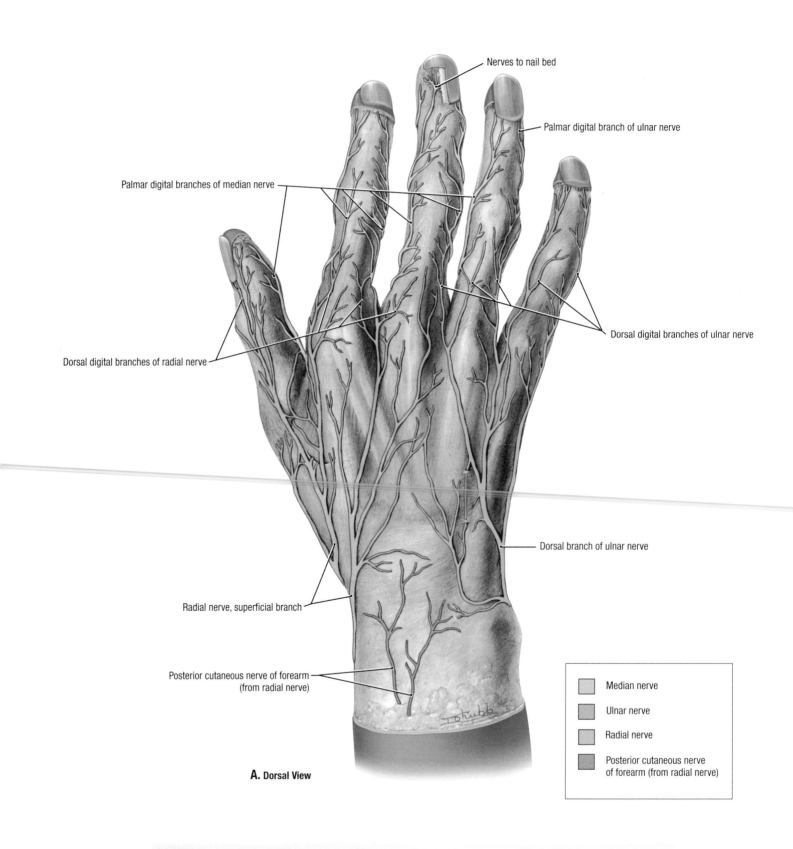

Nerves to nail bed

Palmar digital branch of ulnar nerve

Palmar digital branches of median nerve

Dorsal digital branches of ulnar nerve

Dorsal digital branches of radial nerve

Dorsal branch of ulnar nerve

Radial nerve, superficial branch

Posterior cutaneous nerve of forearm
(from radial nerve)

A. Dorsal View

Median nerve

Ulnar nerve

Radial nerve

Posterior cutaneous nerve
of forearm (from radial nerve)

6.86 CUTANEOUS INNERVATION OF HAND

A. Dissection of nerves of dorsum of hand.

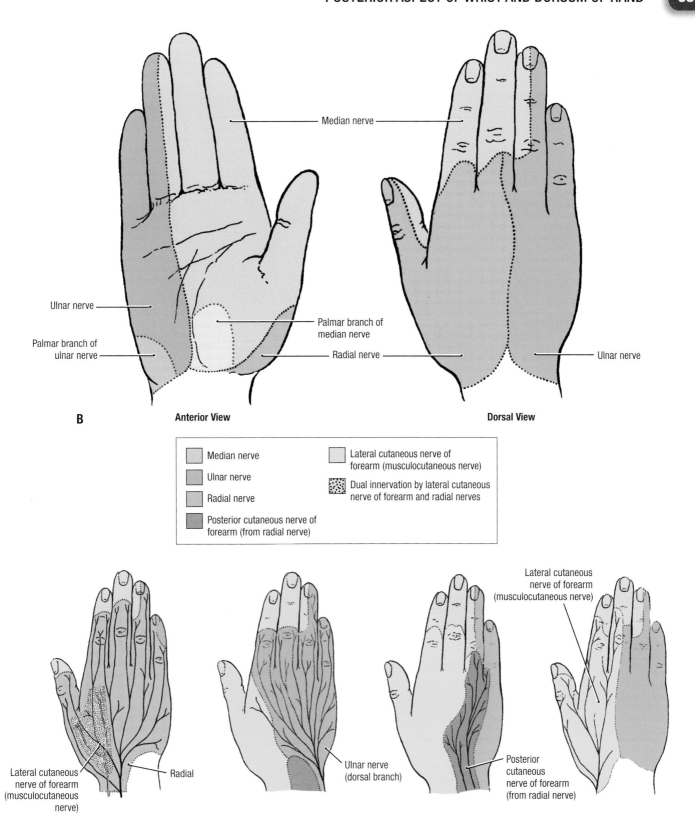

B Anterior View Dorsal View

Median nerve

Ulnar nerve

Palmar branch of ulnar nerve

Palmar branch of median nerve

Radial nerve

Ulnar nerve

Median nerve

Ulnar nerve

Radial nerve

Posterior cutaneous nerve of forearm (from radial nerve)

Lateral cutaneous nerve of forearm (musculocutaneous nerve)

Dual innervation by lateral cutaneous nerve of forearm and radial nerves

Lateral cutaneous nerve of forearm (musculocutaneous nerve)

Radial

Ulnar nerve (dorsal branch)

Posterior cutaneous nerve of forearm (from radial nerve)

Lateral cutaneous nerve of forearm (musculocutaneous nerve)

C. Dorsal Views

6.86 CUTANEOUS INNERVATION OF HAND *(CONTINUED)*

B. Distribution of the cutaneous nerves to the palm and dorsum of the hand, schematic illustration. **C.** Variations in pattern of cutaneous nerves in dorsum of hand.

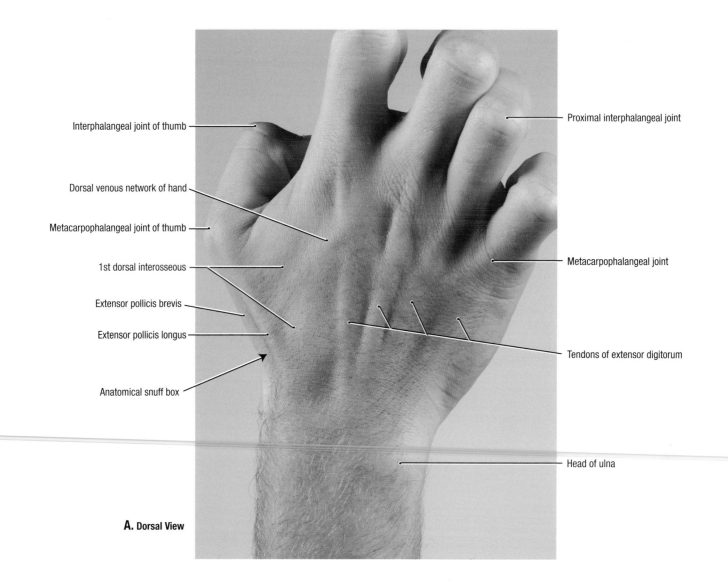

Interphalangeal joint of thumb

Dorsal venous network of hand

Metacarpophalangeal joint of thumb

1st dorsal interosseous

Extensor pollicis brevis

Extensor pollicis longus

Anatomical snuff box

Proximal interphalangeal joint

Metacarpophalangeal joint

Tendons of extensor digitorum

Head of ulna

A. Dorsal View

6.87   DORSUM OF HAND

A. Surface anatomy. The interphalangeal joints are flexed, and the metacarpophalangeal joints are hyper-extended to demonstrate the extensor digitorum tendons. **B.** Tendinous (synovial) sheaths distended with blue fluid. **C.** Transverse section of distal forearm (*numbers* refer to structures labeled in B). **D.** Sites of bony attachments.

- Six tendinous sheaths occupy the six osseofibrous tunnels deep to the extensor retinaculum. They contain nine tendons: tendons for the thumb in sheaths 1 and 3, tendons for the extensors of the wrist in sheaths 2 and 6, and tendons for the extensors of the wrist and fingers in sheaths 4 and 5.
- The tendon of the extensor pollicis longus hooks around the dorsal tubercle of radius to pass obliquely across the tendons of the extensor carpi radialis longus and brevis to the thumb.

The tendons of the abductor pollicis longus and extensor pollicis brevis are in the same tendinous sheath on the dorsum of the wrist. Excessive friction of these tendons results in fibrous thickening of the sheath and stenosis of the osseofibrous tunnel, **Quervain tenovaginitis stenosans.** This condition causes pain in the wrist that radiates proximally to the forearm and distally to the thumb.

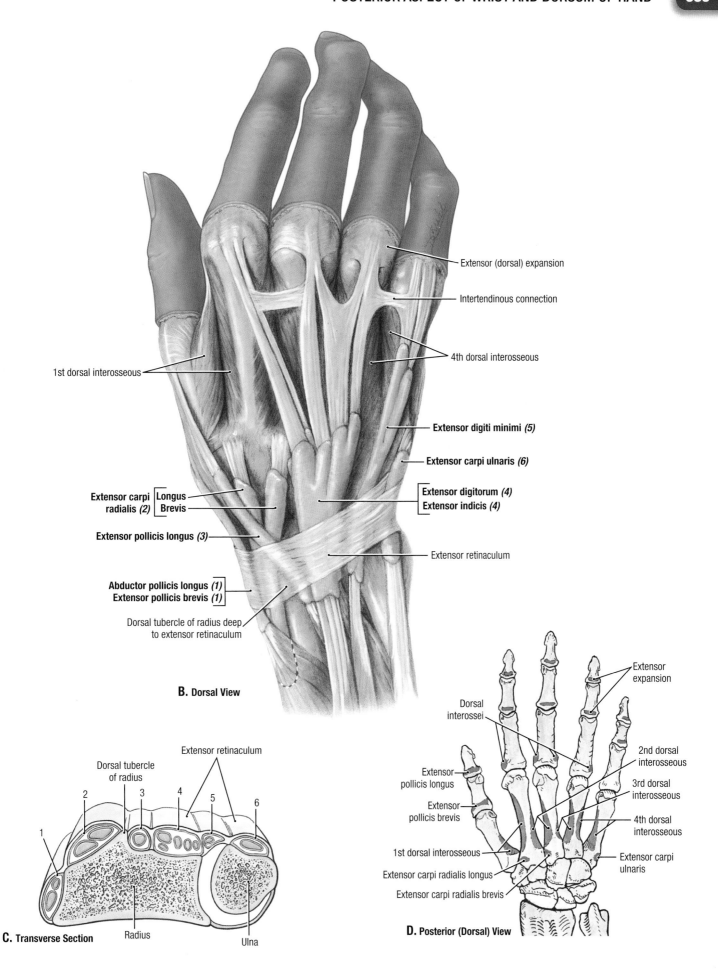

Extensor (dorsal) expansion

Intertendinous connection

4th dorsal interosseous

1st dorsal interosseous

Extensor digiti minimi *(5)*

Extensor carpi ulnaris *(6)*

Extensor carpi | **Longus**
radialis *(2)* | **Brevis**

Extensor digitorum *(4)*
Extensor indicis *(4)*

Extensor pollicis longus *(3)*

Extensor retinaculum

Abductor pollicis longus *(1)*
Extensor pollicis brevis *(1)*

Dorsal tubercle of radius deep
to extensor retinaculum

B. Dorsal View

Extensor retinaculum

Dorsal tubercle
of radius

2
1
3
4
5
6

C. Transverse Section

Radius

Ulna

Extensor
expansion

Dorsal
interossei

Extensor
pollicis longus

2nd dorsal
interosseous

3rd dorsal
interosseous

Extensor
pollicis brevis

4th dorsal
interosseous

1st dorsal interosseous

Extensor carpi
ulnaris

Extensor carpi radialis longus

Extensor carpi radialis brevis

D. Posterior (Dorsal) View

Extensor expansion

Extensor indicis

Body of 2nd metacarpal

1st dorsal interosseous

Intertendinous connections
(between tendons of
extensor digitorum)

Radial artery

Extensor carpi radialis longus

Extensor carpi radialis brevis

Superficial branch
of radial nerve

Extensor pollicis longus

Extensor pollicis brevis

Abductor pollicis longus

Dorsal digital vein

Extensor digiti minimi

Dorsal branch
of ulnar nerve

Extensor retinaculum

Extensor carpi ulnaris

Extensor indicis

Extensor digiti minimi

Extensor digitorum

E. Dorsal View

6.87 DORSUM OF HAND *(CONTINUED)*

E. Tendons on dorsum of hand and extensor retinaculum.
- The deep fascia is thickened to form the extensor retinaculum.
- Proximal to the knuckles, intertendinous connections extend between the tendons of the digital extensors and, thereby, restrict the independent action of the fingers.

"Ganglion" cyst. Sometimes a nontender cystic swelling appears on the hand, most commonly on the dorsum of the wrist. The thin-walled cyst contains clear mucinous fluid. Clinically, this type of swelling is called a "ganglion" (G. swelling or knot). These synovial cysts are close to and often communicate with the synovial sheaths. The distal attachment of the extensor carpi radialis brevis tendon is a common site for such a cyst.

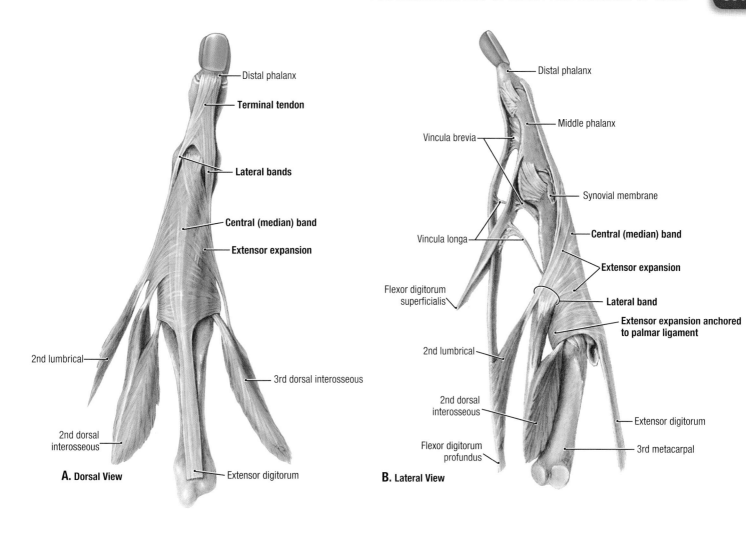

A. Dorsal View

- Distal phalanx
- **Terminal tendon**
- **Lateral bands**
- **Central (median) band**
- **Extensor expansion**
- 2nd lumbrical
- 3rd dorsal interosseous
- 2nd dorsal interosseous
- Extensor digitorum

B. Lateral View

- Distal phalanx
- Vincula brevia
- Middle phalanx
- Synovial membrane
- **Central (median) band**
- Vincula longa
- **Extensor expansion**
- Flexor digitorum superficialis
- **Lateral band**
- **Extensor expansion anchored to palmar ligament**
- 2nd lumbrical
- 2nd dorsal interosseous
- Extensor digitorum
- Flexor digitorum profundus
- 3rd metacarpal

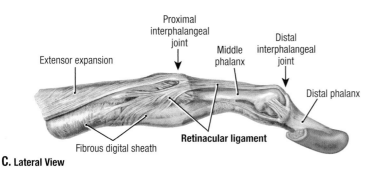

C. Lateral View

- Extensor expansion
- Proximal interphalangeal joint
- Middle phalanx
- Distal interphalangeal joint
- Distal phalanx
- **Retinacular ligament**
- Fibrous digital sheath

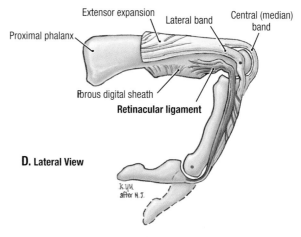

D. Lateral View

- Extensor expansion
- Lateral band
- Central (median) band
- Proximal phalanx
- Fibrous digital sheath
- **Retinacular ligament**

kyu
after N.J.

6.88   EXTENSOR (DORSAL) EXPANSION OF THIRD DIGIT

A. Dorsal aspect. **B.** Lateral aspect. **C.** Retinacular ligaments of extended digit. **D.** Retinacular ligaments of flexed digit.

- The hood covering the head of the metacarpal is attached to the palmar ligament.
- Contraction of the muscles attaching to the lateral band will produce flexion of the metacarpophalangeal joint and extension of the interphalangeal joints.

- The retinacular ligament is a fibrous band that runs from the proximal phalanx and fibrous digital sheath obliquely across the middle phalanx and two interphalangeal joints to join the extensor (dorsal) expansion, and then to the distal phalanx.
- On flexion of the distal interphalangeal joint, the retinacular ligament becomes taut and pulls the proximal joint into flexion; on extension of the proximal joint, the distal joint is pulled by the ligament into nearly complete extension.

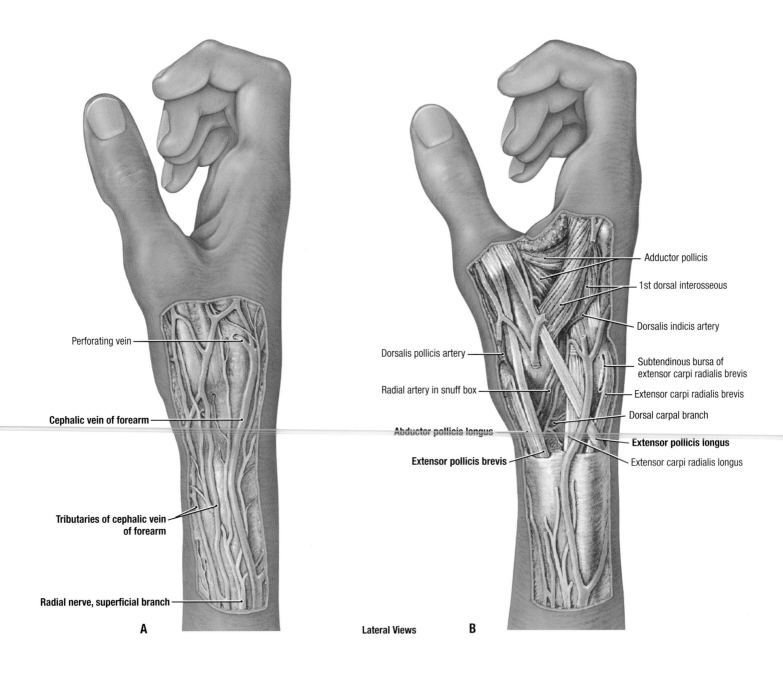

Perforating vein

Cephalic vein of forearm

Tributaries of cephalic vein of forearm

Radial nerve, superficial branch

Adductor pollicis

1st dorsal interosseous

Dorsalis indicis artery

Dorsalis pollicis artery

Subtendinous bursa of extensor carpi radialis brevis

Radial artery in snuff box

Extensor carpi radialis brevis

Dorsal carpal branch

Abductor pollicis longus

Extensor pollicis longus

Extensor pollicis brevis

Extensor carpi radialis longus

A

Lateral Views

B

6.89 LATERAL ASPECT OF WRIST AND HAND

A. Anatomical snuff box—I. **B.** Anatomical snuff box—II.

In **A**:
- The depression at the base of the thumb, the "anatomical snuff box," retains its name from an archaic habit.
- Note the superficial veins, including the cephalic vein of forearm and/or its tributaries, and cutaneous nerves crossing the snuff box.

In **B**:
- Three long tendons of the thumb form the boundaries of the snuff box; the extensor pollicis longus forms the medial boundary and the abductor pollicis longus and extensor pollicis brevis the lateral boundary.
- The radial artery crosses the floor of the snuff box and travels between the two heads of the 1st dorsal interosseous.
- The adductor pollicis and 1st dorsal interosseous are supplied by the ulnar nerve.

1st dorsal interosseous

Extensor (dorsal) expansion

Adductor pollicis (1)

Extensor digitorum (6)

1st metacarpal

1st dorsal interosseous (2)

Extensor pollicis brevis (5)

Opponens pollicis

Radial artery

Abductor pollicis longus (4)

Extensor pollicis longus (3)

Joint capsule of
1st carpometacarpal joint

Midcarpal joint

Scaphoid bone

Extensor carpi radialis brevis

Wrist joint

Styloid process of radius

Extensor carpi radialis longus

Radial artery

Flexor carpi radialis

Extensor digitorum (6)

Brachioradialis

C. Lateral View

D. Lateral View

Distal Extents of:	
EPL	Extensor pollicis longus
EPB	Extensor pollicis brevis
APL	Abductor pollicis longus

6.89   **LATERAL ASPECT OF WRIST AND HAND** *(CONTINUED)*

C. Anatomical snuff box—III. **D.** Surface anatomy.
In **C**: Note the scaphoid bone, the wrist joint proximal to the scaphoid, and the midcarpal joint distal to it.

    Fracture of the scaphoid often results from a fall on the palm with the hand abducted. The fracture occurs across the narrow part ("waist") of the scaphoid. Pain occurs primarily on the lateral side of the wrist, especially during dorsiflexion and abduction of the hand. Initial radiographs

of the wrist may not reveal a fracture, but radiographs taken 10 to 14 days later reveal a fracture because bone resorption has occurred. Owing to the poor blood supply to the proximal part of the scaphoid, union of the fractured parts may take several months. **Avascular necrosis of the proximal fragment of the scaphoid** (pathological death of bone resulting from poor blood supply) may occur and produce degenerative joint disease of the wrist.

E. Bony hand showing muscle attachments.

Extensor pollicis longus

Adductor pollicis

Extensor pollicis brevis

1st metacarpal

Abductor pollicis longus

Trapezium

Scaphoid

Styloid process

Grooves for:

Abductor pollicis longus
Extensor pollicis brevis

Extensor carpi radialis longus
Extensor carpi radialis brevis

1st dorsal interosseous

1st dorsal interosseous

Extensor carpi radialis longus

Trapezoid

Dorsal tubercle of radius

Groove for extensor pollicis longus

E

Distal phalanx of 2nd digit

Proximal phalanx of thumb

1st metacarpal

Thenar eminence

Hypothenar eminence

Trapezium

Scaphoid

Lunate

Radius

F

Lateral Views, Right Hand

6.89   LATERAL ASPECT OF WRIST AND HAND *(CONTINUED)*

E. Bony hand showing muscle attachments. **F.** Radiograph.

- The anatomical snuff box is limited proximally by the styloid process of the radius and distally by the base of the 1st metacarpal; aspects of the two lateral bones of the carpus (scaphoid and trapezium) form the floor of the snuff box.

Medial Views

A. Superficial dissection labels:

5th metacarpal

Opponens digiti minimi

Abductor digiti minimi

Extensor carpi ulnaris

Pisiform

Extensor retinaculum

Dorsal carpal branch of ulnar artery

Subcutaneous part of ulna

Flexor carpi ulnaris

Extensor carpi ulnaris

Dorsal branch of ulnar nerve

Basilic vein of forearm

Flexor carpi ulnaris

Dorsal branch of ulnar nerve

Basilic vein of forearm

Abductor digiti minimi

Opponens digiti minimi

5th metacarpal

Pisometacarpal ligament

Opponens / Flexor brevis] Digiti minimi

Pisohamate ligament

Abductor digiti minimi

Flexor carpi ulnaris

Pisiform

Lunate

Extensor carpi ulnaris

Hamate

Triquetrum

Styloid process of ulna

6.90 **MEDIAL ASPECT OF WRIST AND HAND**

A. Superficial dissection. **B.** Deep dissection. **C.** Bony hand showing sites of muscular and ligamentous attachments. The extensor carpi ulnaris is inserted directly into the base of the fifth metacarpal, but the flexor carpi ulnaris inserts indirectly to the base of the fifth metacarpal via the pisiform and pisohamate and pisometacarpal ligaments. These ligaments are often considered to be a part of the distal attachment of flexor carpi ulnaris.

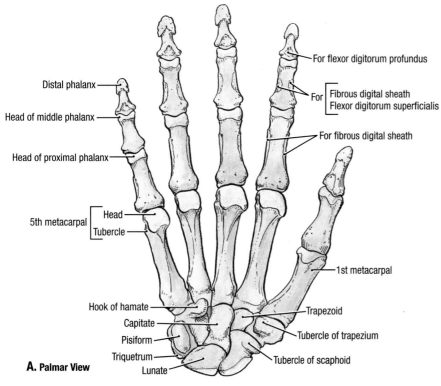

Distal phalanx

Head of middle phalanx

Head of proximal phalanx

For flexor digitorum profundus

For Fibrous digital sheath
Flexor digitorum superficialis

For fibrous digital sheath

5th metacarpal — Head
Tubercle

1st metacarpal

Hook of hamate
Capitate
Pisiform
Triquetrum
Lunate

Trapezoid
Tubercle of trapezium
Tubercle of scaphoid

A. Palmar View

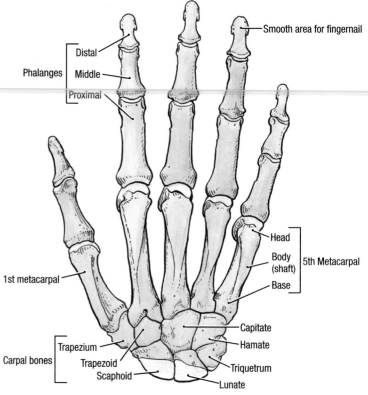

Smooth area for fingernail

Phalanges — Distal
Middle
Proximal

1st metacarpal

Head
Body (shaft) 5th Metacarpal
Base

Carpal bones — Trapezium
Trapezoid
Scaphoid

Capitate
Hamate
Triquetrum
Lunate

B. Dorsal View

6.91 BONES OF HAND

A. Palmar view. **B.** Dorsal view.

The eight carpal bones form two rows: in the distal row, the hamate, cap-itate, trapezoid, and trapezium, the trapezium forming a saddle-shaped joint with the 1st metacarpal, and in the proximal row, the scaphoid, lunate, and pisiform, the pisiform being superimposed on the triquetrum.

Severe **crushing injuries of the hand** may produce multiple metacarpal fractures, resulting in instability of the hand. Similar inju-ries of the distal phalanges are common (e.g., when a finger is caught in a car door).

A **fracture of a distal phalanx** is usually comminuted, and a painful **hematoma** (collection of blood) develops. **Fractures of the proximal and middle phalanges** are usually the result of crushing or hypertension injuries.

A. Anterior View

Phalanges
- Distal (D)
- Middle (M)
- Proximal (Pr)

Metacarpal
- Head
- Shaft (body)
- Base

Hook of hamate (H)
Pisiform (P)
Triquetrum (Tq)
Styloid process of ulna (Su)
Head of ulna (Hu)

Distal interphalangeal (DIP) joint
Proximal interphalangeal (PIP) joint
Metacarpophalangeal (MCP) joint
Distal phalanx (D)
Proximal phalanx (Pr)
Sesamoid bone (F)
Muscle and soft tissue
Trapezoid (Td)
Trapezium (Tz)
Capitate (C)
Scaphoid (S)
Lunate (L)
Styloid process of radius (Sr)
Ulnar notch of radius

B. Anterior View

6.92   IMAGING OF BONES OF WRIST AND HAND

A. Radiograph. **B.** Three-dimensional computer-generated image of wrist and hand (letters correspond to structures labeled in **A**).

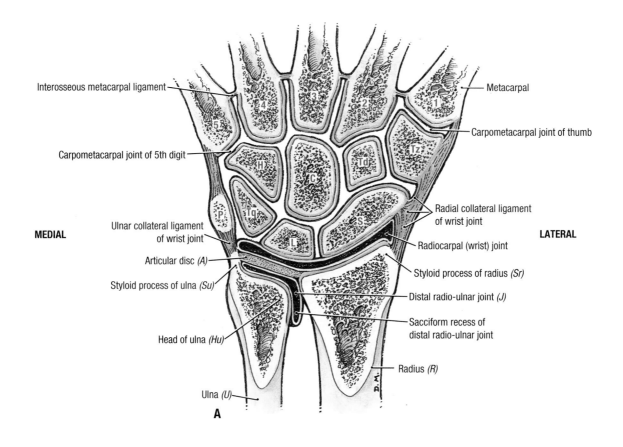

Interosseous metacarpal ligament

Metacarpal

Carpometacarpal joint of thumb

Carpometacarpal joint of 5th digit

Radial collateral ligament of wrist joint

MEDIAL

Ulnar collateral ligament of wrist joint

LATERAL

Radiocarpal (wrist) joint

Articular disc (A)

Styloid process of radius (Sr)

Styloid process of ulna (Su)

Distal radio-ulnar joint (J)

Sacciform recess of distal radio-ulnar joint

Head of ulna (Hu)

Radius (R)

Ulna (U)

A

B

6.93   CORONAL SECTION OF WRIST

A. Schematic illustration. **B.** Coronal MRI. *EL,* epiphysial line; letters correspond to structures labeled in **A.**

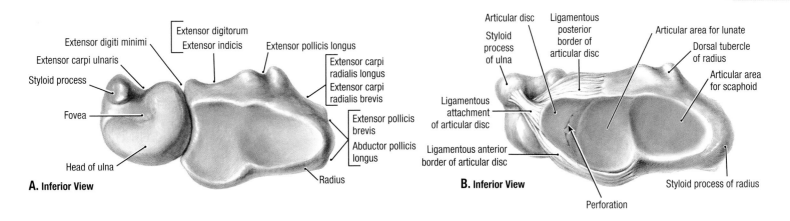

A. Inferior View

Extensor digiti minimi
Extensor carpi ulnaris
Styloid process
Fovea
Head of ulna
Extensor digitorum
Extensor indicis
Extensor pollicis longus
Extensor carpi radialis longus
Extensor carpi radialis brevis
Extensor pollicis brevis
Abductor pollicis longus
Radius

B. Inferior View

Articular disc
Styloid process of ulna
Ligamentous posterior border of articular disc
Articular area for lunate
Dorsal tubercle of radius
Articular area for scaphoid
Ligamentous attachment of articular disc
Ligamentous anterior border of articular disc
Styloid process of radius
Perforation

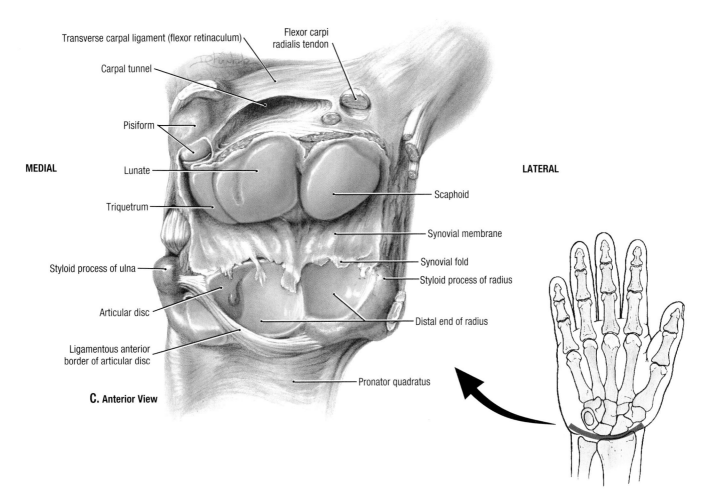

C. Anterior View

Transverse carpal ligament (flexor retinaculum)
Carpal tunnel
Pisiform
Lunate
Triquetrum
Styloid process of ulna
Articular disc
Ligamentous anterior border of articular disc
Flexor carpi radialis tendon
MEDIAL
LATERAL
Scaphoid
Synovial membrane
Synovial fold
Styloid process of radius
Distal end of radius
Pronator quadratus

6.94 **RADIOCARPAL (WRIST) JOINT**

A. Distal ends of radius and ulna showing grooves for tendons on the posterior aspects. **B.** Articular disc. The articular disc unites the distal ends of the radius and ulna; it is fibrocartilaginous at the triangular area between the head of the ulna and the lunate bone, but ligamentous and pliable elsewhere. The cartilaginous part of the articular disc commonly has a fissure or perforation, as shown here, associated with a roughened surface of the lunate. **C.** Articular surface of the radiocarpal joint, which is opened anteriorly. The lunate articulates with the radius and articular disc; only during adduction of the wrist does the triquetrum come into articulation with the disc.

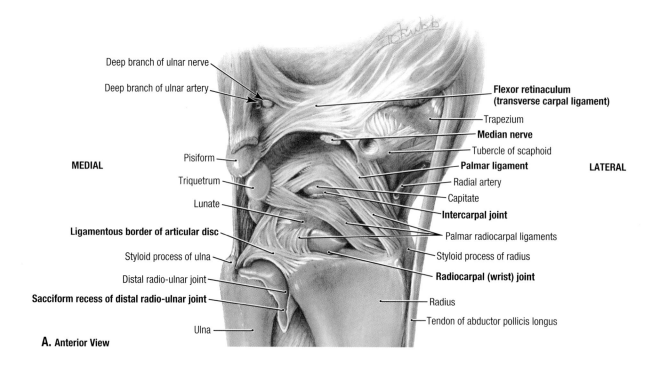

A. Anterior View

Deep branch of ulnar nerve
Deep branch of ulnar artery
MEDIAL
Pisiform
Triquetrum
Lunate
Ligamentous border of articular disc
Styloid process of ulna
Distal radio-ulnar joint
Sacciform recess of distal radio-ulnar joint
Ulna

Flexor retinaculum (transverse carpal ligament)
Trapezium
Median nerve
Tubercle of scaphoid
Palmar ligament
Radial artery
Capitate
Intercarpal joint
Palmar radiocarpal ligaments
Styloid process of radius
Radiocarpal (wrist) joint
Radius
Tendon of abductor pollicis longus
LATERAL

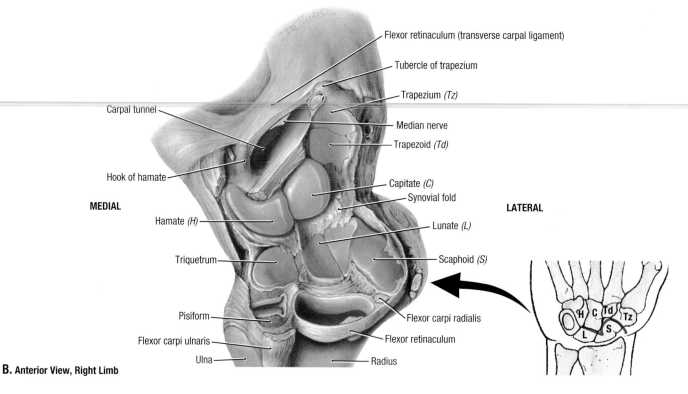

B. Anterior View, Right Limb

Carpal tunnel
MEDIAL
Hook of hamate
Hamate (H)
Triquetrum
Pisiform
Flexor carpi ulnaris
Ulna

Flexor retinaculum (transverse carpal ligament)
Tubercle of trapezium
Trapezium (Tz)
Median nerve
Trapezoid (Td)
Capitate (C)
Synovial fold
Lunate (L)
Scaphoid (S)
Flexor carpi radialis
Flexor retinaculum
Radius
LATERAL

6.95 RADIOCARPAL (WRIST) AND MIDCARPAL (TRANSVERSE CARPAL) JOINT

A. Ligaments. The hand is forcibly extended. The palmar radiocarpal ligaments pass from the radius to the two rows of carpal bones; they are strong and directed so that the hand moves with the radius during supination.
B. Articular surfaces of midcarpal (transverse carpal) joint, opened anteriorly.
• The flexor retinaculum (transverse carpal ligament) is cut; the proximal part of the ligament, which spans from the pisiform to the scaphoid, is

relatively weak; the distal part, which passes from the hook of the hamate to the tubercle of the trapezium, is strong.
• The opposed bones have sinuous surfaces: the trapezium and trapezoid together form a concave, oval surface for the scaphoid, and the capitate and hamate together form a convex surface for the scaphoid, lunate, and triquetrum.

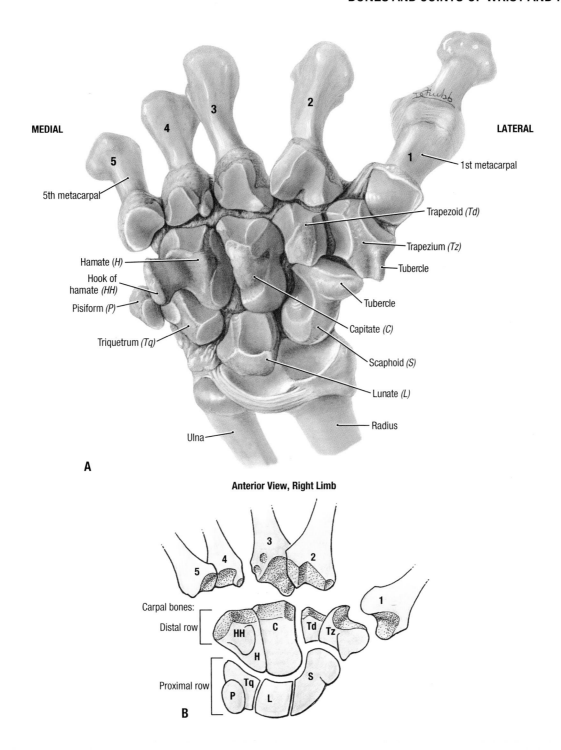

MEDIAL

LATERAL

3

2

4

5

1

5th metacarpal

1st metacarpal

Trapezoid *(Td)*

Trapezium *(Tz)*

Hamate *(H)*

Tubercle

Hook of
hamate *(HH)*

Pisiform *(P)*

Tubercle

Capitate *(C)*

Triquetrum *(Tq)*

Scaphoid *(S)*

Lunate *(L)*

Radius

Ulna

A

Anterior View, Right Limb

3

4

2

5

1

Carpal bones:

Distal row

HH

C

Td

Tz

H

Proximal row

Tq

S

P

L

B

6.96   CARPAL BONES AND BASES OF METACARPALS

A. Open intercarpal and carpometacarpal (CMC) joints. The dorsal ligaments remain intact, and all the joints have been hyperextended, permitting study of articular facets. **B.** Diagram of the articular surfaces of the CMC joints (*letters* refer to structures labeled in **A**).

- The capitate articulates with three metacarpals (2nd, 3rd, and 4th).
- The 2nd metacarpal articulates with three carpals (trapezium, trapezoid, and capitate).
- The 1st CMC joint is saddle-shaped and especially mobile, allowing opposition of the thumb; the 2nd and 3rd CMC joints have interlocking surfaces

and are practically immobile; and the 4th and 5th are hinge-shaped synovial joints with limited movement.

Anterior dislocation of the lunate is a serious injury that usually results from a fall on the extended wrist. The lunate is pushed to the palmar surface of the wrist and may compress the median nerve and lead to carpal tunnel syndrome. Because of poor blood supply, **avascular necrosis of the lunate** may occur.

Proximal interphalangeal joint

Middle phalanx

Collateral ligament

Distal phalanx

Collateral ligament

Distal interphalangeal joint

Proximal phalanx

Collateral ligament — "Cordlike" part

"Fanlike" part

Palmar ligament (plate)

Collateral ligament

Palmar ligament (plate)

Metacarpal

A   B   C

Lateral Views of Right 3rd Digit

6.97   COLLATERAL LIGAMENTS OF METACARPOPHALANGEAL AND INTERPHALANGEAL JOINTS OF THIRD DIGIT

A. Extended metacarpophalangeal (MCP) and distal interphalangeal (IP) joints. **B.** Flexed interphalangeal joints. **C.** Flexed MCP joint.

- A fibrocartilaginous plate, the palmar ligament, hangs from the base of the proximal phalanx; is fixed to the head of the metacarpal by the weaker, fanlike part of the collateral ligament (**A**); and moves like a visor across the metacarpal head (**C**). The IP joints have similar palmar ligaments.
- The extremely strong, cordlike parts of the collateral ligaments of this joint (**A** and **B**) are eccentrically attached to the metacarpal heads; they are slack during extension and taut during flexion (**C**), so the fingers cannot be spread (abducted) unless the hand is open; the IP joints have similar collateral ligaments.

Skier's thumb refers to the rupture or chronic laxity of the collateral ligament of the 1st metacarpophalangeal joint. The injury results from hyperextension of the joint, which occurs when the thumb is held by the ski pole while the rest of the hand hits the ground or enters the snow.

TABLE 6.16 LESIONS OF NERVES OF UPPER LIMB

Nerve Injury	Injury Description	Impairments	Clinical Aspect
Long thoracic nerve	Stab wound Mastectomy	Abduction of shoulder joint and protraction of the scapula is compromised	Test: Pushing against a wall causes winging of scapula
Axillary nerve	Surgical neck fracture of humerus Anterior dislocation of shoulder joint	Abduction of shoulder joint to horizontal is compromised; sensory loss on lateral side of upper arm	Test: Abduct shoulder joint to horizontal and ask patient to hold position against a downward pull
Radial nerve	Midshaft fracture of humerus Badly fitted crutch Arm draped over a chair	Extension at wrist and joints of digits is lost; supination of forearm is compromised; sensory loss on posterior arm and forearm, and lateral aspect of dorsum of hand	Wrist drop
Median nerve at elbow	Supra-epicondylar fracture of humerus	Flexion of wrist joint is weakened; hand will deviate to ulnar side during flexion of wrist joint; flexion of DIP, PIP and MP joints of index and middle digits is lost; abduction, opposition and flexion of thumb joints are lost; sensory loss on palmar and dorsal aspects of index, middle, and lateral half of ring fingers and palmar aspect of thumb	Absence of thumb opposition Hand of benediction
Median nerve at wrist	Slashing of wrist Carpal tunnel syndrome	Weakened flexion of MP joints of index and middle fingers; opposition and abduction of CMC and MP joint of thumb lost; sensory loss same as for median nerve injury at elbow	Test: Make an "O" with thumb and index finger
Ulnar nerve at elbow	Fracture of medial epicondyle of humerus	Hand will deviate to radial side during flexion of wrist joint; flexion of DIP joints of ring and little finger lost; flexion at MP joint and extension at PIP and DIP joints of little and ring finger are lost; adduction and abduction of MP joints of digits 2–5 lost; adduction of thumb lost; sensory loss on palmar and dorsal aspects of little and medial half of ring fingers	Claw hand
Ulnar nerve at wrist	Slashing of wrist	Flexion at MP joint and extension at PIP and DIP joints of little and ring fingers lost; adduction and abduction of MP joints of digits 2–5 lost; adduction of thumb lost; sensory loss same as for ulnar nerve injury at elbow	Test: Hold paper between middle and ring fingers

CMC, carpometacarpal joint; MP, metacarpophalangeal joint; PIP, proximal interphalangeal joint; DIP, distal interphalangeal joint.

A. Lateral view

B. Anterior view

C. Medial view

D. Medial view

E. Medial view

F. Medial view

I. Lateral view

G. Anterior view

H. Anterior view

6.98 FUNCTIONAL POSITIONS OF HAND

A. Cylindrical (power) grasp. When grasping an object, the metacarpophalangeal and interphalangeal joints are flexed, but the radiocarpal joints are extended. Without wrist extension the grip is weak and insecure. **B.** Hook grasp. This grasp involves primarily the long flexors of the fingers, which are flexed to a varying degree depending on the size of the object. **C.** Tripod (three-jaw chuck) pinch. **D. and E.** Fingertip pinch. **F.** Rest position of hand. Casts for fractures are applied most often with the hand in this position. **G.** Loose cylindrical grasp. **H.** Firm cylindrical (power) grasp. **I.** Disc (power) grasp.

ANTERIOR

POSTERIOR

A

ANTERIOR

POSTERIOR

B

ANTERIOR

POSTERIOR

C

Key for A, B, and C:	
BB	Biceps brachii
BC	Brachialis
BR	Brachioradialis
BS	Basilic Vein
BV	Brachial vessels and nerves
CV	Cephalic vein
D	Deltoid
F	Fat in axilla
H	Humerus
L	Lung
LAT	Lateral head of triceps brachii
LHB	Long head of biceps brachii
LI	Lateral intermuscular septum
LT	Long head of triceps brachii
MI	Medial intermuscular septum
MT	Medial head of triceps brachii
PMi	Pectoralis minor
PMj	Pectoralis major
SA	Serratus anterior
SC	Subscapularis
SHB	Short head of biceps brachii
T	Deltoid tuberosity
TL	Teres major and latissimus dorsi
TM	Teres minor
TR	Triceps brachii

6.99   TRANSVERSE (AXIAL) MRIs OF ARM

A. Transverse MRI through the proximal arm. **B.** Transverse MRI though the middle of the arm. **C.** Transverse MRI through the distal arm.

POSTERIOR

Radius

Ulna

Interosseous membrane

Extensor–supinator compartment
Flexor–pronator compartment

A. Anterosuperior View

ANTERIOR

Flexors:

1 Pronator teres
2 Flexor carpi radialis
3 Palmaris longus
4 Flexor carpi ulnaris
5 Flexor digitorum superficialis
6 Flexor digitorum profundus
7 Flexor pollicis longus

Extensors:

8 Brachioradialis
9 Extensor carpi radialis longus
10 Extensor carpi radialis brevis
11 Extensor digitorum
12 Extensor digiti minimi
13 Extensor carpi ulnaris
14 Abductor pollicis longus
15 Extensor pollicis brevis
16 Extensor pollicis longus and extensor indicis

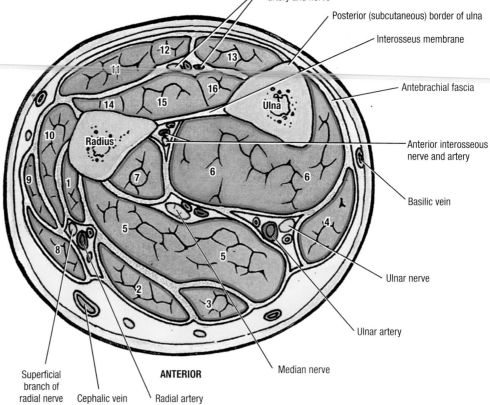

POSTERIOR

Posterior interosseous artery and nerve

Posterior (subcutaneous) border of ulna

Interosseus membrane

Antebrachial fascia

Ulna

Anterior interosseous nerve and artery

Basilic vein

Radius

Ulnar nerve

Ulnar artery

Median nerve

ANTERIOR

Superficial branch of radial nerve

Cephalic vein

Radial artery

A and B

B. Transverse Section

6.100   TRANSVERSE SECTIONS AND TRANSVERSE (AXIAL) MRIs OF FOREARM

A. Stepped transverse sections of the anterior and posterior compartments. **B.** Contents of the anterior and posterior compartments.

Key for C, D, and E:

AN	Anconeus
APL	Abductor pollicis longus
AV	Anterior interosseous vessels and nerve
BB	Biceps brachii
BR	Brachioradialis
BV	Brachial vessels
CV	Cephalic vein
ECRB	Extensor carpi radialis brevis
ECRL	Extensor carpi radialis longus
ECU	Extensor carpi ulnaris
ED	Extensor digitorum
EPB	Extensor pollicis brevis
EPL	Extensor pollicis longus
FCR	Flexor carpi radialis
FCU	Flexor carpi ulnaris
FDP	Flexor digitorum profundus
FDS	Flexor digitorum superficialis
FPL	Flexor pollicis longus
INT	Interosseous membrane
PQ	Pronator quadratus
PT	Pronator teres
R	Radius
RV	Radial vessels
SP	Supinator
U	Ulnar
UN	Ulnar vessels and nerve

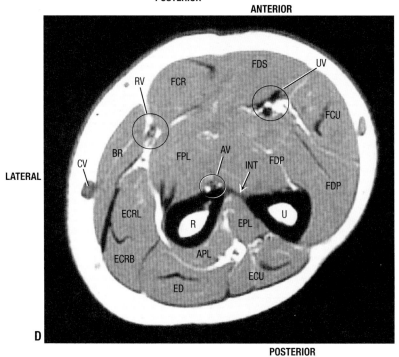

6.100 TRANSVERSE SECTIONS AND TRANSVERSE (AXIAL) MRIs OF FOREARM
(CONTINUED)

C. Transverse MRI through the proximal forearm. **D.** Transverse MRI through the middle forearm. **E.** Transverse MRI through the distal forearm.

A. Transverse MRI

B. Coronal MRI

6.101 TRANSVERSE (AXIAL) SECTION AND MRIs THROUGH CARPAL TUNNEL

A. Transverse MRI through the proximal carpal tunnel (*numbers* and *letters* in MRIs refer to structures in **D**).
B. Coronal MRI of wrist and hand showing the course of the long flexor tendons in the carpal tunnel (*numbers* and *letters* in MRIs refer to structures in **D**). *FT*, long flexor tendons in carpal tunnel; *TH*, thenar muscles; *P*, pisiform; *H*, hook of hamate; *Tm*, trapezium; *I*, interossei, *A–E*, proximal phalanges.

C. Transverse MRI

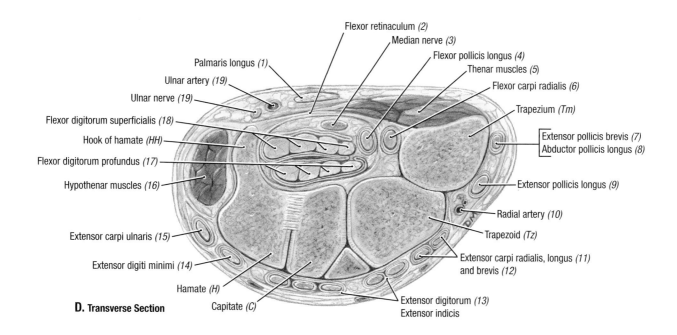

Palmaris longus (1)
Ulnar artery (19)
Ulnar nerve (19)
Flexor digitorum superficialis (18)
Hook of hamate (HH)
Flexor digitorum profundus (17)
Hypothenar muscles (16)
Extensor carpi ulnaris (15)
Extensor digiti minimi (14)
Hamate (H)
Capitate (C)

Flexor retinaculum (2)
Median nerve (3)
Flexor pollicis longus (4)
Thenar muscles (5)
Flexor carpi radialis (6)
Trapezium (Tm)
Extensor pollicis brevis (7)
Abductor pollicis longus (8)
Extensor pollicis longus (9)
Radial artery (10)
Trapezoid (Tz)
Extensor carpi radialis, longus (11) and brevis (12)
Extensor digitorum (13)
Extensor indicis

D. Transverse Section

6.101 **TRANSVERSE (AXIAL) SECTION AND MRIs THROUGH CARPAL TUNNEL**
(CONTINUED)

C. Transverse MRI through the distal carpal tunnel (*numbers* and *letters* in MRIs refer to structures in **D**).
D. Transverse section of carpal tunnel through the distal row of carpal bones.

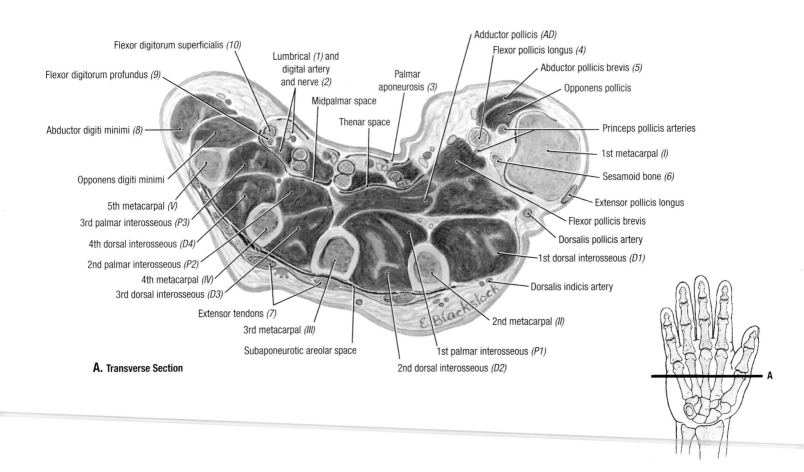

Flexor digitorum superficialis (10)

Flexor digitorum profundus (9)

Lumbrical (1) and
digital artery
and nerve (2)

Midpalmar space

Palmar
aponeurosis (3)

Thenar space

Adductor pollicis (AD)

Flexor pollicis longus (4)

Abductor pollicis brevis (5)

Opponens pollicis

Abductor digiti minimi (8)

Opponens digiti minimi

5th metacarpal (V)

3rd palmar interosseous (P3)

4th dorsal interosseous (D4)

2nd palmar interosseous (P2)

4th metacarpal (IV)

3rd dorsal interosseous (D3)

Extensor tendons (7)

3rd metacarpal (III)

Subaponeurotic areolar space

2nd dorsal interosseous (D2)

Princeps pollicis arteries

1st metacarpal (I)

Sesamoid bone (6)

Extensor pollicis longus

Flexor pollicis brevis

Dorsalis pollicis artery

1st dorsal interosseous (D1)

Dorsalis indicis artery

2nd metacarpal (II)

1st palmar interosseous (P1)

E. Blackstock

A. Transverse Section

B. Transverse MRI

6.102 TRANSVERSE SECTION AND MRI THROUGH PALM (METACARPALS) AT LEVEL OF ADDUCTOR POLLICIS

Head

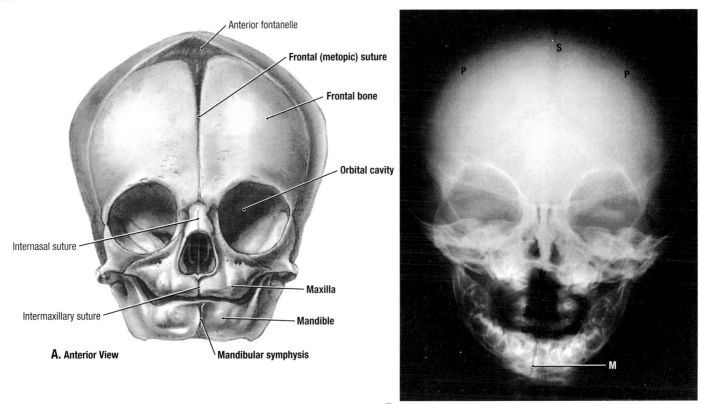

Anterior fontanelle

Frontal (metopic) suture

Frontal bone

Orbital cavity

Internasal suture

Maxilla

Intermaxillary suture

Mandible

A. Anterior View

Mandibular symphysis

B. Anteroposterior View

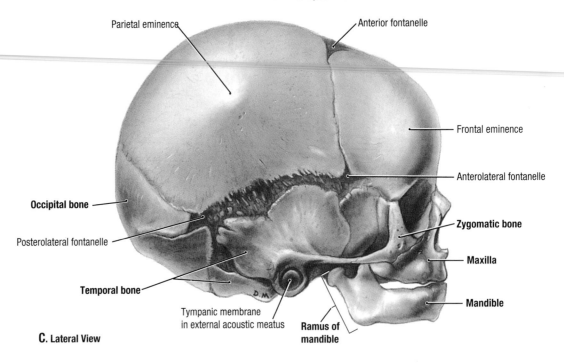

Parietal eminence

Anterior fontanelle

Frontal eminence

Anterolateral fontanelle

Occipital bone

Zygomatic bone

Posterolateral fontanelle

Maxilla

Temporal bone

Mandible

Tympanic membrane
in external acoustic meatus

**Ramus of
mandible**

C. Lateral View

| **7.1** | **CRANIUM AT BIRTH AND IN EARLY CHILDHOOD** |

A. Cranium at birth, anterior aspect. **B.** Radiograph of 6½-month-old child. **C.** Cranium at birth, lateral aspect.

Compared with the adult skull (Figs. 7.2–7.4):

- The maxilla and mandible are proportionately small.

- The mandibular symphysis, which closes during the second year, and the frontal suture, which closes during the sixth year, are still open (unfused).

- The orbital cavities are proportionately large, but the face is small; the facial skeleton forming only one eighth of the whole cranium, while in the adult, it forms one third.

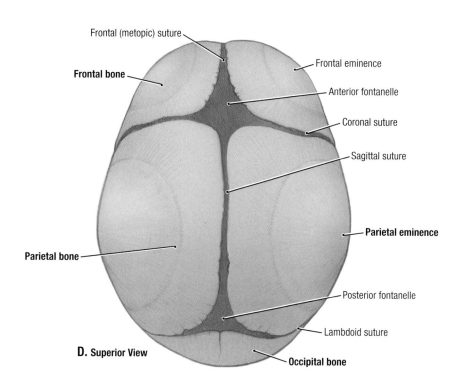

D. Superior View

Key for B, E and F

A	Angle of mandible
B	Body of mandible
C	Coronal suture
F	Frontal bone
L	Lambdoid suture
M	Mandibular symphysis
O	Occipital bone
P	Parietal eminence
S	Sagittal suture
SP	Sphenoid
T	Temporal bone
X	Maxilla
Y	Mastoid process
Z	Zygomatic bone

Arrowheads = Membranous outline of parietal bone

Labels in D (Superior View): Frontal (metopic) suture, Frontal bone, Frontal eminence, Anterior fontanelle, Coronal suture, Sagittal suture, Parietal eminence, Parietal bone, Posterior fontanelle, Lambdoid suture, Occipital bone

E. Lateral View

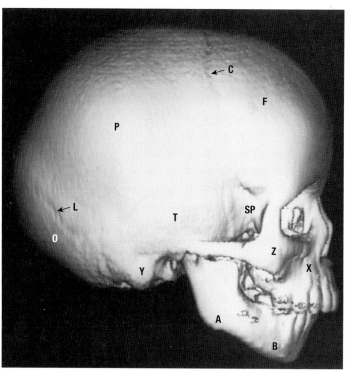

F. Lateral View

7.1   CRANIUM AT BIRTH AND IN EARLY CHILDHOOD (CONTINUED)

D. Cranium at birth, superior aspect. **E.** Radiograph of 6½-month-old child. **F.** Three-dimensional computer-generated images of 3-year-old child's cranium.

• The parietal eminence is a shallow, rounded cone. Ossification, which starts at the eminences, has not yet reached the ultimate four angles of the parietal bone; accordingly, these regions are membranous, and the membrane is blended with the pericranium externally and the dura mater internally to form the fontanelles. The fontanelles are usually closed by the second year. There is no mastoid process until the second year.

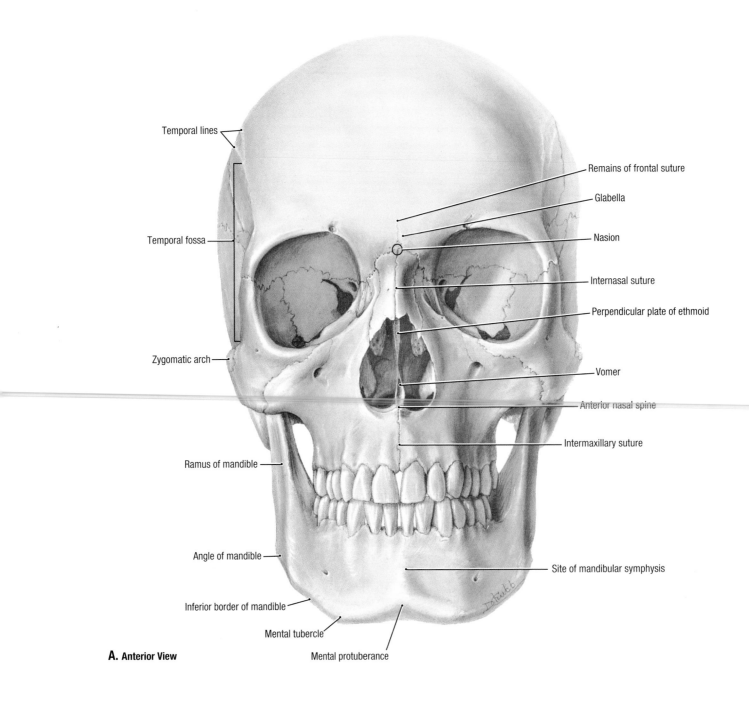

Temporal lines

Remains of frontal suture

Glabella

Nasion

Temporal fossa

Internasal suture

Perpendicular plate of ethmoid

Zygomatic arch

Vomer

Anterior nasal spine

Intermaxillary suture

Ramus of mandible

Angle of mandible

Site of mandibular symphysis

Inferior border of mandible

Mental tubercle

A. Anterior View

Mental protuberance

7.2   CRANIUM, FACIAL (FRONTAL) ASPECT

A. Formations of the bony cranium. **B.** Bones of cranium and their features. The individual bones forming the cranium are color coded. For the orbital cavity, see also Figure 7.36A.

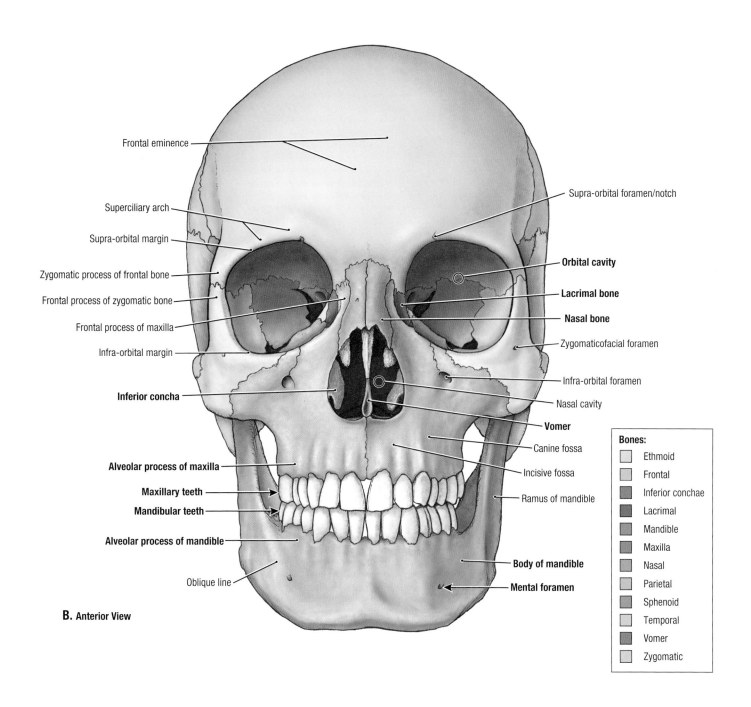

Frontal eminence

Superciliary arch

Supra-orbital margin

Zygomatic process of frontal bone

Frontal process of zygomatic bone

Frontal process of maxilla

Infra-orbital margin

Inferior concha

Alveolar process of maxilla

Maxillary teeth

Mandibular teeth

Alveolar process of mandible

Oblique line

Supra-orbital foramen/notch

Orbital cavity

Lacrimal bone

Nasal bone

Zygomaticofacial foramen

Infra-orbital foramen

Nasal cavity

Vomer

Canine fossa

Incisive fossa

Ramus of mandible

Body of mandible

Mental foramen

Bones:

Ethmoid

Frontal

Inferior conchae

Lacrimal

Mandible

Maxilla

Nasal

Parietal

Sphenoid

Temporal

Vomer

Zygomatic

B. Anterior View

7.2   CRANIUM, FACIAL (FRONTAL) ASPECT *(CONTINUED)*

Extraction of teeth causes the alveolar bone to resorb in the affected regions(s). Following complete loss or extraction of maxillary teeth, the sockets begin to fill in with bone, and the alveolar process begins to resorb. Similarly, extraction of mandibular teeth causes the bone of the alveolar process to resorb. The mental foramen may eventually lie near the superior border of the body of the mandible. In some cases, the mental foramina disappear, exposing the mental nerves to injury.

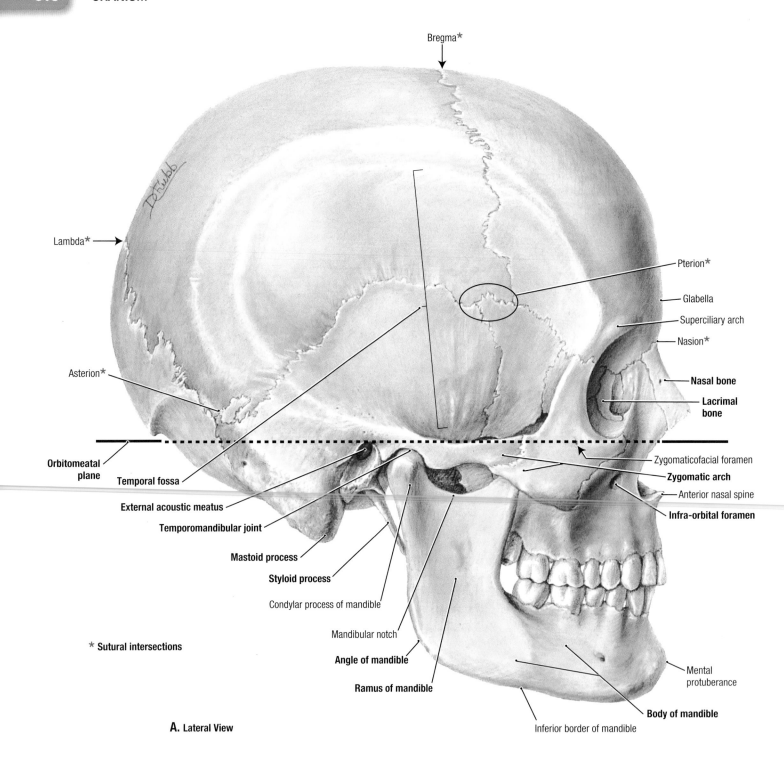

Bregma*

Lambda*

Pterion*

Glabella

Superciliary arch

Nasion*

Nasal bone

Lacrimal bone

Asterion*

Orbitomeatal plane

Zygomaticofacial foramen

Zygomatic arch

Anterior nasal spine

Infra-orbital foramen

Temporal fossa

External acoustic meatus

Temporomandibular joint

Mastoid process

Styloid process

Condylar process of mandible

Mandibular notch

* **Sutural intersections**

Angle of mandible

Ramus of mandible

Body of mandible

Mental protuberance

Inferior border of mandible

A. Lateral View

7.3 CRANIUM, LATERAL ASPECT

A. Bony cranium. **B.** Cranium with bones color coded. The cranium is in the anatomical position when the orbitomeatal plane is horizontal. **C.** Buttresses of cranium. The buttresses are thicker portions of cranial bones that transfer forces around the weaker regions of the orbits and nasal cavity.

The convexity of the neurocranium (braincase) distributes and thereby minimizes the effects of a blow to it. However, hard blows to the head in thin areas of the cranium (e.g., in the temporal fossa) are likely to produce **depressed fractures**, in which a fragment of bone is depressed inward, compressing and/or injuring the brain. In **comminuted fractures**, the bone is broken into several pieces. **Linear fractures**, the most frequent type, usually occur at the point of impact, but fracture lines often radiate away from it in two or more directions.

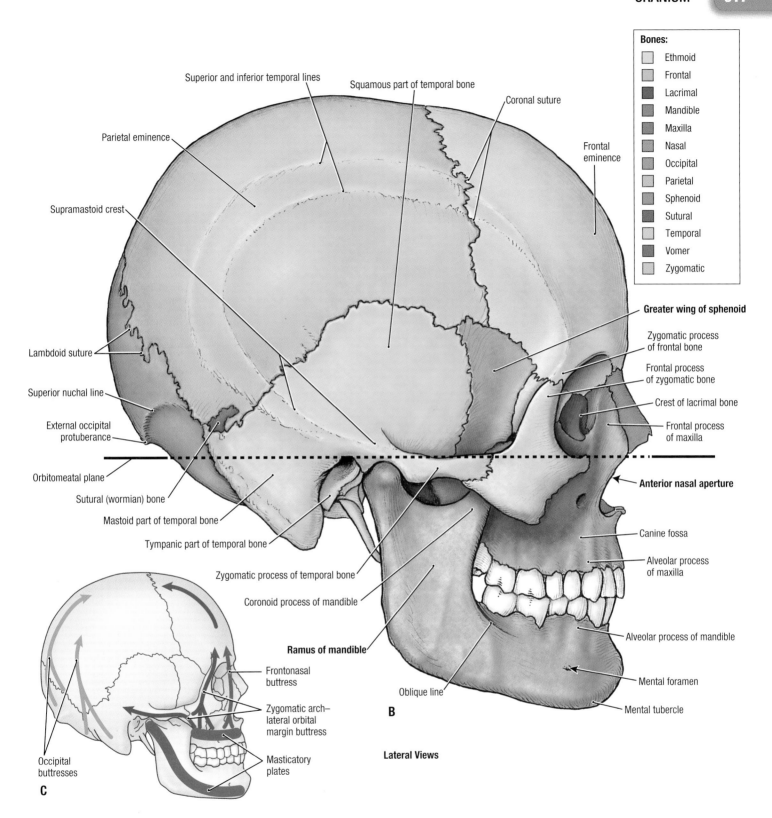

Bones:
- Ethmoid
- Frontal
- Lacrimal
- Mandible
- Maxilla
- Nasal
- Occipital
- Parietal
- Sphenoid
- Sutural
- Temporal
- Vomer
- Zygomatic

Superior and inferior temporal lines

Squamous part of temporal bone

Coronal suture

Parietal eminence

Frontal eminence

Supramastoid crest

Greater wing of sphenoid

Zygomatic process of frontal bone

Frontal process of zygomatic bone

Lambdoid suture

Crest of lacrimal bone

Superior nuchal line

Frontal process of maxilla

External occipital protuberance

Anterior nasal aperture

Orbitomeatal plane

Sutural (wormian) bone

Canine fossa

Mastoid part of temporal bone

Alveolar process of maxilla

Tympanic part of temporal bone

Zygomatic process of temporal bone

Coronoid process of mandible

Alveolar process of mandible

Ramus of mandible

Frontonasal buttress

Oblique line

Mental foramen

Zygomatic arch–lateral orbital margin buttress

Mental tubercle

B

Masticatory plates

Occipital buttresses

C

Lateral Views

7.3 **CRANIUM, LATERAL ASPECT** *(CONTINUED)*

If the area of the neurocranium is thick at the site of impact, the bone usually bends inward without fracturing; however, a fracture may occur some distance from the site of direct trauma where the calvaria is thinner. In a **contrecoup (counterblow) fracture**, the fracture occurs on the opposite side of the cranium rather than at the point of impact. One or more sutural (accessory) bones may be located at the lambda or near the mastoid process.

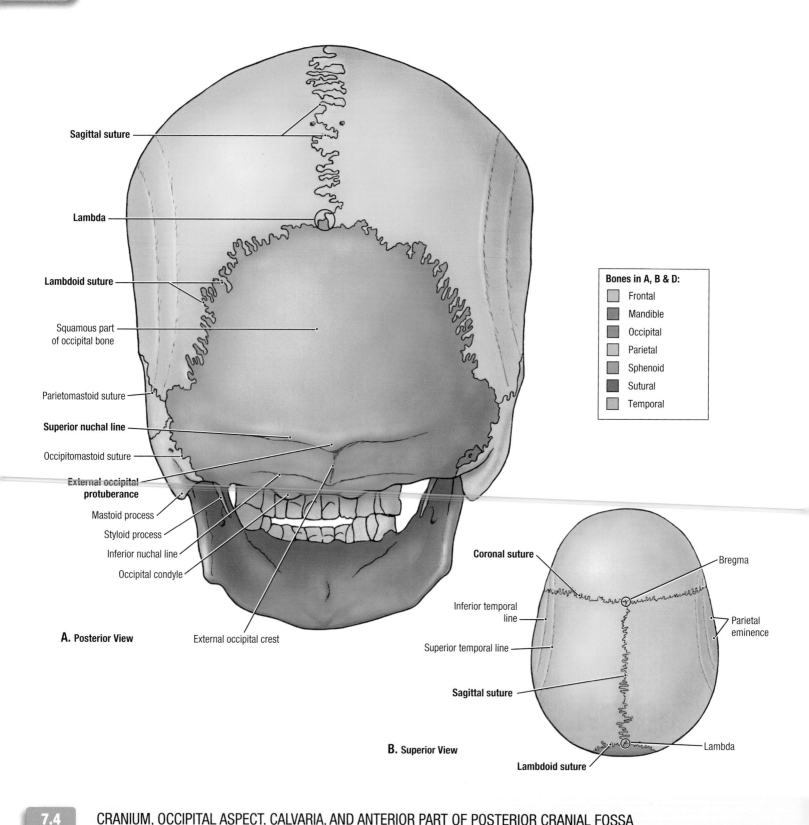

Sagittal suture

Lambda

Lambdoid suture

Squamous part
of occipital bone

Parietomastoid suture

Superior nuchal line

Occipitomastoid suture

**External occipital
protuberance**

Mastoid process

Styloid process

Inferior nuchal line

Occipital condyle

A. Posterior View

External occipital crest

Bones in A, B & D:
- Frontal
- Mandible
- Occipital
- Parietal
- Sphenoid
- Sutural
- Temporal

Coronal suture

Inferior temporal
line

Superior temporal line

Sagittal suture

Lambdoid suture

Bregma

Parietal
eminence

Lambda

B. Superior View

7.4   **CRANIUM, OCCIPITAL ASPECT, CALVARIA, AND ANTERIOR PART OF POSTERIOR CRANIAL FOSSA**

A. The lambda, near the center of this convex surface, is located at the junction of the sagittal and lambdoid sutures. **B.** The roof of the neurocranium, or calvaria (skullcap), is formed primarily by the paired parietal bones, the frontal bone, and the occipital bone.

Premature closure of the coronal suture results in a high, tower-like cranium, called **oxycephaly** or **turricephaly**. Premature closure of sutures usually does not affect brain development. When premature closure occurs on one side only, the cranium is asymmetrical, a condition known as **plagiocephaly**.

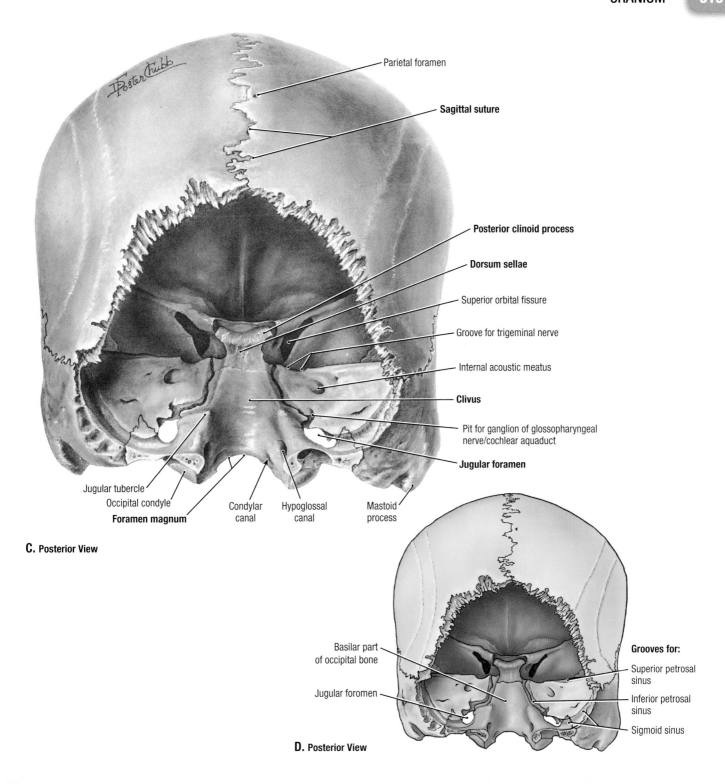

Parietal foramen

Sagittal suture

Posterior clinoid process

Dorsum sellae

Superior orbital fissure

Groove for trigeminal nerve

Internal acoustic meatus

Clivus

Pit for ganglion of glossopharyngeal nerve/cochlear aquaduct

Jugular foramen

Jugular tubercle

Occipital condyle

Foramen magnum

Condylar canal

Hypoglossal canal

Mastoid process

C. **Posterior View**

Basilar part of occipital bone

Jugular foromen

Grooves for:

Superior petrosal sinus

Inferior petrosal sinus

Sigmoid sinus

D. **Posterior View**

7.4   CRANIUM, OCCIPITAL ASPECT, CALVARIA, AND ANTERIOR PART OF POSTERIOR CRANIAL FOSSA *(CONTINUED)*

C. and D. Cranium after removal of squamous part of occipital bone.
- The dorsum sellae projects from the body of the sphenoid; the posterior clinoid processes form its superolateral corners.
- The clivus is the slope descending from the dorsum sellae to the foramen magnum.
- The grooves for the sigmoid sinus and inferior petrosal sinus lead inferiorly to the jugular foramen.

Premature closure of the sagittal suture, in which the anterior fontanelle is small or absent, results in a long, narrow, wedge-shaped cranium, a condition called **scaphocephaly**.

A. Inferior View

7.5 CRANIUM, INFERIOR ASPECT

A. Bony cranium. **B.** Diagram of cranium with bones color coded.

TABLE 7.1 FORAMINA AND OTHER APERTURES OF CRANIAL FOSSAE, AND CONTENTS (SEE FIGS. 7.2–7.6)

Foramen cecum: Nasal emissary vein (1% of population)	Optic canals: Optic nerve (CN II) and ophthalmic arteries
Cribriform plate: Olfactory nerves (CN I)	Superior orbital fissure: Ophthalmic veins; ophthalmic nerve (CN V$_1$); CN III, IV and VI; and sympathetic fibers
Anterior and posterior ethmoidal foramina: Vessels and nerves with same names	Foramen rotundum: Maxillary nerve (CN V$_2$)

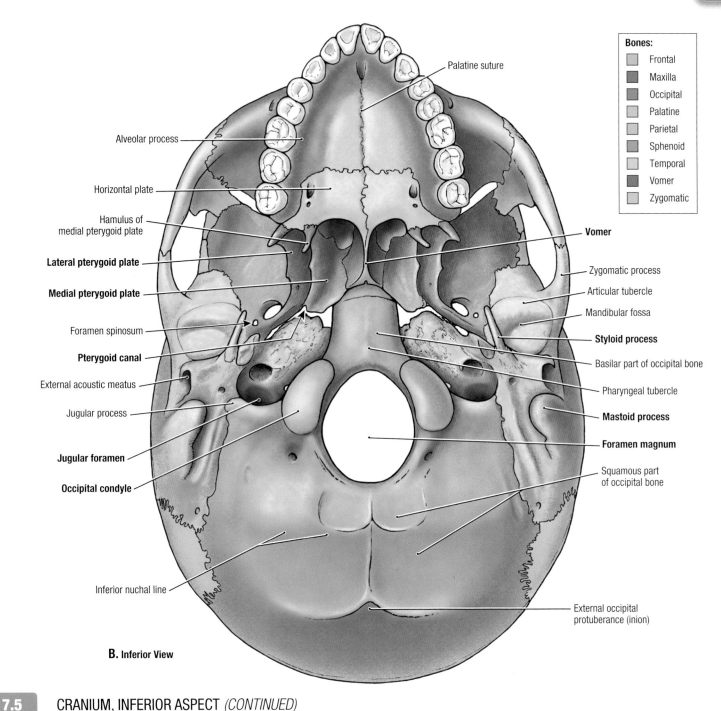

Palatine suture

Alveolar process

Horizontal plate

Hamulus of
medial pterygoid plate

Lateral pterygoid plate

Medial pterygoid plate

Foramen spinosum

Pterygoid canal

External acoustic meatus

Jugular process

Jugular foramen

Occipital condyle

Inferior nuchal line

Vomer

Zygomatic process

Articular tubercle

Mandibular fossa

Styloid process

Basilar part of occipital bone

Pharyngeal tubercle

Mastoid process

Foramen magnum

Squamous part
of occipital bone

External occipital
protuberance (inion)

Bones:
- Frontal
- Maxilla
- Occipital
- Palatine
- Parietal
- Sphenoid
- Temporal
- Vomer
- Zygomatic

B. Inferior View

7.5   CRANIUM, INFERIOR ASPECT *(CONTINUED)*

TABLE 7.1 FORAMINA AND OTHER APERTURES OF CRANIAL FOSSAE, AND CONTENTS (SEE FIGS. 7.2–7.6) (CONTINUED)

Foramen ovale: Mandibular nerve (CN V₃) and accessory meningeal artery	Jugular foramen: CN IX, X, and XI; superior bulb of internal jugular vein; inferior petrosal and sigmoid sinuses; meningeal branches of ascending pharyngeal and occipital arteries.
Foramen spinosum: Middle meningeal artery/vein and meningeal branch of CN V₃	Hypoglossal canal: Hypoglossal nerve (CN XII)
Foramen lacerum[a]: Deep petrosal nerve, some meningeal arterial branches and small veins.	Foramen magnum: Spinal cord; spinal accessory nerve (CN XI); vertebral arteries; internal vertebral venous plexus.
Groove of greater petrosal nerve: Greater petrosal nerve and petrosal branch of middle meningeal artery	Condylar canal: Condyloid emissary vein (passes from sigmoid sinus to vertebral veins in neck)
Carotid canal: Internal carotid artery and accompanying sympathetic and venous plexuses	Stylomastoid foramen: Facial nerve (CN VII)
Internal acoustic meatus: Facial nerve/ intermediate nerve (CN VII); vestibulocochlear nerve (CN VIII); labyrinthine artery	Mastoid foramina: Mastoid emissary vein from sigmoid sinus and meningeal branch of occipital artery

[a]The internal carotid artery and its accompanying sympathetic and venous plexuses actually pass horizontally across (rather than vertically through) the area of the foramen lacerum, an artifact of dry crania, which is closed by cartilage in life.

The foramen ovale subscript V₃ is rendered as $CN\ V_3$.

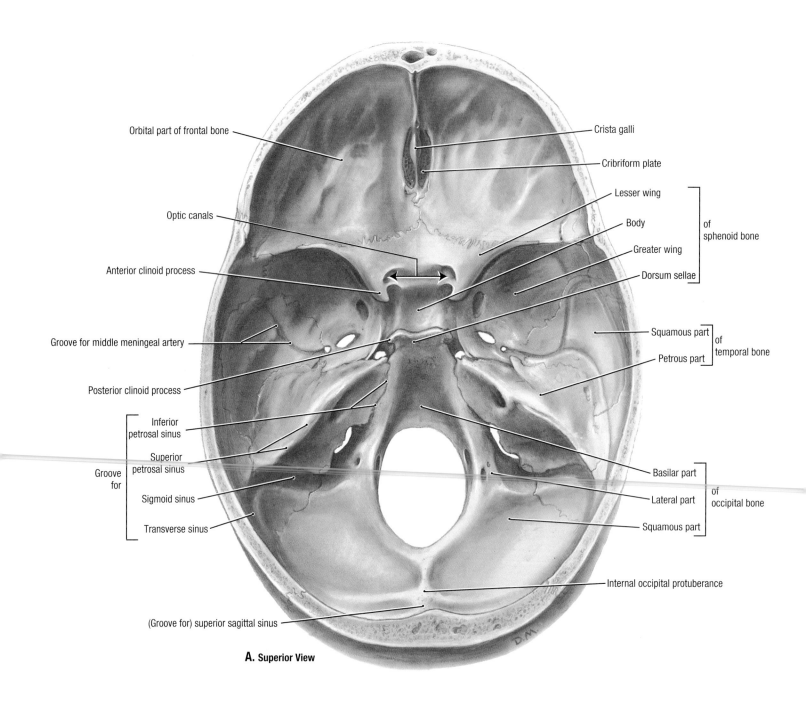

Orbital part of frontal bone

Optic canals

Anterior clinoid process

Groove for middle meningeal artery

Posterior clinoid process

Inferior petrosal sinus

Superior petrosal sinus

Groove for

Sigmoid sinus

Transverse sinus

(Groove for) superior sagittal sinus

Crista galli

Cribriform plate

Lesser wing

Body   of sphenoid bone

Greater wing

Dorsum sellae

Squamous part   of temporal bone

Petrous part

Basilar part

Lateral part   of occipital bone

Squamous part

Internal occipital protuberance

A. Superior View

7.6   INTERIOR OF THE CRANIAL BASE

A. Bony cranial base. **B.** Diagrammatic cranial base with bones color coded.
In **A:**

- Three bones contribute to the anterior cranial fossa: the orbital part of the frontal bone, the cribriform plate of the ethmoid, and the lesser wing of the sphenoid.
- The four parts of the occipital bone are the basilar, right and left lateral, and squamous.
- **Fractures in the floor of the anterior cranial fossa** may involve the cribriform plate of the ethmoid, resulting in leakage of CSF through the nose (CSF rhinorrhea). **CSF rhinorrhea** may be a primary indication of a cranial base fracture which increases the risk of meningitis, because an infection could spread to the meninges from the ear or nose.

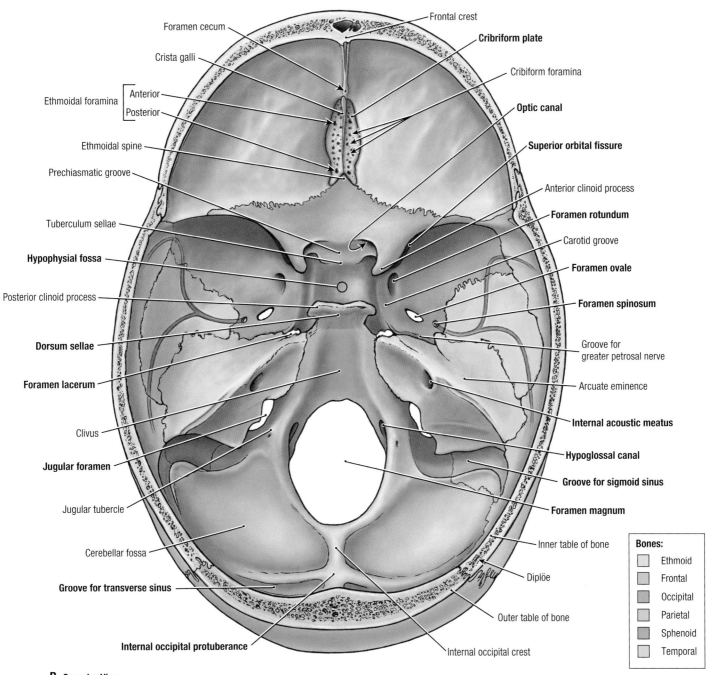

Foramen cecum

Frontal crest

Cribriform plate

Crista galli

Cribiform foramina

Ethmoidal foramina { Anterior / Posterior

Optic canal

Ethmoidal spine

Superior orbital fissure

Prechiasmatic groove

Anterior clinoid process

Tuberculum sellae

Foramen rotundum

Hypophysial fossa

Carotid groove

Posterior clinoid process

Foramen ovale

Dorsum sellae

Foramen spinosum

Foramen lacerum

Groove for greater petrosal nerve

Clivus

Arcuate eminence

Jugular foramen

Internal acoustic meatus

Jugular tubercle

Hypoglossal canal

Cerebellar fossa

Groove for sigmoid sinus

Groove for transverse sinus

Foramen magnum

Inner table of bone

Diplöe

Outer table of bone

Internal occipital protuberance

Internal occipital crest

Bones:
☐	Ethmoid
☐	Frontal
☐	Occipital
☐	Parietal
☐	Sphenoid
☐	Temporal

B. Superior View

7.6   **INTERIOR OF THE CRANIAL BASE** *(CONTINUED)*

In **B,** note the following midline features:
- In the anterior cranial fossa, the frontal crest and crista galli for anterior attachment of the falx cerebri have between them the foramen cecum, which, during development, transmits a vein connecting the superior sagittal sinus with the veins of the frontal sinus and root of the nose.
- In the middle cranial fossa, the tuberculum sellae, hypophysial fossa, dorsum sellae, and posterior clinoid processes constitute the sella turcica (L. Turkish saddle).
- In the posterior cranial fossa, note the clivus, foramen magnum, internal occipital crest for attachment of the falx cerebelli, and the internal occipital protuberance, from which the grooves for the transverse sinuses course laterally.

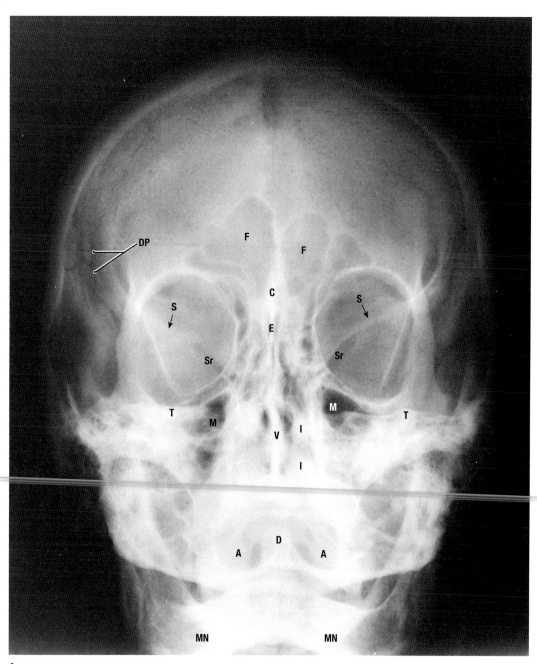

A. Anteroposterior View

7.7 RADIOGRAPHS OF THE CRANIUM

A. Postero-anterior (*Caldwell*) radiograph. This view places the orbits centrally in the head and is used to examine the orbits and paranasal sinuses. Observe in **A:**
- The labeled features include the superior orbital fissure *(Sr)*, lesser wing of the sphenoid *(S)*, superior surface of the petrous part of the temporal bone *(T)*, crista galli *(C)*, frontal sinus *(F)*, mandible *(MN)*, maxillary sinus *(M)*, and diploic veins *(DP)*.
- The nasal septum is formed by the perpendicular plate of the ethmoid *(E)* and the vomer *(V)*; note the inferior and middle conchae *(I)* of the lateral wall of the nose.
- Superimposed on the facial skeleton are the dens *(D)* and lateral masses of the atlas *(A)*.

Beam

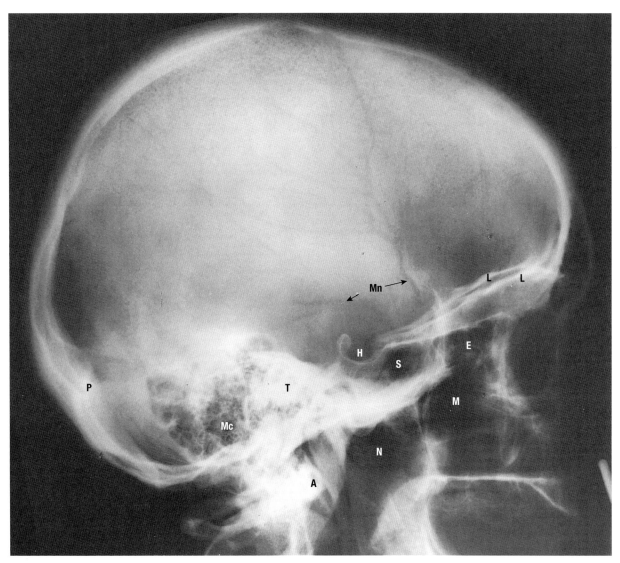

B. Lateral View

7.7   RADIOGRAPHS OF THE CRANIUM *(CONTINUED)*

B. Lateral radiograph of the cranium. Most of the relatively thin bone of the facial skeleton (viscerocranium) is radiolucent (appears *black*).

- The labeled features include the ethmoidal cells (*E*), sphenoidal (*S*) and maxillary (*M*) sinuses, the hypophysial fossa (*H*) for the pituitary gland, the petrous part of the temporal bone (*T*), mastoid cells (*Mc*), grooves for the branches of the middle meningeal vessels (*Mn*), anterior arch of the atlas (*A*), internal occipital protuberance (*P*), and the nasopharynx (*N*).
- The right and left orbital plates of the frontal bone are not superimposed; thus, the floor of the anterior cranial fossa appears as two lines (*L*).

A. Inferior View

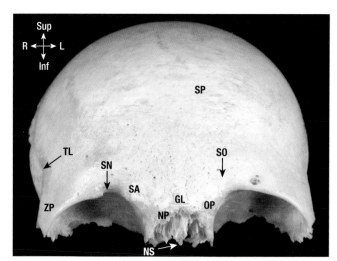

B. Anterior View

Key for A and B: Frontal Bone

EN	Ethmoidal notch	NP	Nasal part	SA	Superciliary arch	SU	Supra-orbital margin
FL	Fossa for lacrimal gland	NS	Nasal spine	SM	Sphenoidal margin	TL	Temporal line
FS	Opening of frontal sinus	OP	Orbital part	SN	Supra-orbital notch	TS	Temporal surface
GL	Glabella	RE	Root of ethmoid cells	SO	Supra-orbital foramen	ZP	Zygomatic process
				SP	Squamous part		

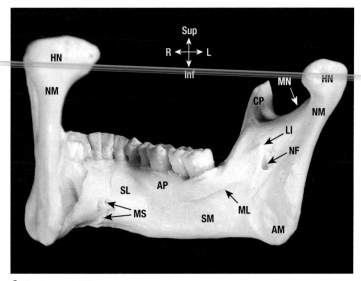

C. Posteromedial View

D. Lateral View

Key for C and D: Mandible

AM	Angle of mandible	ML	Mylohyoid groove	NM	Neck of mandible
AP	Alveolar part	MN	Mandibular notch	PF	Pterygoid fovea
CP	Coronoid process	MS	Mental (genial) spines	RM	Ramus of mandible
HM	Head of mandible	MT	Mental foramen	SL	Sublingual fossa
LI	Lingula	NF	Mandibular foramen	SM	Submandibular fossa

7.8 MANDIBLE, MAXILLA, FRONTAL, ETHMOID, AND LACRIMAL BONES

A. and B. Frontal bone. **C. and D.** Mandible.

E. Anterior View

F. Posterior View

G. Superior View

H. Anterior View

Key for H: Palatine Bone

HP	Horizontal plate	PP	Perpendicular plate
NC	Nasal crest	PY	Pyramidal process
OP	Orbital process		

I. Lateral View

Key for I: Maxilla and Nasal Bone

AN	Anterior nasal spine	LG	Lacrimal groove
AP	Alveolar part	NB	Nasal bone
AS	Anterior surface	OS	Orbital surface
FP	Frontal process	TM	Tuberosity
IT	Infratemporal surface	ZP	Zygomatic process

Key for E-G: Ethmoid Bone

AC	Ala of crista galli	EB	Ethmoidal bulla	OP	Orbital plate
CG	Crista galli	EL	Ethmoidal labyrinth (cells)	PP	Perpendicular plate
CP	Cribriform plate	MC	Middle nasal concha	SC	Superior nasal concha

7.8

MANDIBLE, MAXILLA, FRONTAL, ETHMOID, AND LACRIMAL BONES *(CONTINUED)*

E.–G. Ethmoid bone. **H.** Lacrimal bone. **I.** Maxilla

A. Lateral Wall of Nose, Medial View

Key for A: Lateral Wall of Nose

CO	Choana (posterior nasal aperture)
HP	Horizontal plate of palatine bone
IC	Inferior nasal concha
IS	Incisive canal
IM	Inferior nasal meatus
MC	Middle nasal concha
MM	Middle nasal meatus
PH	Pterygoid hamulus
PM	Palatine process of maxilla
OS	Orbital surface of frontal bone
PA	Piriform aperture
PM	Palatine process of maxilla
SC	Superior nasal concha
SE	Spheno-ethmoidal recess
SF	Sphenopalatine foramen
SM	Superior nasal meatus
SS	Sphenoidal sinus

B. Infratemporal Region, Inferolateral View

Key for B: Infratemporal Region

PF	Pterygopalatine fossa
MF	Mandibular fossa
AT	Articular tubercle
ZPT	Zygomatic process of temporal bone
CC	Carotid canal
FL	Foramen lacerum
ZF	Zygomaticofacial foramen
PQ	Petrosquamous fissure
TG	Tegmen tympani
TT	Temporal bone (tympanic part)
ZB	Zygomatic bone
MX	Maxilla
IOF	Inferior orbital fissure
PMF	Pterygomaxillary fissure
ZPM	Zygomatic process of maxilla
EM	External acoustic meatus
GW	Greater wing of sphenoid
LP	Lateral pterygoid plate
MP	Medial pterygoid plate
SY	Stylomastoid foramen

7.9 LATERAL WALL OF NOSE AND INFRATEMPORAL REGION

A. Lateral wall of nose. **B.** Infratemporal region.

A. Lateral View

B. Medial View

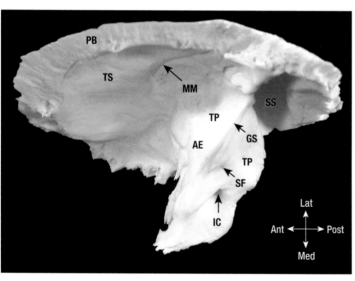

C. Superior View

D. Inferior View

Key for A-D: Temporal Bone

AE	Arcuate eminence	MF	Mandibular fossa	SM	Sphenoid margin
AT	Articular tubercle	MM	Groove for middle meningeal artery	SP	Styloid process
CC	Carotid canal	MN	Mastoid notch	SS	Groove for sigmoid sinus
CO	Cochlear canaliculus	MP	Mastoid process	SY	Stylomastoid foramen
EM	External acoustic meatus	OB	Occipital border	TC	Tympanic canaliculus
GM	Groove for middle temporal artery	PB	Parietal border	TP	Temporal bone (petrous part)
GP	Hiatus for greater petrosal nerve	PN	Parietal notch	TS	Temporal bone (squamous part)
GS	Groove for superior petrosal sinus	PT	Petrotympanic fissure	TT	Temporal bone (tympanic part)
IC	Internal acoustic meatus	SC	Supramastoid crest	VC	Vestibular canaliculus
JF	Jugular fossa	SF	Subarcuate fossa	ZP	Zygomatic process

A. Posterior View

B. Anterior View

Key for A-D: Sphenoid Bone

AC	Anterior clinoid process	FO	Foramen ovale	GWO	Greater wing (orbital surface)
CG	Carotid sulcus	FR	Foramen rotundum	GWT	Greater wing (temporal surface)
CS	Prechiasmatic sulcus	FS	Foramen spinosum	H	Hypophysial fossa
DS	Dorsum sellae	GWC	Greater wing (cerebral surface)	LP	Lateral pterygoid plate
ES	Ethmoidal spine	GWI	Greater wing (infratemporal surface)	LW	Lesser wing

C. Superior View

D. Inferior View

Key for A-D: Sphenoid Bone (Continued)

MP	Medial pterygoid plate	PL	Posterior clinoid process	SP	Spine of sphenoid bone
OC	Optic canal	PN	Pterygoid notch	SS	Sphenoidal sinus (in body of sphenoid)
PC	Pterygoid canal	PP	Pterygoid process	TS	Tuberculum sellae
PF	Pterygoid fossa	SC	Scaphoid fossa	VP	Vaginal process
PH	Pterygoid hamulus	SF	Superior orbital fissure		

7.11 SPHENOID BONE *(CONTINUED)*

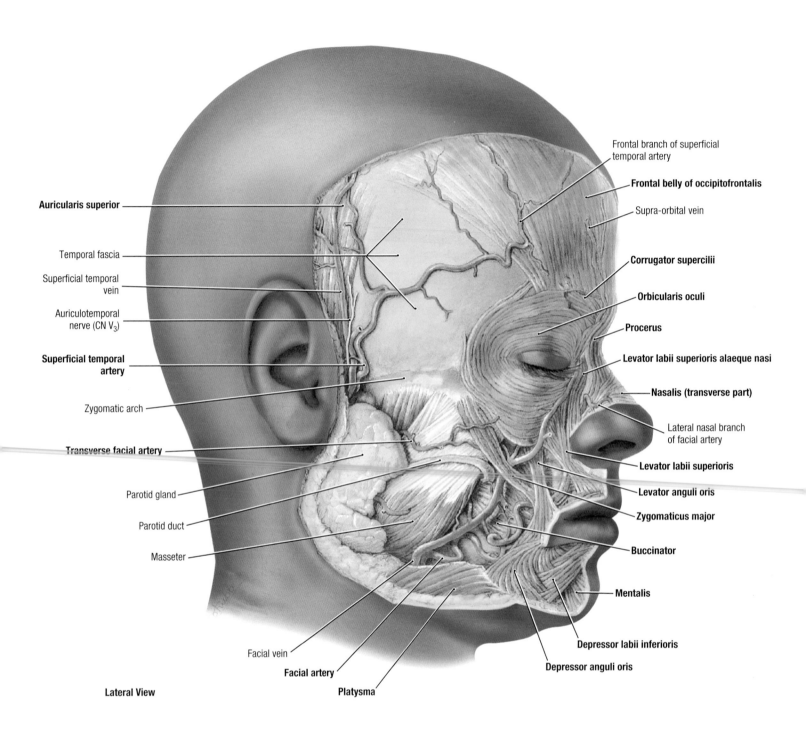

Auricularis superior

Temporal fascia

Superficial temporal vein

Auriculotemporal nerve (CN V₃)

Superficial temporal artery

Zygomatic arch

Transverse facial artery

Parotid gland

Parotid duct

Masseter

Facial vein

Facial artery

Platysma

Lateral View

Frontal branch of superficial temporal artery

Frontal belly of occipitofrontalis

Supra-orbital vein

Corrugator supercilii

Orbicularis oculi

Procerus

Levator labii superioris alaeque nasi

Nasalis (transverse part)

Lateral nasal branch of facial artery

Levator labii superioris

Levator anguli oris

Zygomaticus major

Buccinator

Mentalis

Depressor labii inferioris

Depressor anguli oris

| 7.12 | MUSCLES OF FACIAL EXPRESSION AND ARTERIES OF THE FACE |

- The muscles of facial expression are the superficial sphincters and dilators of the openings of the head; all are supplied by the facial nerve (CN VII). The masseter and temporalis (the latter covered here by temporal fascia) are muscles of mastication that are innervated by the trigeminal nerve (CN V).
- **Superficial temporal and facial artery pulses.** Anesthesiologists, usually stationed at the head of the operating table, take these pulses. The superficial temporal pulse is palpated anterior to the auricle as the artery crosses the zygomatic arch. The facial pulse is palpated where the facial artery crosses the inferior border of the mandible immediately anterior to the masseter.

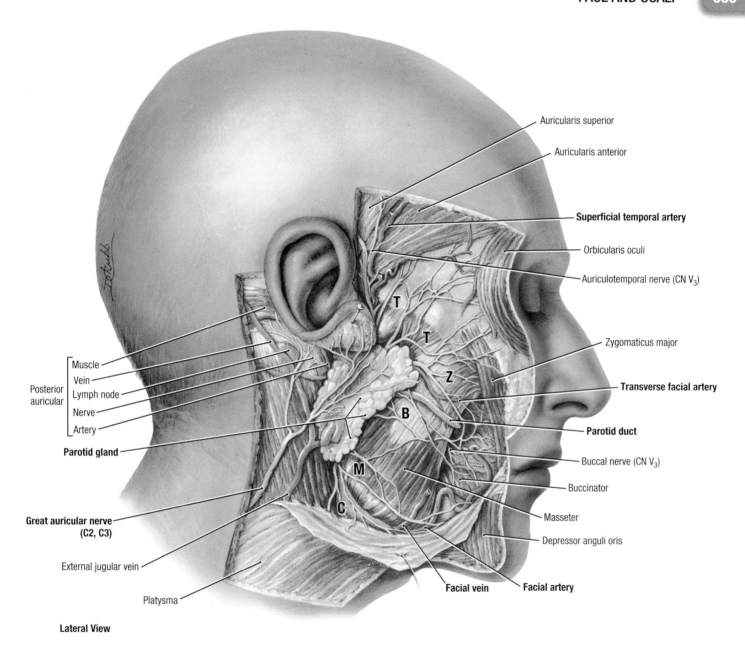

Auricularis superior

Auricularis anterior

Superficial temporal artery

Orbicularis oculi

Auriculotemporal nerve (CN V₃)

Zygomaticus major

Transverse facial artery

Parotid duct

Buccal nerve (CN V₃)

Buccinator

Masseter

Depressor anguli oris

Facial vein   Facial artery

Posterior auricular
- Muscle
- Vein
- Lymph node
- Nerve
- Artery

Parotid gland

Great auricular nerve (C2, C3)

External jugular vein

Platysma

Lateral View

| | | |

<table></table>

7.13 RELATIONSHIPS OF BRANCHES OF FACIAL NERVE AND VESSELS TO THE PAROTID GLAND AND DUCT

- The parotid duct extends across the masseter muscle just inferior to the zygomatic arch; the duct turns medially to pierce the buccinator and opens into the oral vestibule.
- The facial nerve (CN VII) innervates the muscles of facial expression. After emerging from the stylomastoid foramen, the main stem of the facial nerve has posterior auricular, digastric, and stylohyoid branches; the parotid plexus gives rise to temporal (T), zygomatic (Z), buccal (B), marginal mandibular (M), cervical (C), and posterior auricular branches. These branches form a plexus within the parotid gland, the branches of which radiate over the face, anastomosing with each other and the branches of the trigeminal nerve.
- During **parotidectomy** (surgical excision of the parotid gland), identification, dissection, and preservation of the branches of the facial nerve are critical.
- The parotid gland may become infected by infectious agents that pass through the bloodstream, as occurs in mumps, an acute communicable viral disease. Infection of the gland causes inflammation, **parotiditis**, and swelling of the gland. Severe pain occurs because the parotid sheath, innervated by the great auricular nerve, is distended by swelling.

Nose (N)

A   B   C

Occipitofrontalis

Corrugator supercilii

Procerus + transverse part of nasalis

Orbicularis oculi

Lev. labii sup. alaeque nasi + alar part of nasalis

Buccinator + orbicularis oris

Zygomaticus major + minor

Risorius

Risorius + depressor labii inferioris

Levator labii sup. + depressor labii

Dilators of mouth:
Risorious plus levator labii superioris
+ depressor labii inferioris

Orbicularis oris

Depressor anguli oris

Mentalis

Platysma

D

Anterior Views

| 7.14 | MUSCLES OF FACIAL EXPRESSION |

A. Orbicularis oculi: palpebral (P) and orbital (O) parts. Eyelids close lateral to medial washing lacrimal fluid across the cornea. **B.** Gentle closure of eyelid—palpebral part. **C.** Tight closure of eyelid—orbital part. **D.** Actions of selected muscles of facial expression.

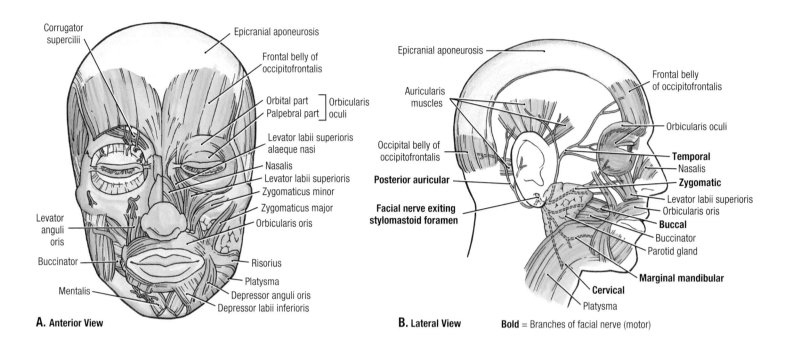

Corrugator supercilii
Epicranial aponeurosis
Frontal belly of occipitofrontalis
Orbital part | Orbicularis
Palpebral part | oculi
Levator labii superioris alaeque nasi
Nasalis
Levator labii superioris
Zygomaticus minor
Zygomaticus major
Orbicularis oris
Levator anguli oris
Buccinator
Risorius
Mentalis
Platysma
Depressor anguli oris
Depressor labii inferioris

A. Anterior View

Epicranial aponeurosis
Auricularis muscles
Occipital belly of occipitofrontalis
Posterior auricular
Facial nerve exiting stylomastoid foramen
Frontal belly of occipitofrontalis
Orbicularis oculi
Temporal
Nasalis
Zygomatic
Levator labii superioris
Orbicularis oris
Buccal
Buccinator
Parotid gland
Marginal mandibular
Cervical
Platysma

B. Lateral View

Bold = Branches of facial nerve (motor)

7.15   BRANCHES OF FACIAL NERVE AND MUSCLES OF FACIAL EXPRESSION

A. Muscles. **B.** Branches of facial nerve.

TABLE 7.2 MAIN MUSCLES OF FACIAL EXPRESSION [a]

Muscle[a]	Origin	Insertion	Action
Occipitofrontalis, frontal belly	Epicranial aponeurosis	Skin of and subcutaneous tissue of eyebrows and forehead	Elevates eyebrows and wrinkles skin of forehead; protracts scalp (indicating surprise or curiosity)
Occipitofrontalis, occipital belly	Lateral two-thirds of superior nuchal line	Epicranial aponeurosis	Retracts scalp; increasing effectiveness of frontal belly
Orbicularis oculi	Medial orbital margin, medial palpebral ligament; lacrimal bone	Skin around margin of orbit; superior and inferior tarsal plates	Closes eyelids; palpebral part does so gently; orbital part tightly (winking)
Orbicularis oris	Medial maxilla and mandible; deep surface of perioral skin; angle of mouth (modiolus)	Mucous membrane of lips	Tonus closes oral fissure; phasic contraction compresses and protrudes lips (kissing) or resists distension (when blowing)
Levator labii superioris	Infra-orbital margin (maxilla)	Skin of upper lip	Part of dilators of mouth; retract (elevate) and/or evert upper lip; deepen nasolabial sulcus (showing sadness)
Zygomaticus minor	Anterior aspect, zygomatic bone		
Buccinator	Mandible, alveolar processes of maxilla and mandible; pterygomandibular raphe	Angle of mouth (modiolus); orbicularis oris	Presses cheek against molar teeth; works with tongue to keep food between occlusal surfaces and out of oral vestibule; resists distension (when blowing)
Zygomaticus major	Lateral aspect of zygomatic bone	Angle of mouth (modiolus)	Part of dilators of mouth; elevate labial commissure—bilaterally to smile (happiness); unilaterally to sneer (disdain)
Rizorius	Parotid fascia and buccal skin (highly variable)		Part of dilators of mouth; widens oral fissure
Platysma	Subcutaneous tissue of infraclavicular and supraclavicular regions	Base of mandible; skin of cheek and lower lip; angle of mouth (modiolus); orbicularis oris	Depresses mandible (against resistance); tenses skin of inferior face and neck (conveying tension and stress)

[a]All of these muscles are supplied by the facial nerve (CN VII).

Supratrochlear nerve (CN V₁)
Supra-orbital nerve (CN V₁)
Orbital septum
Lacrimal nerve (CN V₁)
Superior tarsal plate
Inferior tarsal plate
Orbital septum
Zygomaticofacial nerve (CN V₂)
Infra-orbital nerve (CN V₂)
Parotid duct
Buccal nerve (CN V₃)
Buccinator
Platysma
Depressor anguli oris
Mental nerve (CN V₃)
Mentalis

Infratrochlear nerve (CN V₁)
Procerus
Corrugator supercilii
Frontal belly of occipitofrontalis
Medial palpebral ligament
Levator palpebrae superioris
Lacrimal gland
Lateral palpebral ligament
Levator labii superioris alaeque nasi
Levator labii superioris
Zygomaticus minor
Levator anguli oris
Buccal fat pad
Orbicularis oris
Masseter
Depressor anguli oris reflected

Anterior View

7.16 | CUTANEOUS BRANCHES OF TRIGEMINAL NERVE, MUSCLES OF FACIAL EXPRESSION, AND EYELID

Injury to the facial nerve (CN VII) or its branches produces paralysis of some or all of the facial muscles on the affected side (Bell palsy). The affected area sags, and facial expression is distorted. The loss of tonus of the orbicularis oculi causes the inferior lid to evert (fall away from the surface of the eyeball). As a result, the lacrimal fluid is not spread over the cornea, preventing adequate lubrication, hydration, and flushing of the cornea. This makes the cornea vulnerable to ulceration. If the injury weakens or paralyzes the buccinator and orbicularis oris, food will accumulate in the oral vestibule during chewing, usually requiring continual removal with a finger. When the sphincters or dilators of the mouth are affected, displacement of the mouth (drooping of the corner) is produced by gravity and contraction of unopposed contralateral facial muscles, resulting in food and saliva dribbling out of the side of the mouth. Weakened lip muscles affect speech. Affected people cannot whistle or blow a wind instrument effectively. They frequently dab their eyes and mouth with a handkerchief to wipe the fluid (tears and saliva) that runs from the drooping lid and mouth.

Because the face does not have a distinct layer of deep fascia and the subcutaneous tissue is loose between the attachments of facial muscles, **facial lacerations** tend to gap (part widely). Consequently, the skin must be sutured carefully to prevent scarring. The looseness of the subcutaneous tissue also enables fluid and blood to accumulate in the loose connective tissue after **bruising of the face**.

A. Anterior view

B. Lateral View (Cervical plexus)

7.17 NERVES OF FACE AND SCALP

TABLE 7.3 NERVES OF FACE AND SCALP

Nerve	Origin	Course	Distribution
Frontal	Ophthalmic nerve (CN V_1)	Crosses orbit on superior aspect of levator palpebrae superioris; divides into supra-orbital and supratrochlear branches	Skin of forehead, scalp, superior eyelid, and nose; conjunctiva of superior lid and mucosa of frontal sinus
Supra-orbital	Continuation of frontal nerve (CN V_1)	Emerges through supra-orbital notch, or foramen, and breaks up into small branches	Mucous membrane of frontal sinus and conjunctiva (lining) of superior eyelid; skin of forehead as far as vertex
Supratrochlear	Frontal nerve (CN V_1)	Continues anteromedially along roof of orbit, passing lateral to trochlea	Skin in middle of forehead to hairline
Infratrochlear	Nasociliary nerve (CN V_1)	Follows medial wall of orbit passing inferior to trochlea to superior eyelid	Skin and conjunctiva (lining) of superior eye lid
Lacrimal	Ophthalmic nerve (CN V_1)	Passes through palpebral fascia of superior eyelid near lateral angle (canthus) of eye	Lacrimal gland and small area of skin and conjunctiva of lateral part of superior eyelid
External nasal	Anterior ethmoidal nerve (CN V_1)	Runs in nasal cavity and emerges on face between nasal bone and lateral nasal cartilage	Skin on dorsum of nose, including tip of nose
Zygomatic	Maxillary nerve (CN V_2)	Arises in floor of orbit, divides into zygomaticofacial and zygomaticotemporal nerves, which traverse foramina of same name	Skin over zygomatic arch and anterior temporal region
Infra-orbital	Terminal branch of maxillary nerve (CN V_2)	Runs in floor of orbit and emerges at infra-orbital foramen	Skin of cheek, inferior lid, lateral side of nose and inferior septum and superior lip, upper premolar incisors and canine teeth; mucosa of maxillary sinus and superior lip
Auriculotemporal	Mandibular nerve (CN V_3)	From posterior division of CN V_3, it passes between neck of mandible and external acoustic meatus to accompany superficial temporal artery	Skin anterior to ear and posterior temporal region, tragus and part of helix of auricle, and roof of external acoustic meatus and upper tympanic membrane
Buccal	Mandibular nerve (CN V_3)	From the anterior division of CN V_3 in infratemporal fossa, it passes anteriorly to reach cheek	Skin and mucosa of cheek, buccal gingiva adjacent to 2nd and 3rd molar teeth
Mental	Terminal branch of inferior alveolar nerve (CN V_3)	Emerges from mandibular canal at mental foramen	Skin of chin and inferior lip and mucosa of lower lip

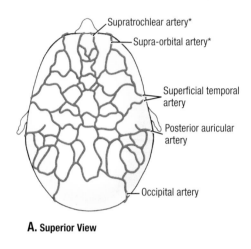

Supratrochlear artery*

Supra-orbital artery*

Superficial temporal artery

Posterior auricular artery

Occipital artery

A. Superior View

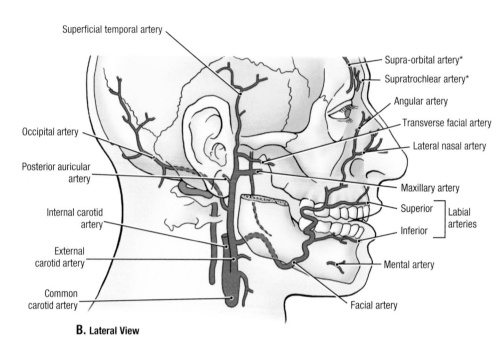

Superficial temporal artery

Occipital artery

Posterior auricular artery

Internal carotid artery

External carotid artery

Common carotid artery

Supra-orbital artery*

Supratrochlear artery*

Angular artery

Transverse facial artery

Lateral nasal artery

Maxillary artery

Superior | Labial
Inferior | arteries

Mental artery

Facial artery

B. Lateral View

*Source= internal carotid artery (ophthalmic artery); all other labeled arteries are from external carotid

7.18   ARTERIES OF FACE AND SCALP

TABLE 7.4 ARTERIES OF SUPERFICIAL FACE AND SCALP

Artery	Origin	Course	Distribution
Facial	External carotid artery	Ascends deep to submandibular gland, winds around inferior border of mandible and enters face	Muscles of facial expression and face
Inferior labial	Facial artery near angle of mouth	Runs medially in lower lip	Lower lip and chin
Superior labial		Runs medially in upper lip	Upper lip and ala (side) and septum of nose
Lateral nasal	Facial artery as it ascends alongside nose	Passes to ala of nose	Skin on ala and dorsum of nose
Angular	Terminal branch of facial artery	Passes to medial angle (canthus) of eye	Superior part of cheek and lower eyelid
Occipital	External carotid artery	Passes medial to posterior belly of digastric and mastoid process; accompanies occipital nerve in occipital region	Scalp of back of head, as far as vertex
Posterior auricular		Passes posteriorly, deep to parotid, along styloid process between mastoid and ear	Scalp posterior to auricle and auricle
Superficial temporal	Smaller terminal branch of external carotid artery	Ascends anterior to ear to temporal region and ends in scalp	Facial muscles and skin of frontal and temporal regions
Transverse facial	Superficial temporal artery within parotid gland	Crosses face superficial to masseter and inferior to zygomatic arch	Parotid gland and duct, muscles and skin of face
Mental	Terminal branch of inferior alveolar artery	Emerges from mental foramen and passes to chin	Facial muscles and skin of chin
***Supra-orbital**	Terminal branch of ophthalmic artery, a branch of internal carotid	Passes superiorly from supra-orbital foramen	Muscles and skin of forehead and scalp
***Supratrochlear**		Passes superiorly from supratrochlear notch	Muscles and skin of scalp

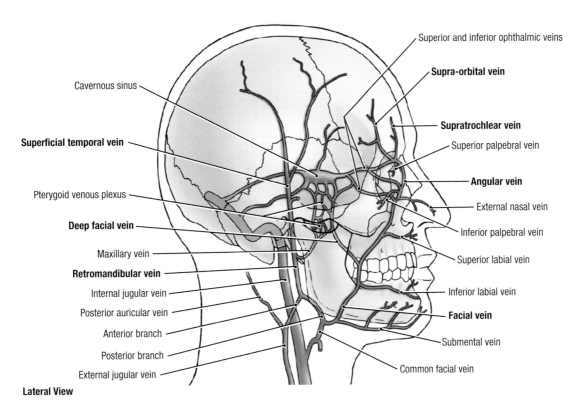

Superior and inferior ophthalmic veins

Supra-orbital vein

Supratrochlear vein

Superior palpebral vein

Angular vein

External nasal vein

Inferior palpebral vein

Superior labial vein

Inferior labial vein

Facial vein

Submental vein

Common facial vein

Cavernous sinus

Superficial temporal vein

Pterygoid venous plexus

Deep facial vein

Maxillary vein

Retromandibular vein

Internal jugular vein

Posterior auricular vein

Anterior branch

Posterior branch

External jugular vein

Lateral View

7.19   VEINS OF FACE

TABLE 7.5 VEINS OF FACE

Vein	Origin	Course	Termination	Area Drained
Supratrochlear	Begins from a venous plexus on the forehead and scalp, through which it communicates with the frontal branch of the superficial temporal vein, its contra-lateral partner, and the supra-orbital vein	Descends near the midline of the forehead to the root of the nose where it joins the supra-orbital vein	Angular vein at the root of the nose	Anterior part of scalp and forehead
Supra-orbital	Begins in the forehead by anastomosing with a frontal tributary of the superficial temporal vein	Passes medially superior to the orbit and joins the supratrochlear vein; a branch passes through the supra-orbital notch and joins with the superior ophthalmic vein		
Angular	Begins at root of nose by union of supra-trochlear and supra-orbital veins	Descends obliquely along the root and side of the nose to the inferior margin of the orbit	Becomes the facial vein at the inferior margin of the orbit	In addition to above, drains upper and lower lids and conjunctiva; may receive drainage from cavernous sinus
Facial	Continuation of angular vein past inferior margin of orbit	Descends along lateral border of the nose, receiving external nasal and inferior palpebral veins, then obliquely across face to mandible; receives anterior division of retromandibular vein, after which it is sometimes called the common facial vein	Internal jugular vein at or inferior to the level of the hyoid bone	Anterior scalp and forehead, eyelids, external nose, and anterior cheek, lips, chin, and submandibular gland
Deep facial	Pterygoid venous plexus	Runs anteriorly on maxilla above buccinator and deep to masseter, emerging medial to anterior border of masseter onto face	Enters posterior aspect of facial vein	Infratemporal fossa (most areas supplied by maxillary artery)
Superficial temporal	Begins from a widespread plexus of veins on the side of the scalp and along the zygomatic arch	Its frontal and parietal tributaries unite anterior to the auricle; it crosses the temporal root of the zygomatic arch to pass from the temporal region and enters the substance of the parotid gland	Joins the maxillary vein posterior to the neck of the mandible to form the retromandibular vein	Side of the scalp, superficial aspect of the temporal muscle, and external ear
Retromandibular	Formed anterior to the ear by the union of the superficial temporal and maxillary veins	Runs posterior and deep to the ramus of the mandible through the substance of the parotid gland; communicates at its inferior end with the facial vein	*Anterior branch* unites with facial vein to form common facial vein; *posterior branch* unites with the posterior auricular vein to form the external jugular vein	Parotid gland and masseter muscle

A. Superolateral view

B.

C. Superior View

D. Lateral View

A. Layers of scalp. **B.** Occipitofrontalis and temporal muscles and fascia. **C.** Sensory nerves and arteries of the scalp. **D.** Diploic veins. The outer layer of the compact bone of the cranium has been filed away, exposing the channels for the diploic veins in the cancellous bone that composes the diploë (see Fig. 7.7).

Scalp injuries and infections. The loose areolar tissue layer is the danger area of the scalp because pus or blood spreads easily in it. Infection in this layer can pass into the cranial cavity through emissary veins, which pass through parietal foramina in the calvaria and reach intracranial structures such as the meninges. An infection cannot pass into the neck because the occipital belly of the occipitofrontalis attaches to the occipital bone and mastoid parts of the temporal bones. Neither can a scalp infection spread laterally beyond the zygomatic arches because the epicranial aponeurosis is continuous with the temporalis fascia that attaches to these arches. An infection or fluid (e.g., pus or blood) can enter the eyelids and the root of the nose because the frontal belly of the occipitofrontalis inserts into the skin and dense subcutaneous tissue and does not attach to the bone. **Ecchymoses**, or purple patches, develop as a result of extravasation of blood into the subcutaneous tissue and skin of the eyelids and surrounding regions.

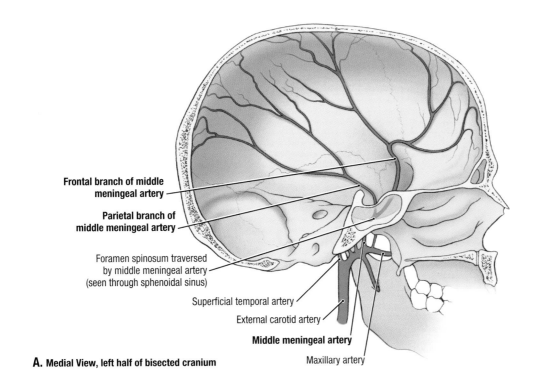

Frontal branch of middle meningeal artery

Parietal branch of middle meningeal artery

Foramen spinosum traversed by middle meningeal artery (seen through sphenoidal sinus)

Superficial temporal artery

External carotid artery

Middle meningeal artery

Maxillary artery

A. Medial View, left half of bisected cranium

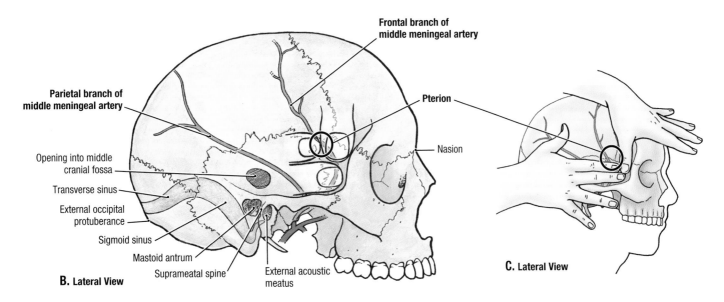

Frontal branch of middle meningeal artery

Parietal branch of middle meningeal artery

Opening into middle cranial fossa

Transverse sinus

External occipital protuberance

Sigmoid sinus

Mastoid antrum

Suprameatal spine

External acoustic meatus

B. Lateral View

Pterion

Nasion

C. Lateral View

7.21   MIDDLE MENINGEAL ARTERY AND PTERION

A. Course of the middle meningeal artery in the cranium. **B.** Surface projections of internal features of the neurocranium. **C.** Locating the pterion. The pterion is located two fingers breadth superior to the zygomatic arch and one thumb breadth posterior to the frontal process of the zygomatic bone (approximately 4 cm superior to the midpoint of the zygomatic arch); the anterior branch of the middle meningeal artery crosses the pterion.

A hard blow to the side of the head may fracture the thin bones forming the pterion, rupturing the anterior branch of the middle meningeal artery crossing the pterion. The resulting **extradural (epidural) hematoma** exerts pressure on the underlying cerebral cortex. Untreated middle meningeal artery hemorrhage may cause death in a few hours.

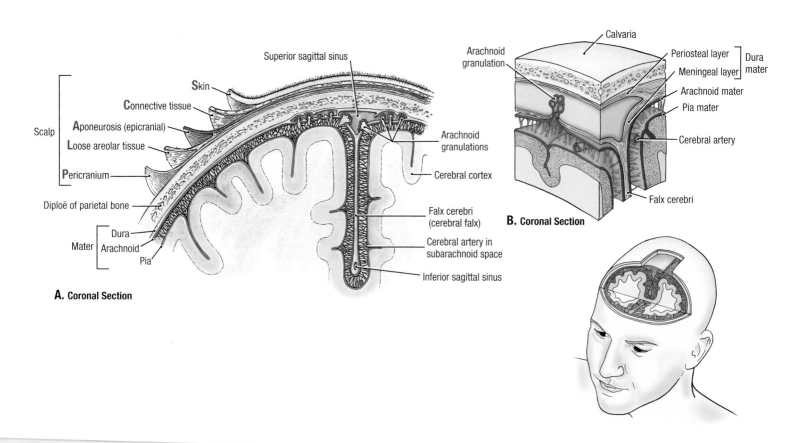

A. Coronal Section

B. Coronal Section

C. Coronal Section

D. Coronal Section

E. Coronal Section

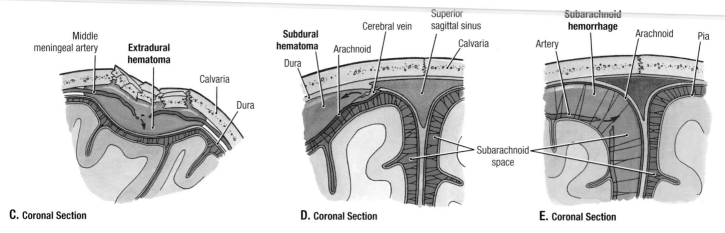

7.22   LAYERS OF THE SCALP AND MENINGES

A. Scalp, cranium, and meninges. **B.** Meninges and their relationship to the calvaria. The three meningeal spaces include the extradural (epidural) space between the cranial bones and dura, which is a potential space normally (it becomes a real space pathologically if blood accumulates in it); the similarly potential subdural space between the dura and arachnoid; and the subarachnoid space, the normal realized space between the arachnoid and pia, which contains cerebrospinal fluid (CSF). **C. Extradural (epidural) hematomas** result from bleeding from a torn middle meningeal artery. **D. Subdural hematomas** commonly result from tearing of a cerebral vein as it enters the superior sagittal sinus. **E. Subarachnoid hemorrhage** results from bleeding within the subarachnoid space, e.g., from rupture of an aneurysm.

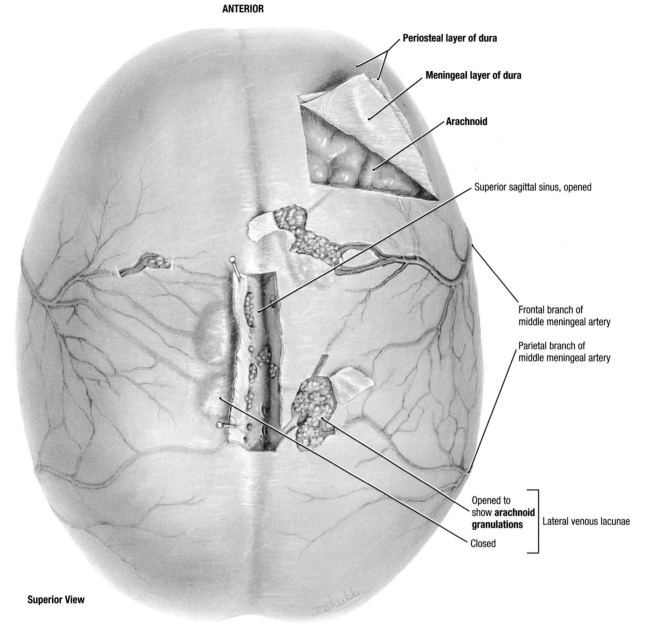

ANTERIOR

Periosteal layer of dura

Meningeal layer of dura

Arachnoid

Superior sagittal sinus, opened

Frontal branch of
middle meningeal artery

Parietal branch of
middle meningeal artery

Opened to
show **arachnoid
granulations**   Lateral venous lacunae

Closed

Superior View

POSTERIOR

7.23   DURA MATER AND ARACHNOID GRANULATIONS

- The calvaria is removed. In the median plane, the thick roof of the superior sagittal sinus is partly pinned aside, and laterally, the thin roofs of two lateral lacunae are reflected.
- The middle meningeal artery lies in a venous channel (middle meningeal vein), which enlarges superiorly into a lateral lacunae. Other channels drain the lateral lacunae into the superior sagittal sinus.
- Arachnoid granulations in the lacunae are responsible for absorption of CSF from the subarachnoid space into the venous system.
- The dura is sensitive to pain, especially where it is related to the dural venous sinuses and meningeal arteries. Although the causes of **headache** are numerous, distention of the scalp or meningeal vessels (or both) is believed to be one cause of headache. Many headaches appear to be dural in origin, such as the headache occurring after a lumbar spinal puncture for removal of CSF. These headaches are thought to result from stimulation of sensory nerve endings in the dura.

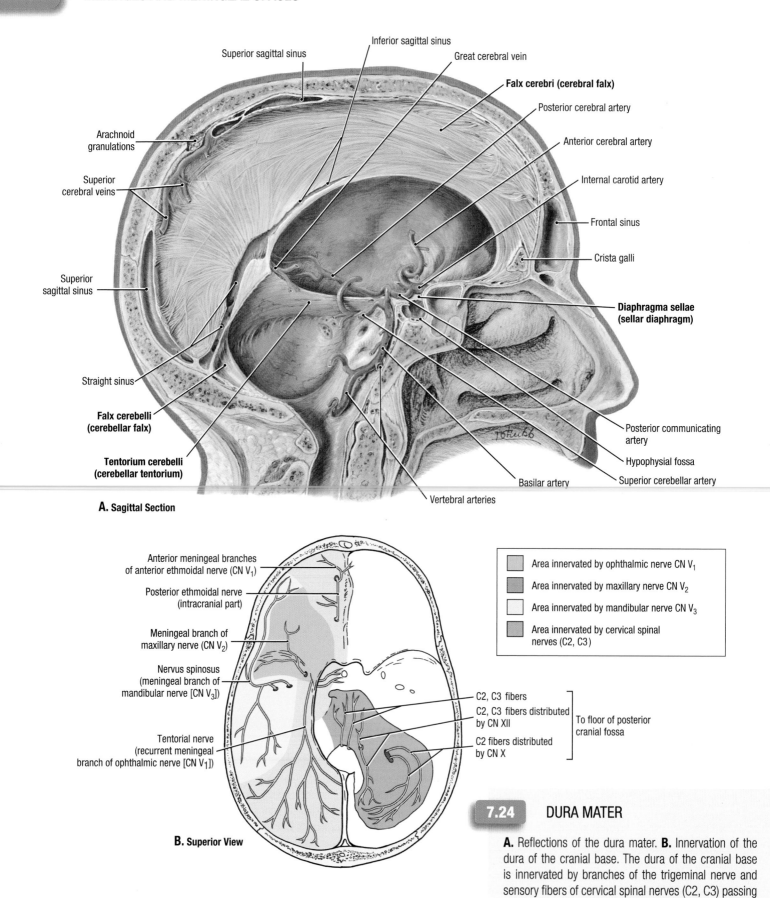

Superior sagittal sinus

Inferior sagittal sinus

Great cerebral vein

Falx cerebri (cerebral falx)

Posterior cerebral artery

Anterior cerebral artery

Internal carotid artery

Frontal sinus

Crista galli

Diaphragma sellae (sellar diaphragm)

Arachnoid granulations

Superior cerebral veins

Superior sagittal sinus

Straight sinus

Falx cerebelli (cerebellar falx)

Tentorium cerebelli (cerebellar tentorium)

Posterior communicating artery

Hypophysial fossa

Basilar artery

Superior cerebellar artery

Vertebral arteries

A. Sagittal Section

Anterior meningeal branches of anterior ethmoidal nerve (CN V$_1$)

Posterior ethmoidal nerve (intracranial part)

Meningeal branch of maxillary nerve (CN V$_2$)

Nervus spinosus (meningeal branch of mandibular nerve [CN V$_3$])

Tentorial nerve (recurrent meningeal branch of ophthalmic nerve [CN V$_1$])

Area innervated by ophthalmic nerve CN V$_1$

Area innervated by maxillary nerve CN V$_2$

Area innervated by mandibular nerve CN V$_3$

Area innervated by cervical spinal nerves (C2, C3)

C2, C3 fibers

C2, C3 fibers distributed by CN XII

C2 fibers distributed by CN X

To floor of posterior cranial fossa

B. Superior View

7.24 **DURA MATER**

A. Reflections of the dura mater. **B.** Innervation of the dura of the cranial base. The dura of the cranial base is innervated by branches of the trigeminal nerve and sensory fibers of cervical spinal nerves (C2, C3) passing directly from those nerves or via meningeal branches of the vagus (CN X) and hypoglossal (CN XII) nerves.

Superior sagittal sinus

Falx cerebri (cerebral falx)

Inferior sagittal sinus

Great cerebral vein

Straight sinus

Tentorium cerebelli
(cerebellar tentorium)

Transverse sinus

Superior petrosal sinus

Inferior petrosal sinus

Falx cerebelli (cerebellar falx)

Occipital sinus

Sigmoid sinus

Supra-orbital vein

Superior ophthalmic vein

Cavernous sinus

Inferior ophthalmic vein

Pterygoid venous plexus

Maxillary vein

Facial vein

Basilar venous plexus (sinus)

Internal vertebral venous plexus

A. Medial View

7.25   VENOUS SINUSES OF DURA MATER

A. Schematic of left half of cranial cavity and right facial skeleton. **B.** Venous sinuses of the cranial base.

- The superior sagittal sinus is at the superior border of the falx cerebri, and the inferior sagittal sinus is in its free border. The great cerebral vein joins the inferior sagittal sinus to form the straight sinus.

- The superior sagittal sinus usually becomes the right transverse sinus, which drains into the right sigmoid sinus, and next into the right internal jugular vein; the straight sinus similarly drains through the left transverse sinus, left sigmoid sinus, and left internal jugular vein.

- The cavernous sinus communicates with the veins of the face through the ophthalmic veins and pterygoid plexus of veins and with the sigmoid sinus through the superior and inferior petrosal sinuses.

- **Metastasis of tumor cells to dural sinuses.** The basilar and occipital sinuses communicate through the foramen magnum with the internal vertebral venous plexuses. Because these venous channels are valveless, increased intra-abdominopelvic or intrathoracic pressure, as occurs during heavy coughing and straining, may force venous blood from these regions into the internal vertebral venous system and from it into the dural venous sinuses. As a result, pus in abscesses and tumor cells in these regions may spread to the vertebrae and brain.

Superior ophthalmic vein

Sphenoparietal sinus

Cavernous sinus

Superior petrosal sinus

Inferior petrosal sinus

Sigmoid sinus

Straight sinus

Intercavernous sinus

Basilar venous plexus (sinus)

Great cerebral vein

Transition of sigmoid sinus into internal jugular vein

Tentorial notch

Tentorium cerebelli

Right transverse sinus

Inferior sagittal sinus

Superior sagittal sinus

B. Superior View

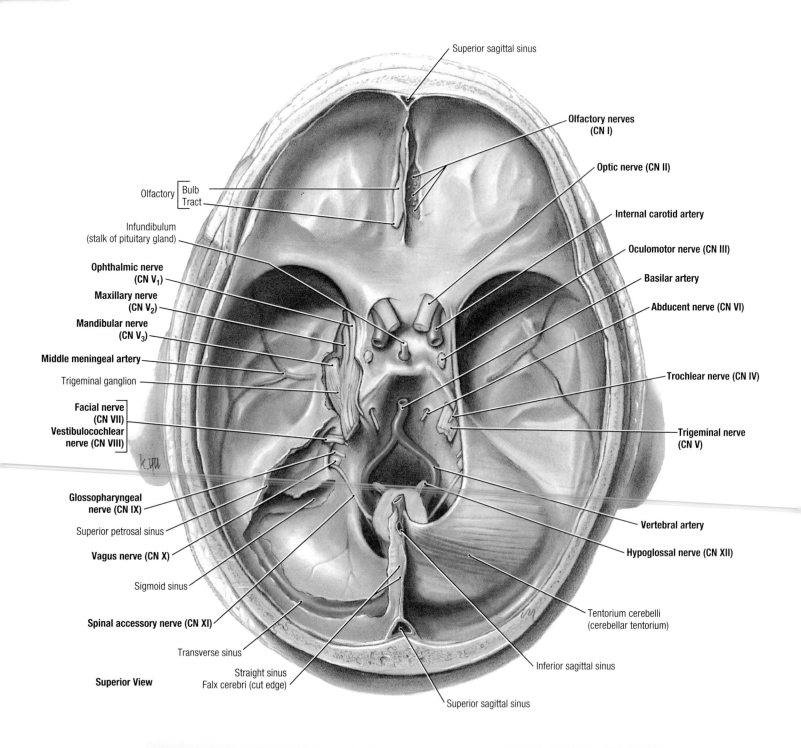

Superior sagittal sinus

Olfactory nerves
(CN I)

Optic nerve (CN II)

Olfactory [Bulb
Tract

Internal carotid artery

Infundibulum
(stalk of pituitary gland)

Oculomotor nerve (CN III)

**Ophthalmic nerve
(CN V₁)**

Basilar artery

Abducent nerve (CN VI)

**Maxillary nerve
(CN V₂)**

**Mandibular nerve
(CN V₃)**

Middle meningeal artery

Trigeminal ganglion

Trochlear nerve (CN IV)

**Facial nerve
(CN VII)**
**Vestibulocochlear
nerve (CN VIII)**

Trigeminal nerve
(CN V)

**Glossopharyngeal
nerve (CN IX)**

Superior petrosal sinus

Vertebral artery

Vagus nerve (CN X)

Hypoglossal nerve (CN XII)

Sigmoid sinus

Spinal accessory nerve (CN XI)

Tentorium cerebelli
(cerebellar tentorium)

Transverse sinus

Inferior sagittal sinus

Superior View

Straight sinus
Falx cerebri (cut edge)

Superior sagittal sinus

7.26   NERVES AND VESSELS OF THE INTERIOR OF THE BASE OF CRANIUM

- On the left of the specimen, the dura mater forming the roof of the trigeminal cave is cut away to expose the trigeminal ganglion and its three branches. The tentorium cerebelli is removed to reveal the transverse and superior petrosal sinuses.
- The frontal lobes of the cerebrum are located in the anterior cranial fossa, the temporal lobes in the middle cranial fossa, and the brainstem and cerebellum in the posterior cranial fossa; the occipital lobes rest on the tentorium cerebelli.
- The sites where the 12 cranial nerves and the internal carotid, vertebral, basilar, and middle meningeal arteries penetrate the dura mater are shown.

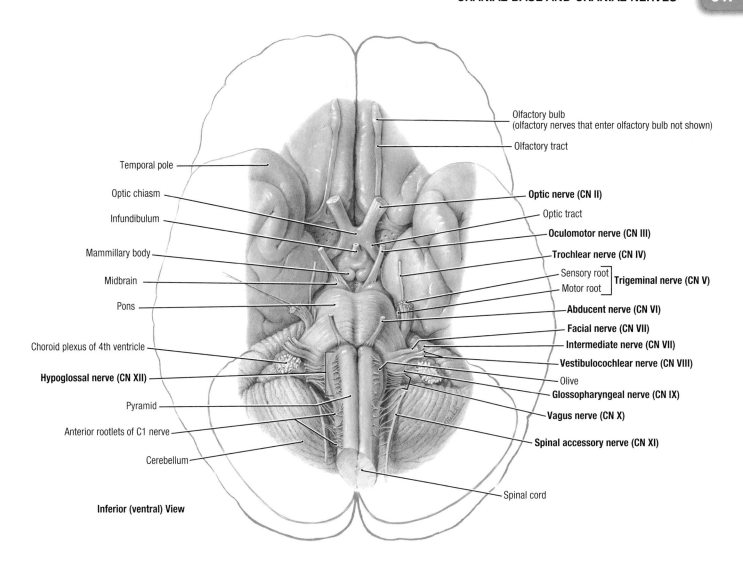

Olfactory bulb
(olfactory nerves that enter olfactory bulb not shown)

Olfactory tract

Temporal pole

Optic chiasm

Infundibulum

Mammillary body

Midbrain

Pons

Choroid plexus of 4th ventricle

Hypoglossal nerve (CN XII)

Pyramid

Anterior rootlets of C1 nerve

Cerebellum

Inferior (ventral) View

Optic nerve (CN II)

Optic tract

Oculomotor nerve (CN III)

Trochlear nerve (CN IV)

Sensory root ⎤
                  Trigeminal nerve (CN V)
Motor root ⎦

Abducent nerve (CN VI)

Facial nerve (CN VII)

Intermediate nerve (CN VII)

Vestibulocochlear nerve (CN VIII)

Olive

Glossopharyngeal nerve (CN IX)

Vagus nerve (CN X)

Spinal accessory nerve (CN XI)

Spinal cord

7.27   BASE OF BRAIN AND SUPERFICIAL ORIGINS OF CRANIAL NERVES

Foramina of skull and their associated cranial nerve(s) are listed below.

TABLE 7.6 *OPENINGS BY WHICH CRANIAL NERVES EXIT CRANIAL CAVITY*

Foramina/Apertures	Cranial nerve
Anterior cranial fossa	
Cribriform foramina in cribriform plate	Axons of olfactory cells in olfactory epithelium form olfactory nerves (CN I)
Middle cranial fossa	
Optic canal	Optic nerve (CN II)
Superior orbital fissure	Ophthalmic nerve (CN V₁), oculomotor nerve (CN III), trochlear nerve (CN IV), abducent nerve (CN VI) and branches of ophthalmic nerve (CN V₁)
Foramen rotundum	Maxillary nerve (CN V₂)
Foramen ovale	Mandibular nerve (CN V₃)
Posterior cranial fossa	
Foramen magnum	Spinal accessory nerve (CN XI)
Jugular foramen	Glossopharyngeal nerve (CN IX), vagus nerve (CN X), and spinal accessory nerve (CN XI)
Hypoglossal canal	Hypoglossal nerve (CN XII)

Inferior colliculus

Floor of
fourth ventricle

Trochlear nerve (CN IV)

**Facial nerve
(CN VII)**

Trigeminal nerve (CN V)

**Vestibulocochlear
nerve (CN VIII)**

**Glossopharyngeal
nerve (CN IX)**

**Vagus
nerve (CN X)**

**Spinal accessory
nerve (CN XI)**

Jugular process
of occipital bone

Atlanto-occipital
joint

Rectus capitis lateralis

Anterior ramus (C1)

**Posterior
ramus (C1)**

Transverse process
of atlas

Atlas

Intertransversarius

Atlanto-axial joint

Capsule of atlanto-axial joint

Vertebral artery

Anterior ramus

C2

Posterior ramus
(Greater occipital nerve)

Dura mater

Axis

Spinal ganglion of C2

A. Posterior View

7.28

POSTERIOR EXPOSURES OF CRANIAL NERVES

A. and B. Squamous part of occipital bone has been removed posterior to foramen magnum to reveal posterior cranial fossa. **A.** Brainstem in situ. **B.** Right side, with brainstem removed. The trochlear nerves (CN IV) arise from the dorsal aspect of the midbrain, just inferior to the inferior colliculi.

- The sensory and motor roots of the trigeminal nerves (CN V) pass anterolaterally to enter the mouth of the trigeminal cave.
- The facial (CN VII) and vestibulocochlear (CN VIII) nerves course laterally to enter the internal acoustic meatus.
- The glossopharyngeal nerve (CN IX) pierces the dura mater separately but passes with the vagus (CN X) and spinal accessory (CN XI) nerves through the jugular foramen.
- An **acoustic neuroma** (neurofibroma) is a slow-growing benign tumor of the neurolemma (Schwann) cells. The tumor begins in the vestibulocochlear nerve (CN VIII) while it is in the internal acoustic meatus. The early symptom of an acoustic neuroma is usually loss of hearing. Dysequilibrium and tinnitus also may occur.

Oculomotor nerve
(CN III)

Trochlear nerve (CN IV)

**Internal acoustic
meatus**

Cavernous sinus

Superior petrosal
sinus

**Trigeminal nerve
(CN V)**

Abducent nerve
(CN VI)

Inferior
petrosal sinus

**Glossopharyngeal (CN IX),
vagus (CN X) nerves**

**Spinal accessory
nerve (CN XI)**

Mastoid air
cells

Sigmoid sinus

B. Posterior View

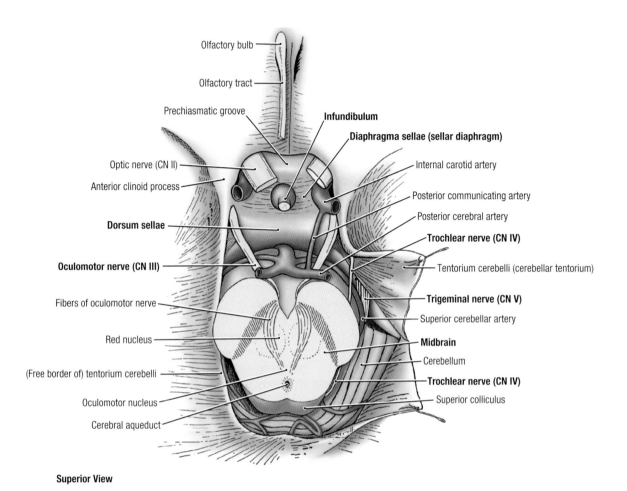

Olfactory bulb
Olfactory tract
Prechiasmatic groove
Infundibulum
Diaphragma sellae (sellar diaphragm)
Optic nerve (CN II)
Internal carotid artery
Anterior clinoid process
Posterior communicating artery
Posterior cerebral artery
Dorsum sellae
Trochlear nerve (CN IV)
Oculomotor nerve (CN III)
Tentorium cerebelli (cerebellar tentorium)
Fibers of oculomotor nerve
Trigeminal nerve (CN V)
Superior cerebellar artery
Red nucleus
Midbrain
Cerebellum
(Free border of) tentorium cerebelli
Trochlear nerve (CN IV)
Oculomotor nucleus
Superior colliculus
Cerebral aqueduct

Superior View

7.29   TENTORIAL NOTCH

- The brain has been removed by cutting through the midbrain, revealing the tentorial notch through which the brainstem extends from the posterior into the middle cranial fossa.
- On the right side of the specimen, the tentorium cerebelli is divided and reflected. The trochlear nerve (CN IV) passes around the midbrain under the free edge of the tentorium cerebelli; the roots of the trigeminal nerve (CN V) enter the mouth of the trigeminal cave.
- There is a circular opening in the diaphragma sellae for the infundibulum, the stalk of the pituitary gland.
- The oculomotor nerve (CN III) passes between the posterior cerebral and superior cerebellar arteries and then laterally around the posterior clinoid process.
- The tentorial notch is the opening in the tentorium cerebelli for the brainstem, which is slightly larger than is necessary to accommodate the midbrain. Hence, space-occupying lesions, such as tumors in the supratentorial compartment, produce increased intracranial pressure that may cause part of the adjacent temporal lobe of the brain to herniate through the tentorial notch. During **tentorial herniation**, the temporal lobe may be lacerated by the tough tentorium cerebelli, and the oculomotor nerve (CN III) may be stretched, compressed, or both. Oculomotor lesions may produce paralysis of the extrinsic eye muscles supplied by CN III.

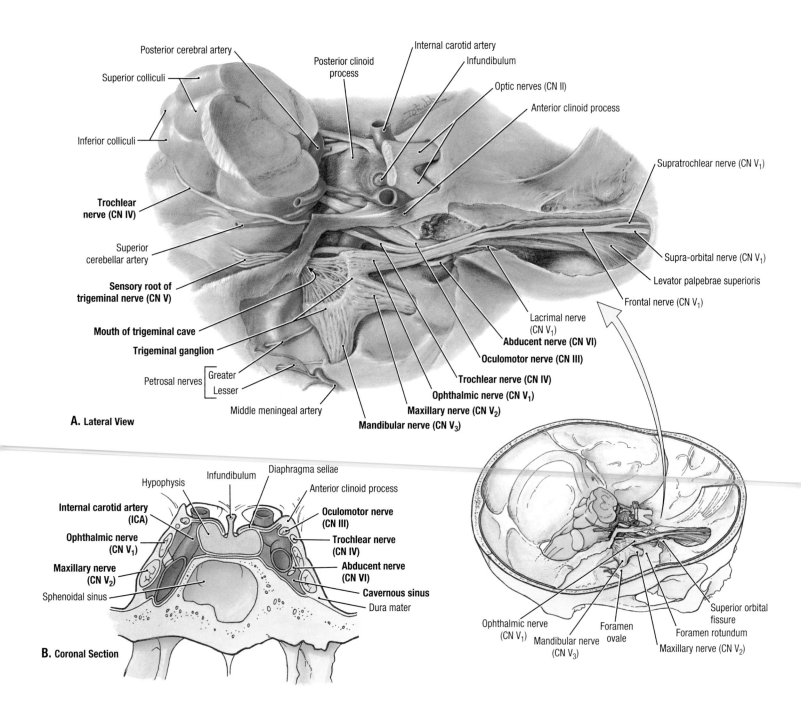

A. Lateral View

Posterior cerebral artery

Superior colliculi

Inferior colliculi

Posterior clinoid process

Internal carotid artery

Infundibulum

Optic nerves (CN II)

Anterior clinoid process

Supratrochlear nerve (CN V$_1$)

Supra-orbital nerve (CN V$_1$)

Levator palpebrae superioris

Frontal nerve (CN V$_1$)

Lacrimal nerve (CN V$_1$)

Abducent nerve (CN VI)

Oculomotor nerve (CN III)

Trochlear nerve (CN IV)

Ophthalmic nerve (CN V$_1$)

Maxillary nerve (CN V$_2$)

Mandibular nerve (CN V$_3$)

Middle meningeal artery

Petrosal nerves [Greater / Lesser]

Trigeminal ganglion

Mouth of trigeminal cave

Sensory root of trigeminal nerve (CN V)

Superior cerebellar artery

Trochlear nerve (CN IV)

B. Coronal Section

Hypophysis

Infundibulum

Diaphragma sellae

Anterior clinoid process

Internal carotid artery (ICA)

Ophthalmic nerve (CN V$_1$)

Maxillary nerve (CN V$_2$)

Sphenoidal sinus

Oculomotor nerve (CN III)

Trochlear nerve (CN IV)

Abducent nerve (CN VI)

Cavernous sinus

Dura mater

Ophthalmic nerve (CN V$_1$)

Mandibular nerve (CN V$_3$)

Foramen ovale

Superior orbital fissure

Foramen rotundum

Maxillary nerve (CN V$_2$)

7.30 NERVES AND VESSELS OF MIDDLE CRANIAL FOSSA I

A. Superficial dissection. The tentorium cerebelli is cut away. The dura mater is largely removed from the middle cranial fossa. The roof of the orbit is partly removed. **B.** Coronal section through the cavernous sinus.

In **fractures of the cranial base**, the internal carotid artery may be torn, producing an arteriovenous fistula within the cavernous sinus. Arterial blood rushes into the sinus, enlarging it and forcing retrograde blood flow into its venous tributaries, especially the ophthalmic veins. As a result, the eyeball protrudes (**exophthalmos**) and the conjunctiva becomes engorged (**chemosis**). Because CN III, CN IV, CN VI, CN V$_1$, and CN V$_2$ lie in or close to the lateral wall of the cavernous sinus, these nerves may also be affected.

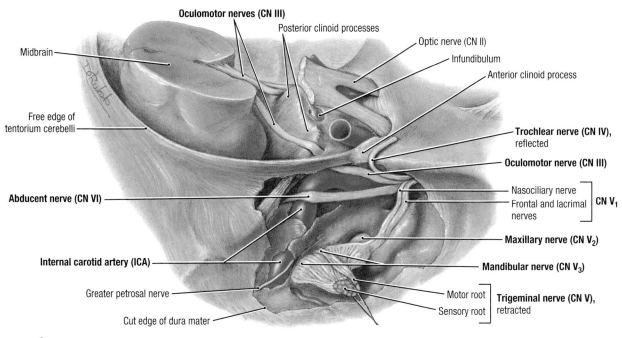

A. Lateral View

Oculomotor nerves (CN III)

Posterior clinoid processes

Optic nerve (CN II)

Infundibulum

Anterior clinoid process

Midbrain

Free edge of tentorium cerebelli

Trochlear nerve (CN IV), reflected

Oculomotor nerve (CN III)

Nasociliary nerve

Frontal and lacrimal nerves

CN V₁

Abducent nerve (CN VI)

Maxillary nerve (CN V₂)

Internal carotid artery (ICA)

Mandibular nerve (CN V₃)

Greater petrosal nerve

Motor root

Sensory root

Trigeminal nerve (CN V), retracted

Cut edge of dura mater

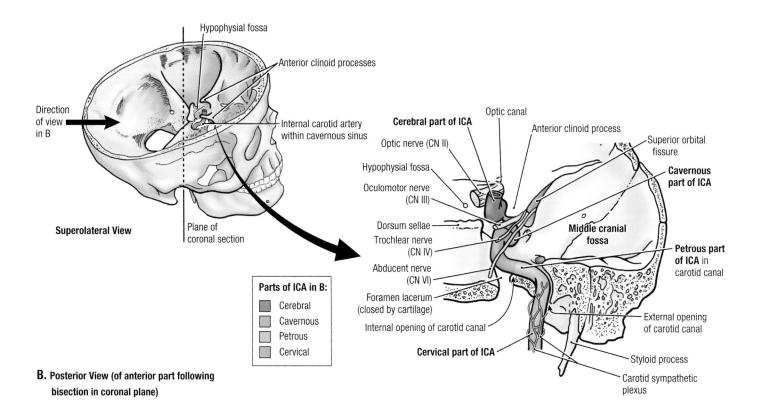

Hypophysial fossa

Anterior clinoid processes

Direction of view in B

Internal carotid artery within cavernous sinus

Superolateral View

Plane of coronal section

Optic canal

Cerebral part of ICA

Anterior clinoid process

Optic nerve (CN II)

Superior orbital fissure

Hypophysial fossa

Cavernous part of ICA

Oculomotor nerve (CN III)

Middle cranial fossa

Dorsum sellae

Trochlear nerve (CN IV)

Petrous part of ICA in carotid canal

Abducent nerve (CN VI)

Foramen lacerum (closed by cartilage)

Internal opening of carotid canal

External opening of carotid canal

Parts of ICA in B:

Cerebral

Cavernous

Petrous

Cervical

Cervical part of ICA

Styloid process

Carotid sympathetic plexus

B. Posterior View (of anterior part following bisection in coronal plane)

| 7.31 | **NERVES AND VESSELS OF MIDDLE CRANIAL FOSSA II** |

A. Deep dissection. The roots of the trigeminal nerve are divided, withdrawn from the mouth of the trigeminal cave, and turned anteriorly. The trochlear nerve is reflected anteriorly. **B.** Course of the internal carotid artery.

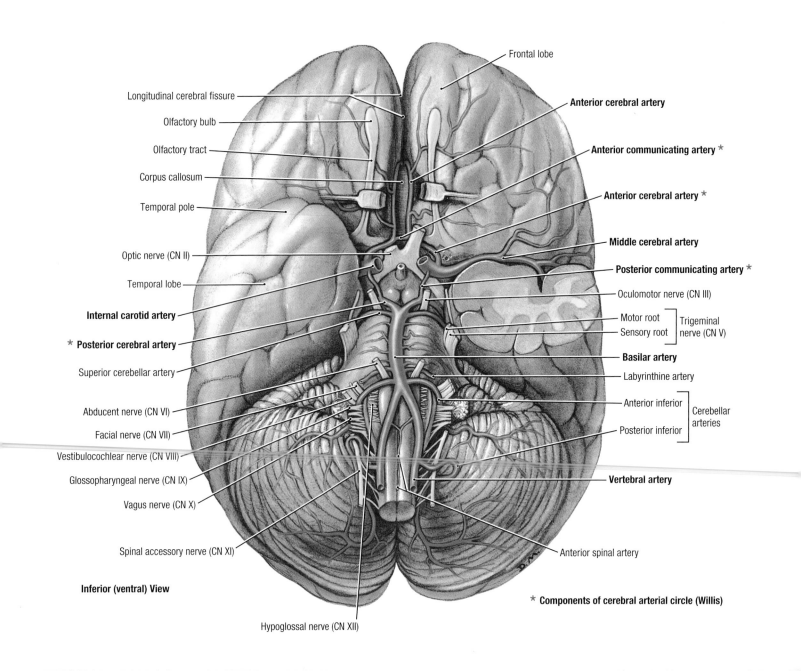

Longitudinal cerebral fissure

Olfactory bulb

Olfactory tract

Corpus callosum

Temporal pole

Optic nerve (CN II)

Temporal lobe

Internal carotid artery

* **Posterior cerebral artery**

Superior cerebellar artery

Abducent nerve (CN VI)

Facial nerve (CN VII)

Vestibulocochlear nerve (CN VIII)

Glossopharyngeal nerve (CN IX)

Vagus nerve (CN X)

Spinal accessory nerve (CN XI)

Inferior (ventral) View

Hypoglossal nerve (CN XII)

Frontal lobe

Anterior cerebral artery

Anterior communicating artery *

Anterior cerebral artery *

Middle cerebral artery

Posterior communicating artery *

Oculomotor nerve (CN III)

Motor root ⎤ Trigeminal
Sensory root ⎦ nerve (CN V)

Basilar artery

Labyrinthine artery

Anterior inferior ⎤ Cerebellar
Posterior inferior ⎦ arteries

Vertebral artery

Anterior spinal artery

* Components of cerebral arterial circle (Willis)

7.32 BASE OF BRAIN AND CEREBRAL ARTERIAL CIRCLE

The anterior part of the left temporal lobe is removed to enable visualization of the middle cerebral artery in the lateral fissure. The frontal lobes are separated to expose the anterior cerebral arteries and corpus callosum.

An **ischemic stroke** denotes the sudden development of neurological deficits that are consequences of impaired cerebral blood flow. The most common causes of strokes are spontaneous cerebrovascular accidents such as cerebral embolism, cerebral thrombosis, cerebral hemorrhage, and subarachnoid hemorrhage (Rowland, 2000). The cerebral arterial circle is an important means of collateral circulation in the event of gradual obstruction of one of the major arteries forming the circle. Sudden occlusion, even if only partial, results in neurological deficits. In elderly persons, the anastomoses are often inadequate when a large artery (e.g., internal carotid) is occluded, even if the occlusion is gradual. In such cases function is impaired at least to some degree.

Hemorrhagic stroke follows the rupture of an artery or a saccular aneurysm, a saclike dilation on a weak part of the arterial wall. The most common type of saccular aneurysm is a berry aneurysm, occurring in the vessels of or near the cerebral arterial circle. In time, especially in people with hypertension (high blood pressure), the weak part of the arterial wall expands and may rupture, allowing blood to enter the subarachnoid space.

A. Inferior (Ventral) View   * Components of cerebral arterial circle (Willis)

B. Lateral View

Blood is supplied to the cerebral hemispheres by the:
- Anterior cerebral artery
- Middle cerebral artery
- Posterior cerebral artery

C. Medial View

7.33   ARTERIES OF BRAIN

A. Schematic overview. **B and C.** Distribution of cerebral arteries.

TABLE 7.7 ARTERIAL SUPPLY TO BRAIN

Artery	Origin	Distribution
Vertebral	Subclavian artery	Cranial meninges and cerebellum
Posterior inferior cerebellar	Vertebral artery	Postero-inferior aspect of cerebellum
Basilar	Formed by junction of vertebral arteries	Brainstem, cerebellum, and cerebrum
Pontine		Numerous branches to brainstem
Anterior inferior cerebellar	Basilar artery	Inferior aspect of cerebellum
Superior cerebellar		Superior aspect of cerebellum
Internal carotid	Common carotid artery at superior border of thyroid cartilage	Gives branches in cavernous sinus and provides supply to brain
Anterior cerebral	Internal carotid artery	Cerebral hemispheres, except for occipital lobes
Middle cerebral	Continuation of the internal carotid artery distal to anterior cerebral artery	Most of lateral surface of cerebral hemispheres
Posterior cerebral	Terminal branch of basilar artery	Inferior aspect of cerebral hemisphere and occipital lobe
Anterior communicating	Anterior cerebral artery	Cerebral arterial circle
Posterior communicating	Internal carotid artery	

A. Postero-anterior View

B. Lateral View

C. Lateral View

Key for A, B and C:

A   Anterior cerebral artery
M   Middle cerebral artery
C   Internal carotid artery
0   Ophthalmic artery
1   Vertebral artery on posterior arch of atlas
2   Vertebral artery entering skull through foramen magnum
3   Posterior inferior cerebellar artery
4   Anterior inferior cerebellar artery
5   Basilar artery
6   Superior cerebellar artery
7   Posterior cerebellar artery
8   Posterior communicating artery

7.34   ARTERIOGRAMS

A. and B. Carotid arteriogram. The four *C*s indicate the parts of the internal carotid artery: cervical, before entering the cranium; petrous, within the temporal bone; cavernous, within the sinus; and cerebral, within the cranial subarachnoid space. **C.** Vertebral arteriogram. **Transient ischemic attacks (TIAs)** refer to neurological symptoms resulting from ischemia (deficient blood supply) of the brain. The symptoms of a TIA may be ambiguous: staggering, dizziness, light-headedness, fainting, and paresthesias (e.g., tingling in a limb). Most TIAs last a few minutes, but some persist longer. Individuals with TIAs are at increased risk for myocardial infarction and *ischemic stroke* (Brust, 2000).

A. Anterior View

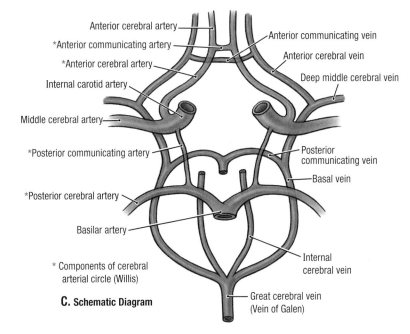

B. Anterior View

Anterior cerebral artery
*Anterior communicating artery
*Anterior cerebral artery
Internal carotid artery
Middle cerebral artery
*Posterior communicating artery
*Posterior cerebral artery
Basilar artery
* Components of cerebral arterial circle (Willis)

Anterior communicating vein
Anterior cerebral vein
Deep middle cerebral vein
Posterior communicating vein
Basal vein
Internal cerebral vein
Great cerebral vein (Vein of Galen)

C. Schematic Diagram

Key for A and B:

ACM	Anterior communicating artery	BT	Brachiocephalic trunk	LC	Left common carotid artery	PCM	Posterior communicating artery
ACA	Anterior cerebral artery	CS	Carotid siphon	LS	Left subclavian artery	RC	Right common carotid artery
AR	Arch of aorta	ECA	External carotid artery	MCA	Middle cerebral artery	RS	Right subclavian artery
BA	Basilar artery	ICA	Internal carotid artery	PCA	Posterior cerebral artery	VA	Vertebral artery

7.35 **BLOOD SUPPLY OF HEAD AND NECK**

A. CT angiogram of arteries of head and neck. **B.** CT angiogram of cerebral arterial circle (circle of Willis).
C. Schematic diagram of cerebral arterial circle and veins of cerebral base.

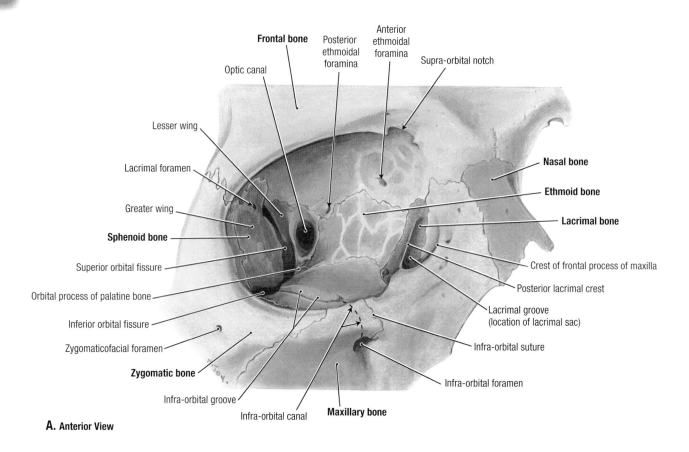

Frontal bone

Optic canal

Posterior ethmoidal foramina

Anterior ethmoidal foramina

Supra-orbital notch

Lesser wing

Lacrimal foramen

Greater wing

Sphenoid bone

Superior orbital fissure

Orbital process of palatine bone

Inferior orbital fissure

Zygomaticofacial foramen

Zygomatic bone

Infra-orbital groove

Infra-orbital canal

Maxillary bone

Nasal bone

Ethmoid bone

Lacrimal bone

Crest of frontal process of maxilla

Posterior lacrimal crest

Lacrimal groove (location of lacrimal sac)

Infra-orbital suture

Infra-orbital foramen

A. Anterior View

Corneoscleral junction

Iris

Pupil

Semilunar conjunctival fold

Lacrimal caruncle in lacus lacrimalis

Medial angle of eye

Lateral angle of eye

Bulbar conjunctiva covering sclera

Superior (upper) eyelid

Iris as seen through cornea

Conjunctival blood vessel

Lateral angle of eye

Bulbar conjunctiva covering sclera

Palpebral conjunctiva of inferior eyelid reflecting onto eyeball at inferior conjunctival fornix, becoming bulbar conjunctiva

B. Anterior View

C. Lateral View

7.36   ORBITAL CAVITY AND SURFACE ANATOMY OF THE EYE

A. Bones and features of the orbital cavity. **B. and C.** Surface anatomy of the eye. In **B,** the inferior eyelid is everted to demonstrate the palpebral conjunctiva. When powerful blows impact directly on the bony rim of the orbit, the resulting **orbital fractures** usually occur at the sutures between the bones forming the orbital margin. Fractures of the medial wall may involve the ethmoidal and sphenoidal sinuses, whereas fractures in the inferior wall may involve the maxillary sinus. Although the superior wall is stronger than the medial and inferior walls, it is thin enough to be translucent and may be readily penetrated. Thus, a sharp object may pass through it into the frontal lobe of the brain. Orbital fractures often result in intraorbital bleeding, which exerts pressure on the eyeball, causing **exophthalmos** (protrusion of the eyeball).

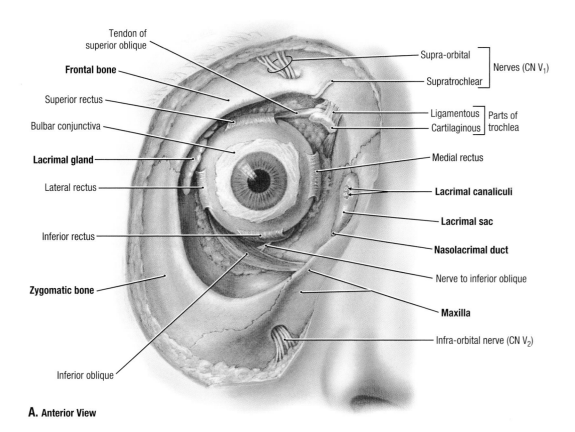

Tendon of
superior oblique

Frontal bone

Superior rectus

Bulbar conjunctiva

Lacrimal gland

Lateral rectus

Inferior rectus

Zygomatic bone

Inferior oblique

Supra-orbital

Supratrochlear

Nerves (CN V₁)

Ligamentous

Cartilaginous

Parts of
trochlea

Medial rectus

Lacrimal canaliculi

Lacrimal sac

Nasolacrimal duct

Nerve to inferior oblique

Maxilla

Infra-orbital nerve (CN V₂)

A. Anterior View

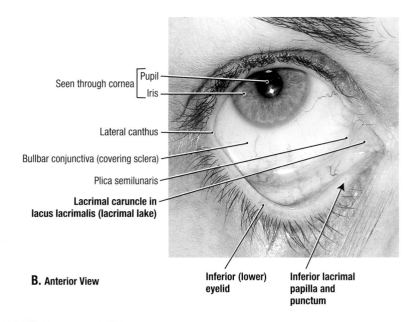

Seen through cornea

Pupil

Iris

Lateral canthus

Bullbar conjunctiva (covering sclera)

Plica semilunaris

**Lacrimal caruncle in
lacus lacrimalis (lacrimal lake)**

**Inferior (lower)
eyelid**

**Inferior lacrimal
papilla and
punctum**

B. Anterior View

C. Anterior View

7.37 **EYE AND LACRIMAL APPARATUS**

A. Anterior dissection of orbital cavity. The eyelids, orbital septum, levator palpebrae superioris, and some fat are removed. **B.** Surface features, with the inferior eyelid everted. **C.** Surface projection of lacrimal apparatus. Tears, secreted by the lacrimal gland *(L)* in the superolateral angle of the bony orbit, pass across the eyeball and enter the lacus lacrimalis (lacrimal lake) at the medial angle of the eye; from here they drain through the lacrimal puncta and lacrimal canaliculi *(C)* to the lacrimal sac *(S)*. The lacrimal sac drains into the nasolacrimal duct *(N)*, which empties into the inferior meatus *(I)* of the nose.

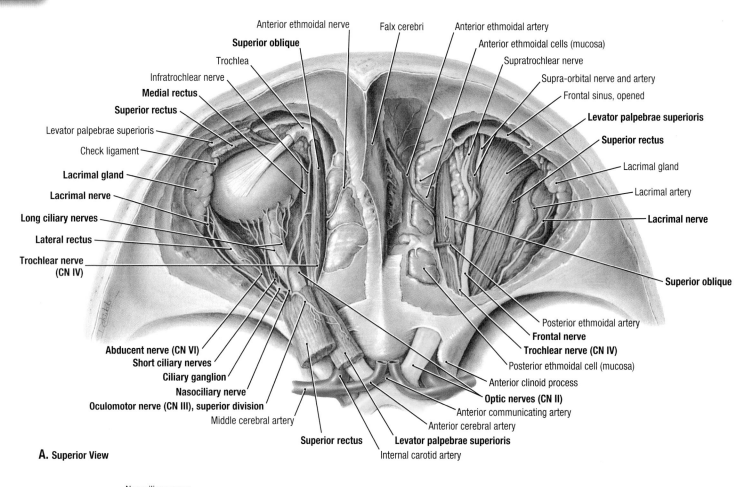

Anterior ethmoidal nerve
Falx cerebri
Anterior ethmoidal artery
Superior oblique
Anterior ethmoidal cells (mucosa)
Trochlea
Supratrochlear nerve
Infratrochlear nerve
Supra-orbital nerve and artery
Medial rectus
Frontal sinus, opened
Superior rectus
Levator palpebrae superioris
Levator palpebrae superioris
Superior rectus
Check ligament
Lacrimal gland
Lacrimal gland
Lacrimal artery
Lacrimal nerve
Lacrimal nerve
Long ciliary nerves
Lateral rectus
Trochlear nerve (CN IV)
Superior oblique
Posterior ethmoidal artery
Frontal nerve
Abducent nerve (CN VI)
Trochlear nerve (CN IV)
Short ciliary nerves
Posterior ethmoidal cell (mucosa)
Ciliary ganglion
Anterior clinoid process
Nasociliary nerve
Optic nerves (CN II)
Oculomotor nerve (CN III), superior division
Anterior communicating artery
Middle cerebral artery
Anterior cerebral artery
Superior rectus
Levator palpebrae superioris
Internal carotid artery

A. Superior View

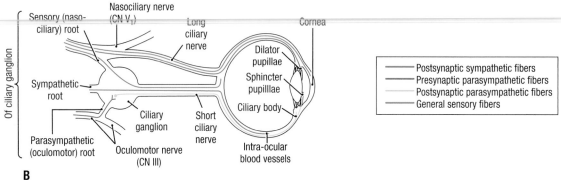

Sensory (naso-ciliary) root
Nasociliary nerve (CN V₁)
Long ciliary nerve
Cornea
Dilator pupillae
Sphincter pupilllae
Ciliary body
Sympathetic root
Of ciliary ganglion
Ciliary ganglion
Short ciliary nerve
Parasympathetic (oculomotor) root
Oculomotor nerve (CN III)
Intra-ocular blood vessels

— Postsynaptic sympathetic fibers
— Presynaptic parasympathetic fibers
— Postsynaptic parasympathetic fibers
— General sensory fibers

B

7.38   ORBITAL CAVITY, SUPERIOR APPROACH

A. Superficial dissection. On the right side of figure **A,** the orbital plate of the frontal bone is removed. On the left side of figure **A,** the levator palpebrae and superior rectus muscles are reflected.

- The trochlear nerve (CN IV) lies on the medial side of the superior oblique muscle, and the abducent nerve (CN VI) on the medial side of the lateral rectus muscle.
- The lacrimal nerve runs superior to the lateral rectus muscle supplying sensory fibers to the conjunctiva and skin of the superior eyelid; it receives a communicating branch of the zygomaticotemporal nerve carrying secretory motor fibers from the pterygopalatine ganglion to the lacrimal gland.

- The parasympathetic ciliary ganglion, placed between the lateral rectus muscle and the optic nerve (CN II), gives rise to many short ciliary nerves; the nasociliary nerve gives rise to two long ciliary nerves that anastomose with each other and the short ciliary nerves.

B. Distribution of nerve fibers to ciliary ganglion and eyeball.

    Horner syndrome results from interruption of a cervical sympathetic trunk and is manifest by the absence of sympathetically stimulated functions on the ipsilateral side of the head. The syndrome includes the following signs: constriction of the pupil (*miosis*), drooping of the superior eyelid (**ptosis**), redness and increased temperature of the skin (**vasodilatation**), and absence of sweating (**anhydrosis**).

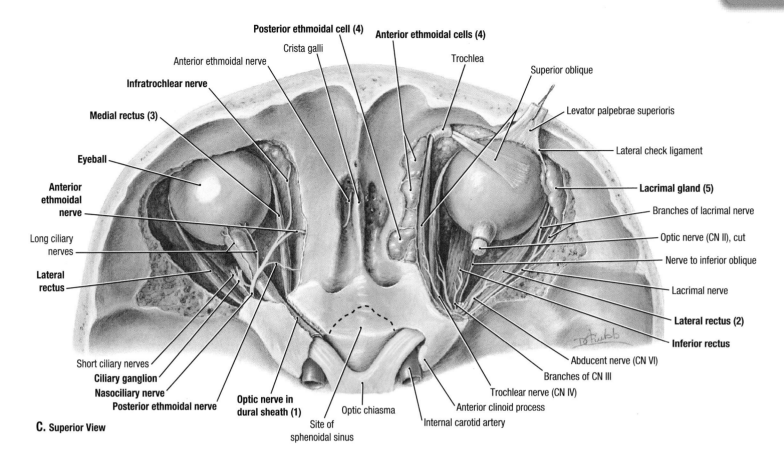

Posterior ethmoidal cell (4)   Anterior ethmoidal cells (4)

Crista galli

Posterior ethmoidal cell (4)

Anterior ethmoidal cells (4)

Anterior ethmoidal nerve

Trochlea

Superior oblique

Infratrochlear nerve

Levator palpebrae superioris

Medial rectus (3)

Lateral check ligament

Eyeball

Lacrimal gland (5)

Anterior ethmoidal nerve

Branches of lacrimal nerve

Optic nerve (CN II), cut

Long ciliary nerves

Nerve to inferior oblique

Lateral rectus

Lacrimal nerve

Lateral rectus (2)

Inferior rectus

Short ciliary nerves

Abducent nerve (CN VI)

Ciliary ganglion

Branches of CN III

Nasociliary nerve

Trochlear nerve (CN IV)

Posterior ethmoidal nerve

Optic nerve in dural sheath (1)

Anterior clinoid process

Optic chiasma

Internal carotid artery

Site of sphenoidal sinus

C. Superior View

7.38   **ORBITAL CAVITY, SUPERIOR APPROACH** *(CONTINUED)*

C. Deep dissection before *(left side of specimen)* and after *(right side of specimen)* section of the optic nerve (CN II). **D.** Transverse (axial) MRI of orbital cavity. (The *numbers* refer to structures labeled in **C**).

Observe on the right side of figure **C:**

- The eyeball occupies the anterior half of the orbital cavity.
  Observe on the left of figure **C:**
- The parasympathetic ciliary ganglion lies posteriorly between the lateral rectus muscle and the sheath of the optic nerve.
- The nasociliary nerve (CN V₁) sends a branch to the ciliary ganglion and crosses the optic nerve (CN II), where it gives off two long ciliary nerves (sensory to the eyeball and cornea) and the posterior ethmoidal nerve (to the sphenoidal sinus and posterior ethmoidal cells). The nasociliary nerve then divides into the anterior ethmoidal and infratrochlear nerves.
- The ciliary ganglion receives sensory fibers from the nasociliary branches of CN VI, postsynaptic sympathetic fibers from the continuation of the internal carotid plexus extending along the ophthalmic artery, and presynaptic parasympathetic fibers from the inferior branch of the oculomotor nerve; only the latter synapse in the ganglion.
- Complete **oculomotor nerve palsy** affects most of the ocular muscles, the levator palpebrae superioris, and the sphincter pupillae. The superior eyelid droops (**ptosis**) and cannot be raised voluntarily because of the unopposed activity of the orbicularis oculi (supplied by the facial nerve). The pupil is also fully dilated and nonreactive because of the unopposed dilator pupillae. The pupil is fully abducted and depressed ("down and out") because of the unopposed activity of the lateral rectus and superior oblique, respectively.
- A **lesion of the abducent nerve** results in loss of lateral gaze to the ipsilateral side because of paralysis of the lateral rectus muscle. On forward gaze, the eye is diverted medially because of the lack of normal resting tone in the lateral rectus, resulting in diplopia (double vision).

D. Axial MRI

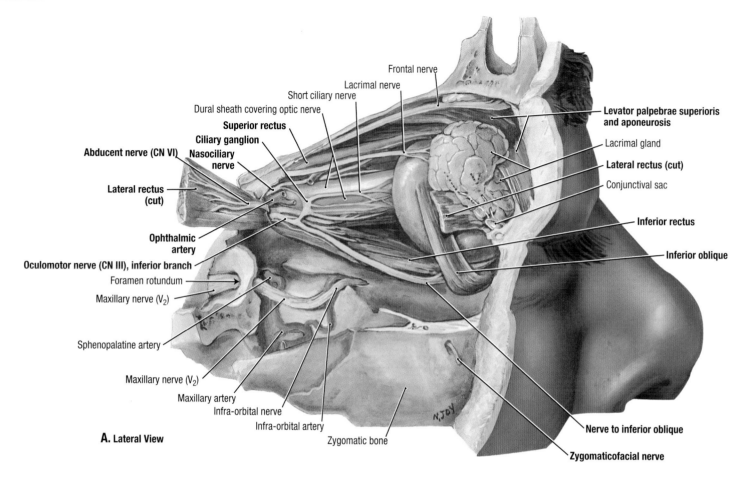

Frontal nerve

Lacrimal nerve

Short ciliary nerve

Dural sheath covering optic nerve

Superior rectus

Ciliary ganglion

Abducent nerve (CN VI)

Nasociliary nerve

Lateral rectus (cut)

Ophthalmic artery

Oculomotor nerve (CN III), inferior branch

Foramen rotundum

Maxillary nerve (V₂)

Sphenopalatine artery

Maxillary nerve (V₂)

Maxillary artery

Infra-orbital nerve

Infra-orbital artery

Zygomatic bone

A. Lateral View

Levator palpebrae superioris and aponeurosis

Lacrimal gland

Lateral rectus (cut)

Conjunctival sac

Inferior rectus

Inferior oblique

Nerve to inferior oblique

Zygomaticofacial nerve

Trochlear nerve (CN IV)

Ophthalmic nerve (CN V₁)

Maxillary nerve (CN V₂)

Nasociliary nerve

Frontal nerve

Medulla oblongata

Pons

Root of trigeminal nerve (CN V)

Medial rectus

Superior rectus

Levator palpebrae superioris

Superior oblique

Trochlea

Lacrimal gland

Lacrimal nerve (CN V₁)

Lateral rectus

Superior palpebral nerve

Ciliary ganglion

Abducent nerve (CN VI)

Inferior palpebral nerve

Infra-orbital nerve

Oculomotor nerve (CN III)

Superior branch

Inferior branch

Nerve of pterygoid canal

Pterygopalatine ganglion

Zygomatic nerve (CN V₂)

Inferior rectus

Inferior oblique

B. Lateral View

LATERAL ASPECT OF THE ORBIT AND STRUCTURE OF THE EYELID

A. Dissection. **B.** Nerves. **C.** Sagittal and cross section through optic nerve. The subarachnoid space around the optic nerve is continuous with the sub-arachnoid space around the brain. **D.** Sagittal MRI. The *numbers* refer to structures labeled in *C*; *S,* superior ophthalmic vein; *M,* maxillary sinus; *circled,* optic foramen. **E.** Structure of eyelid.

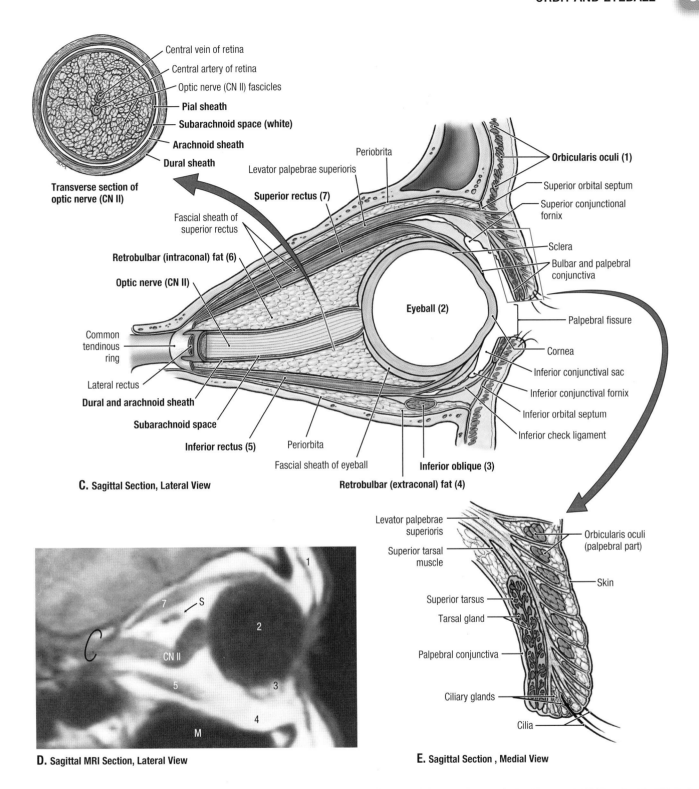

Transverse section of optic nerve (CN II)

Central vein of retina
Central artery of retina
Optic nerve (CN II) fascicles
Pial sheath
Subarachnoid space (white)
Arachnoid sheath
Dural sheath

Periobrita
Levator palpebrae superioris
Superior rectus (7)

Fascial sheath of superior rectus
Retrobulbar (intraconal) fat (6)
Optic nerve (CN II)

Common tendinous ring
Lateral rectus
Dural and arachnoid sheath
Subarachnoid space
Inferior rectus (5)
Periorbita
Fascial sheath of eyeball
Inferior oblique (3)
Retrobulbar (extraconal) fat (4)

Orbicularis oculi (1)
Superior orbital septum
Superior conjunctional fornix
Sclera
Bulbar and palpebral conjunctiva
Eyeball (2)
Palpebral fissure
Cornea
Inferior conjunctival sac
Inferior conjunctival fornix
Inferior orbital septum
Inferior check ligament

C. Sagittal Section, Lateral View

D. Sagittal MRI Section, Lateral View

Levator palpebrae superioris
Superior tarsal muscle
Superior tarsus
Tarsal gland
Palpebral conjunctiva
Ciliary glands
Cilia
Orbicularis oculi (palpebral part)
Skin

E. Sagittal Section , Medial View

7.39   LATERAL ASPECT OF THE ORBIT AND STRUCTURE OF THE EYELID *(CONTINUED)*

- Foreign objects, such as sand or metal filings, produce **corneal abrasions** that cause sudden, stabbing eye pain and tears. Opening and closing the eyelids is also painful. **Corneal lacerations** are caused by sharp objects such as fingernails or the corner of a page of a book.
- Any of the glands in the eyelid may become inflamed and swollen from infection or obstruction of their ducts. If the ducts of the ciliary glands are obstructed, a painful red suppurative (pus-producing) swelling, a sty (hordeolum), develops on the eyelid. **Obstruction of a tarsal gland** produces inflammation, a tarsal chalazion, that protrudes toward the eyeball and rubs against it as the eyelids blink.

A

B. Anterior View of Right and Left Eyes

7.40 EXTRA-OCULAR MUSCLES AND THEIR MOVEMENTS

A. The line of pull of the muscles relative to the eyeball and the axes around which movements occur. The orientation of the orbit is important in understanding the actions of the extra-ocular muscles. The common tendinous ring (origin of the recti), the origin of the inferior oblique, and the trochlea of the superior oblique all lie medial to the eyeball and to the A-P and vertical axes **(a)** The medial and lateral recti are the primary adductors and abductors of the eyeball. However, when movements begin from the primary position (gaze directed anteriorly along the A-P axis): (1) the line of pull of the superior and inferior rectus muscles passes medial and anterior to the vertical axis, resulting in secondary actions of a̲dduction; and (2) the line of pull of the superior and inferior oblique muscles passes medial and posterior to the vertical axis, resulting in secondary actions of a̲bduction. **(b)** Pulling in opposite directions relative to the transverse axis, the superior rectus and inferior oblique muscles are synergistic elevators, and the inferior rectus and superior oblique are synergistic depressors. **(c)** Medial pull produced by the muscles attaching to the superior eyeball (superior rectus and oblique) produces secondary actions of medial rotation (intorsion), and that produced by muscles attaching to the inferior eyeball (inferior rectus and oblique) produces lateral rotation (extorsion). **B.** Movements produced by isolated contraction of the four rectus and two oblique muscles, starting from the primary position. Large arrows indicate prime movers for the six cardinal movements. Movements in directions between large arrows (e.g., vertical elevation or depression) require synergistic actions of adjacent muscles. Contralaterally-paired muscles that work synergistically to direct parallel binocular gaze are called yoke muscles. For example, the right LR and left MR act as yoke muscles in directing gaze to the right.

TABLE 7.8 *ACTIONS OF MUSCLES OF ORBIT STARTING FROM PRIMARY POSITION*[a]

Muscle	Main Action		
	Vertical Axis (A)	**Horizontal Axis (B)**	**Anteroposterior Axis (C)**
Superior rectus (SR)	Elevates	Adducts	Rotates medially (intorsion)
Inferior rectus (IR)	Depresses	Adducts	Rotates laterally (extorsion)
Superior oblique (SO)	Depresses	Abducts	Rotates medially (intorsion)
Inferior oblique (IO)	Elevates	Abducts	Rotates laterally (extorsion)
Medial rectus (MR)	N/A	Adducts	N/A
Lateral rectus (LR)	N/A	Abducts	N/A

[a]Primary position, gaze directed anteriorly.

A. Binocular movements of eyeball from primary position, and muscles and nerves producing them. B. Muscles of eyeball.

7.41 **EXTRA-OCULAR MUSCLES AND THEIR MOVEMENTS** *(CONTINUED)*

A. Binocular movements of eyeball from primary position, and muscles and nerves producing them. **B.** Muscles of eyeball.

TABLE 7.9 MUSCLES OF ORBIT

Muscle	Origin	Insertion	Innervation	Main Action(s)[a]
Levator palpebrae superioris	Lesser wing of sphenoid bone, superior and anterior to optic canal	Superior tarsus and skin of superior eyelid	Oculomotor nerve; deep layer (superior tarsal muscle) supplied by sympathetic fibers	Elevates superior eyelid
Superior oblique (SO)	Body of sphenoid bone	Tendon passes through trochlea to insert into sclera, deep to SR	Trochlear nerve (CN IV)	Abducts, depresses, and rotates eyeball medially (intorsion)
Inferior oblique (IO)	Anterior part of floor of orbit	Sclera deep to lateral rectus muscle		Abducts, elevates, and rotates eyeball laterally (extorsion)
Superior rectus (SR)			Oculomotor nerve (CN III)	Elevates, adducts, and (SR) rotates eyeball medially (intorsion)
Inferior rectus (IR)	Common tendinous ring	Sclera just posterior to corneoscleral junction		Depresses, adducts, and rotates eyeball laterally (extorsion)
Medial rectus (MR)				Adducts eyeball
Lateral rectus (LR)			Abducent nerve (CN VI)	Abducts eyeball

[a]It is essential to appreciate that all muscles are continuously involved in eyeball movements; thus the individual actions are not usually tested clinically.

Angle of gaze coinciding with angle of muscle
ELEVATION ONLY

Angle of gaze coinciding with angle of muscle
DEPRESSION ONLY

Angle of gaze coinciding with angle of muscle
DEPRESSION ONLY

Angle of gaze coinciding with angle of muscle
ELEVATION ONLY

A. Superior Rectus

B. Inferior Rectus

C. Superior Oblique

D. Inferior Oblique

ELEVATION

ABDUCTION / ADDUCTION

SR IO
LR MR
IR SO

DEPRESSION

E. Pattern of movement of pupil used for clinical testing of extra-ocular muscles. Patient is asked to follow movement of examiner's finger, tracing and "H" pattern.

7.42 CLINICAL TESTING OF EXTRA-OCULAR MUSCLES AND MOTOR NERVES (CN III, IV, AND VI)

Most movements from the primary position involve synergists. When testing muscles (usually to determine the integrity of the involved motor nerve), it is desirable to isolate muscle activity. If the pupil is first adducted (MR—CN III) so that the direction of gaze coincides with the line of pull of the oblique muscles, only the SO (CN IV) can depress and only the IO (CN III) can elevate the pupil. If the pupil is first abducted (LR—CN VI) so that the direction of gaze coincides with the line of pull of the superior and inferior recti, only these muscles can elevate and depress the pupil (superior and inferior divisions of CN III)

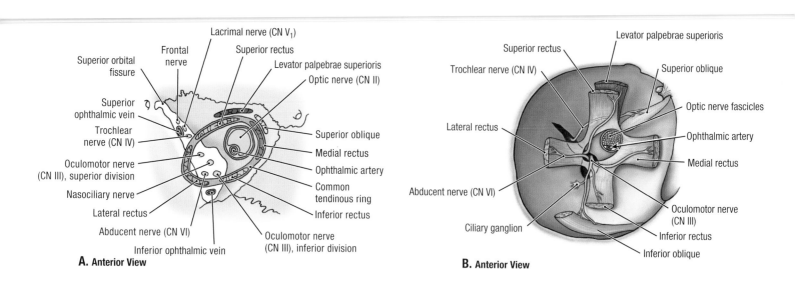

A. Anterior View

Superior orbital fissure
Frontal nerve
Lacrimal nerve (CN V$_1$)
Superior rectus
Levator palpebrae superioris
Optic nerve (CN II)
Superior ophthalmic vein
Trochlear nerve (CN IV)
Oculomotor nerve (CN III), superior division
Nasociliary nerve
Lateral rectus
Abducent nerve (CN VI)
Inferior ophthalmic vein
Superior oblique
Medial rectus
Ophthalmic artery
Common tendinous ring
Inferior rectus
Oculomotor nerve (CN III), inferior division

B. Anterior View

Superior rectus
Levator palpebrae superioris
Trochlear nerve (CN IV)
Superior oblique
Lateral rectus
Optic nerve fascicles
Ophthalmic artery
Medial rectus
Abducent nerve (CN VI)
Oculomotor nerve (CN III)
Ciliary ganglion
Inferior rectus
Inferior oblique

7.43 NERVES OF ORBIT

A. Overview. **B.** Relationships at apex of orbit. **C.** Common tendinous ring, structural relationships.

Orbital tumors. Because of the closeness of the optic nerve to the sphenoidal and posterior ethmoidal sinuses, a malignant tumor in these sinuses may erode the thin bony walls of the orbit and compress the optic nerve and orbital contents. Tumors in the orbit produce **exophthalmos** (protrusion of eyeball). Tumors in the middle cranial fossa enter the orbital cavity through the superior orbital fissure. Tumors in the temporal or infratemporal fossae enter the orbit through the inferior orbital fissure.

A. Superior View

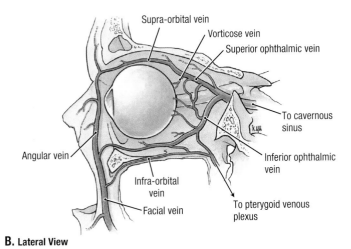

B. Lateral View

7.44 ARTERIES AND VEINS OF ORBIT

A. Arteries.

Blockage of central retinal artery. The terminal branches of the central retinal artery are end arteries. Obstruction of the artery by an embolus results in instant and total blindness. Blockage of the artery is usually unilateral and occurs in older people. **B.** Veins. The superior and inferior ophthalmic veins receive the vorticose veins from the eyeball and drain into the cavernous sinus posteriorly and the pterygoid plexus inferiorly. They communicate with the facial and supra-orbital veins anteriorly.

- The facial veins make clinically important connections with the cavernous sinus through the superior ophthalmic veins. **Cavernous sinus thrombosis** usually results from infections in the orbit, nasal sinuses, and superior part of the face (the danger triangle). In persons with thrombophlebitis of the facial vein, pieces of an infected thrombus may extend into the cavernous sinus, producing **thrombophlebitis of the cavernous sinus.** The infection usually involves only one sinus initially but may spread to the opposite side through the intercavernous sinuses.

- **Blockade of central retinal vein.** The central retinal vein enters the cavernous sinus. Thrombophlebitis of this sinus may result in passage of a thrombus to the central retinal vein and produce a blockage in one of the small retinal veins. Occlusion of a branch of the central vein of the retina usually results in slow, painless loss of vision.

TABLE 7.10 ARTERIES OF ORBIT

Artery	Origin	Course and Distribution
Ophthalmic	Internal carotid artery	Traverses optic foramen to reach orbital cavity
Central retinal	Ophthalmic artery	Runs in dural sheath of optic nerve, entering nerve near eyeball; appears at center of optic disc; supplies optic retina (except cones and rods)
Supra-orbital		Passes superiorly and posteriorly from supra-orbital foramen to supply forehead and scalp
Supratrochlear		Passes from supra-orbital margin to forehead and scalp
Lacrimal		Passes along superior border of lateral rectus muscle to supply lacrimal gland, conjunctiva, and eyelids
Dorsal nasal		Courses along dorsal aspect of nose and supplies its surface
Short posterior ciliary		Pierces sclera at periphery of optic nerve to supply choroid, which, in turn, supplies cones and rods of optic retina
Long posterior ciliary		Pierces sclera to supply ciliary body and iris
Posterior ethmoidal		Passes through posterior ethmoidal foramen to posterior ethmoidal cells
Anterior ethmoidal		Passes through anterior ethmoidal foramen to anterior cranial fossa; supplies anterior and middle ethmoidal cells, frontal sinus, nasal cavity, and skin on dorsum of nose
Anterior ciliary	Muscular rami of the opthalmic and infra-orbital arteries	Pierces sclera at attachments of rectus muscles and forms network in iris and ciliary body
Infra-orbital	Third part of maxillary artery	Passes along infra-orbital groove and exits through infra-orbital foramen to face

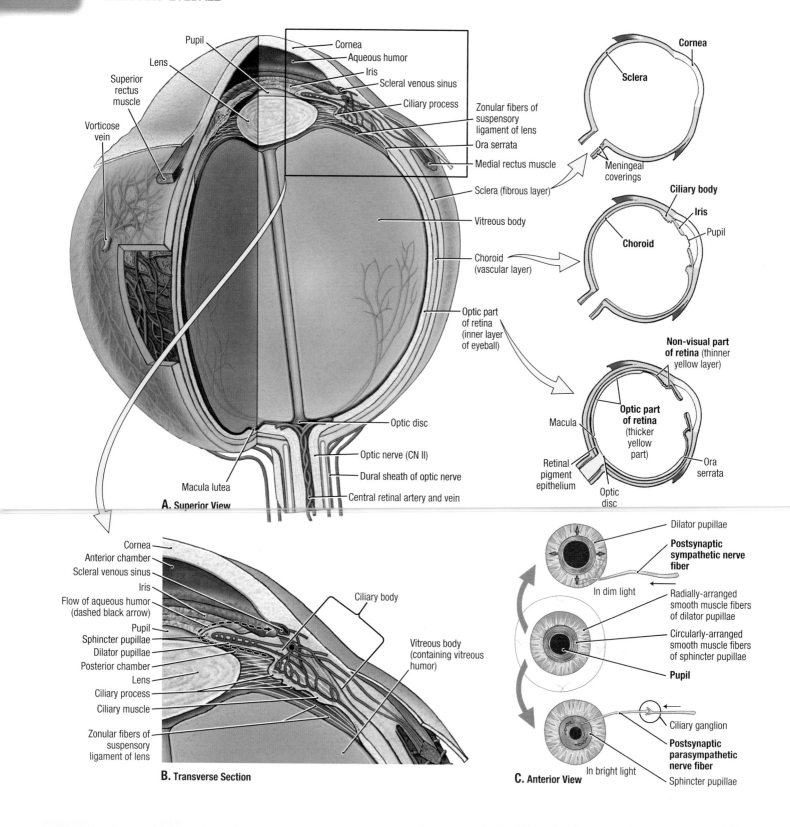

A. Superior View

B. Transverse Section

C. Anterior View

7.45   ILLUSTRATION OF A DISSECTED EYEBALL

A. Parts of the eyeball. **B.** Ciliary region. **C.** Structure and function of iris. The aqueous humor is produced by the ciliary processes and provides nutrients for the avascular cornea and lens; the aqueous humor drains into the scleral venous sinus (also called the sinus venosus sclerae or canal of Schlemm). **Glaucoma.**

If drainage of the aqueous humor is reduced significantly, pressure builds up in the chambers of the eye (glaucoma). Blindness can result from compression of the inner layer of the retina and retinal arteries if aqueous humor production is not reduced to maintain normal intraocular pressure.

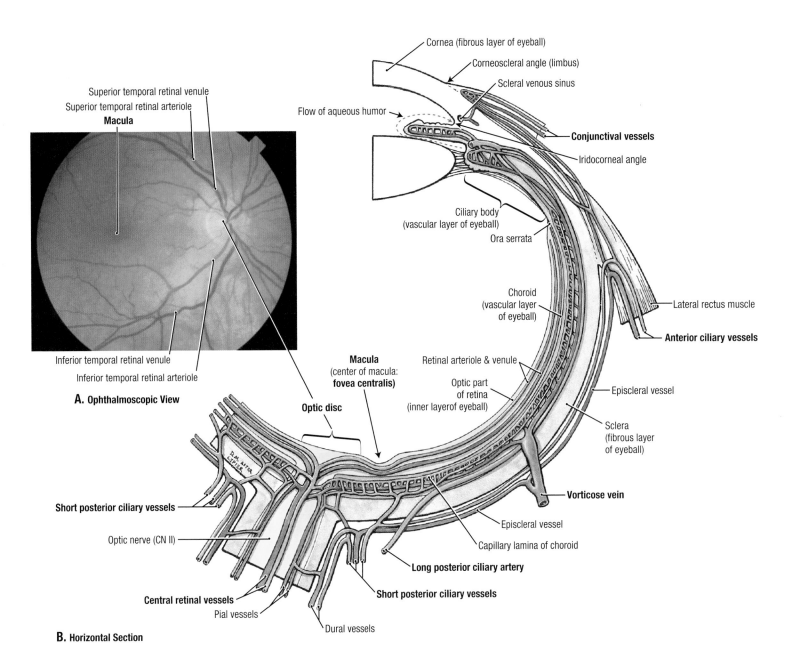

Cornea (fibrous layer of eyeball)

Corneoscleral angle (limbus)

Scleral venous sinus

Flow of aqueous humor

Conjunctival vessels

Iridocorneal angle

Superior temporal retinal venule
Superior temporal retinal arteriole
Macula

Inferior temporal retinal venule

Inferior temporal retinal arteriole

A. Ophthalmoscopic View

Ciliary body
(vascular layer of eyeball)

Ora serrata

Choroid
(vascular layer
of eyeball)

Lateral rectus muscle

Anterior ciliary vessels

Macula
(center of macula:
fovea centralis)

Optic disc

Retinal arteriole & venule

Optic part
of retina
(inner layerof eyeball)

Episcleral vessel

Sclera
(fibrous layer
of eyeball)

Short posterior ciliary vessels

Optic nerve (CN II)

Central retinal vessels

Pial vessels

Dural vessels

Capillary lamina of choroid

Long posterior ciliary artery

Short posterior ciliary vessels

Episcleral vessel

Vorticose vein

B. Horizontal Section

7.46   OCULAR FUNDUS AND BLOOD SUPPLY TO THE EYEBALL

A. Right ocular fundus, ophthalmoscopic view. Retinal venules (wider) and retinal arterioles (narrower) radiate from the center of the oval optic disc, formed in relation to the entry of the optic nerve into the eyeball. The round, dark area lateral to the disc is the macula; branches of vessels extend to this area, but do not reach its center, the fovea centralis, a depressed spot that is the area of most acute vision. It is avascular but, like the rest of the outermost (cones and rods) layer of the retina, is nourished by the adjacent choriocapillaris. Increased intracranial pressure is transmitted through the CSF in the subarachnoid space surrounding the optic nerve, causing the optic disc to protrude. The protrusion, called **papilledema,** is apparent during ophthalmoscopy. **B.** Blood supply to eyeball. The eyeball has three layers: (1) the external, fibrous layer is the sclera and cornea; (2) the middle, vascular layer is the choroid, ciliary body, and iris; and (3) the internal, neural layer or retina consists of a pigment cell layer and a neural layer. The central artery of the retina, a branch of the ophthalmic artery, is an end artery. Of the eight posterior ciliary arteries, six are short posterior ciliary arteries and supply the choroid, which in turn nourishes the outer, nonvascular layer of the retina. Two long posterior ciliary arteries, one on each side of the eyeball, run between the sclera and choroid to anastomose with the anterior ciliary arteries, which are derived from muscular branches. The choroid is drained by posterior ciliary veins, and four to five vorticose veins drain into the ophthalmic veins.

Superficial temporal artery

Orbicularis oculi

Auriculotemporal nerve (CN V₃)

Zygomatic branches (CN VII)

Zygomaticus major

Transverse facial artery

Parotid duct

Buccal branches (CN VII)

Buccal nerve (CN V₃)

Buccinator

Depressor anguli oris

Masseter

Facial artery

Facial vein

Temporal branches (CN VII)

Posterior auricular
- Muscle
- Vein
- Lymph node
- Nerve (CN VII)
- Artery

Parotid gland
Parotid lymph nodes
Great auricular nerve

External jugular vein

Cervical branch (CN VII)
Marginal mandibular branch (CN VII)

A. Lateral View

Auriculotemporal nerve (CN V₃)

Superficial temporal vein

Superficial temporal artery

Temporal branches of facial nerve (CN VII)

Transverse facial artery

Parotid duct

Parotid gland

Cervical branch of facial nerve

Masseter

Hypoglossal nerve (CN XII)

External carotid artery

Pre-auricular lymph nodes

Facial nerve (CN VII)

Posterior auricular nerve

Nerve to posterior belly of digastric

Posterior auricular artery

Sternocleidomastoid

Digastric, posterior belly

Retromandibular vein

Internal jugular vein

Spinal accessory nerve (CN XI)

Vagus nerve (CN X)

Internal carotid artery

B. Lateral View

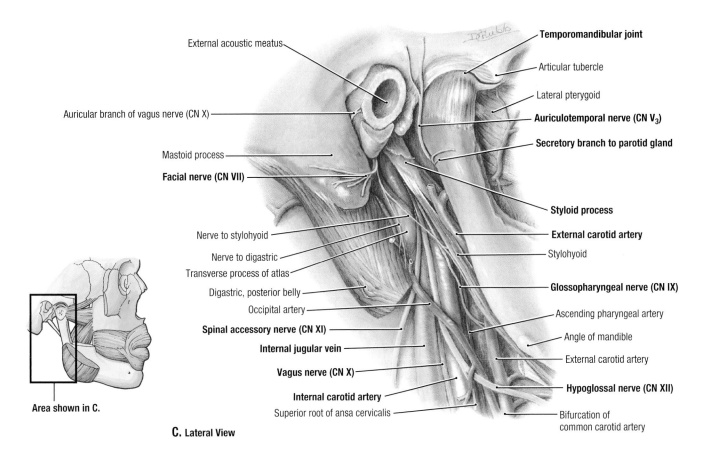

External acoustic meatus

Auricular branch of vagus nerve (CN X)

Mastoid process

Facial nerve (CN VII)

Nerve to stylohyoid

Nerve to digastric

Transverse process of atlas

Digastric, posterior belly

Occipital artery

Spinal accessory nerve (CN XI)

Internal jugular vein

Vagus nerve (CN X)

Internal carotid artery

Superior root of ansa cervicalis

Area shown in C.

C. Lateral View

Temporomandibular joint

Articular tubercle

Lateral pterygoid

Auriculotemporal nerve (CN V₃)

Secretory branch to parotid gland

Styloid process

External carotid artery

Stylohyoid

Glossopharyngeal nerve (CN IX)

Ascending pharyngeal artery

Angle of mandible

External carotid artery

Hypoglossal nerve (CN XII)

Bifurcation of common carotid artery

7.47   PAROTID REGION

A. Superficial dissection. **B.** Deep dissection with part of the gland removed. During **parotidectomy** (surgical excision of the parotid gland), identification, dissection, and preservation of the facial nerve are critical. The parotid gland has superficial and deep parts. In parotidectomy the superficial part is removed, then the plexus may be retracted to remove the deep part. **C.** Deep dissection following removal of the parotid gland. The facial nerve, posterior belly of the digastric muscle, and its nerve are retracted; the external carotid artery, stylohyoid muscle, and the nerve to the stylohyoid remain in situ. The internal jugular vein, internal carotid artery, and glossopharyngeal (CN IX), vagus (CN X), accessory (CN XI), and hypoglossal (CN XII) nerves cross anterior to the transverse process of the atlas and deep to the styloid process.

Trauma, such as a **fractured mandible,** may injure the hypoglossal nerve (CN XII), resulting in paralysis and eventual atrophy of one side of the tongue. The tongue deviates to the paralyzed side during protrusion.

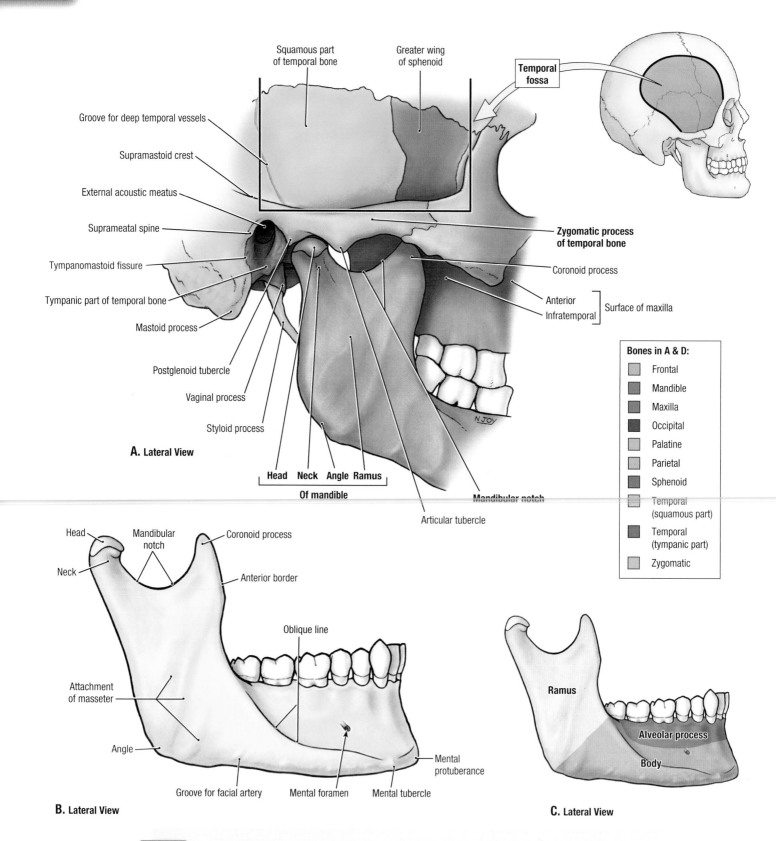

A. Lateral View

B. Lateral View

C. Lateral View

Bones in A & D:

	Frontal
	Mandible
	Maxilla
	Occipital
	Palatine
	Parietal
	Sphenoid
	Temporal (squamous part)
	Temporal (tympanic part)
	Zygomatic

7.48   TEMPORAL AND INFRATEMPORAL FOSSAE AND MANDIBLE

A. Bones and bony features. Note that superficially the zygomatic process of the temporal bone is the boundary between the temporal fossa superiorly and the infratemporal fossa inferiorly. **B.** External surface of the mandible. **C.** Parts of mandible.

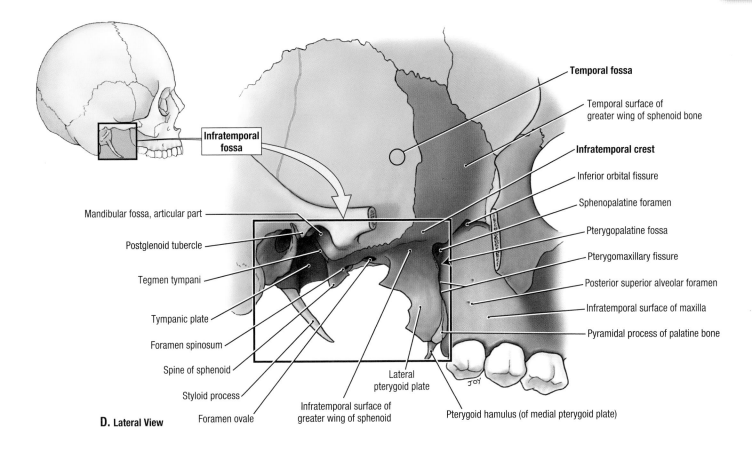

Temporal fossa

Temporal surface of greater wing of sphenoid bone

Infratemporal crest

Inferior orbital fissure

Sphenopalatine foramen

Pterygopalatine fossa

Pterygomaxillary fissure

Posterior superior alveolar foramen

Infratemporal surface of maxilla

Pyramidal process of palatine bone

Mandibular fossa, articular part

Postglenoid tubercle

Tegmen tympani

Tympanic plate

Foramen spinosum

Spine of sphenoid

Styloid process

Foramen ovale

Infratemporal surface of greater wing of sphenoid

Lateral pterygoid plate

Pterygoid hamulus (of medial pterygoid plate)

D. Lateral View

7.48

TEMPORAL AND INFRATEMPORAL FOSSAE AND MANDIBLE *(CONTINUED)*

D. Bones and bony features of the infratemporal fossa. The mandible and part of the zygomatic arch have been removed. Deeply, the infratemporal crest separates the temporal and infratemporal fossae. **E.** Internal surface of the mandible.

- The temporal region is the region of the head that includes the lateral area of the scalp and the deeper soft tissues overlying the temporal fossa of the cranium, superior to the zygomatic arch. The temporal fossa, occupied primarily by the upper portion of the temporalis muscle, is bounded by the inferior temporal lines (see Fig. 7.3B).
- The infratemporal fossa is an irregularly shaped space deep and inferior to the zygomatic arch, deep to the ramus of the mandible and posterior to the maxilla. It communicates with the temporal fossa through the interval between the zygomatic arch and the cranial bones.

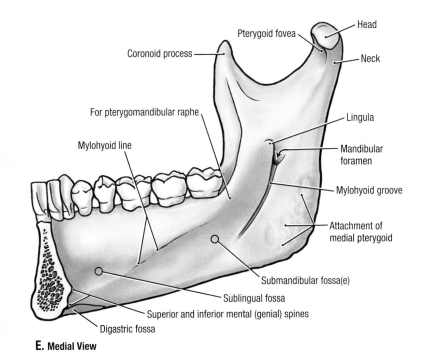

Pterygoid fovea

Head

Coronoid process

Neck

For pterygomandibular raphe

Lingula

Mylohyoid line

Mandibular foramen

Mylohyoid groove

Attachment of medial pterygoid

Submandibular fossa(e)

Sublingual fossa

Superior and inferior mental (genial) spines

Digastric fossa

E. Medial View

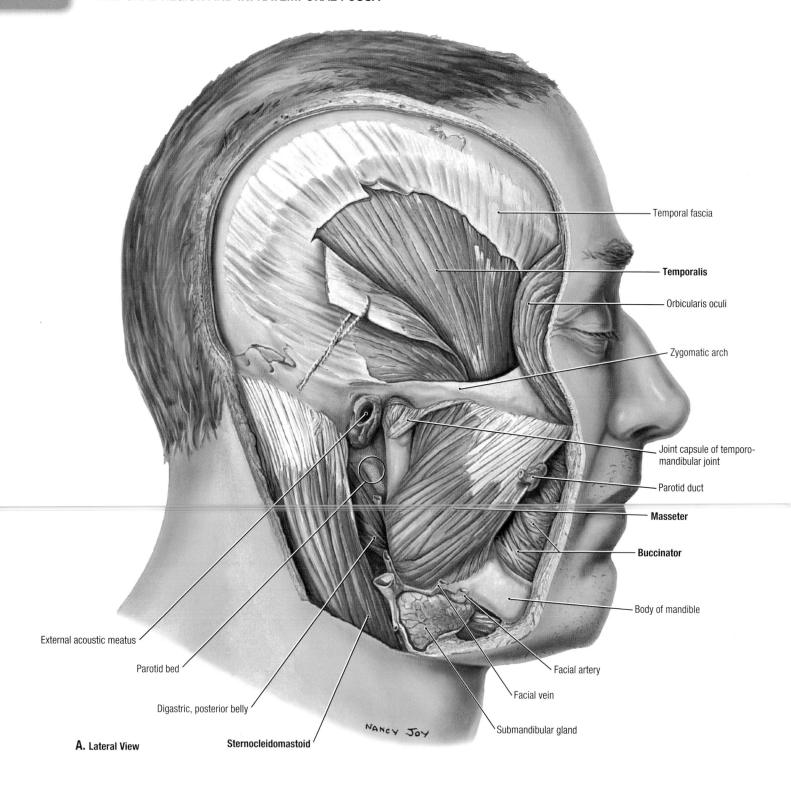

Temporal fascia

Temporalis

Orbicularis oculi

Zygomatic arch

Joint capsule of temporo-
mandibular joint

Parotid duct

Masseter

Buccinator

Body of mandible

Facial artery

Facial vein

Submandibular gland

External acoustic meatus

Parotid bed

Digastric, posterior belly

Sternocleidomastoid

NANCY JOY

A. Lateral View

7.49   **TEMPORALIS AND MASSETER**

A. Superficial dissection.

- The temporalis and masseter muscles are supplied by the trigeminal nerve (CN V), and both elevate the mandible. The buccinator muscle, supplied by the facial nerve (CN VII), functions during chewing to keep food between the teeth but does not act on the mandible.
- The sternocleidomastoid muscle, supplied by the spinal accessory nerve (CN XI), is the chief flexor of the head and neck; it forms the lateral part of the posterior boundary of the parotid region/parotid bed.

Branch of superficial temporal artery

Branch of posterior auricular artery

Branch of great auricular nerve (C2/C3)

Auricular branches of vagus nerve (CN X)

Lateral (temporomandibular) ligament

Styloid process

Mastoid process

Lateral pterygoid

Stylohyoid

Posterior belly of digastric

Spinal accessory nerve (CN XI)

Internal jugular vein

Sternocleidomastoid branch of occipital artery

Vagus nerve (CN X)

Internal carotid artery

Superior root of ansa cervicalis on internal carotid artery

B. Lateral View

External carotid artery

Temporalis

Zygomaticotemporal nerve (CN V₂)

Zygomatic process of temporal bone (cut)

Zygomatic bone (cut surface)

Masseteric nerve

Masseteric artery

Coronoid process of mandible

Parotid duct

Masseter

Facial artery

Lingual artery

Mylohyoid

Hypoglossal nerve (CN XII)

7.49   TEMPORALIS AND MASSETER *(CONTINUED)*

B. Deep dissection.

- Parts of the zygomatic arch and the attached masseter muscle have been removed to expose the attachment of the temporalis muscle to the coronoid process of the mandible.
- The carotid sheath surrounding the internal jugular vein, internal carotid artery, and the vagus nerve (CN X) has been removed. The external carotid artery and its lingual, facial, and occipital branches, and the spinal accessory (CN XI) and hypoglossal (CN XII) nerves pass deep to the posterior belly of the digastric muscle.

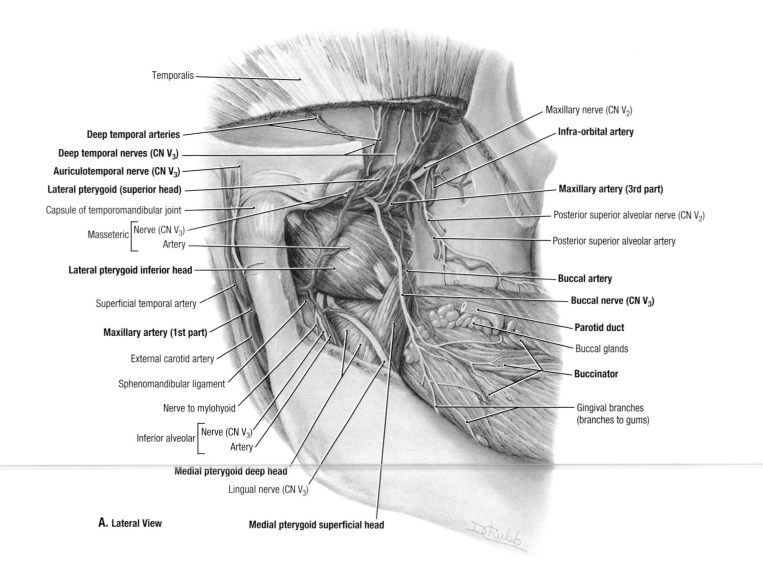

Temporalis

Maxillary nerve (CN V₂)

Infra-orbital artery

Deep temporal arteries

Deep temporal nerves (CN V₃)

Auriculotemporal nerve (CN V₃)

Lateral pterygoid (superior head)

Capsule of temporomandibular joint

Masseteric ⎡ Nerve (CN V₃)
⎣ Artery

Maxillary artery (3rd part)

Posterior superior alveolar nerve (CN V₂)

Posterior superior alveolar artery

Lateral pterygoid inferior head

Superficial temporal artery

Maxillary artery (1st part)

External carotid artery

Sphenomandibular ligament

Nerve to mylohyoid

Inferior alveolar ⎡ Nerve (CN V₃)
⎣ Artery

Buccal artery

Buccal nerve (CN V₃)

Parotid duct

Buccal glands

Buccinator

Gingival branches
(branches to gums)

Medial pterygoid deep head

Lingual nerve (CN V₃)

A. Lateral View

Medial pterygoid superficial head

7.50   INFRATEMPORAL REGION

A. Superficial dissection.

- The maxillary artery, the larger of two terminal branches of the external carotid, is divided into three parts relative to the lateral pterygoid muscle.
- The buccinator is pierced by the parotid duct, the ducts of the buccal glands, and sensory branches of the buccal nerve.
- The lateral pterygoid muscle arises by two heads (parts), one head from the roof, and the other head from the medial wall of the infratemporal fossa; both heads insert in relation to the temporomandibular joint— the superior head attaching primarily to the articular disc of the joint and the inferior head primarily to the anterior aspect of the neck of the mandible (pterygoid fovea).
- Because of the close relationship of the facial and auriculotemporal nerves to the temporomandibular joint (TMJ), care must be taken during **surgical procedures on the temporomandibular joint** to preserve both the branches of the facial nerve overlying it and the articular branches of the auriculotemporal nerve that enter the posterior part of the joint. Injury to articular branches of the auriculotemporal nerve supplying the TMJ—associated with traumatic dislocation and rupture of the joint capsule and lateral ligament—leads to laxity and instability of the TMJ.

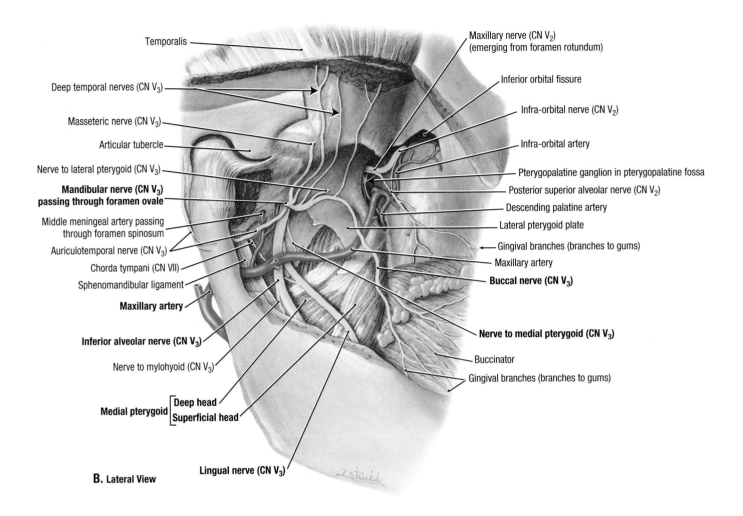

Temporalis

Deep temporal nerves (CN V$_3$)

Masseteric nerve (CN V$_3$)

Articular tubercle

Nerve to lateral pterygoid (CN V$_3$)

Mandibular nerve (CN V$_3$) passing through foramen ovale

Middle meningeal artery passing through foramen spinosum

Auriculotemporal nerve (CN V$_3$)

Chorda tympani (CN VII)

Sphenomandibular ligament

Maxillary artery

Inferior alveolar nerve (CN V$_3$)

Nerve to mylohyoid (CN V$_3$)

Medial pterygoid [**Deep head** / **Superficial head**]

B. Lateral View

Lingual nerve (CN V$_3$)

Maxillary nerve (CN V$_2$) (emerging from foramen rotundum)

Inferior orbital fissure

Infra-orbital nerve (CN V$_2$)

Infra-orbital artery

Pterygopalatine ganglion in pterygopalatine fossa

Posterior superior alveolar nerve (CN V$_2$)

Descending palatine artery

Lateral pterygoid plate

Gingival branches (branches to gums)

Maxillary artery

Buccal nerve (CN V$_3$)

Nerve to medial pterygoid (CN V$_3$)

Buccinator

Gingival branches (branches to gums)

7.50   INFRATEMPORAL REGION (CONTINUED)

B. Deeper dissection.

- The lateral pterygoid muscle and most of the branches of the maxillary artery have been removed to expose the mandibular nerve (CN V$_3$) entering the infratemporal fossa through the foramen ovale and the middle meningeal artery passing through the foramen spinosum.

- The deep head of the medial pterygoid muscle arises from the medial surface of the lateral pterygoid plate and the pyramidal process of the palatine bone. It has a small, superficial head that arises from the tuberosity of the maxilla.

- The inferior alveolar and lingual nerves descend on the medial pterygoid muscle. The inferior alveolar nerve gives off the nerve to mylohyoid and nerve to anterior belly of the digastric muscle, and the lingual nerve receives the chorda tympani, which carries secretory parasympathetic fibers and fibers of taste.

- Motor nerves arising from CN V$_3$ supply the four muscles of mastication: the masseter, temporalis, and lateral and medial pterygoids. The buccal nerve from the mandibular nerve is sensory; the buccal branch of the facial nerve is the motor supply to the buccinator muscle.

- To perform a **mandibular nerve block,** an anesthetic agent is injected near the mandibular nerve where it enters the infratemporal fossa. This block usually anesthetizes the auriculotemporal, inferior alveolar, lingual, and buccal branches of the mandibular nerve.

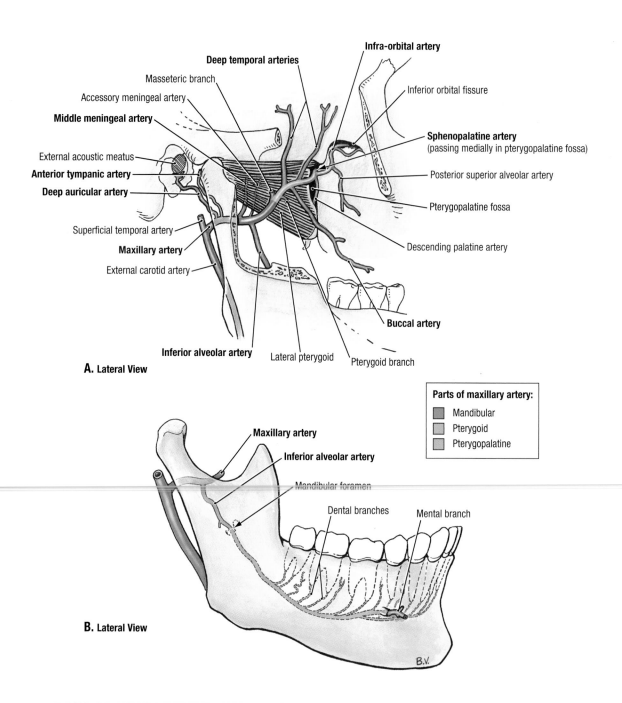

A. Lateral View

Parts of maxillary artery:
- Mandibular
- Pterygoid
- Pterygopalatine

B. Lateral View

7.51 BRANCHES OF MAXILLARY ARTERY

A. Infratemporal region. **B.** Mandible.

- The maxillary artery arises at the neck of the mandible and is divided into three parts (mandibular, pterygoid, and pterygopalatine) by the lateral pterygoid; it can pass medial or lateral to the lateral pterygoid.
- The branches of the *first (mandibular) part* pass through foramina or canals: the deep auricular to the external acoustic meatus, the anterior tympanic to the tympanic cavity, the middle and accessory meningeal to the cranial cavity, and the inferior alveolar to the mandible and teeth.
- The branches of the *second (pterygoid) part*, directly related to the lateral pterygoid, supply muscles via the masseteric, deep temporal, pterygoid, and buccal branches.
- The branches of the *third (pterygopalatine) part* (posterior superior alveolar, infra-orbital, descending palatine, and sphenopalatine arteries) arise immediately proximal to and within the pterygopalatine fossa.

A. Lateral View

B

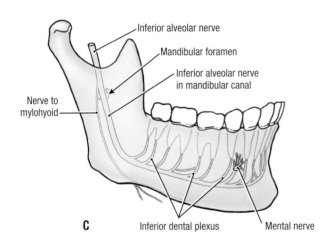

C

7.52 BRANCHES OF MAXILLARY AND MANDIBULAR NERVES

A. Infratemporal region and pterygopalatine fossa. Branches of the maxillary (CN V$_2$) and mandibular (CN V$_3$) nerves accompany branches from the three parts of the maxillary artery. **B.** Nerves of infratemporal fossa and otic ganglion. **C.** Mandible and inferior alveolar nerve.

An **alveolar nerve block**—commonly used by dentists when repairing mandibular teeth—anesthetizes the inferior alveolar nerve, a branch of CN V$_3$. The anesthetic agent is injected around the mandibular foramen, the opening into the mandibular canal on the medial aspect of the ramus of the mandible. This canal gives passage to the inferior alveolar nerve, artery, and vein. When this nerve block is successful, all mandibular teeth are anesthetized to the median plane. The skin and mucous membrane of the lower lip, the labial alveolar mucosa and gingiva, and the skin of the chin are also anesthetized because they are supplied by the mental branch of this nerve.

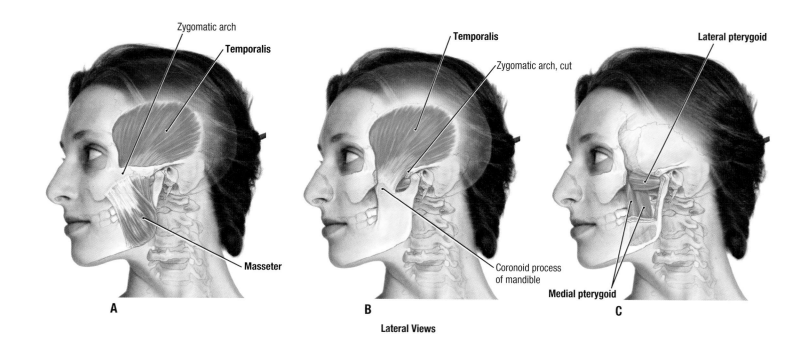

A

B

C

Lateral Views

7.53 MUSCLES OF MASTICATION

A. Temporalis and masseter. **B.** Temporalis. Zygomatic arch has been removed. **C.** Medial and lateral pterygoid.

TABLE 7.11 MUSCLES OF MASTICATION (ACTING ON TEMPOROMANDIBULAR JOINT)

Muscle	Origin	Insertion	Innervation	Main Action
Temporalis	Floor of temporal fossa and deep surface of temporal fascia	Tip and medial surface of coronoid process and anterior border of ramus of mandible	Deep temporal branches of mandibular nerve (CN V$_3$)	Elevates mandible, closing jaws; posterior fibers retrude mandible after protrusion
Masseter	Inferior border and medial surface of zygomatic arch	Lateral surface of ramus of mandible and coronoid process	Mandibular nerve (CN V$_3$) through masseteric nerve that enters deep surface of the muscle	Elevates and protrudes mandible, thus closing jaws; deep fibers retrude it
Lateral pterygoid	*Superior head:* infratemporal surface and infratemporal crest of greater wing of sphenoid bone *Inferior head:* lateral surface of lateral pterygoid plate	Neck of mandible, articular disc, and capsule of temporomandibular joint	Mandibular nerve (CN V$_3$) through lateral pterygoid nerve which enters its deep surface	*Acting bilaterally,* protrude mandible and depress chin; *Acting unilaterally* alternately, they produce side-to-side movements of mandible
Medial pterygoid	*Deep head:* medial surface of lateral pterygoid plate and pyramidal process of palatine bone *Superficial head:* tuberosity of maxilla	Medial surface of ramus of mandible, inferior to mandibular foramen	Mandibular nerve (CN V$_3$) through medial pterygoid nerve	Helps elevate mandible, closing jaws; *acting bilaterally* protrude mandible; *acting unilaterally,* protrudes side of jaw; acting alternately, they produce a grinding motion

A. Elevation of mandible

B. Depression of mandible

C. Retrusion

D. Protrusion

Lateral Views

E. Protrusion

F. Lateral movement to right side

G. Lateral movement to left side

Anterior Views

7.54 MOVEMENTS OF TEMPOROMANDIBULAR JOINT

TABLE 7.12 MOVEMENTS OF TEMPOROMANDIBULAR JOINT

Movements	Muscles
Elevation (close mouth) (A)	Temporalis, masseter, and medial pterygoid
Depression (open mouth) (B)	Lateral pterygoid; suprahyoid and infrahyoid muscles; gravity
Retrusion (retrude chin) (C)	Temporalis (posterior oblique and near horizontal fibers) and masseter
Protrusion (protrude chin) (D and E)	Lateral pterygoid, masseter, and medial pterygoid
Lateral movements (grinding and chewing) (F and G)	Temporalis of same side, pterygoids of opposite side, and masseter

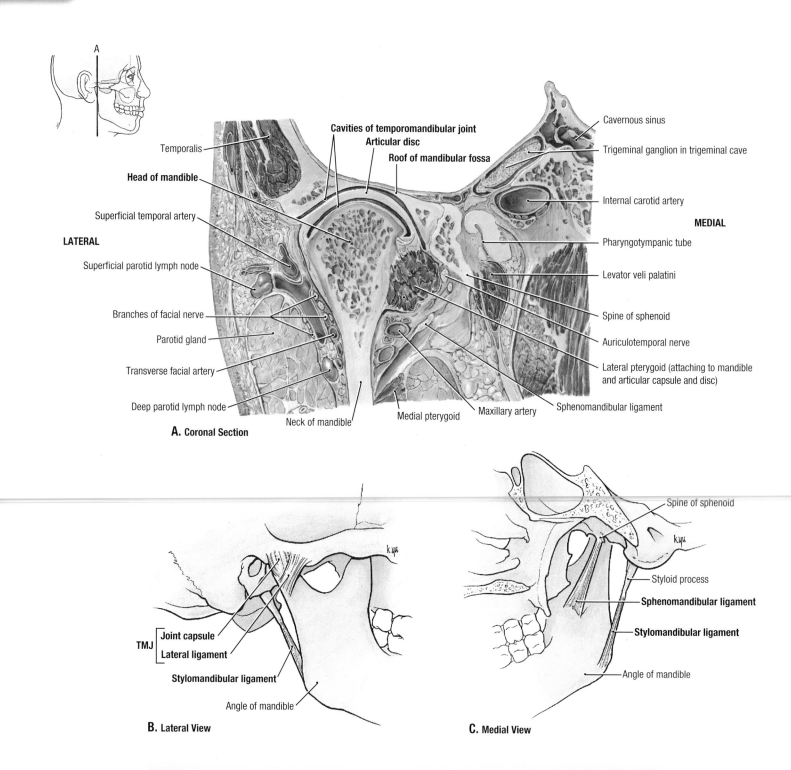

A. Coronal Section

- Temporalis
- **Head of mandible**
- Superficial temporal artery
- **LATERAL**
- Superficial parotid lymph node
- Branches of facial nerve
- Parotid gland
- Transverse facial artery
- Deep parotid lymph node
- Neck of mandible

Cavities of temporomandibular joint
Articular disc
Roof of mandibular fossa

- Cavernous sinus
- Trigeminal ganglion in trigeminal cave
- Internal carotid artery
- **MEDIAL**
- Pharyngotympanic tube
- Levator veli palatini
- Spine of sphenoid
- Auriculotemporal nerve
- Lateral pterygoid (attaching to mandible and articular capsule and disc)
- Sphenomandibular ligament
- Maxillary artery
- Medial pterygoid

B. Lateral View

- **TMJ** { Joint capsule / Lateral ligament }
- **Stylomandibular ligament**
- Angle of mandible

C. Medial View

- Spine of sphenoid
- Styloid process
- **Sphenomandibular ligament**
- **Stylomandibular ligament**
- Angle of mandible

7.55   TEMPOROMANDIBULAR JOINT

A. Coronal section. **B.** Temporomandibular joint and stylomandibular ligament. The joint capsule of the temporomandibular joint attaches to the margins of the mandibular fossa and articular tubercle of the temporal bone and around the neck of the mandible; the lateral (temporomandibular) ligament strengthens the lateral aspect of the joint. **C.** Stylomandibular and sphenomandibular ligaments. The strong sphenomandibular ligament descends from near the spine of the sphenoid to the lingula of the mandible and is the "swinging hinge" by which the mandible is suspended; the weaker stylomandibular ligament is a thickened part of the parotid sheath that joins the styloid process to the angle of the mandible.

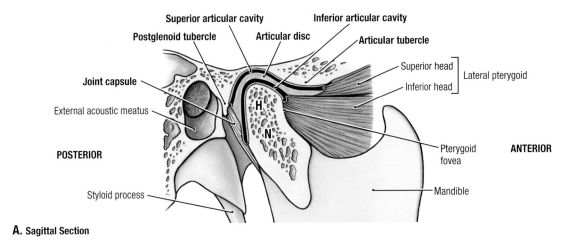

Superior articular cavity   Inferior articular cavity

Postglenoid tubercle   Articular disc   Articular tubercle

Superior head ⎱ Lateral pterygoid
Inferior head ⎰

Joint capsule

External acoustic meatus

H

N

POSTERIOR

Pterygoid fovea   ANTERIOR

Styloid process

Mandible

A. Sagittal Section

Mandibular fossa
of temporal bone (M)

**Posterior and anterior
bands of articular disc (AD)**

Articular
tubercle (AT)

Postglenoid
tubercle

Of condylar
process of ⎱ Head (H)
mandible ⎰ Neck (N)

Joint capsule

Lateral
pterygoid

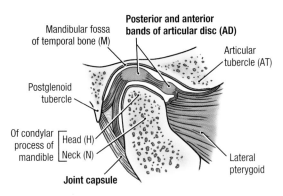

B. Closed Mouth, Sagittal Section

Sagittal CT

Sagittal MRI

Mandibular fossa
of temporal bone (M)

**Posterior and anterior
bands of articular disc (AD)**

Articular
tubercle (AT)

Postglenoid
tubercle

Of condylar
process of ⎱ Head (H)
mandible ⎰ Neck (N)

Joint capsule

Lateral
pterygoid

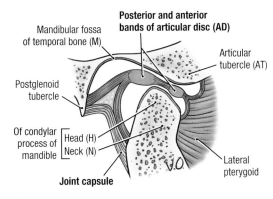

C. Open Mouth, Sagittal Section

Sagittal CT

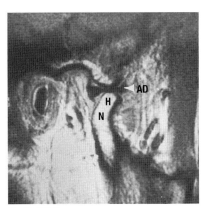

Sagittal MRI

7.56   SECTIONAL ANATOMY OF TEMPOROMANDIBULAR JOINT

A. TMJ and related structures, sagittal section. **B.** Sagittal orientation figure, CT, and MRI—mouth closed.
C. Sagittal orientation figure, CT, and MRI—mouth opened widely. The articular disc divides the articular cavity
into superior and inferior compartments, each lined by a separate synovial membrane.

Dislocation of mandible. During yawning or taking large bites, excessive contraction of the lateral
pterygoids can cause the head of the mandible to dislocate (pass anterior to the articular tubercle). In
this position, the mouth remains wide open, and the person cannot close it without manual distraction.

A. Superior View

- Epiglottis
- Palatopharyngeus
- Palatine tonsil
- Palatoglossus
- Palatoglossal arch
- Lingual nodules of **lingual tonsil**
- **Foramen cecum**
- **Terminal sulcus**
- **Root of tongue**
- Vallate
- Foliate
- Midline groove of tongue
- Filiform
- **Lingual papillae**
- **Body of tongue**
- Fungiform
- Apex

B. Superior View

- Internal branch of superior laryngeal nerve
- Glossopharyngeal nerve (CN IX, general and special sensory)
- Palatoglossus (vagus nerve, CN X)
- Overlapping nerve supply
- All other muscles of tongue (hypoglossal nerve, CN XII)
- Lingual nerve (CN V₃, general sensory)
- Chorda tympani (CN VII, special sensory)
- **Motor nerves**
- **Sensory nerves**

C. Superior View

- To superior deep cervical lymph nodes
- To inferior deep cervical lymph nodes
- To submandibular lymph nodes
- To submental lymph nodes

D. Lateral View

- Internal jugular vein (IJV)

Retropharyngeal	Submental
Deep cervical	Submandibular
Jugulo-omohyoid	Infrahyoid
Jugulodigastric	

7.57   TONGUE

A. Features of dorsum of the tongue. The foramen cecum is the upper end of the primitive thyroglossal duct; the arms of the V-shaped terminal sulcus diverge from the foramen, demarcating the posterior third of the tongue from the anterior two thirds. **B.** General sensory, special sensory (taste), and motor innervation of tongue. **C.** Lymphatic drainage of dorsum of tongue. **D.** Lymphatic drainage of tongue, mouth, nasal cavity, and nose.

Carcinoma of tongue. Malignant tumors in the posterior part of the tongue metastasize to the superior deep cervical lymph nodes on both sides. In contrast, tumors in the apex and anterolateral parts usually do not metastasize to the inferior deep cervical nodes until late in the disease. Because the deep nodes are closely related to the internal jugular vein, metastases from the carcinoma may spread to the submental and submandibular regions and along the IJV into the neck.

Gag reflex. One may touch the anterior part of the tongue without feeling discomfort; however, when the posterior part is touched, one usually gags. CN IX and CN X are responsible for the muscular contraction of each side of the pharynx. Glossopharyngeal branches (CN IX) provide the afferent limb of the gag reflex.

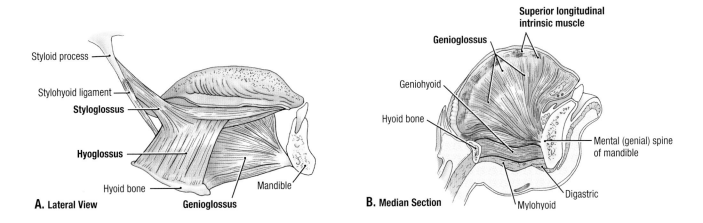

A. Lateral View

B. Median Section

C. Coronal Section

7.58 MUSCLES OF TONGUE

The extrinsic muscles of the tongue originate outside the tongue and attach to it, whereas the intrinsic muscles have their attachments entirely within the tongue and are not attached to bone.

TABLE 7.13 MUSCLES OF TONGUE

Extrinsic Muscles				
Muscle	**Origin**	**Insertion**	**Innervation**	**Main Action**
Genioglossus	Superior part of mental spine of mandible	Dorsum of tongue and body of hyoid bone	Hypoglossal nerve (CN XII)	Depresses tongue; its posterior part pulls tonguew anteriorly for protrusion[a]
Hyoglossus	Body and greater horn of hyoid bone	Side and inferior aspect of tongue		Depresses and retracts tongue
Styloglossus	Styloid process of temporal bone and stylohyoid ligament	Side and inferior aspect of tongue		Retracts tongue and draws it up to create a trough for swallowing
Palatoglossus	Palatine aponeurosis of soft palate	Side of tongue	CN X and pharyngeal plexus	Elevates posterior part of tongue plexus

Intrinsic Muscles				
Muscle	**Origin**	**Insertion**	**Innervation**	**Main Action**
Superior longitudinal	Submucous fibrous layer and lingual septum	Margins and mucous membrane of tongue	Hypoglossal nerve (CN XII)	Curls tip and sides of tongue superiorly and shortens tongue
Inferior longitudinal	Root of tongue and body of hyoid bone	Apex of tongue		Curls tip of tongue inferiorly and shortens tongue
Transverse	Lingual septum	Fibrous tissue at margins of tongue		Narrows and elongates the tongue[a]
Vertical	Superior surface of borders of tongue	Inferior surface of borders of tongue		Flattens and broadens the tongue[a]

[a]Acts simultaneously to protrude tongue.

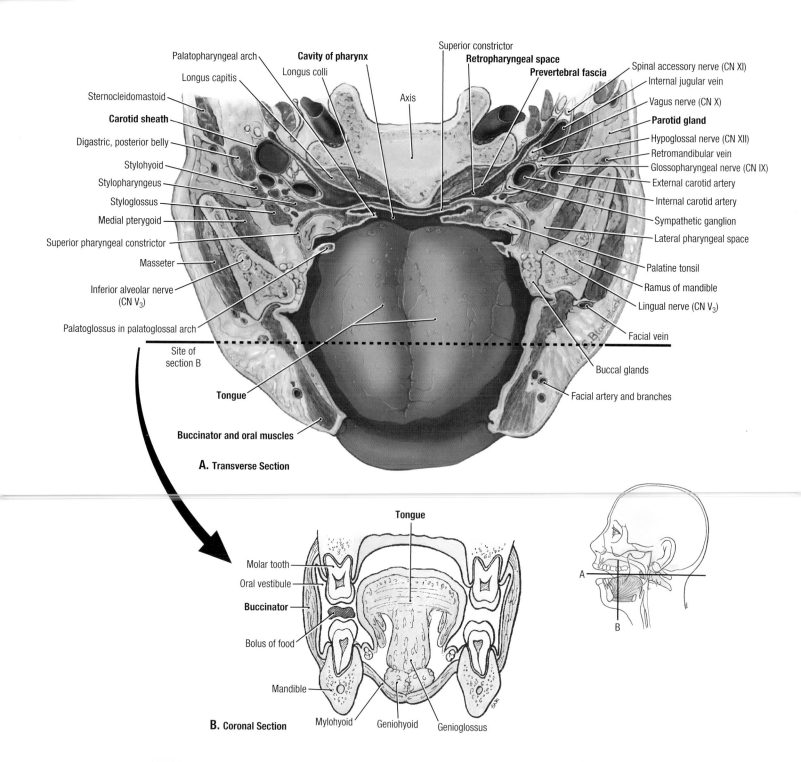

Palatopharyngeal arch
Longus capitis
Sternocleidomastoid
Carotid sheath
Digastric, posterior belly
Stylohyoid
Stylopharyngeus
Styloglossus
Medial pterygoid
Superior pharyngeal constrictor
Masseter
Inferior alveolar nerve (CN V₃)
Palatoglossus in palatoglossal arch
Site of section B
Tongue
Buccinator and oral muscles

Cavity of pharynx
Longus colli
Axis

Superior constrictor
Retropharyngeal space
Prevertebral fascia

Spinal accessory nerve (CN XI)
Internal jugular vein
Vagus nerve (CN X)
Parotid gland
Hypoglossal nerve (CN XII)
Retromandibular vein
Glossopharyngeal nerve (CN IX)
External carotid artery
Internal carotid artery
Sympathetic ganglion
Lateral pharyngeal space
Palatine tonsil
Ramus of mandible
Lingual nerve (CN V₃)
Facial vein
Buccal glands
Facial artery and branches

A. Transverse Section

Tongue
Molar tooth
Oral vestibule
Buccinator
Bolus of food
Mandible
Mylohyoid   Geniohyoid   Genioglossus

B. Coronal Section

7.59   SECTIONS THROUGH MOUTH

A. The viscerocranium has been sectioned at the C1 vertebral level, the plane of section passing through the oral fissure anteriorly. The retropharyngeal space (opened up in this specimen) allows the pharynx to contract and relax during swallowing; the retropharyngeal space is closed laterally at the carotid sheath and limited posteriorly by the prevertebral fascia. The beds of the parotid glands are also demonstrated. **B.** Schematic coronal section demonstrating how the tongue and buccinator (or, anteriorly, the orbicularis oris) work together to retain food between the teeth when chewing. The buccinator and superior part of the orbicularis oris are innervated by the buccal branch of the facial nerve (CN VII).

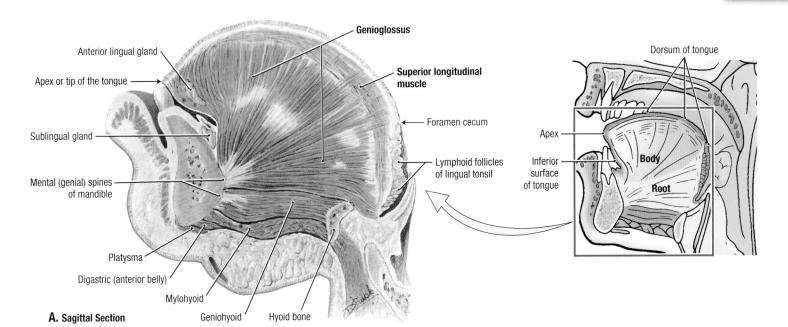

A. Sagittal Section

Anterior lingual gland

Apex or tip of the tongue

Sublingual gland

Mental (genial) spines of mandible

Platysma

Digastric (anterior belly)

Mylohyoid

Geniohyoid

Hyoid bone

Genioglossus

Superior longitudinal muscle

Foramen cecum

Lymphoid follicles of lingual tonsil

Dorsum of tongue

Apex

Inferior surface of tongue

Body

Root

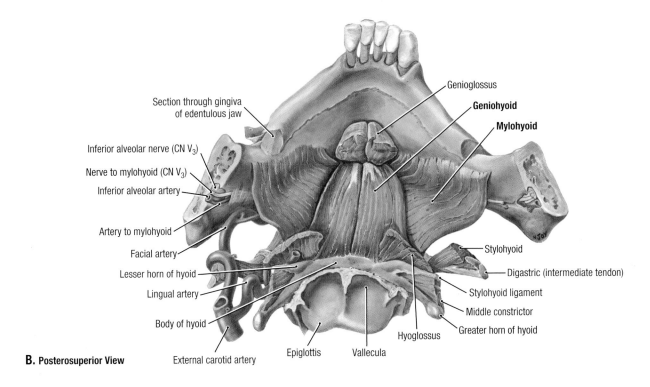

Section through gingiva of edentulous jaw

Inferior alveolar nerve (CN V₃)

Nerve to mylohyoid (CN V₃)

Inferior alveolar artery

Artery to mylohyoid

Facial artery

Lesser horn of hyoid

Lingual artery

Body of hyoid

External carotid artery

Epiglottis

Vallecula

Hyoglossus

Greater horn of hyoid

Middle constrictor

Stylohyoid ligament

Digastric (intermediate tendon)

Stylohyoid

Mylohyoid

Geniohyoid

Genioglossus

B. Posterosuperior View

7.60   **TONGUE AND FLOOR OF MOUTH**

A. Median section though the tongue and lower jaw. The tongue is composed mainly of muscle; extrinsic muscles alter the position of the tongue, and intrinsic muscles alter its shape. The genioglossus is the extrinsic muscle apparent in this plane, and the superior longitudinal muscle is the intrinsic muscle. **B.** Muscles of the floor of the mouth viewed posterosuperiorly. The mylohyoid muscle extends between the two mylohyoid lines of the mandible. It has a thick, free posterior border and becomes thinner anteriorly.

Genioglossus paralysis. When the genioglossus is paralyzed, the tongue mass has a tendency to shift posteriorly, obstructing the airway and presenting the risk of suffocation. Total relaxation of the genioglossus muscles occurs during general anesthesia; therefore, the tongue of an anesthetized patient must be prevented from relapsing by inserting an airway.

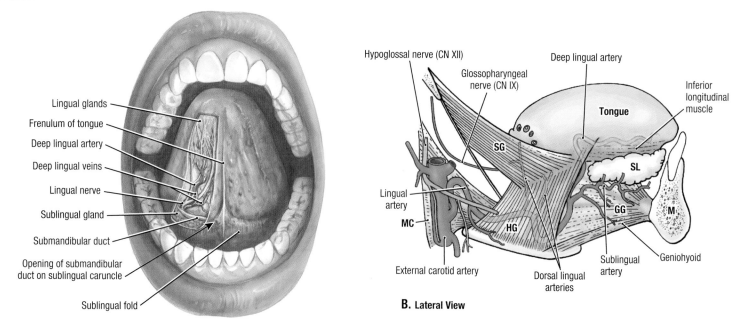

Lingual glands

Frenulum of tongue

Deep lingual artery

Deep lingual veins

Lingual nerve

Sublingual gland

Submandibular duct

Opening of submandibular duct on sublingual caruncle

Sublingual fold

A. Anterior View

Hypoglossal nerve (CN XII)

Glossopharyngeal nerve (CN IX)

Deep lingual artery

Inferior longitudinal muscle

Tongue

SG

Lingual artery

SL

MC

HG

GG

M

External carotid artery

Dorsal lingual arteries

Sublingual artery

Geniohyoid

B. Lateral View

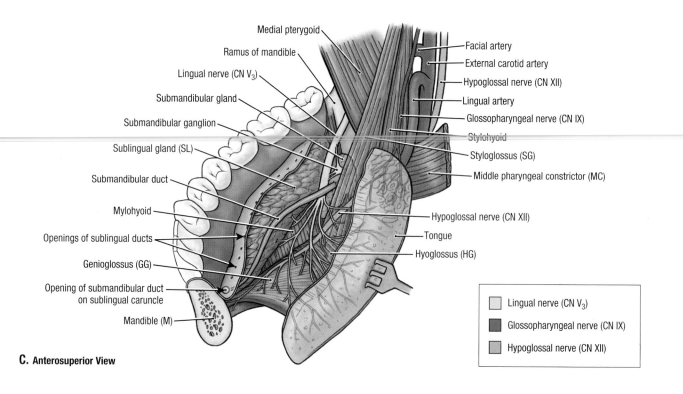

Medial pterygoid

Ramus of mandible

Lingual nerve (CN V₃)

Submandibular gland

Submandibular ganglion

Sublingual gland (SL)

Submandibular duct

Mylohyoid

Openings of sublingual ducts

Genioglossus (GG)

Opening of submandibular duct on sublingual caruncle

Mandible (M)

Facial artery

External carotid artery

Hypoglossal nerve (CN XII)

Lingual artery

Glossopharyngeal nerve (CN IX)

Stylohyoid

Styloglossus (SG)

Middle pharyngeal constrictor (MC)

Hypoglossal nerve (CN XII)

Tongue

Hyoglossus (HG)

Lingual nerve (CN V₃)

Glossopharyngeal nerve (CN IX)

Hypoglossal nerve (CN XII)

C. Anterosuperior View

7.61   ARTERIES AND NERVES OF THE TONGUE

A. Inferior surface of the tongue and floor of the mouth. The thin sublingual mucosa has been removed on the left side. **B.** Course and distribution of the lingual artery. **C.** Dissection of right side of floor of mouth. Letters in parentheses refer to **B**.

Sialography. The parotid and submandibular salivary glands may be examined radiographically after the injection of a contrast medium into their ducts. This special type of radiograph (sialogram) demonstrates the salivary ducts and some secretory units. Because of the small size and number of sublingual ducts of the sublingual glands, one cannot usually inject contrast medium into them.

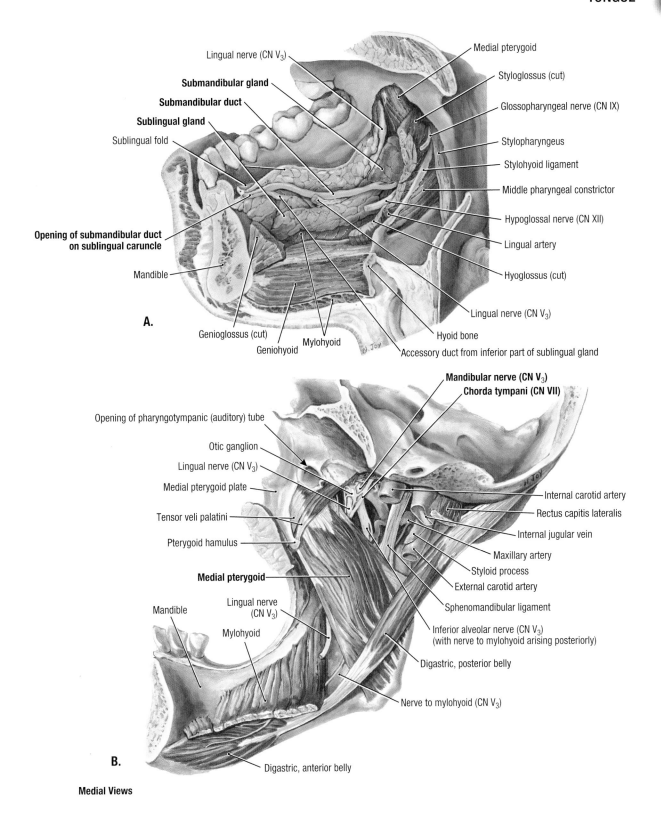

Lingual nerve (CN V₃)
Submandibular gland
Submandibular duct
Sublingual gland
Sublingual fold
Opening of submandibular duct on sublingual caruncle
Mandible
Genioglossus (cut)
Geniohyoid
Mylohyoid

Medial pterygoid
Styloglossus (cut)
Glossopharyngeal nerve (CN IX)
Stylopharyngeus
Stylohyoid ligament
Middle pharyngeal constrictor
Hypoglossal nerve (CN XII)
Lingual artery
Hyoglossus (cut)
Lingual nerve (CN V₃)
Hyoid bone
Accessory duct from inferior part of sublingual gland

A.

Mandibular nerve (CN V₃)
Chorda tympani (CN VII)

Opening of pharyngotympanic (auditory) tube
Otic ganglion
Lingual nerve (CN V₃)
Medial pterygoid plate
Tensor veli palatini
Pterygoid hamulus
Medial pterygoid
Mandible
Lingual nerve (CN V₃)
Mylohyoid

Internal carotid artery
Rectus capitis lateralis
Internal jugular vein
Maxillary artery
Styloid process
External carotid artery
Sphenomandibular ligament
Inferior alveolar nerve (CN V₃) (with nerve to mylohyoid arising posteriorly)
Digastric, posterior belly
Nerve to mylohyoid (CN V₃)

B.
Digastric, anterior belly

Medial Views

7.62

MUSCLES, GLANDS, AND VESSELS OF FLOOR OF MOUTH AND MEDIAL ASPECT OF MANDIBLE

A. Sublingual and submandibular glands. The tongue has been excised. **B.** Structures related to the medial surface of the mandible. The otic ganglion lies medial to the mandibular nerve (CN V₃) and between the foramen ovale superiorly and the medial pterygoid muscle inferiorly.

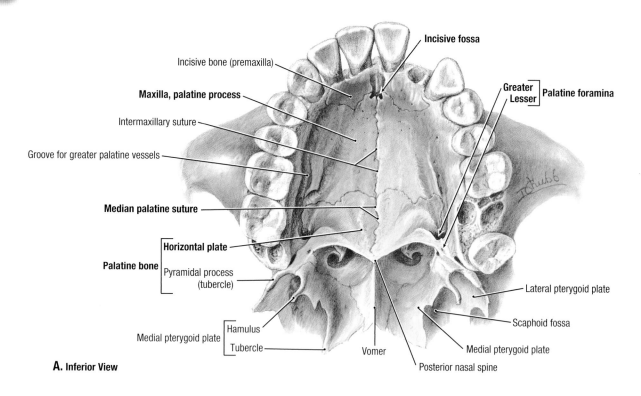

Incisive fossa

Incisive bone (premaxilla)

Maxilla, palatine process

Intermaxillary suture

Groove for greater palatine vessels

Greater
Lesser **Palatine foramina**

Median palatine suture

Horizontal plate

Palatine bone

Pyramidal process
(tubercle)

Lateral pterygoid plate

Scaphoid fossa

Medial pterygoid plate | Hamulus

Tubercle

Vomer

Medial pterygoid plate

Posterior nasal spine

A. Inferior View

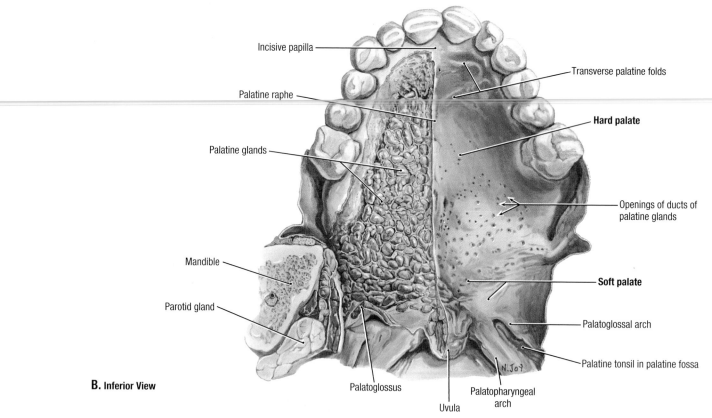

Incisive papilla

Transverse palatine folds

Palatine raphe

Hard palate

Palatine glands

Openings of ducts of
palatine glands

Mandible

Parotid gland

Soft palate

Palatoglossal arch

Palatine tonsil in palatine fossa

B. Inferior View

Palatoglossus

Palatopharyngeal
arch

Uvula

7.63   PALATE

A. Bones of the hard palate. The palatine aponeurosis, which forms the fibrous "skeleton" of the soft palate,
stretches between the hamuli of the medial pterygoid plates. **B.** Mucous membrane and glands of palate.

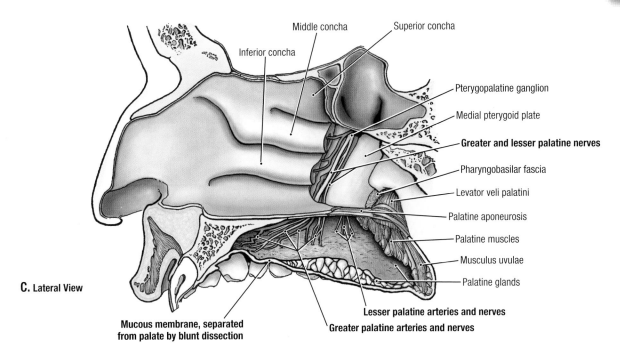

Middle concha
Superior concha
Inferior concha
Pterygopalatine ganglion
Medial pterygoid plate
Greater and lesser palatine nerves
Pharyngobasilar fascia
Levator veli palatini
Palatine aponeurosis
Palatine muscles
Musculus uvulae
Palatine glands

C. Lateral View

Mucous membrane, separated
from palate by blunt dissection

Lesser palatine arteries and nerves
Greater palatine arteries and nerves

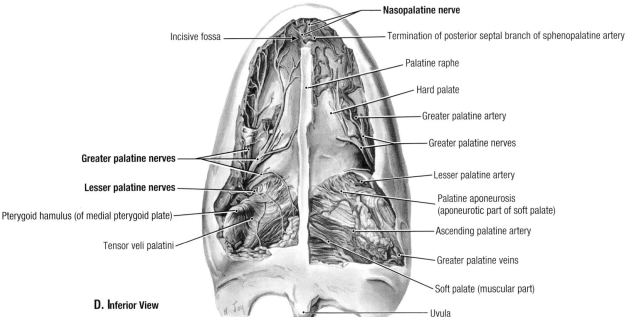

Nasopalatine nerve
Incisive fossa
Termination of posterior septal branch of sphenopalatine artery
Palatine raphe
Hard palate
Greater palatine artery
Greater palatine nerves
Greater palatine nerves
Lesser palatine artery
Lesser palatine nerves
Palatine aponeurosis
(aponeurotic part of soft palate)
Pterygoid hamulus (of medial pterygoid plate)
Ascending palatine artery
Tensor veli palatini
Greater palatine veins
Soft palate (muscular part)
D. Inferior View
Uvula

| 7.63 | **PALATE** *(CONTINUED)* |

C. Nerves and vessels of palatine canal. The lateral wall of the nasal cavity is shown. The posterior ends of the middle and inferior conchae are excised along with the mucoperiosteum; the thin, perpendicular plate of the palatine bone is removed to expose the palatine nerves and arteries. **D.** Dissection of an edentulous palate. The greater palatine nerve supplies the gingivae and hard palate, the nasopalatine nerve the incisive region, and the lesser palatine nerves the soft palate. **Anesthesia of palatine nerves.** The nasopalatine nerves can be anesthetized by injecting anesthetic into the mouth of the incisive fossa in the hard palate. The anesthetized tissues are the palatal mucosa, the lingual gingivae, the six anterior maxillary teeth, and associated alveolar bone. The greater palatine nerve can be anesthetized by injecting anesthetic into the greater palatine foramen. The nerve emerges between the second and third maxillary molar teeth. This nerve block anesthetizes the palatal mucosa and lingual gingivae posterior to the maxillary canine teeth, and the underlying bone of the palate.

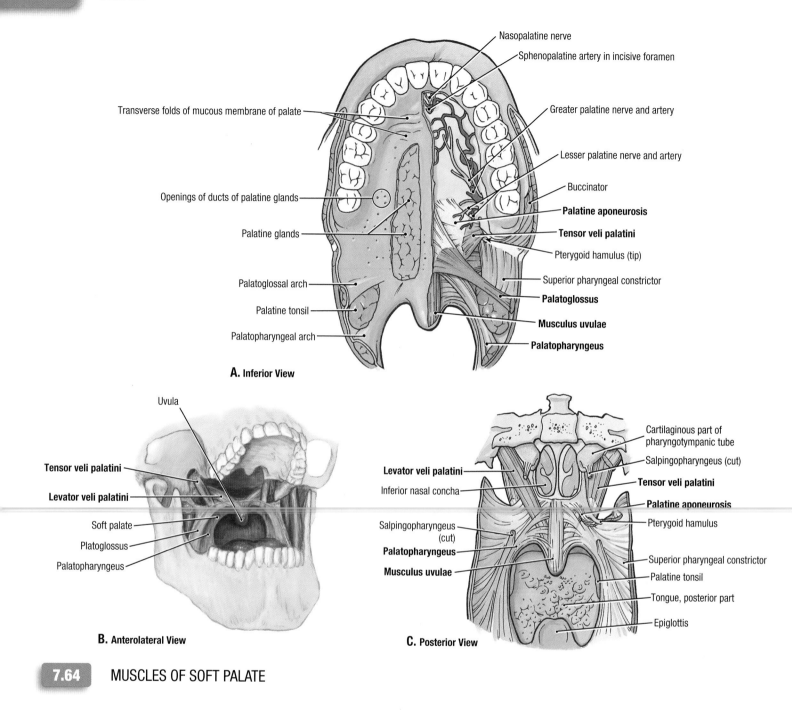

Nasopalatine nerve

Sphenopalatine artery in incisive foramen

Transverse folds of mucous membrane of palate

Greater palatine nerve and artery

Lesser palatine nerve and artery

Buccinator

Openings of ducts of palatine glands

Palatine aponeurosis

Tensor veli palatini

Palatine glands

Pterygoid hamulus (tip)

Superior pharyngeal constrictor

Palatoglossal arch

Palatoglossus

Palatine tonsil

Musculus uvulae

Palatopharyngeal arch

Palatopharyngeus

A. Inferior View

Uvula

Tensor veli palatini

Levator veli palatini

Soft palate

Platoglossus

Palatopharyngeus

B. Anterolateral View

Cartilaginous part of pharyngotympanic tube

Salpingopharyngeus (cut)

Levator veli palatini

Inferior nasal concha

Tensor veli palatini

Palatine aponeurosis

Salpingopharyngeus (cut)

Pterygoid hamulus

Palatopharyngeus

Superior pharyngeal constrictor

Musculus uvulae

Palatine tonsil

Tongue, posterior part

Epiglottis

C. Posterior View

7.64   MUSCLES OF SOFT PALATE

TABLE 7.14 MUSCLES OF SOFT PALATE

Muscle	Superior Attachment	Inferior Attachment	Innervation	Main Action(s)
Levator veli palatini	Cartilage of pharyngotympanic tube and petrous part of temporal bone		Pharyngeal branch of vagus nerve through pharyngeal plexus	Elevates soft palate during swallowing and yawning
Tensor veli palatini	Scaphoid fossa of medial pterygoid plate, spine of sphenoid bone, and cartilage of pharyngotympanic tube	Palatine aponeurosis	Medial pterygoid nerve (CN V$_3$) through otic ganglion	Tenses soft palate and opens mouth of pharyngotympanic tube during swallowing and yawning
Palatoglossus	Palatine aponeurosis	Side of tongue		Elevates posterior part of tongue and draws soft palate onto tongue
Palatopharyngeus	Hard palate and palatine aponeurosis	Lateral wall of pharynx	Pharyngeal branch of vagus nerve (CN X) via pharyngeal plexus	Tenses soft palate and pulls walls of pharynx superiorly, anteriorly, and medially during swallowing
Musculus uvulae	Posterior nasal spine and palatine aponeurosis	Mucosa of uvula		Shortens uvula and pulls it superiorly

A. Lateral View

B. Lateral Radiograph

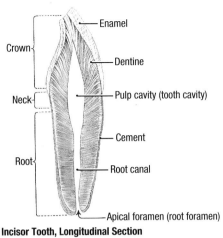

Incisor Tooth, Longitudinal Section

- Enamel
- Crown
- Dentine
- Pulp cavity (tooth cavity)
- Neck
- Cement
- Root
- Root canal
- Apical foramen (root foramen)

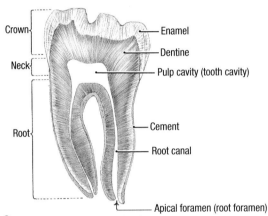

C. Molar Tooth, Longitudinal Section

- Crown
- Enamel
- Dentine
- Neck
- Pulp cavity (tooth cavity)
- Root
- Cement
- Root canal
- Apical foramen (root foramen)

D. Pantomographic Radiograph

7.65

PERMANENT TEETH I

A. Teeth in situ with roots exposed. Incisors *(I1, I2)*, canine *(C1)*, premolars *(PM1, PM2)*, and molars *(M1, M2, M3)*. The roots of the 2nd lower molar have been removed. **B.** Lateral radiograph. *(1)* enamel, *(2)* dentin, *(3)* pulp chamber, *(4)* pulp canal, *(5)* buccal cusp, *(6)* alveolar bone, and *(7)* root apex. **C.** Longitudinal sections of an incisor and a molar tooth. **D.** Pantomographic radiograph of mandible and maxilla. The left lower third molar is not present.

Decay of the hard tissues of a tooth results in the formation of **dental caries** (cavities). Invasion of the pulp of the tooth by a carious lesion (cavity) results in infection and irritation of the tissues in the pulp cavity. This condition causes an inflammatory process (pulpitis). Because the pulp cavity is a rigid space, the swollen pulpal tissues cause pain (toothache).

A. Vestibular View

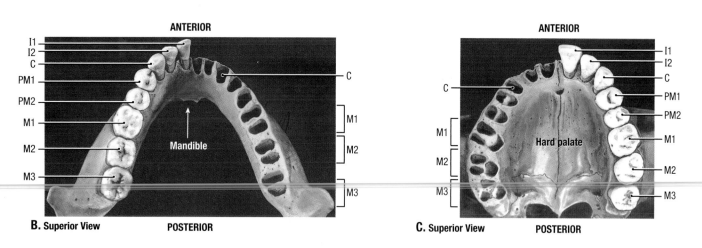

B. Superior View   POSTERIOR

C. Superior View   POSTERIOR

D. Anterolateral View

E. Anterior View

7.66   PERMANENT TEETH II

A. Removed teeth, displaying roots. There are 32 permanent teeth; 8 are on each side of each dental arch on the top (maxillary teeth) and bottom (mandibular teeth): 2 incisors *(I1–2)*, 1 canine *(C)*, 2 premolars *(PM1–2)*, and 3 molars *(M1–3)*. **B.** Permanent mandibular teeth and their sockets. **C.** Permanent maxillary teeth and their sockets. **D.** Teeth in occlusion. **E.** Vestibule and gingivae of the maxilla

A. Lateral view

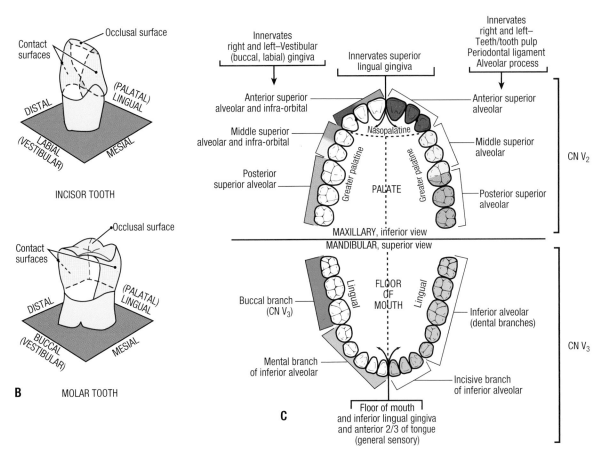

INCISOR TOOTH

B   MOLAR TOOTH

MAXILLARY, inferior view

MANDIBULAR, superior view

C

Floor of mouth
and inferior lingual gingiva
and anterior 2/3 of tongue
(general sensory)

7.67   INNERVATION OF TEETH

A. Superior and inferior alveolar nerves. **B.** Surfaces of an incisor and molar tooth. **C.** Innervation of the mouth and teeth.

Improper oral hygiene results in food deposits in tooth and gingival crevices, which may cause inflammation of the gingivae, **gingivitis**. If untreated, the disease spreads to other supporting structures (including the alveolar bone), producing **periodontitis**. Periodontitis results in inflammation of the gingivae and may result in absorption of alveolar bone and gingival recession. Gingival recession exposes the sensitive cement of the teeth.

MAXILLARY TEETH

MANDIBULAR TEETH

A. Vestibular View

2nd molar   1st molar   Canine   Lateral incisor   Central incisor

INFERIOR VIEW OF MAXILLARY TEETH

Hard palate

SUPERIOR VIEW OF MANDIBULAR TEETH

Mandible

B

M1
M2
Socket for M1
Canine
Alveolus for permanent incisor
Central and lateral incisors
Canine
M1
M2
M1
M2

7.68   PRIMARY TEETH

A. Removed teeth. There are 20 primary (deciduous) teeth, 5 in each half of the mandible and 5 in each maxilla. They are named central incisor, lateral incisor, canine, 1st molar *(M1)*, and 2nd molar *(M2)*. Primary teeth differ from permanent teeth in that the primary teeth are smaller and whiter; the molars also have more bulbous crowns and more divergent roots. **B.** Teeth in situ, younger than 2 years of age. Permanent teeth are colored orange; the crowns of the unerupted first and second permanent molars are partly visible.

TABLE 7.15 PRIMARY AND SECONDARY DENTITION

Deciduous Teeth	Central Incisor	Lateral Incisor	Canine	First Molar	Second Molar
Eruption (months)[a]	6–8	8–10	16–20	12–16	20–24
Shedding (years)	6–7	7–8	10–12	9–11	10–12

[a]In some normal infants, the first teeth (medial incisors) may not erupt until 12 to 13 months of age

Age: 6–7 years

The 1st molars (6-year molars) have fully erupted, the primary central incisor has been shed, the lower central incisor is almost fully erupted, and the upper central incisor is descending into the vacated socket.

Age: 8 years

All of the permanent incisors have erupted; however, the lower lateral incisor is only partially erupted.

Age: 12 years

The primary teeth have been replaced by 20 permanent teeth, and the 1st and 2nd molars (12-year molars) have erupted; the canines, 2nd premolars, and 2nd molars (especially those in the upper jaw) have not erupted fully, nor have their bony sockets closed around them. By age 12, 28 permanent teeth are in evidence; the last 4 teeth, the 3rd molars, may erupt any time after this, or never.

Permanent Teeth	Central Incisor	Lateral Incisor	Canine	First Premolar	Second Premolar	First Molar	Second Molar	Third Molar
Eruption (years)	7–8	8–9	10–12	10–11	11–12	6–7	12	13–25

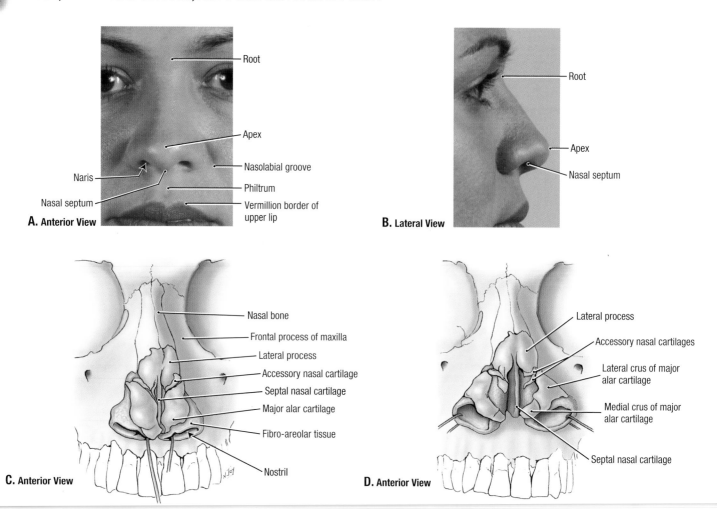

A. Anterior View

Root

Apex

Nasolabial groove

Naris

Philtrum

Nasal septum

Vermillion border of upper lip

B. Lateral View

Root

Apex

Nasal septum

Nasal bone

Frontal process of maxilla

Lateral process

Accessory nasal cartilage

Septal nasal cartilage

Major alar cartilage

Fibro-areolar tissue

Nostril

C. Anterior View

Lateral process

Accessory nasal cartilages

Lateral crus of major alar cartilage

Medial crus of major alar cartilage

Septal nasal cartilage

D. Anterior View

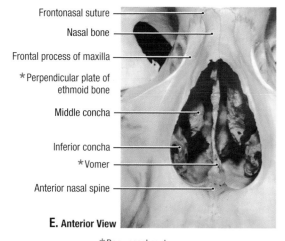

Frontonasal suture

Nasal bone

Frontal process of maxilla

*Perpendicular plate of ethmoid bone

Middle concha

Inferior concha

*Vomer

Anterior nasal spine

E. Anterior View

*Bony nasal septum

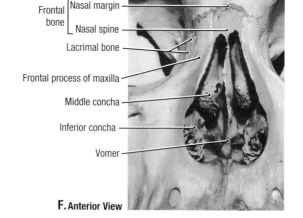

Frontal bone { Nasal margin

Nasal spine

Lacrimal bone

Frontal process of maxilla

Middle concha

Inferior concha

Vomer

F. Anterior View

7.69   SURFACE ANATOMY, CARTILAGES, AND BONES OF NOSE

A. Surface features of anterior aspect of nose. **B.** Surface features of lateral aspect of nose. **C.** Nasal cartilages, with the septum pulled inferiorly. **D.** Nasal cartilages, separated and retracted laterally. **E.** Lower conchae and bony septum seen through the piriform aperture. The margin of the piriform aperture is sharp and formed by the maxillae and nasal bones. **F.** Nasal bones removed. The areas of the frontal processes of the maxillae (yellow) and of the frontal bone (blue) that articulate with the nasal bones can be seen.

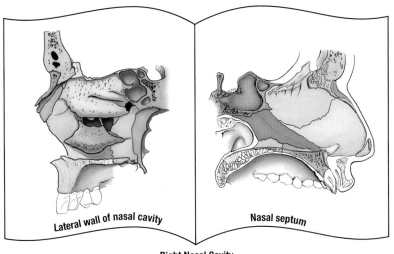

Lateral wall of nasal cavity   Nasal septum

Right Nasal Cavity

ANTERIOR   POSTERIOR

Frontal sinus
Nasal spine
Superior concha
Superior meatus
Middle concha
Frontal process
Middle meatus
Inferior concha
Inferior meatus
Anterior nasal spine

Cribriform plate

Sphenopalatine foramen
Pterygoid tubercle
Perpendicular plate of palatine
Pterygoid spine
Medial pterygoid plate
Horizontal plate
Pterygoid hamulus
Lesser } Palatine foramina
Greater

Bones:
- Ethmoid
- Frontal
- Inferior concha
- Lacrimal
- Maxilla
- Nasal
- Palatine
- Sphenoid
- Vomer

Other tissue:
- Lateral wall of maxillary sinus
- Nasal cartilage

A. Medial View of Lateral Wall

Crista galli
Sphenoidal crest
Perpendicular plate
Nasal spine of frontal bone
Septal nasal cartilage
Major alar cartilage, medial crus
Vomeronasal cartilage
Nasal crest
Anterior nasal spine

B. Lateral View of Nasal Septum

7.70   BONES OF THE NASAL WALL AND SEPTUM

A. Lateral wall of nose. The superior and middle conchae are parts of the ethmoid bone, whereas the inferior concha is itself a bone. **B.** Nasal septum.

   Deformity of the external nose usually is present with a fracture, particularly when a lateral force is applied by someone's elbow, for example. When the injury results from a direct blow (e.g., from a hockey stick), the cribriform plate of the ethmoid bone may fracture, resulting in CSF rhinorrhea.

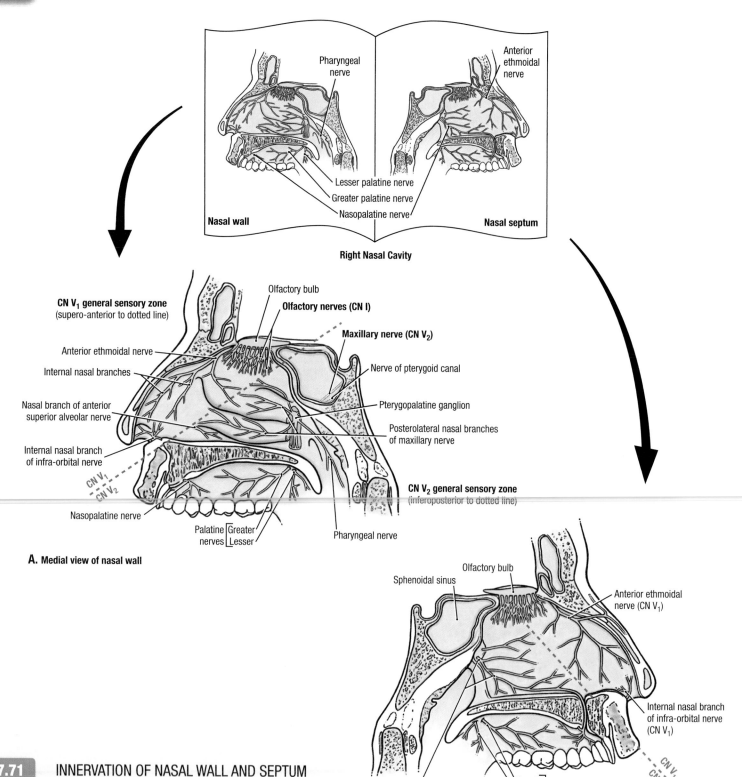

Right Nasal Cavity

A. Medial view of nasal wall

B. Lateral view of nasal septum

7.71   INNERVATION OF NASAL WALL AND SEPTUM

A. Lateral wall of nose. *Dashed diagonal lines* demarcate CN V_1 and CN V_2 general sensory zones. The olfactory neuroepithelium is in the superior part of the lateral and septal walls of the nasal cavity. The central processes of the olfactory neurosensory cells of each side form approximately 20 bundles that together form an olfactory nerve (CN I). **B.** Nasal septum. The nasopalatine nerve from the pterygopalatine ganglion supplies the posteroinferior septum, and the anterior ethmoidal nerve (branch of V_1) supplies the anterosuperior septum.

Posterior ethmoidal arteries

Anterior ethmoidal arteries

Sphenopalatine artery traversing sphenopalatine foramen

Maxillary artery

Lateral nasal branches of facial artery

Greater palatine artery

Nasal wall

Branches of sphenopalatine artery

External
Internal
Common

Carotid artery

Posterior ethmoidal arteries

Anterior ethmoidal arteries

Kiesselbach area (orange)

Incisive canal

Nasal septal branch of superior labial branch

Greater palatine artery

Nasal septum

Frontal sinus

Anterior ethmoidal artery

Lateral nasal branches of anterior ethmoidal artery

Lateral nasal branches of posterior ethmoidal artery

Sphenoidal sinus

Posterior septal branch

Sphenopalatine artery in sphenopalatine foramen

Posterior lateral nasal arteries

Lateral nasal branches of facial artery

Ascending palatine artery

A. Medial View of nasal wall

Frontal sinus

Anterior ethmoidal artery

Posterior ethmoidal artery

Kiesselbach area

Sphenoidal sinus

Posterior septal branch of **sphenopalatine artery**

Nasal septal branch of superior labial branch

Greater palatine artery

Superior labial branch of facial artery

B. Lateral View of Nasal Septum

7.72 ARTERIES OF NASAL WALL AND SEPTUM

A. Lateral wall of nose. **B.** Nasal septum.

Epistaxis. On the anterior part of the nasal septum is an area rich in capillaries (Kiesselbach area) where all five arteries (sphenopalatine, anterior and posterior ethmoidal, greater palatine and superior labial and lateral nasal branches of the facial artery) supplying the nasal septum anastomose. This area is often where profuse bleeding from the nose (epistaxis) occurs.

Frontal sinus

Corpus callosum

Third ventricle

Superior concha

Midbrain

Ethmoidal crest of maxilla

Sphenoidal sinus

Middle concha

Hypophysis

Fourth ventricle

Atrium

Pons

Inferior concha

Basilar artery

Medulla oblongata

Atlas (C1 vertebra)

Nasal vestibule

Posterior cerebellomedullary cistern (cisterna magna)

Axis (C2 vertebra)

Inferior meatus

Middle meatus

Superior meatus

Spinal cord

Spheno-ethmoidal recess

Medial View

Pharyngeal opening of pharyngotympanic tube

7.73

RIGHT HALF OF HEMISECTED HEAD DEMONSTRATING UPPER RESPIRATORY TRACT

- The vestibule is superior to the nostril and anterior to the inferior meatus; hairs grow from its skin-lined surface. The atrium is superior to the vestibule and anterior to the middle meatus.
- The inferior and middle conchae curve inferiorly and medially from the lateral wall, dividing it into three nearly equal parts and covering the inferior and middle meatuses, respectively. The middle concha ends inferior to the sphenoidal sinus, and the inferior concha ends inferior to the middle concha, just anterior to the orifice of the auditory tube. The superior concha is small and anterior to the sphenoidal sinus.
- The roof comprises an anterior sloping part corresponding to the bridge of the nose; an intermediate horizontal part; a perpendicular part anterior to the sphenoidal sinus; and a curved part, inferior to the sinus, that is continuous with the roof of the nasopharynx.

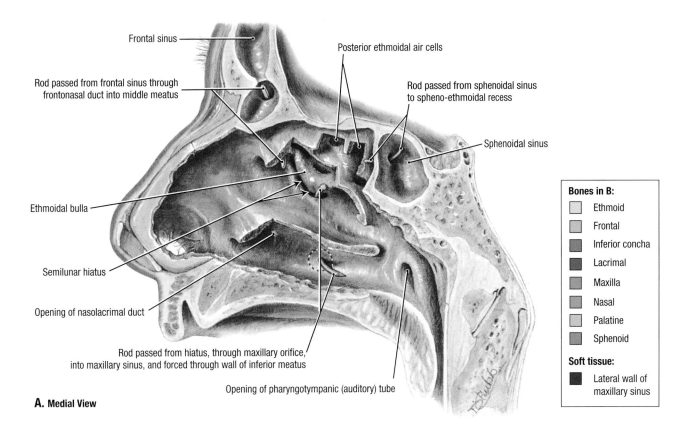

Frontal sinus

Rod passed from frontal sinus through frontonasal duct into middle meatus

Posterior ethmoidal air cells

Rod passed from sphenoidal sinus to spheno-ethmoidal recess

Sphenoidal sinus

Ethmoidal bulla

Semilunar hiatus

Opening of nasolacrimal duct

Rod passed from hiatus, through maxillary orifice, into maxillary sinus, and forced through wall of inferior meatus

Opening of pharyngotympanic (auditory) tube

A. Medial View

Bones in B:
- Ethmoid
- Frontal
- Inferior concha
- Lacrimal
- Maxilla
- Nasal
- Palatine
- Sphenoid

Soft tissue:
- Lateral wall of maxillary sinus

7.74

COMMUNICATIONS THROUGH NASAL WALL

A. Dissection. Parts of the superior, middle, and inferior conchae are cut away to reveal the openings of the air sinuses. **B.** Diagrams of the bones and openings of the lateral wall of nasal cavity following dissection. Note one *arrow* passing from the frontal sinus through the frontonasal duct into the middle meatus and another *arrow* coming from the anteromedial orbit via the nasolacrimal canal.

Rhinits. The nasal mucosa becomes swollen and inflamed (rhinitis) during upper respiratory infections and allergic reactions (e.g., hay fever). Swelling of this mucous membrane occurs readily because of its vascularity and abundant mucosal glands. Infections of the nasal cavities may spread to the anterior cranial fossa through the cribriform plate, nasopharynx and retropharyngeal soft tissues, middle ear through the pharyngotympanic (auditory) tube, paranasal sinuses, lacrimal apparatus, and conjunctiva.

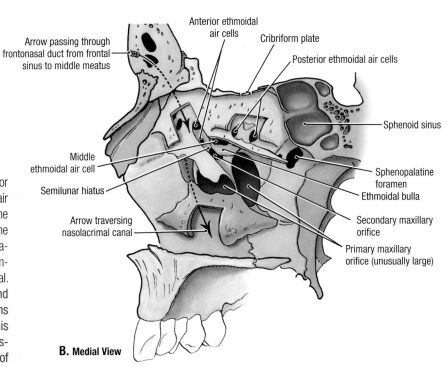

Arrow passing through frontonasal duct from frontal sinus to middle meatus

Anterior ethmoidal air cells

Cribriform plate

Posterior ethmoidal air cells

Sphenoid sinus

Middle ethmoidal air cell

Semilunar hiatus

Arrow traversing nasolacrimal canal

Sphenopalatine foramen

Ethmoidal bulla

Secondary maxillary orifice

Primary maxillary orifice (unusually large)

B. Medial View

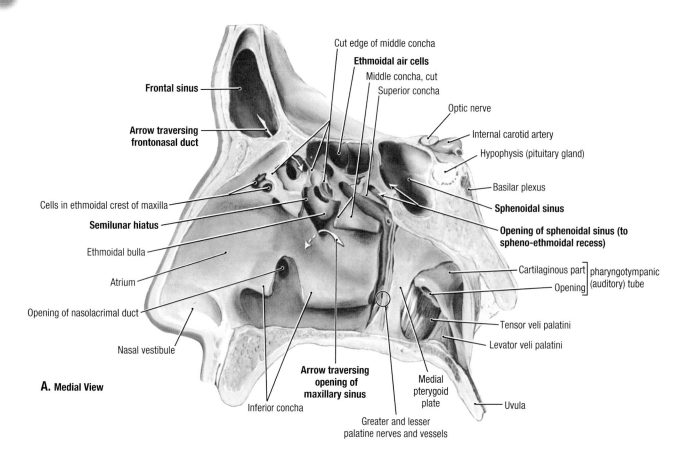

A. Medial View

Cut edge of middle concha
Ethmoidal air cells
Middle concha, cut
Superior concha
Optic nerve
Internal carotid artery
Hypophysis (pituitary gland)
Basilar plexus
Sphenoidal sinus
Opening of sphenoidal sinus (to spheno-ethmoidal recess)
Cartilaginous part ⎤ pharyngotympanic
Opening ⎦ (auditory) tube
Tensor veli palatini
Levator veli palatini
Uvula
Medial pterygoid plate
Greater and lesser palatine nerves and vessels
Arrow traversing opening of maxillary sinus
Inferior concha
Nasal vestibule
Opening of nasolacrimal duct
Atrium
Ethmoidal bulla
Semilunar hiatus
Cells in ethmoidal crest of maxilla
Arrow traversing frontonasal duct
Frontal sinus

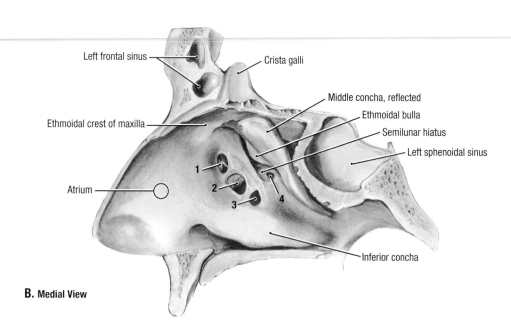

B. Medial View

Left frontal sinus
Crista galli
Middle concha, reflected
Ethmoidal bulla
Semilunar hiatus
Left sphenoidal sinus
Ethmoidal crest of maxilla
Atrium
Inferior concha
1
2
3
4

7.75 PARANASAL SINUSES, OPENINGS, AND PALATINE MUSCLES IN NASAL WALL

A. Dissection. Parts of the middle and inferior conchae and lateral wall of the nasal cavity are cut away to expose the nerves and vessels in the palatine canal and the extrinsic palatine muscles. **B.** Accessory maxillary orifices. In addition to the primary, or normal, ostium (not shown), there are four secondary, or acquired, ostia (numbered 1 to 4).

A. Posterior View

B. Posterior View

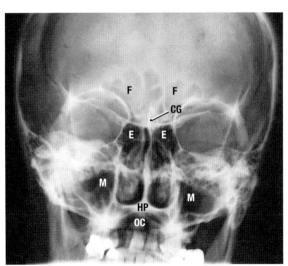

C. Anteroposterior View

7.76   PARANASAL SINUSES AND NASAL CAVITY

A. Coronal section of right side of the head. **B.** CT scan. **C.** Radiograph of cranium. Letters in **B** and **C** refer to structures labeled in **A**.

If nasal drainage is blocked, **infections of the ethmoidal cells** of the ethmoidal sinuses may break through the fragile medial wall of the orbit. Severe infections from this source may cause blindness but could also affect the dural sheath of the optic nerve, causing **optic neuritis**.

During **removal of a maxillary molar tooth,** a fracture of a root may occur. If proper retrieval methods are not used, a piece of the root may be driven superiorly into the maxillary sinus.

Radiographs/CT scans of the frontal sinuses may be used for forensic identification of unknown individuals. The frontal sinuses are unique to each person, much like fingerprints.

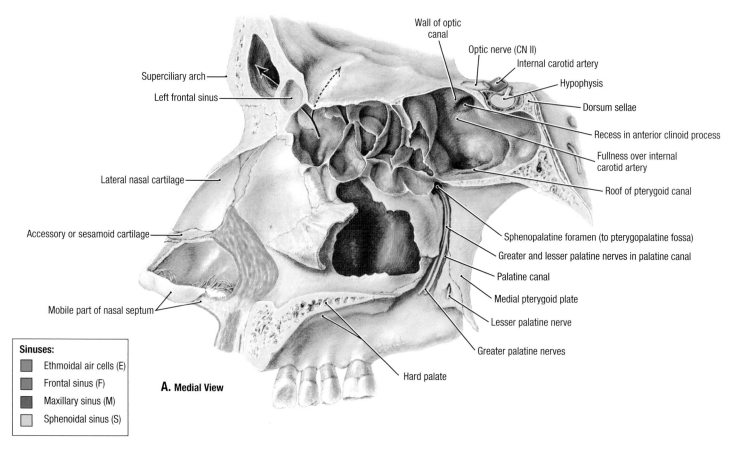

A. Medial View

Wall of optic canal

Optic nerve (CN II)

Internal carotid artery

Hypophysis

Dorsum sellae

Recess in anterior clinoid process

Fullness over internal carotid artery

Roof of pterygoid canal

Sphenopalatine foramen (to pterygopalatine fossa)

Greater and lesser palatine nerves in palatine canal

Palatine canal

Medial pterygoid plate

Lesser palatine nerve

Greater palatine nerves

Hard palate

Superciliary arch

Left frontal sinus

Lateral nasal cartilage

Accessory or sesamoid cartilage

Mobile part of nasal septum

Sinuses:
- Ethmoidal air cells (E)
- Frontal sinus (F)
- Maxillary sinus (M)
- Sphenoidal sinus (S)

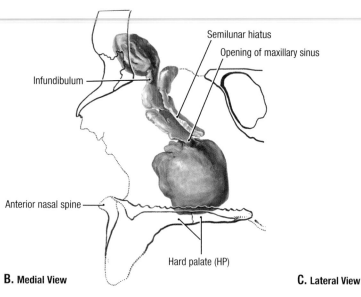

Infundibulum

Anterior nasal spine

Semilunar hiatus

Opening of maxillary sinus

Hard palate (HP)

B. Medial View

C. Lateral View

7.77 PARANASAL SINUSES

A. Opened sinuses, color coded. **B.** Cast of frontal and maxillary sinuses. **C.** Radiograph of cranium. *P*, pharynx; *dotted lines*, pterygopalatine fossa. Letters refer to structures labeled in **B. Maxillary sinusitis.** The maxillary sinuses are the most commonly infected, probably because their ostia are small and located high on their superomedial walls, a poor location for natural drainage of the sinus. When the mucous membrane of the sinus is congested, the maxillary ostia often are obstructed. The maxillary sinus can be cannulated and drained by passing a canula from the nares through the maxillary ostium into the sinus.

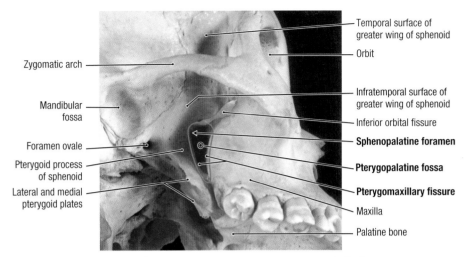

A. Inferolateral and slightly posterior view, looking into infratemporal and pterygopalatine fossae

B

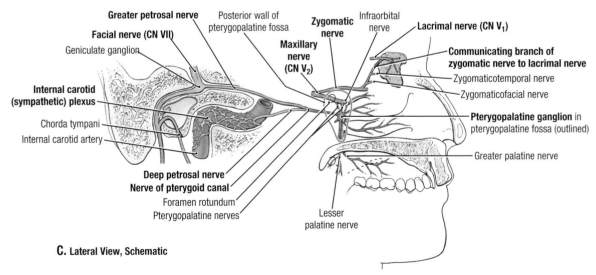

C. Lateral View, Schematic

7.78   PTERYGOPALATINE FOSSA

A. Bony relationships. The pterygopalatine fossa is a small pyramidal space inferior to the apex of the orbit. It lies between the pterygoid process of the sphenoid and the posterior aspect of the maxilla anteriorly. **B.** Communications. **C.** Pterygopalatine ganglion and related nerves.

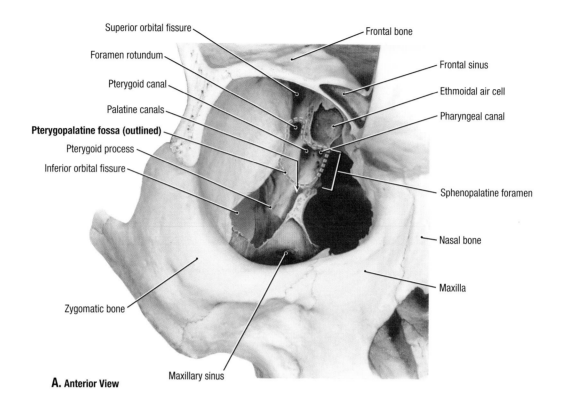

Superior orbital fissure
Foramen rotundum
Pterygoid canal
Palatine canals
Pterygopalatine fossa (outlined)
Pterygoid process
Inferior orbital fissure
Zygomatic bone
Maxillary sinus

Frontal bone
Frontal sinus
Ethmoidal air cell
Pharyngeal canal
Sphenopalatine foramen
Nasal bone
Maxilla

A. Anterior View

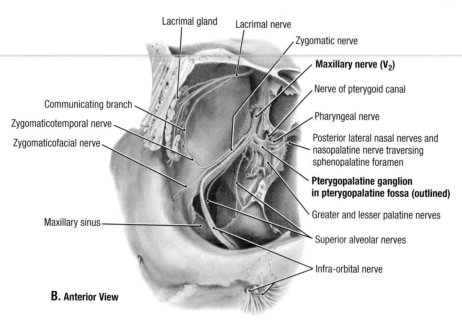

Lacrimal gland   Lacrimal nerve
Zygomatic nerve
Maxillary nerve (V₂)
Nerve of pterygoid canal
Pharyngeal nerve
Posterior lateral nasal nerves and
nasopalatine nerve traversing
sphenopalatine foramen
**Pterygopalatine ganglion
in pterygopalatine fossa (outlined)**
Greater and lesser palatine nerves
Superior alveolar nerves
Infra-orbital nerve

Communicating branch
Zygomaticotemporal nerve
Zygomaticofacial nerve
Maxillary sinus

B. Anterior View

7.79   NERVES OF THE PTERYGOPALATINE FOSSA

A. Bones and foramina, orbital approach. **B.** Vessels and nerves, orbital approach. In **A** and **B,** the pterygo-palatine fossa has been exposed through the floor of the orbit and maxillary sinus.

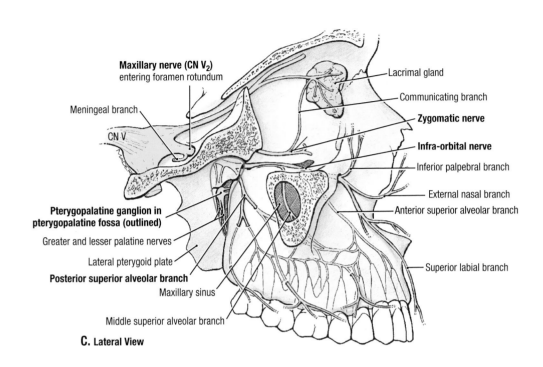

Maxillary nerve (CN V₂) entering foramen rotundum

Meningeal branch

CN V

Pterygopalatine ganglion in pterygopalatine fossa (outlined)

Greater and lesser palatine nerves

Lateral pterygoid plate

Posterior superior alveolar branch

Maxillary sinus

Middle superior alveolar branch

Lacrimal gland

Communicating branch

Zygomatic nerve

Infra-orbital nerve

Inferior palpebral branch

External nasal branch

Anterior superior alveolar branch

Superior labial branch

C. Lateral View

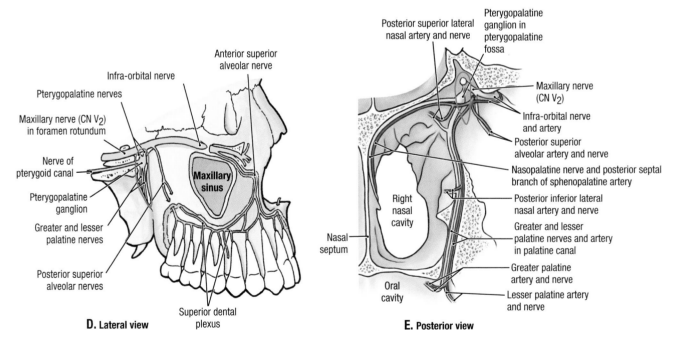

Infra-orbital nerve

Pterygopalatine nerves

Maxillary nerve (CN V₂) in foramen rotundum

Nerve of pterygoid canal

Pterygopalatine ganglion

Greater and lesser palatine nerves

Posterior superior alveolar nerves

Anterior superior alveolar nerve

Maxillary sinus

Superior dental plexus

D. Lateral view

Posterior superior lateral nasal artery and nerve

Pterygopalatine ganglion in pterygopalatine fossa

Maxillary nerve (CN V₂)

Infra-orbital nerve and artery

Posterior superior alveolar artery and nerve

Nasopalatine nerve and posterior septal branch of sphenopalatine artery

Posterior inferior lateral nasal artery and nerve

Greater and lesser palatine nerves and artery in palatine canal

Greater palatine artery and nerve

Lesser palatine artery and nerve

Right nasal cavity

Nasal septum

Oral cavity

E. Posterior view

7.79   NERVES OF THE PTERYGOPALATINE FOSSA *(CONTINUED)*

C. Maxillary nerve (CN V₂) and branches. **D.** The fossa is viewed laterally. Part of the wall of the maxillary sinus has been removed. **E.** Nasopalatine and greater and lesser palatine nerves.

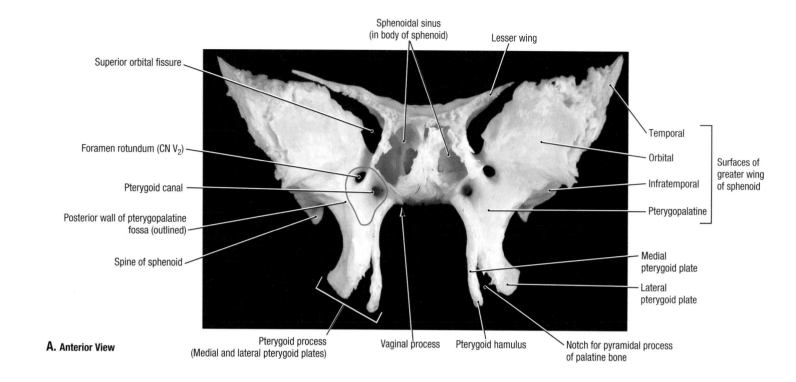

A. Anterior View

Labels (clockwise):
- Superior orbital fissure
- Foramen rotundum (CN V₂)
- Pterygoid canal
- Posterior wall of pterygopalatine fossa (outlined)
- Spine of sphenoid
- Pterygoid process (Medial and lateral pterygoid plates)
- Vaginal process
- Pterygoid hamulus
- Notch for pyramidal process of palatine bone
- Lateral pterygoid plate
- Medial pterygoid plate
- Pterygopalatine
- Infratemporal
- Orbital
- Temporal
- Surfaces of greater wing of sphenoid
- Lesser wing
- Sphenoidal sinus (in body of sphenoid)

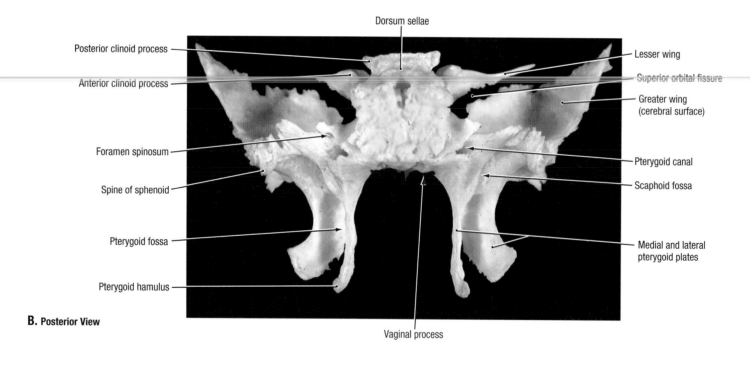

B. Posterior View

Labels:
- Posterior clinoid process
- Anterior clinoid process
- Foramen spinosum
- Spine of sphenoid
- Pterygoid fossa
- Pterygoid hamulus
- Vaginal process
- Dorsum sellae
- Lesser wing
- Superior orbital fissure
- Greater wing (cerebral surface)
- Pterygoid canal
- Scaphoid fossa
- Medial and lateral pterygoid plates

7.80   SPHENOID BONE: FEATURES AND RELATIONSHIP TO PTERYGOPALATINE FOSSA

A. The pterygopalatine fossa communicates posterosuperiorly with the middle cranial fossa through the foramen rotundum and pterygoid canal. **B.** Bony features and tensor veli palatini.

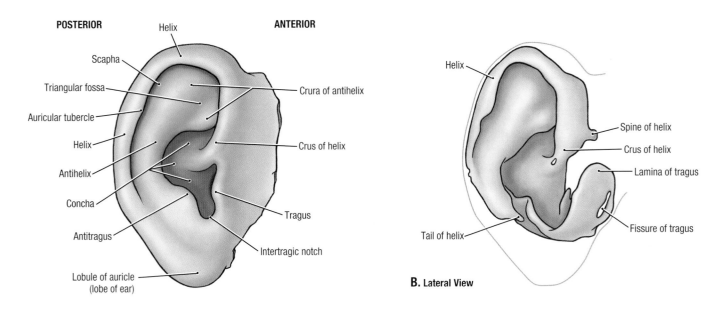

POSTERIOR Helix ANTERIOR

Scapha

Triangular fossa

Auricular tubercle Crura of antihelix

Helix

Antihelix Crus of helix

Concha

Antitragus Tragus

Lobule of auricle Intertragic notch
(lobe of ear)

A. Lateral View

Helix

Spine of helix

Crus of helix

Lamina of tragus

Tail of helix Fissure of tragus

B. Lateral View

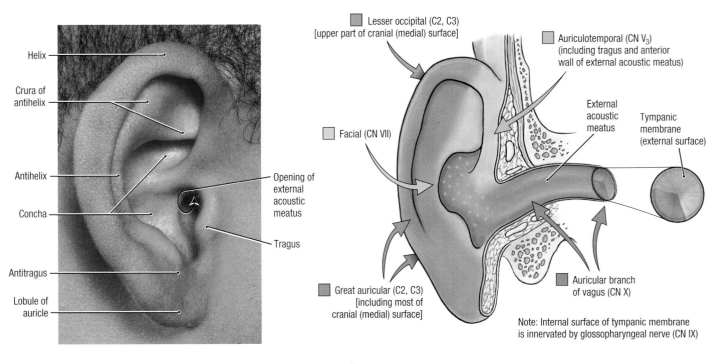

Helix

Crura of
antihelix

Antihelix

Concha

Antitragus

Lobule of
auricle

Opening of
external
acoustic
meatus

Tragus

C. Lateral View

Lesser occipital (C2, C3)
[upper part of cranial (medial) surface]

Auriculotemporal (CN V₃)
(including tragus and anterior
wall of external acoustic meatus)

Facial (CN VII)

External
acoustic
meatus

Tympanic
membrane
(external surface)

Great auricular (C2, C3)
[including most of
cranial (medial) surface]

Auricular branch
of vagus (CN X)

Note: Internal surface of tympanic membrane
is innervated by glossopharyngeal nerve (CN IX)

D. Schematic Section

7.81   AURICLE

A. Features of auricle. **B.** Cartilage of auricle. **C.** Surface anatomy of auricle. **D.** Sensory innervation.

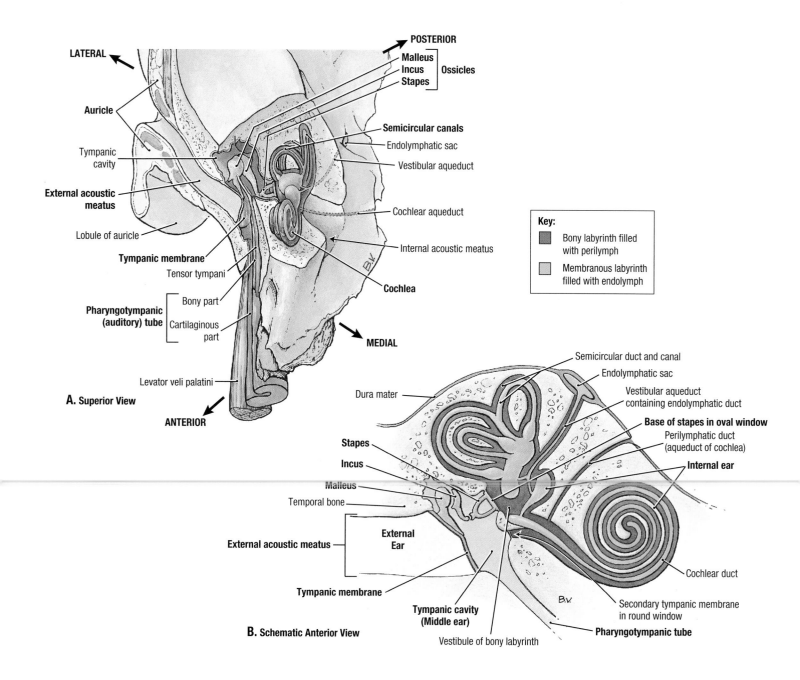

LATERAL

POSTERIOR

Malleus
Incus   Ossicles
Stapes

Auricle

Semicircular canals

Tympanic
cavity

Endolymphatic sac

Vestibular aqueduct

**External acoustic
meatus**

Cochlear aqueduct

Lobule of auricle

Internal acoustic meatus

Tympanic membrane

Tensor tympani

Cochlea

Bony part

**Pharyngotympanic
(auditory) tube**   Cartilaginous
part

MEDIAL

Levator veli palatini

A. Superior View

ANTERIOR

Key:

Bony labyrinth filled
with perilymph

Membranous labyrinth
filled with endolymph

Semicircular duct and canal

Endolymphatic sac

Vestibular aqueduct
containing endolymphatic duct

Dura mater

Base of stapes in oval window

Perilymphatic duct
(aqueduct of cochlea)

Stapes

Internal ear

Incus

Malleus

Temporal bone

External acoustic meatus

**External
Ear**

Cochlear duct

Tympanic membrane

Secondary tympanic membrane
in round window

**Tympanic cavity
(Middle ear)**

Pharyngotympanic tube

Vestibule of bony labyrinth

B. Schematic Anterior View

7.82 **EXTERNAL, MIDDLE, AND INTERNAL EAR I: OVERVIEWS**

A. Right temporal bone and auricle, sectioned in planes of (1) externa acoustic meatus and (2) pharyngotympanic tube. **B.** Schematic section of petrous temporal bone.

- The external ear comprises the auricle and external acoustic (auditory) meatus.
- The middle ear (tympanum) lies between the tympanic membrane and internal ear. Three ossicles extend from the lateral to the medial walls of the tympanum. Of these, the malleus is attached to the tympanic membrane. The stapes is attached by the anular ligament to the oval window, and the incus connects to the malleus and stapes. The pharyngotympanic tube, extending from the nasopharynx, opens into the anterior wall of the tympanic cavity.
- The membranous labyrinth comprises a closed system of membranous tubes and bulbs filled with fluid, endolymph (*orange* in **A** and **B**) and bathed in surrounding fluid, called perilymph *(purple* in **A** and **B**); both membranous labyrinth and perilymph are contained within the bony labyrinth.

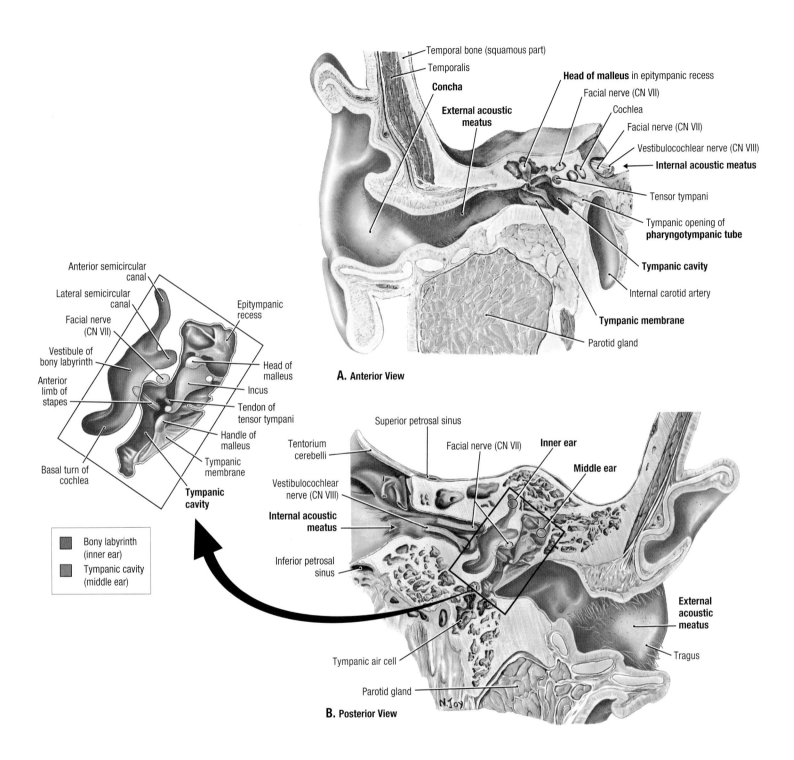

Temporal bone (squamous part)

Temporalis

Concha

Head of malleus in epitympanic recess

Facial nerve (CN VII)

External acoustic meatus

Cochlea

Facial nerve (CN VII)

Vestibulocochlear nerve (CN VIII)

Internal acoustic meatus

Tensor tympani

Tympanic opening of **pharyngotympanic tube**

Tympanic cavity

Internal carotid artery

Tympanic membrane

Parotid gland

A. Anterior View

Anterior semicircular canal

Lateral semicircular canal

Facial nerve (CN VII)

Vestibule of bony labyrinth

Anterior limb of stapes

Epitympanic recess

Head of malleus

Incus

Tendon of tensor tympani

Handle of malleus

Tympanic membrane

Basal turn of cochlea

Tympanic cavity

| | Bony labyrinth (inner ear) |
| Tympanic cavity (middle ear) |

Superior petrosal sinus

Tentorium cerebelli

Facial nerve (CN VII)

Inner ear

Middle ear

Vestibulocochlear nerve (CN VIII)

Internal acoustic meatus

Inferior petrosal sinus

External acoustic meatus

Tympanic air cell

Tragus

Parotid gland

N. Joy

B. Posterior View

7.83   **EXTERNAL, MIDDLE, AND INTERNAL EAR II: CORONALLY SECTIONED**

A. Anterior portion. **B.** Posterior portion. The inset *(outlined by the box)* is an enlargement of the structures of the middle and internal ear as they appear in **B.**

- The external acoustic meatus is about 3 cm long; half is cartilaginous and half is bony. It is narrowest at the isthmus, near the junction of the cartilaginous and bony parts.

- The external acoustic meatus is innervated by the auriculotemporal branch of the mandibular nerve (CN V$_3$) and the auricular branches of the vagus nerve (CN X); the middle ear is innervated by the glossopharyngeal nerve (CN IX).

- The cartilaginous part of the external acoustic meatus is lined with thick skin; the bony part is lined with thin skin that adheres to the periosteum and forms the outermost layer of the tympanic membrane.

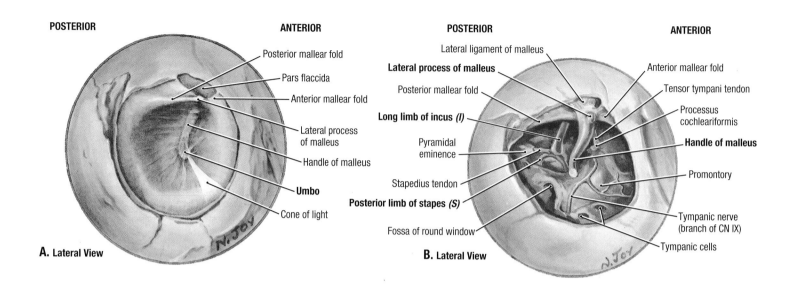

A. Lateral View

POSTERIOR — ANTERIOR

- Posterior mallear fold
- Pars flaccida
- Anterior mallear fold
- Lateral process of malleus
- Handle of malleus
- **Umbo**
- Cone of light

B. Lateral View

POSTERIOR — ANTERIOR

- Lateral ligament of malleus
- **Lateral process of malleus**
- Posterior mallear fold
- **Long limb of incus (I)**
- Pyramidal eminence
- Stapedius tendon
- **Posterior limb of stapes (S)**
- Fossa of round window
- Anterior mallear fold
- Tensor tympani tendon
- Processus cochleariformis
- **Handle of malleus**
- Promontory
- Tympanic nerve (branch of CN IX)
- Tympanic cells

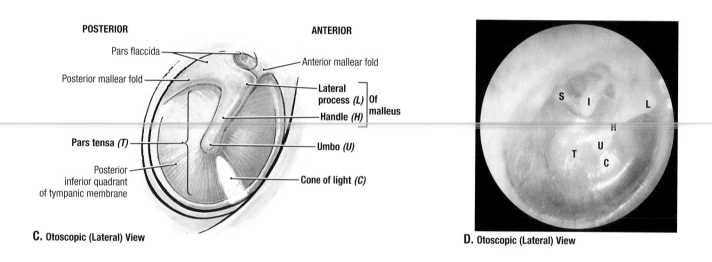

C. Otoscopic (Lateral) View

POSTERIOR — ANTERIOR

- Pars flaccida
- Posterior mallear fold
- Anterior mallear fold
- Lateral process (L) | Of malleus
- Handle (H) |
- **Pars tensa (T)**
- Posterior inferior quadrant of tympanic membrane
- Umbo (U)
- **Cone of light (C)**

D. Otoscopic (Lateral) View

7.84 TYMPANIC MEMBRANE

A. External (lateral) surface of tympanic membrane. **B.** Tympanic membrane removed, demonstrating structures that lie medially. **C.** Diagram of otoscopic view of tympanic membrane. **D.** Otoscopic view of tympanic membrane. Letter labels are identified in **C.**

- The oval tympanic membrane is a shallow cone deepest at the central apex, the umbo, where the membrane is attached to the tip of the handle of the malleus. The handle of the malleus is attached to the membrane along its entire length as it extends anterosuperiorly toward the periphery of the membrane.
- Superior to the lateral process of the malleus, the membrane is thin (pars flaccida); the flaccid part lacks the radial and circular fibers present in the remainder of the membrane (pars tensa). The junction between the two parts is marked by anterior and posterior mallear folds.

- The lateral surface of the tympanic membrane is innervated by the auricular branch of the auriculotemporal nerve (CN V₃) and the auricular branch of the vagus nerve (CN X); the medial surface is innervated by tympanic branches of CN IX.

Examination of the external acoustic meatus and tympanic membrane begins by straightening the meatus. In adults, the helix is grasped and pulled posterosuperiorly (up, out, and back). These movements reduce the curvature of the external acoustic meatus, facilitating insertion of the otoscope. The external acoustic meatus is relatively short in infants; therefore, extra care must be taken to prevent damage to the tympanic membrane.

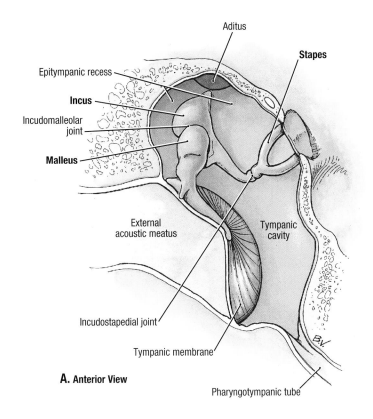

A. Anterior View

Labels in figure A:
Aditus
Stapes
Epitympanic recess
Incus
Incudomalleolar joint
Malleus
External acoustic meatus
Tympanic cavity
Incudostapedial joint
Tympanic membrane
Pharyngotympanic tube
B.v.

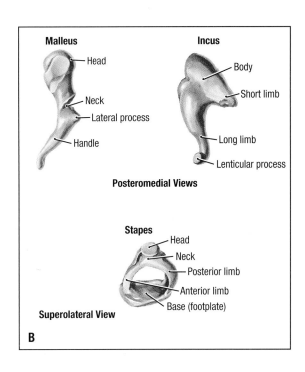

Malleus — Head, Neck, Lateral process, Handle

Incus — Body, Short limb, Long limb, Lenticular process

Posteromedial Views

Stapes — Head, Neck, Posterior limb, Anterior limb, Base (footplate)

Superolateral View

B

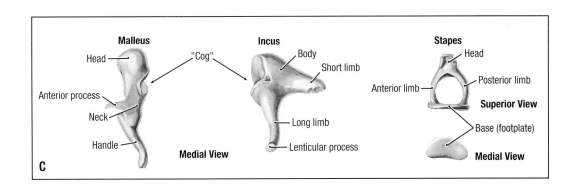

Malleus — Head, Anterior process, Neck, Handle — "Cog" — **Medial View**

Incus — Body, Short limb, Long limb, Lenticular process — **Medial View**

Stapes — Head, Anterior limb, Posterior limb, Base (footplate) — **Superior View**, **Medial View**

C

7.85 **OSSICLES OF THE MIDDLE EAR**

A. Ossicles in situ, as revealed by a coronal section of the temporal bone.
B. and C. Isolated ossicles.
- The head of the malleus and body and short process of the incus lie in the epitympanic recess, and the handle of the malleus is embedded in the tympanic membrane.
- The saddle-shaped articular surface of the head of the malleus and the reciprocally shaped articular surface of the body of the incus form the incudomalleolar synovial joint.
- A convex articular facet at the end of the long process of the incus articulates with the head of the stapes to compose the incudostapedial synovial joint.

- An earache and bulging red tympanic membrane may indicate pus or fluid in the middle ear, a sign of **otitis media.** Infection of the middle ear often is secondary to upper respiratory infections. Inflammation and swelling of the mucous membrane lining the tympanic cavity may cause partial or complete blockage of the pharyngotympanic tube. The tympanic membrane becomes red and bulges, and the person may complain of "ear popping." If untreated, otitis media may produce impaired hearing as the result of scarring of the auditory ossicles, limiting the ability of these bones to move in response to sound.

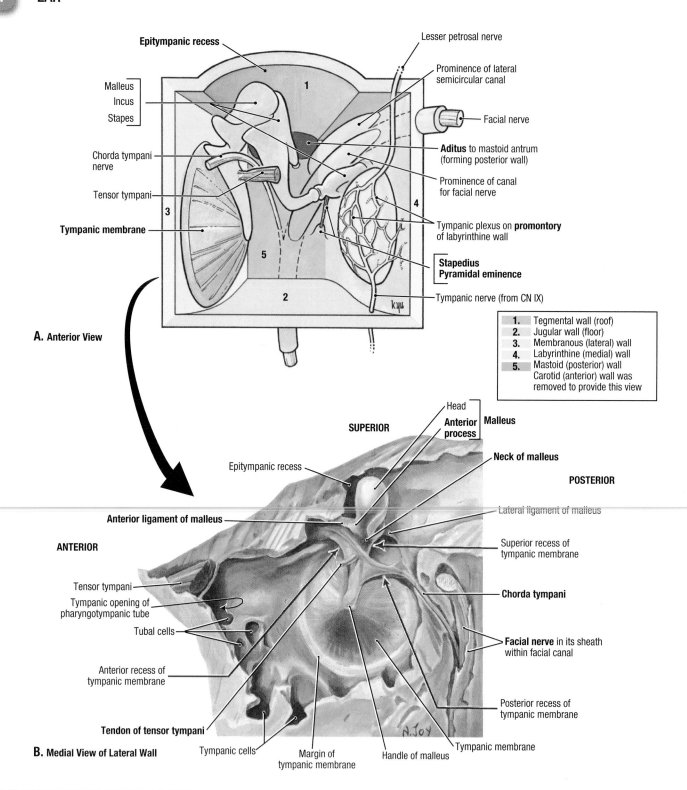

A. Anterior View

Epitympanic recess

Malleus
Incus
Stapes

Chorda tympani nerve

Tensor tympani

Tympanic membrane

Lesser petrosal nerve

Prominence of lateral semicircular canal

Facial nerve

Aditus to mastoid antrum (forming posterior wall)

Prominence of canal for facial nerve

Tympanic plexus on **promontory** of labyrinthine wall

Stapedius
Pyramidal eminence

Tympanic nerve (from CN IX)

1. Tegmental wall (roof)
2. Jugular wall (floor)
3. Membranous (lateral) wall
4. Labyrinthine (medial) wall
5. Mastoid (posterior) wall
   Carotid (anterior) wall was removed to provide this view

B. Medial View of Lateral Wall

SUPERIOR

Head
Anterior process | **Malleus**

Neck of malleus

POSTERIOR

Epitympanic recess

Anterior ligament of malleus

ANTERIOR

Lateral ligament of malleus

Superior recess of tympanic membrane

Tensor tympani

Tympanic opening of pharyngotympanic tube

Tubal cells

Anterior recess of tympanic membrane

Chorda tympani

Facial nerve in its sheath within facial canal

Posterior recess of tympanic membrane

Tendon of tensor tympani

Tympanic cells

Margin of tympanic membrane

Handle of malleus

Tympanic membrane

7.86   STRUCTURES OF THE TYMPANIC CAVITY

A. Schematic illustration of the tympanic cavity with the anterior wall removed. **B.** Lateral wall of the tympanic cavity. The facial nerve lies within the facial canal surrounded by a tough periosteal tube; the chorda tympani leaves the facial nerve and lies within two crescentic folds of mucous membrane, crossing the neck of the malleus superior to the tendon of tensor tympani.

Perforation of the tympanic membrane (ruptured eardrum) may result from otitis media. Perforation may also result from foreign bodies in the external acoustic meatus, trauma, or excessive pressure. Because the superior half of the tympanic membrane is much more vascular than the inferior half, incisions are made posteroinferiorly through the membrane. This incision also avoids injury to the chorda tympani nerve and auditory ossicles.

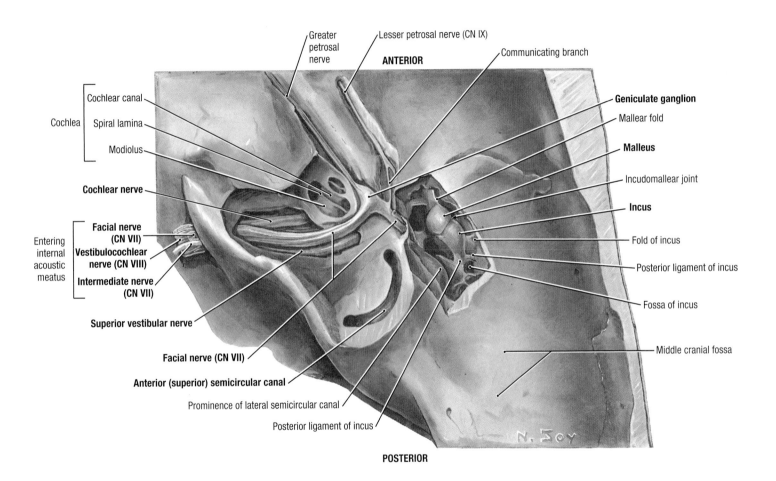

Greater petrosal nerve

Lesser petrosal nerve (CN IX)

ANTERIOR

Communicating branch

Cochlea
- Cochlear canal
- Spiral lamina
- Modiolus

Cochlear nerve

Entering internal acoustic meatus
- **Facial nerve (CN VII)**
- **Vestibulocochlear nerve (CN VIII)**
- **Intermediate nerve (CN VII)**

Superior vestibular nerve

Facial nerve (CN VII)

Anterior (superior) semicircular canal

Prominence of lateral semicircular canal

Posterior ligament of incus

Geniculate ganglion

Mallear fold

Malleus

Incudomallear joint

Incus

Fold of incus

Posterior ligament of incus

Fossa of incus

Middle cranial fossa

POSTERIOR

7.87   MIDDLE AND INNER EAR IN SITU

The tegmen tympani has been removed to expose the middle ear, the arcuate eminence has been removed to expose the anterior semicircular canal, and the course of the facial and vestibulocochlear nerves through the internal acoustic meatus and internal ear is demonstrated. At the geniculate ganglion, the facial nerve executes a sharp bend, called the genu, and then curves posteroinferiorly within the bony facial canal; the thin lateral wall of the facial canal separates the facial nerve from the tympanic cavity of the middle ear.

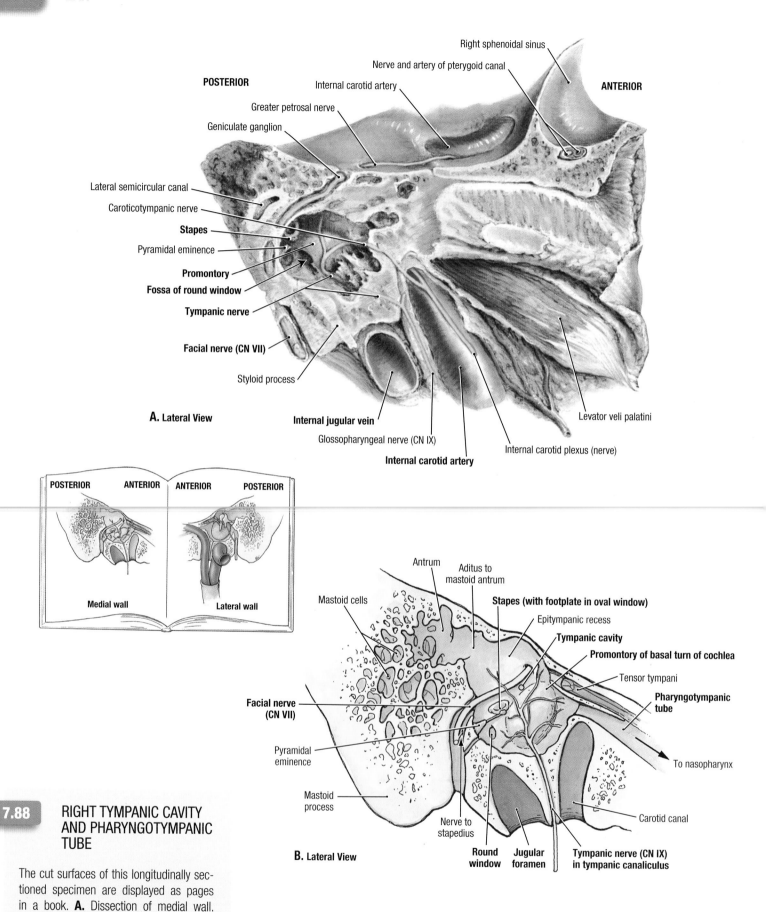

A. Lateral View

Right sphenoidal sinus
Nerve and artery of pterygoid canal
POSTERIOR
Internal carotid artery
Greater petrosal nerve
Geniculate ganglion
ANTERIOR

Lateral semicircular canal
Caroticotympanic nerve
Stapes
Pyramidal eminence
Promontory
Fossa of round window
Tympanic nerve

Facial nerve (CN VII)

Styloid process

Internal jugular vein
Glossopharyngeal nerve (CN IX)
Internal carotid artery
Internal carotid plexus (nerve)
Levator veli palatini

POSTERIOR   ANTERIOR   ANTERIOR   POSTERIOR

Medial wall   **Lateral wall**

Antrum
Aditus to mastoid antrum
Mastoid cells
Stapes (with footplate in oval window)
Epitympanic recess
Tympanic cavity
Promontory of basal turn of cochlea
Tensor tympani
Pharyngotympanic tube
Facial nerve (CN VII)
To nasopharynx
Pyramidal eminence
Mastoid process
Nerve to stapedius
Carotid canal
Round window **Jugular foramen** **Tympanic nerve (CN IX) in tympanic canaliculus**

B. Lateral View

7.88

RIGHT TYMPANIC CAVITY AND PHARYNGOTYMPANIC TUBE

The cut surfaces of this longitudinally sectioned specimen are displayed as pages in a book. **A.** Dissection of medial wall. **B.** Schematic illustration of medial wall.

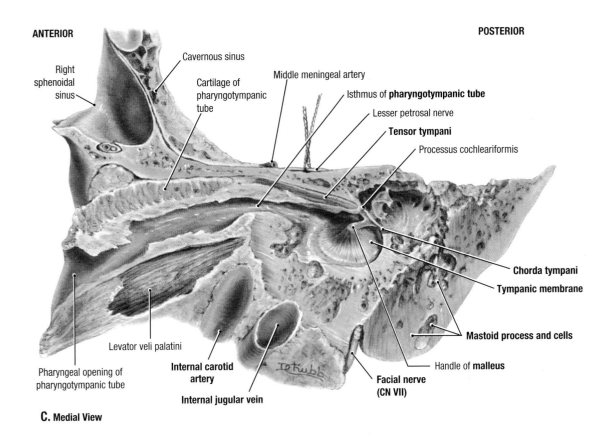

ANTERIOR

POSTERIOR

Right sphenoidal sinus

Cavernous sinus

Cartilage of pharyngotympanic tube

Middle meningeal artery

Isthmus of **pharyngotympanic tube**

Lesser petrosal nerve

Tensor tympani

Processus cochleariformis

Chorda tympani

Tympanic membrane

Mastoid process and cells

Handle of **malleus**

Levator veli palatini

Pharyngeal opening of pharyngotympanic tube

Internal carotid artery

Internal jugular vein

Facial nerve (CN VII)

C. Medial View

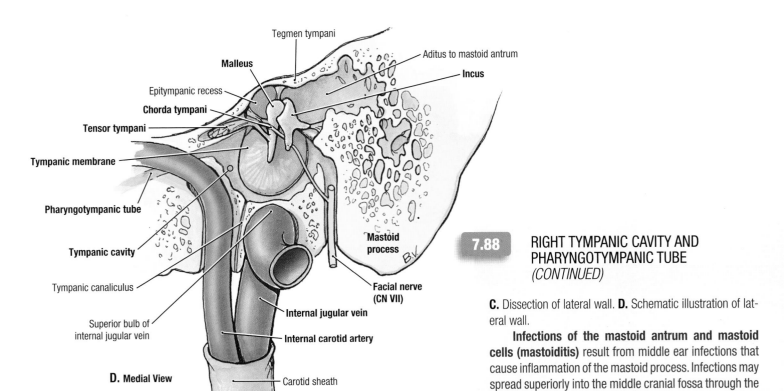

Tegmen tympani

Malleus

Aditus to mastoid antrum

Incus

Epitympanic recess

Chorda tympani

Tensor tympani

Tympanic membrane

Pharyngotympanic tube

Tympanic cavity

Tympanic canaliculus

Superior bulb of internal jugular vein

Internal jugular vein

Internal carotid artery

Carotid sheath

Mastoid process

Facial nerve (CN VII)

D. Medial View

7.88 RIGHT TYMPANIC CAVITY AND PHARYNGOTYMPANIC TUBE *(CONTINUED)*

C. Dissection of lateral wall. **D.** Schematic illustration of lateral wall.

Infections of the mastoid antrum and mastoid cells (mastoiditis) result from middle ear infections that cause inflammation of the mastoid process. Infections may spread superiorly into the middle cranial fossa through the petrosquamous fissure in children or may cause osteomyelitis (bone infection) of the tegmen tympani. Since the advent of antibiotics, mastoiditis is uncommon.

Membranous part*

Bony part, opened*

Cartilaginous part*

* Parts of pharyngotympani
(auditory) tube

Posterior superior
alveolar artery

Levator veli
palatini

Lateral pterygoid
plate

Buccinator

Palatine tonsil

Superior pharyngeal
constrictor

Tympanic membrane

Facial nerve

Internal jugular vein

Internal carotid artery

Styloid process

Middle meningeal artery

Emissary veins in foramen ovale

Ascending palatine vessels

A. Lateral View

Malleus

External
acoustic
meatus

Incus

Semicircular canals

Stapes

Cochlea

Tympanic cavity

Pharyngotympanic
tube:

Bony part

Cartilaginous
part

Tympanic
membrane

Isthmus

Tensor veli palatini

Pharyngo-
tympanic
tube

Levator veli
palatini

Pterygoid hamulus

B. Anterior view

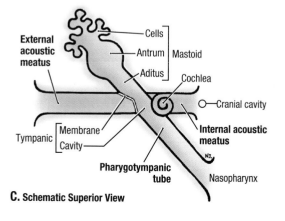

Cells

External
acoustic
meatus

Antrum   Mastoid

Aditus

Cochlea

Cranial cavity

Tympanic

Membrane

Cavity

**Internal acoustic
meatus**

**Pharyngotympanic
tube**

Nasopharynx

C. Schematic Superior View

7.89   RIGHT TYMPANIC CAVITY AND PHARYNGOTYMPANIC
TUBE

A. Dissection demonstrating lateral aspect of pharyngotympanic tube and structures located medially. **B.** Right pharyngotympanic tube. **C.** Schematic illustration demonstrating relationship between internal and external acoustic meatuses.

- The general direction of the pharyngotympanic tube is superior, posterior, and lateral from the nasopharynx to the tympanic cavity.
- The cartilaginous part of the tube rests throughout its length on the levator veli palatini muscle.
- The line of the meatuses and the line of the airway, from nasopharynx to mastoid cells, intersect at the tympanic cavity.
- The tegmen tympani forms the roof of the tympanic cavity and mastoid antrum.

The **function of the pharyngotympanic tube** is to equalize pressure in the middle ear with the atmospheric pressure, thereby allowing free movement of the tympanic membrane. By allowing air to enter and leave the tympanic cavity, this tube balances the pressure on both sides of the membrane. Because the walls of the cartilaginous part of the tube are normally in apposition, the tube must be actively opened. The tube is opened by the expanding girth of the belly of the levator veli palatini as it contracts longitudinally, pushing against one wall while the tensor veli palatini pulls on the other. Because these are muscles of the soft palate, equalizing pressure (popping the eardrums) is commonly associated with activities such as yawning and swallowing.

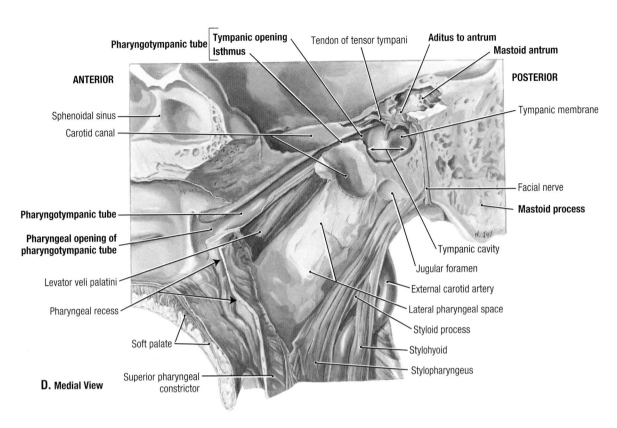

Pharyngotympanic tube — **Tympanic opening** — Tendon of tensor tympani — **Aditus to antrum**

Isthmus — **Mastoid antrum**

ANTERIOR

POSTERIOR

Sphenoidal sinus

Carotid canal

Tympanic membrane

Pharyngotympanic tube

Facial nerve

Pharyngeal opening of pharyngotympanic tube

Mastoid process

Levator veli palatini

Tympanic cavity

Jugular foramen

Pharyngeal recess

External carotid artery

Lateral pharyngeal space

Soft palate

Styloid process

Stylohyoid

Superior pharyngeal constrictor

Stylopharyngeus

D. Medial View

SUPERIOR

Facial nerve (CN VII)

Tegmen tympani

Mastoid antrum

Tendon of tensor tympani

ANTERIOR

Tympanic opening of pharyngotympanic (auditory) tube

Internal carotid artery in carotid canal

Superior bulb of internal jugular vein

Sigmoid sinus

E. Medial View

Mastoid

Tegmen tympani — Tympanic cavity — **Aditus** **Antrum** **Cells**

Pharyngotympanic tube

Nasopharynx

Styloid process

Mastoid process

F. Schematic illustration

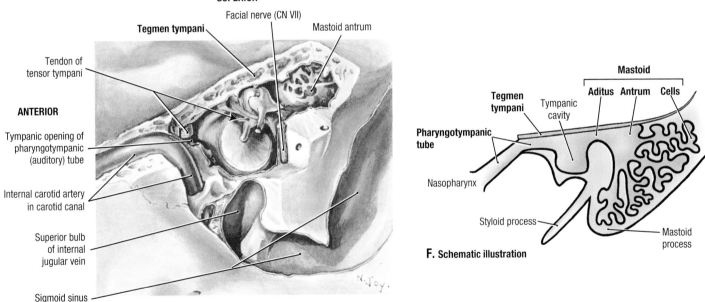

| 7.89 | RIGHT TYMPANIC CAVITY AND PHARYNGOTYMPANIC TUBE *(CONTINUED)* |

D. Spaces of tympanic bone. **E.** Relationship of tympanic cavity to internal carotid artery, sigmoid sinus, and middle cranial fossa. **F.** Diagram of tegmen tympani.

- The internal carotid artery is the primary relationship of the anterior wall, the internal jugular vein is the primary relationship of the floor, and the facial nerve is the primary relationship of the posterior wall.

A. Superior View

B. Posterosuperior View

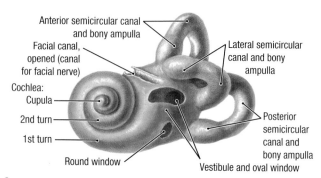

C. Anterolateral view of left otic capsule

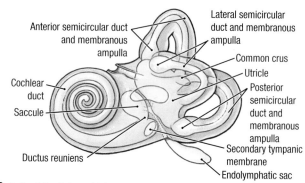

D. Anterolateral view of left membranous labyrinth (through transparent otic capsule)

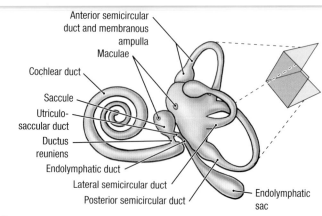

E. Anterolateral view of left membranous labyrinth

7.90 BONY AND MEMBRANOUS LABYRINTHS

A. Location and orientation of bony labyrinth within petrous temporal bone. **B.** Semicircular canals and aqueducts *in situ*. The tegmen tympani has been excised, and the softer bone surrounding the harder bone of the otic capsule has been drilled away. **C.** Walls of left bony labyrinth (otic capsule). The bony labyrinth is the fluid-filled space contained within this formation. **D.** Membranous labyrinth as it lies within the surrounding bony labyrinth. **E.** Isolated left membranous labyrinth.

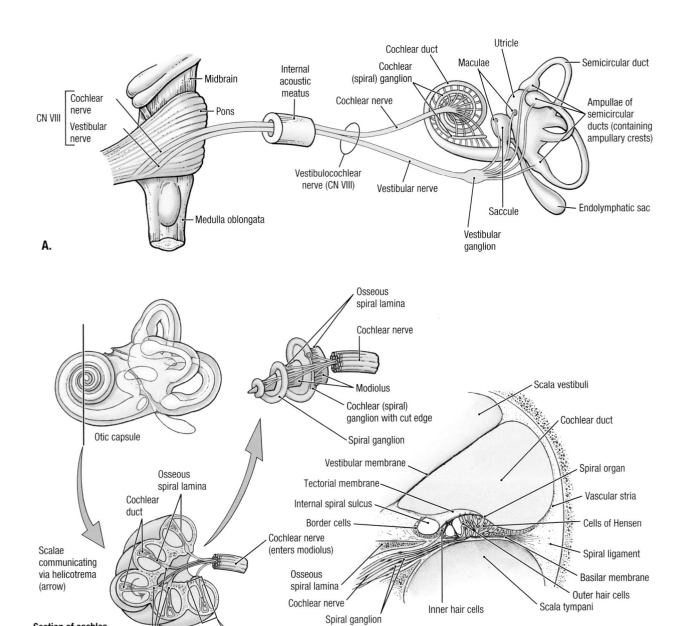

A. Distribution of vestibulocochlear nerve (schematic). **B.** Structure of cochlea. The cochlea has been sectioned along the bony core of the cochlea (modiolus), the axis about which the cochlea winds. An isolated modiolus is shown after the turns of the cochlea are removed, leaving only the spiral lamina winding around it. The *large drawing* shows the details of the *area enclosed in the rectangle,* including a cross section of the cochlear duct of the membranous labyrinth.

- The maculae of the membranous labyrinth are primarily static organs, which have small dense particles (otoliths) embedded among the hair

cells. Under the influence of gravity, the otoliths cause bending of the hair cells, which stimulate the vestibular nerve and provide awareness of the position of the head in space; the hairs also respond to quick tilting movements and to linear acceleration and deceleration. **Motion sickness** results mainly from discordance between vestibular and visual stimuli.

- Persistent exposure to excessively loud sound causes degenerative changes in the spiral organ, resulting in **high-tone deafness.** This type of hearing loss commonly occurs in workers who are exposed to loud noises and do not wear protective earmuffs.

7.91   **VESTIBULOCOCHLEAR NERVE (CN VIII) AND STRUCTURE OF COCHLEA**

A. Lateral View

Superficial temporal vein

Posterior auricular vein

Retromandibular vein:
Posterior branch
Anterior branch

Right external jugular vein

PG

SM

Facial vein

Anterior jugular vein

Right subclavian vein

B. Anterior View

SM

H

SM

TC   TC

TG   TG

T

Right jugular lymphatic trunk

Right subclavian vein

Right lymphatic duct

Left internal jugular vein

Left jugular lymphatic trunk

Left subclavian vein

Thoracic duct

C. Anterior View

From head and neck

Bronchomediastinal lymphatic trunk

Right jugular lymphatic trunk
Right internal jugular vein
Subclavian lymphatic trunk
Right lymphatic duct
Right subclavian vein
Right venous angle
Right brachiocephalic vein
Superior vena cava

Left jugular lymphatic trunk
Left internal jugular vein
Thoracic duct
Subclavian lymphatic trunk
Left venous angle
Left subclavian vein
Left brachiocephalic vein
Bronchomediastinal lymphatic trunk
Thoracic duct

D. Lateral View

Ph

SM

P

Right jugular lymphatic trunk

Right subclavian vein

Right internal jugular vein

Right lymphatic duct

Lymph nodes:

Buccinator	Paratracheal	Superficial cervical
Inferior deep cervical	Parotid	Superior deep cervical
Infrahyoid	Prelaryngeal	**Structures:**
Jugulodigastric	Pretracheal	→ Initial drainage
Jugulo-omohyoid	Retropharyngeal	➡ Secondary (subsequent) drainage
Mastoid (retro-auricular)	Submandibular	
Occipital	Submental	H Hyoid

SM   Sternocleidomastoid
T   Trachea
TC   Thyroid cartilage
TG   Thyroid gland
P   Palatine tonsil
PG   Parotid gland
Ph   Pharyngeal tonsil

7.92   LYMPHATIC AND VENOUS DRAINAGE OF HEAD AND NECK

A. Superficial drainage. **B.** Drainage of the trachea, thyroid gland, larynx, and floor of mouth. **C.** Termination of right and left jugular lymphatic trunks. **D.** Deep drainage.

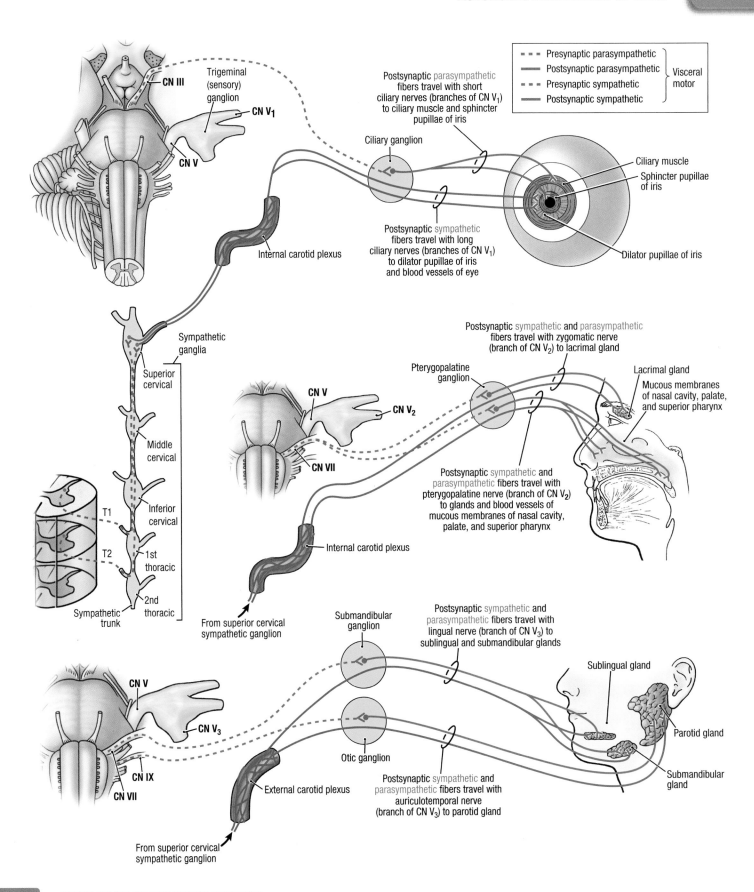

CN III

Trigeminal
(sensory)
ganglion

CN V₁

CN V

Internal carotid plexus

Presynaptic parasympathetic
Postsynaptic parasympathetic
Presynaptic sympathetic
Postsynaptic sympathetic

Visceral
motor

Postsynaptic parasympathetic
fibers travel with short
ciliary nerves (branches of CN V₁)
to ciliary muscle and sphincter
pupillae of iris

Ciliary ganglion

Ciliary muscle

Sphincter pupillae
of iris

Postsynaptic sympathetic
fibers travel with long
ciliary nerves (branches of CN V₁)
to dilator pupillae of iris
and blood vessels of eye

Dilator pupillae of iris

Sympathetic
ganglia

Superior
cervical

Middle
cervical

T1

T2

Inferior
cervical

1st
thoracic

2nd
thoracic

Sympathetic
trunk

CN V

CN V₂

CN VII

Postsynaptic sympathetic and parasympathetic
fibers travel with zygomatic nerve
(branch of CN V₂) to lacrimal gland

Pterygopalatine
ganglion

Lacrimal gland

Mucous membranes
of nasal cavity, palate,
and superior pharynx

Postsynaptic sympathetic and
parasympathetic fibers travel with
pterygopalatine nerve (branch of CN V₂)
to glands and blood vessels of
mucous membranes of nasal cavity,
palate, and superior pharynx

Internal carotid plexus

From superior cervical
sympathetic ganglion

CN V

CN V₃

CN IX

CN VII

External carotid plexus

From superior cervical
sympathetic ganglion

Submandibular
ganglion

Postsynaptic sympathetic and
parasympathetic fibers travel with
lingual nerve (branch of CN V₃) to
sublingual and submandibular glands

Sublingual gland

Parotid gland

Otic ganglion

Submandibular
gland

Postsynaptic sympathetic and
parasympathetic fibers travel with
auriculotemporal nerve
(branch of CN V₃) to parotid gland

7.93 AUTONOMIC INNERVATION OF HEAD

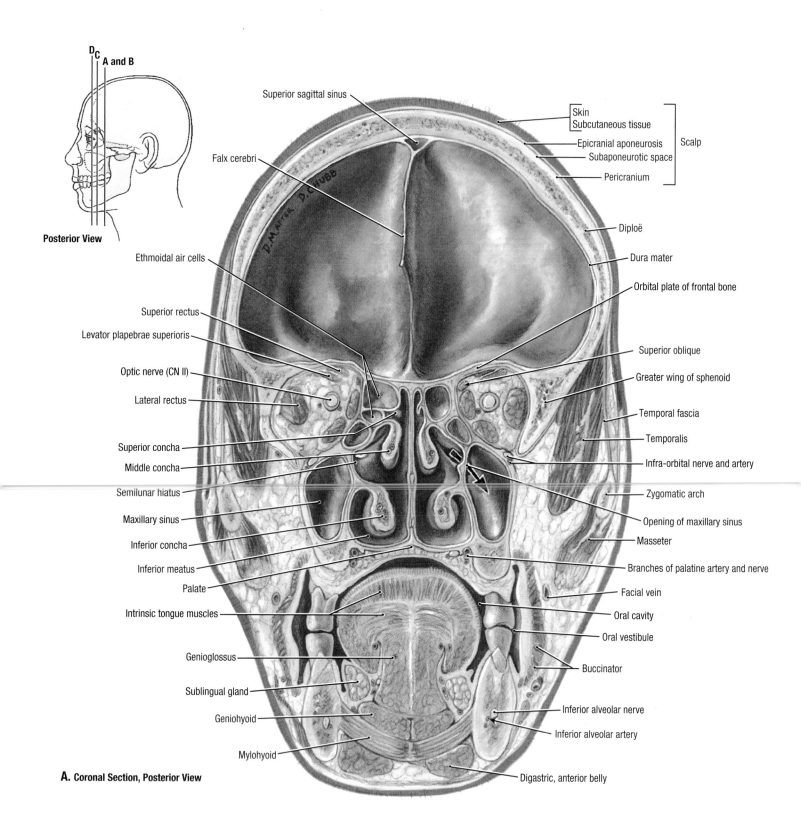

D C
A and B

Posterior View

Superior sagittal sinus

Skin
Subcutaneous tissue
Epicranial aponeurosis
Subaponeurotic space   Scalp
Pericranium

Falx cerebri

Diploë

Dura mater

Ethmoidal air cells

Orbital plate of frontal bone

Superior rectus

Levator plapebrae superioris

Superior oblique

Optic nerve (CN II)

Greater wing of sphenoid

Lateral rectus

Temporal fascia

Temporalis

Superior concha

Middle concha

Infra-orbital nerve and artery

Semilunar hiatus

Zygomatic arch

Maxillary sinus

Opening of maxillary sinus

Inferior concha

Masseter

Inferior meatus

Branches of palatine artery and nerve

Palate

Facial vein

Intrinsic tongue muscles

Oral cavity

Oral vestibule

Genioglossus

Buccinator

Sublingual gland

Geniohyoid

Inferior alveolar nerve

Inferior alveolar artery

Mylohyoid

Digastric, anterior belly

A. Coronal Section, Posterior View

7.94   CORONAL SECTION AND MRI IMAGING OF NASOPHARYNX AND ORAL CAVITY

A. Coronal section. B.–D. Coronal MRIs.

B

C

Posterior
Views

D

1	Levator palpebrae superioris
2	Superior rectus
3	Lateral rectus
4	Inferior rectus
5	Medial rectus
6	Superior oblique
7	Inferior oblique
8	Optic nerve
9	Olfactory bulb
10	Crista galli
11	Nasal septum
12	Superior concha
13	Middle concha
14	Inferior concha
15	Lacrimal gland
16	Eyeball
17	Frontal lobe
18	Tongue
19	Infra-orbital vessels and nerve
20	Hard palate
21	Intrinsic muscles of tongue
22	Mandible
23	Temporalis
24	Masseter
25	Zygomatic arch
26	Molar teeth
27	Genioglossus
28	Sublingual gland
M	Maxillary sinus
E	Ethmoidal air cell

7.94   CORONAL SECTION AND MRI IMAGING OF NASOPHARYNX AND ORAL CAVITY *(CONTINUED)*

Lateral nasal cartilage
Septal cartilage
Middle concha
Nasolacrimal duct
Inferior meatus
Inferior concha
Vomer
Pharyngeal tonsil
Greater palatine canal
Lateral pterygoid plate
Medial pterygoid muscle
Tensor veli palatini
Pharyngotympanic tube
Pharyngeal recess
Lateral pharyngeal space
Glossopharyngeal nerve (CN IX)
Accessory nerve (CN XI)
Hypoglossal nerve (CN XII)
Vagus nerve (CN X)
Sympathetic trunk

Nasolacrimal duct
Infra-orbital artery and nerve
Maxillary sinus
Buccal fat pad
Temporalis
Coronoid process
Masseter
Lateral pterygoid
Maxillary artery
Branches of mandibular nerve
Branch of facial nerve
Neck of mandible
Superficial temporal artery
Retromandibular vein
Parotid gland
Tip of mastoid process

Dens of axis
Atlas
Internal carotid artery
Internal jugular vein
Facial nerve
Styloid process and stylopharyngeus

A. Inferior View

Nasal septum
Inferior concha
Nasopharynx
Medial pterygoid
Tensor veli palatini
Pharyngotympanic tube
Pharyngeal recess
Internal carotid artery
Internal jugular vein
Vertebral artery

Maxillary sinus
Buccal fat pad
Coronoid process of mandible
Temporalis
Lateral pterygoid plate
Masseter
Lateral pterygoid
Maxillary artery
Branches of mandibular nerve
Neck of mandible
Superficial temporal vessels
Mastoid cells

B. Inferior View

7.95   TRANSVERSE SECTION AND MRI IMAGE OF NASAL CAVITY AND NASOPHARYNX

A. Transverse section of left side of head. **B.** Transverse (axial) MRI scan.

A. Transverse Section and Transverse (axial) MRI Scan

Key							
1	Nasal bones	7	Posterior ethmoidal air cell	13	Retrobulbar fat	19	Optic tract
2	Angular artery	8	Sphenoid sinus	14	Anterior chamber	20	Temporalis muscle
3	Frontal process of maxilla	9	Orbicularis oculi muscle	15	Lens	21	Superficial temporal vessels
4	Nasal septum	10	Medial rectus muscle	16	Vitreous body	22	Greater wing of sphenoid
5	Anterior ethmoidal cell	11	Lateral rectus muscle	17	Optic nerve	23	Squamous part of temporal bone
6	Middle ethmoidal cell	12	Cornea	18	Optic chiasm		

B. Transverse Section and Transverse (axial) MRI Scan

Key							
1	Orbicularis oris muscle	12	Ramus of mandible	23	Transverse ligament of atlas		
2	Levator anguli oris muscle	13	Lateral pterygoid muscle	24	Spinal cord		
3	Facial artery and vein	14	Parotid gland	25	Vertebral artery in foramina transversaria		
4	Zygomaticus major muscle	15	Superficial temporal vessels	26	Longus colli muscle		
5	Buccinator muscle	16	Region of pharyngeal tubercle	27	Longus capitis muscle		
6	Maxilla	17	Sphenoid bone	28	Internal carotid artery		
7	Alveolar process of maxilla	18	Stylohyoid ligament and muscle	29	Internal jugular vein		
8	Dorsum of tongue	19	Posterior belly of digastric muscle	30	Inferior portion of helix of auricle		
9	Soft palate (uvula apparent in image)	20	Occipital artery	a	Hard palate		
10	Masseter muscle	21	First cervical vertebrae (atlas)	b	Palatoglossus muscle		
11	Retromandibular vein	22	Dens (axis)	c	Palatopharyngeus muscle		

7.96   IMAGING OF ORBIT AND ORAL CAVITY/MAXILLARY REGION

A. Transverse section and MRI through in plane of optic nerve. **B.** Transverse section and MRI at level of atlas/dens.

Central sulcus

Precentral gyrus (motor area)

Postcentral gyrus (sensory area)

Parietal lobe

Lateral sulcus (fissure)

Frontal lobe

Sensory speech area

Motor speech area

Occipital lobe

Transverse cerebral fissure

Temporal lobe

Cerebellum

Pons

A. Lateral View

Opening of lateral aperture (of Luschka)

Medulla oblongata

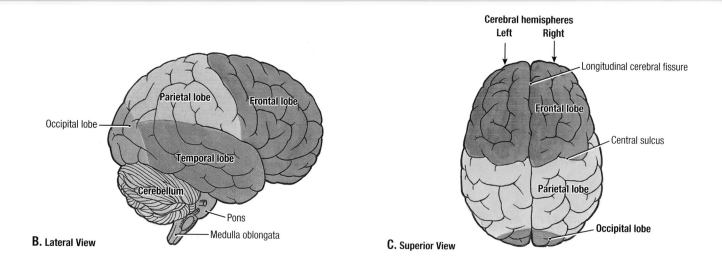

Parietal lobe

Frontal lobe

Occipital lobe

Temporal lobe

Cerebellum

Pons

Medulla oblongata

B. Lateral View

Cerebral hemispheres
Left   Right

Longitudinal cerebral fissure

Frontal lobe

Central sulcus

Parietal lobe

Occipital lobe

C. Superior View

| 7.97 | BRAIN |

A. Cerebrum, cerebellum, and brainstem, lateral aspect. **B.** Lobes of the cerebral hemispheres, lateral aspect. **C.** Lobes of the cerebral hemispheres, superior aspect.

Cerebral contusion (bruising) results from brain trauma in which the pia is stripped from the injured surface of the brain and may be torn, allowing blood to enter the subarachnoid space. The bruising results from the sudden impact of the moving brain against the stationary cranium or from the suddenly moving cranium against the stationary brain. Cerebral contusion may result in an extended loss of consciousness.

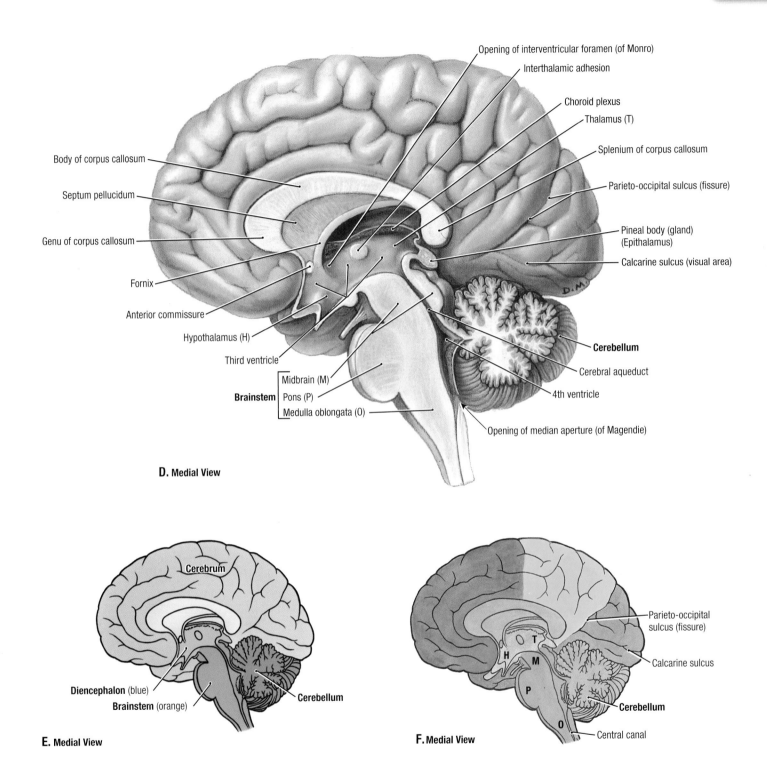

Opening of interventricular foramen (of Monro)
Interthalamic adhesion
Choroid plexus
Thalamus (T)
Splenium of corpus callosum
Parieto-occipital sulcus (fissure)
Pineal body (gland) (Epithalamus)
Calcarine sulcus (visual area)
Cerebellum
Cerebral aqueduct
4th ventricle
Opening of median aperture (of Magendie)

Body of corpus callosum
Septum pellucidum
Genu of corpus callosum
Fornix
Anterior commissure
Hypothalamus (H)
Third ventricle
Brainstem { Midbrain (M)
Pons (P)
Medulla oblongata (O) }

D. Medial View

Cerebrum
Diencephalon (blue)
Brainstem (orange)
Cerebellum

E. Medial View

Parieto-occipital sulcus (fissure)
Calcarine sulcus
Cerebellum
Central canal
T
H
M
P
O

F. Medial View

7.97   BRAIN *(CONTINUED)*

D. Cerebrum, cerebellum, and brainstem, median section. **E.** Parts of the brain, median section. **F.** Lobes of the cerebral hemisphere, median section. See **D** for labeling key.

Cerebral compression may be produced by intracranial collections of blood, obstruction of CSF circulation or absorption, intracranial tumors or abscesses, and brain swelling caused by brain edema, an increase in brain volume resulting from an increase in water and sodium content.

KEY for A:

1 Right and left lateral ventricles
2 Interventricular foramen
3 Third ventricle
4 Cerebral aqueduct
5 Fourth ventricle
6 Median aperture
7 Lateral apertures
8 Central canal
9 Subarachnoid space
10 Arachnoid granulations
11 Superior sagittal sinus
12 Great cerebral vein
13 Straight sinus
14 Confluence of sinuses

A. Lateral View, Schematic

B. Superior View

- Anterior horn*
- **Third ventricle**
- Inferior horn
- Body*
- Trigone
- Cerebral aqueduct
- **Fourth ventricle**
- Posterior horn*
- Lateral aperture
- *** Lateral ventricle**

C. Medial View

- Septum pellucidum
- Subarachnoid space
- Corpus callosum
- Third ventricle
- Choroid plexus
- Pineal body
- **Quadrigeminal cistern**
- Cerebral aqueduct
- Tentorium cerebelli
- Choroid plexus
- **Posterior cerebello-medullary cistern**
- **Chiasmatic cistern**
- **Interpeduncular cistern**
- **Pontocerebellar cistern**
- Subarachnoid space

7.98 VENTRICULAR SYSTEM

A. Circulation of cerebrospinal fluid (CSF). **B.** Ventricles: lateral, third, and fourth.

- The ventricular system consists of two lateral ventricles located in the cerebral hemispheres, a third ventricle located between the right and left halves of the diencephalon, and a fourth ventricle located in the posterior parts of the pons and medulla.
- CSF secreted by choroid plexus in the ventricles drains via the interventricular foramen from the lateral to the third ventricle, via the cerebral aqueduct from the third to the fourth ventricle, and via median and lateral apertures into the subarachnoid space. CSF is absorbed by arachnoid granulations into the venous sinuses (especially the superior sagittal sinus).
- **Hydrocephalus.** Overproduction of CSF, obstruction of its flow, or interference with its absorption results in an excess of CSF in the ventricles and enlargement of the head, a condition known as hydrocephalus. Excess CSF dilates the ventricles; thins the brain; and, in infants, separates the bones of the calvaria because the sutures and fontanelles are still open.

A. Lateral View

B. Lateral View

7.99 SERIAL DISSECTIONS OF LATERAL ASPECT OF CEREBRAL HEMISPHERE

The dissections begin from the lateral surface of the cerebral hemisphere **(A)** and proceed sequentially medially **(B.–F.)**.

A. Sulci and gyri of the lateral surface of one cerebral hemisphere. Each gyrus is a fold of cerebral cortex with a core of white matter. The furrows are called *sulci*. The pattern of sulci and gyri, formed shortly before birth,

is recognizable in some adult brains, as shown in this specimen. Usually the expanding cortex acquires secondary foldings, which make identification of this basic pattern more difficult. **B.** Superior longitudinal fasciculus, transverse temporal gyri, and insula. The cortex and short association fiber bundles around the lateral fissure have been removed.

C. Lateral View

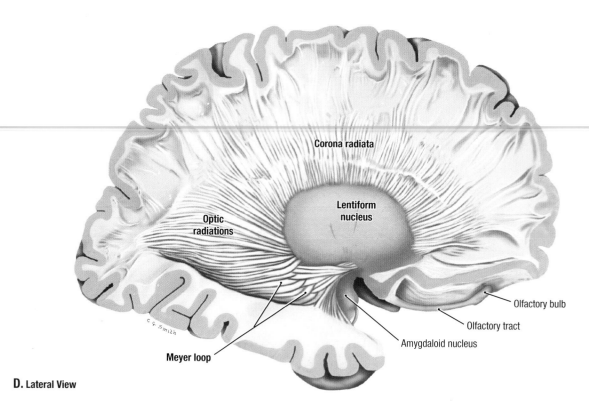

D. Lateral View

7.99   SERIAL DISSECTIONS OF LATERAL ASPECT OF CEREBRAL HEMISPHERE *(CONTINUED)*

C. Uncinate and inferior fronto-occipital fasciculi and external capsule. The external capsule consists of projection fibers that pass between the claustrum laterally and the lentiform nucleus medially. **D.** Lentiform nucleus and corona radiata. The inferior longitudinal and uncinate fasciculi, claustrum, and external capsule have been removed. The fibers of the optic radiations convey impulses from the right half of the retina of each eye; the fibers extending closest to the temporal pole (Meyer's loop) carry impulses from the lower portion of each retina.

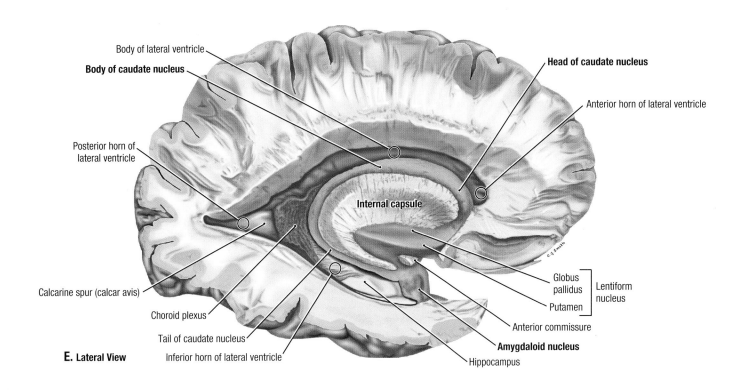

Body of lateral ventricle

Body of caudate nucleus

Head of caudate nucleus

Anterior horn of lateral ventricle

Posterior horn of lateral ventricle

Internal capsule

Calcarine spur (calcar avis)

Globus pallidus ⎱ Lentiform
Putamen ⎰ nucleus

Choroid plexus

Anterior commissure

Tail of caudate nucleus

Amygdaloid nucleus

E. Lateral View

Inferior horn of lateral ventricle

Hippocampus

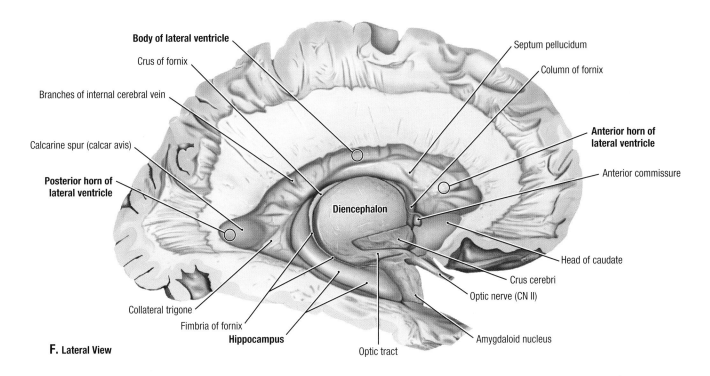

Body of lateral ventricle

Septum pellucidum

Crus of fornix

Column of fornix

Branches of internal cerebral vein

Anterior horn of lateral ventricle

Calcarine spur (calcar avis)

Anterior commissure

Posterior horn of lateral ventricle

Diencephalon

Head of caudate

Crus cerebri

Optic nerve (CN II)

Collateral trigone

Fimbria of fornix

Hippocampus

Amygdaloid nucleus

F. Lateral View

Optic tract

7.99   SERIAL DISSECTIONS OF LATERAL ASPECT OF CEREBRAL HEMISPHERE *(CONTINUED)*

E. Caudate and amygdaloid nuclei and internal capsule. The lateral wall of the lateral ventricle, the marginal part of the internal capsule, the anterior commissure, and the superior part of the lentiform nucleus have been removed. **F.** Lateral ventricle, hippocampus, and diencephalon. The inferior parts of the lentiform nucleus, internal capsule, and caudate nucleus have been removed.

Cingulate sulcus

Paracentral lobule

Marginal sulcus

Callosal sulcus

Superior frontal gyrus

Cingulate gyrus

Precuneus

Parieto-occipital sulcus

Septum pellucidum

Corpus callosum

Cuneus

Fornix

3rd ventricle

Lingual gyrus

Calcarine sulcus

Frontal pole

Occipital lobe

Subcallosal area

Uncus

Anterior commissure

Parahippocampal gyrus

Hippocampal sulcus

Olfactory tract

Optic chiasma

Optic nerve

Occipitotemporal gyri

A. Medial View

Collateral sulcus

Interventricular foramen

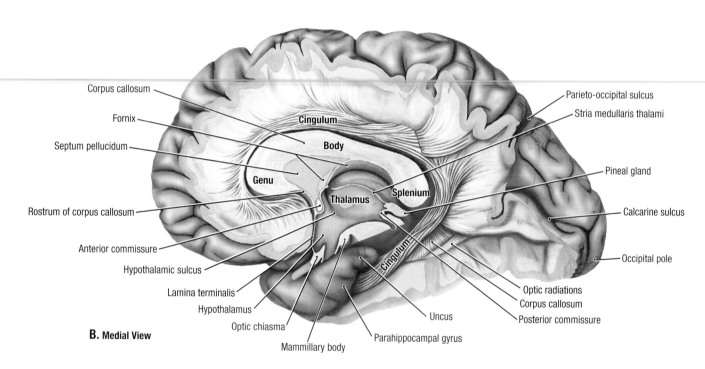

Corpus callosum

Parieto-occipital sulcus

Fornix

Cingulum

Stria medullaris thalami

Septum pellucidum

Body

Genu

Pineal gland

Rostrum of corpus callosum

Thalamus

Splenium

Calcarine sulcus

Anterior commissure

Cingulum

Occipital pole

Hypothalamic sulcus

Lamina terminalis

Optic radiations

Hypothalamus

Corpus callosum

Optic chiasma

Uncus

Posterior commissure

Mammillary body

Parahippocampal gyrus

B. Medial View

7.100 ## SERIAL DISSECTIONS OF MEDIAL ASPECT OF CEREBRAL HEMISPHERE

The dissections begin from the medial surface of the cerebral hemisphere **(A)** and proceed sequentially laterally **(B.–D)**.

A. Sulci and gyri of medial surface of cerebral hemisphere. The corpus callosum consists of the rostrum, genu, body, and splenium; the cingulate and parahippocampal gyri from the limbic lobe. **B.** Cingulum. The cortex and short association fibers were removed from the medial aspect of the hemisphere. The cingulum is a long association fiber bundle that lies in the core of the cingulate and parahippocampal gyri.

C. Median View

Interventricular foramen
Anterior commissure
Mammillothalamic fasciculus
Septum pellucidum
Pineal gland
Fornix
Corpus callosum
Fornix
Forceps minor
Forceps major
Mammillary body
Infundibulum
Cerebral aqueduct
Crus cerebri
Fornix
Uncus
Parahippocampal gyrus
Choroid plexus of lateral ventricle
Hippocampal sulcus
Hippocampus
Dentate gyrus
Ependyma of lateral wall of inferior horn of lateral ventricle

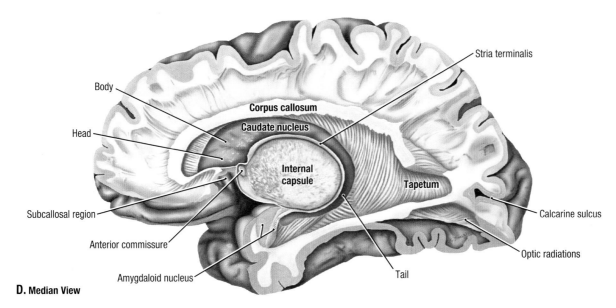

D. Median View

Stria terminalis
Body
Corpus callosum
Caudate nucleus
Head
Internal capsule
Tapetum
Subcallosal region
Anterior commissure
Calcarine sulcus
Amygdaloid nucleus
Optic radiations
Tail

7.100

SERIAL DISSECTIONS OF THE MEDIAL ASPECT OF CEREBRAL HEMISPHERE *(CONTINUED)*

C. Fornix, mammillothalamic fasciculus, and forceps major and minor. The cingulum and a portion of the wall of the third ventricle have been removed. The fornix begins at the hippocampus and terminates in the mammillary body by passing anterior to the interventricular foramen and posterior to the anterior commissure. The mammillothalamic fasciculus emerges from the mammillary body and terminates in the anterior nucleus of the thalamus. **D.** Caudate nucleus and internal capsule. The diencephalon was removed, along with the ependyma of the lateral ventricle, except where it covers the caudate and amygdaloid nuclei. **E.** Corpus callosum. The body of the corpus callosum connects the two cerebral hemispheres; the minor (frontal) forceps (at the genu of corpus callosum) connects the frontal lobes, and the major (occipital) forceps (at splenium) connects the occipital lobes.

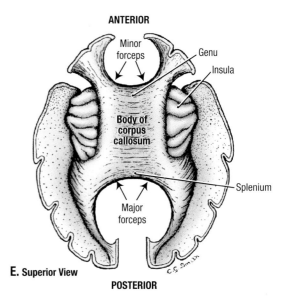

ANTERIOR
Minor forceps
Genu
Insula
Body of corpus callosum
Splenium
Major forceps

E. Superior View
POSTERIOR

A. Posterosuperior View

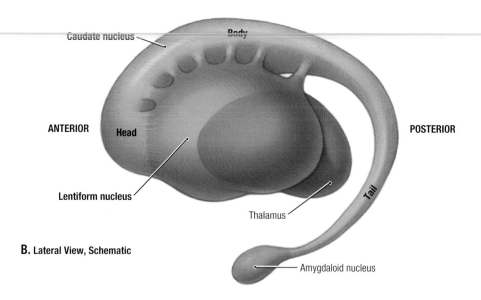

B. Lateral View, Schematic

7.101   CAUDATE AND LENTIFORM NUCLEI

A. Relationship to the lateral ventricles and internal capsule. The dorsal surface of the diencephalon has been exposed by dissecting away the two cerebral hemispheres, except the anterior part of the corpus callosum, the inferior part of the septum pellucidum, the internal capsule, and the caudate and lentiform nuclei. On the right side of the specimen, the thalamus, caudate, and lentiform nuclei have been cut horizontally at the level of the interventricular foramen. The parts of the internal capsule include the anterior, posterior, retrolenticular sublenticular limbs, and genu. **B.** Schematic illustration of nuclei.

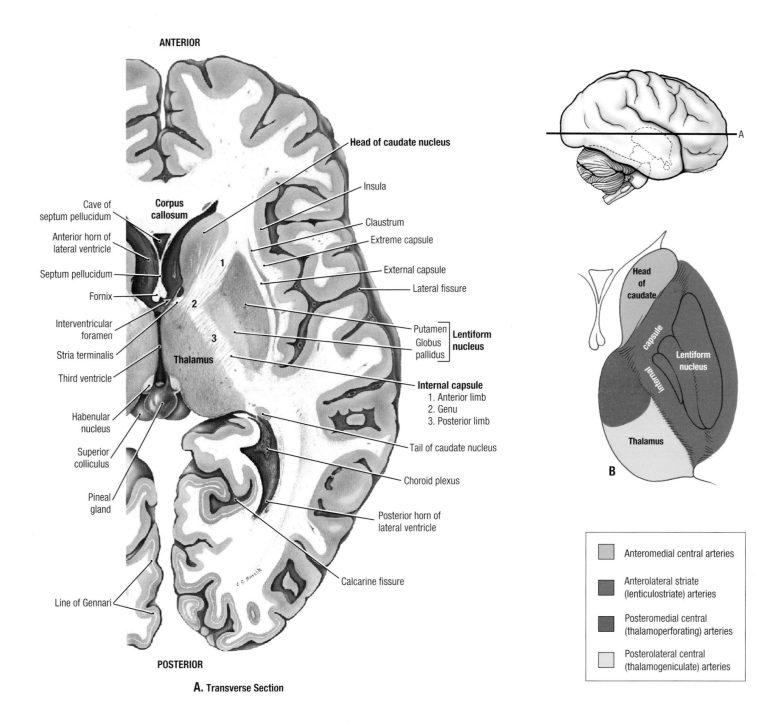

ANTERIOR

Head of caudate nucleus

Insula

Cave of
septum pellucidum

Corpus
callosum

Anterior horn of
lateral ventricle

Septum pellucidum

Fornix

Interventricular
foramen

Stria terminalis

Third ventricle

Habenular
nucleus

Superior
colliculus

Pineal
gland

Line of Gennari

POSTERIOR

Claustrum

Extreme capsule

External capsule

Lateral fissure

Putamen   Lentiform
Globus   nucleus
pallidus

Internal capsule
1. Anterior limb
2. Genu
3. Posterior limb

Tail of caudate nucleus

Choroid plexus

Posterior horn of
lateral ventricle

Calcarine fissure

1
2
3
Thalamus

A. Transverse Section

A

Head
of
caudate

Internal capsule

Lentiform
nucleus

Thalamus

B

Anteromedial central arteries

Anterolateral striate
(lenticulostriate) arteries

Posteromedial central
(thalamoperforating) arteries

Posterolateral central
(thalamogeniculate) arteries

7.102   AXIAL SECTIONS THROUGH THALAMUS, CAUDATE NUCLEUS, AND LENTIFORM NUCLEUS

A. Relationships of the internal capsule. **B.** Blood supply of region.

AXIAL (TRANSVERSE) MRIs THROUGH CEREBRAL HEMISPHERES

See orientation drawing for sites of scans **A.–F. A** is T2 weighted, and **B.–F.** are T1 weighted.

Transverse (Axial) Sections

AC	Anterior commissure	GL	Globus pallidus
ACA	Anterior cerebral artery	GR	Gyrus rectus
AH	Anterior horn of lateral ventricle	HB	Habenular commissure
		HC	Head of caudate nucleus
C1	Anterior limb of internal capsule	IN	Insular cortex
		L	Lentiform nucleus
C2	Genu of internal capsule	LF	Lateral fissure
C3	Posterior limb of internal capsule	LV	Lateral ventricle
		M	Mammillary body
C4	Retrolenticular limb of internal capsule	MCA	Middle cerebral artery
		OL	Occipital lobe
CC	Collicular cistern	ON	Optic nerve
CD	Cerebral peduncle	OR	Optic radiations
CH	Choroid plexus	OT	Optic tract
CL	Claustrum	P	Putamen
CN	Caudate nucleus	PL	Pulvinar
CV	Great cerebral vein	RN	Red nucleus
ET	External capsule	SP	Septum pellucidum
EX	Extreme capsule	ST	Straight sinus
F	Fornix	T	Thalamus
FC	Falx cerebri	TC	Tail of caudate nucleus
FL	Frontal lobe	TR	Trigone of lateral ventricle
FM	Interventricular foramen	TU	Tuber cinereum
FMa	Forceps major	TV	Third ventricle
FMi	Forceps minor	W	White matter
G	Gray matter		

7.103 AXIAL (TRANSVERSE) MRIs THROUGH CEREBRAL HEMISPHERES *(CONTINUED)*

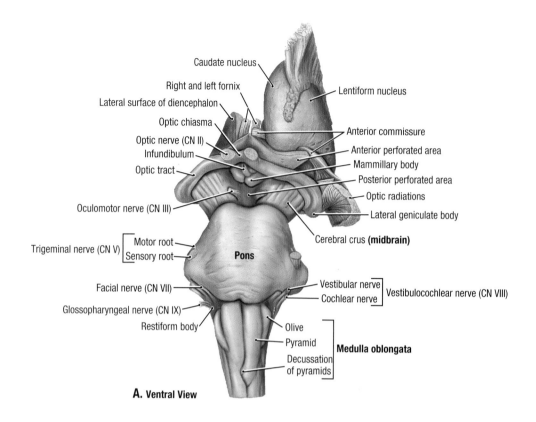

Caudate nucleus
Right and left fornix
Lateral surface of diencephalon
Optic chiasma
Optic nerve (CN II)
Infundibulum
Optic tract
Oculomotor nerve (CN III)
Trigeminal nerve (CN V) { Motor root / Sensory root }
Facial nerve (CN VII)
Glossopharyngeal nerve (CN IX)
Restiform body

Lentiform nucleus
Anterior commissure
Anterior perforated area
Mammillary body
Posterior perforated area
Optic radiations
Lateral geniculate body
Cerebral crus (**midbrain**)
Pons
Vestibular nerve / Cochlear nerve } Vestibulocochlear nerve (CN VIII)
Olive
Pyramid } **Medulla oblongata**
Decussation of pyramids

A. Ventral View

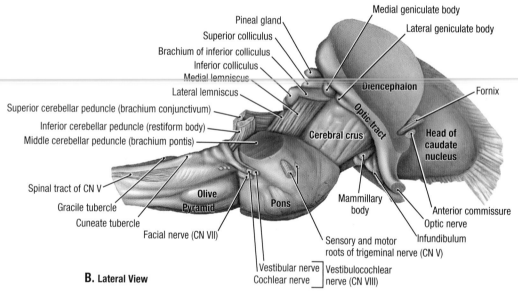

Pineal gland
Superior colliculus
Brachium of inferior colliculus
Inferior colliculus
Medial lemniscus
Lateral lemniscus
Superior cerebellar peduncle (brachium conjunctivum)
Inferior cerebellar peduncle (restiform body)
Middle cerebellar peduncle (brachium pontis)
Spinal tract of CN V
Gracile tubercle
Cuneate tubercle
Facial nerve (CN VII)

Medial geniculate body
Lateral geniculate body
Diencephalon
Fornix
Optic tract
Cerebral crus
Head of caudate nucleus
Olive
Pyramid
Pons
Mammillary body
Anterior commissure
Optic nerve
Infundibulum
Sensory and motor roots of trigeminal nerve (CN V)
Vestibular nerve / Cochlear nerve } Vestibulocochlear nerve (CN VIII)

B. Lateral View

7.104   BRAINSTEM

The brainstem has been exposed by removing the cerebellum, all of the right cerebral hemisphere, and the major portion of the left hemisphere. **A.** Ventral aspect.

- The brainstem consists of the medulla oblongata, pons, and midbrain.
- The pyramid is on the ventral surface of the medulla; the decussation of the pyramids is formed by the decussating (crossing) lateral corticospinal tract.
- The trigeminal nerve (CN V) emerges as sensory and motor roots.
- The crus cerebri are part of the midbrain.
- The oculomotor nerve emerges from the interpeduncular fossa.

B. Lateral aspect.

- The vestibulocochlear nerve (CN VIII) consists of two nerves, the vestibular and cochlear nerves.
- The spinal tract of the trigeminal nerve is exposed where it comes to the surface of the medulla to form the tuber cinereum.
- The three are cerebellar peduncles: superior, middle, and inferior.
- The medial and lateral lemnisci on the lateral aspect of the midbrain

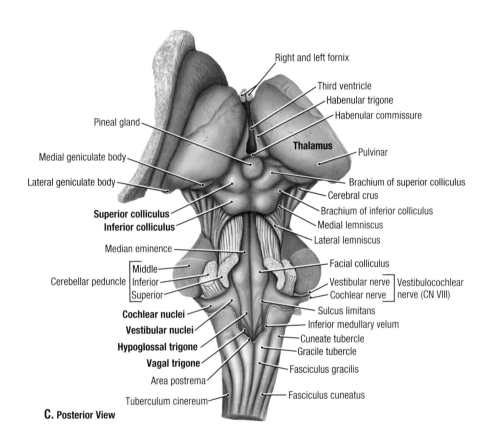

Right and left fornix
Third ventricle
Habenular trigone
Habenular commissure
Pineal gland
Thalamus
Pulvinar
Medial geniculate body
Lateral geniculate body
Brachium of superior colliculus
Cerebral crus
Brachium of inferior colliculus
Superior colliculus
Medial lemniscus
Inferior colliculus
Lateral lemniscus
Median eminence
Facial colliculus
Middle
Inferior
Superior
Cerebellar peduncle
Vestibular nerve ⎤ Vestibulocochlear
Cochlear nerve ⎦ nerve (CN VIII)
Cochlear nuclei
Sulcus limitans
Vestibular nuclei
Inferior medullary velum
Hypoglossal trigone
Cuneate tubercle
Vagal trigone
Gracile tubercle
Area postrema
Fasciculus gracilis
Tuberculum cinereum
Fasciculus cuneatus

C. Posterior View

| 7.104 | **BRAINSTEM** *(CONTINUED)* |

C. Dorsal aspect.
- Ridges are formed by the fasciculus gracilis and cuneatus.
- The gracile and cuneate tubercles are the sites of the nucleus gracilis and nucleus cuneatus.
- The diamond-shaped floor of the fourth ventricle; lateral to the sulcus limitans are the vestibular and cochlear nuclei and medially are the hypoglossal and vagal trigones and the facial colliculus.
- The superior and inferior colliculi form the dorsal surface of the midbrain.

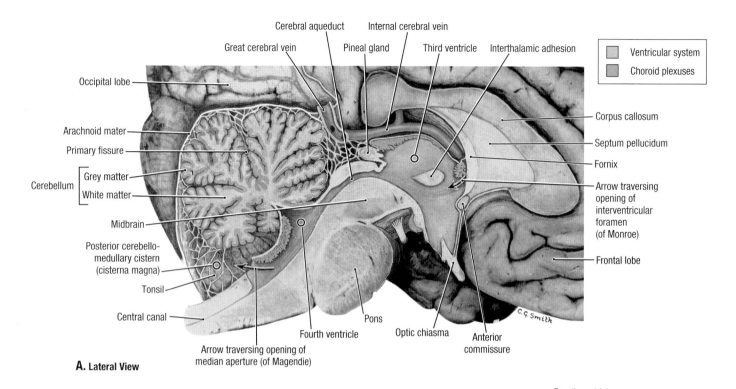

Cerebral aqueduct
Internal cerebral vein
Great cerebral vein
Pineal gland
Third ventricle
Interthalamic adhesion
Occipital lobe

Ventricular system
Choroid plexuses

Arachnoid mater
Primary fissure
Cerebellum
Grey matter
White matter
Midbrain
Posterior cerebello-
medullary cistern
(cisterna magna)
Tonsil
Central canal

Corpus callosum
Septum pellucidum
Fornix
Arrow traversing
opening of
interventricular
foramen
(of Monroe)
Frontal lobe

Fourth ventricle
Pons
Optic chiasma
Anterior
commissure

Arrow traversing opening of
median aperture (of Magendie)

A. Lateral View

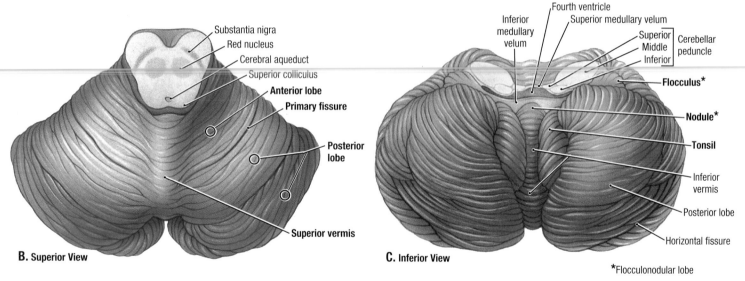

Substantia nigra
Red nucleus
Cerebral aqueduct
Superior colliculus
Anterior lobe
Primary fissure

**Posterior
lobe**

Superior vermis

B. Superior View

Fourth ventricle
Inferior
medullary
velum
Superior medullary velum
Superior
Middle
Inferior
Cerebellar
peduncle
Flocculus*
Nodule*
Tonsil
Inferior
vermis
Posterior lobe
Horizontal fissure

C. Inferior View

*Flocculonodular lobe

7.105   CEREBELLUM

A. Median section. The arachnoid mater was removed except where it covered the cerebellum and the occipital lobe. **Cisternal puncture.** CSF may be obtained, for diagnostic purposes, from the posterior cerebellomedullary cistern, using a procedure known as cisternal puncture. The subarachnoid space or the ventricular system may also be entered for measuring or monitoring CSF pressure, injecting antibiotics, or administering contrast media for radiography. **B.** Superior view of the cerebellum. The right and left cerebellar hemispheres are united by the superior vermis; the anterior and posterior lobes are separated by the primary fissure. **C.** Inferior view of cerebellum. The flocculonodular lobe, the oldest part of the cerebellum, consists of the flocculus and nodule; the cerebellar tonsils typically extend into the foramen magnum.

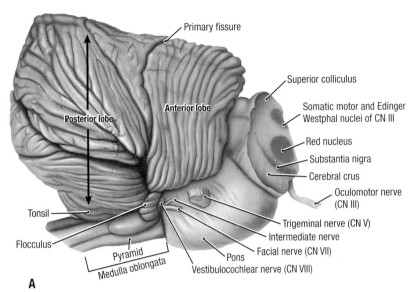

A. Cerebellum and brainstem

- Primary fissure
- **Posterior lobe**
- **Anterior lobe**
- Superior colliculus
- Somatic motor and Edinger Westphal nuclei of CN III
- Red nucleus
- Substantia nigra
- Cerebral crus
- Oculomotor nerve (CN III)
- Tonsil
- Trigeminal nerve (CN V)
- Intermediate nerve
- Flocculus
- Facial nerve (CN VII)
- Pyramid
- Pons
- Medulla oblongata
- Vestibulocochlear nerve (CN VIII)

A

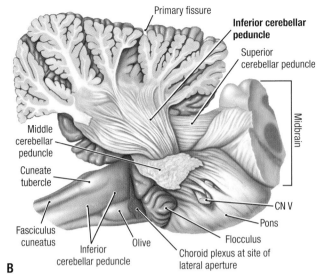

- Primary fissure
- **Inferior cerebellar peduncle**
- Superior cerebellar peduncle
- Middle cerebellar peduncle
- Cuneate tubercle
- Midbrain
- Fasciculus cuneatus
- Inferior cerebellar peduncle
- Olive
- CN V
- Pons
- Flocculus
- Choroid plexus at site of lateral aperture

B

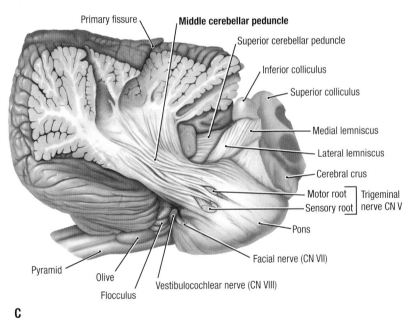

- Primary fissure
- **Middle cerebellar peduncle**
- Superior cerebellar peduncle
- Inferior colliculus
- Superior colliculus
- Medial lemniscus
- Lateral lemniscus
- Cerebral crus
- Motor root
- Sensory root
- Trigeminal nerve CN V
- Pons
- Facial nerve (CN VII)
- Pyramid
- Olive
- Flocculus
- Vestibulocochlear nerve (CN VIII)

C

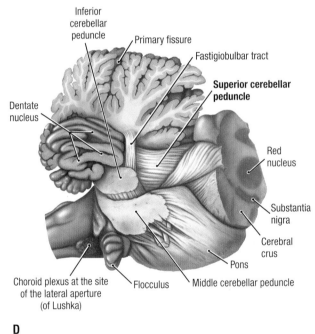

- Inferior cerebellar peduncle
- Primary fissure
- Fastigiobulbar tract
- **Superior cerebellar peduncle**
- Dentate nucleus
- Red nucleus
- Substantia nigra
- Cerebral crus
- Pons
- Choroid plexus at the site of the lateral aperture (of Lushka)
- Flocculus
- Middle cerebellar peduncle

D

Lateral Views

7.106 SERIAL DISSECTIONS OF THE CEREBELLUM

The series begins with the lateral surface of the cerebellar hemispheres **(A)** and proceeds medially in sequence **(B–D)**.

A. Cerebellum and brainstem. **B.** Inferior cerebellar peduncle. The fibers of the middle cerebellar peduncle were cut dorsal to the trigeminal nerve and peeled away to expose the fibers of the inferior cerebellar peduncle. **C.** Middle cerebellar peduncle. The fibers of the middle cerebellar peduncle were exposed by peeling away the lateral portion of the lobules of the cerebellar hemisphere. **D.** Superior cerebellar peduncle and dentate nucleus. The fibers of the inferior cerebellar peduncle were cut just dorsal to the previously sectioned middle cerebellar peduncle and peeled away until the gray matter of the dentate nucleus could be seen.

Blood Supply:

- Posterior cerebral
- Superior cerebellar
- Anterior inferior cerebellar
- Posterior inferior cerebellar
- Vertebral
- Anterior spinal
- Posterior spinal

Basilar:
- Long circumferential branches
- Short circumferential branches
- Paramedian branches

AICA	Anterior inferior cerebellar artery
AM	Internal acoustic meatus
BA	Basilar artery
C	Cerebral crus
CA	Cerebral aqueduct
CB	Ciliary body
CC	Common carotid artery
CI	Colliculi
CL	Left cerebellar hemisphere
CP	Cochlear perilymph
CR	Right cerebellar hemisphere
CSF	CSF in subarachnoid space
DS	Dorsum sellae
EB	Eyeball
F	CN VII and CN VIII
FC	Facial colliculus
FI	Fat in infratemporal fossa
FL	Flocculus
FV	Fourth ventricle
G	Gray matter
HF	Hypophysial fossa
HP	Hippocampus
IN	Infundibulum
IC	Interpeduncular cistern
ICA	Internal carotid artery
ICP	Inferior cerebellar peduncle
IF	Inferior concha
IH	Inferior horn (lateral ventricle)
IJV	Internal jugular vein
IP	Interpeduncular fossa
IV	Inferior vermis
L	Lens
LP	Lateral pterygoid
MA	Mastoid air cells
MB	Mandible
MC	Middle concha
MCP	Middle cerebellar peduncle
MD	Midbrain
MO	Medulla oblongata
MS	Maxillary sinus
MT	Masseter
MX	Maxilla
ND	Nodule of cerebellum
NS	Nasal septum
OB	Occipital bone
OC	Optic chiasm

Site of transverse (axial) scans

Transverse section through lower medulla oblongata (Part A)

Transverse section through upper medulla oblongata (Part B)

7.107   AXIAL (TRANSVERSE) MRIs THROUGH BRAINSTEM, INFERIOR VIEWS

Images on left side of the page are T1 weighted, and images on the right side are T2 weighted.

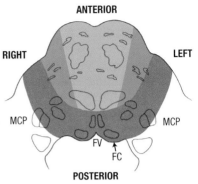

Transverse section through pons (Parts C & D)

OL	Occipital lobe
ON	Optic nerve (CN II)
P	Pons
PA	Pharynx
PCA	Posterior cerebral artery
PF	Parapharyngeal fat
PG	Parotid gland
PH	Posterior horn (lateral ventricle)
PN	Pinna
PY	Pyramid
RN	Red nucleus
SC	Semicircular canal
SCP	Superior cerebellar peduncle
SE	Suprasellar cistern
SH	Superior concha
SN	Substantia nigra
SS	Superior sagittal sinus
ST	Straight sinus
SV	Superior vermis
TG	Tongue
TL	Temporal lobe
TP	Temporalis
UN	Uncus
VA	Vertebral artery
VP	Vestibular perilymph
VT	Vitreous body
W	White matter

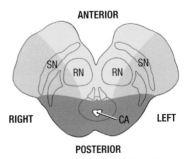

Transverse section through midbrain (Part E)

7.107 AXIAL (TRANSVERSE) MRIs THROUGH BRAINSTEM, INFERIOR VIEWS *(CONTINUED)*

AA	Anterior communicating artery
AC	Anterior commissure
ACA	Anterior cerebral artery
AH	Anterior horn of lateral ventricle
BC	Body of caudate nucleus
BV	Body of lateral ventricle
C	Cerebellum
CC	Corpus callosum
CH	Choroid plexus
CS	Cavernous sinus
CT	Corticospinal tract
CV	Great cerebral vein
DN	Dentate nucleus
DS	Diaphragma sellae
F	Fornix
FV	Fourth ventricle
G	Gray matter
HC	Head of caudate nucleus
HP	Hippocampus
IC	Interpeduncular cistern
ICA	Internal carotid artery
IH	Interior horn of lateral ventricle
IN	Insular cortex
INC	Internal capsule
IR	Intervertebral vein
IV	Inferior vermis
L	Lentiform nucleus
L1	Putamen
L2	External (lateral) segment of globus pallidus
L3	Internal (medial) segment of globus pallidus
LF	Lateral fissure
LGF	Longitudinal fissure
MCA	Middle cerebral artery
MD	Midbrain
OT	Optic tract
P	Pons
PCA	Posterior cerebral artery
PH	Posterior horn of lateral ventricle
PICA	Posterior inferior cerebellar artery
PY	Pyramid
S	Carotid siphon
SC	Supracellebellar cistern
SCA	Superior cerebellar artery
SN	Substantia nigra
SP	Septum pellucidum
SS	Superior sagittal sinus
ST	Straight sinus
SV	Superior vermis
T	Thalamus
TC	Tail of caudate nucleus
TL	Temporal lobe
To	Cerebellar tonsil
TR	Trigone of lateral ventricle
TT	Tentorium cerebelli
TV	Third ventricle
VA	Vertebral artery
W	White matter
Y	Hypophysis

7.108 CORONAL MRIs (T2 WEIGHTED) AND SECTIONS OF BRAIN

A.–F. Coronal MRIs. **G.–H.** Coronal sections, posterior views.

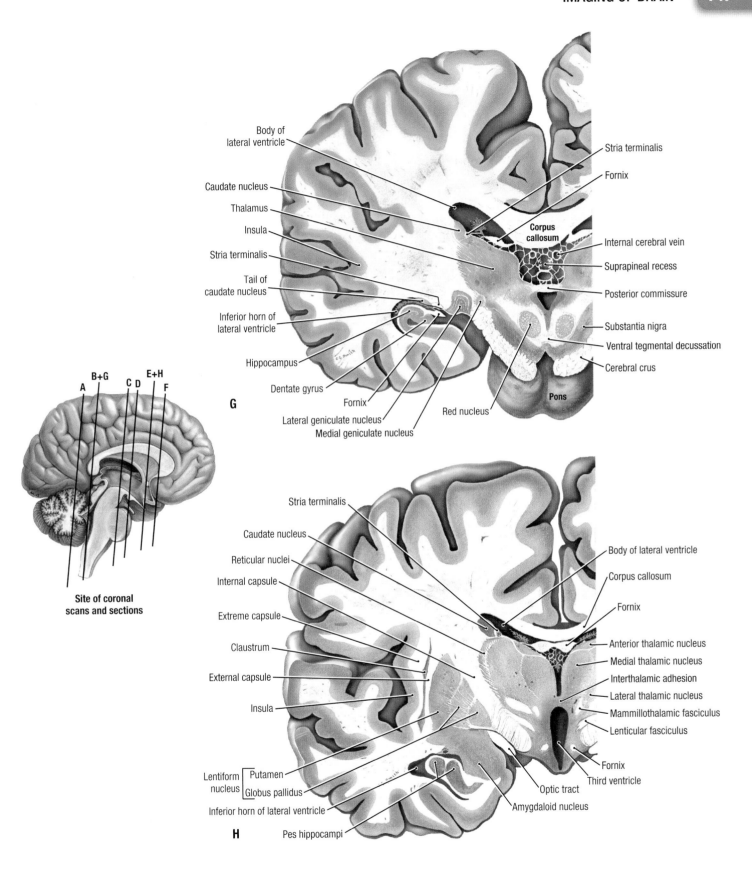

G

- Body of lateral ventricle
- Caudate nucleus
- Thalamus
- Insula
- Stria terminalis
- Tail of caudate nucleus
- Inferior horn of lateral ventricle
- Hippocampus
- Dentate gyrus
- Fornix
- Lateral geniculate nucleus
- Medial geniculate nucleus
- Red nucleus
- Stria terminalis
- Fornix
- **Corpus callosum**
- Internal cerebral vein
- Suprapineal recess
- Posterior commissure
- Substantia nigra
- Ventral tegmental decussation
- Cerebral crus
- **Pons**

Site of coronal scans and sections

A B+G C D E+H F

H

- Stria terminalis
- Caudate nucleus
- Reticular nuclei
- Internal capsule
- Extreme capsule
- Claustrum
- External capsule
- Insula
- Lentiform nucleus
  - Putamen
  - Globus pallidus
- Inferior horn of lateral ventricle
- Pes hippocampi
- Amygdaloid nucleus
- Optic tract
- Fornix
- Third ventricle
- Lenticular fasciculus
- Mammillothalamic fasciculus
- Lateral thalamic nucleus
- Interthalamic adhesion
- Medial thalamic nucleus
- Anterior thalamic nucleus
- Fornix
- Corpus callosum
- Body of lateral ventricle

A

B

C

ACA	Anterior cerebral artery
AH	Anterior horn of lateral ventricle
B	Body of corpus callosum
BA	Basilar artery
BV	Body of lateral ventricle
C	Colliculi
C1	Anterior tubercle of atlas
Cal	Calcarine sulcus
Cb	Cerebellum
CG	Cingulate nucleus
CQ	Cerebral aqueduct
CS	Cingulate sulcus
D	Dens (odontoid process)
F	Fornix
FM	Foramen magnum
FP	Frontal pole
FV	Fourth ventricle
G	Cerebral cortex (gray matter)
GC	Genus of corpus callosum
H	Hypothalamus
HC	Head of caudate nucleus
I	Infundibulum
IN	Insular cortex
M	Mammillary body
MCA	Middle cerebral artery
MD	Midbrain
OP	Occipital pole
P	Pons
PA	Pharynx
PD	Cerebral peduncle
PI	Pineal
PO	Parieto-occipital fissure
R	Rostrum of corpus callosum
S	Splenium of corpus callosum
SC	Spinal cord
SF	Superior frontal sulcus
ST	Straight sinus
STS	Superior temporal sulcus
SV	Superior medullary vellum
T	Thalamus
To	Cerebellar tonsil
TP	Temporal pole
TS	Transverse sinus
W	White matter
Y	Hypophysis

Sagittal Sections

Superior cerebral vein

Skin

Subcutaneous tissue

Epicranial aponeurosis

Great cerebral vein

Pericranium

Midbrain

Tentorium cerebelli

Pons

Cerebellum

External occipital protuberance

Internal occipital protuberance

Fourth ventricle

Falx cerebelli

Medulla oblongata

Cerebellar tonsil (herniated)

Atlas (posterior arch)

Dens of axis

Axis

Epiglottis

Posterior wall of pharynx

Vertebral body C6

Superior sagittal sinus

Falx cerebri

Corpus callosum

Fornix

Septum pellucidum

Frontal sinus

Anterior cerebral artery

Cribriform plate of ethmoid bone

Nasal septum

Pharyngeal tonsil

Foramen magnum

Soft palate

Hard palate

Tongue

Geniohyoid

Mylohyoid

Mandible

Hyoid

Thyroid cartilage

Vocal fold

D. Median Section

7.109 **SAGITTAL MRIs (T1 WEIGHTED) AND MEDIAN SECTION OF BRAIN**

See orientation drawing for sites of scans **A.–C.**

Increased intracranial pressure (e.g., due to a tumor) may cause displacement of the cerebellar tonsils through the foramen magnum, resulting in a foraminal (tonsillar) herniation. Compression of the brainstem, if severe, may result in respiratory and cardiac arrest.

Neck

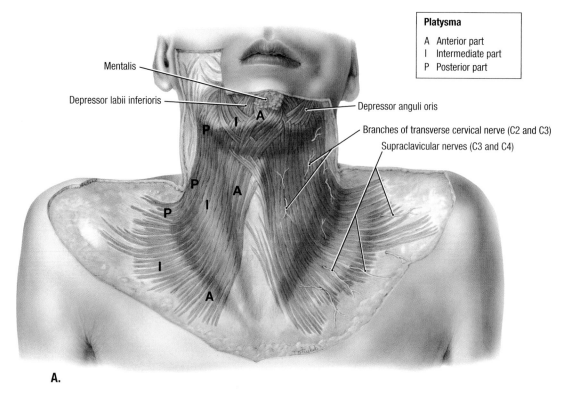

Platysma
A Anterior part
I Intermediate part
P Posterior part

Mentalis

Depressor labii inferioris

Depressor anguli oris

Branches of transverse cervical nerve (C2 and C3)

Supraclavicular nerves (C3 and C4)

A.

Anterior Views

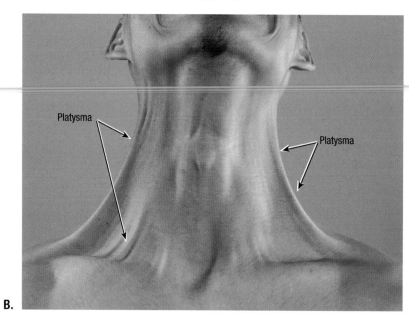

Platysma

Platysma

B.

8.1 PLATYSMA

A. Parts of platysma. **B.** Surface anatomy.

TABLE 8.1 PLATYSMA

Muscle	Superior Attachment	Inferior Attachment	Innervation	Main Action
Platysma	*Anterior part:* Fibers interlace with contralateral muscle *Intermediate part:* Fibers pass deep to depressors anguli oris and labii inferioris to attach to inferior border of mandible *Posterior part:* Skin/subcutaneous tissue of lower face lateral to mouth	Subcutaneous tissue overlying superior parts of pectoralis major and sometimes deltoid muscles	Cervical branch of facial nerve (CN VII)	Draws corner of mouth inferiorly and widens it as in expressions of sadness and fright; draws the skin of the neck superiorly, forming tense vertical and oblique ridges over the anterior neck

Occipital bone

Pharynx

Mandible

Hyoid

Investing layer of deep cervical fascia

Larynx

Thyroid isthmus

Esophagus

Suprasternal space

Trachea

Manubrium of sternum

A. Medial View

Plane of section for parts **B** and **C**

Anterior longitudinal ligament

Buccopharyngeal fascia*

Alar fascia

Retropharyngeal space †

Intervertebral disc

Prevertebral fascia

Body of vertebra

Longus colli

Pharyngeal muscle

Pharynx

B. Anterosuperior View of Part C

Nuchal ligament

Vertebral arch of cervical vertebra

Trapezius

Middle scalene

Longus colli

Phrenic nerve

Sympathetic trunk

Omohyoid

Platysma

Sternocleidomastoid (SCM)

Sternothyroid

Sternohyoid

POSTERIOR

Skin

Retropharyngeal † space

Alar fascia

Lymph node

Anterior scalene

Carotid sheath

Vagus nerve

Internal jugular vein

External jugular vein

Common carotid artery

Thyroid gland**

Esophagus**

Trachea**

ANTERIOR

C. Superior View of Transverse Section (at level of C7 vertebra)

☐ **Subcutaneous tissue of neck** (superficial cervical fascia)

Deep cervical fascia:

Investing layer

Pretracheal layer *

Prevertebral layer

Alar fascia and carotid sheath

* Buccopharyngeal fascia is a component of the pretracheal layer

** In visceral compartment of neck

† Retropharyngeal "space" is normally a potential space only – actually a loose areolar plane enabling pharyngeal/upper esophageal movement

8.2

SUBCUTANEOUS TISSUE AND DEEP FASCIA OF NECK

Sectional demonstrations of the fasciae of the neck. **A.** Fasciae of the neck are continuous inferiorly and superiorly with thoracic and cranial fasciae. The *inset* illustrates the fascia of the retropharyngeal region. **B.** Relationship of the main layers of deep cervical fascia and the carotid sheath. Midline access to the cervical viscera is possible with minimal disruption of tissues. **C.** The concentric layers of fascia are apparent in this transverse section of neck at the level indicated in **A.**

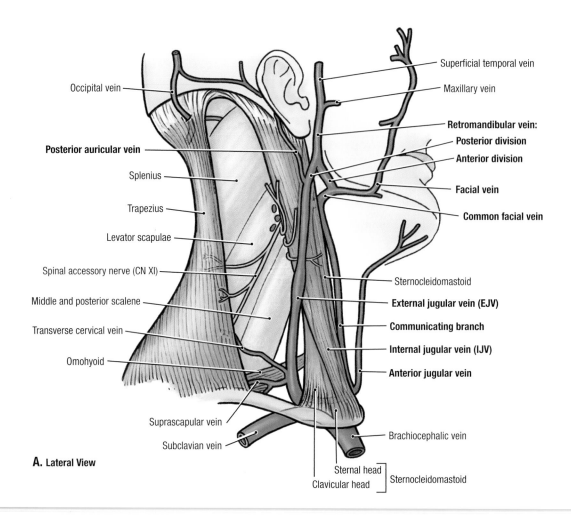

A. Lateral View

8.3 ## SUPERFICIAL VEINS OF NECK

A. Schematic illustration of superficial veins of the neck. The superficial temporal and maxillary veins merge to form the retromandibular vein. The posterior division of the retromandibular vein unites with the posterior auricular vein to form the external jugular vein (EJV). The facial vein receives the anterior division of the retromandibular vein, forming the common facial vein that empties into the internal jugular vein. Variations are common. **B.** Surface anatomy of the external jugular vein and the muscles bounding the lateral cervical region (posterior triangle) of the neck.

External jugular vein (EJV). The EJV may serve as an "internal barometer." When venous pressure is in the normal range, the EJV is usually visible superior to the clavicle for only a short distance. However, when venous pressure rises (e.g., as in heart failure) the vein is prominent throughout its course along the side of the neck. Consequently, routine observation for distention of the EJVs during physical examinations may reveal diagnostic signs of heart failure, obstruction of the superior vena cava, enlarged supraclavicular lymph nodes, or increased intrathoracic pressure.

B. Right Anterolateral View

C	Cricoid cartilage
H	Hyoid bone
IP	Inferior pole of thyroid gland
LL	Left lobe of thyroid gland
P	Laryngeal prominence
RL	Right lobe of thyroid gland
S	Isthmus
SP	Superior pole of thyroid gland
T	Thyroid cartilage
★	Tracheal rings

A. Anterior View

Incision in trachea after retracting infrahyoid muscles and incising isthmus of thyroid gland

8.4   SURFACE ANATOMY OF HYOID AND CARTILAGES OF ANTERIOR NECK

A. Surface anatomy. **B.** Tracheostomy. The U-shaped hyoid bone lies superior to the thyroid cartilage at the level of the C4 and C5 vertebrae. The laryngeal prominence is produced by the fused laminae of the thyroid cartilage, which meet in the median plane. The cricoid cartilage can be felt inferior to the laryngeal prominence. It lies at the level of the C6 vertebra. The cartilaginous tracheal rings are palpable in the inferior part of the neck. The 2nd to 4th rings cannot be felt because the isthmus of the thyroid, connecting its right and left lobes, covers them. The first tracheal ring is just superior to the isthmus.

Tracheostomy. A transverse incision through the skin of the neck and anterior wall of the trachea (*tracheostomy*) establishes an airway in patients with upper airway obstruction or respiratory failure. The infrahyoid muscles are retracted laterally, and the isthmus of the thyroid gland is either divided or retracted superiorly. An opening is made in the trachea between the 1st and 2nd tracheal rings or through the 2nd through 4th rings. A *tracheostomy tube* is then inserted into the trachea and secured. To avoid complications during a tracheostomy, the following anatomical relationships are important:

- The inferior thyroid veins arise from a venous plexus on the thyroid gland and descend anterior to the trachea (see Fig. 8.10).
- A small thyroid ima artery is present in approximately 10% of people; it ascends from the brachiocephalic trunk or the arch of the aorta to the isthmus of the thyroid gland (see Fig. 8.21).
- The left brachiocephalic vein, jugular venous arch, and pleurae may be encountered, particularly in infants and children.
- The thymus covers the inferior part of the trachea in infants and children.
- The trachea is small, mobile, and soft in infants, making it easy to cut through its posterior wall and damage the esophagus.

Tracheostomy tube inserted in tracheal opening

B. Tracheostomy

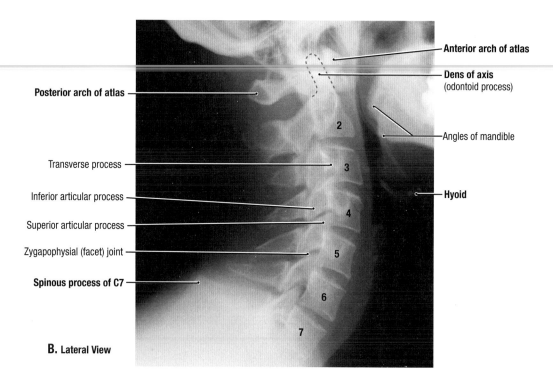

8.5   BONES AND CARTILAGES OF NECK

A. Bony and cartilaginous landmarks of the neck. **B.** Radiograph of hyoid bone and cervical vertebrae. Because the upper cervical vertebrae lie posterior to the upper and lower jaws and teeth, they are best seen radiographically in lateral views.

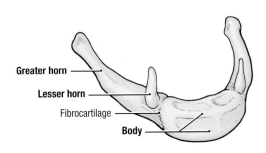

C. Right Anterolateral View of Hyoid

- Greater horn
- Lesser horn
- Fibrocartilage
- Body

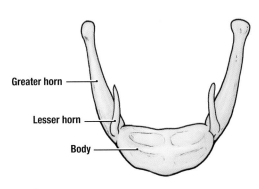

D. Anterosuperior View of Hyoid

- Greater horn
- Lesser horn
- Body

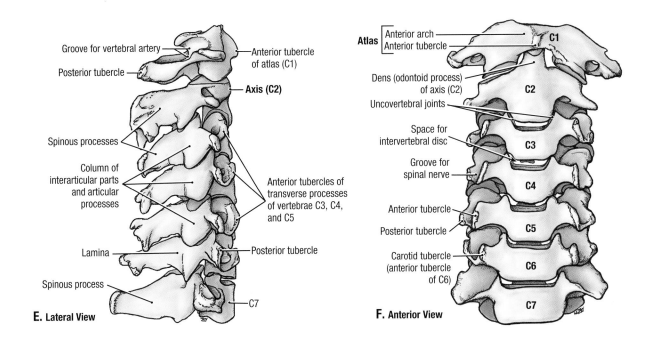

E. Lateral View

- Groove for vertebral artery
- Posterior tubercle
- Anterior tubercle of atlas (C1)
- Axis (C2)
- Spinous processes
- Column of interarticular parts and articular processes
- Anterior tubercles of transverse processes of vertebrae C3, C4, and C5
- Lamina
- Posterior tubercle
- Spinous process
- C7

F. Anterior View

- Atlas
  - Anterior arch
  - Anterior tubercle
- C1
- Dens (odontoid process) of axis (C2)
- C2
- Uncovertebral joints
- Space for intervertebral disc
- C3
- Groove for spinal nerve
- C4
- Anterior tubercle
- Posterior tubercle
- C5
- Carotid tubercle (anterior tubercle of C6)
- C6
- C7

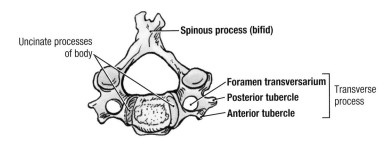

G. Superior View of Typical Cervical Vertebra (e.g., C4)

- Uncinate processes of body
- Spinous process (bifid)
- Foramen transversarium
- Posterior tubercle
- Anterior tubercle
- Transverse process

8.5 BONES AND CARTILAGES OF NECK *(CONTINUED)*

C. and D. Features of hyoid bone. **E. and F.** Articulated cervical vertebrae. **G.** Features of typical cervical vertebrae.

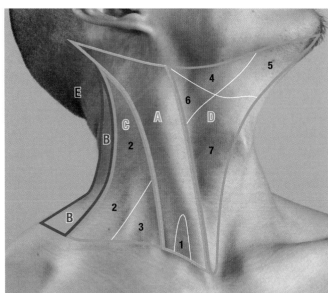

A. Anterolateral view

KEY for A and B:

A	Sternocleidomastoid region
B	Posterior cervical region
C	Lateral cervical region
D	Anterior cervical region
E	Suboccipital region
SCM	Sternocleidomastoid
	CH Clavicular head
	SH Sternal head
TRAP	Trapezius

B. Lateral view

Parotid region

Digastric, posterior belly

Submandibular (digastric) triangle

Digastric, anterior belly

Submental triangle (5)

Carotid triangle

Superior belly of omohyoid

Muscular (omotracheal) triangle (7)

Lesser supraclavicular fossa (1)

Omoclavicular (subclavian) triangle (3)

Trapezius

Occipital triangle (2)

Spinal accessory n. (CN XI)

Inferior belly of omohyoid

C. Lateral view

8.6   CERVICAL REGIONS

A. Surface anatomy. **B. and C.** Regions and triangles of neck.

TABLE 8.2   CERVICAL REGIONS AND CONTENTS[a]

Region	Main Contents and Underlying Structures
Sternocleidomastoid region (A)	Sternocleidomastoid (SCM) muscle; superior part of the external jugular vein; greater auricular nerve; transverse cervical nerve
Lesser supraclavicular fossa (1)	Inferior part of internal jugular vein
Posterior cervical region (B)	Trapezius muscle; cutaneous branches of posterior rami of cervical spinal nerves; suboccipital region (E) lies deep to superior part of this region
Lateral cervical region (posterior triangle) (C) Occipital triangle (2)	Part of external jugular vein; posterior branches of cervical plexus of nerves; spinal accessory nerve; trunks of brachial plexus; transverse cervical artery; cervical lymph nodes
Omoclavicular triangle (3)	Subclavian artery; part of subclavian vein (variable); suprascapular artery; supraclavicular lymph nodes
Anterior cervical region (anterior triangle) (D) Submandibular (digastric) triangle (4)	Submandibular gland almost fills triangle; submandibular lymph nodes; hypoglossal nerve; mylohyoid nerve; parts of facial artery and vein
Submental triangle (5)	Submental lymph nodes and small veins that unite to form anterior jugular vein
Carotid triangle (6)	Common carotid artery and its branches; internal jugular vein and its tributaries; vagus nerve; external carotid artery and some of its branches; hypoglossal nerve and superior root of ansa cervicalis; spinal accessory nerve; thyroid gland, larynx, and pharynx; deep cervical lymph nodes; branches of cervical plexus
Muscular (omotracheal) triangle (7)	Sternothyroid and sternohyoid muscles; thyroid and parathyroid glands

[a]Letters and numbers in parentheses refer to Figures A, B and C.

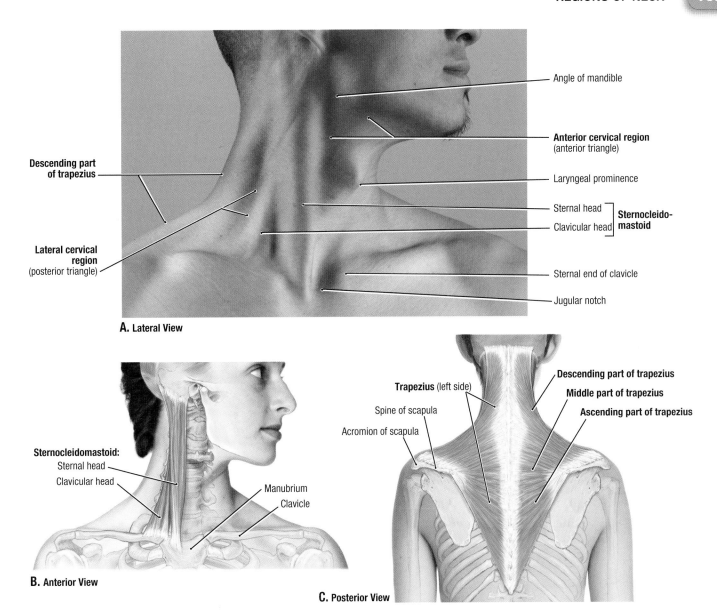

A. Lateral View

- Angle of mandible
- **Anterior cervical region** (anterior triangle)
- Laryngeal prominence
- Sternal head ⎤ **Sternocleido-**
- Clavicular head ⎦ **mastoid**
- Sternal end of clavicle
- Jugular notch
- Descending part of trapezius
- Lateral cervical region (posterior triangle)

B. Anterior View

- Sternocleidomastoid:
  - Sternal head
  - Clavicular head
- Manubrium
- Clavicle

C. Posterior View

- Trapezius (left side)
- Spine of scapula
- Acromion of scapula
- **Descending part of trapezius**
- **Middle part of trapezius**
- **Ascending part of trapezius**

8.7   STERNOCLEIDOMASTOID AND TRAPEZIUS.

A. Surface anatomy. **B.** Sternocleidomastoid. **C.** Trapezius.

TABLE 8.3 STERNOCLEIDOMASTOID AND TRAPEZIUS

Muscle	Superior Attachment	Inferior Attachment	Innervation	Main Action
Sternocleidomastoid	Lateral surface of mastoid process of temporal bone; lateral half of superior nuchal line	*Sternal head:* anterior surface of manubrium of sternum *Clavicular head:* superior surface of medial third of clavicle	Spinal accessory nerve (CN XI) [motor] and C2 and C3 nerves (pain and proprioception)	*Unilateral contraction:* laterally flexes neck; rotates neck so face is turned superiorly toward opposite side; *Bilateral contraction:* (1) extends neck at atlanto-occipital joints, (2) flexes cervical vertebrae so that chin approaches manubrium, or (3) extends superior cervical vertebrae while flexing inferior vertebrae, so chin is thrust forward with head kept level; with cervical vertebrae fixed, may elevate manubrium and medial end of clavicles, assisting deep respiration
Trapezius	Medial third of superior nuchal line, external occipital protuberance, nuchal ligament, spinous processes of C7–T12 vertebrae, lumbar and sacral spinous processes	Lateral third of clavicle, acromion, spine of scapula	Spinal accessory nerve (CN XI) [motor] and C2 and C3 nerves (pain and proprioception)	*Descending fibers* elevate pectoral girdle, maintain level of shoulders against gravity or resistance; *middle fibers* retract scapula; and *ascending fibers* depress shoulders; *superior* and *inferior fibers* work together to rotate scapula upward; *when shoulders are fixed,* bilateral contraction extends neck; unilateral contraction produces lateral flexion to same side

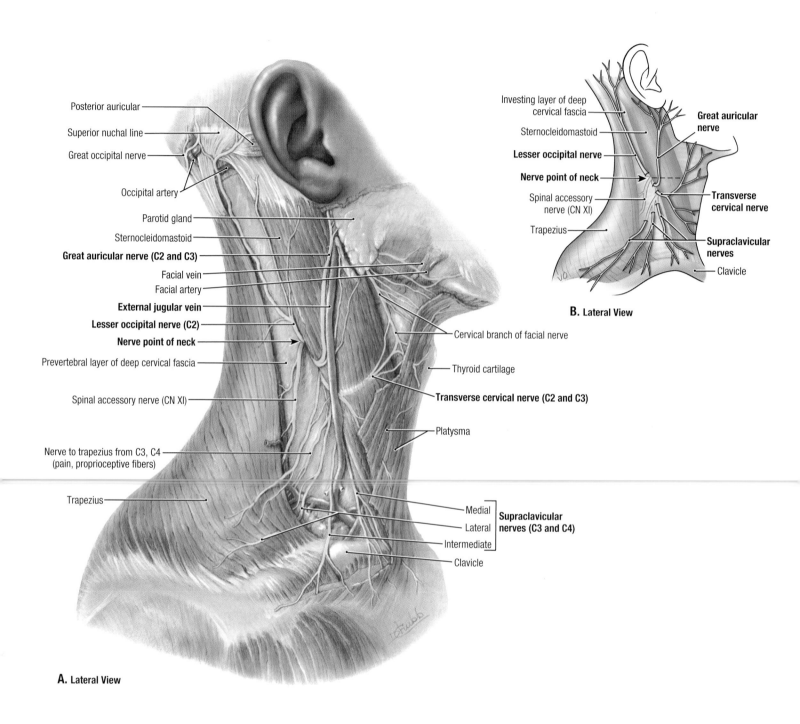

Posterior auricular

Superior nuchal line

Great occipital nerve

Occipital artery

Parotid gland

Sternocleidomastoid

Great auricular nerve (C2 and C3)

Facial vein

Facial artery

External jugular vein

Lesser occipital nerve (C2)

Nerve point of neck

Prevertebral layer of deep cervical fascia

Spinal accessory nerve (CN XI)

Nerve to trapezius from C3, C4
(pain, proprioceptive fibers)

Trapezius

Cervical branch of facial nerve

Thyroid cartilage

Transverse cervical nerve (C2 and C3)

Platysma

Medial
Lateral } **Supraclavicular nerves (C3 and C4)**
Intermediate
Clavicle

A. Lateral View

Investing layer of deep
cervical fascia

Sternocleidomastoid

Lesser occipital nerve

Nerve point of neck

Spinal accessory
nerve (CN XI)

Trapezius

**Great auricular
nerve**

**Transverse
cervical nerve**

**Supraclavicular
nerves**

Clavicle

B. Lateral View

8.8 SERIAL DISSECTIONS OF LATERAL CERVICAL REGION (POSTERIOR TRIANGLE OF NECK)

A. External jugular vein and cutaneous branches of cervical plexus. Subcutaneous fat, the part of the plasma overlying the inferior part of the lateral cervical region, and the investing layer of deep cervical fascia have all been removed. The external jugular vein descends vertically across the sternocleidomastoid and pierces the prevertebral layer of deep cervical fascia superior to the clavicle.

B. and C. Branches of the cervical plexus.
• Branches arising from the nerve loop between the anterior rami of C2 and C3 are the lesser occipital, great auricular, and transverse cervical nerves.

• Branches arising from the loop formed between the anterior rami of C3 and C4 are the supraclavicular nerves, which emerge as a common trunk under cover of the SCM.

Regional anesthesia is often used for surgical procedures in the neck region or upper limb. In a **cervical plexus block,** an anesthetic agent is injected at several points along the posterior border of the SCM, mainly at its midpoint, the nerve point of the neck.

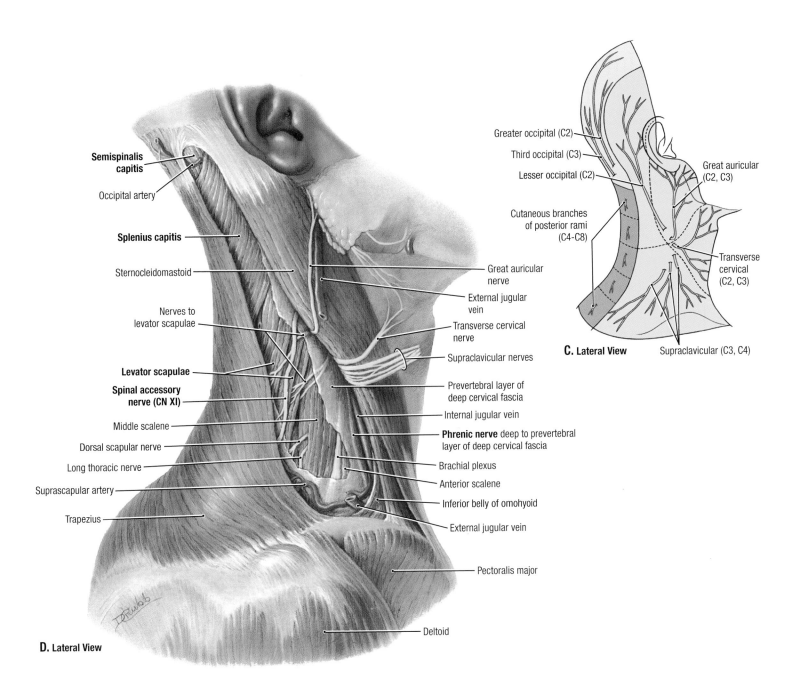

Semispinalis capitis

Occipital artery

Splenius capitis

Sternocleidomastoid

Nerves to levator scapulae

Levator scapulae

Spinal accessory nerve (CN XI)

Middle scalene

Dorsal scapular nerve

Long thoracic nerve

Suprascapular artery

Trapezius

D. Lateral View

Great auricular nerve

External jugular vein

Transverse cervical nerve

Supraclavicular nerves

Prevertebral layer of deep cervical fascia

Internal jugular vein

Phrenic nerve deep to prevertebral layer of deep cervical fascia

Brachial plexus

Anterior scalene

Inferior belly of omohyoid

External jugular vein

Pectoralis major

Deltoid

Greater occipital (C2)

Third occipital (C3)

Lesser occipital (C2)

Great auricular (C2, C3)

Cutaneous branches of posterior rami (C4–C8)

Transverse cervical (C2, C3)

C. Lateral View

Supraclavicular (C3, C4)

8.8

SERIAL DISSECTIONS OF LATERAL CERVICAL REGION *(CONTINUED)*

D. Muscles forming the floor of the lateral cervical region. The prevertebral layer of deep cervical fascia has been partially removed, and the motor nerves and most of the floor of the region are exposed.

- The spinal accessory nerve (CN XI) supplies the SCM and trapezius muscles; between them, it courses along the levator scapulae muscle but is separated from it by the prevertebral layer of deep cervical fascia.
- The phrenic nerve (C3, C4, C5) supplies the diaphragm and is located deep to the prevertebral layer of deep cervical fascia on the anterior surface of the anterior scalene muscle.

Severance of a phrenic nerve results in an ipsilateral paralysis of the diaphragm. A phrenic nerve block produces a short period of paralysis of the diaphragm on one side (e.g., for a lung operation). The anesthetic agent is injected around the nerve where it lies on the anterior surface of the anterior scalene muscle.

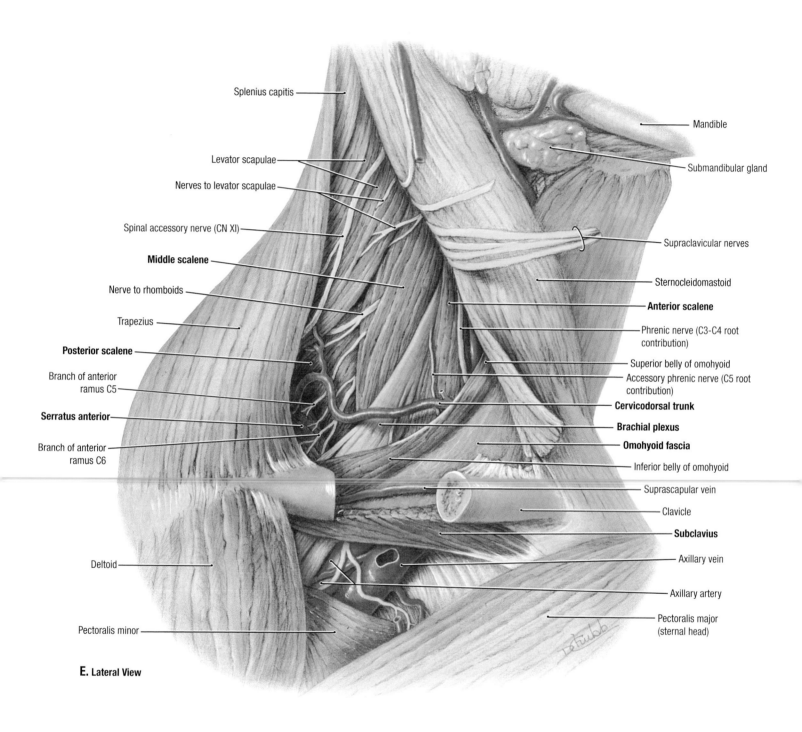

Splenius capitis

Levator scapulae

Nerves to levator scapulae

Spinal accessory nerve (CN XI)

Middle scalene

Nerve to rhomboids

Trapezius

Posterior scalene

Branch of anterior ramus C5

Serratus anterior

Branch of anterior ramus C6

Deltoid

Pectoralis minor

Mandible

Submandibular gland

Supraclavicular nerves

Sternocleidomastoid

Anterior scalene

Phrenic nerve (C3-C4 root contribution)

Superior belly of omohyoid

Accessory phrenic nerve (C5 root contribution)

Cervicodorsal trunk

Brachial plexus

Omohyoid fascia

Inferior belly of omohyoid

Suprascapular vein

Clavicle

Subclavius

Axillary vein

Axillary artery

Pectoralis major (sternal head)

E. Lateral View

8.8 SERIAL DISSECTIONS OF LATERAL CERVICAL REGION (CONTINUED)

E. Vessels and motor nerves of the lateral cervical region. The clavicular head of the pectoralis major muscle and part of the clavicle have been removed.

The muscles that form the floor of the region are the semispinalis capitis, splenius capitis and levator scapulae superiorly and the anterior, middle and posterior scalenes and serratus anterior inferiorly.

• The brachial plexus emerges between the anterior and middle scalene muscles.

A **supraclavicular brachial plexus block** may be utilized for anesthesia of the upper limb. The anesthetic agent is injected around the supraclavicular part of the brachial plexus. The main injection site is superior to the midpoint of the clavicle.

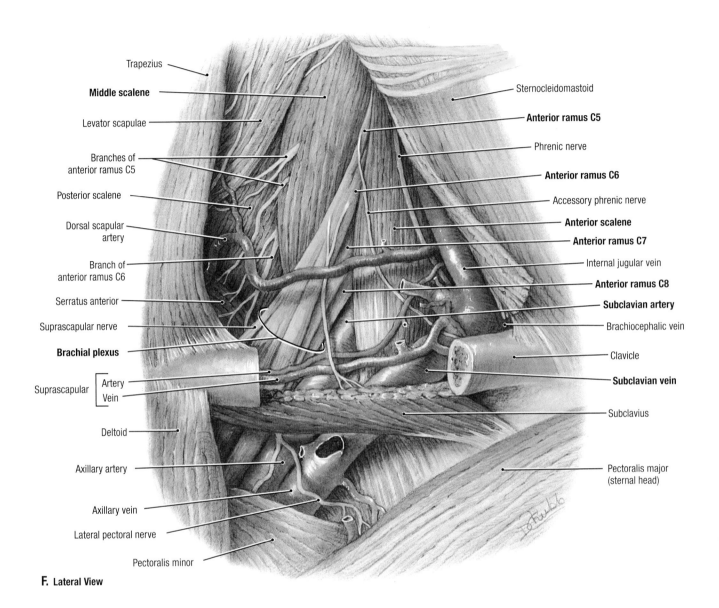

Trapezius

Middle scalene

Levator scapulae

Branches of
anterior ramus C5

Posterior scalene

Dorsal scapular
artery

Branch of
anterior ramus C6

Serratus anterior

Suprascapular nerve

Brachial plexus

Suprascapular { Artery / Vein }

Deltoid

Axillary artery

Axillary vein

Lateral pectoral nerve

Pectoralis minor

Sternocleidomastoid

Anterior ramus C5

Phrenic nerve

Anterior ramus C6

Accessory phrenic nerve

Anterior scalene

Anterior ramus C7

Internal jugular vein

Anterior ramus C8

Subclavian artery

Brachiocephalic vein

Clavicle

Subclavian vein

Subclavius

Pectoralis major
(sternal head)

F. Lateral View

8.8   SERIAL DISSECTIONS OF LATERAL CERVICAL REGION *(CONTINUED)*

F. Structures of the omoclavicular (subclavian) triangle. The omohyoid muscle and fascia have been removed, exposing the brachial plexus and subclavian vessels.

- The anterior rami of C5–T1 form the brachial plexus; the anterior ramus of T1 lies posterior to the subclavian artery.
- The brachial plexus and subclavian artery emerge between the middle and anterior scalene muscles.
- The anterior scalene muscle lies between the subclavian artery and vein.

The right or left subclavian vein is often the site of **placement for a central venous catheter**, used to insert intravenous tubes ("central venous lines") for the administration of parenteral nutritional fluids or medications, for testing blood chemistry or central venous pressure, or inserting electrode wires for heart pacemaker devices. The relationships of the subclavian vein to the sternocleidomastoid muscle, clavicle, sternoclavicular joint and 1st rib are of clinical importance in line placement, and there is danger of puncture of the pleura or subclavian artery if the procedure is not performed correctly.

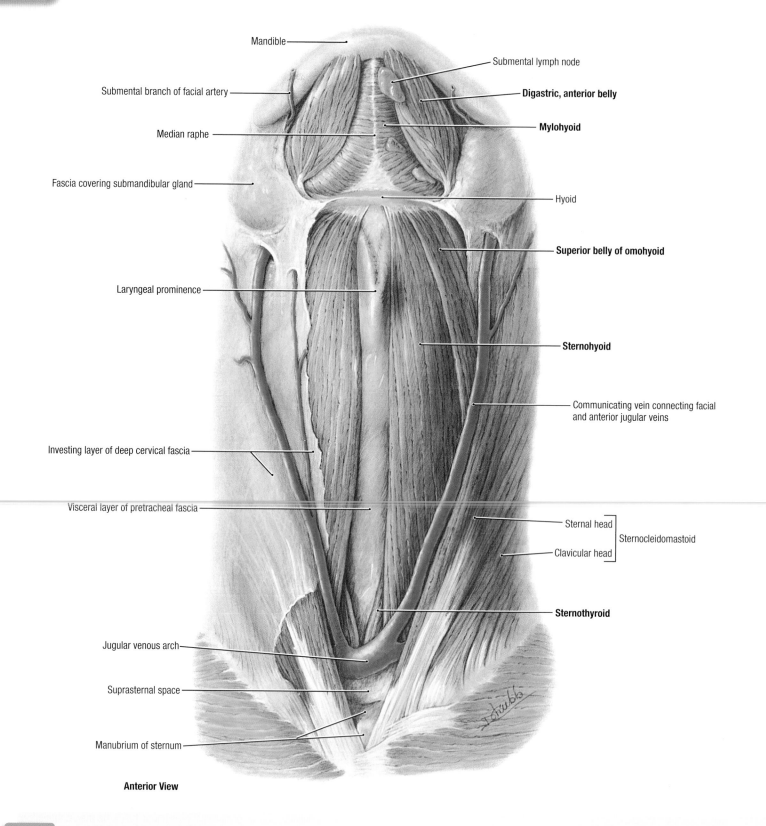

Mandible

Submental lymph node

Submental branch of facial artery

Digastric, anterior belly

Mylohyoid

Median raphe

Fascia covering submandibular gland

Hyoid

Superior belly of omohyoid

Laryngeal prominence

Sternohyoid

Communicating vein connecting facial and anterior jugular veins

Investing layer of deep cervical fascia

Visceral layer of pretracheal fascia

Sternal head

Sternocleidomastoid

Clavicular head

Sternothyroid

Jugular venous arch

Suprasternal space

Manubrium of sternum

Anterior View

8.9   SUPRAHYOID AND INFRAHYOID MUSCLES

Much of the investing layer of deep cervical fascia has been removed.

- The anterior bellies of the digastric muscles form the sides of the suprahyoid part of the anterior cervical region, or submental triangle (floor of mouth). The hyoid bone forms the triangle's base, and the mylohyoid muscles are its floor.

- The infrahyoid part of the anterior cervical region is shaped like an elongated diamond bounded by the sternohyoid muscle superiorly and sternothyroid muscle inferiorly.

Mylohyoid

Body of hyoid

Thyrohyoid membrane

Superior belly of omohyoid

Thyroid cartilage

Sternohyoid

Median cricothyroid ligament

Cricothyroid

Arch of cricoid cartilage

1st tracheal ring

Communicating vein connecting facial and anterior jugular veins

Right lobe of thyroid gland

Left lobe of thyroid gland

Inferior thyroid vein

Sternocleidomastoid

Anterior jugular vein

Clavicle

Sternothyroid

Thymus

Jugular (suprasternal) notch of sternum

Anterior View

8.10   INFRAHYOID REGION, SUPERFICIAL MUSCULAR LAYER

A. Muscular attachments onto the hyoid bone. **B.** The pretracheal fascia, right anterior jugular vein, and jugular venous arch have been removed.

- A persistent thymus projects superiorly from the thorax.
- The two superficial depressors of the larynx ("strap muscles") are the omohyoid (only the superior belly of which is seen here) and sternohyoid.

Fracture of the hyoid. This results in depression of the body of the hyoid onto the thyroid cartilage. Inability to elevate the hyoid and move it anteriorly beneath the tongue makes swallowing and maintenance of the separation of the alimentary and respiratory tracts difficult and may result in **aspiration pneumonia.**

Mandible

Submental lymph node

Submental branch of facial artery

Digastric, anterior belly

Mylohyoid

Median raphe

Fascia covering submandibular gland

Hyoid

Laryngeal prominence of thyroid cartilage

Superior belly of omohyoid

Sternohyoid

A. Anterior View, Head Extended

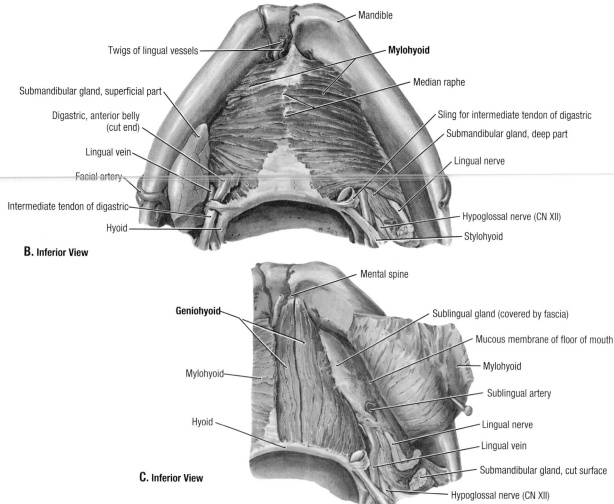

Mandible

Twigs of lingual vessels

Mylohyoid

Submandibular gland, superficial part

Median raphe

Digastric, anterior belly (cut end)

Sling for intermediate tendon of digastric

Submandibular gland, deep part

Lingual vein

Lingual nerve

Facial artery

Intermediate tendon of digastric

Hypoglossal nerve (CN XII)

Hyoid

Stylohyoid

B. Inferior View

Mental spine

Geniohyoid

Sublingual gland (covered by fascia)

Mucous membrane of floor of mouth

Mylohyoid

Mylohyoid

Sublingual artery

Hyoid

Lingual nerve

Lingual vein

Submandibular gland, cut surface

C. Inferior View

Hypoglossal nerve (CN XII)

8.11 SUPRAHYOID REGION (SUBMENTAL TRIANGLE)

A. Superficial layer—anterior belly of digastric. **B.** Intermediate layer—mylohyoid muscles. **C.** Deep layer—geniohyoid muscles.

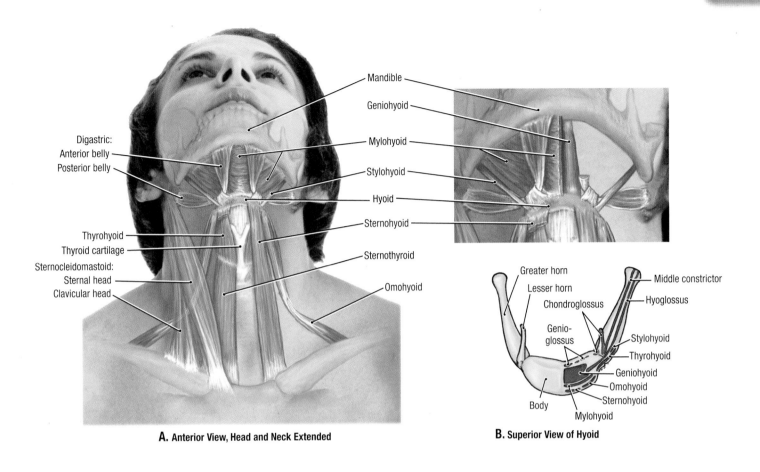

A. Anterior View, Head and Neck Extended

B. Superior View of Hyoid

8.12   SUPRAHYOID AND INFRAHYOID MUSCLES

A. Overview. **B.** Muscular attachments onto the hyoid bone.

TABLE 8.4 SUPRAHYOID AND INFRAHYOID MUSCLES

Muscle	Superior Attachment	Inferior Attachment	Innervation	Main Action
Suprahyoid muscles				
Mylohyoid	Mylohyoid line of mandible	Raphe and body of hyoid bone	Nerve to mylohyoid, a branch of inferior alveolar nerve (CN V³)	Elevates hyoid bone, floor of mouth and tongue during swallowing and speaking
Digastric	*Anterior belly:* digastric fossa of mandible *Posterior belly:* mastoid notch of temporal bone	Intermediate tendon to body and greater horn of hyoid bone	*Anterior belly:* nerve to mylohyoid, a branch of inferior alveolar nerve (CN V³) *Posterior belly:* facial nerve (CN VII)	Elevates hyoid bone and steadies it during swallowing and speaking; depresses mandible against resistance
Geniohyoid	Inferior mental spine of mandible	Body of hyoid bone	C1 via the hypoglossal nerve (CN XII)	Pulls hyoid bone anterosuperiorly, shortens floor of mouth, and widens pharynx
Stylohyoid	Styloid process of temporal bone		Cervical branch of facial nerve (CN VII)	Elevates and retracts hyoid bone, thereby elongating floor of mouth
Infrahyoid muscles				
Sternohyoid	Body of hyoid bone	Manubrium of sternum and medial end of clavicle	C1–C3 by a branch of ansa cervicalis	Depresses hyoid bone after it has been elevated during swallowing
Omohyoid	Inferior border of hyoid bone	Superior border of scapula near suprascapular notch		Depresses, retracts, and steadies hyoid bone
Sternothyroid	Oblique line of thyroid cartilage	Posterior surface of manubrium of sternum	C2 and C3 by a branch of ansa cervicalis	Depresses hyoid bone and larynx
Thyrohyoid	Inferior border of body and greater horn of hyoid bone	Oblique line of thyroid cartilage	C1 via hypoglossal nerve (CN XII)	Depresses hyoid bone and elevates larynx

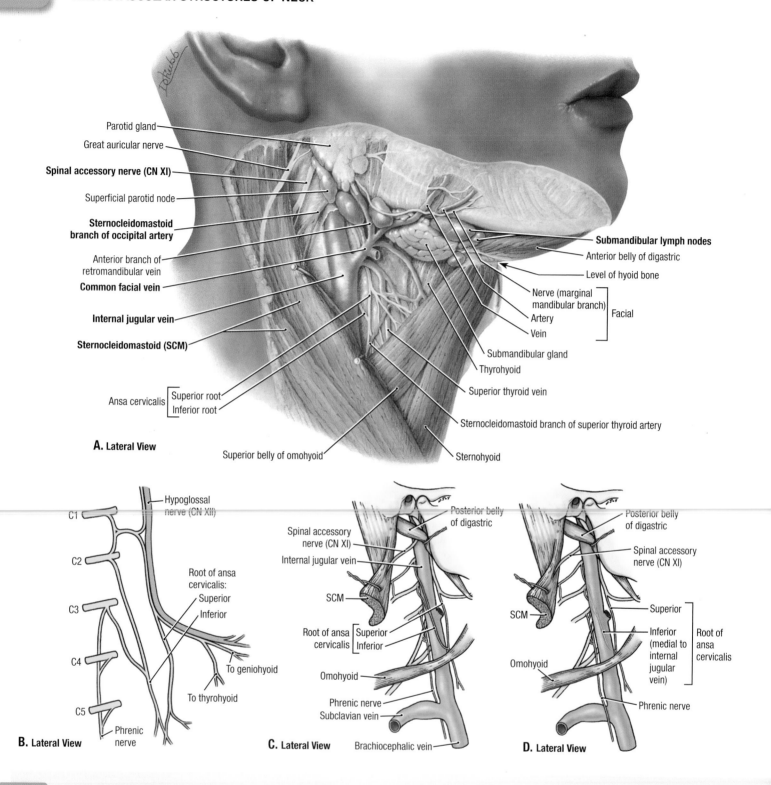

Parotid gland
Great auricular nerve
Spinal accessory nerve (CN XI)
Superficial parotid node
Sternocleidomastoid branch of occipital artery
Anterior branch of retromandibular vein
Common facial vein
Internal jugular vein
Sternocleidomastoid (SCM)
Ansa cervicalis — Superior root / Inferior root

A. Lateral View
Superior belly of omohyoid

Submandibular lymph nodes
Anterior belly of digastric
Level of hyoid bone
Nerve (marginal mandibular branch) | Artery | Vein | Facial
Submandibular gland
Thyrohyoid
Superior thyroid vein
Sternocleidomastoid branch of superior thyroid artery
Sternohyoid

B. Lateral View
C1
Hypoglossal nerve (CN XII)
C2
Root of ansa cervicalis: Superior / Inferior
C3
C4
To geniohyoid
To thyrohyoid
C5
Phrenic nerve

C. Lateral View
Spinal accessory nerve (CN XI)
Internal jugular vein
Posterior belly of digastric
SCM
Root of ansa cervicalis Superior / Inferior
Omohyoid
Phrenic nerve
Subclavian vein
Brachiocephalic vein

D. Lateral View
Posterior belly of digastric
Spinal accessory nerve (CN XI)
SCM
Superior
Inferior (medial to internal jugular vein) | Root of ansa cervicalis
Omohyoid
Phrenic nerve

8.13 **SUPERFICIAL DISSECTION OF CAROTID TRIANGLE**

A. The skin, subcutaneous tissue (with platysma), and the investing layer of deep cervical fascia, including the sheaths of the parotid and submandibular glands, have been removed.

- The spinal accessory nerve (CN XI) enters the deep surface of the sternocleidomastoid muscle and is joined along its anterior border by the sternocleidomastoid branch of the occipital artery.
- The (common) facial vein joins the internal jugular vein near the level of the hyoid bone; here, the facial vein is joined by several other veins.

- The submandibular lymph nodes lie deep to the investing layer of deep cervical fascia in the submandibular triangle; some of the nodes lie deep in the submandibular gland.

B. Diagram of the motor branches of cervical plexus. **C.** Typical relationships of ansa cervicalis, spinal accessory nerve (CN XI), and phrenic nerve to the internal jugular and subclavian veins. **D.** Atypical relationships.

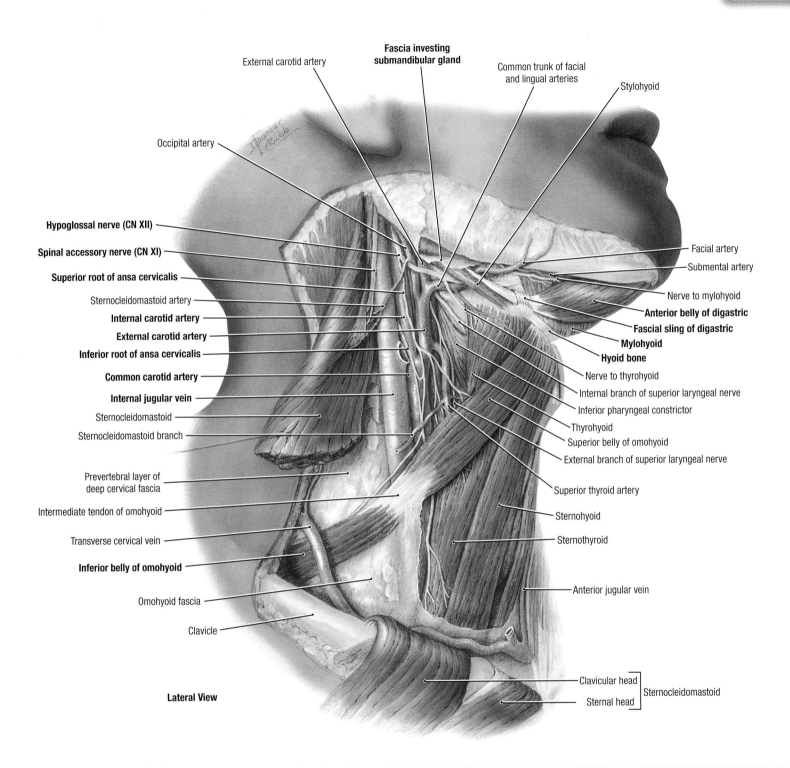

External carotid artery

Fascia investing
submandibular gland

Common trunk of facial
and lingual arteries

Stylohyoid

Occipital artery

Hypoglossal nerve (CN XII)

Spinal accessory nerve (CN XI)

Superior root of ansa cervicalis

Sternocleidomastoid artery

Internal carotid artery

External carotid artery

Inferior root of ansa cervicalis

Common carotid artery

Internal jugular vein

Sternocleidomastoid

Sternocleidomastoid branch

Prevertebral layer of
deep cervical fascia

Intermediate tendon of omohyoid

Transverse cervical vein

Inferior belly of omohyoid

Omohyoid fascia

Clavicle

Lateral View

Facial artery

Submental artery

Nerve to mylohyoid

Anterior belly of digastric

Fascial sling of digastric

Mylohyoid

Hyoid bone

Nerve to thyrohyoid

Internal branch of superior laryngeal nerve

Inferior pharyngeal constrictor

Thyrohyoid

Superior belly of omohyoid

External branch of superior laryngeal nerve

Superior thyroid artery

Sternohyoid

Sternothyroid

Anterior jugular vein

Clavicular head
Sternocleidomastoid
Sternal head

8.14 **DEEP DISSECTION OF CAROTID TRIANGLE**

The sternocleidomastoid muscle has been severed; the inferior portion reflected inferiorly and superior portion posteriorly.

- The tendon of the digastric muscle is connected to the hyoid bone by a fascial sling derived from the muscular part of the pretracheal layer of deep cervical fascia; the tendon of the omohyoid muscle is similarly tethered to the clavicle.
- In this specimen, the facial and lingual arteries arise from a common trunk and pass deep to the stylohyoid and digastric muscles.

- The hypoglossal nerve (CN XII) crosses the internal and external carotid arteries and gives off two branches, the superior root of the ansa cervicalis and the nerve to the thyrohyoid, before passing anteriorly deep to the mylohyoid muscle. In this specimen, the inferior root of the ansa cervicalis lies deep to the internal jugular vein and emerges at its medial aspect.

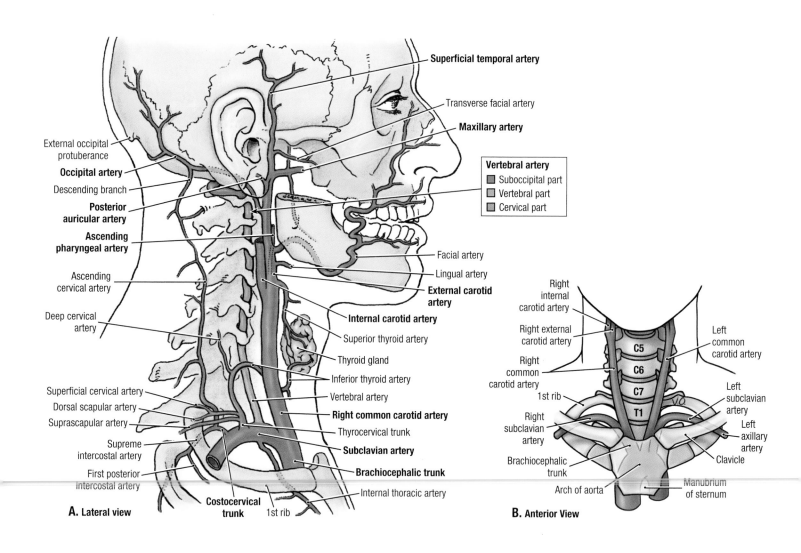

A. Lateral view

B. Anterior View

8.15   ARTERIES OF NECK

A. Overview. **B.** Common carotid and subclavian arteries.

TABLE 8.5 ARTERIES OF NECK

Artery	Origin	Course and Distribution
Right common carotid	Bifurcation of brachiocephalic trunk	Ascends in neck within carotid sheath with the internal jugular vein and vagus nerve (CN X). Terminates at superior border of thyroid cartilage (C4 vertebral level) by dividing into internal and external carotid arteries
Left common carotid	Arch of aorta	
Right and left internal carotid	Right and left common carotid	No branches in the neck. Enters cranium via carotid canal to supply brain and orbits. Proximal part location of carotid sinus, a baroreceptor that reacts to change in arterial blood pressure. The carotid body, a chemoreceptor that monitors oxygen level in blood, is located in bifurcation of common carotid
Right and left external carotid		Supplies most structures external to cranium; the orbit, part of forehead, and scalp are major exceptions (supplied by ophthalmic artery from intra-cranial internal carotid artery)
Ascending pharyngeal	External carotid	Ascends on pharynx to supply pharynx, prevertebral muscles, middle ear, and cranial meninges
Occipital		Passes posteriorly, medial and parallel to the posterior belly of digastric, ending in the posterior scalp
Posterior auricular		Ascends posteriorly between external acoustic meatus and mastoid process to supply adjacent muscles, parotid gland, facial nerve, auricle, and scalp

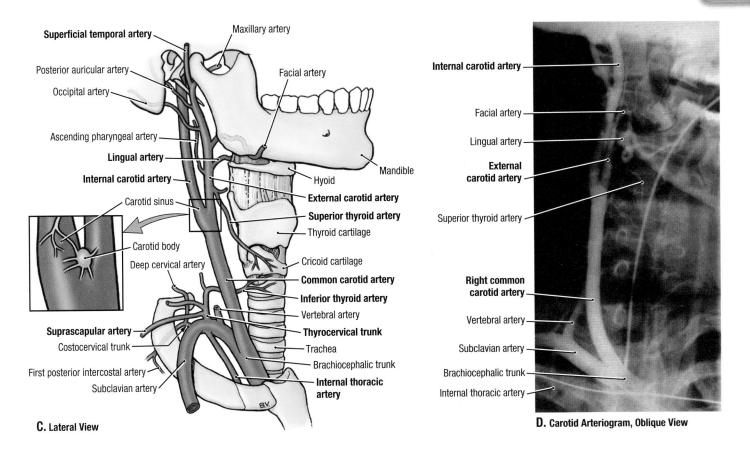

C. Lateral View

D. Carotid Arteriogram, Oblique View

8.15   ARTERIES OF NECK *(CONTINUED)*

C. Branches of external carotid and subclavian arteries. The carotid sinus is a baroreceptor that reacts to changes in arterial blood pressure and is located in the dilatation of the proximal part of the internal carotid artery. The carotid body is an ovoid mass of tissue that lies at the bifurcation of the common carotid artery. It is a chemoreceptor that monitors the level of oxygen in the blood.

TABLE 8.5 ARTERIES OF NECK (CONTINUED)

Artery	Origin	Course and Distribution
Superior thyroid	External carotid	Runs antero-inferiorly deep to infrahyoid muscles to reach thyroid gland. Supplies thyroid gland, infrahyoid muscles, SCM, and larynx via *superior laryngeal artery*
Lingual		Lies on middle constrictor muscle of pharynx; arches supero-anteriorly and passes deep to CN XII, stylohyoid muscle, and posterior belly of digastric then passes deep to hyoglossus, giving branches to the posterior tongue and bifurcating into *deep lingual* and *sublingual arteries*
Facial		After giving rise to *ascending palatine artery* and a tonsillar branch, it passes superiorly under cover of the angle of the mandible. It then loops anteriorly to supply the submandibular gland and give rise to the *submental artery* to the floor of the mouth before entering the face
Maxillary	Terminal branches of external carotid	Passes posterior to neck of mandible, enters infratemporal fossa then pterygopalatine fossa to supply teeth, nose, ear, and face
Superficial temporal		Ascends anterior to auricle to temporal region and ends in scalp
Vertebral	Subclavian	Passes through the foramina transversaria of the transverse processes of vertebrae C1–C6, runs in a groove on the posterior arch of the atlas, and enters the cranial cavity through the foramen magnum
Internal thoracic		No branches in neck; enters thorax
Thyrocervical trunk		Has two branches: the *inferior thyroid artery*, the main visceral artery of the neck; the cervicodorsal trunk sending branches to the lateral cervical region, trapezius, and medial scapular arteries
Costocervical trunk		Trunk passes posterosuperiorly and divides into *superior intercostal* and *deep cervical arteries* to supply the 1st and 2nd intercostal spaces and posterior deep cervical muscles, respectively

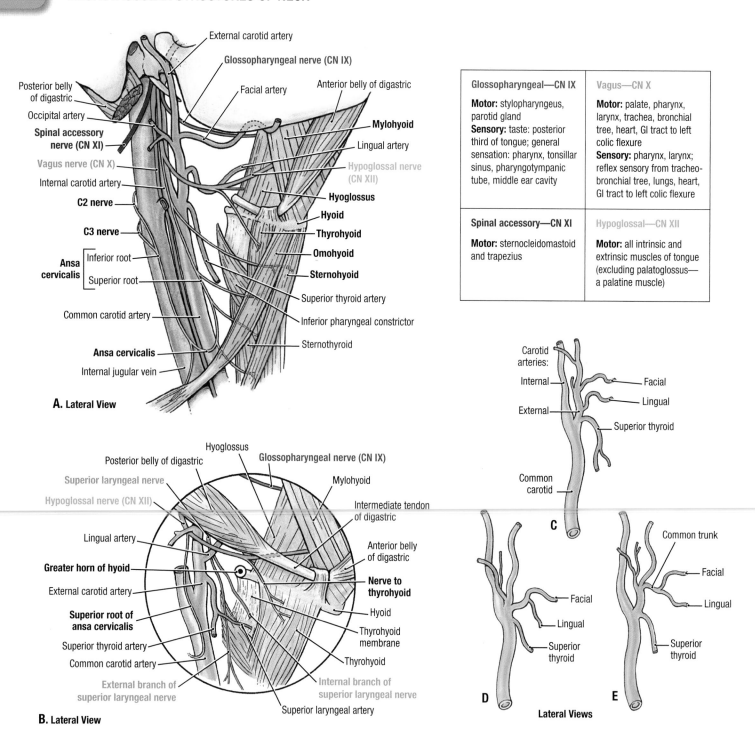

A. Lateral View

Glossopharyngeal—CN IX	Vagus—CN X
Motor: stylopharyngeus, parotid gland **Sensory:** taste: posterior third of tongue; general sensation: pharynx, tonsillar sinus, pharyngotympanic tube, middle ear cavity	**Motor:** palate, pharynx, larynx, trachea, bronchial tree, heart, GI tract to left colic flexure **Sensory:** pharynx, larynx; reflex sensory from tracheobronchial tree, lungs, heart, GI tract to left colic flexure
Spinal accessory—CN XI **Motor:** sternocleidomastoid and trapezius	**Hypoglossal—CN XII** **Motor:** all intrinsic and extrinsic muscles of tongue (excluding palatoglossus—a palatine muscle)

B. Lateral View

Lateral Views

8.16

RELATIONSHIPS OF NERVES AND VESSELS IN CAROTID TRIANGLE OF NECK

A. Ansa cervicalis and the strap muscles. **B.** Hypoglossal nerve (CN XII) and internal and external branches of superior laryngeal nerve (CN X). The tip of the greater hyoid bone, indicated with a *circle* is the reference point for many structures. **C.–E.** Variation in the origin of the lingual artery as studied by Dr. Grant in 211 specimens. In 80%, the superior thyroid, lingual, and facial arteries arose separately **(C)**; in 20%, the lingual and facial arteries arose from a common stem inferiorly **(D)** or high on the external carotid artery **(E)**. In one specimen, the superior thyroid and lingual arteries arose from a common stem.

Carotid occlusion, causing stenosis (narrowing), can be relieved by opening the artery at its origin and stripping off the atherosclerotic plaque with the artery's lining (intima). This procedure is called carotid endarterectomy. Because of the relationships of the internal carotid artery, there is a risk of cranial nerve injury during the procedure involving one or more of the following nerves: CN IX, CN X (or its branch, the superior laryngeal nerve), CN XI, or CN XII.

Superficial temporal vein

Pterygoid venous plexus

Occipital vein

Posterior auricular vein

Transverse facial vein

Retromandibular vein

Ascending pharyngeal vein

Deep facial vein

Maxillary vein

Posterior branch

Retromandibular vein

Anterior branch

Facial vein

Mandible

Common facial vein

External jugular vein

Submental vein

Deep cervical vein

Lingual vein

Superior thyroid vein

Vertebral vein

Thyroid gland

Middle thyroid vein

Internal jugular vein

Inferior thyroid vein

External jugular vein

Anterior jugular vein

Transverse cervical vein

Suprascapular vein

Right brachiocephalic vein

First posterior intercostal vein

Right subclavian vein

Internal thoracic vein

A. Lateral View

8.17   DEEP VEINS OF NECK

A. Overview. The IJV begins at the jugular foramen as the continuation of the sigmoid sinus. From a dilated origin, the superior bulb of the IJV, the vein runs inferiorly through the neck in the carotid sheath. Posterior to the sternal end of the clavicle the vein merges perpendicularly with the subclavian vein, forming the "venous angle" that marks the origin of the brachiocephalic vein. The inferior end of the IJV dilates superior to its terminal valve, forming the inferior bulb of the IJV. The valve permits blood to flow toward the heart while preventing backflow into the IJV. The external jugular vein drains blood from the occipital region and posterior neck to the subclavian vein, and the anterior jugular vein the anterior aspect of the neck. **B. Internal jugular vein puncture**. A needle and catheter may be inserted into the IJV, using ultrasonic guidance, for diagnostic or therapeutic purposes. The right internal jugular vein is preferable to the left because it is usually larger and straighter. During this procedure, the clinician palpates the common carotid artery and inserts the needle into the IJV just lateral to it at a 30° angle, aiming at the apex of the triangle between the sternal and clavicular heads of the SCM. The needle is then directed inferolaterally toward the ipsilateral nipple.

Sterno-cleidomastoid

Internal jugular vein

Subclavian vein

Superior vena cava

B. Internal jugular vein puncture

Internal branch of superior laryngeal nerve

External carotid artery

External branch of superior laryngeal nerve

Superior thyroid artery

Accessory thyroid gland

Sternocleidomastoid branch

Sternothyroid

Superior pole of thyroid gland

Superior thyroid vein

Superior thyroid artery

Internal jugular vein

Middle thyroid vein

Inferior pole of thyroid gland

Vagus nerve (CN X)

Common carotid artery

Subclavian artery

Sternothyroid

Inferior thyroid vein

Brachiocephalic trunk

Sternohyoid, reflected superiorly

Hyoid bone

Thyrohyoid membrane

Thyrohyoid

Thyroid cartilage

Cricothyroid ligament

Cricothyroid

Cricoid cartilage

Sternothyroid

Isthmus of thyroid gland

Inferior thyroid veins

Sternohyoid, reflected inferiorly

A. Anterior View

8.18 ENDOCRINE LAYER OF VISCERAL COMPARTMENT I

A. On the left side of the specimen, the sternohyoid and omohyoid muscles are reflected, exposing the sternothyroid and the thyrohyoid muscles; on the right side of the specimen, the sternothyroid muscle is largely excised. **B.** Schematic illustration of the venous drainage of the thyroid gland. Except for the superior thyroid veins, the thyroid veins are not paired with arteries of corresponding names.

The **carotid pulse (neck pulse)** is easily felt by palpating the common carotid artery in the side of the neck, where it lies in a groove between the trachea and the infrahyoid muscles. It is usually easily palpated just deep to the anterior border of the SCM at the level of the superior border of the thyroid cartilage. It is routinely checked during cardiopulmonary resuscitation (CPR). Absence of a carotid pulse indicates cardiac arrest.

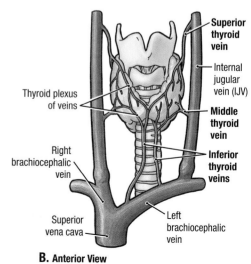

Superior thyroid vein

Internal jugular vein (IJV)

Thyroid plexus of veins

Middle thyroid vein

Right brachiocephalic vein

Inferior thyroid veins

Superior vena cava

Left brachiocephalic vein

B. Anterior View

A. Anterior View

Anterosuperior View

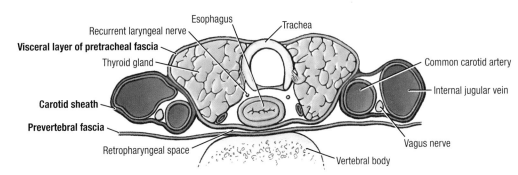

B. Transverse Section, Inferior View

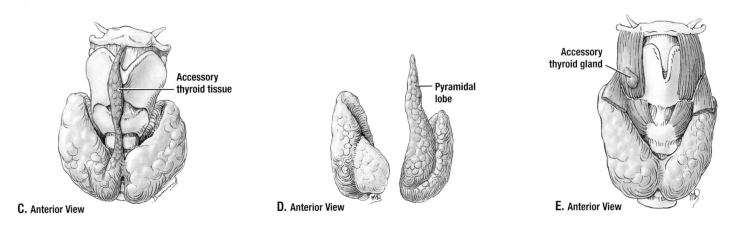

C. Anterior View   **D. Anterior View**   **E. Anterior View**

8.19   ENDOCRINE LAYER OF VISCERAL COMPARTMENT II

A. Relations of thyroid gland with transverse section showing alimentary, respiratory, and endocrine layers of visceral compartment. **B.** Fascia. **C.** Accessory thyroid tissue along the course of the thyroglossal duct, which was the path of migration of thyroid tissue from its embryonic site of development.

D. Approximately 50% of glands have a pyramidal lobe that extends from near the isthmus to or toward the hyoid bone; the isthmus is occasionally absent, in which case the gland is in two parts. **E.** An accessory thyroid gland can occur between the suprahyoid region and arch of the aorta (see Fig. 8.18A).

Internal branch of superior laryngeal nerve

Thyrohyoid membrane

Superior laryngeal artery

Inferior pharyngeal constrictor

Thyroid cartilage

External branch of superior laryngeal nerve

Sternothyroid, reflected

Superior thyroid artery

Superior thyroid vein

Cricothyroid ligament

Right and left cricothyroids

Cricotracheal ligament

Cricoid cartilage

Fascial band

Thyroid gland, left lobe

Thyroid gland, right lobe

Trachea

Left recurrent laryngeal nerve

Inferior thyroid vein

Inferior parathyroid gland

Vagus nerve (CN X)

Vagus nerve (CN X)

Common carotid artery

Internal jugular vein

Internal jugular vein

Thoracic duct

Right subclavian artery

Clavicle

Sternothyroid

Jugular notch

A. Anterolateral View

8.20 RESPIRATORY LAYER OF VISCERAL COMPARTMENT

A. The isthmus of the thyroid gland is divided, and the left lobe is retracted. The left recurrent laryngeal nerve ascends on the lateral aspect of the trachea between the trachea and esophagus. The internal branch of the superior laryngeal nerve runs along the superior border of the inferior pharyngeal constrictor muscle and pierces the thyrohyoid membrane. The external branch of the superior laryngeal nerve lies adjacent to the inferior pharyngeal constrictor muscle and supplies its lower portion; it continues to run along the anterior border of the superior thyroid artery, passing deep to the superior attachment of the sternothyroid muscle, and then supplies the cricothyroid muscle. **B.** Blood supply of the parathyroid glands and courses of the left and right recurrent laryngeal nerves.

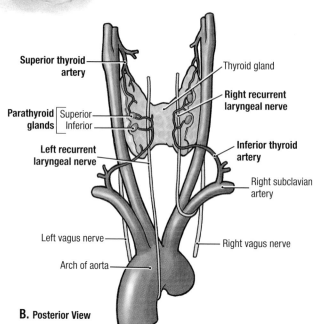

Superior thyroid artery

Thyroid gland

Right recurrent laryngeal nerve

Parathyroid glands { Superior / Inferior }

Left recurrent laryngeal nerve

Inferior thyroid artery

Right subclavian artery

Left vagus nerve

Right vagus nerve

Arch of aorta

B. Posterior View

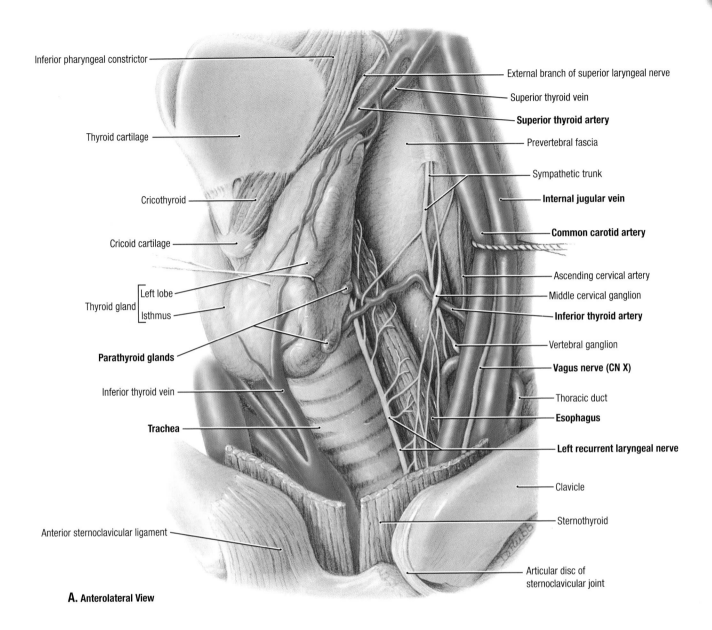

Inferior pharyngeal constrictor

External branch of superior laryngeal nerve

Superior thyroid vein

Superior thyroid artery

Thyroid cartilage

Prevertebral fascia

Sympathetic trunk

Cricothyroid

Internal jugular vein

Cricoid cartilage

Common carotid artery

Ascending cervical artery

Middle cervical ganglion

Left lobe

Inferior thyroid artery

Thyroid gland

Isthmus

Vertebral ganglion

Parathyroid glands

Vagus nerve (CN X)

Inferior thyroid vein

Thoracic duct

Esophagus

Trachea

Left recurrent laryngeal nerve

Clavicle

Sternothyroid

Anterior sternoclavicular ligament

Articular disc of
sternoclavicular joint

A. Anterolateral View

8.21 ALIMENTARY LAYER OF VISCERAL COMPARTMENT

A. Dissection of the left side of the root of the neck. The three structures contained in the carotid sheath (internal jugular vein, common carotid artery, and vagus nerve) are retracted. The left recurrent laryngeal nerve ascends on the lateral aspect of the trachea, just anterior to the recess between the trachea and esophagus. **B.** Arterial supply of thyroid gland. The thyroid ima artery is infrequent (10%) and variable in its origin.

During a **total thyroidectomy** (e.g., excision of a malignant thyroid gland), the parathyroid glands are in danger of being inadvertently damaged or removed. These glands are safe during **subtotal thyroidectomy** because the most posterior part of the thyroid gland usually is preserved. Variability in the position of the parathyroid glands, especially the inferior ones, puts them in danger of being removed during surgery on the thyroid gland. If the parathyroid glands are inadvertently removed during surgery, the patient suffers from **tetany,** a severe convulsive disorder. The generalized convulsive muscle spasms result from a fall in blood calcium levels.

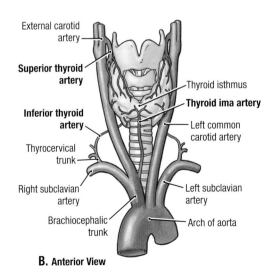

External carotid artery

Superior thyroid artery

Thyroid isthmus

Thyroid ima artery

Inferior thyroid artery

Left common carotid artery

Thyrocervical trunk

Right subclavian artery

Left subclavian artery

Brachiocephalic trunk

Arch of aorta

B. Anterior View

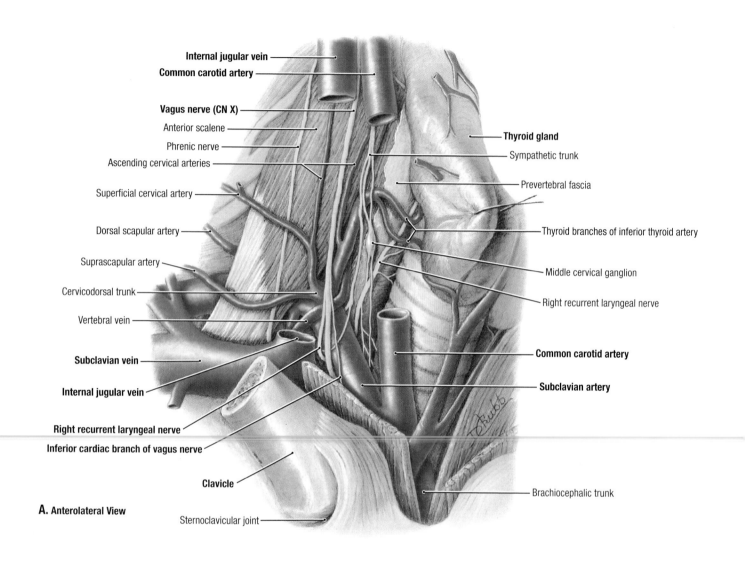

Internal jugular vein
Common carotid artery
Vagus nerve (CN X)
Anterior scalene
Phrenic nerve
Ascending cervical arteries
Superficial cervical artery
Dorsal scapular artery
Suprascapular artery
Cervicodorsal trunk
Vertebral vein
Subclavian vein
Internal jugular vein
Right recurrent laryngeal nerve
Inferior cardiac branch of vagus nerve
Clavicle

Thyroid gland
Sympathetic trunk
Prevertebral fascia
Thyroid branches of inferior thyroid artery
Middle cervical ganglion
Right recurrent laryngeal nerve
Common carotid artery
Subclavian artery
Brachiocephalic trunk

A. Anterolateral View

Sternoclavicular joint

8.22 ROOT OF NECK

A. Dissection of the right side of the root of the neck. The clavicle is cut, sections of the common carotid artery and internal jugular vein are removed, and the right lobe of the thyroid gland is retracted. The right vagus nerve crosses the first part of the subclavian artery and gives off an inferior cardiac branch and the right recurrent laryngeal nerve. The right recurrent laryngeal nerve loops inferior to the subclavian artery and passes posterior to the common carotid artery on its way to the posterolateral aspect of the trachea.

- The **recurrent laryngeal nerves are vulnerable to injury** during thyroidectomy and other surgeries in the anterior cervical region of the neck. Because the terminal branch of this nerve, the inferior laryngeal nerve, innervates the muscles moving the vocal folds, injury to the nerve results in **paralysis of the vocal folds.**

- A non-neoplastic and noninflammatory enlargement of the thyroid gland, other than the variable enlargement that may occur during menstruation and pregnancy, is called a goiter. A **goiter** results from a lack of iodine. It is common in certain parts of the world where the soil and water are deficient in iodine and iodized salt is unavailable. The enlarged gland causes a swelling in the neck that may compress the trachea, esophagus, and recurrent laryngeal nerves. When the gland enlarges, it may do so anteriorly, posteriorly, inferiorly, or laterally. It cannot move superiorly because of the superior attachments of the sternothyroid and sternohyoid muscles. Substernal extension of a goiter is also common.

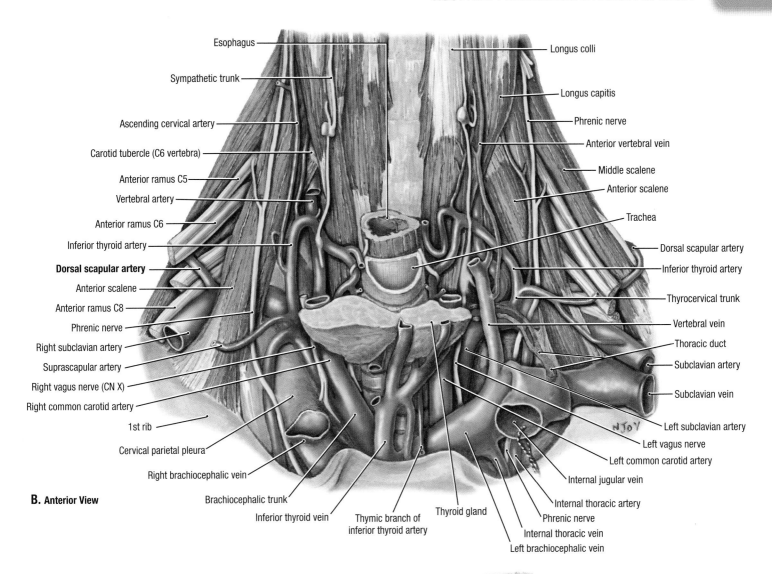

Esophagus

Sympathetic trunk

Ascending cervical artery

Carotid tubercle (C6 vertebra)

Anterior ramus C5

Vertebral artery

Anterior ramus C6

Inferior thyroid artery

Dorsal scapular artery

Anterior scalene

Anterior ramus C8

Phrenic nerve

Right subclavian artery

Suprascapular artery

Right vagus nerve (CN X)

Right common carotid artery

1st rib

Cervical parietal pleura

Right brachiocephalic vein

B. Anterior View

Inferior thyroid vein

Brachiocephalic trunk

Thymic branch of
inferior thyroid artery

Thyroid gland

Longus colli

Longus capitis

Phrenic nerve

Anterior vertebral vein

Middle scalene

Anterior scalene

Trachea

Dorsal scapular artery

Inferior thyroid artery

Thyrocervical trunk

Vertebral vein

Thoracic duct

Subclavian artery

Subclavian vein

Left subclavian artery

Left vagus nerve

Left common carotid artery

Internal jugular vein

Internal thoracic artery

Phrenic nerve

Internal thoracic vein

Left brachiocephalic vein

8.22　　**ROOT OF NECK** *(CONTINUED)*

B. Deep anterior dissection. Note that the right dorsal scapular artery arises directly from the subclavian artery, a common variation. **C.** Dissection of termination of the thoracic duct. The sternocleidomastoid muscle is removed, the sternohyoid muscle is resected, and the omohyoid portion of the pretracheal fascia is partially removed. The thoracic duct arches laterally in the neck, passing posterior to the carotid sheath and anterior to the vertebral artery, thyrocervical trunk, and subclavian arteries; it enters the angle formed by the junction of the left subclavian and internal jugular veins to form the left brachiocephalic vein (the left venous angle).

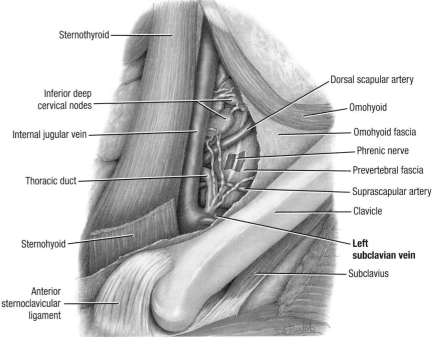

Sternothyroid

Inferior deep
cervical nodes

Internal jugular vein

Thoracic duct

Sternohyoid

Anterior
sternoclavicular
ligament

Dorsal scapular artery

Omohyoid

Omohyoid fascia

Phrenic nerve

Prevertebral fascia

Suprascapular artery

Clavicle

**Left
subclavian vein**

Subclavius

C. Anterolateral View

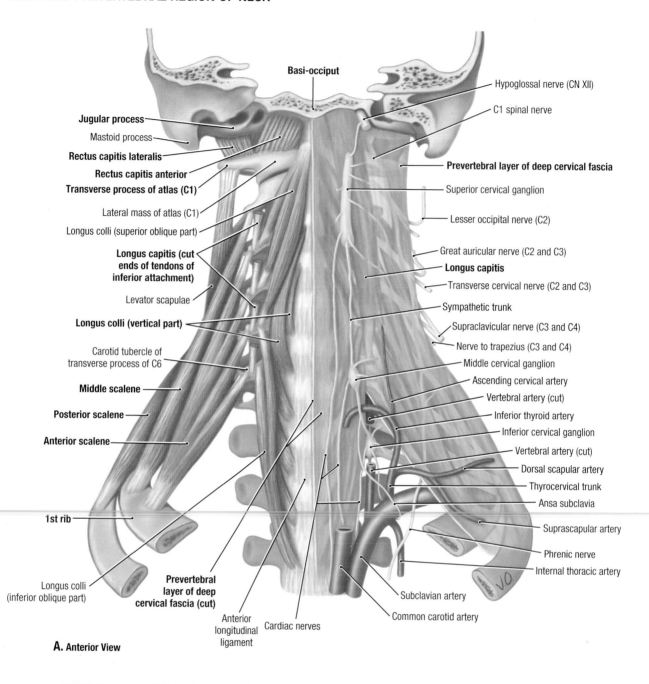

A. Anterior View

8.23 PREVERTEBRAL REGION

A. and B. Overview of muscles, nerves and vessels.

TABLE 8.6 PREVERTEBRAL AND SCALENE MUSCLES

Muscle	Superior Attachment	Inferior Attachment	Innervation	Main Action
Longus colli				
Superior oblique part	Anterior tubercle of atlas (C1)	Anterior tubercles of TVP C3–C5	Anterior rami of C2–C6 spinal nerves (cervical plexus)	Rotation of cervical spine to opposite side (acting unilaterally)
Vertical part	Vertebral bodies of C2–C4	Vertebral bodies C5–T3		
Inferior oblique part	Anterior tubercles of TVP C5–C6	Vertebral bodies T1–T3		Flexion of cervical spine (acting bilaterally)
Longus capitis	Basilar part of occipital bone	Anterior tubercles of TVP C3–C6	Anterior rami of C1–C3 spinal nerves (cervical plexus)	Flexion of head (atlanto-occipital joints)

TVP, transverse process

Cranial nerves
XII XI X and IX

Base of cranium (basiocciput)

Anterior tubercle of atlas

Internal jugular vein

Facial nerve (CN VII)

Jugular process

Rectus capitis lateralis

Longus capitis

Anterior ramus C1

Posterior belly of digastric

Superior cervical ganglion

Anterior ramus C2

Anterior ramus C3

Sympathetic trunk

Anterior ramus C4

Longus capitis

Phrenic nerve

Anterior ramus C5

Anterior scalene

Sympathetic ganglion

C6
Anterior rami C7
C8
T1

Right subclavian artery

Inferior cervical ganglion

Ansa subclavia

Right subclavian artery

Right common carotid artery

Brachiocephalic trunk

Rectus capitis anterior

Mastoid process

Rectus capitis lateralis

Transverse process of atlas

Intertransversarii

Longus colli (superior oblique part)

Levator scapulae

Longus capitis

Middle scalene

Longus colli (vertical part)

Carotid tubercle (transverse process of C6)

Anterior scalene

Vertebral artery

Inferior thyroid artery

Ascending cervical artery

Dorsal scapular artery

Costocervical trunk

Suprascapular artery

Thyrocervical trunk

Recurrent laryngeal nerve

Internal thoracic artery

1st rib

Left subclavian artery

Left common carotid artery

B. Anterior View

8.23

PREVERTEBRAL REGION *(CONTINUED)*

TABLE 8.6 PREVERTEBRAL AND SCALENE MUSCLES

Muscle	Superior Attachment	Inferior Attachment	Innervation	Main Action
Rectus capitis anterior	Base of cranium, just anterior to occipital condyle	Anterior surface of lateral mass of atlas (C1)	Branches from loop between C1 and C2 spinal nerves	Lateral flexion at atlanto-occipital joints (acting unilaterally)
Rectus capitis lateralis	Base of cranium just lateral to occipital condyle	Transverse process of atlas (C1)		Flexion at atlanto-occipital joints (acting bilaterally)
Anterior scalene	Anterior tubercles of TVP C3–C6	Scalene tubercle of 1st rib	Anterior rami of C3–C8 (cervical and brachial plexus)	Forced inspiration (ribs mobile): elevate superior ribs
Middle scalene	TVP C1–C2	Superior surface of 1st rib; posterior to groove for subclavian artery		Ribs fixed: lateral flexion of cervical spine (acting unilaterally) Flexes neck (acting bilaterally)
	Posterior tubercles of TVP C3–C7			
Posterior scalene	Posterior tubercles of TVP C5–C7	External border of 2nd rib		

TVP, Transverse process.

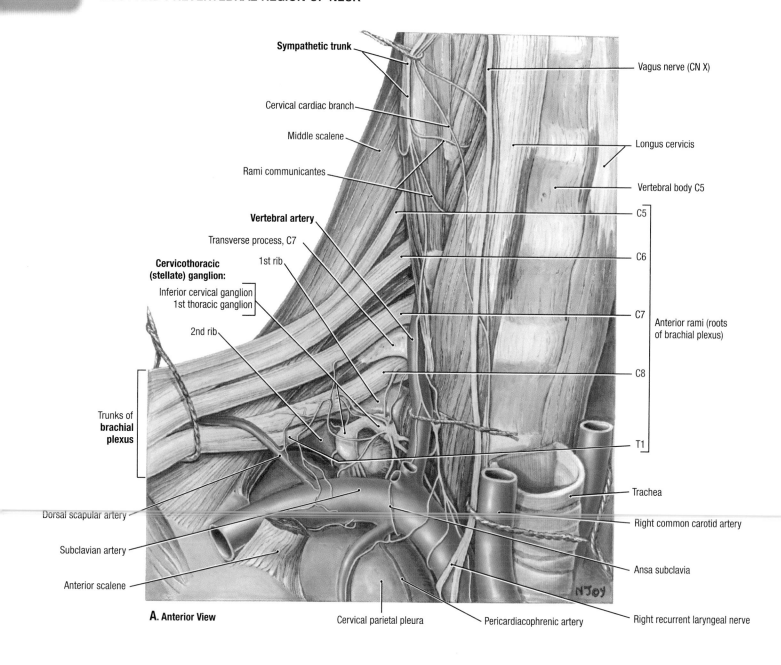

Sympathetic trunk

Cervical cardiac branch

Middle scalene

Rami communicantes

Vertebral artery

Transverse process, C7

1st rib

Cervicothoracic (stellate) ganglion:

Inferior cervical ganglion
1st thoracic ganglion

2nd rib

Trunks of **brachial plexus**

Dorsal scapular artery

Subclavian artery

Anterior scalene

Vagus nerve (CN X)

Longus cervicis

Vertebral body C5

C5

C6

C7 — Anterior rami (roots of brachial plexus)

C8

T1

Trachea

Right common carotid artery

Ansa subclavia

Right recurrent laryngeal nerve

Cervical parietal pleura

Pericardiacophrenic artery

A. Anterior View

8.24 BRACHIAL PLEXUS AND SYMPATHETIC TRUNK IN ROOT OF NECK

A. Dissection of right side of specimen. The pleura has been depressed, the vertebral artery retracted medially, and the brachial plexus retracted superiorly to reveal the cervicothoracic (stellate) ganglion (the combined inferior cervical and 1st thoracic ganglia). Anesthetic injected around the cervicothoracic (stellate) ganglion blocks transmission of stimuli through the cervical and superior thoracic ganglia. This **stellate ganglion block** may relieve vascular spasms involving the brain and upper limb. It is also useful when deciding if surgical resection of the ganglion would be beneficial to a person with excess vasoconstriction of the ipsilateral limb. **B.** Relation of brachial plexus and subclavian artery to anterior and middle scalene muscles.

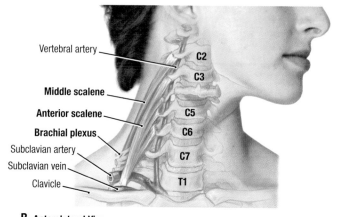

Vertebral artery

Middle scalene

Anterior scalene

Brachial plexus

Subclavian artery

Subclavian vein

Clavicle

C2

C3

C5

C6

C7

T1

B. Anterolateral View

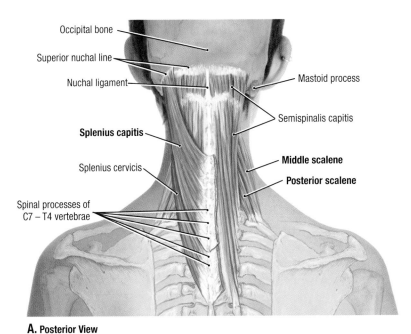

Occipital bone

Superior nuchal line

Nuchal ligament

Mastoid process

Semispinalis capitis

Splenius capitis

Middle scalene

Splenius cervicis

Posterior scalene

Spinal processes of
C7 – T4 vertebrae

A. Posterior View

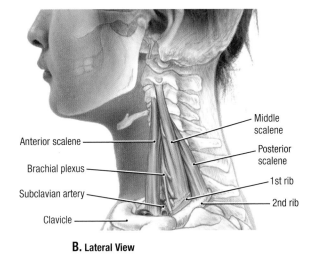

Anterior scalene

Middle
scalene

Brachial plexus

Posterior
scalene

Subclavian artery

1st rib

2nd rib

Clavicle

B. Lateral View

Transverse process, C1

Superior angle
of scapula

Levator scapulae

C. Posterior View

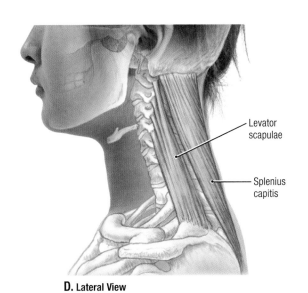

Levator
scapulae

Splenius
capitis

D. Lateral View

8.25   LATERAL VERTEBRAL MUSCLES

A. Overview. **B.** Scalene muscles. **C.** Levator scapulae. **D.** Levator scapulae and splenius capitis.

TABLE 8.7 *LATERAL VERTEBRAL MUSCLES*

Muscle	Superior Attachment	Inferior Attachment	Innervation	Main Action
Splenius capitis	Inferior half of nuchal ligament and spinous processes of C7 and superior 3–4 thoracic vertebrae	Lateral aspect of mastoid process and lateral third of superior nuchal line	Posterior rami of middle cervical spinal nerves	Laterally flexes and rotates head and neck to same side; acting bilaterally, extends head and neck[a]
Levator scapulae	Posterior tubercles of transverse processes of C1–C4 vertebrae See Table 8.6.	Superior part of medial border of scapula	Dorsal scapular nerve (C5) and cervical spinal nerves C3 and C4	Elevates scapula and tilts glenoid cavity inferiorly by rotating scapula
Middle scalene				
Posterior scalene				

[a]Rotation of head occurs at atlanto-axial joints.

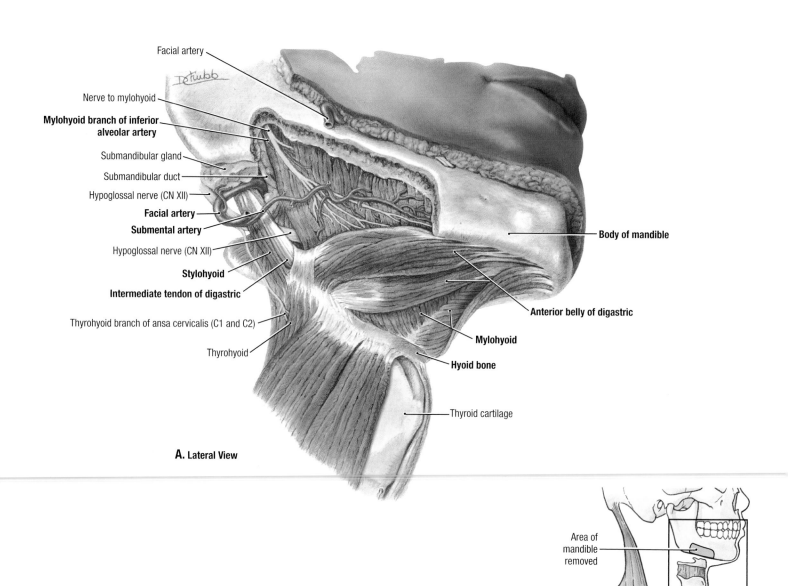

Facial artery

Nerve to mylohyoid

Mylohyoid branch of inferior alveolar artery

Submandibular gland

Submandibular duct

Hypoglossal nerve (CN XII)

Facial artery

Submental artery

Hypoglossal nerve (CN XII)

Stylohyoid

Intermediate tendon of digastric

Thyrohyoid branch of ansa cervicalis (C1 and C2)

Thyrohyoid

Body of mandible

Anterior belly of digastric

Mylohyoid

Hyoid bone

Thyroid cartilage

A. Lateral View

Area of mandible removed

8.26 SERIAL DISSECTION OF SUBMANDIBULAR REGION AND FLOOR OF MOUTH I

Mylohyoid and digastric muscles. **A.** Structures overlying the mandible and a portion of the body of the mandible have been removed.

- The stylohyoid and posterior belly and intermediate tendon of the digastric muscle form the posterior border of the submandibular triangle; the facial artery passes superficial to these muscles.
- The anterior belly of the digastric muscle forms the anterior border of the submandibular triangle. In this specimen, the anterior belly has an additional origin from the hyoid bone; the mylohyoid muscle forms the medial wall of the triangle and has a thick, free posterior border.
- The nerve to mylohyoid, which supplies the mylohyoid muscle and anterior belly of the digastric muscle, is accompanied by the mylohyoid branch of the inferior alveolar artery posteriorly and the submental artery from the facial artery anteriorly.

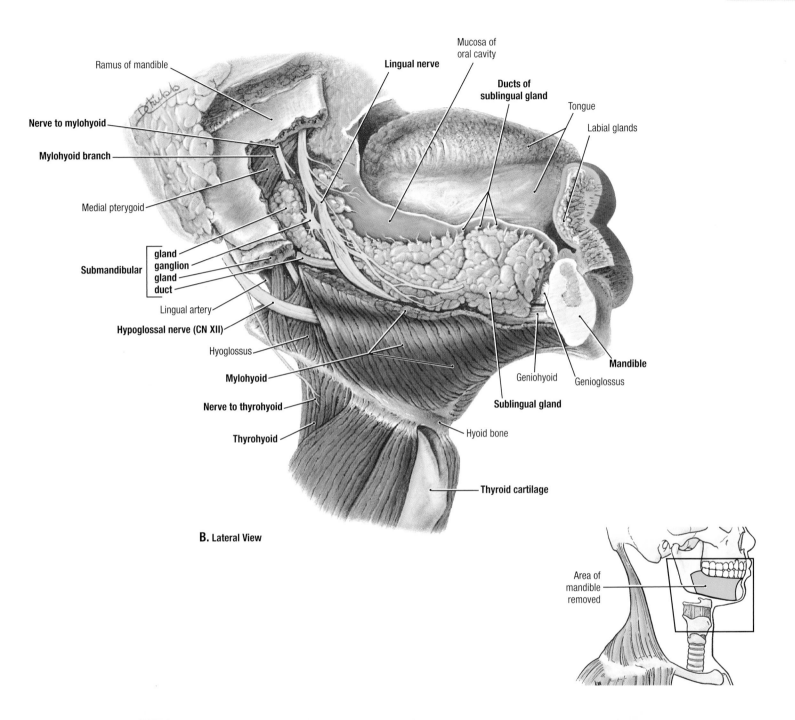

B. Lateral View

8.26   **SERIAL DISSECTION OF SUBMANDIBULAR REGION AND FLOOR OF MOUTH II**

B. Sublingual and submandibular glands. The body and adjacent portion of the ramus of the mandible have been removed.

- The sublingual salivary gland lies posterior to the mandible and is in contact with the deep part of the submandibular gland posteriorly.
- Numerous fine ducts pass from the superior border of the sublingual gland to open on the sublingual fold of the overlying mucosa.
- The lingual nerve lies between the sublingual gland and the deep part of the submandibular gland; the submandibular ganglion is suspended from this nerve.
- Spinal nerve C1 fibers, conveyed by the hypoglossal nerve (CN XII), pass to the thyrohyoid muscle before the hypoglossal nerve passes deep to the mylohyoid muscle.

Stylohyoid
Ramus of mandible
Posterior belly of digastric
Facial artery
Hypoglossal nerve (CN XII)
Sternocleidomastoid artery
External jugular vein
Intermediate tendon of digastric
Superior root of ansa cervicalis
Lingual artery
External carotid artery
Nerve to thyrohyoid
Superior thyroid artery
Thyrohyoid
Sternocleidomastoid

Tonsillar branch of facial artery
Styloglossus (longitudinal part)
Lingual nerve
Submandibular ganglion
Styloglossus (oblique part)
Opening of submandibular duct
Submandibular duct
Genioglossus
Mandible
Sublingual artery
Geniohyoid
Mylohyoid
Hyoglossus
Hyoid bone
Sternohyoid
Superior belly of omohyoid

Area of mandible removed

C. Lateral View

8.26 SERIAL DISSECTION OF SUBMANDIBULAR REGION AND FLOOR OF MOUTH III

C. Hyoglossus muscle, lingual (CN V₃) and hypoglossal nerves (CN XII). All of the right half of the mandible, except the superior part of the ramus, has been removed. The stylohyoid muscle is reflected superiorly, and the posterior belly of the digastric muscle is left in situ.

- The hyoglossus muscle ascends from the greater horn and body of the hyoid bone to the side of the tongue.
- The styloglossus muscle is crossed by the tonsillar branch of the facial artery posterosuperiorly, and its oblique part interdigitates with bundles of the hyoglossus muscle inferiorly.

- The hypoglossal nerve (CN XII) supplies all of the muscles of the tongue, both extrinsic and intrinsic, except the palatoglossus (a palatine muscle, innervated by CN X).
- The submandibular duct runs anteriorly in contact with the hyoglossus and genioglossus muscles to its opening on the side of the frenulum of the tongue.
- The lingual nerve is in contact with the mandible posteriorly, looping inferior to the submandibular duct and ending in the tongue. The submandibular ganglion is suspended from the lingual nerve; twigs leave the nerve to supply the mucous membrane.

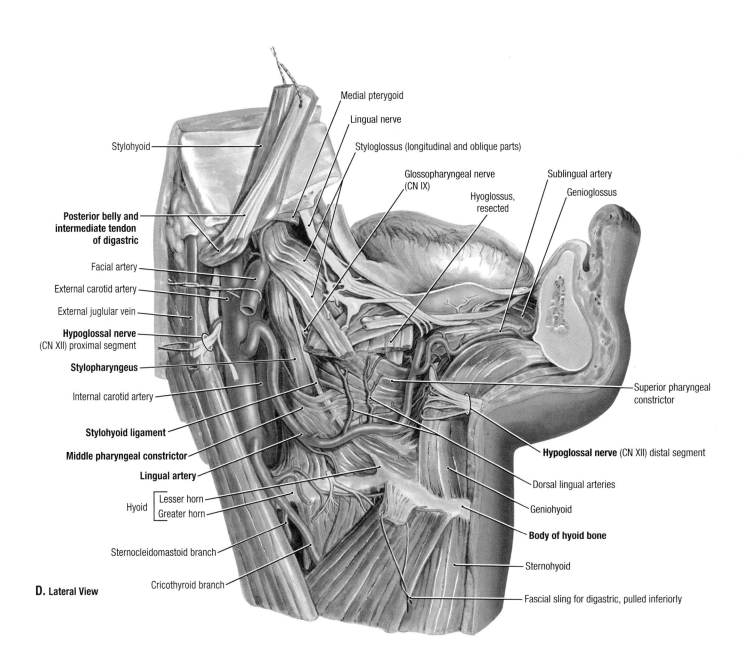

Medial pterygoid

Lingual nerve

Styloglossus (longitudinal and oblique parts)

Stylohyoid

Glossopharyngeal nerve
(CN IX)

Sublingual artery

Genioglossus

Hyoglossus,
resected

**Posterior belly and
intermediate tendon
of digastric**

Facial artery

External carotid artery

External jugular vein

Hypoglossal nerve
(CN XII) proximal segment

Stylopharyngeus

Internal carotid artery

Superior pharyngeal
constrictor

Stylohyoid ligament

Middle pharyngeal constrictor

Hypoglossal nerve (CN XII) distal segment

Lingual artery

Dorsal lingual arteries

Hyoid ⎡ Lesser horn
      ⎣ Greater horn

Geniohyoid

Body of hyoid bone

Sternocleidomastoid branch

Sternohyoid

D. Lateral View

Cricothyroid branch

Fascial sling for digastric, pulled inferiorly

8.26   SERIAL DISSECTION OF SUBMANDIBULAR REGION AND FLOOR OF MOUTH IV

D. Genioglossus and geniohyoid muscles. The stylohyoid, posterior belly and intermediate tendon of the digastric muscle are reflected superiorly, the hypoglossal nerve (CN XII) is divided, and the hyoglossus muscle is mostly removed.

• The lingual artery passes deep to the hyoglossus muscle (resected here), close to the greater horn of the hyoid, and then passes lateral to the middle pharyngeal constrictor muscle, stylohyoid ligament, and genioglossus muscle and turns into the tongue as the deep lingual arteries.

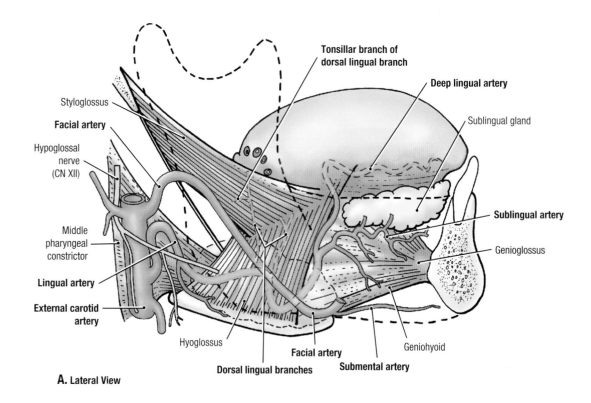

Tonsillar branch of
dorsal lingual branch

Deep lingual artery

Styloglossus

Sublingual gland

Facial artery

Hypoglossal
nerve
(CN XII)

Sublingual artery

Genioglossus

Middle
pharyngeal
constrictor

Lingual artery

**External carotid
artery**

Hyoglossus

Geniohyoid

Facial artery

Dorsal lingual branches

Submental artery

A. Lateral View

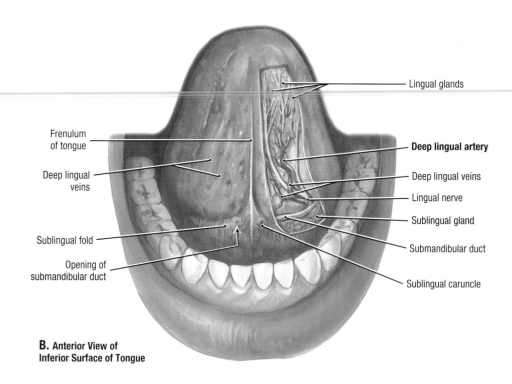

Lingual glands

Frenulum
of tongue

Deep lingual artery

Deep lingual
veins

Deep lingual veins

Lingual nerve

Sublingual gland

Sublingual fold

Submandibular duct

Opening of
submandibular duct

Sublingual caruncle

**B. Anterior View of
Inferior Surface of Tongue**

8.27 LINGUAL AND FACIAL ARTERIES IN SUBMANDIBULAR REGION AND FLOOR OF MOUTH

A. Course of the lingual artery. **B.** Inferior surface of the tongue and floor of the mouth.

In **A**: The lingual artery arises from the anterior aspect of the external carotid artery, where it lies on the middle pharyngeal constrictor. Then it arches supero-anteriorly, passes deep to CN XII and disappears deep to the hyoglossus muscle, giving branches to the posterior tongue (dorsal lingual branches). It then turns superiorly at the anterior border of hyoglossus, bifurcating into the deep lingual and sublingual arteries.

In **B**: The inferior (sublingual) surface of the tongue is covered by mucous membrane through which the underlying deep lingual veins can be seen.

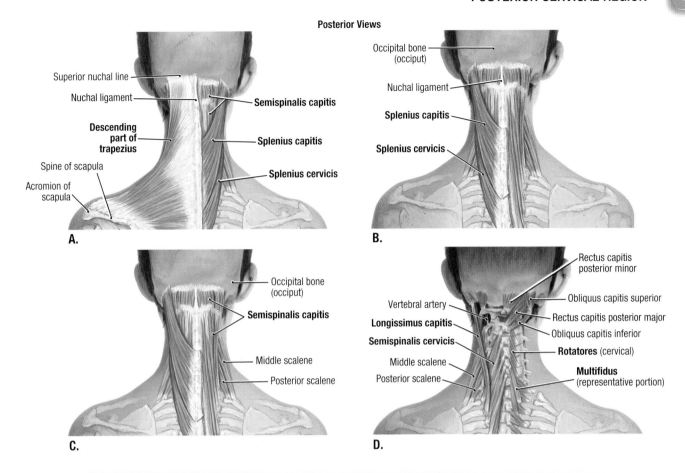

Posterior Views

A.
- Superior nuchal line
- Nuchal ligament
- **Semispinalis capitis**
- **Descending part of trapezius**
- **Splenius capitis**
- Spine of scapula
- **Splenius cervicis**
- Acromion of scapula

B.
- Occipital bone (occiput)
- Nuchal ligament
- **Splenius capitis**
- **Splenius cervicis**

C.
- Occipital bone (occiput)
- **Semispinalis capitis**
- Middle scalene
- Posterior scalene

D.
- Rectus capitis posterior minor
- Vertebral artery
- Obliquus capitis superior
- **Longissimus capitis**
- Rectus capitis posterior major
- **Semispinalis cervicis**
- Obliquus capitis inferior
- **Rotatores** (cervical)
- Middle scalene
- **Multifidus** (representative portion)
- Posterior scalene

8.28 **MUSCLES OF POSTERIOR CERVICAL REGION**

A. Trapezius. **B.** Splenius. **C.** Semispinalis. **D.** Deep muscles.

TABLE 8.8 MUSCLES OF POSTERIOR CERVICAL REGION

Muscle	Superior Attachment	Inferior Attachment	Innervation	Main Action
Extrinsic muscle of back (superior axioappendicular muscle)				
Descending part of trapezius	Medial third of superior nuchal line; external occipital protuberance; nuchal ligament	Lateral third of clavicle and lateral aspect of acromion of scapula	Spinal accessory nerve (CN XI)	Elevates scapulae and works with other parts of muscle to retract scapulae; with shoulder fixed, contributes to extension of head, side bending (lateral flexion) of neck
Intrinsic muscles of back—superficial layer				
Splenius	Nuchal ligament and spinous processes of C7 to T3–T4 vertebrae	*Splenius capitis:* fibers run superolaterally to mastoid process of temporal bone and lateral third of superior nuchal line of occipital bone *Splenius cervicis:* Tubercles of transverse processes of C1–C4 vertebrae	Posterior rami of spinal nerves	*Acting unilaterally:* laterally flex and rotate head to side of active muscle *Acting bilaterally:* extend head and neck
Intrinsic muscles of back—intermediate layer				
Longissimus	Transverse processes of T1–T5 vertebrae	*Longissimus capitis:* posterior mastoid process *Longissimus cervicis:* transverse processes of C2–C6	Posterior rami of spinal nerves	Extends vertebral column; longissimus capitis turns face ipsilaterally
Intrinsic muscles of back—deep layer				
Semispinalis	Transverse processes of C4–T5 vertebrae	*Semispinalis capitis:* Superior nuchal line of occipital bone *Semispinalis cervicis:* Spinous processes of cervical vertebrae		*Acting unilaterally:* contribute to contralateral rotation; *Acting bilaterally:* extend head and neck
Multifidus of cervical region	Transverse processes of T1–T3 Articular processes of C4–C7 vertebrae	Spinous processes 2–4 segments inferior to attachment	Posterior rami of spinal nerves	Stabilizes vertebrae during local movements of vertebral column
Rotatores	Transverse processes	Junction of lamina and transverse process, or spinous process of vertebra immediately (brevis) or two segments (longus) superior to origin		Stabilize, assist with local extension and rotatory movements; may function as proprioceptive organs

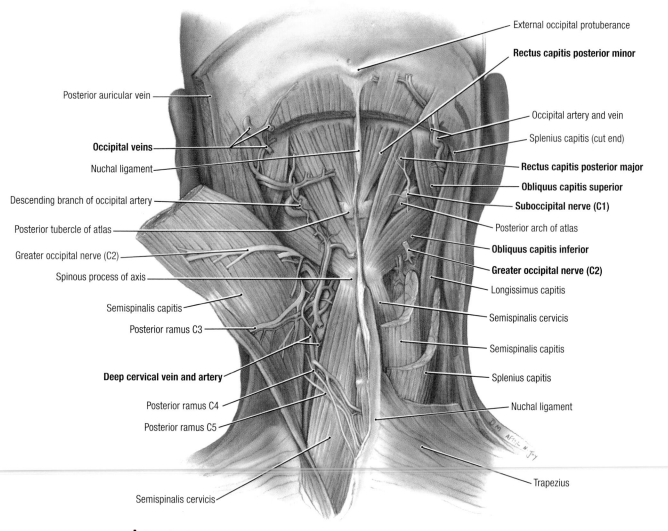

Posterior auricular vein

Occipital veins

Nuchal ligament

Descending branch of occipital artery

Posterior tubercle of atlas

Greater occipital nerve (C2)

Spinous process of axis

Semispinalis capitis

Posterior ramus C3

Deep cervical vein and artery

Posterior ramus C4

Posterior ramus C5

Semispinalis cervicis

External occipital protuberance

Rectus capitis posterior minor

Occipital artery and vein

Splenius capitis (cut end)

Rectus capitis posterior major

Obliquus capitis superior

Suboccipital nerve (C1)

Posterior arch of atlas

Obliquus capitis inferior

Greater occipital nerve (C2)

Longissimus capitis

Semispinalis cervicis

Semispinalis capitis

Splenius capitis

Nuchal ligament

Trapezius

A. Posterior View

8.29

SUBOCCIPITAL REGION

A. Dissection. **B.** Schematic illustration.

- The suboccipital triangle is bounded by three muscles: obliquus capitis inferior and superior, and rectus capitis posterior major.
- The suboccipital nerve (posterior ramus of C1 spinal nerve) emerges through the suboccipital triangle to innervate the muscles forming the triangle.

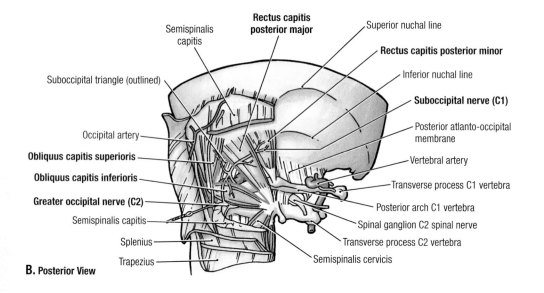

Semispinalis capitis

Rectus capitis posterior major

Superior nuchal line

Rectus capitis posterior minor

Inferior nuchal line

Suboccipital nerve (C1)

Suboccipital triangle (outlined)

Occipital artery

Obliquus capitis superioris

Obliquus capitis inferioris

Greater occipital nerve (C2)

Semispinalis capitis

Splenius

Trapezius

Posterior atlanto-occipital membrane

Vertebral artery

Transverse process C1 vertebra

Posterior arch C1 vertebra

Spinal ganglion C2 spinal nerve

Transverse process C2 vertebra

Semispinalis cervicis

B. Posterior View

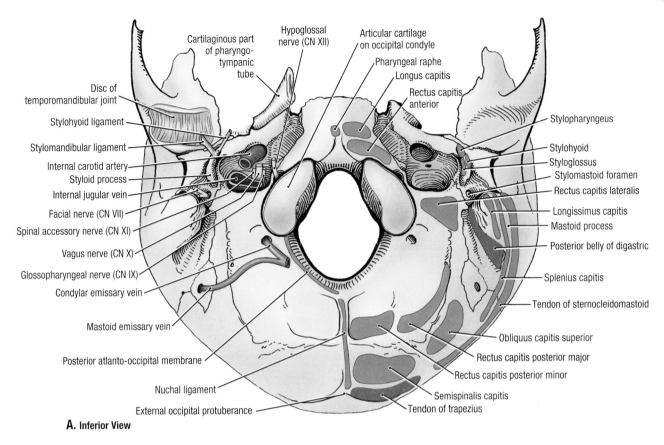

Disc of temporomandibular joint
Stylohyoid ligament
Stylomandibular ligament
Internal carotid artery
Styloid process
Internal jugular vein
Facial nerve (CN VII)
Spinal accessory nerve (CN XI)
Vagus nerve (CN X)
Glossopharyngeal nerve (CN IX)
Condylar emissary vein
Mastoid emissary vein
Posterior atlanto-occipital membrane
Nuchal ligament
External occipital protuberance

Cartilaginous part of pharyngo-tympanic tube
Hypoglossal nerve (CN XII)
Articular cartilage on occipital condyle
Pharyngeal raphe
Longus capitis
Rectus capitis anterior

Stylopharyngeus
Stylohyoid
Styloglossus
Stylomastoid foramen
Rectus capitis lateralis
Longissimus capitis
Mastoid process
Posterior belly of digastric
Splenius capitis
Tendon of sternocleidomastoid
Obliquus capitis superior
Rectus capitis posterior major
Rectus capitis posterior minor
Semispinalis capitis
Tendon of trapezius

A. Inferior View

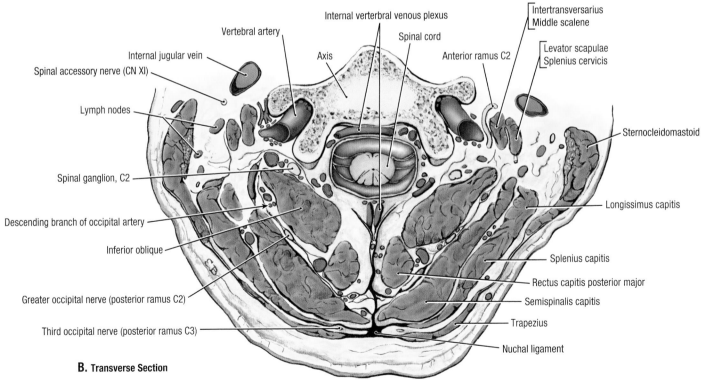

Spinal accessory nerve (CN XI)
Lymph nodes
Spinal ganglion, C2
Descending branch of occipital artery
Inferior oblique
Greater occipital nerve (posterior ramus C2)
Third occipital nerve (posterior ramus C3)

Internal jugular vein
Vertebral artery
Internal verterbral venous plexus
Axis
Spinal cord
Anterior ramus C2
Intertransversarius
Middle scalene
Levator scapulae
Splenius cervicis

Sternocleidomastoid
Longissimus capitis
Splenius capitis
Rectus capitis posterior major
Semispinalis capitis
Trapezius
Nuchal ligament

B. Transverse Section

8.30   POSTERIOR CERVICAL REGION—BASE OF SKULL AND TRANSVERSE SECTION

A. Muscular attachments to and neurovascular relationships at the base of the skull. **B.** Transverse section through the axis (C2 vertebra).

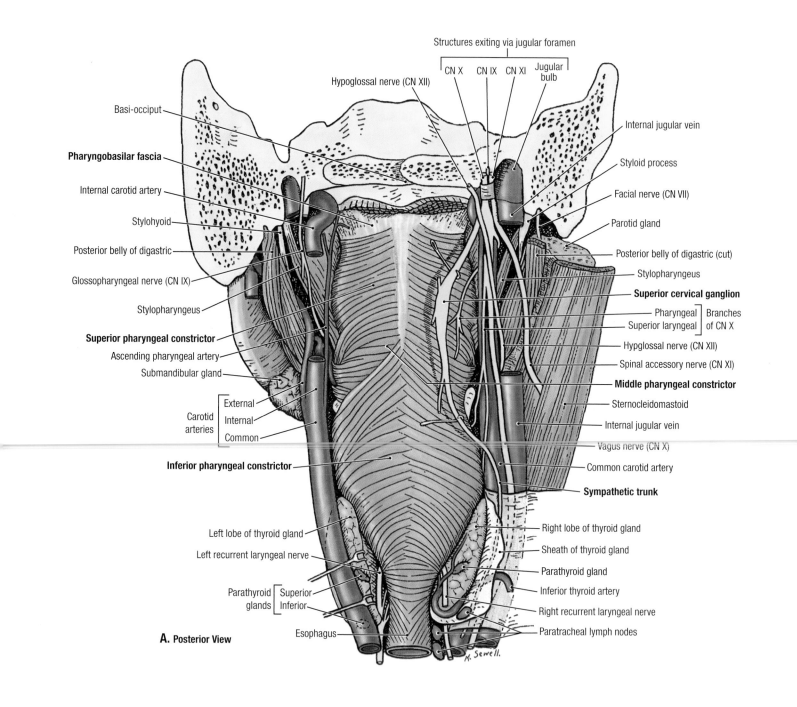

Structures exiting via jugular foramen

CN X CN IX CN XI Jugular bulb

Hypoglossal nerve (CN XII)

Basi-occiput

Internal jugular vein

Pharyngobasilar fascia

Styloid process

Internal carotid artery

Facial nerve (CN VII)

Stylohyoid

Parotid gland

Posterior belly of digastric

Posterior belly of digastric (cut)

Glossopharyngeal nerve (CN IX)

Stylopharyngeus

Stylopharyngeus

Superior cervical ganglion

Pharyngeal — Branches
Superior laryngeal — of CN X

Superior pharyngeal constrictor

Hypglossal nerve (CN XII)

Ascending pharyngeal artery

Spinal accessory nerve (CN XI)

Submandibular gland

Middle pharyngeal constrictor

External

Sternocleidomastoid

Carotid
arteries   Internal

Internal jugular vein

Common

Vagus nerve (CN X)

Inferior pharyngeal constrictor

Common carotid artery

Sympathetic trunk

Left lobe of thyroid gland

Right lobe of thyroid gland

Left recurrent laryngeal nerve

Sheath of thyroid gland

Parathyroid gland

Parathyroid   Superior
glands   Inferior

Inferior thyroid artery

Right recurrent laryngeal nerve

Esophagus

Paratracheal lymph nodes

M. Sewell.

A. Posterior View

8.31 EXTERNAL PHARYNX—POSTERIOR VIEWS

A. Illustration of a dissection similar to **B.** The sympathetic trunk (including the superior cervical ganglion), which normally lies posterior to the internal carotid artery, has been retracted medially.

- The pharyngobasilar fascia, between the superior pharyngeal constrictor muscle and the base of the skull, attaches the pharynx to the

occipital bone and forms the wall of the noncollapsible pharyngeal recesses.

- As they exit the jugular foramen, CN IX lies anterior to CN X, and CN XI; CN XII, exiting the hypoglossal canal, lies medially.

Glossopharyngeal nerve (CN IX)

Spinal accessory nerve (CN XI)

Hypoglossal nerve (CN XII)

Superior pharyngeal constrictor

Pharyngeal raphe attaching to pharyngeal tubercle

Pharyngobasilar fascia

Internal jugular vein

Internal carotid artery

Glossopharyngeal nerve (CN IX)

Styloid process

Stylohyoid

Digastric, posterior belly

Stylopharyngeus

Medial pterygoid

Intermediate tendon of digastric

Middle pharyngeal constrictor

Greater horn of hyoid bone

Pharyngeal branches of CN IX and CN X forming pharyngeal plexus

Inferior pharyngeal constrictor (thyropharyngeus)

Thyroid gland

Inferior thyroid artery

Inferior pharyngeal constrictor (cricopharyngeus)

Right recurrent laryngeal nerve

Esophagus

Spinal accessory nerve (CN XI)

Sternocleidomastoid (retracted)

Parotid gland

External carotid artery

Hypoglossal nerve (CN XII)

Superior cervical ganglion

Superior laryngeal nerve

Common carotid artery

Sympathetic plexus

Sympathetic trunk

Vagus nerve (CN X)

Middle cervical ganglion

Inferior cervical ganglion

Left recurrent laryngeal nerve

B. Posterior View

8.31   **EXTERNAL PHARYNX—POSTERIOR VIEWS** *(CONTINUED)*

B. Dissection. A large wedge of occipital bone (including the foramen magnum) and the articulated cervical vertebrae have been separated from the remainder (anterior portion) of the head and cervical viscera at the retropharyngeal space and removed.

- The pharynx is a unique portion of the alimentary tract, having a circular layer of muscle externally and a longitudinal layer internally.
- The circular layer of the pharynx consists of the three pharyngeal constrictor muscles (superior, middle, and inferior), which overlap one another.
- On the right side of the specimen, the stylopharyngeus muscle and glossopharyngeal nerve (IX) pass from the medial side of the styloid

process anteromedially through the interval between the superior and middle pharyngeal constrictor muscles to become part of the internal longitudinal layer. The stylohyoid muscle passes from the lateral side of the styloid process anterolaterally and splits on its way to the hyoid bone to accommodate passage of the intermediate tendon of the digastric.

- Pharyngeal branches of the glossopharyngeal nerve (CN IX) and the vagus nerve (CN X) form the pharyngeal plexus, which provides most of the pharyngeal innervation. The glossopharyngeal nerve supplies the sensory component, while the vagus supplies motor innervation.

A. Lateral View

8.32   EXTERNAL PHARYNX—LATERAL VIEWS

A. Illustration of a dissection similar to **B.**

TABLE 8.9 MUSCLES OF PHARYNX

Muscle	Origin	Insertion	Innervation	Main Action(s)
Superior pharyngeal constrictor	Pterygoid hamulus, pterygo-mandibular raphe, posterior end of mylohyoid line of mandible, and side of tongue	Pharyngeal raphe	Pharyngeal and superior laryngeal branches of vagus (CN X) through pharyngeal plexus	Constrict wall of pharynx during swallowing
Middle pharyngeal constrictor	Stylohyoid ligament and superior (greater) and inferior (lesser) horns of hyoid bone			
Inferior pharyngeal constrictor	Oblique line of thyroid cartilage			
Thyropharyngeus				
Cricopharyngeus (see Fig. 8.20B)	Side of cricoid cartilage	Contralateral side of cricoid cartilage	Pharyngeal and superior laryngeal branches of vagus (CN X) through pharyngeal plexus + external laryngeal plexus	Serves as superior esophageal sphincter
Palatopharyngeus (see Fig. 8.31B)	Hard palate and palatine aponeurosis	Posterior border of lamina of thyroid cartilage and side of pharynx and esophagus	Pharyngeal and superior laryngeal branches of vagus (CN X) through pharyngeal plexus	Elevate pharynx and larynx during swallowing and speaking
Salpingopharyngeus (see Fig. 8.33B)	Cartilaginous part of pharyngotympanic tube	Blends with palatopharyngeus		
Stylopharyngeus	Styloid process of temporal bone	Posterior and superior borders of thyroid cartilage with palatopharyngeus	Glossopharyngeal nerve (CN IX)	

Maxillary artery

Lateral pterygoid plate

Pterygomaxillary fissure

Tensor veli palatini

Mandibular nerve (V₃)

Middle meningeal artery

Levator veli palatini

Superior pharyngeal constrictor

Styloglossus

Glossopharyngeal nerve (CN IX)

Stylopharyngeus

Hypoglossal nerve (CN XII)

Middle pharyngeal constrictor

Digastric tendon

Greater horn of hyoid bone

Vagus nerve (CN X)

Internal branch of superior laryngeal nerve

Inferior pharyngeal constrictor

External branch of superior laryngeal nerve

Right recurrent laryngeal nerve

Trachea

B. Lateral View

Pterygomandibular raphe

Buccinator

Lingual nerve

Mylohyoid

Hyoglossus

Stylohyoid

Thyrohyoid membrane

Lamina of thyroid cartilage

Cricothyroid

Cricoid cartilage

Pterygomandibular raphe

Superior pharyngeal constrictor

Middle pharyngeal constrictor

Thyropharyngeus ⎫ Inferior pharyngeal constrictor
Cricopharyngeus ⎭

Esophagus

C. Lateral View

8.32 **EXTERNAL PHARYNX—LATERAL VIEWS** *(CONTINUED)*

B. Dissection. **C.** Observe that there are gaps in the pharyngeal musculature (1-4 in **C**) allowing the entry of structures:

1. Superior to the superior constrictor muscle: levator veli palatini muscle and pharyngotympanic (auditory) tube (see Fig. 8.33B)

2. Between the superior and middle constrictors: stylopharyngeus muscle, CN IX, and stylohyoid ligament

3. Between the middle and inferior constrictors: internal branch of superior laryngeal nerve and superior laryngeal artery and nerve (not shown)

4. Inferior to the inferior constrictor muscle: recurrent laryngeal nerve

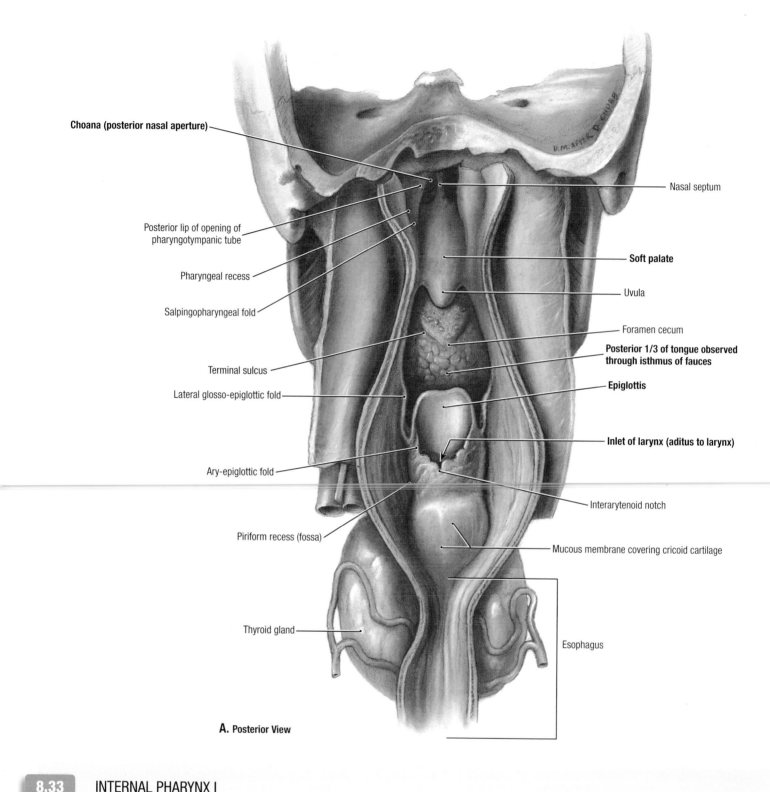

Choana (posterior nasal aperture)

Posterior lip of opening of
pharyngotympanic tube

Pharyngeal recess

Salpingopharyngeal fold

Terminal sulcus

Lateral glosso-epiglottic fold

Ary-epiglottic fold

Piriform recess (fossa)

Thyroid gland

Nasal septum

Soft palate

Uvula

Foramen cecum

**Posterior 1/3 of tongue observed
through isthmus of fauces**

Epiglottis

Inlet of larynx (aditus to larynx)

Interarytenoid notch

Mucous membrane covering cricoid cartilage

Esophagus

A. Posterior View

8.33   INTERNAL PHARYNX I

A. Dissection. The posterior wall of the pharynx has been split in the midline and the halves retracted laterally to reveal the internal aspect of the anterior wall of the pharynx, occupied by communications that define three parts of the pharynx: (1) the nasal part (nasopharynx), superior to the level of the soft palate, communicates anteriorly through the choanae with the nasal cavities; (2) the oral part (oropharynx), between the soft palate and the epiglottis, communicates anteriorly through the isthmus of the fauces with the oral cavity; and (3) the laryngeal part (laryngopharynx), posterior to the larynx, communicates with the vestibule of the larynx through the inlet of (aditus to) the larynx. The pharynx extends from the cranial base to the inferior border of the cricoid cartilage. Inferiorly, it is narrowed by the encircling cricopharyngeus.

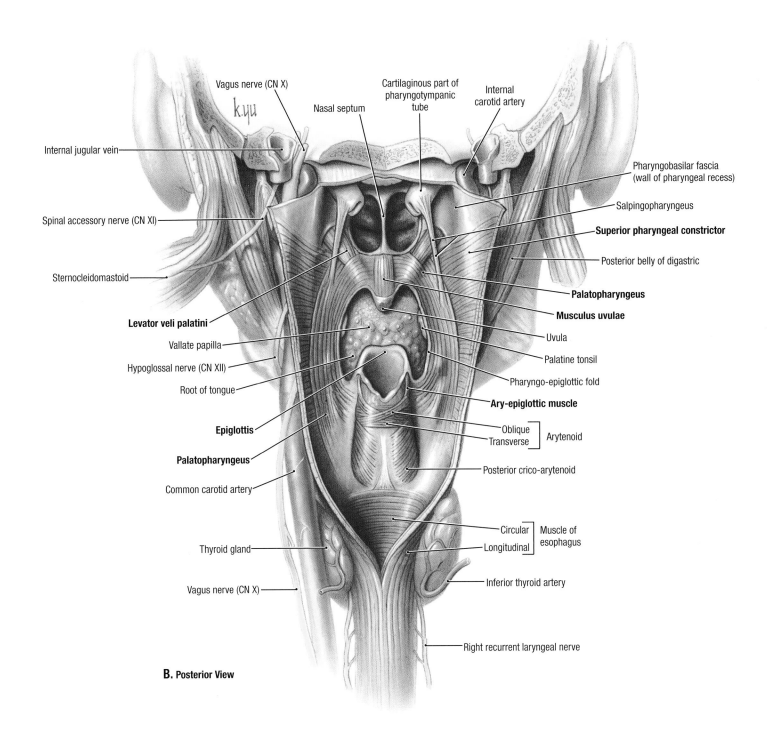

Vagus nerve (CN X)

k.yu

Nasal septum

Cartilaginous part of pharyngotympanic tube

Internal carotid artery

Internal jugular vein

Spinal accessory nerve (CN XI)

Sternocleidomastoid

Levator veli palatini

Vallate papilla

Hypoglossal nerve (CN XII)

Root of tongue

Epiglottis

Palatopharyngeus

Common carotid artery

Thyroid gland

Vagus nerve (CN X)

Pharyngobasilar fascia (wall of pharyngeal recess)

Salpingopharyngeus

Superior pharyngeal constrictor

Posterior belly of digastric

Palatopharyngeus

Musculus uvulae

Uvula

Palatine tonsil

Pharyngo-epiglottic fold

Ary-epiglottic muscle

Oblique
Transverse   Arytenoid

Posterior crico-arytenoid

Circular   Muscle of
Longitudinal   esophagus

Inferior thyroid artery

Right recurrent laryngeal nerve

B. Posterior View

| 8.33 | INTERNAL PHARYNX II |

B. Illustration. The posterior wall of the pharynx has been split in the midline and reflected laterally as in **A**; then, the mucous membrane was removed to expose the underlying musculature. The muscles of the soft palate, pharynx, and larynx work together during swallowing, elevating the soft palate, narrowing the pharyngeal isthmus (passageway between the nasal and oral parts of the pharynx) and laryngeal inlet, retracting the epiglottis, and closing the glottis, to keep food and drink out of the nasopharynx and larynx as they pass from oral cavity to esophagus. At other times, as when blowing one's nose, the palatopharyngeus muscles, partially encircling the opening to the oral cavity, constrict this opening and depress the soft palate, working with placement and expansion of the posterior tongue to direct expired air through the nasal cavity.

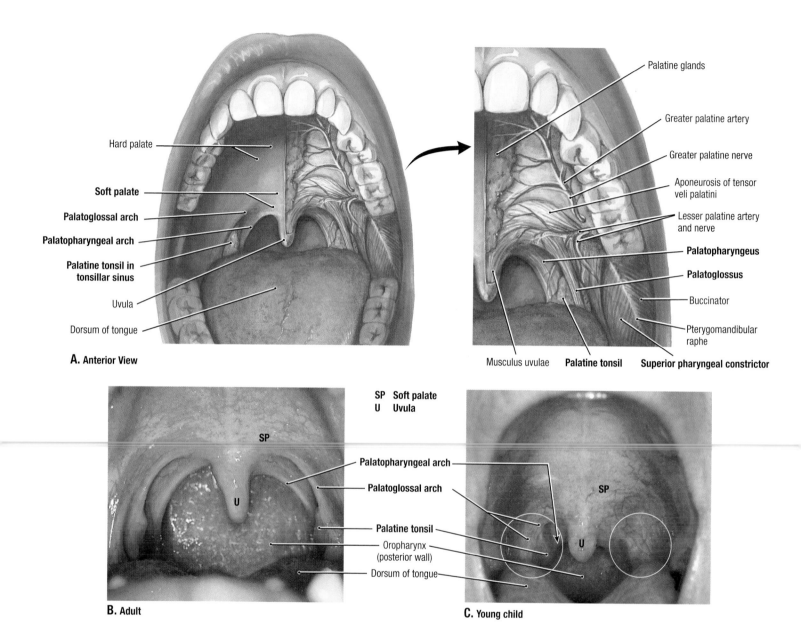

A. Anterior View

Hard palate
Soft palate
Palatoglossal arch
Palatopharyngeal arch
Palatine tonsil in tonsillar sinus
Uvula
Dorsum of tongue

Palatine glands
Greater palatine artery
Greater palatine nerve
Aponeurosis of tensor veli palatini
Lesser palatine artery and nerve
Palatopharyngeus
Palatoglossus
Buccinator
Pterygomandibular raphe
Musculus uvulae **Palatine tonsil** **Superior pharyngeal constrictor**

SP Soft palate
U Uvula

B. Adult

C. Young child

Palatopharyngeal arch
Palatoglossal arch
Palatine tonsil
Oropharynx (posterior wall)
Dorsum of tongue

8.34 SURFACE ANATOMY OF ISTHMUS OF THE FAUCES (OROPHARYNGEAL ISTHMUS)

A. Oral cavity and isthmus demonstrating the sinus (bed) of the tonsils. **B. and C.** Tonsillar sinuses with palatine tonsils in situ, and oropharynx in adult **(B)** and young child **(C)**.

- The fauces (throat), the passage from the mouth to the pharynx, is bounded superiorly by the soft palate, inferiorly by the root (base) of the tongue, and laterally by the palatoglossal and palatopharyngeal arches.
- The palatine tonsils are located between the palatoglossal and palatopharyngeal arches, formed by mucosa overlying the similarly named muscles;

the arches form the boundaries, and the superior pharyngeal constrictor the floor, of the tonsillar sinuses.

- **Normal palatine tonsils.** In the adult the palatine tonsils are normally involuted, with little glandular tissue in the tonsillar sinuses (B). In contrast in young children the palatine tonsils are large relative to the adult, since most of the development of the lymphoid system occurs prior to puberty. Despite their large size, as long as the tonsils are not inflamed and not interfering with swallowing/breathing they are considered normal.

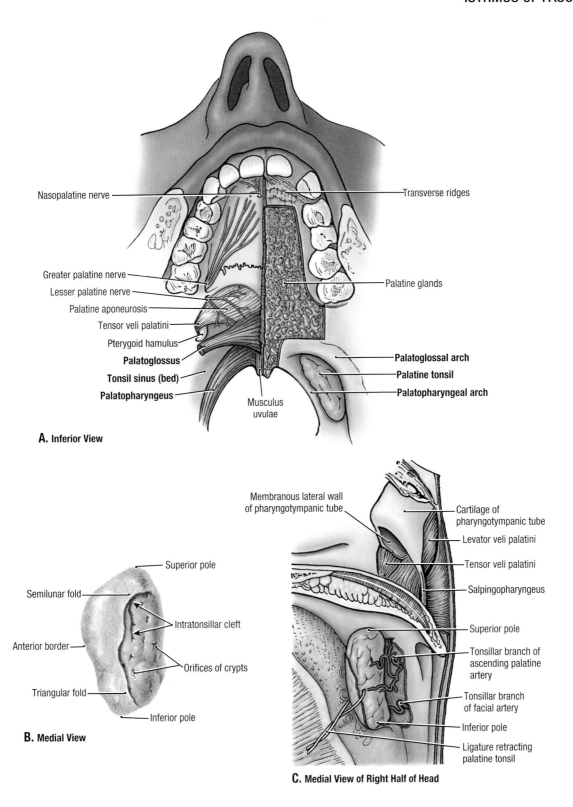

A. Inferior View

Nasopalatine nerve

Transverse ridges

Greater palatine nerve

Lesser palatine nerve

Palatine aponeurosis

Tensor veli palatini

Pterygoid hamulus

Palatoglossus

Tonsil sinus (bed)

Palatopharyngeus

Musculus uvulae

Palatine glands

Palatoglossal arch

Palatine tonsil

Palatopharyngeal arch

B. Medial View

Superior pole

Semilunar fold

Intratonsillar cleft

Anterior border

Orifices of crypts

Triangular fold

Inferior pole

C. Medial View of Right Half of Head

Membranous lateral wall of pharyngotympanic tube

Cartilage of pharyngotympanic tube

Levator veli palatini

Tensor veli palatini

Salpingopharyngeus

Superior pole

Tonsillar branch of ascending palatine artery

Tonsillar branch of facial artery

Inferior pole

Ligature retracting palatine tonsil

8.35   PALATINE TONSIL

A. Left side: Palatine tonsil in situ and glands of palatine mucosa. Right side: Palatine mucosa and tonsils removed demonstrating palatine nerves and muscles. **B.** Isolated palatine tonsil. **C. Tonsillectomy.** The procedure involves removal of the tonsil and the fascial sheet covering the tonsillar sinus. Because of the rich blood supply of the tonsil, bleeding commonly arises from the large external palatine vein or less commonly from the tonsillar artery or other arterial twigs. The glossopharyngeal nerve accompanies the tonsillar artery on the lateral wall of the pharynx and is vulnerable to injury because this wall is thin. The internal carotid artery is especially vulnerable when it is tortuous, as it lies directly lateral to the tonsil.

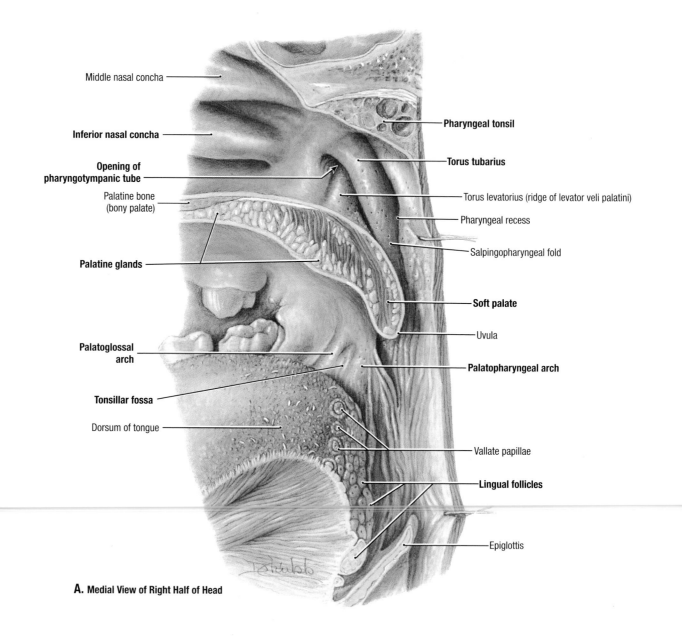

Middle nasal concha

Inferior nasal concha

Opening of pharyngotympanic tube

Palatine bone (bony palate)

Palatine glands

Palatoglossal arch

Tonsillar fossa

Dorsum of tongue

Pharyngeal tonsil

Torus tubarius

Torus levatorius (ridge of levator veli palatini)

Pharyngeal recess

Salpingopharyngeal fold

Soft palate

Uvula

Palatopharyngeal arch

Vallate papillae

Lingual follicles

Epiglottis

A. Medial View of Right Half of Head

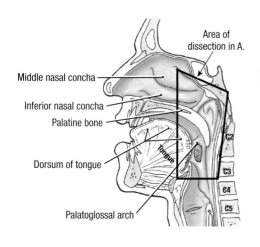

Area of dissection in A.

Middle nasal concha

Inferior nasal concha

Palatine bone

Dorsum of tongue

Palatoglossal arch

8.36 SERIAL DISSECTION OF ISTHMUS OF FAUCES AND LATERAL WALL OF NASOPHARYNX I

- The pharyngeal opening of the pharyngotympanic tube is located approximately 1 cm posterior to the inferior concha.
- The numerous pinpoint orifices of the ducts of the mucous glands can be seen in the mucosa of the torus.
- The pharyngeal tonsil lies in the mucous membrane of the roof and posterior wall of the nasopharynx.
- The palatine glands lie in the soft palate.
- The palatine tonsil lies in the tonsillar sinus between the palatoglossal and palatopharyngeal arches.
- Each lingual follicle has the duct of a mucous gland opening onto its surface; collectively, the follicles are known as the lingual tonsil.

Opening of pharyngotympanic tube

Tensor veli palatini

Ascending palatine
branch of facial artery

Palatoglossus

External palatine (paratonsillar) vein

Tonsillar branch of facial artery

Tongue retracted

B. Medial View of Right Half of Head

Basilar part of occipital bone (basi-occiput)

Cartilage of pharyngotympanic tube

Pharyngobasilar fascia

Levator veli palatini

Salpingopharyngeus

Musculus uvulae

Superior pharyngeal constrictor

Axis (C2)

Palatopharyngeus

Middle pharyngeal constrictor

Vertebral body C3

Area of
dissection in B

8.36   **SERIAL DISSECTION OF ISTHMUS OF FAUCES AND LATERAL WALL OF NASOPHARYNX II**

Muscles underlying tonsillar sinus and wall of nasopharynx. The palatine and pharyngeal tonsils and mucous membrane have been removed. The pharyngobasilar fascia, which attaches the pharynx to the basilar part of the occipital bone was also removed, except at the superior, arched border of the superior pharyngeal constrictor.

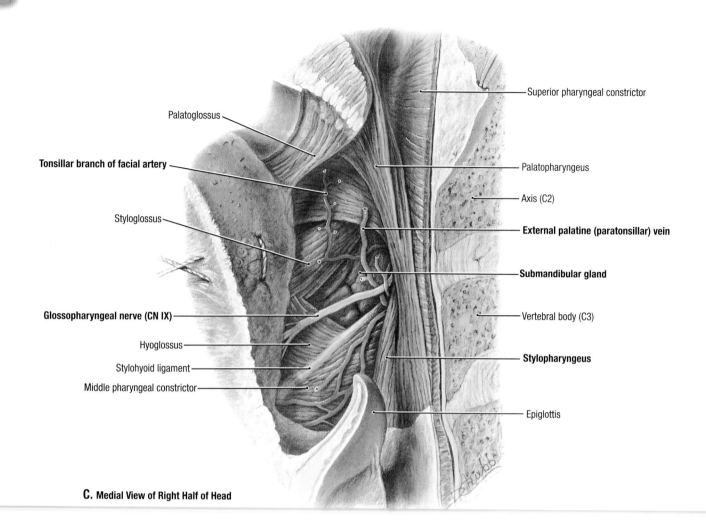

Palatoglossus

Tonsillar branch of facial artery

Styloglossus

Glossopharyngeal nerve (CN IX)

Hyoglossus

Stylohyoid ligament

Middle pharyngeal constrictor

Superior pharyngeal constrictor

Palatopharyngeus

Axis (C2)

External palatine (paratonsillar) vein

Submandibular gland

Vertebral body (C3)

Stylopharyngeus

Epiglottis

C. Medial View of Right Half of Head

Area of dissection in C

8.36

SERIAL DISSECTION OF ISTHMUS OF FAUCES AND LATERAL WALL OF NASOPHARYNX III

Neurovascular structures of tonsillar sinus and longitudinal muscles of the pharynx.
- In this deeper dissection, the tongue was pulled anteriorly, and the inferior part of the origin of the superior pharyngeal constrictor muscle was cut away.
- The glossopharyngeal nerve passes to the posterior one third of the tongue and lies anterior to the stylopharyngeus muscle.
- The tonsillar branch of the facial artery sends a branch (cut short here) to accompany the glosso-pharyngeal nerve to the tongue; the submandibular gland is seen lateral to the artery and external palatine (paratonsillar) vein.

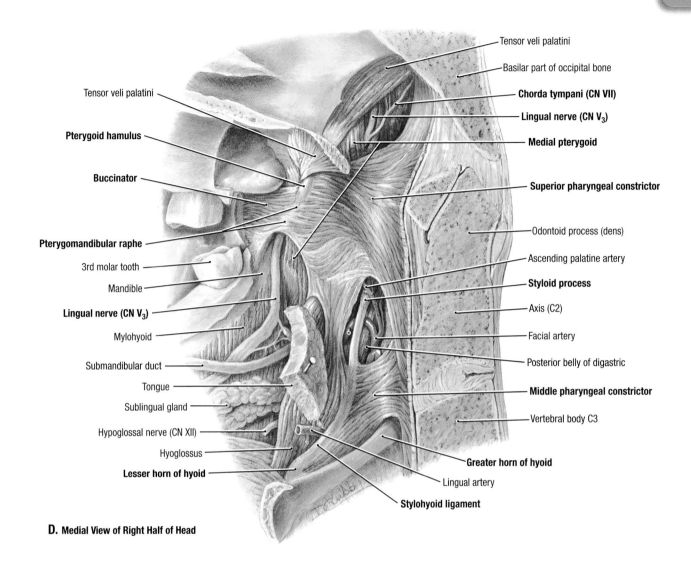

Tensor veli palatini

Basilar part of occipital bone

Chorda tympani (CN VII)

Lingual nerve (CN V₃)

Medial pterygoid

Superior pharyngeal constrictor

Odontoid process (dens)

Ascending palatine artery

Styloid process

Axis (C2)

Facial artery

Posterior belly of digastric

Middle pharyngeal constrictor

Vertebral body C3

Greater horn of hyoid

Lingual artery

Tensor veli palatini

Pterygoid hamulus

Buccinator

Pterygomandibular raphe

3rd molar tooth

Mandible

Lingual nerve (CN V₃)

Mylohyoid

Submandibular duct

Tongue

Sublingual gland

Hypoglossal nerve (CN XII)

Hyoglossus

Lesser horn of hyoid

Stylohyoid ligament

D. Medial View of Right Half of Head

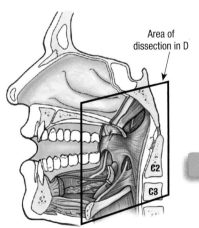

Area of dissection in D

C2

C3

8.36

SERIAL DISSECTION OF ISTHMUS OF FAUCES AND LATERAL WALL OF NASOPHARYNX IV

- The superior pharyngeal constrictor muscle arises from (1) the pterygomandibular raphe, which unites it to the buccinator muscle; (2) the bones at each end of the raphe, the hamulus of the medial pterygoid plate superiorly and the mandible inferiorly; and (3) the root (posterior part) of the tongue.
- The middle pharyngeal constrictor muscle arises from the angle formed by the greater and lesser horns of the hyoid bone and from the stylohyoid ligament; in this specimen, the styloid process is long and, therefore, a lateral relation of the tonsil.
- The lingual nerve is joined by the chorda tympani, disappears at the posterior border of the medial pterygoid muscle, and reappears at the anterior border to follow the mandible.

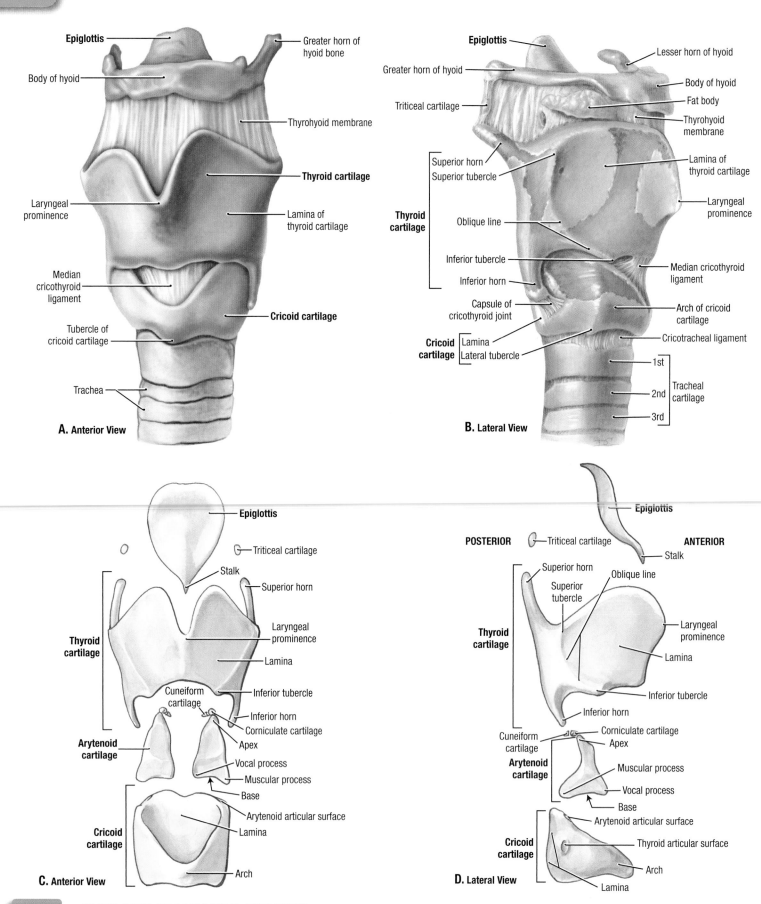

Epiglottis

Greater horn of hyoid bone

Body of hyoid

Thyrohyoid membrane

Thyroid cartilage

Laryngeal prominence

Lamina of thyroid cartilage

Median cricothyroid ligament

Cricoid cartilage

Tubercle of cricoid cartilage

Trachea

A. Anterior View

Epiglottis

Lesser horn of hyoid

Greater horn of hyoid

Body of hyoid

Triticeal cartilage

Fat body

Thyrohyoid membrane

Superior horn

Superior tubercle

Lamina of thyroid cartilage

Thyroid cartilage

Laryngeal prominence

Oblique line

Inferior tubercle

Median cricothyroid ligament

Inferior horn

Capsule of cricothyroid joint

Arch of cricoid cartilage

Cricotracheal ligament

Cricoid cartilage Lamina

Lateral tubercle

1st

2nd Tracheal cartilage

3rd

B. Lateral View

Epiglottis

Triticeal cartilage

Stalk

Superior horn

Thyroid cartilage

Laryngeal prominence

Lamina

Cuneiform cartilage

Inferior tubercle

Inferior horn

Corniculate cartilage

Arytenoid cartilage

Apex

Vocal process

Muscular process

Base

Arytenoid articular surface

Cricoid cartilage

Lamina

Arch

C. Anterior View

Epiglottis

POSTERIOR   Triticeal cartilage   ANTERIOR

Stalk

Superior horn

Oblique line

Superior tubercle

Thyroid cartilage

Laryngeal prominence

Lamina

Inferior tubercle

Inferior horn

Cuneiform cartilage

Corniculate cartilage

Apex

Arytenoid cartilage

Muscular process

Vocal process

Base

Arytenoid articular surface

Cricoid cartilage

Thyroid articular surface

Arch

Lamina

D. Lateral View

8.37   CARTILAGES OF LARYNGEAL SKELETON

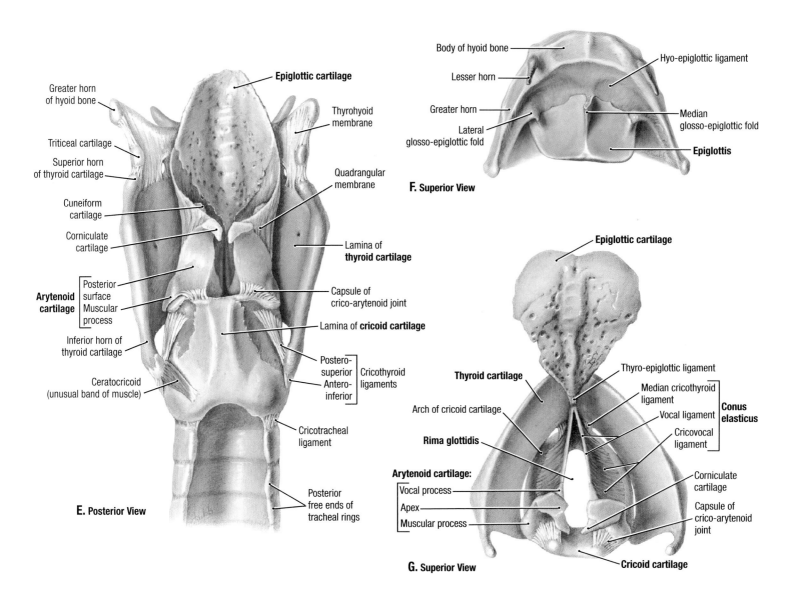

Epiglottic cartilage

Greater horn of hyoid bone

Thyrohyoid membrane

Triticeal cartilage

Superior horn of thyroid cartilage

Cuneiform cartilage

Corniculate cartilage

Arytenoid cartilage — Posterior surface, Muscular process

Quadrangular membrane

Lamina of **thyroid cartilage**

Capsule of crico-arytenoid joint

Lamina of **cricoid cartilage**

Inferior horn of thyroid cartilage

Ceratocricoid (unusual band of muscle)

Postero-superior / Antero-inferior — Cricothyroid ligaments

Cricotracheal ligament

E. Posterior View

Posterior free ends of tracheal rings

Body of hyoid bone

Lesser horn

Greater horn

Lateral glosso-epiglottic fold

Hyo-epiglottic ligament

Median glosso-epiglottic fold

Epiglottis

F. Superior View

Epiglottic cartilage

Thyroid cartilage

Arch of cricoid cartilage

Rima glottidis

Arytenoid cartilage: Vocal process, Apex, Muscular process

Thyro-epiglottic ligament

Median cricothyroid ligament

Vocal ligament

Cricovocal ligament

Conus elasticus

Corniculate cartilage

Capsule of crico-arytenoid joint

Cricoid cartilage

G. Superior View

8.37   **CARTILAGES OF THE LARYNGEAL SKELETON** *(CONTINUED)*

A., B. and E. Articulated laryngeal skeleton. **C. and D.** Cartilages disarticulated and separated. **F.** Epiglottis and hyo-epiglottic ligament. **G.** Conus elasticus and rima glottidis.

- The larynx extends vertically from the tip of the epiglottis to the inferior border of the cricoid cartilage. The hyoid bone is generally not regarded as part of the larynx.
- The cricoid cartilage is the only cartilage that totally encircles the airway.
- The rima glottidis is the aperture between the vocal folds. During normal respiration, it is narrow and wedge shaped; during forced respiration, it is wide. Variations in the tension and length of the vocal folds, in the width

of the rima glottidis, and in the intensity of the expiratory effort produce changes in the pitch of the voice.

- **Laryngeal fractures** may result from blows received in sports such as kickboxing and hockey or from compression by a shoulder strap during an automobile accident. Laryngeal fractures produce submucous hemorrhage and edema, respiratory obstruction, hoarseness, and sometimes a temporary inability to speak. The thyroid, cricoid, and most of the arytenoid cartilages often ossify as age advances, commencing at approximately 25 years of age in the thyroid cartilage.

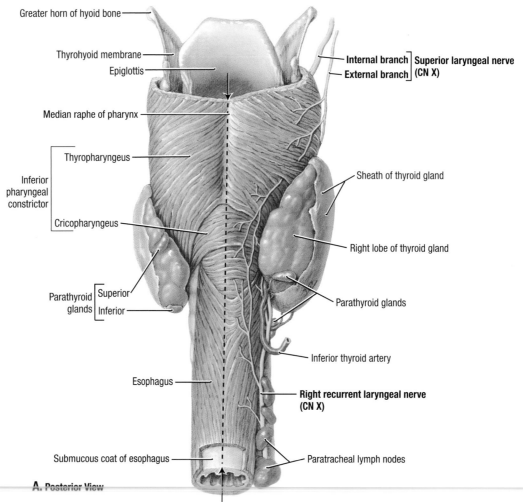

Greater horn of hyoid bone

Thyrohyoid membrane

Epiglottis

Internal branch ⌉ **Superior laryngeal nerve**
External branch ⌋ **(CN X)**

Median raphe of pharynx

Thyropharyngeus

Inferior pharyngeal constrictor

Cricopharyngeus

Sheath of thyroid gland

Right lobe of thyroid gland

Parathyroid glands ⌈ Superior
glands ⌊ Inferior

Parathyroid glands

Inferior thyroid artery

Esophagus

Right recurrent laryngeal nerve (CN X)

Submucous coat of esophagus

Paratracheal lymph nodes

A. Posterior View

Incision to open posterior wall of larynx and trachea (Fig. 8.39A)

Thyrohyoid membrane

Superior laryngeal nerve (CN X)

Internal branch

External branch

Cricopharyngeus

Laryngocele (enlarged laryngeal saccule)

Muscle band

Lamina of thyroid cartilage

Anterior tubercle of cricoid cartilage

Recurrent laryngeal nerve

B. Lateral View Before Removal of the Right Thyroid Cartilage

8.38   EXTERNAL LARYNX AND LARYNGEAL NERVES

A. Posterior aspect.

- The internal branch of the superior laryngeal nerve innervates the mucous membrane superior to the vocal folds, and the external laryngeal branch supplies the inferior pharyngeal constrictor and cricothyroid muscles.
- The recurrent laryngeal nerve supplies the esophagus, trachea, and inferior pharyngeal constrictor muscle. It supplies sensory innervation inferior to the vocal folds and motor innervation to the intrinsic muscles of the larynx, except the cricothyroid.

B. Laryngocele. A laryngocele (enlarged laryngeal saccule) projects through the thyrohyoid membrane and communicates with the larynx through the ventricle. This air sac can form a bulge in the neck, especially on coughing. The inferior laryngeal nerves are vulnerable to injury during operations in the anterior triangles of the neck. **Injury of the inferior laryngeal nerve** results in paralysis of the vocal fold. The voice is initially poor because the paralyzed fold cannot adduct to meet the normal vocal fold. In a bilateral paralysis, the voice is almost absent. **Injury to the external branch of the superior laryngeal nerve** results in a voice that is monotonous in character because the cricothyroid muscle is unable to vary the tension of the vocal fold. Hoarseness is the most common symptom of serious disorders of the larynx.

Epiglottis

Ary-epiglottic fold

Cuneiform tubercle

Corniculate tubercle

Arytenoid (cut)

Vestibular fold

Ventricle

Vocal fold

Lamina of cricoid cartilage (cut)

Mucous membrane

Epiglottic cartilage

Quadrangular membrane

Vestibular ligament

Cuneiform cartilage

Superior horn

Corniculate cartilage

Arytenoid cartilage, medial surface

Thyroid cartilage

Posterior crico-arytenoid ligament

Vocal process of arytenoid cartilage

Vocal ligament

Cricothyroid ligament

Surgical needle spreading cricoid cartilage

Tracheal ring

A. Posterior View
After incision and retraction (spreading)
of posterior wall of larynx and trachea

8.39   INTERNAL LARYNX

A. The posterior wall of the larynx is split in the median plane (see Fig. 8.29A), and the two sides held apart. On the left side of the specimen, the mucous membrane, which is the innermost coat of the larynx, is intact; on the right side of the specimen, the mucous and submucous coats are peeled off, and the next coat, consisting of cartilages, ligaments, and fibro-elastic membrane, is uncovered.
B. Interior of the larynx superior to the vocal folds. The larynx is sectioned near the median plane to reveal the interior of its left side. Inferior to this level, the right side of the intact larynx is dissected.

- The three compartments of the larynx are (1) the superior compartment of the vestibule, superior to the level of the vestibular folds (false cords); (2) the middle, between the levels of the vestibular and vocal folds; and (3) the inferior, or infraglottic, cavity, inferior to the level of the vocal folds.
- The quadrangular membrane underlies the ary-epiglottic fold superiorly and is thickened inferiorly to form the vestibular ligament. The cricothyroid ligament (conus elasticus) begins inferiorly as the strong median cricothyroid ligament and is thickened superiorly as the vocal ligament. The lateral recess between the vocal and vestibular ligaments, lined with mucous membrane, is the ventricle.

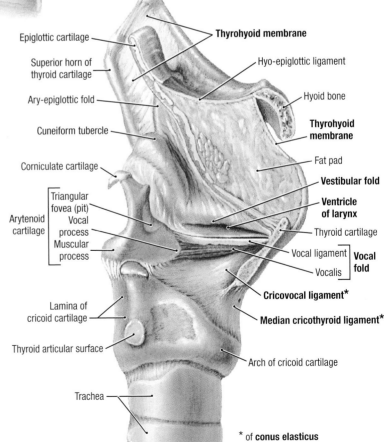

Epiglottic cartilage

Superior horn of thyroid cartilage

Ary-epiglottic fold

Cuneiform tubercle

Corniculate cartilage

Arytenoid cartilage
- Triangular fovea (pit)
- Vocal process
- Muscular process

Lamina of cricoid cartilage

Thyroid articular surface

Trachea

Thyrohyoid membrane

Hyo-epiglottic ligament

Hyoid bone

Thyrohyoid membrane

Fat pad

Vestibular fold

Ventricle of larynx

Thyroid cartilage

Vocal ligament } **Vocal fold**
Vocalis

Cricovocal ligament*

Median cricothyroid ligament*

Arch of cricoid cartilage

* of **conus elasticus**

B. Lateral View After Removal of the Right Thyroid Cartilage

MUSCLES OF LARYNX

TABLE 8.10 MUSCLES OF LARYNX

Muscle	Origin	Insertion	Innervation	Main Action(s)
Cricothyroid	Anterolateral part of cricoid cartilage	Inferior margin and inferior horn of thyroid cartilage	External branch of superior laryngeal nerve (CN X)	Tenses vocal fold
Posterior cricoarytenoid	Posterior surface of laminae of cricoid cartilage	Muscular process of arytenoid cartilage	Recurrent laryngeal nerve (CN X)	Abducts vocal fold
Lateral cricoarytenoid	Arch of cricoid cartilage			Adducts vocal fold
Thyroarytenoid[a]	Posterior surface of thyroid cartilage			Relaxes vocal fold
Transverse and oblique arytenoids[b]	One arytenoid cartilage	Opposite arytenoid cartilage		Close inlet of larynx by approximating arytenoid cartilages
Vocalis[c]	Angle between laminae of thyroid cartilage	Vocal ligament, between origin and vocal process of arytenoid cartilage		Alters vocal fold during phonation

[a]Superior fibers of the thyroarytenoid muscle pass into the aryepiglottic fold, and some of them reach the epiglottic cartilage. These fibers constitute the thyroepiglottic muscle, which widens the inlet of the larynx.
[b]Some fibers of the oblique arytenoid muscle continue as the aryepiglottic muscle.
[c]This slender muscular slip is derived from inferior deeper fibers of the thyroarytenoid muscle.

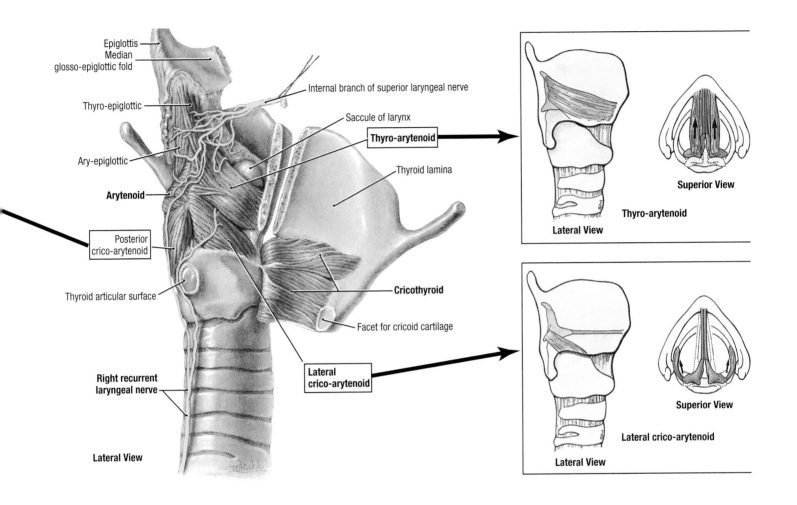

Epiglottis
Median
glosso-epiglottic fold

Thyro-epiglottic

Ary-epiglottic

Arytenoid

Posterior
crico-arytenoid

Thyroid articular surface

**Right recurrent
laryngeal nerve**

Lateral View

Internal branch of superior laryngeal nerve

Saccule of larynx

Thyro-arytenoid

Thyroid lamina

Cricothyroid

Facet for cricoid cartilage

**Lateral
crico-arytenoid**

Superior View

Thyro-arytenoid

Lateral View

Superior View

Lateral crico-arytenoid

Lateral View

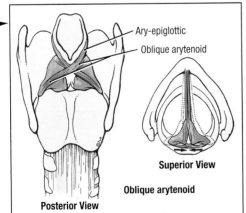

Ary-epiglottic
Oblique arytenoid

Superior View

Oblique arytenoid

Posterior View

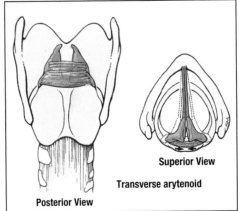

Superior View

Transverse arytenoid

Posterior View

8.40   MUSCLES OF LARYNX *(CONTINUED)*

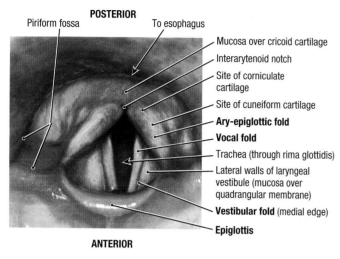

POSTERIOR

Piriform fossa   To esophagus

Mucosa over cricoid cartilage

Interarytenoid notch

Site of corniculate cartilage

Site of cuneiform cartilage

Ary-epiglottic fold

Vocal fold

Trachea (through rima glottidis)

Lateral walls of laryngeal vestibule (mucosa over quadrangular membrane)

Vestibular fold (medial edge)

Epiglottis

ANTERIOR

A. Laryngoscopic Examination

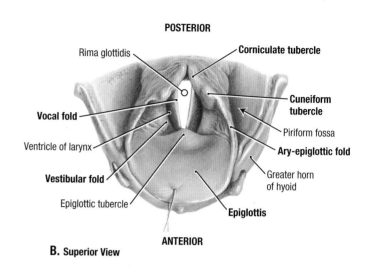

POSTERIOR

Rima glottidis   **Corniculate tubercle**

Vocal fold

Cuneiform tubercle

Ventricle of larynx

Piriform fossa

Ary-epiglottic fold

Vestibular fold

Greater horn of hyoid

Epiglottic tubercle

Epiglottis

ANTERIOR

B. Superior View

Pre-epiglottic fat   Tongue

1
2
3   4
5

C. Coronal MRI

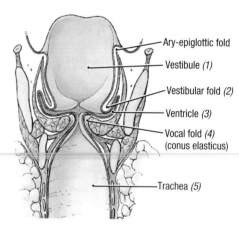

Ary-epiglottic fold

Vestibule (1)

Vestibular fold (2)

Ventricle (3)

Vocal fold (4) (conus elasticus)

Trachea (5)

D. Posterior View

8.41   LARYNGOSCOPIC EXAMINATION AND MRI IMAGING OF LARYNX

A. Laryngoscopic examination. Laryngoscopy is the procedure used to examine the interior of the larynx. The larynx may be examined visually by indirect laryngoscopy using a laryngeal mirror or it may be viewed by direct laryngoscopy using a tubular and endoscopic instrument, a laryngoscope. The vestibular and vocal folds can be observed. **B.** Vocal folds and rima glottidis. The inlet, or aditus, to the larynx is bounded anteriorly by the epiglottis; posteriorly by the arytenoid cartilages, the corniculate cartilages that cap them, and the interarytenoid fold that unites them; and on each side by the ary-epiglottic fold, which contains the superior end of the cuneiform cartilage. The vocal apparatus of the larynx, the glottis, includes the vocal folds, vocal processes of the arytenoid cartilages and the rima glottidis, the aperture between the vocal folds. **C.** Coronal MRI. **D.** Coronal section. Numbers in parentheses on diagram refer to numbered structures on MRI.

A foreign object, such as a piece of steak, may accidentally aspirate through the laryngeal inlet into the vestibule of the larynx, where it becomes trapped superior to the vestibular folds. When a foreign object enters the vestibule, the laryngeal muscles go into spasm, tensing the vocal folds. The rima glottidis closes and no air enters the trachea. **Asphyxiation** occurs, and the person will die in approximately 5 minutes from lack of oxygen if the obstruction is not removed. Emergency therapy must be given to open the airway. The procedure used depends on the condition of the patient, the facilities available, and the experience of the person giving first aid. Because the lungs still contain air, sudden compression of the abdomen **(Heimlich maneuver)** causes the diaphragm to elevate and compress the lungs, expelling air from the trachea into the larynx. This maneuver may dislodge the food or other material from the larynx.

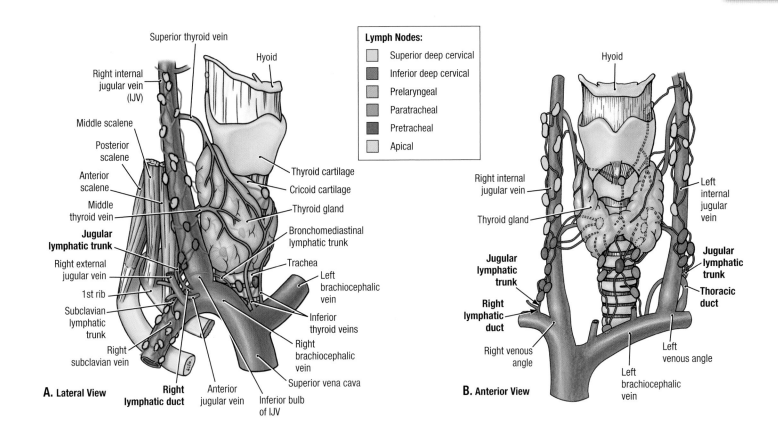

A. Lateral View

Superior thyroid vein
Hyoid
Right internal jugular vein (IJV)
Middle scalene
Posterior scalene
Anterior scalene
Middle thyroid vein
Jugular lymphatic trunk
Right external jugular vein
1st rib
Subclavian lymphatic trunk
Right subclavian vein
Right lymphatic duct
Anterior jugular vein
Inferior bulb of IJV

Thyroid cartilage
Cricoid cartilage
Thyroid gland
Bronchomediastinal lymphatic trunk
Trachea
Left brachiocephalic vein
Inferior thyroid veins
Right brachiocephalic vein
Superior vena cava

Lymph Nodes:
- Superior deep cervical
- Inferior deep cervical
- Prelaryngeal
- Paratracheal
- Pretracheal
- Apical

B. Anterior View

Hyoid
Right internal jugular vein
Thyroid gland
Jugular lymphatic trunk
Right lymphatic duct
Right venous angle
Left brachiocephalic vein

Left internal jugular vein
Jugular lymphatic trunk
Thoracic duct
Left venous angle

| 8.42 | LYMPHATIC DRAINAGE OF THYROID GLAND, LARYNX, AND TRACHEA |

Radical neck dissections are performed when cancer invades the lymphatics. During the procedure, the deep cervical lymph nodes and the tissues around them are removed as completely as possible. Although major arteries, the brachial plexus, CN X, and the phrenic nerve are preserved, most cutaneous branches of the cervical plexus are removed. The aim of the dissection is to remove all tissue that contains lymph nodes in one piece.

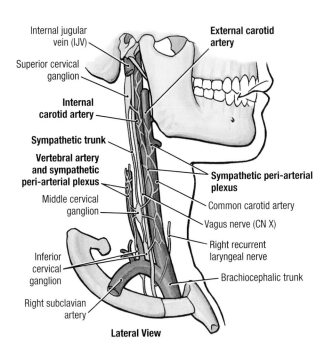

Internal jugular vein (IJV)
Superior cervical ganglion
Internal carotid artery
Sympathetic trunk
Vertebral artery and sympathetic peri-arterial plexus
Middle cervical ganglion
Inferior cervical ganglion
Right subclavian artery

External carotid artery
Sympathetic peri-arterial plexus
Common carotid artery
Vagus nerve (CN X)
Right recurrent laryngeal nerve
Brachiocephalic trunk

Lateral View

| 8.43 | SYMPATHETIC TRUNK AND SYMPATHETIC PERIARTERIAL PLEXUS |

A **lesion of a sympathetic trunk** in the neck results in a sympathetic disturbance called **Horner syndrome,** which is characterized by the following:

- Pupillary constriction resulting from paralysis of the dilator pupillae muscle.
- Ptosis (drooping of the superior eyelid), resulting from paralysis of the smooth (tarsal) muscle intermingled with striated muscle of the levator palpebrae superioris.
- Sinking in of the eyeball (enophthalmos), possibly caused by paralysis of smooth (orbitalis) muscle in the floor of the orbit.
- Vasodilation and absence of sweating on the face and neck (anhydrosis), caused by a lack of sympathetic (vasoconstrictive) nerve supply to the blood vessels and sweat glands.

A

B

Inferior Views

C

1	Tooth	16	Semispinalis cervicis
2	Cricoid cartilage	17	Semispinalis capitis
3	Pharynx	18	Splenius capitis
4	Vertebral artery	19	Trapezius
5	Spinal cord	20	Sternocleidomastoid
6	Cerebrospinal fluid in subarachnoid space	21	Internal jugular vein
		22	Bifurcation of common carotid artery
7	Body of mandible	23	Levator scapulae
8	Mylohyoid	24	External jugular vein
9	Hyoglossus	25	Common carotid artery
10	Genioglossus	26	Rima glottidis
11	Buccal fat pad	27	Vocal fold
12	Submandibular gland	28	Strap muscles
13	Intrinsic muscles of tongue	29	Thyroid cartilage
14	Vertebral body	30	Sublingual gland
15	Lamina of vertebra	31	Inferior pharyngeal constrictor

8.44   TRANSVERSE MRIs OF NECK

The orientation figure indicates the vertebral level of the MRI sections.

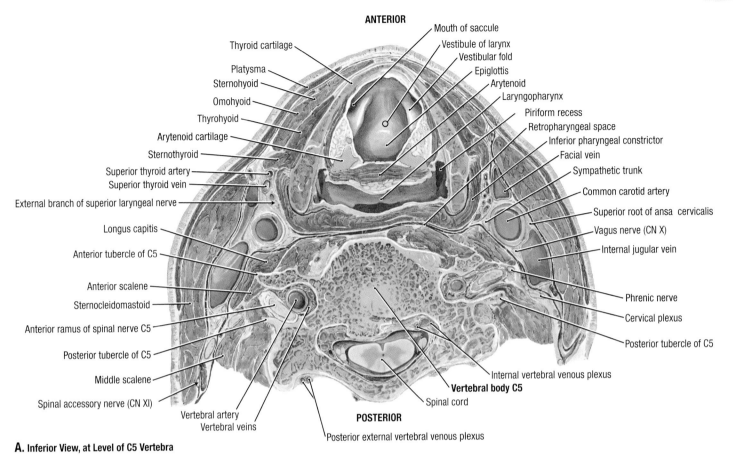

A. Inferior View, at Level of C5 Vertebra

Labels (clockwise):
ANTERIOR
Thyroid cartilage
Platysma
Sternohyoid
Omohyoid
Thyrohyoid
Arytenoid cartilage
Sternothyroid
Superior thyroid artery
Superior thyroid vein
External branch of superior laryngeal nerve
Longus capitis
Anterior tubercle of C5
Anterior scalene
Sternocleidomastoid
Anterior ramus of spinal nerve C5
Posterior tubercle of C5
Middle scalene
Spinal accessory nerve (CN XI)
Vertebral artery
Vertebral veins
Posterior external vertebral venous plexus
POSTERIOR
Spinal cord
Vertebral body C5
Internal vertebral venous plexus
Posterior tubercle of C5
Cervical plexus
Phrenic nerve
Internal jugular vein
Vagus nerve (CN X)
Superior root of ansa cervicalis
Common carotid artery
Sympathetic trunk
Facial vein
Inferior pharyngeal constrictor
Retropharyngeal space
Piriform recess
Laryngopharynx
Arytenoid
Epiglottis
Vestibular fold
Vestibule of larynx
Mouth of saccule

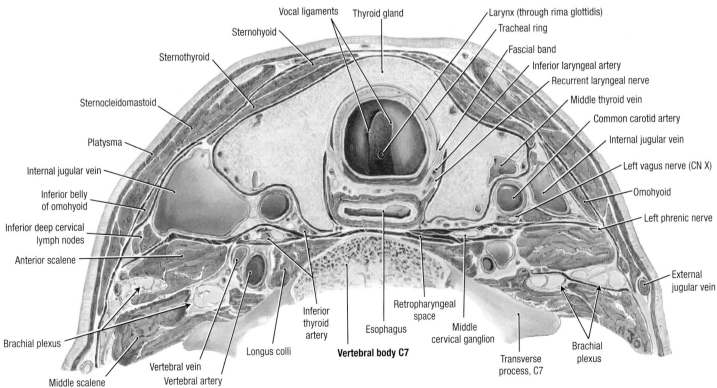

B. Inferior View, at Level of C7 Vertebra

Labels:
Vocal ligaments
Thyroid gland
Sternohyoid
Sternothyroid
Sternocleidomastoid
Platysma
Internal jugular vein
Inferior belly of omohyoid
Inferior deep cervical lymph nodes
Anterior scalene
Brachial plexus
Middle scalene
Vertebral vein
Vertebral artery
Longus colli
Inferior thyroid artery
Esophagus
Vertebral body C7
Retropharyngeal space
Middle cervical ganglion
Transverse process, C7
Brachial plexus
External jugular vein
Left phrenic nerve
Omohyoid
Left vagus nerve (CN X)
Internal jugular vein
Common carotid artery
Middle thyroid vein
Recurrent laryngeal nerve
Inferior laryngeal artery
Fascial band
Tracheal ring
Larynx (through rima glottidis)

8.45 TRANSVERSE ANATOMICAL SECTIONS OF NECK

Hypophysis (pituitary gland)

Pons

Cerebellum

Cribriform plate of ethmoid bone

Nasal septum

External occipital protuberance

Internal occipital protuberance

Apical recess

Cerebellar falx

Medulla oblongata

Pharyngeal tonsil

Cerebellar tonsil

Palate

Atlas (posterior arch)

Tongue

Dens of axis (C2)

Geniohyoid

Axis (C2)

Mylohyoid

Epiglottis

Mandible

Posterior wall of pharynx

Hyoid

Retropharyngeal space

Thyroid cartilage

Vocal fold

Vertebral body C6

Larynx

Lamina of cricoid cartilage

Arch of cricoid cartilage

Trachea

Thyroid gland

Suprasternal space

Thymus

Spinal cord

Brachiocephalic trunk

Vertebral body T2

Left brachiocephalic vein

Esophagus

Manubrium

Sternal angle

Pericardial cavity

Aorta

Ligamentum flavum

Pleural cavity

Right bronchus

A. Median Section

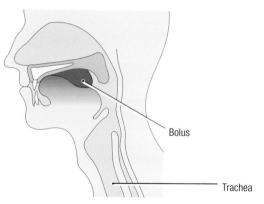

Bolus

Trachea

(1) The bolus of food is squeezed to the back of the mouth by pushing the tongue against the palate.

C.

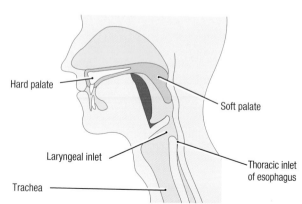

Hard palate

Soft palate

Laryngeal inlet

Thoracic inlet of esophagus

Trachea

(2) The nasopharynx is sealed off, and the larynx is elevated, enlarging the pharynx to receive food.

B. Median MRI Scan

AA	Anterior arch of C1
Ar	Arytenoid cartilage
C3-T4	Vertebral bodies
Cb	Cerebellum
Cr	Cricoid cartilage
CSF	Cerebrospinal fluid in subarachnoid space
Ct	Tonsil of cerebellum
D	Dens
E	Esophagus
Ep	Epiglottis
G	Genioglossus
H	Hyoid
IC	Inferior concha
IV	Intervertebral disc
M	Medulla oblongata
Ma	Mandible
MS	Manubrium of sternum
N	Nuchal ligament
Ph	Pharyngeal tonsil (adenoid)
PT	Posterior tubercle of C1
SC	Spinal cord
So	Soft palate
SP	Spinous process
St	Strap muscles
T	Trachea
Ton	Tongue
1	Nasopharynx
2	Oropharynx
3	Laryngopharynx

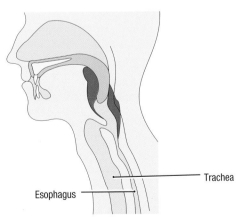

(3) The pharyngeal sphincters contract sequentially, squeezing food into the esophagus. The epiglottis deflects the bolus from but does not close the inlet to the larynx and trachia.

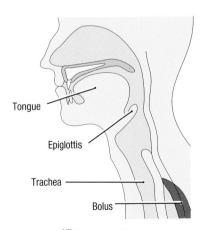

(4) The bolus of food moves down the esophagus by peristaltic contractions.

8.46   **MEDIAN SECTION AND MRI SCAN OF HEAD AND NECK**

A. Median anatomical section. **B.** Median MRI scan. **C.** (1–4) Swallowing.

Anterior View

Key

AR	Arch of aorta
BA	Basilar artery
BT	Brachiocephalic trunk
ECA	External carotid artery
ICA	Internal carotid artery
LC	Left common carotid artery
LS	Left subclavian artery
RC	Right common carotid artery
RS	Right subclavian artery
VA	Vertebral artery

8.47   DOPPLER US COLOR FLOW STUDY OF CAROTID ARTERY

Ultrasonography is a useful diagnostic imaging technique for studying soft tissues of the neck. Ultrasound provides images of many abnormal conditions noninvasively, at relatively low cost, and with minimal discomfort. Ultrasound is useful for distinguishing solid from cystic masses, for example, which may be difficult to determine during physical examination. Vascular imaging of arteries and veins of the neck is possible using intravascular ultrasonography. The images are produced by placing the transducer over the blood vessel. Doppler ultrasound techniques help evaluate blood flow through a vessel (e.g., for detecting stenosis [narrowing] of a carotid artery).

Cranial Nerves

Longitudinal cerebral fissure

Olfactory bulb — Site of termination of olfactory nerves (CN I)

Olfactory tract

Temporal pole

Optic nerve (CN II)

Lateral cerebral sulcus (fissure)

Optic tract

Anterior perforated substance

Oculomotor nerve (CN III)

Optic chiasm

Infundibulum

Trochlear nerve (CN IV)

Mammillary body

Midbrain

Sensory root — Trigeminal nerve (CN V)
Motor root

Pons

Abducent nerve (CN VI)

Middle cerebellar peduncle

Facial nerve (CN VII)

Choroid plexus of 4th ventricle

Intermediate nerve (CN VII)

Hypoglossal nerve (CN XII)

Vestibulocochlear nerve (CN VIII)

Lateral aperture of 4th ventricle

Glossopharyngeal nerve (CN IX)

Vagus nerve (CN X)

Medulla oblongata — Olive / Pyramid

Anterior rootlets of C1 nerve

Spinal accessory nerve (CN XI)

Cerebellum

Inferior View

Spinal cord

9.1   CRANIAL NERVES IN RELATION TO THE BASE OF THE BRAIN

Cranial nerves are nerves that exit from the cranial cavity through openings in the cranium. There are 12 pairs of cranial nerves that are named and numbered in rostrocaudal sequence of their superficial origins from the brain, brainstem, and superior spinal cord. The olfactory nerves (CN I, not shown) end in the olfactory bulb. The entire origin of the spinal accessory nerve (CN XI) from the spinal cord is not included here; it extends inferiorly as far as the C6 spinal cord segment.

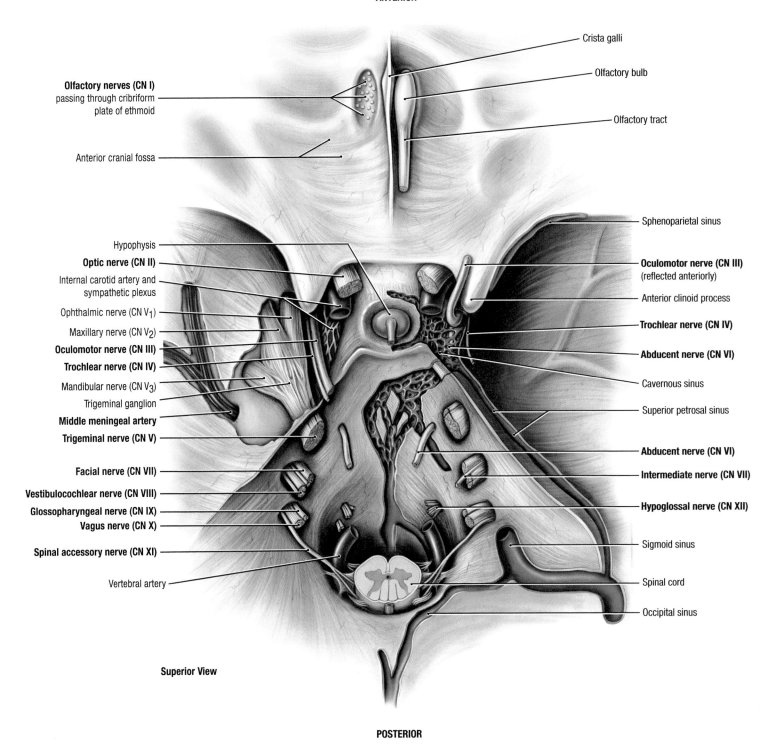

ANTERIOR

Crista galli

Olfactory bulb

Olfactory nerves (CN I) passing through cribriform plate of ethmoid

Olfactory tract

Anterior cranial fossa

Sphenoparietal sinus

Hypophysis

Optic nerve (CN II)

Oculomotor nerve (CN III) (reflected anteriorly)

Internal carotid artery and sympathetic plexus

Anterior clinoid process

Ophthalmic nerve (CN V₁)

Trochlear nerve (CN IV)

Maxillary nerve (CN V₂)

Oculomotor nerve (CN III)

Abducent nerve (CN VI)

Trochlear nerve (CN IV)

Cavernous sinus

Mandibular nerve (CN V₃)

Superior petrosal sinus

Trigeminal ganglion

Middle meningeal artery

Abducent nerve (CN VI)

Trigeminal nerve (CN V)

Facial nerve (CN VII)

Intermediate nerve (CN VII)

Vestibulocochlear nerve (CN VIII)

Glossopharyngeal nerve (CN IX)

Hypoglossal nerve (CN XII)

Vagus nerve (CN X)

Spinal accessory nerve (CN XI)

Sigmoid sinus

Vertebral artery

Spinal cord

Occipital sinus

Superior View

POSTERIOR

9.2   CRANIAL NERVES IN RELATION TO THE INTERNAL ASPECT OF THE CRANIAL BASE

The venous sinuses have been opened on the right side. The ophthalmic division of the trigeminal nerve (CN V₁) and the trochlear (CN IV) and oculomotor (CN III) nerves have been dissected from the lateral wall of the cavernous sinus. Although there are no sympathetic fibers in cranial nerves as they leave the brain, postsynaptic sympathetic nerve fibers "hitch-hike" onto branches of cranial nerves having traveled to the region via major blood vessels.

Trochlear—CN IV

Motor: superior oblique muscle of eye

Abducent—CN VI

Motor: lateral rectus muscle of eye

Oculomotor—CN III

Motor: ciliary muscles, sphincter of pupil, all extrinsic muscles of eye except those listed for CN IV and VI

Optic—CN II

Sensory: vision

Cranial nerve fibers

— Motor (efferent)
— Sensory (afferent)

Facial—CN VII
Primary root

Motor: muscles of facial expression and 3 other muscles (see table 9.1)

Olfactory—CN I

Sensory: smell

Trigeminal—CN V
Sensory root

Sensory: face; oral, nasal and sinus mucosa; teeth and anterior two thirds of tongue

Facial—CN VII
Intermediate nerve

Motor: lacrimal, nasal, palatine, submandibular, and sublingual glands
Sensory: taste to anterior two thirds of tongue, soft palate

Trigeminal—CN V
Motor root

Motor: muscles of mastication and 4 other muscles (see table 9.1)

Vestibulocochlear—CN VIII

Vestibular nerve, sensory: orientation, motion
Cochlear nerve, sensory: hearing

Hypoglossal—CN XII

Motor: all intrinsic and extrinsic muscles of tongue (excluding palatoglossus—a palatine muscle)

Spinal accessory—CN XI

Motor: sternocleidomastoid and trapezius

Vagus—CN X

Motor: palate, pharynx, larynx, trachea, bronchial tree, heart, GI tract to left colic flexure
Sensory : pharynx, larynx; reflex sensory from tracheo-bronchial tree, lungs, heart, GI tract to left colic flexure; taste to epiglottis, palate

Glossopharyngeal—CN IX

Motor: stylopharyngeus, parotid gland
Sensory: pharynx, tonsillar sinus, pharyngotympanic tube, middle ear cavity; taste to posterior third of tongue

CN I · CN II · CN III · CN IV · CN VI · CN V · CN V · CN VII · CN VII · CN VIII · CN VII · CN X · CN IX · CN XII · CN XI

9.3 SUMMARY OF CRANIAL NERVES

TABLE 9.1   SUMMARY OF CRANIAL NERVES

Nerve	Components	Location of Nerve Cell Bodies	Cranial Exit	Function
Olfactory (CN I)	Special sensory	Olfactory epithelium (olfactory cells)	Foramina in cribriform plate of ethmoid bone	Smell from nasal mucosa of roof of each nasal cavity, superior sides of nasal septum and superior concha
Optic (CN II)	Special sensory	Retina (ganglion cells)	Optic canal	Vision from retina
Oculomotor (CN III)	Somatic motor	Midbrain (nucleus of CN III)	Superior orbital fissure	Motor to superior, inferior, and medial rectus, inferior oblique, and levator palpebrae superioris that raise upper eyelid and direct gaze superiorly, inferiorly, and medially
	Visceral motor	Presynaptic: midbrain (Edinger-Westphal nucleus); Postsynaptic: ciliary ganglion		Parasympathetic innervation to sphincter pupillae and ciliary muscles that constrict pupil and accommodate lens of eye
Trochlear (CN IV)	Somatic motor	Midbrain (nucleus of CN IV)		Motor to superior oblique that assists in directing gaze inferolaterally
Trigeminal (CN V) Ophthalmic division (CN V^1)	Somatic (general) sensory	Trigeminal ganglion Synapse: sensory nucleus of CN V		Sensation from cornea, skin of forehead, scalp, eyelids, nose, and mucosa of nasal cavity and paranasal sinuses
Maxillary division (CN V^2)			Foramen rotundum	Sensation from skin of face over maxilla including upper lip, maxillary teeth, mucosa of nose, maxillary sinuses, and palate
Mandibular division (CN V^3)	Somatic (branchial) motor	Pons (motor nucleus of CN V)	Foramen ovale	Sensation from the skin over mandible, including lower lip and side of head, mandibular teeth, temporomandibular joint, and mucosa of mouth and anterior two thirds of tongue
				Motor to muscles of mastication, mylohyoid, anterior belly of digastric, tensor veli palatini, and tensor tympani
Abducent (CN VI)	Somatic motor	Pons (nucleus of CN VI)	Superior orbital fissure	Motor to lateral rectus to direct gaze laterally
Facial (CN VII)	Somatic (branchial) motor	Pons (motor nucleus of CN VII)	Internal acoustic meatus, facial canal, and stylomastoid foramen	Motor to muscles of facial expression and scalp; also supplies stapedius of middle ear, stylohyoid, and posterior belly of digastric
	Special sensory	Geniculate ganglion Synapse: nuclei of solitary tract		
	General sensory	Geniculate ganglion Synapse: sensory nucleus of CN V		Taste from anterior two thirds of tongue, and palate
				Sensation from skin of external acoustic meatus
	Visceral motor	Presynaptic: pons (superior salivatory nucleus); Postsynaptic: pterygopalatine ganglion and submandibular ganglion		Parasympathetic innervation to submandibular and sublingual salivary glands, lacrimal gland, and glands of nose and palate
Vestibulocochlear (CN VIII) Vestibular	Special sensory	Vestibular ganglion Synapse: vestibular nuclei	Internal acoustic meatus	Vestibular sensation from semicircular ducts, utricle, and saccule related to position and movement of head
Cochlear	Special sensory	Spiral ganglion Synapse: cochlear nuclei		Hearing from spiral organ
Glossopharyngeal (CN IX)	Somatic (branchial) motor	Medulla (nucleus ambiguus)	Jugular foramen	Motor to stylopharyngeus that assists with swallowing
	Visceral motor	Presynaptic: medulla (inferior salivatory nucleus); Postsynaptic: otic ganglion		Parasympathetic innervation to parotid gland
	Visceral sensory	Inferior ganglion		Visceral sensation from parotid gland, carotid body and sinus, pharynx, and middle ear
	Special sensory	Inferior ganglion Synapse: nuclei of solitary tract		Taste from posterior third of tongue
	General sensory	Superior ganglion Synapse: sensory nucleus of CN V		Cutaneous sensation from external ear
Vagus (CN X)	Somatic (branchial) motor	Medulla (nucleus ambiguus)		Motor to constrictor muscles of pharynx, intrinsic muscles of larynx, muscles of palate (except tensor veli palatini), and striated muscle in superior two thirds of esophagus
	Visceral motor	Presynaptic: medulla; Postsynaptic: neurons in, on, or near viscera		Smooth muscle of trachea, bronchi, and digestive tract, cardiac muscle
	Visceral sensory	Inferior ganglion Synapse: nuclei of solitary tract		Visceral sensation from base of tongue, pharynx, larynx, trachea, bronchi, heart, esophagus, stomach, and intestine
	Special sensory	Inferior ganglion Synapse: nuclei of solitary tract		Taste from epiglottis and palate
	Somatic (general) sensory	Superior ganglion Synapse: sensory nucleus of trigeminal nerve		Sensation from auricle, external acoustic meatus, and dura mater of posterior cranial fossa
Spinal accessory nerve (CN XI)	Somatic motor	Cervical spinal cord		Motor to sternocleidomastoid and trapezius
Hypoglossal (CN XII)	Somatic motor	Medulla (Nucleus of CN XII)	Hypoglossal canal	Motor to muscles of tongue (except palatoglossus)

Edinger-Westphal nucleus
of oculomotor nerve (CN III)

Superior colliculus (midbrain)

Nucleus of oculomotor nerve (CN III)

Mesencephalic nucleus of trigeminal nerve (CN V)*

Nucleus of trochlear nerve (CN IV)

Motor nucleus of trigeminal nerve (CN V)

Principal sensory nucleus of trigeminal nerve (CN V)*

Middle cerebellar peduncle

Nucleus of abducent nerve (CN VI)

Motor nucleus of facial nerve (CN VII)

Vestibular nuclei (CN VIII)

Superior salivatory nucleus (CN VII)

Cochlear nuclei (CN VIII)

Sulcus limitans (on floor of fourth ventricle)

Gustatory nucleus

Inferior salivatory nucleus (CN IX)

Nuclei of solitary tract
(CNs VII, IX, and X)

Nucleus ambiguus (CNs IX, X)

Cardiorespiratory nucleus

Posterior (motor) nucleus of vagus nerve (CN X)

Spinal nucleus of trigeminal nerve (CN V)*

Nucleus of hypoglossal nerve (CN XII)

* Sensory nucleus of CN V

Motor Nuclei:

- ■ Somatic motor (including
  - ■ Branchial motor)
- ■ Visceral motor
  (Parasympathetic)

Fasciculus gracilis
of medulla oblongata

Nucleus of spinal
accessory nerve (CN XI)

Sensory Nuclei:

- ■ Somatic (general) sensory
- ■ Special sensory
- ■ Visceral sensory

A. Posterior (Dorsal) View

9.4   CRANIAL NERVE NUCLEI

The fibers of the cranial nerves are connected to nuclei (groups of nerve cell bodies in the central nervous system), in which afferent (sensory) fibers terminate and from which efferent (motor) fibers originate. Nuclei of common functional types (motor, sensory, parasympathetic, and special sensory nuclei) have a generally columnar placement within the brainstem, with the sulcus limitans demarcating motor and sensory columns.

Somatic motor: motor fibers innervating voluntary (striated muscle). For the muscles derived from the embryonic pharyngeal arches, their somatic motor innervation can be referred to more specifically as *branchial motor.*

Red nucleus

Edinger-Westphal nucleus of oculomotor nerve (CN III)

Nucleus of oculomotor nerve (CN III)

Nucleus of trochlear nerve (CN IV)

Oculomotor nerve (CN III)

Trochlear nerve (CN IV)

Mesencephalic nucleus of trigeminal nerve (CN V)*

Pons

Motor nucleus of trigeminal nerve (CN V)

Principal sensory nucleus of trigeminal nerve (CN V)*

Trigeminal ganglion

Fourth ventricle

Trigeminal nerve (CN V) [Sensory / Motor]

Nucleus of abducent nerve (CN VI)

Vestibular nuclei (CN VIII)

Motor nucleus of facial nerve (CN VII)

Superior salivatory nucleus (CN VII)

Cochlear nuclei (CN VIII)

Nuclei of solitary tract (CNs VII, IX, and X)

Abducent nerve (CN VI)

Inferior salivatory nucleus (CN IX)

Vestibulocochlear nerve (CN VIII)

Nucleus ambiguus (CNs IX, X)

Facial nerve (CN VII)

Posterior (motor) nucleus of vagus nerve (CN X)

Glossopharyngeal nerve (CN IX)

Inferior olivary complex

Nucleus of hypoglossal nerve (CN XII)

Vagus nerve (CN X)

Spinal nucleus of trigeminal nerve (CN V)*

Spinal accessory nerve (CN XI)

Hypoglossal nerve (CN XII)

* Sensory nucleus of CN V

Motor Nuclei:

- Somatic motor (including Branchial motor)
- Visceral motor (Parasympathetic)

Nucleus of spinal accessory nerve (CN XI)

Central canal

B. Lateral View

Sensory Nuclei:

- Somatic (general) sensory
- Special sensory
- Visceral sensory

V.O.

9.4   CRANIAL NERVE NUCLEI *(CONTINUED)*

Visceral motor: Parasympathetic innervation to glands and involuntary (smooth) muscle.

Somatic (general) sensory: Fibers transmitting general sensation from skin and membranes (e.g., touch, pressure, heat, cold).

Visceral sensory: Fibers conveying sensation from viscera (organs) and mucous membranes.

Special sensory: Taste, smell, vision, hearing, and balance.

A. Medial View of Lateral Wall of Nasal Cavity

B. Medial View of Sagittal Section through Cribriform Plate of Ethmoid Bone

9.5   OLFACTORY NERVE (CN I)

A. Relationship of olfactory mucosa to olfactory bulb. **B.** Olfactory epithelium.

TABLE 9.2   OLFACTORY NERVE (CN I)

Nerve	Functional Components	Cells of Origin/Termination	Cranial Exit	Distribution and Functions
Olfactory	Special sensory	Olfactory epithelium (olfactory cells/olfactory bulb)	Foramina in cribriform plate of ethmoid bone	Smell from nasal mucosa of roof and superior sides of nasal septum and superior concha of each nasal cavity

Left visual field
Right visual field

Eyeball
Retina
Optic nerve (CN II)
Optic canal
Anterior clinoid process
Optic chiasm
Optic tract
Lateral geniculate nucleus
Optic radiations
Visual cortex (occipital lobe)

A

Left visual field
Right visual field

Macula

1
3
4
2

T   N   N   T
2   2
1   1
4   3

Left retinal representations of visual field
Right retinal representations of visual field

Optic chiasm

1 2
3 4
Left lateral geniculate nucleus

Parieto-occipital sulcus

Left visual cortex

2
4
3 1

Calcarine sulcus

C

Optic disc

Axons of retinal ganglion cells
Ganglion cell layer
Bipolar cell layer
Layer of rods and cones
Sclera
Central retinal artery and vein
Optic nerve (CN II)

B. Schematic Superior View

9.6   OPTIC NERVE (CN II)

A. Origin and course of visual pathway. **B.** Rods and cones in retina. **C.** Right visual field representation on retinae, left lateral geniculate nucleus, and left visual cortex.

TABLE 9.3   OPTIC NERVE (CN II)

Nerve	Functional Components	Cells of Origin/Termination	Cranial Exit	Distribution and Functions
Optic	Special sensory	Retina (ganglion cells)/lateral geniculate body (nucleus)	Optic canal	Vision from retina

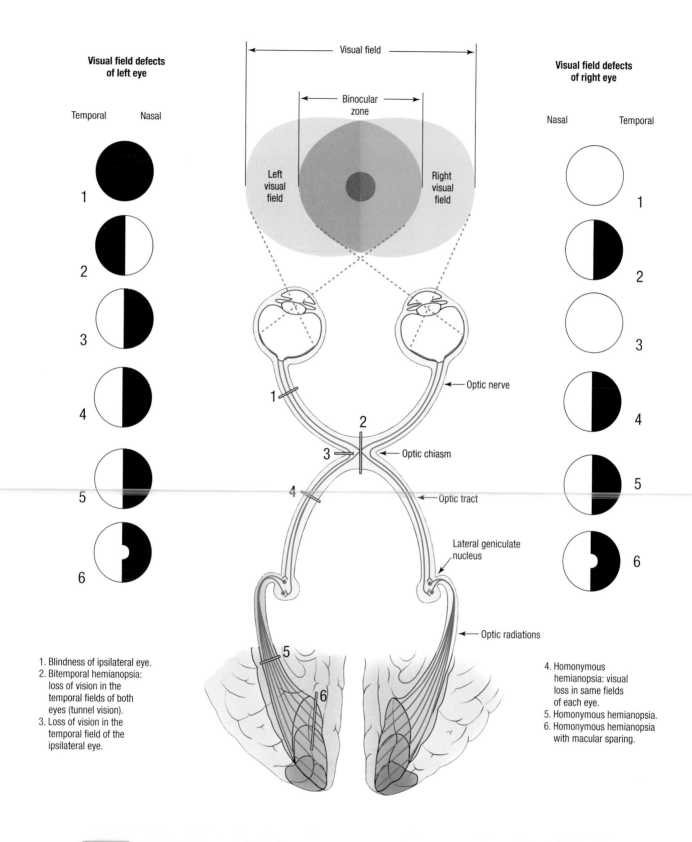

Visual field defects of left eye

Temporal   Nasal

1
2
3
4
5
6

Visual field

Binocular zone

Left visual field

Right visual field

Optic nerve

Optic chiasm

Optic tract

Lateral geniculate nucleus

Optic radiations

Visual field defects of right eye

Nasal   Temporal

1
2
3
4
5
6

1. Blindness of ipsilateral eye.
2. Bitemporal hemianopsia: loss of vision in the temporal fields of both eyes (tunnel vision).
3. Loss of vision in the temporal field of the ipsilateral eye.

4. Homonymous hemianopsia: visual loss in same fields of each eye.
5. Homonymous hemianopsia.
6. Homonymous hemianopsia with macular sparing.

9.7   VISUAL FIELD DEFECTS (CN II)

Visual field defects may result from a large number of neurologic diseases. It is clinically important to be able to link the defects to a likely location of the lesion.

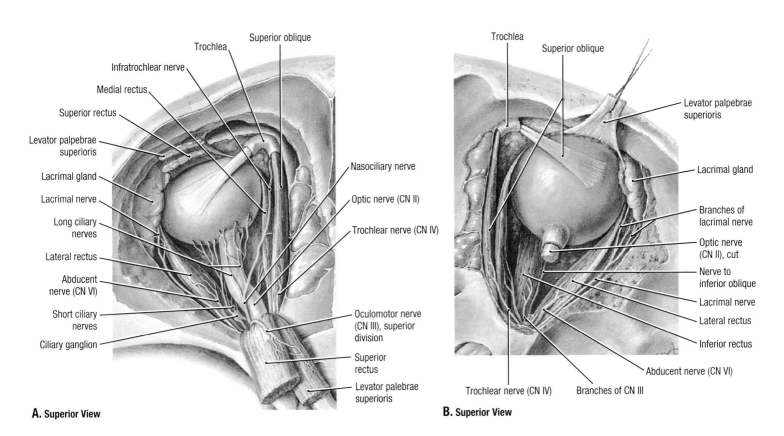

Trochlea
Superior oblique
Infratrochlear nerve
Medial rectus
Superior rectus
Levator palpebrae superioris
Lacrimal gland
Lacrimal nerve
Long ciliary nerves
Lateral rectus
Abducent nerve (CN VI)
Short ciliary nerves
Ciliary ganglion
Nasociliary nerve
Optic nerve (CN II)
Trochlear nerve (CN IV)
Oculomotor nerve (CN III), superior division
Superior rectus
Levator palebrae superioris

A. Superior View

Trochlea
Superior oblique
Levator palpebrae superioris
Lacrimal gland
Branches of lacrimal nerve
Optic nerve (CN II), cut
Nerve to inferior oblique
Lacrimal nerve
Lateral rectus
Inferior rectus
Abducent nerve (CN VI)
Trochlear nerve (CN IV)   Branches of CN III

B. Superior View

Oculomotor nerve (CN III), superior division
Superior rectus (SR)
Levator palpebrae superioris (LP)
Trochlea
Superior oblique (SO)
Optic nerve (CN II) fascicles
Ophthalmic artery
Medial rectus (MR)
Lacrimal fossa
Oculomotor nerve (CN III), inferior division
Trochlear nerve (CN IV)
Lateral rectus (LR)
Abducent nerve (CN VI)
Common tendinous ring
Ciliary ganglion
Inferior rectus (IR)
Inferior oblique

C. Anterior View

Frontal nerve
Lacrimal nerve
SR
LP
SO
Superior orbital fissure
Superior ophthalmic vein
CN IV
CN III, superior division
Nasociliary nerve
LR
CN VI
Inferior ophthalmic vein
CN II
MR
Ophthalmic artery
Common tendinous ring
IR
CN III, inferior division

D. Anterior View

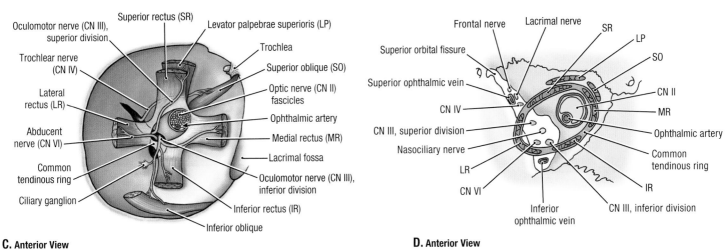

9.8   OVERVIEW OF MUSCLES AND NERVES OF ORBIT

A. and B. Orbital cavities, dissected from a superior approach. The optic nerve is intact in **A** and cut away in
B., C. and D. Relationship of muscle attachments and nerves at apex of orbit.

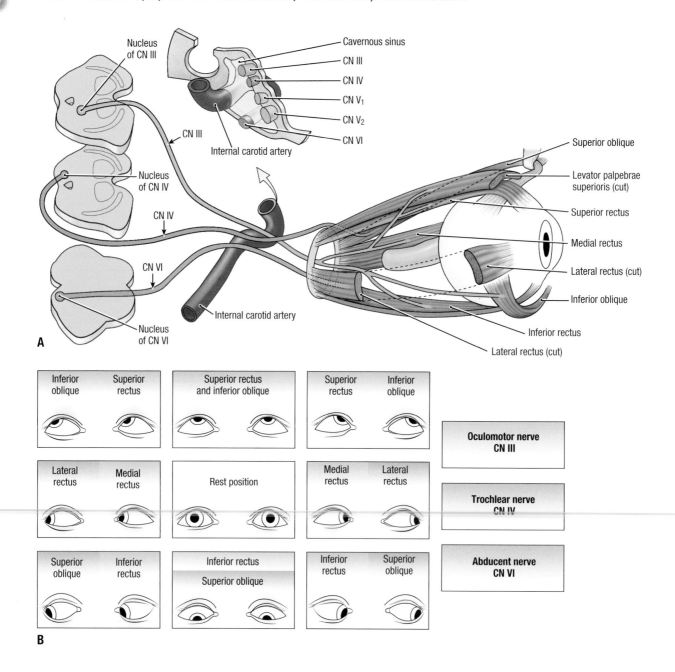

9.9 OCULOMOTOR (CN III), TROCHLEAR (CN IV), AND ABDUCENT (CN VI) NERVES

A. Schematic overview. **B.** Binocular movements and muscles producing them. All movements start from the rest (primary) position.

TABLE 9.4 *OCULOMOTOR (CN III), TROCHLEAR (CN IV), AND ABDUCENT (CN VI) NERVES*[a]

Nerve	Functional Components	Cells of Origin/Termination	Cranial Exit	Distribution and Functions
Oculomotor	Somatic motor	Nucleus of CN III	Superior orbital fissure	Motor to superior, inferior, and medial recti, inferior oblique, and levator palpebrae superioris muscles; raises upper eyelid, directing gaze superiorly, inferiorly, and medially
	Visceral motor (parasympathetic)	Presynaptic: midbrain (Edinger-Westphal nucleus); Postsynaptic: ciliary ganglion		Motor to sphincter pupillae and ciliary muscle that constrict pupil and accommodate lens of eyeball
Trochlear	Somatic motor	Nucleus of CN IV		Motor to superior oblique that assists in directing gaze inferolaterally
Abducent	Somatic motor	Nucleus of CN VI		Motor to lateral rectus that directs gaze laterally

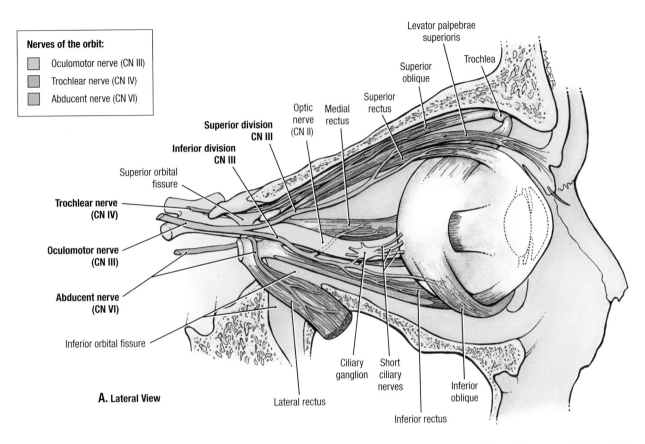

Nerves of the orbit:

- Oculomotor nerve (CN III)
- Trochlear nerve (CN IV)
- Abducent nerve (CN VI)

Levator palpebrae superioris

Trochlea

Superior oblique

Superior rectus

Optic nerve (CN II)

Medial rectus

Superior division CN III

Inferior division CN III

Superior orbital fissure

Trochlear nerve (CN IV)

Oculomotor nerve (CN III)

Abducent nerve (CN VI)

Inferior orbital fissure

Ciliary ganglion

Short ciliary nerves

Inferior oblique

Lateral rectus

Inferior rectus

A. Lateral View

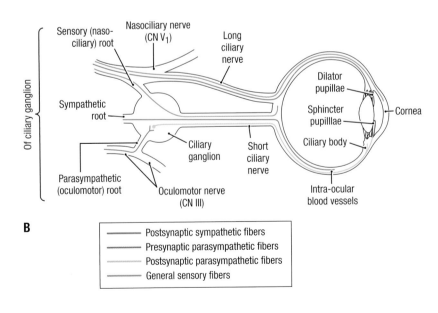

Sensory (naso-ciliary) root

Nasociliary nerve (CN V$_1$)

Long ciliary nerve

Of ciliary ganglion

Sympathetic root

Parasympathetic (oculomotor) root

Oculomotor nerve (CN III)

Ciliary ganglion

Short ciliary nerve

Dilator pupillae

Sphincter pupilllae

Cornea

Ciliary body

Intra-ocular blood vessels

B

- Postsynaptic sympathetic fibers
- Presynaptic parasympathetic fibers
- Postsynaptic parasympathetic fibers
- General sensory fibers

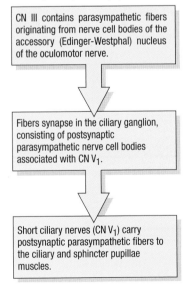

Visceral (parasympathetic) motor innervation of ciliary and sphincter pupillae muscles

CN III contains parasympathetic fibers originating from nerve cell bodies of the accessory (Edinger-Westphal) nucleus of the oculomotor nerve.

Fibers synapse in the ciliary ganglion, consisting of postsynaptic parasympathetic nerve cell bodies associated with CN V$_1$.

Short ciliary nerves (CN V$_1$) carry postsynaptic parasympathetic fibers to the ciliary and sphincter pupillae muscles.

9.10   **INNERVATION OF EYEBALL**

A. Nerves of orbit. **B.** Somatic and autonomic innervation of eyeball.

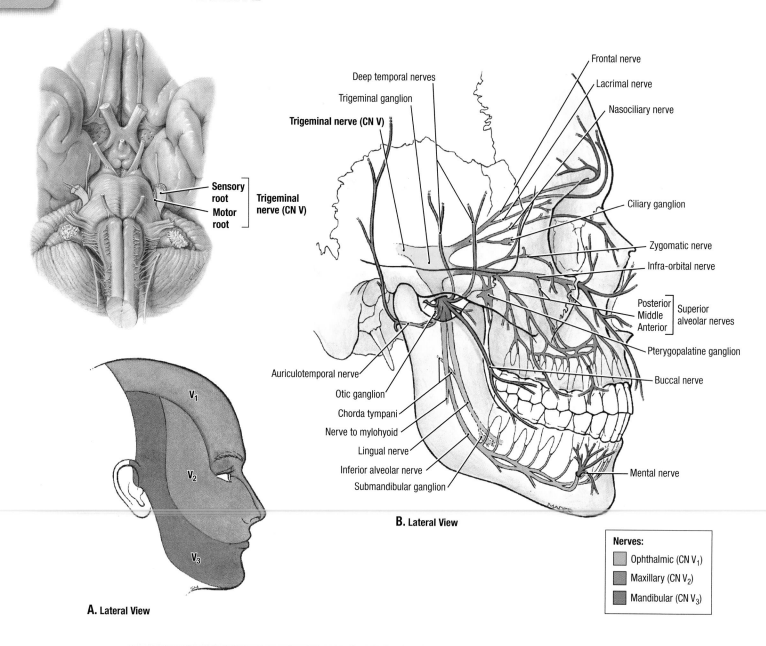

A. Lateral View

B. Lateral View

Nerves:
- ☐ Ophthalmic (CN V₁)
- ☐ Maxillary (CN V₂)
- ☐ Mandibular (CN V₃)

9.11   TRIGEMINAL NERVE (CN V)

A. Cutaneous (somatic sensory) distribution. **B.** Branches of ophthalmic (CN V₁), maxillary (CN V₂), and mandibular (CN V₃) divisions.

TABLE 9.5   TRIGEMINAL NERVE (CN V)

Nerve	Functional Components	Cells of Origin/Termination	Cranial Exit	Distribution and Functions
Ophthalmic division (CN V₁)	Somatic (general sensory)	Trigeminal ganglion/spinal, principal and mesencephalic nucleus of CN V	Superior orbital fissure	Sensation from cornea, skin of forehead, scalp, eyelids, nose, and mucosa of nasal cavity and paranasal sinuses
Maxillary division (CN V₂)			Foramen rotundum	Sensation from skin of face over maxilla including upper lip, maxillary teeth, mucosa of nose, maxillary sinuses, and palate
Mandibular division (CN V₃)			Foramen ovale	Sensation from the skin over mandible, including lower lip and side of head, mandibular teeth, temporomandibular joint, and mucosa of mouth and anterior two thirds of tongue
	Somatic (branchial) motor	Motor nucleus of CN V		Motor to muscles of mastication, mylohyoid, anterior belly of digastric, tensor veli palatini, and tensor tympani

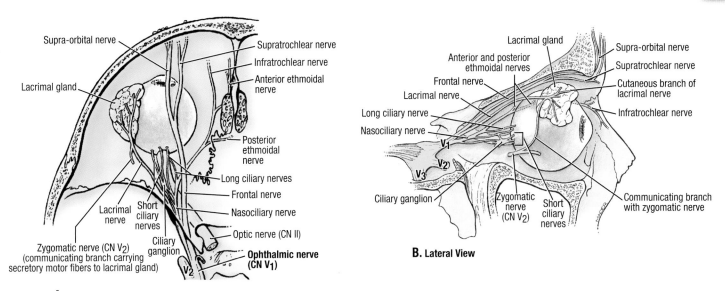

A. Superior View

B. Lateral View

C. Lateral View

9.12   OPHTHALMIC NERVE (CN V₁)

A. and B. Overview. **C.** Course through cavernous sinus.

TABLE 9.6   *BRANCHES OF OPHTHALMIC NERVE (CN V₁)*

Function	Branches

Ophthalmic nerve (CN V₁)
Somatic sensory only at origin from trigeminal ganglion
Visceral motor: extracranially, conveys (1) postsynaptic parasympathetic fibers from ciliary ganglion to ciliary body and sphincter of pupillae; (2) postsynaptic parasympathetic fibers from communicating branch of zygomatic nerve (CN V₂) to lacrimal gland; and (3) postsynaptic sympathetic fibers from internal carotid plexus to dilator pupillae and intra-ocular blood vessels.
Passes through superior orbital fissure to enter orbit
Supplies general sensory innervation to cornea, superior bulbar and palpebral conjunctiva, mucosa of anterosuperior nasal cavity, frontal, ethmoidal, and sphenoidal sinuses, anterior and supratentorial dura mater, skin of dorsum of external nose, superior eyelid, forehead and anterior scalp.
	Somatic sensory branches:
	Tentorial nerve (an intracranial meningeal branch)
	Lacrimal nerve [terminal portion also receives postsynaptic parasympathetic fibers from zygomatic nerve (CN V₂) and conveys them to lacrimal gland]
	Frontal nerve
	  Supra-orbital nerve
	  Supratrochlear nerve
	Nasociliary nerve
	  Sensory root of ciliary ganglion
	  Long and short ciliary nerves [also convey postsynaptic sympathetic fibers (from internal carotid plexus to eyeball additionally, short ciliary nerves convey postsynaptic parasympathetic fibers from ciliary ganglion to eyeball]
	  Anterior and posterior ethmoidal nerves
	    Anterior meningeal nerves
	    Internal and external nasal branches
	Infratrochlear nerve

Somatic sensory CN V₁

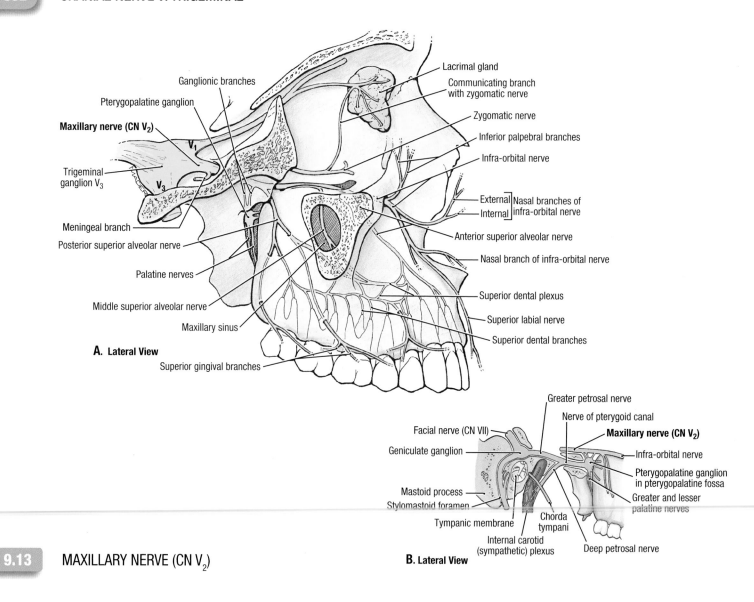

A. Lateral View

Maxillary nerve (CN V₂) labels (panel A):
Ganglionic branches · Pterygopalatine ganglion · Maxillary nerve (CN V₂) · V₁ · Trigeminal ganglion V₃ · V₃ · Meningeal branch · Posterior superior alveolar nerve · Palatine nerves · Middle superior alveolar nerve · Maxillary sinus · Superior gingival branches

Lacrimal gland · Communicating branch with zygomatic nerve · Zygomatic nerve · Inferior palpebral branches · Infra-orbital nerve · External / Internal Nasal branches of infra-orbital nerve · Anterior superior alveolar nerve · Nasal branch of infra-orbital nerve · Superior dental plexus · Superior labial nerve · Superior dental branches

B. Lateral View labels:
Greater petrosal nerve · Nerve of pterygoid canal · Maxillary nerve (CN V₂) · Facial nerve (CN VII) · Geniculate ganglion · Infra-orbital nerve · Pterygopalatine ganglion in pterygopalatine fossa · Greater and lesser palatine nerves · Mastoid process · Stylomastoid foramen · Tympanic membrane · Chorda tympani · Internal carotid (sympathetic) plexus · Deep petrosal nerve

9.13   MAXILLARY NERVE (CN V₂)

TABLE 9.7   BRANCHES OF MAXILLARY NERVE (CN V₂)

Function	Branches

Maxillary nerve (CN V₂)
  Somatic sensory only (proximally, at origin from trigeminal ganglion)
  Visceral motor: distally, conveys (1) postsynaptic parasympathetic fibers from pterygopalatine ganglion (presynaptic fibers are from CN VII via greater petrosal nerve and nerve of pterygoid canal); and (2) postsynaptic sympathetic fibers from superior cervical ganglion via internal carotid plexus (presynaptic fibers are from intermediolateral column of gray matter, spinal cord segments T1–T3).
  Passes through foramen rotundum to enter pterygopalatine fossa
  Supplies dura mater of anterior aspect of lateral part of middle cranial fossa; conjunctiva of inferior eyelid; mucosa of postero-inferior nasal cavity, maxillary sinus, palate, and anterior part of superior oral vestibule; maxillary teeth; and skin of lateral external nose, inferior eyelid, anterior cheek, and upper lip.
	Meningeal branch
	Zygomatic branch
	  Zygomaticofacial branch
	  Zygomaticotemporal branch
	  Communicating branch to lacrimal nerve
	Ganglionic branches to (sensory root of) pterygopalatine ganglion
	Infra-orbital nerve
	  Posterior, middle, and anterior superior alveolar branches
	    Superior dental plexus and branches
	    Superior gingival branches
	  Inferior palpebral branches
	  External and internal nasal branches
	  Superior labial branches
	Greater palatine nerve
	  Posterior inferior lateral nasal nerves
	Lesser palatine nerves
	Posterior superior lateral and medial nasal branches
	Nasopalatine nerve
	Pharyngeal nerve

Somatic sensory CN V₂

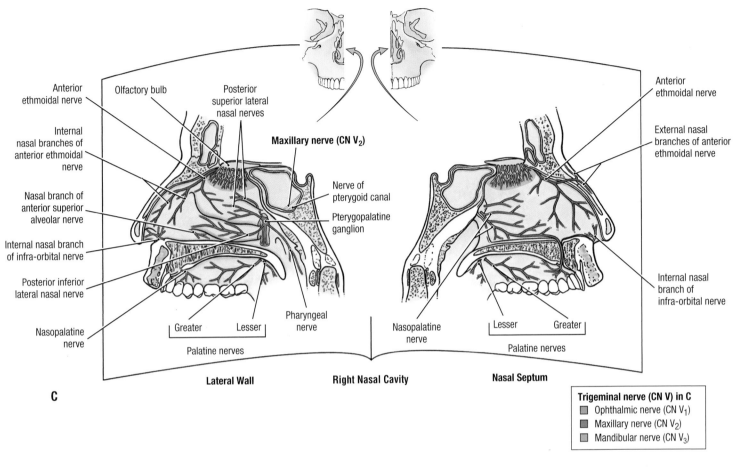

Anterior ethmoidal nerve

Olfactory bulb

Posterior superior lateral nasal nerves

Maxillary nerve (CN V₂)

Anterior ethmoidal nerve

Internal nasal branches of anterior ethmoidal nerve

Nerve of pterygoid canal

External nasal branches of anterior ethmoidal nerve

Nasal branch of anterior superior alveolar nerve

Pterygopalatine ganglion

Internal nasal branch of infra-orbital nerve

Posterior inferior lateral nasal nerve

Pharyngeal nerve

Internal nasal branch of infra-orbital nerve

Nasopalatine nerve

Greater   Lesser

Nasopalatine nerve

Lesser   Greater

Palatine nerves

Palatine nerves

Lateral Wall   **Right Nasal Cavity**   **Nasal Septum**

C

Trigeminal nerve (CN V) in C
- Ophthalmic nerve (CN V₁)
- Maxillary nerve (CN V₂)
- Mandibular nerve (CN V₃)

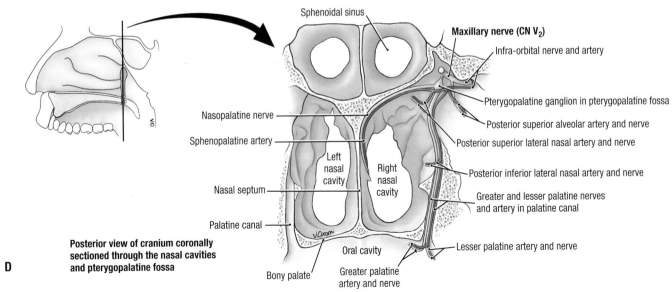

Sphenoidal sinus

Maxillary nerve (CN V₂)

Infra-orbital nerve and artery

Pterygopalatine ganglion in pterygopalatine fossa

Nasopalatine nerve

Posterior superior alveolar artery and nerve

Sphenopalatine artery

Posterior superior lateral nasal artery and nerve

Left nasal cavity

Right nasal cavity

Posterior inferior lateral nasal artery and nerve

Nasal septum

Greater and lesser palatine nerves and artery in palatine canal

Palatine canal

Posterior view of cranium coronally sectioned through the nasal cavities and pterygopalatine fossa

Lesser palatine artery and nerve

D

Oral cavity

Bony palate

Greater palatine artery and nerve

9.13   MAXILLARY NERVE (CN V₂) *(CONTINUED)*

A. Overview. **B.** Nerves of pterygopalatine fossa. **C. and D.** Innervation of lateral wall and septum of nasal cavity and palate.

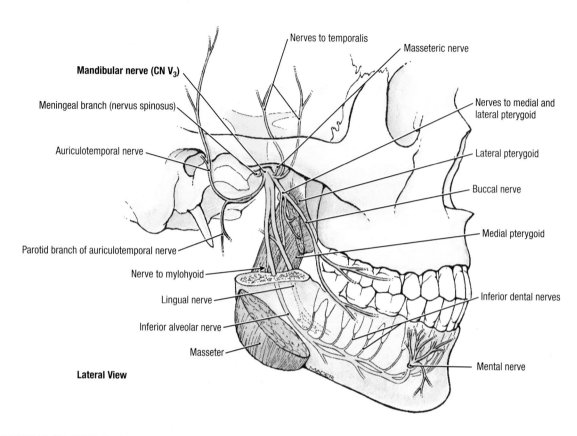

Nerves to temporalis

Masseteric nerve

Mandibular nerve (CN V₃)

Meningeal branch (nervus spinosus)

Nerves to medial and lateral pterygoid

Auriculotemporal nerve

Lateral pterygoid

Buccal nerve

Parotid branch of auriculotemporal nerve

Medial pterygoid

Nerve to mylohyoid

Lingual nerve

Inferior dental nerves

Inferior alveolar nerve

Masseter

Mental nerve

Lateral View

9.14   MANDIBULAR NERVE (CN V₃)

TABLE 9.8   BRANCHES OF MANDIBULAR NERVE (CN V₃)

Function	Branches

Maxillary nerve (CN V₃)
Somatic sensory and somatic (branchial) motor
Special sensory: extracranially, conveys taste fibers (from CN VII via chorda tympani nerve) to anterior 2/3 of tongue
Visceral motor: extracranially, conveys (1) presynaptic parasympathetic fibers to submandibular ganglion
(presynaptic fibers are from CN VII via chorda tympani nerve); (2) postsynaptic parasympathetic fibers from submandibular ganglion to submandibular and sublingual glands; and (3) postsynaptic parasympathetic fibers from otic ganglion to parotid gland.
Passes through foramen ovale to enter infratemporal fossa
Supplies general sensory innervation to mucosa of anterior 2/3 of tongue, floor of mouth, and posterior and anterior inferior oral vestibule; mandibular teeth; and skin of lower lip, buccal and temporal regions of face, and external ear (anterior superior auricle, upper external auditory meatus, and tympanic membrane).
Supplies motor innervation to all 4 muscles of mastication, mylohyoid, anterior belly of digastric, tensor tympani and tensor veli palatin
	Somatic sensory branches:
	  Meningeal branch (nervus spinosum)
	  Buccal nerve
	  Auriculotemporal nerve (also conveys *visceral motor fibers*)
	    Superficial temporal branches
	    Parotid branches
	  Lingual nerve (also conveys *visceral motor* and *special sensory fibers*)
	  Inferior alveolar nerve
	    Nerve to mylohyoid
	    Inferior dental plexus
	      Inferior dental branches
	      Inferior gingival branches
	  Mental nerve
	Somatic (branchial) motor branches:
	  Masseteric nerve
	  Medial and lateral pterygoid branches
	  Deep temporal nerves
	  Nerve to mylohyoid
	  Nerve to tensor tympani
	  Nerve to tensor veli palatini

Somatic sensory CN V₃

Somatic motor CN V₃

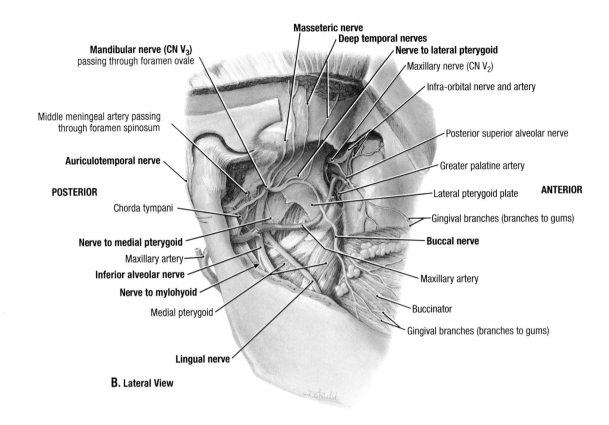

Masseteric nerve
Deep temporal nerves
Mandibular nerve (CN V₃)
passing through foramen ovale
Nerve to lateral pterygoid
Maxillary nerve (CN V₂)
Infra-orbital nerve and artery
Middle meningeal artery passing
through foramen spinosum
Posterior superior alveolar nerve
Auriculotemporal nerve
Greater palatine artery
POSTERIOR   Lateral pterygoid plate   **ANTERIOR**
Chorda tympani
Gingival branches (branches to gums)
Nerve to medial pterygoid
Buccal nerve
Maxillary artery
Inferior alveolar nerve
Maxillary artery
Nerve to mylohyoid
Buccinator
Medial pterygoid
Gingival branches (branches to gums)
Lingual nerve

B. Lateral View

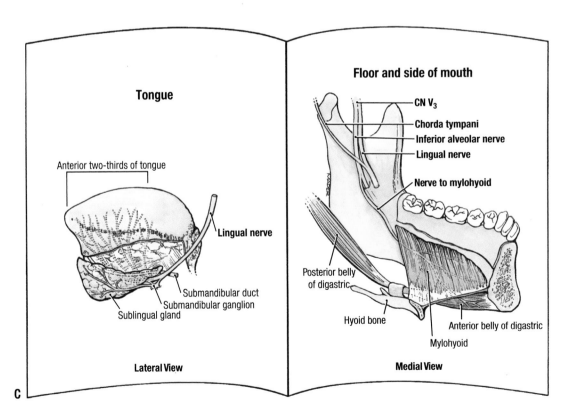

Tongue

Floor and side of mouth

CN V₃
Chorda tympani
Inferior alveolar nerve
Lingual nerve

Anterior two-thirds of tongue

Nerve to mylohyoid

Lingual nerve

Posterior belly
of digastric

Submandibular duct
Submandibular ganglion
Sublingual gland

Hyoid bone

Anterior belly of digastric

Mylohyoid

Lateral View   **Medial View**

C

9.14   MANDIBULAR NERVE (CN V₃) *(CONTINUED)*

A. Overview. **B.** Deep dissection of CN V₃ and branches at foramen ovale. **C.** Lateral aspect of tongue and medial aspect of mandible displayed as pages in an open book that is, the tongue has been reflected from the mandible.

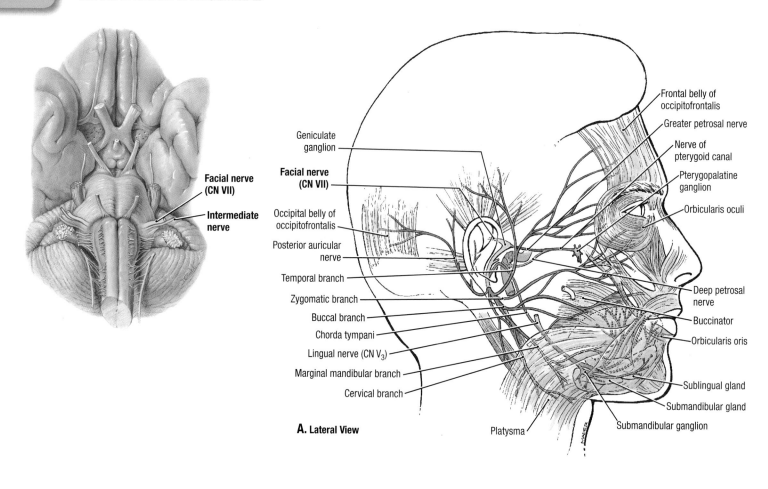

Geniculate ganglion

Facial nerve (CN VII)

Frontal belly of occipitofrontalis

Greater petrosal nerve

Nerve of pterygoid canal

Pterygopalatine ganglion

Orbicularis oculi

Occipital belly of occipitofrontalis

Posterior auricular nerve

Temporal branch

Zygomatic branch

Buccal branch

Chorda tympani

Lingual nerve (CN V₃)

Marginal mandibular branch

Cervical branch

Deep petrosal nerve

Buccinator

Orbicularis oris

Sublingual gland

Submandibular gland

Submandibular ganglion

A. Lateral View

Platysma

Facial nerve (CN VII)

Intermediate nerve

9.15   FACIAL NERVE (CN VII)

A. Overview. **B.** Parasympathetic motor innervation of lacrimal, submandibular, and sublingual glands. **C.** Nerve of pterygoid canal.

TABLE 9.9   FACIAL NERVE (CN VII), INCLUDING MOTOR ROOT AND INTERMEDIATE NERVE[a]

Nerve	Functional Components	Cells of Origin/Termination	Cranial Exit	Distribution and Functions
Temporal, zygomatic, buccal, mandibular, cervical, and posterior auricular nerves, nerve to posterior belly of digastric, nerve to stylohyoid, nerve to stapedius	Somatic (branchial) motor	Motor nucleus of CN VII	Stylomastoid foramen	Motor to muscles of facial expression and scalp;, also supplies stapedius of middle ear, stylohyoid, and posterior belly of digastric
Intermediate nerve through chorda tympani	Special sensory	Geniculate ganglion/solitary nucleus	Internal acoustic meatus/facial canal/petrotympanic fissure	Taste from anterior two thirds of tongue, through chorda tympani floor of mouth, and palate
Intermediate nerve	Somatic (general) sensory	Geniculate ganglion/spinal trigeminal nucleus	Internal acoustic meatus	Sensation from skin of external acoustic meatus
Intermediate nerve through greater petrosal nerve	Visceral sensory	Nuclei of solitary tract	Internal acoustic meatus/facial canal/foramen for greater petrosal nerve	Visceral sensation from mucous membranes of nasopharynx and palate
Greater petrosal nerve Chorda tympani	Visceral motor	Presynaptic: superior salivatory nucleus; Postsynaptic: pterygopalatine ganglion (greater petrosal nerve) and submandibular ganglion (chorda tympani)	Internal acoustic meatus/facial canal/foramen for greater petrosal nerve, (greater petrosal nerve) petrotympanic fissure (chorda tympani)	Parasympathetic innervation to lacrimal gland and glands of the nose and palate (greater petrosal nerve); submandibular and sublingual salivary glands (chorda tympani)

[a]See also Table 9.15.

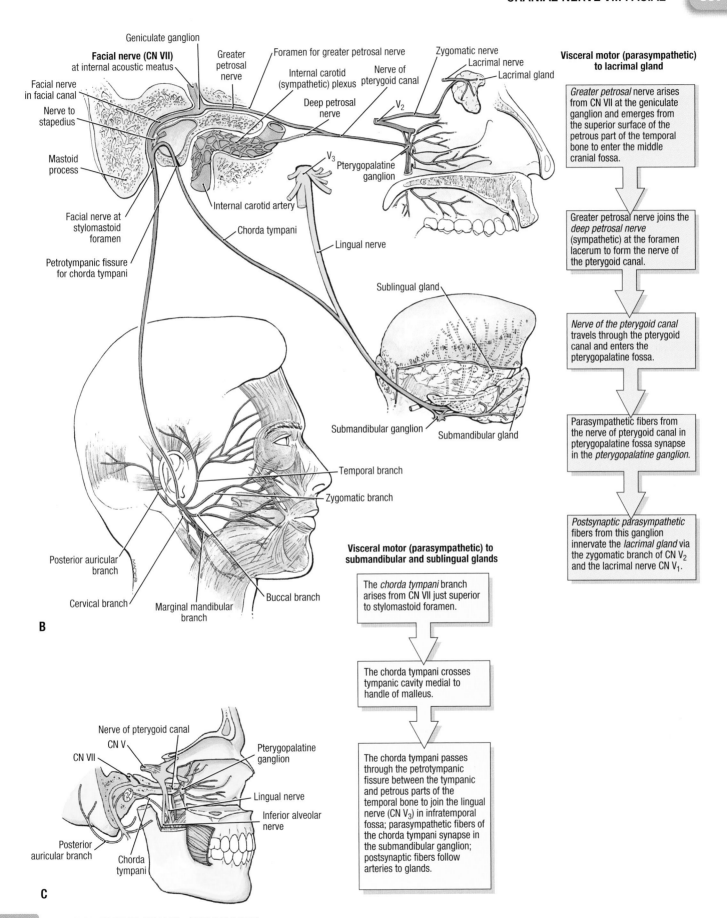

Facial nerve (CN VII) at internal acoustic meatus

Geniculate ganglion

Facial nerve in facial canal

Nerve to stapedius

Mastoid process

Greater petrosal nerve

Foramen for greater petrosal nerve

Internal carotid (sympathetic) plexus

Internal carotid artery

Deep petrosal nerve

Nerve of pterygoid canal

Zygomatic nerve

Lacrimal nerve

Lacrimal gland

V₂

V₃ Pterygopalatine ganglion

Facial nerve at stylomastoid foramen

Petrotympanic fissure for chorda tympani

Chorda tympani

Lingual nerve

Sublingual gland

Submandibular ganglion

Submandibular gland

Temporal branch

Zygomatic branch

Buccal branch

Marginal mandibular branch

Posterior auricular branch

Cervical branch

B

Nerve of pterygoid canal

CN V

CN VII

Pterygopalatine ganglion

Lingual nerve

Inferior alveolar nerve

Posterior auricular branch

Chorda tympani

C

Visceral motor (parasympathetic) to lacrimal gland

Greater petrosal nerve arises from CN VII at the geniculate ganglion and emerges from the superior surface of the petrous part of the temporal bone to enter the middle cranial fossa.

Greater petrosal nerve joins the *deep petrosal nerve* (sympathetic) at the foramen lacerum to form the nerve of the pterygoid canal.

Nerve of the pterygoid canal travels through the pterygoid canal and enters the pterygopalatine fossa.

Parasympathetic fibers from the nerve of pterygoid canal in pterygopalatine fossa synapse in the *pterygopalatine ganglion.*

Postsynaptic parasympathetic fibers from this ganglion innervate the *lacrimal gland* via the zygomatic branch of CN V₂ and the lacrimal nerve CN V₁.

Visceral motor (parasympathetic) to submandibular and sublingual glands

The *chorda tympani* branch arises from CN VII just superior to stylomastoid foramen.

The chorda tympani crosses tympanic cavity medial to handle of malleus.

The chorda tympani passes through the petrotympanic fissure between the tympanic and petrous parts of the temporal bone to join the lingual nerve (CN V₃) in infratemporal fossa; parasympathetic fibers of the chorda tympani synapse in the submandibular ganglion; postsynaptic fibers follow arteries to glands.

9.15   FACIAL NERVE (CN VII) *(CONTINUED)*

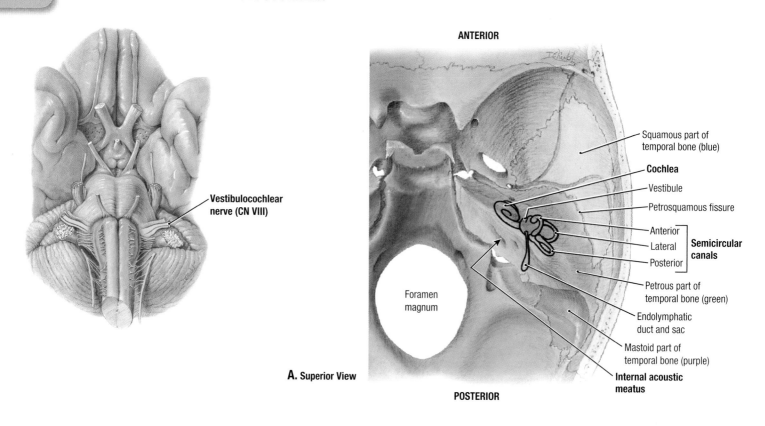

ANTERIOR

Squamous part of temporal bone (blue)

Cochlea

Vestibule

Petrosquamous fissure

Anterior

Lateral — **Semicircular canals**

Posterior

Petrous part of temporal bone (green)

Endolymphatic duct and sac

Mastoid part of temporal bone (purple)

Internal acoustic meatus

Foramen magnum

A. Superior View

POSTERIOR

Vestibulocochlear nerve (CN VIII)

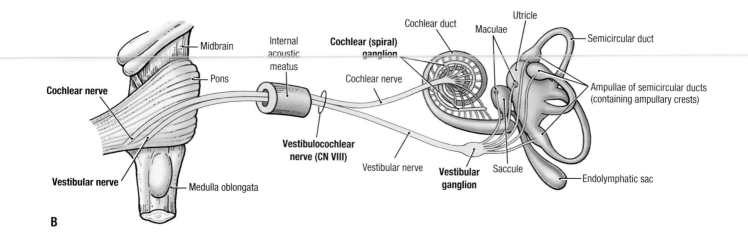

Midbrain

Internal acoustic meatus

Pons

Cochlear nerve

Vestibular nerve

Medulla oblongata

B

Cochlear (spiral) ganglion

Cochlear nerve

Cochlear duct

Maculae

Utricle

Semicircular duct

Ampullae of semicircular ducts (containing ampullary crests)

Vestibulocochlear nerve (CN VIII)

Vestibular nerve

Vestibular ganglion

Saccule

Endolymphatic sac

9.16 VESTIBULOCOCHLEAR NERVE (CN VIII)

A. Cochlea and semicircular canals in situ in the cranium. **B.** Schematic overview of distribution.

TABLE 9.10   VESTIBULOCOCHLEAR NERVE (CN VIII)

Part of Vestibulocochlear Nerve	Functional Components	Cells of Origin/Termination	Cranial Exit	Distribution and Functions
Vestibular nerve	Special sensory	Vestibular ganglion/vestibular nuclei	Internal acoustic meatus	Vestibular sensation from semicircular ducts, utricle, and saccule related to position and movement of head
Cochlear nerve		Spiral ganglion/cochlear nuclei		Hearing from spiral organ

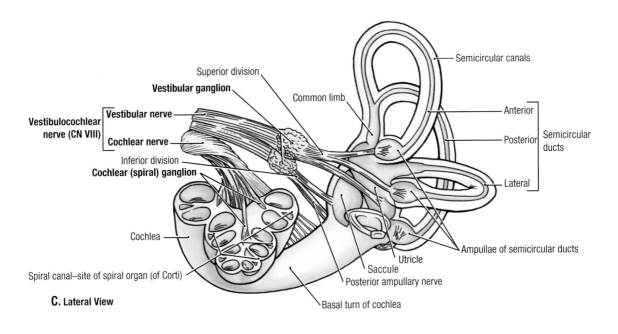

Superior division
Vestibular ganglion
Common limb
Vestibular nerve
Vestibulocochlear nerve (CN VIII)
Cochlear nerve
Inferior division
Cochlear (spiral) ganglion
Semicircular canals
Anterior
Posterior
Semicircular ducts
Lateral
Ampullae of semicircular ducts
Cochlea
Spiral canal–site of spiral organ (of Corti)
Utricle
Saccule
Posterior ampullary nerve
Basal turn of cochlea

C. Lateral View

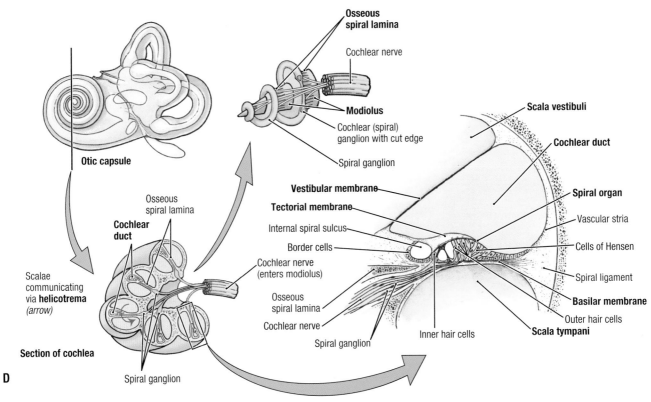

Otic capsule
Osseous spiral lamina
Cochlear nerve
Modiolus
Cochlear (spiral) ganglion with cut edge
Spiral ganglion
Scala vestibuli
Cochlear duct
Vestibular membrane
Tectorial membrane
Internal spiral sulcus
Border cells
Cochlear nerve (enters modiolus)
Osseous spiral lamina
Cochlear nerve
Spiral ganglion
Spiral organ
Vascular stria
Cells of Hensen
Spiral ligament
Basilar membrane
Outer hair cells
Scala tympani
Inner hair cells

Scalae communicating via **helicotrema** (arrow)
Osseous spiral lamina
Cochlear duct

Section of cochlea

D

Spiral ganglion

9.16 **VESTIBULOCOCHLEAR NERVE (CN VIII)** *(CONTINUED)*

C. Labyrinthine and cochlear apparatus, nerves and ganglia. **D.** Structure of cochlea. Observe in **D:**

- The cochlear duct is a spiral tube fixed to the internal and external walls of the cochlear canal by the spiral ligament.
- The triangular cochlear duct lies between the osseous spiral lamina and the external wall of the cochlear canal.
- The roof of the cochlear duct is formed by the vestibular membrane and the floor by the basilar membrane and osseous spiral lamina.

- The receptor of auditory stimuli is the spiral organ (of Corti), situated on the basilar membrane; it is overlaid by the gelatinous tectorial membrane.
- The spiral organ contains hair cells that respond to vibrations induced in the endolymph by sound waves.
- The fibers of the cochlear nerve are axons of neurons in the spiral ganglion; the peripheral processes enter the spiral organ (of Corti).

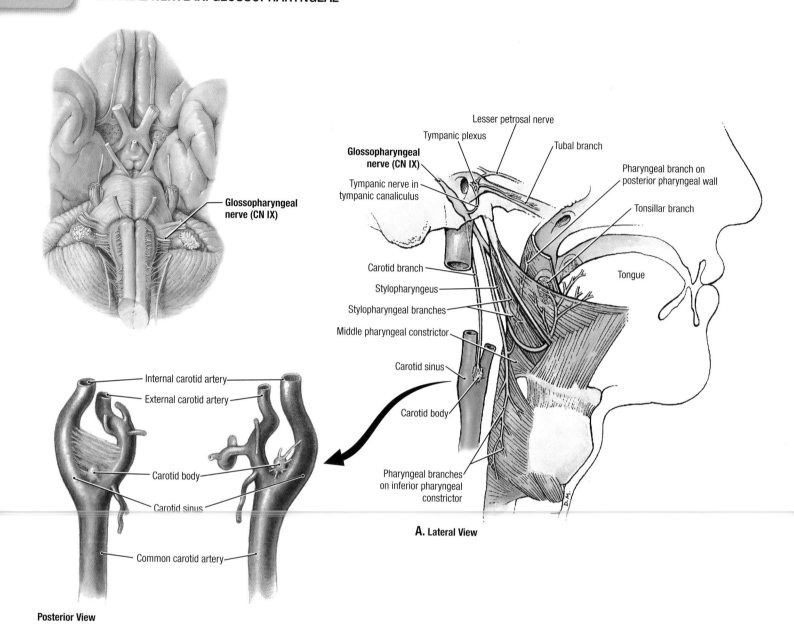

Glossopharyngeal nerve (CN IX)

Lesser petrosal nerve

Tympanic plexus

Tubal branch

Glossopharyngeal nerve (CN IX)

Pharyngeal branch on posterior pharyngeal wall

Tympanic nerve in tympanic canaliculus

Tonsillar branch

Carotid branch

Tongue

Stylopharyngeus

Stylopharyngeal branches

Middle pharyngeal constrictor

Carotid sinus

Carotid body

Pharyngeal branches on inferior pharyngeal constrictor

A. Lateral View

Internal carotid artery

External carotid artery

Carotid body

Carotid sinus

Common carotid artery

Posterior View

9.17   GLOSSOPHARYNGEAL NERVE (CN IX)

A. Overview of distribution. **B. and C.** Parasympathetic innervation.

TABLE 9.11   GLOSSOPHARYNGEAL NERVE (CN IX)[a]

Nerve	Functional Components	Cells of Origin/Termination	Cranial Exit	Distribution and Functions
Glossopharyngeal	Somatic (branchial) motor	Nucleus ambiguus		Motor to stylopharyngeus that assists with swallowing
	Visceral motor	Presynaptic: inferior salivatory nucleus; postsynaptic: otic ganglion		Parasympathetic innervation to parotid gland
	Visceral sensory	Nuclei of solitary tract, spinal trigeminal nucleus/ inferior ganglion	Jugular foramen	Visceral sensation from parotid gland, carotid body, carotid sinus, pharynx, and middle ear
	Special sensory	Nuclei of solitary tract /inferior ganglion		Taste from posterior third of tongue
	General sensory	Spinal trigeminal nucleus/superior ganglion		Cutaneous sensation from external ear

[a]See also Table 9.15.

B

C   **Lateral View**

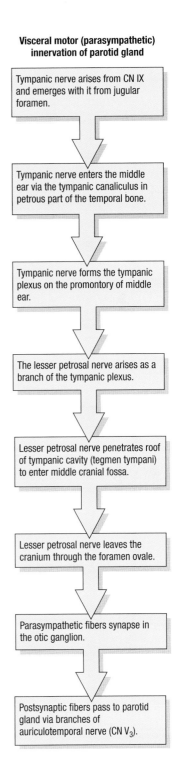

Visceral motor (parasympathetic) innervation of parotid gland

Tympanic nerve arises from CN IX and emerges with it from jugular foramen.

Tympanic nerve enters the middle ear via the tympanic canaliculus in petrous part of the temporal bone.

Tympanic nerve forms the tympanic plexus on the promontory of middle ear.

The lesser petrosal nerve arises as a branch of the tympanic plexus.

Lesser petrosal nerve penetrates roof of tympanic cavity (tegmen tympani) to enter middle cranial fossa.

Lesser petrosal nerve leaves the cranium through the foramen ovale.

Parasympathetic fibers synapse in the otic ganglion.

Postsynaptic fibers pass to parotid gland via branches of auriculotemporal nerve (CN V₃).

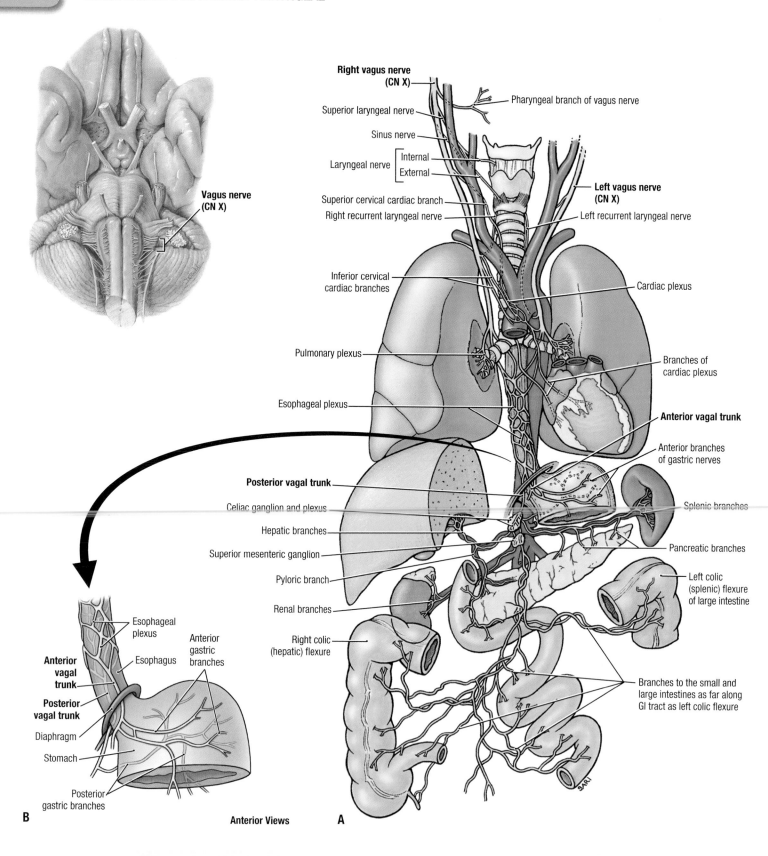

Vagus nerve (CN X)

Right vagus nerve (CN X)

Pharyngeal branch of vagus nerve

Superior laryngeal nerve

Sinus nerve

Laryngeal nerve — Internal / External

Superior cervical cardiac branch

Right recurrent laryngeal nerve

Left vagus nerve (CN X)

Left recurrent laryngeal nerve

Inferior cervical cardiac branches

Cardiac plexus

Pulmonary plexus

Branches of cardiac plexus

Esophageal plexus

Anterior vagal trunk

Anterior branches of gastric nerves

Posterior vagal trunk

Celiac ganglion and plexus

Splenic branches

Hepatic branches

Superior mesenteric ganglion

Pancreatic branches

Pyloric branch

Left colic (splenic) flexure of large intestine

Renal branches

Right colic (hepatic) flexure

Branches to the small and large intestines as far along GI tract as left colic flexure

Esophageal plexus

Anterior gastric branches

Anterior vagal trunk

Esophagus

Posterior vagal trunk

Diaphragm

Stomach

Posterior gastric branches

B

Anterior Views

A

9.18 VAGUS NERVE (CN X)

A. Course in neck, thorax and abdomen. **B.** Anterior and posterior vagal trunks. **C.** Branches in neck.
D. Superior and inferior ganglia of vagus nerve.

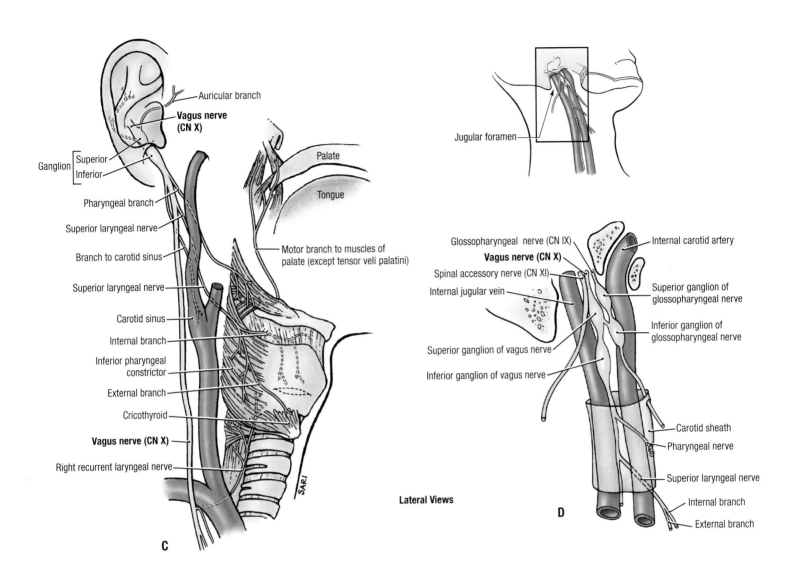

Auricular branch

Vagus nerve (CN X)

Ganglion [Superior / Inferior]

Pharyngeal branch

Superior laryngeal nerve

Branch to carotid sinus

Superior laryngeal nerve

Carotid sinus

Internal branch

Inferior pharyngeal constrictor

External branch

Cricothyroid

Vagus nerve (CN X)

Right recurrent laryngeal nerve

Palate

Tongue

Motor branch to muscles of palate (except tensor veli palatini)

SARI

C

Jugular foramen

Glossopharyngeal nerve (CN IX)

Vagus nerve (CN X)

Spinal accessory nerve (CN XI)

Internal jugular vein

Superior ganglion of vagus nerve

Inferior ganglion of vagus nerve

Internal carotid artery

Superior ganglion of glossopharyngeal nerve

Inferior ganglion of glossopharyngeal nerve

Carotid sheath

Pharyngeal nerve

Superior laryngeal nerve

Internal branch

External branch

Lateral Views

D

9.18 VAGUS NERVE (CN X) *(CONTINUED)*

TABLE 9.12   VAGUS NERVE (CN X)

Nerve	Functional Components	Cells of Origin/Termination	Cranial Exit	Distribution and Functions
Vagus	Branchial motor	Nucleus ambiguus	Jugular foramen	Motor to constrictor muscles of pharynx, intrinsic muscles of larynx, muscles of palate (except tensor veli palatini), and striated muscle in superior two thirds of esophagus
	Visceral motor	Presynaptic: posterior (dorsal) nucleus of CN X; Postsynaptic: neurons in, on, or near viscera		Parasympathetic innervation to smooth muscle of trachea, bronchi, and digestive tract, cardiac muscle
	Visceral sensory	Nuclei of solitary tract, spinal trigeminal nucleus/ inferior ganglion		Visceral sensation from base of tongue, pharynx, larynx, trachea, bronchi, heart, esophagus, stomach, and intestine
	Special sensory	Nuclei of solitary tract/inferior ganglion		Taste from epiglottis and palate
	General sensory	Spinal trigeminal nucleus/superior ganglion		Sensation from auricle, external acoustic meatus, and dura mater of posterior cranial fossa

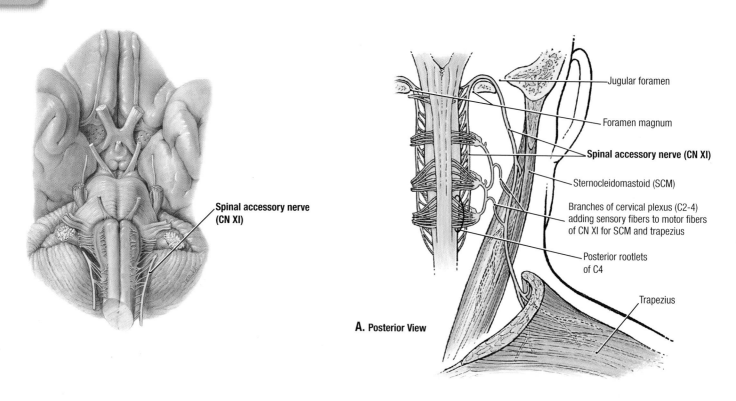

Spinal accessory nerve
(CN XI)

Jugular foramen

Foramen magnum

Spinal accessory nerve (CN XI)

Sternocleidomastoid (SCM)

Branches of cervical plexus (C2-4)
adding sensory fibers to motor fibers
of CN XI for SCM and trapezius

Posterior rootlets
of C4

Trapezius

A. Posterior View

Facial nerve (CN VII)

Vestibulocochlear nerve
(CN VIII)

Jugular foramen

Atlanto-occipital joint

Spinal accessory nerve (CN XI)

Posterior ramus (C1)

Internal acoustic meatus

Glossopharyngeal nerve
(CN IX)

Vagus nerve (CN X)

Spinal accessory nerve (CN XI)

Structures traversing foramen magnum

Anterior ramus (C1)

Transverse process of atlas (C1 vertebra)

Posterior tubercle of atlas (C1 vertebra)

B. Posterior View

9.19   SPINAL ACCESSORY NERVE (CN XI)

A. Schematic illustration of distribution. **B.** Intracranial course.

TABLE 9.13   SPINAL ACCESSORY NERVE (CN XI)

Nerve	Functional Components	Cells of Origin/Termination	Cranial Exit	Distribution and Functions
Spinal accessory	Somatic motor	Accessory nucleus of spinal cord	Jugular foramen	Motor to sternocleidomastoid and trapezius

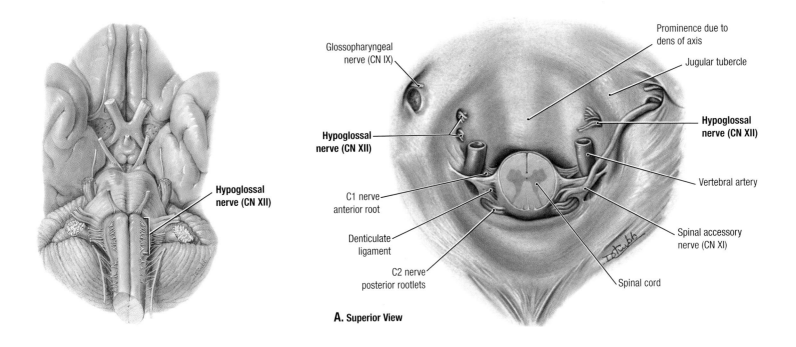

Glossopharyngeal nerve (CN IX)

Prominence due to dens of axis

Jugular tubercle

Hypoglossal nerve (CN XII)

Hypoglossal nerve (CN XII)

C1 nerve anterior root

Denticulate ligament

C2 nerve posterior rootlets

Vertebral artery

Spinal accessory nerve (CN XI)

Spinal cord

A. Superior View

Intrinsic muscles of tongue

Stylogossus

Hypoglossal nerve (CN XII)

Nerve roots of cervical plexus

C1

C2

C3

Internal carotid artery

Hyoglossus

Genioglossus

Geniohyoid

Nerve to thyrohyoid

Thyrohyoid

Ansa cervicalis

Inferior root

Superior root

Sternohyoid

Sternothyroid

B. Lateral View

9.20   HYPOGLOSSAL NERVE (CN XII)

A. Intracranial exit from cranium into hypoglossal canal. **B.** Schematic illustration of distribution.

TABLE 9.14   HYPOGLOSSAL NERVE (CN XII)

Nerve	Functional Components	Cells of Origin/Termination	Cranial Exit	Distribution and Functions
Hypoglossal	Somatic motor	Nucleus of CN XII	Hypoglossal canal	Motor to muscles of tongue (except palatoglossus)

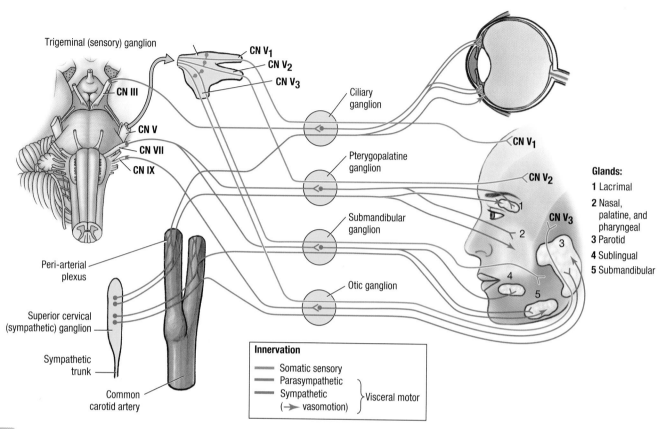

Trigeminal (sensory) ganglion

CN V₁
CN V₂
CN V₃

CN III

CN V
CN VII
CN IX

Ciliary ganglion

Pterygopalatine ganglion

Submandibular ganglion

CN V₁

CN V₂

CN V₃

Peri-arterial plexus

Otic ganglion

Glands:
1 Lacrimal
2 Nasal, palatine, and pharyngeal
3 Parotid
4 Sublingual
5 Submandibular

Superior cervical (sympathetic) ganglion

Sympathetic trunk

Common carotid artery

Innervation
— Somatic sensory
— Parasympathetic ⎫
— Sympathetic ⎬ Visceral motor
(→ vasomotion) ⎭

9.21 SUMMARY OF AUTONOMIC INNERVATION OF HEAD

TABLE 9.15 AUTONOMIC GANGLIA OF HEAD

Ganglion	Location	Parasympathetic Root (Nucleus of Origin)[a]	Sympathetic Root	Main Distribution
Ciliary	Between optic nerve and lateral rectus, close to apex of orbit	Inferior branch of oculomotor nerve (CN III) (Edinger-Westphal nucleus)	Branch from internal carotid plexus in cavernous sinus	Parasympathetic postsynaptic fibers from ciliary ganglion pass to ciliary muscle and sphincter, pupillae of iris; sympathetic postsynaptic fibers from superior cervical ganglion pass to dilator pupillae and blood vessels of eye
Pterygopalatine	In pterygopalatine fossa, where it is attached by pterygopalatine branches of maxillary nerve; located just anterior to opening of pterygoid canal and inferior to CN V₂	Greater petrosal nerve from facial nerve (CN VII) (superior salivatory nucleus)	Deep petrosal nerve, a branch of internal carotid plexus that is continuation of postsynaptic fibers of cervical sympathetic trunk; fibers from superior cervical ganglion pass through pterygopalatine ganglion and enter branches of CN V₂	Parasympathetic postsynaptic fibers from pterygopalatine ganglion innervate lacrimal gland through zygomatic branch of CN V₂; sympathetic postsynaptic fibers from superior cervical ganglion accompany branches of pterygopalatine nerve that are distributed to the nasal cavity, palate, and superior parts of the pharynx
Otic	Between tensor veli palatini and mandibular nerve; lies inferior to foramen ovale	Tympanic nerve from glossopharyngeal nerve (CN IX); tympanic nerve continues from tympanic plexus as lesser petrosal nerve (inferior salivatory nucleus)	Fibers from superior cervical ganglion travel via plexus on middle meningeal artery	Parasympathetic postsynaptic fibers from otic ganglion are distributed to parotid gland through auriculotemporal nerve (branch of CN V₃); sympathetic postsynaptic fibers from superior cervical ganglion pass to parotid gland and supply its blood vessels
Submandibular	Suspended from lingual nerve by two short roots; lies on surface of hyoglossus muscle inferior to submandibular duct	Parasympathetic fibers join facial nerve (CN VII) and leave it in its chorda tympani branch, which unites with lingual nerve (superior salivatory nucleus)	Sympathetic fibers from superior cervical ganglion travel via the plexus on facial artery	Postsynaptic parasympathetic fibers from submandibular ganglion are distributed to the sublingual and submandibular glands; sympathetic fibers supply sublingual and submandibular glands and appear to be secretomotor

[a]For location of nuclei, see Figure 9.3.

Right eye: Downward and outward gaze, dilated pupil, eyelid manually elevated due to ptosis   Left

A. Right oculomotor (CN III) nerve palsy

Direction of gaze →

Right   Left eye: Does not abduct

B. Left abducent (CN VI) nerve palsy

C. Right facial (CN VII) palsy (Bell palsy)

D. Right CN XI lesion

E. Right CN XII lesion

9.22   CRANIAL NERVE LESIONS

TABLE 9.16   SUMMARY OF CRANIAL NERVE LESIONS

Nerve	Lesion Type and/or Site	Abnormal Findings
CN I	Fracture of cribriform plate	Anosmia (loss of smell); cerebrospinal fluid (CSF) rhinorrhea (leakage of CSF through nose)
CN II	Direct trauma to orbit or eyeball; fracture involving optic canal	Loss of pupillary constriction
	Pressure on optic pathway; laceration or intracerebral clot in temporal, parietal, or occipital lobes of brain	Visual field defects
	Increased CSF pressure	Swelling of optic disc (papilledema)
CN III	Pressure from herniating uncus on nerve; fracture involving cavernous sinus; aneurysms	Dilated pupil, ptosis, eye rotates inferiorly and laterally (down and out), pupillary reflex on the side of the lesion will be lost (**A**)
CN IV	Stretching of nerve during its course around brainstem; fracture of orbit	Inability to rotate adducted eye inferiorly
CN V	Injury to terminal branches (particularly CN V$_2$) in roof of maxillary sinus; pathologic processes (tumors, aneurysms, infections) affecting trigeminal nerve	Loss of pain and touch sensations/paresthesia on face; loss of corneal reflex (blinking when cornea touched); paralysis of muscles of mastication; deviation of mandible to side of lesion when mouth is opened
CN VI	Base of brain or fracture involving cavernous sinus or orbit	Inability to rotate eye laterally; diplopia on lateral gaze (**B**)
CN VII	Laceration or contusion in parotid region	Paralysis of facial muscles; eye remains open; angle of mouth droops; forehead does not wrinkle (**C**)
	Fracture of temporal bone	As above, plus associated involvement of cochlear nerve and chorda tympani; dry cornea and loss of taste on anterior two thirds of tongue
	Intracranial hematoma ("stroke")	Weakness (paralysis) of lower facial muscles contralateral to the lesion, upper facial muscles are not affected because they are bilaterally innervated
CN VIII	Tumor of nerve	Progressive unilateral hearing loss; tinnitus (noises in ear); vertigo (loss of balance)
CN IX[a]	Brainstem lesion or deep laceration of neck	Loss of taste on posterior third of tongue; loss of sensation on affected side of soft palate; loss of gag reflex on affected side
CN X	Brainstem lesion or deep laceration of neck	Sagging of soft palate; deviation of uvula to unaffected side; hoarseness owing to paralysis of vocal fold; difficulty in swallowing and speaking
CN XI	Laceration of neck	Paralysis of sternocleidomastoid and superior fibers of trapezius; drooping of shoulder (**D**)
CN XII	Neck laceration; basal skull fractures	Protruded tongue deviates toward affected side; moderate dysarthria, disturbance of articulation (**E**)

[a]Isolated lesions of CN IX are uncommon; usually, CN IX, X, and XI are involved together as they pass through the jugular foramen.

9.23   TRANSVERSE MRIs THROUGH HEAD, SHOWING CRANIAL NERVES

A. Optic nerve (CN II). **B.** Oculomotor nerve (CN III). **C.** Trigeminal nerve (CN V).

9.23 TRANSVERSE MRIs THROUGH HEAD, SHOWING CRANIAL NERVES *(CONTINUED)*

D. Abducent (CN VI), facial (CN VII), and vestibulocochlear (CN VIII) nerves. **E.** Glossopharyngeal (CN IX), vagus (CN X), and spinal accessory (CN XI) nerves. **F.** Hypoglossal nerve (CN XII).

9.24   CORONAL MRIs THROUGH HEAD, SHOWING CRANIAL NERVES

A. Olfactory bulb. **B.** Trigeminal (CN V) nerve. **C.** Oculomotor (CN III) and trigeminal (CN V) nerves.

Tribute to Dr. Grant

1. Robinson C. *Canadian Medical Lives: J.C. Boileau Grant: Anatomist Extraordinary.* Markham, Ontario, Canada: Associated Medical Services Inc./Fithzenry & Whiteside, 1993.
2. Grant JCB. *A Method of Anatomy, Descriptive and Deductive.* Baltimore, MD: Williams & Wilkins Co., 1937 (11th ed., Basmajian J, Slonecker C, 1989).
3. Grant JCB. *Grant's Atlas of Anatomy.* Baltimore, MD: Williams & Wilkins Co., 1943 (10th ed., Agur A, Ming L, 1999).
4. Grant JCB, Cates HA. *Grant's Dissector (A Handbook for Dissectors).* Baltimore, MD: Williams & Wilkins Co., 1940 (12th ed., Sauerland EK, 1999).

Chapter 1

Fig. 1.51: Anson BH. The aortic arch and its branches. *Cardiology.* Vol. 1. New York, NY: McGraw-Hill, 1963.

Chapter 2

Fig. 2.49: Couinaud C. Lobes et segments hepatiques: Note sur l'architecture anatomique et chirurgicale du foie. *Presse Med* 1954;62:709.

Fig. 2.49: Healy JE, Schroy PC. Anatomy of the biliary ducts within the human liver: analysis of the prevailing pattern of branchings and the major variations of the biliary ducts. *Arch Surg* 1953;66:599.

Fig. 2.89B: Campbell M. Ureteral reduplication (double ureter). *Urology.* Vol. 1. Philadelphia, PA: WB Saunders, 1954:309.

Chapter 3

Fig. 3.43A: Oelrich TM. The urethral sphincter muscle in the male. *Am J Anat* 1980;158:229.

Fig. 3.43B: Oelrich TM. The striated urogenital sphincter muscle in the female. *Anat Rec* 1983;205:223.

Chapter 4

Fig. 4.48A: Jit I, Charnakia VM. The vertebral level of the termination of the spinal cord. *J Anat Soc India* 1959;8:93.